ESSENTIALS OF PHARMATOXICOLOGY IN DRUG RESEARCH, VOLUME 1

ADVANCES IN PHARMACEUTICAL PRODUCT DEVELOPMENT AND RESEARCH SERIES

ESSENTIALS OF PHARMATOXICOLOGY IN DRUG RESEARCH, VOLUME 1

TOXICITY AND TOXICODYNAMICS

Edited by

RAKESH TEKADE

National Institute of Pharmaceutical Education and Research (NIPER)- Ahmedabad, An Institute of National Importance, Government of India, Department of Pharmaceuticals, Ministry of Chemicals and Fertilizers, Palaj, Gandhinagar, Gujarat, India

ELSEVIER

ACADEMIC PRESS

An imprint of Elsevier

Academic Press is an imprint of Elsevier
125 London Wall, London EC2Y 5AS, United Kingdom
525 B Street, Suite 1650, San Diego, CA 92101, United States
50 Hampshire Street, 5th Floor, Cambridge, MA 02139, United States
The Boulevard, Langford Lane, Kidlington, Oxford OX5 1GB, United Kingdom

Notices

Knowledge and best practice in this field are constantly changing. As new research and experience broaden our understanding, changes in research methods, professional practices, or medical treatment may become necessary.

Practitioners and researchers must always rely on their own experience and knowledge in evaluating and using any information, methods, compounds, or experiments described herein. In using such information or methods they should be mindful of their own safety and the safety of others, including parties for whom they have a professional responsibility.

To the fullest extent of the law, neither the Publisher nor the authors, contributors, or editors, assume any liability for any injury and/or damage to persons or property as a matter of products liability, negligence or otherwise, or from any use or operation of any methods, products, instructions, or ideas contained in the material herein.

ISBN: 978-0-443-15840-7

For information on all Academic Press publications visit our website at https://www.elsevier.com/books-and-journals

Publisher: Stacy Masucci
Acquisitions Editor: Kattie Washington
Senior Editorial Project Manager: Pat Gonzalez
Production Project Manager: Selvaraj Raviraj
Cover Designer: Mark Rogers

Typeset by TNQ Technologies

Dedication

First of all, I thank Almighty God for giving me this opportunity to serve the scientific fraternity through the book series 'Advances in Pharmaceutical Product Development and Research'. This book, *"Essentials of Pharmatoxicology in Drug Research"* is devoted to my father, Shri Ganpat Rao Tekade—I know you are always watching me and showering your blessings on me from heaven. My dedication goes to my loving mother (Smt. Godavari Tekade), whose prayers have always followed me and clung to me all my life. My dedication goes to my best friend, my support system, and my wife Muktika Tekade, whose words of encouragement and deep faith in me and my ability have always caused the flowers of untiring efforts to blossom in my eyes. Your hope gives me the courageous determination to fight back, even when things go off-track and uphill. My dedication to the twinkles of my eyes: my daughter 😊, my treasure Manyata and my son 😊, my superhero Atharva for being my rock star and my number one fan. Kids, your hugs give me an intense reason to smile, even when worries are around. I hope one day you will comprehend why I spent tireless time on writing. I love you forever! A special gratitude for my sisters and remembrance to my brother. I would also like to thank my friends for their motivation. My superior respect goes toward all my teachers and mentors (Prof. N.K. Jain, Prof. Xiankai Sun, and Prof. Antony D' Emanuele) for being my role models.

Contents

15. Medication errors and approaches for its prevention

Ankit Mishra, Nimeet Desai, Muktika Tekade, Kuldeep Rajpoot, Anuradha Gadeval, Manish Sharma and Rakesh Kumar Tekade

16. Understanding the bioaccumulation of pharmaceuticals and personal care products

Amarjitsing P. Rajput, Madhur Kulkarni, Prashant L. Pingale, Muktika Tekade, Ashok K. Shakya and Rakesh Kumar Tekade

17. Toxicity of dental materials and ways to screen their biosafety

Prashant L. Pingale, Neetu R. Saudagar, Amarjitsing P. Rajput, Kuldeep Rajpoot, Muktika Tekade, Anjali Pingale and Rakesh Kumar Tekade

18. Clinical detoxification of the body from chemical toxicants

Muktika Tekade, Prashant L. Pingale, Sakshi P. Wani, Kuldeep Rajpoot, Nagaraja Sreeharsha, Mrudul Deshpande, Rakesh Kumar Tekade and Mukesh C. Sharma

19. Molecular mechanisms of the chemopreventive role of dietary phytochemicals

Suryanarayana Polaka, Nupur Vasdev, Lakshmi Vineela Nalla, Sivarupa Raji, Muktika Tekade, Nagendra Singh Chauhan, Satyajit D. Sarker and Rakesh Kumar Tekade

20. Toxicity labels

Bhakti Pawar, Anoothi Bain, Nagaraja Sreeharsha, Muktika Tekade, Nupur Vasdev and Rakesh Kumar Tekade

21. Toxic potential indicator

Kuldeep Rajpoot, Muktika Tekade, Bhakti Pawar, Nupur Vasdev, Tanisha Gupta and Rakesh Kumar Tekade

22. Concept of pharmacotherapy and managed care in clinical interventions

Vishakha Tambe, Kuldeep Rajpoot, Nimeet Desai and Rakesh Kumar Tekade

23. Understanding the connection between dietary supplementation and inadvertent doping

Manish Kumar Sharma, Hari Priya Koppisetti, Priyanka Lohar, Rahul Maheshwari, Pinaki Sengupta and Rakesh Kumar Tekade

24. Cells and tissue-based models as a rational substitute in toxicity testing

Mamata Panchal, Vinayak Pawar, Mahi Mhatre, Shweta Ingole, Suryanarayana Polaka, Muktika Tekade, Kuldeep Rajpoot and Rakesh Kumar Tekade

25. Regulatory agencies for toxicological studies

Kuldeep Rajpoot, Anand More, Yogesh Wankhede, Shyam Gomte, Muktika Tekade, Tanisha Gupta, Bhakti Pawar, Sanyam Gandhi and Rakesh Kumar Tekade

26. Key challenges for toxicologists in the 21st century

Havish Shukla, Muktika Tekade, Bhakti Pawar, Kuldeep Rajpoot and Rakesh Kumar Tekade

List of contributors

Nagendra Sai Kumar Achanta University of Campania, Luigi Vanvitelli, Caserta, Italy

Omar Husham Ahmed Al-Attraqchi Centre for Drug Research, Universiti Sains Malaysia, George Town, Penang, Malaysia

Nizar Al-Shar'i Faculty of Pharmacy, Jordan University of Science and Technology, Irbid, Jordan

Neelima Anup National Institute of Pharmaceutical Education and Research (NIPER)-Ahmedabad, An Institute of National Importance, Government of India, Department of Pharmaceuticals, Ministry of Chemicals and Fertilizers, Palaj, Gandhinagar, Gujarat, India

Basel Arafat Faculty of Health, Education, Medicine, and Social Care, Anglia Ruskin University, Chelmsford, United Kingdom

Anoothi Bain National Institute of Pharmaceutical Education and Research (NIPER)-Ahmedabad, An Institute of National Importance, Government of India, Department of Pharmaceuticals, Ministry of Chemicals and Fertilizers, Palaj, Gandhinagar, Gujarat, India

Kuldeep Kumar Bansal Pharmaceutical Sciences Laboratory, Faculty of Science and Engineering, Åbo Akademi University, Turku, Finland

Santosh Kumar Behera National Institute of Pharmaceutical Education and Research (NIPER)- Ahmedabad, An Institute of National Importance, Government of India, Department of Pharmaceuticals, Ministry of Chemicals and Fertilizers, Palaj, Gandhinagar, Gujarat, India

Nagendra Singh Chauhan Drugs Testing Laboratory Avam Anusandhan Kendra, Raipur, Chhattisgarh, India

Dinesh Kumar Chellappan Department of Life Sciences, School of Pharmacy, International Medical University, Kuala Lumpur, Malaysia

Nimeet Desai National Institute of Pharmaceutical Education and Research (NIPER)-Ahmedabad, An Institute of National Importance, Government of India, Department of Pharmaceuticals, Ministry of Chemicals and Fertilizers, Palaj, Gandhinagar, Gujarat, India

Mrudul Deshpande National Institute of Pharmaceutical Education and Research (NIPER)-Ahmedabad, An Institute of National Importance, Government of India, Department of Pharmaceuticals, Ministry of Chemicals and Fertilizers, Palaj, Gandhinagar, Gujarat, India

Sneha A. Dhamne GES's Sir Dr. M. S. Gosavi College of Pharmaceutical Education and Research, Nashik, Maharashtra, India

Pankaj Vinodrao Dixit Indore Institute of Pharmacy, Indore, Madhya Pradesh, India

Anuradha Gadeval National Institute of Pharmaceutical Education and Research (NIPER)-Ahmedabad, An Institute of National Importance, Government of India, Department of Pharmaceuticals, Ministry of Chemicals and Fertilizers, Palaj, Gandhinagar, Gujarat, India

Sanyam Gandhi Takeda Pharmaceuticals, Cambridge, MA, United States

Shyam Gomte National Institute of Pharmaceutical Education and Research (NIPER)- Ahmedabad, An Institute of National Importance, Government of India, Department of Pharmaceuticals, Ministry of Chemicals and Fertilizers, Palaj, Gandhinagar, Gujarat, India

Piyush Gondaliya Department of Transplantation, Mayo Clinic, Jacksonville, FL, United States

Deepak Kumar Gupta Indira Gandhi National Tribal University, Amarkantak, Madhya Pradesh, India

Rachna Gupta National Institute of Pharmaceutical Education and Research (NIPER)-Ahmedabad, An Institute of National Importance, Government of India, Department of Pharmaceuticals, Ministry of Chemicals and Fertilizers, Palaj, Gandhinagar, Gujarat, India

Tanisha Gupta National Institute of Pharmaceutical Education and Research (NIPER)-Ahmedabad, An Institute of National Importance, Government of India, Department of Pharmaceuticals, Ministry of Chemicals and Fertilizers, Palaj, Gandhinagar, Gujarat, India

Shweta Ingole National Institute of Pharmaceutical Education and Research (NIPER)-Ahmedabad, An Institute of National Importance, Government of India, Department of Pharmaceuticals, Ministry of Chemicals and Fertilizers, Palaj, Gandhinagar, Gujarat, India

Megha Joshi Vikram University, Ujjain, Madhya Pradesh, India

Rana Dhwani Kalpeshkumar National Institute of Pharmaceutical Education and Research (NIPER)- Ahmedabad, An Institute of National Importance, Government of India, Department of Pharmaceuticals, Ministry of Chemicals and Fertilizers, Palaj, Gandhinagar, Gujarat, India

Hari Priya Koppisetti National Institute of Pharmaceutical Education and Research (NIPER)-Ahmedabad, An Institute of National Importance, Government of India, Department of Pharmaceuticals, Ministry of Chemicals and Fertilizers, Palaj, Gandhinagar, Gujarat, India

Madhur Kulkarni SCES's Indira College of Pharmacy, Pune, Maharashtra, India

Manoj Kumar Department of Radiology, Stanford University, Stanford, CA, United States

Priyanka Lohar National Institute of Pharmaceutical Education and Research (NIPER)-Ahmedabad, An Institute of National Importance, Government of India, Department of Pharmaceuticals, Ministry of Chemicals and Fertilizers, Palaj, Gandhinagar, Gujarat, India

Rahul Maheshwari School of Pharmacy and Technology Management, SVKM' NMIMS, Hyderabad, Telangana, India

Randa SH. Mansour Faculty of Pharmacy, Philadelphia University, Amman, Jordan

Mahi Mhatre National Institute of Pharmaceutical Education and Research (NIPER)-Ahmedabad, An Institute of National Importance, Government of India, Department of Pharmaceuticals, Ministry of Chemicals and Fertilizers, Palaj, Gandhinagar, Gujarat, India

Ankit Mishra VNS Group of Institutions, Bhopal, Madhya Pradesh, India

Dinesh Kumar Mishra Indore Institute of Pharmacy, Indore, Madhya Pradesh, India

Pranali Mishra VNS Group of Institutions, Bhopal, Madhya Pradesh, India

Farahidah Mohamed Kulliyyah of Pharmacy, International Islamic University Malaysia, Kuantan, Malaysia

Anand More National Institute of Pharmaceutical Education and Research (NIPER)- Ahmedabad, An Institute of National Importance, Government of India, Department of Pharmaceuticals, Ministry of Chemicals and Fertilizers, Palaj, Gandhinagar, Gujarat, India

Lakshmi Vineela Nalla National Institute of Pharmaceutical Education and Research (NIPER)- Ahmedabad, An Institute of National Importance, Government of India, Department of Pharmaceuticals, Ministry of Chemicals and Fertilizers, Palaj, Gandhinagar, Gujarat, India; Department of Pharmacy, Koneru Lakshmaiah Education Foundation, Vaddeswaram, Andhra Pradesh, India

Mamata Panchal National Institute of Pharmaceutical Education and Research (NIPER)-Ahmedabad, An Institute of National Importance, Government of India, Department of Pharmaceuticals, Ministry of Chemicals and Fertilizers, Palaj, Gandhinagar, Gujarat, India

Krutika H. Pardeshi Department of Pharmaceutics, School of Pharmaceutical Sciences, Sandip University, Nashik, Maharashtra, India

Bhakti Pawar National Institute of Pharmaceutical Education and Research (NIPER)-Ahmedabad, An Institute of National Importance, Government of India, Department of Pharmaceuticals, Ministry of Chemicals and Fertilizers, Palaj, Gandhinagar, Gujarat, India

Vinayak Pawar National Institute of Pharmaceutical Education and Research (NIPER)-Ahmedabad, An Institute of National Importance, Government of India, Department of Pharmaceuticals, Ministry of Chemicals and Fertilizers, Palaj, Gandhinagar, Gujarat, India

Prashant L. Pingale Department of Pharmaceutics, GES's Sir Dr. M. S. Gosavi College of Pharmaceutical Education and Research, Nashik, Maharashtra, India

Anjali Pingale Shree Panchavati Education Society's Institute of Pharmacy, Nashik, Maharashtra, India

Suryanarayana Polaka National Institute of Pharmaceutical Education and Research (NIPER)- Ahmedabad, An Institute of National Importance, Government of India, Department of Pharmaceuticals, Ministry of Chemicals and Fertilizers, Palaj, Gandhinagar, Gujarat, India

Sivarupa Raji Redox Biology Lab, National Centre for Cell Science (NCCS), Pune, India

Kuldeep Rajpoot National Institute of Pharmaceutical Education and Research (NIPER)-Ahmedabad, An Institute of National Importance, Government of India, Department of Pharmaceuticals, Ministry of Chemicals and Fertilizers, Palaj, Gandhinagar, Gujarat, India

Amarjitsing P. Rajput Nanomedicine Laboratory, Department of Biosciences and Bioengineering, Indian Institute of Technology Bombay, Mumbai, Maharashtra, India; Department of Pharmaceutics, Poona College of Pharmacy, Bharti Vidyapeeth Deemed University, Pune, Maharashtra, India

Nidhi Raval University of British Columbia, Pharmaceutical Sciences Building, Vancouver, BC, Canada

Maliheh Safavi Department of Biotechnology, Iranian Research Organization for Science and Technology, Tehran, Iran

Satyajit D. Sarker Centre for Natural Products Discovery, School of Pharmacy and Biomolecular Sciences, Liverpool John Moores University, Liverpool, United Kingdom

Neetu R. Saudagar Department of Pharmaceutics, GES's Sir Dr. M. S. Gosavi College of Pharmaceutical Education and Research, Nashik, Maharashtra, India

Adil Ali Sayyed Department of Transplantation, Mayo Clinic, Jacksonville, FL, United States

Pinaki Sengupta National Institute of Pharmaceutical Education and Research (NIPER)-Ahmedabad, An Institute of National Importance, Government of India, Department of Pharmaceuticals, Ministry of Chemicals and Fertilizers, Palaj, Gandhinagar, Gujarat, India

Ashok K. Shakya Pharmacological and Diagnostic Research Center, Faculty of Pharmacy, Al-Ahliyya Amman University, Amman, Jordan

Manish Kumar Sharma National Institute of Pharmaceutical Education and Research (NIPER)-Ahmedabad, An Institute of National Importance, Government of India, Department of Pharmaceuticals, Ministry of Chemicals and Fertilizers, Palaj, Gandhinagar, Gujarat, India; College of Pharmacy, Pharmacy Practice, and Science, University of Nebraska Medical Center, NE, United States

Manish Sharma Dept of Pharmacy Practice, University of Nebraska Medical Center, Omaha, NE, United States

Mukesh C. Sharma School of Pharmacy, Devi Ahilya Vishwavidyalaya, Indore, Madhya Pradesh, India

Anjani Sheth National Institute of Pharmaceutical Education and Research (NIPER) Ahmedabad, An Institute of National Importance, Government of India, Department of Pharmaceuticals, Ministry of Chemicals and Fertilizers, Palaj, Gandhinagar, Gujarat, India

Havish Shukla National Institute of Pharmaceutical Education and Research (NIPER)-Ahmedabad, An Institute of National Importance, Government of India, Department of Pharmaceuticals, Ministry of Chemicals and Fertilizers, Palaj, Gandhinagar, Gujarat, India

Nagaraja Sreeharsha Department of Pharmaceutical Sciences, College of Clinical Pharmacy,

King Faisal University, Al-Ahsa, Saudi Arabia; Department of Pharmaceutics, Vidya Siri College of Pharmacy, Bengaluru, Karnataka, India

Vishakha Tambe National Institute of Pharmaceutical Education and Research (NIPER)-Ahmedabad, An Institute of National Importance, Government of India, Department of Pharmaceuticals, Ministry of Chemicals and Fertilizers, Palaj, Gandhinagar, Gujarat, India

Paritala Sree Teja National Institute of Pharmaceutical Education and Research (NIPER)-Ahmedabad, An Institute of National Importance, Government of India, Department of Pharmaceuticals, Ministry of Chemicals and Fertilizers, Palaj, Gandhinagar, Gujarat, India

Muktika Tekade School of Pharmacy, Devi Ahilya Vishwavidyalaya, Indore, Madhya Pradesh, India

Rakesh Kumar Tekade National Institute of Pharmaceutical Education and Research (NIPER)- Ahmedabad, An Institute of National Importance, Government of India, Department of Pharmaceuticals, Ministry of Chemicals and Fertilizers, Palaj, Gandhinagar, Gujarat, India

Akhilesh Tiwari Indira Gandhi National Tribal University, Amarkantak, Madhya Pradesh, India

Nupur Vasdev National Institute of Pharmaceutical Education and Research (NIPER)-Ahmedabad, An Institute of National Importance, Government of India, Department of Pharmaceuticals, Ministry of Chemicals and Fertilizers, Palaj, Gandhinagar, Gujarat, India

Sakshi P. Wani Department of Pharmaceutics, GES's Sir Dr. M. S. Gosavi College of Pharmaceutical Education and Research, Nashik, Maharashtra, India

Yogesh Wankhede National Institute of Pharmaceutical Education and Research (NIPER)-Ahmedabad, An Institute of National Importance, Government of India, Department of Pharmaceuticals, Ministry of Chemicals and Fertilizers, Palaj, Gandhinagar, Gujarat, India

CHAPTER

1

Understanding pharmacotoxicology

Bhakti Pawar[1], *Tanisha Gupta*[1], *Nupur Vasdev*[1], *Muktika Tekade*[2], *Basel Arafat*[3] *and Rakesh Kumar Tekade*[1]

[1]National Institute of Pharmaceutical Education and Research (NIPER)- Ahmedabad, An Institute of National Importance, Government of India, Department of Pharmaceuticals, Ministry of Chemicals and Fertilizers, Palaj, Gandhinagar, Gujarat, India; [2]School of Pharmacy, Devi Ahilya Vishwavidyalaya, Indore, Madhya Pradesh, India; [3]Faculty of Health, Education, Medicine, and Social Care, Anglia Ruskin University, Chelmsford, United Kingdom

1.1 Introduction

Pharmacotoxicology is the study of the effects of toxic exposure to pharmacological medications, and it also deals with the treatment and prevention of side effects caused by pharmaceuticals. It is categorized into two parts, viz. pharmacodynamics and pharmacokinetics (Rajpoot et al., 2022a; Anup et al., 2021). Pharmacodynamics provides information on how the administered drug affects the organism and describes how the body responds to the drug. The link between drug concentration at the site of action and the subsequent effect, including the time course and severity of therapeutic and unfavorable effects, is referred to as pharmacodynamics (Mealey and Karriker, 2019; Pandey et al., 2022; Gupta et al., 2022a). The binding of a drug to the receptor is like a lock and fundamental model. Receptors may be present in the cardiac muscle (affecting the intensity of contraction), neurons (subsiding the pain sensation), and even within bacteria (disruption of the bacterial cell wall), etc. Signal transduction is an essential mechanism in pharmacodynamics, which leads to a series of events giving therapeutic effects (Tekade et al., 2022).

Pharmacokinetic studies of the administered drug involve absorption, distribution, metabolism, excretion, and toxicology (ADMET) (Chandrasekaran et al., 2018). A compound's pharmacokinetics are influenced by its physicochemical properties, intrinsic clearance, apparent volume of distribution, as well as interactions with different tissue types.

Essentials of Pharmatoxicology in Drug Research, Volume 1
https://doi.org/10.1016/B978-0-443-15840-7.00025-7

Pharmacotoxicology is vital in determining drug toxicity, drug-drug interactions, safety, efficacy, etc. (Schoenmakers and Jones, 2018; Polaka et al., 2022f).

1.1.1 Reasons for drug toxicity

There are multiple factors that can contribute to drug-induced toxicity, such as inherent properties of the drug, drug-drug interaction, drug overdose, improper storage conditions, and drug abuse.

- ***Overdose toxicity*** is when a substance is accidentally overdosed (for instance, due to a mistake made by the doctor, pharmacist, or individual taking medicine). When a drug is intentionally administered at a higher dose level, it is referred to as an intentional overdose (homicide or suicide). An example of the class of drugs that could lead to such overdose toxicity is antidepressant drugs. If a patient is suffering from depression, doctors will prescribe sedatives, antianxiety, and sleep aids. To reduce the risk of toxicity induced by antidepressants, doctors could prescribe drugs of higher therapeutic index. For instance, instead of barbiturates which have a narrow therapeutic index, doctors can prescribe benzodiazepines.
- ***Improper storage conditions*** can change the physical and chemical properties of the drug, causing toxicity. The proper storage condition, explicitly mentioned on the storage label, must be followed. Here are a few examples of drugs that get destroyed and show an adverse effect when kept under improper storage conditions; antibiotics after deterioration cause kidney damage, degraded aspirin leads to stomach upset. Also an insulin and anticoagulants; a slight modification in their doses can make a significant impact on the health, etc.
- ***Drug-drug interactions (DDI)*** are another cause of drug toxicity. Nowadays, polypharmacy approach is used to treat multiple diseases, such as cancer, tuberculosis, and rare diseases. Drug-drug interactions can occur at both pharmacodynamic and pharmacokinetic levels. Examples of drugs showing interaction at the pharmacodynamic level are aspirin and ibuprofen, which are antagonistic when administered simultaneously. At the pharmacokinetic level, DDI could occur at any absorption, metabolism, and elimination stages. Examples of drug interaction at the absorption level are levothyroxine and neutralizing antacids. At the metabolism level, SSRIs and some beta-blockers, and at the elimination level, digoxin and macrolides (Galetin et al., 2022; Kayat et al., 2011).

1.1.2 Types of pharmacotoxicity

The drug-induced toxicity can be categorized as acute, chronic, absolute, and relative toxicity. Exposure to drug substances can happen in different ways and over different lengths of time.

1.1.2.1 Acute toxicity

It is also known as single-dose toxicity. To ascertain the short-term undesirable effects of a drug when taken in a single dose, acute toxicity tests are carried out. Usually, adverse effects related to acute toxicity occur within 14 days. An acute toxicity study helps provide information on a drug's safe dose level, its ability to cause acute toxicity, and possible target organ toxicity. The Median Lethal Dose (LD_{50}), i.e., the dose required to kill 50% of the population, is calculated. An earlier assessment of acute toxicity may be crucial for therapeutic purposes where there is a more considerable risk of overdose in specific patient populations. Phase III clinical studies should have access to data on the acute toxicity of medications, which might be used to forecast the outcomes of human overdose scenarios.

1.1.2.2 *Subacute toxicity*

A subacute toxicity study is performed for a duration of 2–4 weeks. This study establishes the dose level for further subchronic and chronic studies. These investigations can also help evaluate the development and remission of drug-induced lesions. Still, they typically last too short a time to comprehensively cover all potential side effects that can manifest during prolonged clinical usage (Colerangle, 2017; Asati et al., 2022).

1.1.2.3 *Chronic toxicity*

Constant daily exposure to a substance leads to chronic toxicity. A goal of a chronic toxicity study is to ascertain the drug's effect after repeated, long-term exposure (Ghiazza et al., 2014). The leading cause of chronic toxicity is the gradual accumulation of damage in one or more target organs (Combes, 2013). Similar to acute toxicity, the goals of chronic toxicity include: defining the mechanism of action of the administered drug, identification of target organs, safe dose level, no observed adverse effect level (NOAEL) determination, the reversibility of toxicity studies, etc. The duration of the chronic toxicity study is between 6 months and 1 year (Colerangle, 2017). Usually, as per the ICHS4 guidelines, chronic toxicity for a 6-month duration is performed in rodents, whereas a 9-month study is performed in non-rodent species.

1.1.2.4 *Subchronic toxicity*

A rodent and a non-rodent species are frequently used in subchronic toxicity studies, which can be done from 3 to 12 months. These studies provide information on the possible long-term side effects associated with the drug, which will help support clinical trial reports (Dong et al., 2022).

This chapter mainly focuses on the different principles of pharmacotoxicology, routes of exposure and drugs toxicokinetics, diverse sources of toxicity, risk assessment, biomarkers, organ-specific toxicity, site-specific toxicity, and mechanism of drug toxicity.

1.2 The principle applied to pharmacotoxicology

Understanding the fundamentals of pharmacotoxicology is crucial for the drug's rationale use. For instance, the dose-response relationship is studied to evaluate the drug's efficacy, potency, and safety. On the other hand, toxicokinetic studies are performed to evaluate the biodisposition of the drug (Rajpoot et al., 2022b). This section describes concepts including pharmacotoxicology, exposure route, toxicokinetics, therapeutic drug monitoring, risk assessment, biomarkers, and site-specific toxicity.

1.2.1 Dose/response relationship

In toxicology, the dose-response relationship is a crucial concept. It is an outline that underpins dose-response model extrapolations, hazard assessment studies, and the development of environmental legislation. "All things are poison, and nothing is without poison," said Paracelsus (1493–1541), who is sometimes referred to as the "father of toxicology." The dose dictates whether a drug is effective or poisonous. The relationship between drug dose and its response can be obtained by plotting the log of the drug dose against the drug's response, which mainly shows a sigmoidal curve. This means an increase in the drug dose is directly related to the drug response. But at some point, an increase in the dose above this range gives little or minimal extra effect (Mealey and Karriker, 2019).

Several variables can be used to compare the response of different drugs. ***Efficacy:*** The effect of drug response depends on how efficiently the drug occupies the available receptors for binding. Therapeutic effectiveness refers to a drug's ability to achieve a desired biological outcome and can be used to compare drugs with different pharmacological modes of action. ***Potency:*** It describes how much drug is needed to produce a desired biological response. The lower the amount of the drug required, the more potent it is. Most of the time, drugs with high potency possess lower ED_{50} as shown in Fig. 1.1 ***Therapeutic index:*** It indicates drug safety. Most of the time, the drug's adverse effects are dependent on the dose of the drug given. Usually, a drug shows several adverse effects. This can be studied by utilizing the concept of the therapeutic index, which is mainly based on the study of adverse effects; such drugs may need a decrease in dose or withdrawal (Raj and Raveendran, 2019). To avoid adverse effects, the dose of the drug must be titrated according to individual's disease condition. The therapeutic index for most drugs is greater than 100. However, there are a few significant exceptions with therapeutic indices of less than 10, like insulin and phenytoin (Gupta, 2020; Ralston et al., 2018).

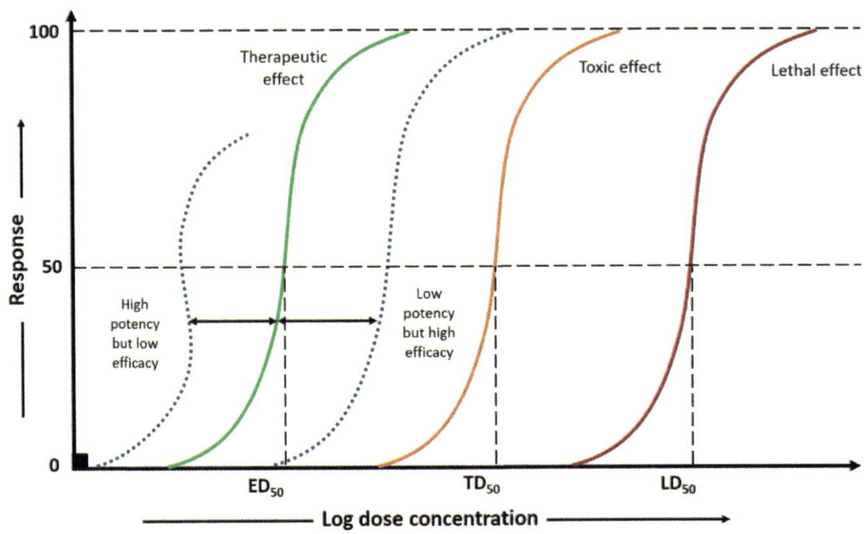

FIGURE 1.1 Dose-response relationship.

1.2.2 Exposure routes and toxicokinetic

The routes by which drugs enter the body have much significance when assessing their toxicity. Inhalation, skin (or eye) absorption, ingestion, and injection are four major routes of chemical exposure to the body (Cohen, 2020).

1.2.2.1 *Inhalation*

This is the primary route of entry for the chemicals for gases, vapors, or mists. After inhalation, these chemicals can either be exhaled or stored in the respiratory tract. Deposition may cause damage to the tissues of the respiratory tract. These chemicals could then diffuse into the blood through the lung-blood interface. This may cause the chemicals to reach circulation and get distributed into the organs with more affinity (Kayat et al., 2011).

1.2.2.2 *Skin absorption*

Skin and eyes are the most exposed body parts. Chemicals can easily be absorbed into the skin tissues, leading to irritation and redness of the skin. Many chemicals can also cross the skin barrier and diffuse into blood circulation. This may also lead to cause internal damage to organs.

1.2.2.3 *Eye absorption*

Retinal pharmacotherapy has become increasingly crucial for the treatment of various retinal disorders. A growing number of drugs, particularly for wet age-related macular degeneration and diabetic macular edema, have been introduced onto the market. Intravitreal injections are used to treat inflammatory, neovascular, and edematous disorders of the macula, retina, and vitreous (Aljundi et al., 2022). Exposure to chemicals in the eyes could result in harmful effects.

Ocular toxicity produced by exposing retinal tissue to high concentrations of drugs for extended periods is still a significant concern when treating retinal disorders with intravitreal injection. Chemicals can easily be absorbed through the eyes, such as sulfuric acid, nitric acid, bisphosphonates, cyclosporin, ethambutol, minocycline, etc. (Jain, 2022; Dave et al., 2022).

1.2.2.4 *Injection*

There are different routes, such as intravenous, intramuscular, subcutaneous, intraperitoneal, etc., through which we can inject the drug into the systemic circulation. However, intravenous injections are the only route in which the chemical is injected directly into the blood circulation, and the amount exposed is absorbed regardless of the chemical provided. It is rare for injections to be contaminated with harmful compounds in their manufacturing sites due to the sterile nature of these facilities. Nonetheless, it can unintentionally happen when chemicals are handled in syringes, glass, or metal contaminated with them. Substances can enter the body if contaminants penetrate or puncture the skin. After penetration, these chemicals can enter the systemic circulation and exhibit adverse effects. Once the chemical enters the systemic circulation, blood is the only vehicle it is exposed. Moreover, the intravenous method is the most rapid method for drug administration. Delivery of any drug through the intravenous method is irreversible; hence, administration in excess can cause severe toxicity (Sawicki et al., 2019).

1.2.2.5 *Ingestion*

Almost 60% of the drugs are administered or swallowed orally, and few have shown an adverse effect on the GIT (Alqahtani et al., 2021). One such example of the drug is Domperidone, an anti-sickness drug that blocks the message from the digestive tract to the brain and gives a healthier feeling to the patient. But the administration of this drug is associated with one severe adverse effect, which is intense abdominal or stomach cramps (Heckert and Parkman, 2018). For such drugs, measuring toxicokinetics is a mandatory task. Insoluble chemicals in the GI fluid are readily excreted from the body. But the soluble chemicals in GI fluid can damage internal organs by diffusing into blood circulation. The toxicokinetics of this exposed compound mostly depends on the metabolic processes that occur after administration, such as metabolism, distribution, and excretion. Certain chemicals may be deposited into specific organs for long durations and hence may result organ failure. For such compounds toxicity evaluation is mandatory to study further dose reduction or excretory pathways.

1.2.3 The therapeutic dose adjustment or monitoring (TDM)

Therapeutic drug monitoring entails determining drug concentrations in the plasma, serum, or blood. This information is used to personalize dosing to keep drug concentrations within a specific range (Vermeire et al., 2020). The concentration of the drug at the desired biological site cannot be quantified, but it can be better correlated with the concentration of the drug in the plasma or blood. Personalizing the dosage regimen for drugs that have shown significant interindividual pharmacokinetic effects is complex. Therapeutic drug monitoring could be helpful, particularly when drugs exhibit time-dependent variations among individuals. Drugs such as digoxin, lithium, valproate, etc., are regulated by therapeutic monitoring. There are certain conditions for a drug to which a TDM can be applied, such as a narrow therapeutic range; an established relationship between plasma concentration and clinically observed effects; imperative pharmacokinetic variations, and availability of a cost-effective drug assay (It would be ideal if the drug having high medicare expenditure possess cost-effective analytical assays, for such drugs TDM can be easily applicable as it will help determine and monitor the concentrations of the drug at the desired biological site) (Eliasson et al., 2013; Ghiculescu, 2008).

There are specific indications to use TDM. It helps to enhance efficacy, reduce toxicity, and study diagnosis. The proper indications to use TDM involves:

- **Toxicity:** To avoid toxicity (e.g., aminoglycosides);
- **Dosing:** Evaluation of loading dose (dose adjustment);
- **Monitoring:** To diagnose failed therapy.

The above section discusses the role of TDM in assessing drug concentration in blood samples. TDM holds promise in the design of personalized medicine. However, more specific justifications of why and when TDM should be used are needed in healthcare, such as identifying patient subpopulations or clinical scenarios where TDM would be especially advantageous to optimize drug treatment for specific patients.

The stepwise risk assessment process and the crucial terms used therein will be highlighted in the next section.

1.3 Risk assessment

In the past, scientists used to assess the risk and level of toxicity of chemicals humans are exposed to by using simple methods or by consulting individuals who have deep knowledge in that field. But nowadays, many techniques are available to assess chemical risks. For a chemical to be toxic, it should possess intrinsic hazardous properties.

There are different terms used while performing a risk assessment.

1.3.1 Occupational exposure level (OEL)

The occupational exposure level is used to assess the toxicity level of chemicals to workers at their workplace. For instance, the risk associated with handling final products, preliminary materials, and process intermediates is all studied with the help of occupational toxicity studies. OELs are based on the No-Observed-Adverse-Effect level (NOAELs) and Lowest-Observed-Adverse-Effect Level (LOAEL) from previous animal studies. Because NOAELs are intended to prevent harmful effects but not all effects, they are preferred to NOELs for setting OELs. This gives the standard for comparison of the measured exposure levels (Greim and Snyder, 2018). The NOAEL is the highest exposure level at which the frequency of an adverse event does not statistically or physiologically differ when compared to a control group. The lowest-observed-adverse-effect level (LOAEL) is the lowest exposure at which there is a marked increase in an observable effect. The LOAEL exposure value is frequently used in risk assessment studies.

An example of an experiment utilizing such risk assessment levels is that of Mišík et al. (2019). Their work evaluated the toxic dose of a chemical causing liver damage in rats. Results from their study indicated that no adverse effect at 1 mg/kg of chemical dosage was observed, and while some adverse effects appeared at 5 mg/kg hence, the 5 mg/kg dosage would be considered as LOAEL, and 1 mg/kg would be NOAEL (Mišík et al., 2019).

1.3.2 Margin of safety

The ratio of no observed adverse effect level (NOAEL) to the predicted human dose. The risk that some persons will get harmed by exposure increases as the ratio decreases. For instance, a drug showing margin of safety (MOS) ≥ 100 is generally considered to be protective (Bright-Ponte et al., 2018).

1.3.3 Point of departure

A point on a dose-response curve studied in toxicology plotted with the help of data generated from experimental animal studies or observational studies is stated as the point of departure (POD). This point is typically associated with a predictable low or no effect level (Farmahin et al., 2017). In the above-discussed example of OELs chemically induced liver damage, the point of departure would be 1 mg/kg daily.

There are three steps by which risk assessment can be studied:

- **Identification of hazard:** This can be done by identifying the source of the hazardous chemicals. Critical endpoints are observed through experimental studies. The route and exposure times are obtained to identify the hazard.
- **Characterization of a hazard:** In this quantitative and semi-quantitative assessment, the nature of the adverse effects that occur after exposing the hazard are studied. While characterizing collected data, the weight of evidence and severity of the adverse effect is evaluated by linking it to the possible adverse effect that the chemical would show. Usually, the dose-response curve is plotted to identify the point of departure from which the LOAEL and NOAEL can be obtained (Tsatsakis, 2021). The threshold value or exposure value can be identified with the help of different available resources such as human epidemiological data, animal data, in vitro, in vivo data, omics data, etc.
- **Evaluation of exposure level:** It involves the determination of the threshold of exposure levels. The no observed adverse effect level and the lowest observed adverse effect level are predicted (Greim and Snyder, 2018).

In the above section, we have briefly discussed the stepwise risk assessment process carried out during toxicity studies. As risk assessment has a significant role in deciding the toxicity of a chemical, there should be some parameters with the help of which we can confirm that the toxicity is due to the same compound. So, in the other section, different biomarkers are mentioned frequently used in testing different organ-specific toxicity.

1.4 Biomarkers

Evaluating the efficacy and safety of the drug is a difficult step in the drug development process. As per the above discussion, risk assessment is a rather critical and time-consuming process. Therefore, researchers have found litmus tests or biomarkers for a specific diseased condition. Biomarkers are used in both the process of drug development, preclinical and clinical. Utilizing biomarkers helps decrease the time and cost of the lengthy development process. Traditionally different biomarkers were used to study organ toxicity. The following section of the chapter describes some of the classic examples of biomarkers (Califf, 2018):

1.4.1 Creatine kinase

Basically, it is a leakage enzyme. Serum levels of creatinine kinase values were found to be high in reversible/irreversible muscle or tissue injury.

1.4.2 Aminotransferases

This is also a leakage enzyme. It leaks out when hepatocyte cell membrane permeability is altered. Amino transferase involves alanine transferase (ALT) and aspartate transferase

(AST). A high level of serum ALT, more than AST, is found when there is damage to hepatocytes. AST is usually present in the liver and muscles. Similar to ALT, damage to liver cells show high levels of AST.

1.4.3 Lactate dehydrogenase

This enzyme is present in the cytoplasm of cells. The increased serum level indicates hemolysis, liver damage, muscle/tissue injury, etc.

1.4.4 Bilirubin

It is a metabolic product of heme catabolism and is used as an indicator for liver damage. Enhance levels of total bilirubin can indicate hemoglobin destruction or cholestasis.

1.4.5 Creatinine and blood urea nitrogen (BUN)

Creatinine shows better specificity than blood urea nitrogen. The filtering capacity of the kidney can be assessed by checking levels of creatinine and BUN. High levels of these markers show kidney damage.

Above-mentioned examples of biomarkers are frequently used in the risk assessment of the chemical. Usually, these biomarkers are organ and disease-specific. So, with the help of scientists can quickly assess the toxicity level of the chemical. The following section provides information on organ-specific, site-specific, and site-non-specific toxicity.

1.5 Organ specificity for toxicity

Organ specificity (or site specificity) involves a chemical interaction between a specific intracellular site and the substance. A xenobiotic frequently interacts with the exact subcellular location in multiple organs; however, one organ is always the first to show signs of toxicity. The central nervous system (CNS) is the critical organ in toxicities that cause generalized loss of energy metabolism, such as cyanide inhibition of cytochrome oxidase, and death due to respiratory arrest occurs due to the respiratory center's greater oxygen sensitivity, even though cytochrome oxidase is inhibited in all tissues. Similarly, manganese shows specific effects on the liver, kidney, and CNS (neurobehavioral disorders) (Haschek et al., 2022).

1.6 Site-specific interaction and toxicity

For site-specific interaction, two things are essential. First, the antigen molecule/ligand, and second, the presence of receptor protein on the cells. The interaction between ligand and receptor is responsible for giving a therapeutic effect. The toxic chemical binds to the receptor and activates the signaling pathway. This section discusses significant interactions such as receptor-enzyme interaction and direct-cascade effects.

1.6.1 Receptor and enzymes

This involves studying the interaction between the receptor and the antigen molecule. A toxic chemical bind to the receptor and mimics the response of an endogenous substance, which usually binds to that receptor. This toxic agent either increases or decreases the effect typically shown by endogenous components (Li et al., 2018). For example, muscarinic antagonist atropine binds to the Ach-binding site at a nerve interval, causing no signal.

1.6.2 Direct and cascade effects

For many substances, the first insult initiates a series of events, such as activating a cAMP-dependent pathway or inducing the gradual build-up of an endogenous metabolite. Similarly, because of a disruption in the equilibrium between triglyceride uptake, synthesis, and release, triglyceride -up is a frequent reaction to various hepatotoxic drugs. So, the normal metabolic pathway is disturbed by the cascade effects (Sassone-Corsi, 2012).

1.7 Nonspecific interaction and toxicity

Narcosis results from nonspecific ways of harmful activity; thus, narcosis is a mode of toxic action. The presence of toxicant molecules in the organism causes narcosis described as a generalized loss in biological activity. The mechanism of action is still unclear, but a few hypotheses state that it causes changes in the cell membrane, such as proteins bound to the cell membranes (Gupta, 2018). In a subsequent section, two modes of action are discussed: (i) electrophiles and covalent binding and (ii) free radicals and lipid peroxidation.

1.7.1 Electrophiles and covalent binding

Some compounds show strong covalent interaction and exhibit toxicity, but this is not the case with all. Although a few compounds bind covalently, they do not show any toxicity. For example, electrophiles that are formed after biological activation of the xenobiotics bind to the macromolecules such as DNA, protein, etc. GSH, nucleophilic in nature, is used by the enzyme GSH S-transferases having an affinity for electrophile compounds (Haschek et al., 2022). Toxicity does not appear until GSH levels have been reduced to less than 20% of normal through conjugation and irreversible covalent binding to cellular components.

1.7.2 Free radicals and lipid peroxidation

When xenobiotic molecules are activated to an intermediate compound, the intermediate compound breaks down, releasing free radicals. Xenobiotics such as paraquat and menadione, which cycle between oxidized and reduced forms and produce oxygen radicals each time they cycle back to the oxidized form, can also cause peroxidation. Some metabolically generated compounds cause cytotoxicity. The compound, such as 4-hydroxynonenal, is cytolytic and destroy the membrane (Recknagel et al., 2020; Reinheckel and Tholen, 2022).

1.8 Mechanisms of toxicity pharmaceutical drugs

Pharmaceutical medications can cause toxicity through a variety of processes. Covalent binding of the drug or its metabolites to specific enzymes or receptors in tissue-specific pathways, which induce toxic reactions, is a typical mechanism. The toxicity mechanism is known to study how chemical or physical factors interact with living organisms to generate toxicity. Knowledge of a substance's toxicity mechanism improves the ability to prevent toxicity and develop more desirable compounds; it also serves as the foundation for overexposure therapy and frequently leads to a better knowledge of underlying biological processes.

1.8.1 On-target toxicity

Mechanism-based toxicity is another term for on-target toxicity. The extent of interaction between the target and therapeutic moiety is responsible for on-target toxicity. Both the therapeutic and harmful targets are the same in this scenario. The drug must often be adjusted to target a different element of the disease or symptoms to avoid toxicity throughout treatment. Statins are a medicine class that can have harmful side effects when used to treat a specific condition (HMG CoA reductase) (Guengerich, 2010).

1.8.2 Immune responses

Immune responses are typical for a few pharmaceutical compounds. One of the most common causes of idiosyncratic toxicity is immune-related drug reactions. For example, penicillin can cause the creation of specific antibodies and trigger an immunological response in some persons. When this response is triggered unnecessarily, it can create serious health problems and inhibit the immune system from functioning correctly. In gilthead seabream, tamoxifen, a selective estrogen receptor modulator, has been demonstrated to modify the humoral adaptive immunological response. Pharmaceuticals can cause harm not just to humans but also to creatures that are unintentionally exposed to this circumstance (Rodenas et al., 2015).

1.8.3 Off-target toxicity

Off-target toxicity can be described as an effect other than desired biological effect. Many nonspecific drugs produce side effects by binding to undesired proteins, receptors, or enzymes, leading to alteration of normal mechanisms and severe side effects. For example, the medicine eplerenone (aldosterone receptor antagonist), which is supposed to boost aldosterone levels, has been proven to cause prostate atrophy (Rudmann, 2013).

1.8.4 Bioactivation

Some drugs are pharmacologically inactive, and such drugs need bioactivation for conversion into their active form. Whereas some drugs do not need this process; instead, they generate reactive forms that start producing adverse effects on their parent drug. Bioactivation can be done by Phase I metabolic enzymes using CYP450 enzymes. This also can lead to the formation of reactive oxygen species.

1.8.5 Drug-drug interactions

Co-administration of two drugs can lead to either synergistic or adverse effects. That means it can give additive (therapeutic effect more significant than single drugs) or no therapeutic effect. Drug-drug interaction is an important point to consider. But this can be extremely dangerous for people on multiple medications (Alam et al., 2016). For example, the co-administration of selective serotonin reuptake inhibitors (SSRIs) such as citalopram and NSAIDs causes gastrointestinal bleeding (Andrade et al., 2010).

1.9 Types of toxic effects

As mentioned earlier, there are many reasons why a chemical is responsible for producing toxic effects like metabolic conversion, drug-drug interaction, etc. So, this toxic effect can be organ-directed or nonorgan-directed. Organ-directed toxicity is related to a specific organ like the liver, kidney, skin, eyes, etc. A specific drug for targeted delivery will show its toxic effect on the targeted organ. So, in further discussion, we have discussed different organ-directed toxicities.

1.9.1 Organ-directed toxicity

Organ toxicity refers to the ability of a chemical substance to cause damage to a specific organ. The different chemical substances act on different body organs such as the liver, kidney, heart, lungs, cardiovascular, hematopoietic, reproductive, and endocrine systems. Fig. 1.2 shows different organ-directed toxicities.

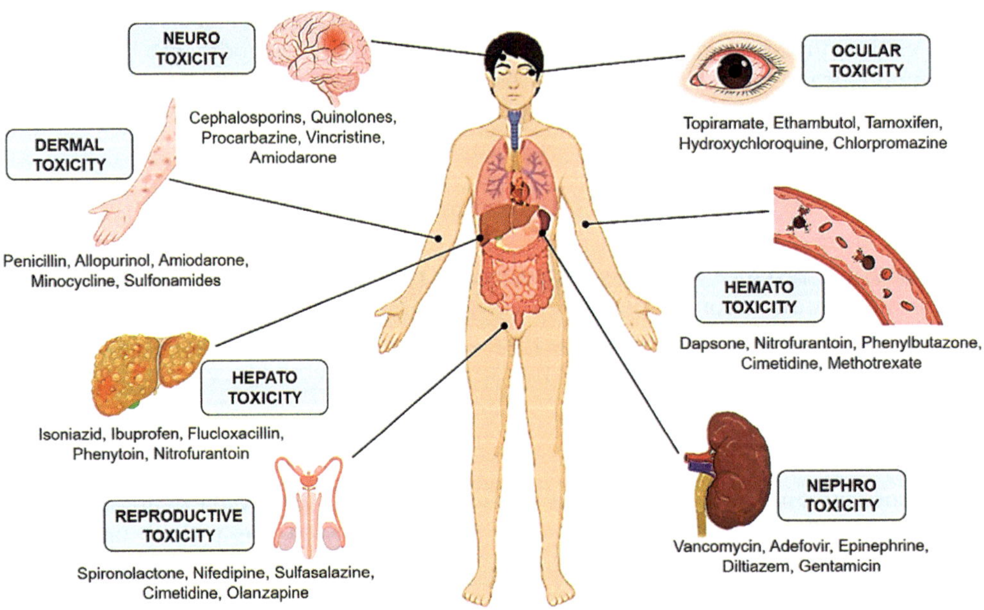

FIGURE 1.2 Organ-directed toxicity.

1.9.1.1 Hepatotoxicity

Hepatotoxicity is a liver injury that includes enlargement and even cirrhosis. Different chemicals, herbal components, solvents, and prescription drugs are all possible causes of liver damage. In patients with acute liver injury with no evident cause, drug-induced liver injury (DILI) is a common differential diagnosis. Hepatotoxicity is responsible for around half of all occurrences of acute liver failure. Among all the over-the-counter drugs, acetaminophen causes severe hepatotoxicity. Other examples are alcohol, cresol, chloroform, nitrosamine, etc. Researchers have studied the effect of ethanol and cerulein on the liver obtained from the white mulberry root bark extract. They have observed tissue infiltration of neutrophils, as shown in Fig. 1.3 (Kavitha and Geetha, 2018).

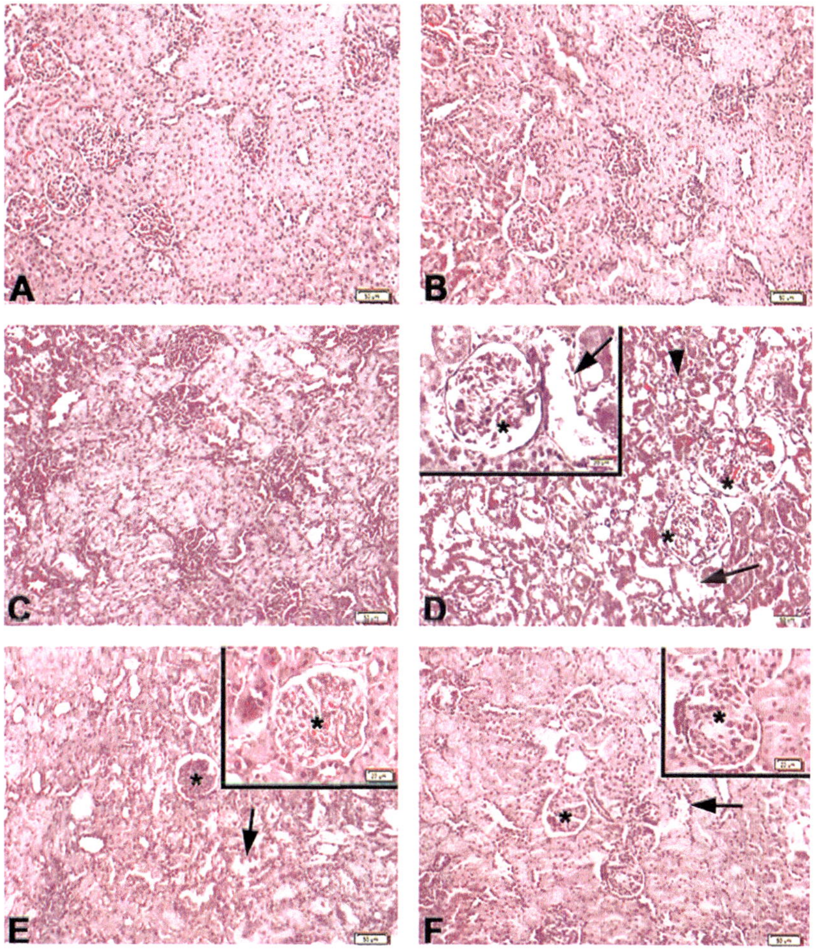

FIGURE 1.3 Histological studies (H and E) were performed in the rat kidney tissues. Normal parenchymal structure of kidney tissue in the control group: (A) saline, (B) Curcumin, and (C) Ferulic acid. (D) Cisplatin-induced toxicity; ("*" indicates blockage of the glomerulus, the arrow indicates destruction of the epithelium of the tubule, and the arrowhead indicates blockage of vessels). (E) Curcumin + cisplatin-treated group ("*" comparatively normal shape of the glomerulus, arrow indicates very less degeneration of epithelium of tubules. (F) Treated group (ferulic acid + cisplatin). *Adopted with the permission from Bami, E., Ozakpinar, O. B., Ozdemir-Kumral, Z. N., Köroglu, K., Ercan, F., Cirakli, Z., Sekerler, T., Izzettin, F. V., Sancar, M., Okuyan, B. 2017. Protective effect of ferulic acid on cisplatin induced nephrotoxicity in rats. Environ. Toxicol. Pharmacol. 54, 105–111.*

1.9.1.2 Nephrotoxicity

A chemical substance that causes a toxic or poisonous effect on kidney function. Acute ethylene glycol poisoning is dangerous, with more than 88% of cases ending in death. Chemicals such as mercury, chloroform, and uranium show nephrotoxicity. Aminoglycosides, amphotericin B, cisplatin, contrast dye, and cyclosporine are among the drugs that are intrinsically nephrotoxic (Schetz et al., 2005). Synergistic nephrotoxicity can occur when numerous nephrotoxins are used together, increasing the risk of kidney damage (Schetz et al., 2005). Researchers have studied the cisplatin-induced nephrotoxicity and protective action of ferulic acid against the nephrotoxicity caused by cisplatin. Saline, curcumin, and ferulic acid were used as control, showing normal kidney structure in histological studies (Bami et al., 2017). Whereas the cisplatin-induced toxicity group has shown infiltration of inflammatory cells, dilation of Bowman's capsule, blockage of the glomerulus, and destruction of the epithelium of the tubule, as shown in Fig. 1.3.

1.9.1.3 Neurotoxicity

Neurotoxins are chemicals that cause damage to both the growing and mature nerves and the central and peripheral nervous systems. These toxins may cause necrosis, changes in behavior, and alteration in muscle coordination. The mechanism of action of neurotoxins involves oxidative stress, apoptotic process, and excitotoxicity. Trigger factors for neurotoxicity involve drug-related (active metabolite, polydrug abuse, substance withdrawal), individual-related (age, gender, antioxidative stress), and environmental-related (chronic stress, temperature).

1.9.1.4 Ocular toxicity

Ocular toxicity occurs due to direct contact or exposure to any toxicant that causes conjunctivitis, corneal injury, or other symptoms. Chemicals such as organic solvents, acids, cresol, bases, etc. have shown ocular toxicity. Because many new pharmaceuticals are launched, systemic drug-induced ocular adverse effects are becoming more common. To help prove causality, reports of drug-induced ocular toxicity must be appropriately documented, and other explanations for these side effects must be ruled out (Alba-Linero and Alba, 2021; Lalu et al., 2017).

In a clinical case study, scientists have documented the ocular damage brought on by a chloroquine overdose. Chloroquine was given to a patient diagnosed with malaria, and the adverse effects that seemed to manifest were impaired vision, decreased distance vision, macular oedema, and variations in color vision, as shown in Fig. 1.4 (Portello, 2000).

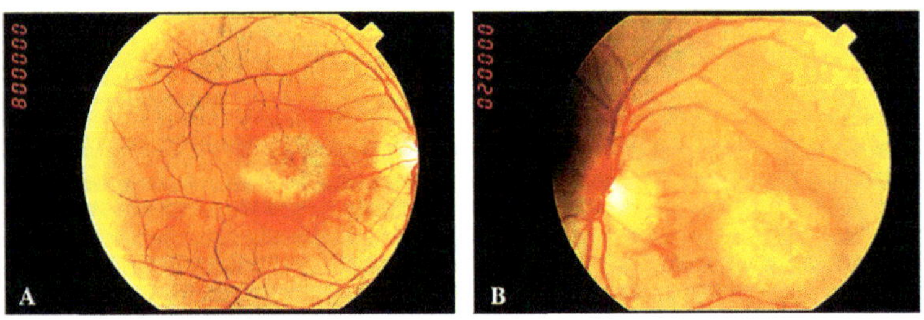

FIGURE 1.4 Representation of an ocular toxicity caused due to the overdosage of chloroquine. (A) Right eye; (B) Left eye. *Adopted with permission from Portello, J.K., 2000. Chloroquine retinopathy and secondary trauma. Clin. Eye Vis. Care 12, 161–165.*

1.9.1.5 Dermatotoxicology

The ability of a drug or poison to have a negative effect on the skin is known as dermal toxicity. The extent of dermal toxicity is mainly dependent on the route of administration. Topically applied medications such as antihistamines, antibiotic ointments, local anesthetics, and paraben esters in cosmetic creams and lotions generally show Type IV immunologic reactions (delayed hypersensitivity) (Amin et al., 2019). When given systemically, agents can elicit nonspecific pruritus or maculopapular eruptions that seem like visual exanthems. Erythema nodosum, fixed drug eruptions, purpura (thrombocytopenic or nonthrombocytopenic), phototoxic and photoallergic reactions, and exfoliative dermatitis or toxic epidermal necrolysis are all examples of cutaneous drug reactions. Various chemicals, such as ketones, alcohol, nickel, phenol, etc., have been reported to be toxic to the skin (Olson, 2020).

1.9.1.6 Hematopoietic (blood) toxicity

Modern drugs have long been associated with the risk of hematologic diseases. Some drugs cause expected blood toxicity, whereas few drugs have shown idiosyncratic reactions. Aplastic anemia, agranulocytosis, megaloblastic anemia, hemolytic anemia, and thrombocytopenia are the most frequent drug-induced hematologic diseases (Greene and Hagemann, 2017). Toxic agents like potassium chlorate, sodium chlorate, benzene, aniline, arsenic, deficiencies of copper, vitamin B12, and folic acid can lead to dermal toxicity.

1.9.1.7 Development and reproductive toxicology

The term "reproductive toxicity" refers to the negative impact on parental generation fertility or offspring development. Developmental toxicology refers to adversely affecting a developing organism from conception to sexual maturity so that developmental toxicology can be regarded as a subset of reproductive toxicology. It seems clear that the intricacy of the reproductive process cannot be examined with a single in vitro model. Hence, the entire process must be divided into steps (gamete maturation, fertilization, implantation, embryogenesis, fetogenesis, and so on) (Rajani et al., 2022). So, it's simple to see why the industry would welcome the employment of quick, safe, and reliable alternative models for testing reproductive toxicity. This developed model can be applied (a) to assess the developmental toxicity potential of a new chemical that is only a minor change of an existing chemical that has already been examined in vivo with that of an existing chemical that has not been tested in vivo, and (b) to assess substances for which testing is not frequently carried out, mainly because the expected exposure is relatively minimal. Different alternative models, such as the whole embryo culture test (WEC), embryonic stem cell test, and micro mass test (MM), have been used to study developmental toxicology (Pamies et al., 2011; Rajani et al., 2022).

1.10 Types of toxicants

The earlier sections of this chapter elaborate on different organ-directed toxicities, but now is the time to look after the sources of toxicities that can be minimized. Any compound in high concentration exhibits its toxic effect. Nowadays, herbal medicines are widely used as therapeutic medicine but are derived from a natural plant source. The toxic compound secreted from the plants may show harmful effects on the body. Similarly, animals and fungi also secrete different toxins, but these toxins can be removed or minimized while performing standardization. Fig. 1.3 shows different types of toxicities arising from various sources. The toxin sources, such as metals, plants, animals, fungi, pesticides, industrial toxicants, etc., have been discussed below:

1.10.1 Metal toxicity

Metal toxicity has recently been identified as one of the most critical mass toxicants, particularly concerning occupational and environmental risks. Researchers are still working on understanding the mechanisms and establishing dose-response relationships for metal-induced reproductive and developmental toxicity. Exposure to metals can cause fertility loss, abortions, skeletal deformities, intrauterine growth retardation, malformations, etc. The extent of toxicity depends on the exposure time of toxicants (Flora and Agrawal, 2017). Male or female reproductive systems can be affected by metal exposure. The influence of metals on intermediate metabolism may directly impact toxicity. Certain metals can build up in mitochondria. In vitro and in vivo studies have revealed that lead, mercury, thallium, and organotin impede oxidative phosphorylation.

Although inorganic lead is hazardous, acute lead poisoning is uncommon. Anemia and hepatic, renal, and neurological complications are all symptoms of lead poisoning. Organic lead poisoning has neurological repercussions, whereas inorganic lead poisoning causes constipation, stomach colic, anemia, and peripheral and motor neuron deficiency (Murphy et al., 2018).

Many studies have reported metals' teratogenic effects, especially arsenic, cadmium, cobalt, mercury, lithium, etc. Disabilities like eye defects, cleft palate, anencephaly, etc. are observed after intoxication, leading to fetal death. The teratogenic effect is dose-dependent; the higher the dose, the greater the effect (Flora and Agrawal, 2017).

1.10.2 Toxins from plants

Plant poisons are metabolites that plants create to defend themselves against various threats, such as insects, predators, and pathogens. Roots, tuber, stems, fruits, buds, and foliage are all parts of the plant that can be harmful. Toxins naturally present in plants are administered as food, leading to food poisoning. Natural toxins such as ricin and N-glycosidase have potential toxicity.

Generally, plants exhibit two types of toxicities: major significant, and minor. Major toxic plants show serious fatal effects, whereas minor toxic plants show less severe symptoms such as diarrhea, vomiting, etc. Usually, plants contain glycosides, alkaloids, tannins, proteins, oxalates, coumarins, volatile oils, etc. Alkaloids (indole alkaloids) beta-carboline-like harmine has activity on CNS (Patel et al., 2012). Pyrrolizidine has a veno-occlusive effect on the liver (Chen and Huo, 2010).

Glycosides such as cardiac glycoside digitoxin in higher doses show cardiac toxicity. Cyanogenic glycosides release prussic acid causing cyanide intoxication; it reduces blood pressure, vomiting, diarrhea, dizziness, etc. (Organization, 1974). Tannins cause the precipitation of proteins making rough skin. Some agents cause Phyto-dermatitis Phyto-photoallergy (Duan et al., 2019).

1.10.3 Toxins from animals

Animal poisons are a complex blend of polypeptides, enzymes, and compounds that can harm cells. Several animal poisons operate on ion channels, causing excitable membranes to polarize or depolarize, affecting the action potential and neuromuscular function. Different animals have different effects on ion channels. For example, Jellyfish, Sea anemone, Ciguatoxin, Palytoxin, Annelid, and Spider activate the sodium ion channel, whereas μ conotoxin, Tetrodotoxin, Saxitoxin, and Gonyautoxin inactivate the sodium ion channel (Sitprija and Suteparak, 2008).

1.10.4 Toxins from fungi

Fungi produce toxins, also known as mycotoxins, which harm plants, animals, and humans. Under several conditions, fungi secrete chemicals that are not useful for their growth. Several species of fungi, such as *Aspergillus, Alternaria, Penicillium*, etc., are known to produce toxins. *Aspergillus* species like *A. flavus* and *A. parasiticus* produce aflatoxins. Aflatoxins mainly act on the liver and cause liver damage. This secreted aflatoxin causes carcinogenicity (Organization, 1974), mutagenicity (Ong, 1975), and immunosuppression. The mode of action of aflatoxin is inhibition of the synthesis of nucleic acid, enzyme, protein, and glycogenesis.

Penicillium citrinum produces citrinin as a potent mycotoxin that causes nephrotoxicity. Fusaric acid is another toxin produced by *Fusarium* species. It has a cytotoxic effect on the colon and a cytostatic effect on human fibroblasts.

1.10.5 Pesticide residue

Due to the increased need for food, pesticides have been used extensively to manage insects, nematodes, rodents, weeds, and fungi. Pesticide residues may be present in the substrate that insects feed on; thus, this factor must also be considered. Grasshoppers and dumplings, for example, are fed entirely or partially with fresh vegetables. These pesticide residues exhibit bioaccumulation. An example of pesticide residue found in food products is honey. Because of its rigorous use, the chances of contamination are more. Pesticides sprayed on crops have the potential to contaminate bees that collect nectar and pollen from flowers, resulting in harmful compounds accumulating in honey. It is reported that pesticides found in honey are known to cause testicular toxicity (El-Nahhal, 2020; Tiwari et al., 2022).

1.10.5.1 Industrial toxicants

Chemical substances ranging from metals and inorganic compounds to complex organic molecules are used in industry. People who work in these fields are at risk of becoming exposed. Exposure levels are higher in fast-industrializing countries, and industrial diseases are more common than in well-developed countries. Toxic substances in the workplace are still a severe hazard in such countries. Some substances can pass through the skin and induce toxicity in other body parts. The insecticide parathion causes lethal toxicity when absorbed

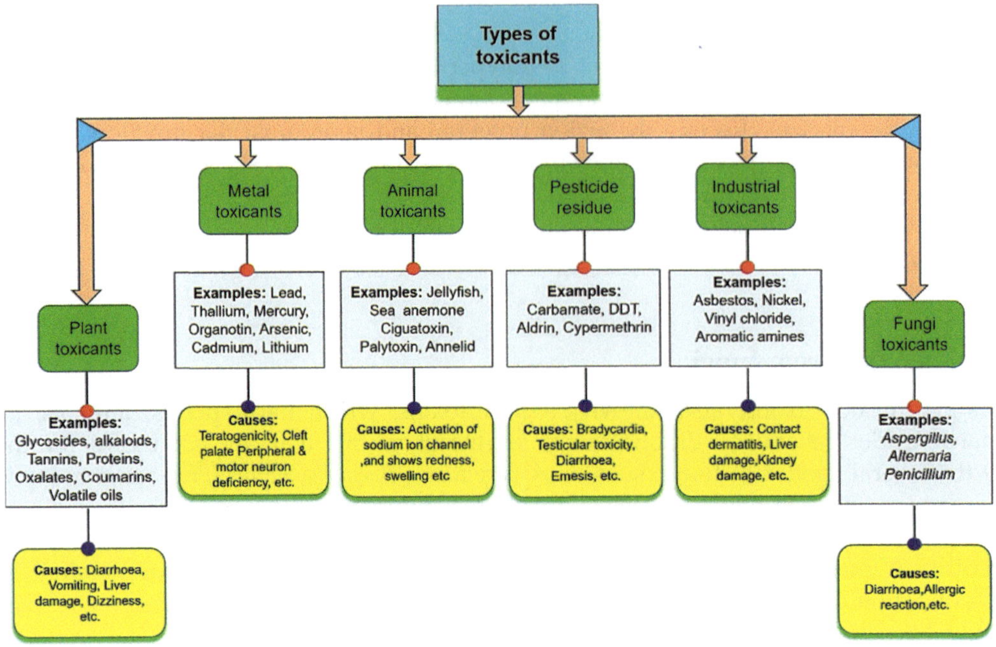

FIGURE 1.5 Different types of toxicants originating from a variety of sources.

via the skin. Other examples of industrial toxicants and their toxicity include asbestos (lung cancer), nickel (contact dermatitis), vinyl chloride (liver damage), cadmium (kidney damage), aromatic amines (carcinogenic), etc. Chemicals naturally mobilized and released into the environment, contaminating water, soil, air, and living beings, including food, are classified as industrial toxicants (Griffith et al., 2015) (Fig. 1.5).

1.11 Types of toxicity tests

The previous discussion expounds on toxic components' sources and how they affect the different organs. But there are specific guidelines to monitor these toxicities. These guidelines will help better understand the types of different toxicity, like acute and chronic. The Food and Drug Administration (FDA), Organisation for Economic Co-operation and Development (OECD), and International Council for Harmonization (ICH) have their guidelines for the evaluation of toxicity. In the following section, a brief description of the above-mentioned guidelines is given:

1.11.1 Guidelines for toxicity tests

OECD guidelines for acute oral toxicity tests can provide preliminary information on a material's toxicity when no further toxicological data is available. Acute toxicity tests involve administering a single dose to every test animal, kept under observation for 1–2 weeks to evaluate a single dose to every test animal kept under observation 1–2 weeks to evaluate any signs or symptoms related to the given treatment. The median lethal dose (LD_{50}) is evaluated in acute oral toxicity. LD_{50} is the dose of a test chemical that causes 50% of the animals in a dose group to die (Buschmann, 2013).

OECD guidelines are used to study the toxic effects of the chemicals. These guidelines include different parts such as 401, 402, and so on. Every single subpart has a different significance. OECD guideline 401 (acute oral toxicity), 402 (acute dermal toxicity), 403 (acute inhalational toxicity), 404 (acute dermal irritation/conversion toxicity), 405 (acute eye irritation/corrosion), 406 (skin sensitization), 407 (repeated dose 28- day oral toxicity study in rodents), 408 (repeated dose 90-day oral toxicity study in rodents), and so on (Buschmann, 2013).

1.11.2 Analysis of statistical method currently used in toxicology

Although statistical approaches are often utilized in toxicology, it is unclear whether the studies' procedures are applied consistently and on acceptable statistical grounds. Although the mean, median, and mode are all valid measures of central tendency, one becomes more appropriate to employ than the others based on the skewness of the distribution of variables. The terms standard deviation (SD) and standard error mean (SEM) are frequently interchanged when discussing data dispersion (Nagele, 2003; Ko et al., 2014). SEM measures sample mean precision, while SD measures individual value variability (Kluxen, 2020).

As the sample size rises, SEM decreases, and the size of SEM is usually less than SD, making the findings appear more consistent and reliable. As a result, the variability of individual parameters may be underestimated when employing SEM (Kluxen, 2020).

1.11.3 Nonprecautionary aspects of toxicology

Empirical toxicological research aims to decipher complex causal linkages, particularly in the context of human disease etiologies. In decision-making based on the precautionary principle, several scientific traditions limit the utility of documentation from current toxicological research (Grandjean, 2005). The concentration on simplified model systems and the consequences of isolated hazards, one by one, are nonprecautionary characteristics of toxicology. As a result, sources of unpredictability and uncertainty, such as individual vulnerability, the effects of mixed and variable exposures, vulnerable life stages, and vulnerable populations, receive less attention. Measurement error, which leads to misclassification, is a significant source of uncertainty, particularly in exposure assessment. The standard statistical analysis assumes that the exposure is accurately recorded and that any inaccuracies will lead to an underestimating of the dose-effect relationship. Toxicology must find its position in the future in this context, and research methods must be created and enhanced to avoid ideological biases.

1.12 Pharmacotoxicology studies

Preclinical studies evaluate the newly designed drug in its dosage form and its toxic effect on animals. To evaluate the toxic effect of a compound in vitro, in vivo techniques are utilized. But before heading toward animal studies, in vitro experiments are performed. Toxicological phenomena studied in nonwhole animal models are referred to as in vitro toxicology. Tissue slices, isolated organs, isolated primary cell cultures, explant cultures, cell lines, and even subcellular fractions like mitochondria, microsomes, and membranes are all included in this comprehensive definition (Gupta et al., 2022b). Whereas in vivo studies are performed on animals, as well as different bioassays are also performed. But by considering ethical issues (Lingayat et al., 2022), it is always better to prefer alternatives for animal studies.

1.12.1 The developing role of In vitro alternative models in pharmacotoxicology

It is widely agreed that, to the extent practicable, animal experimentation should be decreased, refined, or replaced. Various in vitro models are used for screening as an alternative to animal studies. Toxicity testing has typically relied on investigations of adverse health effects observed in appropriate animal models (i.e., toxicological endpoints) at high doses to determine a no-observed-effect level (NOEL)/no-observed-adverse-effect level (NOAEL). Chemical compounds' acute toxicity can be assessed using one of the various in vitro cytotoxicity tests that have been developed. Only a few in vitro procedures have been used thus far. The earliest accepted in vitro test systems were those for genotoxicity testing, which included a test for bacterial reverse mutation using *Salmonella typhimurium* (TA1535, TA1537 or TA97a or TA97, TA98, and TA100) strains as well as *Escherichia coli* WP2 [e.g., *E. coli* WP2 or *E. coli* WP2 (pKM101)] strains, a test for (e.g., phototoxicity, corrosivity) (Webster, 1980).

To establish the level of accuracy of predictivity once produced and validated, it is necessary to determine the value of in vitro test systems (e.g., human tissues, human tissue slices, or primary human cells and cell lines). In terms of in vitro tissue test systems, whole blood, generally from rabbits or humans, was the only tissue frequently employed in regulatory testing in the past. The Hen's Egg Test-Chorioallantoic Membrane, a non-mammalian assay, has also achieved widespread recognition in Europe (Djabari et al., 2002). The development of two-dimensional (2D) and three-dimensional (3D) cell (co)-cultures, which closely imitate cells and tissues in the human body, is one of the most recent developments in cell-based research (İpek et al., 2022). Finally, in vitro pyrogenicity testing (or bacterial endotoxin testing) is an in vitro test used to identify pyrogen in parenteral medications and is one of the biggest success stories for in vitro testing (Spoladore et al., 2021).

1.12.1.1 In vivo studies

The study of the hazardous effects of chemical substances on a living organism, such as a laboratory animal, is known as in vivo toxicology. Different in vivo toxicity assays are performed, such as dose-range finding assay, single and repeat-dose toxicity assay, acute, subchronic, chronic assay, local tolerance assay, genotoxicity assay, carcinogenicity assay, and reproduction toxicity assay (Pour and Sasidharan, 2011).

1.12.2 Zebrafish as a model to study toxicity

The cyprinid schooling teleost zebrafish (*Danio rerio*) is an excellent model for genetic research (Polaka et al., 2022c). The Zebrafish model acts as a bridge between in vitro toxicity testing and in vivo mammalian toxicity testing. Toxic heavy metals are monitored by using the zebrafish model. In the aquatic environment, toxic heavy metals could be detected indirectly by measuring enzyme activity or biomarker gene expression in wild-type embryos or adult zebrafish (Richetti et al., 2011; Polaka et al., 2022b). Zebrafish provides the 3R principle for toxicity testing, i.e., replacement, reduction, and refinement for animal studies.

a) **Replacement:** Zebrafish allows the use of larval zebrafish to establish the applicable model (for tissue organ, target, mechanism, etc.) and replaces the use of the animal model.
b) **Reduction:** Zebrafish larvae could be used to discover harmful drug candidates as a first model for toxicity, enabling safer compounds to be investigated in mammalian models. This would ultimately result in the reduction of animals being used in experimentation.
c) **Refinement:** The use of embryonic zebrafish can be used to refine animal studies because embryos are externally fertilized and remain transparent for the first few days of their initial life.

Zebrafish offers many advantages like its small size, ease of husbandry, rapid organ development, etc. As zebrafish show transparency, we can say it is a noninvasive technique to observe organ development. It has been reported that zebrafish can be used to study different organ toxicities such as ocular toxicity (Cassar et al., 2021), neurotoxicity (Fitzgerald et al., 2021), liver (Katoch and Patial, 2021), and intestinal toxicity (Zhao et al., 2021).

1.13 Pharmacotoxicity examples

Many pharmacological medications can have adverse side effects due to biotransformation, contact with other targets, or drug-drug interactions (Polaka et al., 2022d), herb-drug interaction (Polaka et al., 2022a), food-drug interaction (Polaka et al., 2022e), etc. This section briefly discusses a few examples of the drug's adverse effects after overdosage.

1.13.1 Acetaminophen

After being biotransformed to produce reactive intermediates, high dosages of acetaminophen have been found to cause severe hepatotoxicity. CYP2E1 converts acetaminophen to NAPQI, which produces severe oxidative stress due to increased reactive oxygen species (ROS) (Boelsterli, 2002). ROS causes a reduction in the enzyme glutathione as well as mitochondrial damage. Drug-drug interaction of acetaminophen with other drugs activates a nuclear receptor CAR causing the metabolism of other drugs (Jaeschke et al., 2021).

1.13.2 Venlafaxine

Venlafaxin is an antidepressant drug, and it is a serotonin-norepinephrine reuptake inhibitor. It is reported that an overdose of Venlafaxin causes mild cardiac toxicity (Singh et al., 2019) and also causes hyperexcitation of neurons, tachycardia, hypertension, seizures sometimes suicide (Bruggeman and O'Day, 2021; Blixt et al., 2018).

1.13.3 Aspirin

Aspirin belongs to the category of nonsteroidal anti-inflammatory drugs (NSAIDs). Deliberate or accidental aspirin consumption causes metabolic disturbances, making the treatment difficult. Moreover, the co-administration of any other drug further complicates the treatment (Palmer and Clegg, 2020). Overdose of aspirin shows severe side effects such as vomiting, nausea, bleeding, epigastric pain, etc. Acute toxicity causes oxidative distress and ROS generation, and chronic toxicity causes respiratory damage.

1.13.4 Doxorubicin

Doxorubicin is a widely used anticancer drug for tumors. However, it can cause multi-organ toxicity. Cardiotoxicity caused by doxorubicin is produced in different ways. One of the mechanisms is the generation of oxidative stress. It exhibits its action on mitochondria, leading to the formation of reactive oxygen species (ROS), causing mitochondrial toxicity (Rosa et al., 2016). Stefen et al. reported doxorubicin-induced hematological toxicity, such as anemia, leukopenia, neutropenia, and thrombocytopenia (Sleijfer et al., 2018). The researchers also reported that doxorubicin causes arterial stiffness in cancer patients receiving chemotherapeutic treatment (Bosman et al., 2021).

1.13.5 Phenobarbital

Phenobarbital belongs to the barbiturates category, which is a CNS depressant. Overdosage of phenobarbital leads to neurotoxicity, and sometimes, it may cause hyperexcitation or confusion. A higher than 8 mg/kg dose of phenobarbital causes severe neurological symptoms. It is also reported that phenobarbital also shows cardiovascular toxicities such as tachycardia, hypotension, etc. (Lewis and Adams, 2021).

1.13.6 Haloperidol

Haloperidol is an antipsychotic drug primarily used in the treatment of mental disorders. The most common adverse effects of haloperidol are extrapyramidal effects such as tremor, rigidity, and restlessness. Overdosage of it can cause tardive dyskinesia (Ward and Citrome, 2018). In tardive dyskinesia, the patient suffers from the repeated movement of lips and rolling of the tongue.

1.13.7 Atropine

Atropine belongs to an anticholinergic category of drugs. Usually, it is administered by both the routes topically and parenterally. Anticholinergic drugs are known to cause delirium. Clinicians have reported that atropine administered mainly by the parenteral route has shown central anticholinergic syndrome (CAS). Atropine is a competitive antagonist of the M1 acetylcholine receptor, which is primarily located in the central nervous system (Maravi et al., 2020). The clinicians also reported that atropine given via the intranasal route in pediatric patients had shown severe toxic effects such as tonic-clonic seizures, loss of consciousness, irritability, vomiting, etc. (Alaula et al., 2019).

1.13.8 Etoposide

The anticancer agent etoposide is a podophyllotoxin glycoside. Its mechanism of action is the formation of a ternary complex with DNA and topoisomerase II. However, researchers have reported genotoxic damage caused by the etoposide in cancer cell lines. The oxidative stress of DNA damages DNA strands and generates reactive oxygen species. It also produces mutations in the genetic material and leads to genotoxicity (Atha et al., 2020; Mišík et al., 2019).

1.14 Conclusion

Pharmacotoxicology is a broad branch that deals with drug and their effect on living organisms. Diagnosis of a proper disease and giving an accurate dose at an accurate time through a proper route of administration is a big task for clinicians. To make it easy, one has to understand a thorough process. To understand the exact mechanism in the pharmacodynamics of a drug, a good researcher has to gain a thorough understanding of the principles applied in pharmacology. The principle discussed above plays a significant role in understanding what a drug does to the body. So, it will help study its pharmacotoxicokinetic effects. The drug has broad exposure in a dynamic body, which is the reason behind the toxicity of different organs. Various biomarkers are used to identify the toxicity or status of the disease. Biomarkers are nothing but litmus paper tests for disease identification.

It is also essential to understand the mechanism of a toxic compound, such as on-target toxicity, off-target toxicity, immune response, etc. Once we understand the mechanism of action, we can move forward with studying the effects of these toxins on different organs; simultaneously, the source from which these toxins arise can also be studied. An authorized regulatory body decided on a standardized toxicity determination protocol to give generalized rules for toxicity. FDA, OECD, and ICH regulatory bodies have made different protocols to study acute and chronic toxicities. Furthermore, these toxicity studies can be performed using In vitro and in vivo techniques that help to understand the nature of chemicals and expected toxicity. Finding a source of toxicity will make a researcher study it thoroughly and eliminate the toxic components effectively. Acetaminophen, venlafaxine, doxorubicin, etc., are a few classic examples of harmful drugs available in the market or routinely used for therapeutic benefits. Hence, it is of utmost importance to observe the pharmaco-toxicokinetic of any drug after its administration.

1.15 List of abbreviations

CAR Chimeric antigen receptor
CAS Central anticholinergic syndrome
DILI drug-induced liver injury
FDA Food and Drug Administration
ICH International Council for Harmonization
NOAEL no-observed-adverse-effect level
NOEL no-observed-effect level
NSAID Nonsteroidal anti-inflammatory drugs
OECD Organisation for Economic Co-operation and Development
OEL Occupational exposure level
ROS reactive oxygen species
SD Standard deviation
SEM Standard error mean
SSRIs selective serotonin reuptake inhibitors
TDM Therapeutic drug monitoring

References

Alam, K., Pahwa, S., Wang, X., Zhang, P., Ding, K., Abuznait, A.H., Li, L., Yue, W., 2016. Downregulation of organic anion transporting polypeptide (OATP) 1B1 transport function by lysosomotropic drug chloroquine: implication in OATP-mediated drug-drug interactions. Mol. Pharm. 13, 839–851.

Alaula, L.S., AL-Kadi, M., Almajed, A., Alhedaithy, R., 2019. Atropine toxicity caused by erroneous intranasal administration in a pediatric patient: case report. Ann. Saudi Med. 39, 279–282.

Alba-Linero, C., Alba, E., 2021. Ocular side effects of checkpoint inhibitors. Surv. Ophthalmol. 66, 951–959.

Aljundi, W., Suffo, S., Munteanu, C., Langenbucher, A., Seitz, B., Abdin, A.D., 2022. Intravitreal injection for diabetic macular edema as adjunctive therapy for proliferative diabetic retinopathy: a retrospective study. Clin. Ophthalmol. 16, 135.

Alqahtani, M.S., Kazi, M., Alsenaidy, M.A., Ahmad, M.Z., 2021. Advances in oral drug delivery. Front. Pharmacol. 12, 618411.

Amin, S., Lauerma, A.I., Maibach, H.I., 2019. Diagnostic tests in dermatotoxicology. In: Dermatotoxicology Methods: The Laboratory Worker's Vade Mecum. CRC Press.

Andrade, C., Sandarsh, S., Chethan, K.B., Nagesh, K.S., 2010. Serotonin reuptake inhibitor antidepressants and abnormal bleeding: a review for clinicians and a reconsideration of mechanisms. J. Clin. Psychiatr. 71, 19280.

Anup, N., Rajpoot, K., Tekade, R.K., 2021. Chapter 1 - overview of biopharmaceutics and pharmacokinetics. In: Tekade, R.K. (Ed.), Biopharmaceutics and Pharmacokinetics Considerations. Academic Press.

Asati, S., Pandey, V., Gour, V., Tiwari, R., Soni, V., Rajpoot, K., Tekade, M., Sharma, M.C., Tekade, R.K., 2022. Chapter 16 - toxicity and toxicokinetic considerations in product development and drug research. In: Tekade, R.K. (Ed.), Pharmacokinetics and Toxicokinetic Considerations. Academic Press.

Atha, D.H., Coskun, E., Erdem, O., Tona, A., Reipa, V., Nelson, B.C., 2020. Genotoxic effects of etoposide, bleomycin, and ethyl methanesulfonate on cultured CHO cells: analysis by GC-MS/MS and comet assay. J. Nucleic Acids 2020.

Bami, E., OZAKPınar, O.B., OZDEMIR-Kumral, Z.N., Köroglu, K., Ercan, F., Cirakli, Z., Sekerler, T., Izzettin, F.V., Sancar, M., Okuyan, B., 2017. Protective effect of ferulic acid on cisplatin induced nephrotoxicity in rats. Environ. Toxicol. Pharmacol. 54, 105–111.

Blixt, J., Raheem, S., Bujarski, S., 2018. Severe venlafaxine intoxication with refractory pulseless electrical activity cardiac arrest successfully treated with intravenous lipid emulsion. Int. J. Crit. Care Emerg. Med. 4, 044.

Boelsterli, U.A., 2002. Mechanistic Toxicology: The Molecular Basis of How Chemicals Disrupt Biological Targets. CRC Press.

Bosman, M., Favere, K., Neutel, C.H., Jacobs, G., DE Meyer, G.R., Martinet, W., VAN Craenenbroeck, E.M., Guns, P.-J.D., 2021. Doxorubicin induces arterial stiffness: a comprehensive in vivo and ex vivo evaluation of vascular toxicity in mice. Toxicol. Lett. 346, 23–33.

Bright-Ponte, S.J., Zhou, T., Murphy, M.J., 2018. Regulatory considerations in veterinary toxicology: an FDA perspective. In: Veterinary Toxicology. Elsevier.

Bruggeman, C., O'day, C.S., 2021. Selective Serotonin Reuptake Inhibitor Toxicity. StatPearls.

Buschmann, J., 2013. The OECD guidelines for the testing of chemicals and pesticides. Teratogenicity Testing, pp. 37–56.

Califf, R.M., 2018. Biomarker definitions and their applications. Exp. Biol. Med. 243, 213–221.

Cassar, S., Dunn, C., Ramos, M.F., 2021. Zebrafish as an animal model for ocular toxicity testing: a review of ocular anatomy and functional assays. Toxicol. Pathol. 49, 438–454.

Chandrasekaran, B., Abed, S.N., AL-Attraqchi, O., Kuche, K., Tekade, R.K., 2018. Computer-aided prediction of pharmacokinetic (ADMET) properties. In: Dosage Form Design Parameters. Elsevier.

Chen, Z., Huo, J.-R., 2010. Hepatic veno-occlusive disease associated with toxicity of pyrrolizidine alkaloids in herbal preparations. Neth. J. Med. 68, 252–260.

Cohen, G.M., 2020. Basic principles of target organ toxicity. In: Target Organ Toxicity. CRC Press.

Colerangle, J.B., 2017. Preclinical development of nononcogenic drugs (Small and large molecules). In: A Comprehensive Guide to Toxicology in Nonclinical Drug Development. Elsevier.

Combes, R., 2013. Progress in the Development, Validation and Regulatory Acceptance of in Vitro Methods for Toxicity Testing.

Dave, A., Shah, S., Mistry, Y., Chaturvedi, N., Jariwala, D., 2022. Ocular side effects in tuberculosis patients receiving direct observed therapy containing ethambutol. Natl. J. Physiol. Pharm. Pharmacol. 12, 127–131.

Djabari, Z., Bauza, E., DAL Farra, C., Domloge, N., 2002. The HET-CAM test combined with histological studies for better evaluation of active ingredient innocuity. Int. J. Tissue React. 24, 117–121.

Dong, Z., Tang, S.-S., Li, C.-H., Tang, Z.-S., Yang, Z.-H., Zeng, J.-G., 2022. Safety assessment of MPTA: an oral acute and 90-day sub-chronic toxicity study in Sprague-Dawley rats. Regul. Toxicol. Pharmacol. 105188.

Duan, L., Akakpo, J.Y., Ramachandran, A., Jaeschke, H., 2019. Environmental Liver Toxins. Encyclopedia of Environmental Health, pp. 578–584.

EL-Nahhal, Y., 2020. Pesticide residues in honey and their potential reproductive toxicity. Sci. Total Environ. 741, 139953.

Eliasson, E., Lindh, J.D., Malmström, R.E., Beck, O., Dahl, M.-L., 2013. Therapeutic drug monitoring for tomorrow. Eur. J. Clin. Pharmacol. 69, 25–32.

Farmahin, R., Williams, A., Kuo, B., Chepelev, N.L., Thomas, R.S., BARTON-Maclaren, T.S., Curran, I.H., Nong, A., Wade, M.G., Yauk, C.L., 2017. Recommended approaches in the application of toxicogenomics to derive points of departure for chemical risk assessment. Arch. Toxicol. 91, 2045–2065.

Fitzgerald, J.A., Könemann, S., Krümpelmann, L., Županič, A., VOM Berg, C., 2021. Approaches to test the neurotoxicity of environmental contaminants in the zebrafish model: from behavior to molecular mechanisms. Environ. Toxicol. Chem. 40, 989–1006.

Flora, S.J., Agrawal, S., 2017. Arsenic, cadmium, and lead. Reproductive and Development Toxicology, pp. 537–566 (Elsevier).

Galetin, A., Zhang, L., Rodrigues, A.D., Huang, S.-M., 2022. Drug-drug interactions. Atkinson's Principles of Clinical Pharmacology, pp. 241–265 (Elsevier).

Ghiazza, M., Vietti, G., Fenoglio, I., 2014. Carbon nanotubes: properties, applications, and toxicity. In: Health and Environmental Safety of Nanomaterials. Elsevier.

Ghiculescu, R., 2008. Therapeutic drug monitoring: which drugs, why, when and how to do it. Aust. Prescr. 31, 4.

Grandjean, P., 2005. Non-precautionary aspects of toxicology. Toxicol. Appl. Pharmacol. 207, 652–657.

Greene, E.M., Hagemann, T.M., 2017. Drug-induced hematologic disorders. In: Dipiro, J.T., Talbert, R.L., Yee, G.C., Matzke, G.R., Wells, B.G., Posey, L.M. (Eds.), Pharmacotherapy: A Pathophysiologic Approach, 10e. McGraw-Hill Education, New York, NY.

Greim, H., Snyder, R., 2018. Toxicology and Risk Assessment: A Comprehensive Introduction. John Wiley & Sons.
Griffith, C.M., Baig, N., Seiber, J.N., 2015. Contamination from industrial toxicants 22. Handbook of Food Chemistry, p. 719.
Guengerich, F.P., 2010. Mechanisms of drug toxicity and relevance to pharmaceutical development. Drug Metab. Pharm. 26, 3–14, 1010210090-1010210090.
Gupta, P., 2020. Principles of toxicology. Problem Solving Questions in Toxicology, pp. 27–45 (Springer).
Gupta, P.K., 2018. Illustrated Toxicology: With Study Questions. Academic Press.
Gupta, R., Polaka, S., Rajpoot, K., Tekade, M., Sharma, M.C., Tekade, R.K., 2022a. Chapter 6 - importance of toxicity testing in drug discovery and research. In: Tekade, R.K. (Ed.), Pharmacokinetics and Toxicokinetic Considerations. Academic Press.
Gupta, R., Rajpoot, K., Tekade, M., Sharma, M.C., Tekade, R.K., 2022b. Chapter 7 - methods and models for in vitro toxicity. In: Tekade, R.K. (Ed.), Pharmacokinetics and Toxicokinetic Considerations. Academic Press.
Haschek, W.M., Rousseaux, C.G., Wallig, M.A., Bolon, B., 2022. Toxicologic pathology: an introduction. In: Haschek and Rousseaux's Handbook of Toxicologic Pathology. Elsevier.
Heckert, J., Parkman, H., 2018. Therapeutic response to domperidone in gastroparesis: a prospective study using the GCSI-daily diary. Neuro Gastroenterol. Motil. 30, e13246.
Ipek, S., Üstündağ, A., Can Eke, B., 2022. Three-dimensional (3D) cell culture studies: a review of the field of toxicology. Drug Chem. Toxicol. 1–11.
Jaeschke, H., Murray, F.J., Monnot, A.D., Jacobson-Kram, D., Cohen, S.M., Hardisty, J.F., Atillasoy, E., Hermanowski-Vosatka, A., Kuffner, E., Wikoff, D., 2021. Assessment of the biochemical pathways for acetaminophen toxicity: implications for its carcinogenic hazard potential. Regul. Toxicol. Pharmacol. 120, 104859.
Jain, D., 2022. Ocular effects of systemic medications. Sci. J. Delhi Ophthalmol. Soc. 32, 87–92.
Katoch, S., Patial, V., 2021. Zebrafish: an emerging model system to study liver diseases and related drug discovery. J. Appl. Toxicol. 41, 33–51.
Kavitha, Y., Geetha, A., 2018. Anti-inflammatory and preventive activity of white mulberry root bark extract in an experimental model of pancreatitis. J. Tradit. Complement. Med. 8, 497–505.
Kayat, J., Gajbhiye, V., Tekade, R.K., Jain, N.K., 2011. Pulmonary toxicity of carbon nanotubes: a systematic report. Nanomed. Nanotechnol. Biol. Med. 7, 40–49.
Kluxen, F.M., 2020. "New statistics" in regulatory toxicology? Regul. Toxicol. Pharmacol. 117, 104763.
Ko, W.-R., Hung, W.-T., Chang, H.-C., Lin, L.-Y., 2014. Inappropriate use of standard error of the mean when reporting variability of study samples: a critical evaluation of four selected journals of obstetrics and gynecology. Taiwan. J. Obstet. Gynecol. 53, 26–29.
Lalu, L., Tambe, V., Pradhan, D., Nayak, K., Bagchi, S., Maheshwari, R., Kalia, K., Tekade, R.K., 2017. Novel nanosystems for the treatment of ocular inflammation: current paradigms and future research directions. J. Contr. Release 268, 19–39.
Lewis, C.B., Adams, N., 2021. Phenobarbital. StatPearls. StatPearls Publishing.
Li, X.-N., Zuo, Y.-Z., Qin, L., Liu, W., Li, Y.-H., Li, J.-L., 2018. Atrazine-xenobiotic nuclear receptor interactions induce cardiac inflammation and endoplasmic reticulum stress in quail (*Coturnix coturnix* coturnix). Chemosphere 206, 549–559.
Lingayat, I., Mishra, P., Vasdev, N., Polaka, S., Mishra, A., Tekade, R.K., 2022. Chapter 25 - ethical defilements in clinical research and potential roles of institutional review board. In: Tekade, R.K. (Ed.), Pharmacokinetics and Toxicokinetic Considerations. Academic Press.
Maravi, P., Mishra, D.K., Singh, A., Niranjan, V., 2020. Atropine eye-drop-induced acute delirium: a case report. Gen. Psychiatry 33.
Mealey, K.L., Karriker, M.J., 2019. Comparative pharmacokinetics and pharmacodynamics. In: Pharmacotherapeutics for Veterinary Dispensing, pp. 75–94.
Mišík, M., Filipic, M., Nersesyan, A., Kundi, M., Isidori, M., Knasmueller, S., 2019. Environmental risk assessment of widely used anticancer drugs (5-fluorouracil, cisplatin, etoposide, imatinib mesylate). Water Res. 164, 114953.
Murphy, M.J., Srivastava, R., Deans, K., 2018. Clinical Biochemistry: An Illustrated Colour Text. Elsevier Health Sciences.
Nagele, P., 2003. Misuse of standard error of the mean (SEM) when reporting variability of a sample. A critical evaluation of four anaesthesia journals. Br. J. Anaesth. 90, 514–516.

Olson, C.T., 2020. Evaluation of the dermal irritancy of chemicals. Dermal and Ocular Toxicology 125–251 (CRC Press).

Ong, T.-M., 1975. Aflatoxin mutagenesis. Mutat. Res. Rev. Genet. Toxicol. 32, 35–53.

Organization, W.H., 1974. Toxicological Evaluation of Some Food Additives Including Anticaking Agents, Antimicrobials, Antioxidants, Emulsifiers and Thickening Agents. Joint FAO/WHO Expert Committee on Food Additives Location Geneva.

Palmer, B.F., Clegg, D.J., 2020. Salicylate toxicity. N. Engl. J. Med. 382, 2544–2555.

Pamies, D., Martínez, C.E., Sogorb, M.A., Vilanova, E., 2011. Mechanism-based models in reproductive and developmental toxicology. In: Reproductive and Developmental Toxicology. Elsevier.

Pandey, V., Polaka, S., Nalla, L.V., Tekade, M., Sharma, M.C., Tekade, R.K., 2022. Chapter 18 - excipient toxicity and safety. In: Tekade, R.K. (Ed.), Pharmacokinetics and Toxicokinetic Considerations. Academic Press.

Patel, K., Gadewar, M., Tripathi, R., Prasad, S., Patel, D.K., 2012. A review on medicinal importance, pharmacological activity and bioanalytical aspects of beta-carboline alkaloid "Harmine". Asian Pac. J. Trop. Biomed. 2, 660–664.

Polaka, S., Chaudhari, S., Tekade, M., Sharma, M.C., Malviya, N., Malviya, S., Tekade, R.K., 2022a. Chapter 13 - clinical importance of herb–drug interaction. In: Tekade, R.K. (Ed.), Pharmacokinetics and Toxicokinetic Considerations. Academic Press.

Polaka, S., Koppisetti, H., Pande, S., Tekade, M., Sharma, M.C., Tekade, R.K., 2022b. Chapter 9 - zebrafish models for toxicological screening. In: Tekade, R.K. (Ed.), Pharmacokinetics and Toxicokinetic Considerations. Academic Press.

Polaka, S., Koppisetti, H., Pande, S., Tekade, M., Sharma, M.C., Tekade, R.K., 2022c. Zebrafish Models for Toxicological Screening. Pharmacokinetics and Toxicokinetic Considerations. Elsevier.

Polaka, S., Koppisetti, H.P., Tekade, M., Sharma, M.C., Sengupta, P., Tekade, R.K., 2022d. Chapter 12 - drug–drug interactions and their implications on the pharmacokinetics of the drugs. In: Tekade, R.K. (Ed.), Pharmacokinetics and Toxicokinetic Considerations. Academic Press.

Polaka, S., Rajpoot, K., Tekade, M., Sharma, M.C., Tekade, R.K., 2022e. Chapter 11 - food–drug interactions and their implications on oral drug bioavailability. In: Tekade, R.K. (Ed.), Pharmacokinetics and Toxicokinetic Considerations. Academic Press.

Polaka, S., Vasdev, N., Raji, S., Makwana, V., Rajput, A., Kulkarni, M., Tekade, M., Pingale, P., Sharma, M.C., Tekade, R.K., 2022f. Chapter 4 - toxicogenomics in drug safety assessment. In: Tekade, R.K. (Ed.), Pharmacokinetics and Toxicokinetic Considerations. Academic Press.

Portello, J.K., 2000. Chloroquine retinopathy and secondary trauma. Clin. Eye Vis. Care 12, 161–165.

Pour, B.M., Sasidharan, S., 2011. In vivo toxicity study of Lantana camara. Asian Pac. J. Trop. Biomed. 1, 230–232.

Raj, G.M., Raveendran, R., 2019. Introduction to Basics of Pharmacology and Toxicology: Volume 1: General and Molecular Pharmacology: Principles of Drug Action. Springer.

Rajani, C., Borisa, P., Bagul, S., Shukla, K., Tambe, V., Desai, N., Tekade, R.K., 2022. Chapter 24 - developmental toxicity of nanomaterials used in drug delivery: understanding molecular biomechanics and potential remedial measures. In: Tekade, R.K. (Ed.), Pharmacokinetics and Toxicokinetic Considerations. Academic Press.

Rajpoot, K., Katare, P., Tekade, M., Sharma, M.C., Polaka, S., Sengupta, P., Tekade, R.K., 2022a. Chapter 26 - toxicokinetic and toxicodynamic considerations in drug research. In: Tekade, R.K. (Ed.), Pharmacokinetics and Toxicokinetic Considerations. Academic Press.

Rajpoot, K., Tekade, M., Sharma, M.C., Arafat, B., Tekade, R.K., 2022b. Chapter 1 - principles and concepts in toxicokinetic. In: Tekade, R.K. (Ed.), Pharmacokinetics and Toxicokinetic Considerations. Academic Press.

Ralston, S.H., Penman, I.D., Strachan, M.W., Hobson, R., 2018. Davidson's Principles and Practice of Medicine E-Book. Elsevier Health Sciences.

Recknagel, R.O., Glende, E.A., Britton, R.S., 2020. Free radical damage and lipid peroxidation. Hepatotoxicology. CRC Press.

Reinheckel, T., Tholen, M., 2022. Low-level lysosomal membrane permeabilization for limited release and sublethal functions of cathepsin proteases in the cytosol and nucleus. FEBS Open bio 12, 694–707.

Richetti, S.K., Rosemberg, D.B., VENTURA-Lima, J., Monserrat, J.M., Bogo, M.R., Bonan, C.D., 2011. Acetylcholinesterase activity and antioxidant capacity of zebrafish brain is altered by heavy metal exposure. Neurotoxicology 32, 116–122.

Rodenas, M., Cabas, I., Abellán, E., Meseguer, J., Mulero, V., GARCÍA-Ayala, A., 2015. Tamoxifen persistently disrupts the humoral adaptive immune response of gilthead seabream (*Sparus aurata* L.). Dev. Comp. Immunol. 53, 283–292.

Rosa, G.M., Gigli, L., Tagliasacchi, M.I., DI Iorio, C., Carbone, F., Nencioni, A., Montecucco, F., Brunelli, C., 2016. Update on cardiotoxicity of anticancer treatments. Eur. J. Clin. Invest. 46, 264–284.

Rudmann, D.G., 2013. On-target and off-target-based toxicologic effects. Toxicol. Pathol. 41, 310–314.

Sassone-Corsi, P., 2012. The cyclic AMP pathway. Cold Spring Harbor Perspect. Biol. 4, a011148.

Sawicki, K., Czajka, M., Matysiak-Kucharek, M., Fal, B., Drop, B., Meczyńska-Wielgosz, S., Sikorska, K., Kruszewski, M., Kapka-Skrzypczak, L., 2019. Toxicity of metallic nanoparticles in the central nervous system. Nanotechnol. Rev. 8, 175–200.

Schetz, M., Dasta, J., Goldstein, S., Golper, T., 2005. Drug-induced acute kidney injury. Curr. Opin. Crit. Care 11, 555–565.

Schoenmakers, I., Jones, K.S., 2018. Pharmacology and pharmacokinetics. Vitamins D 635–661. Elsevier).

Singh, H., Dubois, B., AL-Jammali, Z., Barrett, T., 2019. Pharmacogenomics in the clinic: genetic polymorphism contributing to venlafaxine-associated heart failure. Pharmacogenomics 20, 1175–1178.

Sitprija, V., Suteparak, S., 2008. Animal toxins: an overview. Asian Biomed. 2, 451–457.

Sleijfer, S., Rizzo, E., Litière, S., Mathijssen, R.H., Judson, I.R., Gelderblom, H., Van Der Graaf, W.T., Gronchi, A., 2018. Predictors for doxorubicin-induced hematological toxicity and its association with outcome in advanced soft tissue sarcoma patients; a retrospective analysis of the EORTC-soft tissue and bone sarcoma group database. Acta Oncol. 57, 1117–1126.

Spoladore, J., Gimenes, I., Bachinski, R., Negherbon, J.P., Hartung, T., Granjeiro, J.M., Alves, G.G., 2021. Standardized pyrogen testing of medical products with the bacterial endotoxin test (BET) as a substitute for rabbit Pyrogen testing (RPT): a scoping review. Toxicol. Vitro 74, 105160.

Tekade, M., Koppisetti, H., Sharma, M.C., Rajpoot, K., Sengupta, P., Kumar, M., Tekade, R.K., 2022. Chapter 5 - understanding the concept of signal toxicity and its implications on human health. In: Tekade, R.K. (Ed.), Pharmacokinetics and Toxicokinetic Considerations. Academic Press.

Tiwari, A., Joshi, M., Salvi, N., Gupta, D., Gandhi, S., Rajpoot, K., Tekade, R.K., 2022. Toxicity of pharmaceutical azo dyes. Pharmacokinetics and Toxicokinetic Considerations, pp. 569–603 (Elsevier).

Tsatsakis, A.M., 2021. Toxicological Risk Assessment and Multi-System Health Impacts from Exposure. Elsevier.

Vermeire, S., Dreesen, E., Papamichael, K., Dubinsky, M.C., 2020. How, when, and for whom should we perform therapeutic drug monitoring? Clin. Gastroenterol. Hepatol. 18, 1291–1299.

Ward, K.M., Citrome, L., 2018. Antipsychotic-related movement disorders: drug-induced parkinsonism vs. tardive dyskinesia—key differences in pathophysiology and clinical management. Neurol. Ther. 7, 233–248.

Webster, C.J., 1980. Principles of a quantitative assay for bacterial endotoxins in blood that uses Limulus lysate and a chromogenic substrate. J. Clin. Microbiol. 12, 644–650.

Zhao, Y., Qiao, R., Zhang, S., Wang, G., 2021. Metabolomic profiling reveals the intestinal toxicity of different length of microplastic fibers on zebrafish (*Danio rerio*). J. Hazard Mater. 403, 123663.

CHAPTER

2

Toxicology in drug research

Ankit Mishra[1], Pranali Mishra[1], Muktika Tekade[2], Rachna Gupta[3], Kuldeep Rajpoot[3], Farahidah Mohamed[4] and Rakesh Kumar Tekade[3]

[1]VNS Group of Institutions, Bhopal, Madhya Pradesh, India; [2]School of Pharmacy, Devi Ahilya Vishwavidyalaya, Indore, Madhya Pradesh, India; [3]National Institute of Pharmaceutical Education and Research (NIPER)- Ahmedabad, An Institute of National Importance, Government of India, Department of Pharmaceuticals, Ministry of Chemicals and Fertilizers, Palaj, Gandhinagar, Gujarat, India; [4]Kulliyyah of Pharmacy, International Islamic University Malaysia, Kuantan, Malaysia

2.1 Introduction

Toxicology is the study of toxic or drug-related adverse effects of drugs or chemicals possessing therapeutic values when administered to living beings (Rajpoot et al., 2022b; Gupta et al., 2022a). Toxicological testing is considered essential for the advancement of novel drugs as well as for upgrading the prevailing drug's therapeutic potency (Shete et al., 2022). Paracelsus (a pioneer of toxicology) found that a particular substance can exhibit dose-dependent drug toxicity. Elsewhere, researchers explained that every substance has positive and negative effects, but its optimal dose decides whether it will be toxic or therapeutic (Hunter, 2008). Toxicology in drug research was established in the mid-1900s, while environmental toxicological research was developed in the mid of 20th century. For drug toxicity testing, animal models are widely accepted by the United States Food and Drug Administration (USFDA), but still the animal testing needs to be approved by the Institute Animal Ethics Committee (IAEC).

Animal testing provides information regarding drug toxicity and is utilized for human toxicity prediction, as it is very close to clinical toxicity. However, researchers are trying to minimize animal testing via alternative methods such as in vitro and in silico studies because of its expensive and complex protocols and extrapolation of data to humans (Rajpoot et al., 2022a; Gupta et al., 2022a). These alternative methods have some limitations because it is impossible to depend entirely on them. Hence, animal usage in drug toxicity testing has

Essentials of Pharmatoxicology in Drug Research, Volume 1
https://doi.org/10.1016/B978-0-443-15840-7.00020-8

not been completely reduced. Drug toxicity assessment such as analytical toxicology, genomics, proteomics, metabolomics, genotoxicity, toxicologic pathology, structure-activity studies, biomathematics and statistics, epidemiology, and others, can mainly be predicted via in vitro, in vivo, and in silico methods (Polaka et al., 2021; Rajpoot et al., 2022a; Tambe et al., 2021e).

In silico data are accepted by regulatory guidelines in combination with in vitro and in vivo data. In addition, in silico process is helpful for pharmacists and researchers in emerging handling, risk identification, labeling, transportation, and disposal measures of a new drug (Gupta et al., 2022c; Asati et al., 2022). The dose parameters of drugs play a vital role in the drug's safety. Drugs at low or high doses may have therapeutic as well as toxic effects. However, various factors are involved that affect the drug's safety (Parikh et al., 2022; Gupta et al., 2022b), such as patient characteristics, environmental conditions, prescribers or health professional-related factors, pharmaceutical factors, animal factors, administration route, physical and chemical aspects of the drug, application of new tools and technologies (nanotechnology, imaging, omics, bioinformatics, robotics for preparation and distribution of drugs and others), etc. (Schneider, 2018; Slikker et al., 2018; Alshammari, 2016).

However, for understanding the mechanism of action of drug toxicity and exploring the drug's long-term effects in the patient population, in vitro, in vivo, and in silico methods play an essential part in verifying the safety of the new drug. A toxicological study should be designed cautiously to reduce the harmful effects of chemicals in human and clinical trials. Hence, the next sections expound in detail different factors affecting the safety of drugs, toxicology assessment of drugs in toxicity studies (i.e., in silico, in vitro, and in vivo drug toxicity studies), use of zebrafish and drosophila in drug discovery toxicology, and use of various toxicological studies drug development like computational toxicity, organs-on-a-chip for toxicological assessment, toxicogenomic in predictive toxicology. Further sections also describe the role of animal models in predicting human toxicology and drug safety and toxicology in preclinical drug development.

2.2 Understanding of therapeutic targets

Target is the protein molecule in the body that interacts with a drug and produces a therapeutic effect for specific diseases. An adequate understanding of drug-target interaction is needed to discover novel biologically active small molecules. This is possible through investigating drug-target systems, assessing their interaction profiles, and computing the interlinkages between genes and drug targets (Tolani et al., 2021; Yildirim et al., 2007). Manifold drugs, targets, and diseases interact as molecular associations. The on-target and off-target effects of the drug results in both predicted and unpredicted therapeutic effects. Therefore, drug-target identification and knowledge of its interface mechanism are crucial for drug discovery that could be useful in enhancing therapeutic effects and reducing undesired effects.

Target identification can be achieved via direct biochemical approaches, genetic exchanges, or computational interpretation (Tolani et al., 2021). Primarily, these methods are combined to identify drug-target interactions and their mechanisms. Cell or organism-based assays are widely applied to find exact protein targets, but the information can be more accurately determined using computational approaches. Numerous in silico methods like structure-based, ligand-based, and machine learning-based have proved their efficiency in predicting drug-target mechanisms. In direct biochemical methods (such as affinity-based methods), the target protein associated with disease has an active or binding site into which a small biological molecule binds strongly and exhibits therapeutic effects.

In general, enzymes are good target proteins with an active site into which ligands can easily bind and prevent it. Affinity or immunoaffinity purification is the best biochemical process to identify drug-target interactions. Besides, enzymes, G-protein coupled receptors, protein kinases, nuclear hormone receptors, serine proteases, and ion channels are target proteins whose binding affinity with therapeutic drugs differs depending on the protein fold and sequence homology of the binding site. The therapeutic effects of drugs are caused due to the modifying action of target functional proteins. Such modification of functional protein occurs owing to altered gene expression by activation or deactivation of enhancers or suppressors and gene knockout activity (Knight and Shokat, 2007; Lamb et al., 2006).

Altered gene expression in the cells or tissues leads to the development of various diseases. Through signal transduction pathways, transcriptome sequencing, and DNA microarrays, intracellular drug targets can be identified by gene expression profiling (Wacker et al., 2012; Tekade et al., 2022). Gene knockout approach also plays a vital role in identifying drug targets; for example, cathepsin K, a protease, has been identified using this technique and confirmed that the legitimacy of formerly developed drug targets is not similar to newly discovered targets. Furthermore, computational methods are also used to discover new targets for current drugs and provide analytical support for proteomic and genetic practices to explore off-target effects. Computational systems have been classified into structure-based, molecular activity-based, side-effect-based, and multi-omics-based for drug target prediction (Huang et al., 2018).

Structure-based processes depend on the three-dimensional protein structures to identify drug target interactions, while molecular activity-based methods rely on the protein-ligand interactions to predict targets for new drugs. Besides this, the similarity ensemble approach is one of the computational methods used to analyze proteins having ligands with similar chemical activity (Keiser et al., 2007). However, in this case, ligands are similar in chemical structure, but proteins are dissimilar in sequence or structure. For example, ion channels and G-protein coupled receptors are ligand-associated but differ in protein sequence and structure.

2.3 Different factors affecting the safety of drugs

Drugs must be given to a patient at their appropriate dose size to treat the disease better, as these drugs are not safe at higher doses. The most basic concept of drug safety is based on the dose-response curves (Zhang et al., 2021). All the factors affecting a drug's dose also affect the drug's safety. Factors affecting drug safety can be broadly classified into five categories: patient characteristics, environmental conditions, prescribers or health professional-related features, pharmaceutical aspects, and newer tools and technology adapted nowadays (Fig. 2.1) (Schneider, 2018; Slikker et al., 2018). On the other hand, essential patient characteristics include age, weight, gender, the health of an individual (disease state), diet, genetics, physiological condition, and concurrent medications.

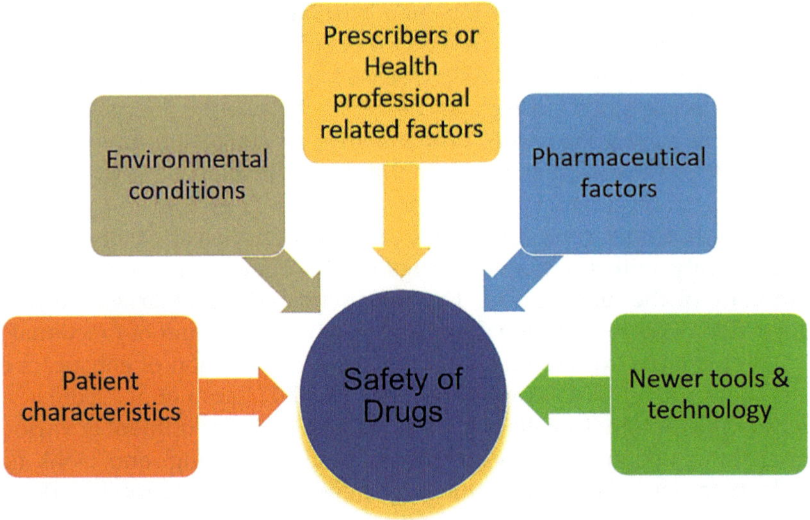

FIGURE 2.1 Factors affecting the safety of drugs.

Environmental characteristics like patient negligence or distraction and interruption influence drug safety. Some environmental factors are indirectly affected by altering patient health (Parikh et al., 2022). Health professional staff (i.e., prescribers, nurses, pharmacists, and others) and their medication knowledge and training are also associated with drug safety. Prescribers or health professional-related factors may arise due to improper collaboration between them, and the possibilities of drug toxicity by these health profession-related factors aggregate through workload and time pressure. Not limited to this, pharmaceutical factors also play a crucial role in drug safety; for instance, routes of administration, medication formula, the pharmacokinetics of the drug, manufacturing procedures, packaging, and labeling are closely associated with the safety of drugs (Tariq et al., 2022; Rajpoot et al., 2021a,b). Adaptation of newer technologies, like the use of computers and barcode systems, helps to reduce drug toxicity. Hi-tech systems like toxicity-reporting systems and potentially inappropriate medication criteria are excellent advancements in detecting drug toxicities. Predicting clinical drug toxicity with the support of an adverse drug event trigger tool is increased several hundred times compared to the conventional method of detecting the same clinical toxicity (Li and Yin, 2019; Rim, 2020).

2.4 Toxicology assessment of drugs

Drug toxicity can be seen by even single or multiple doses of the drug, referred to as acute or chronic toxicity. Even in the body, drug toxicity may vary in various organs. Worldwide regulatory agencies, including the USFDA, requires comprehensive drug toxicological study data. In this regard, the Organization for Economic Cooperation and Development (OCED) issued guidelines to perform these toxicological studies. Drug toxicity assessment is a bit complex, but it can be easy if the scientific approach is used. In the recent era of technologies, a drug toxicity measurement is a systematic approach, which includes different steps like an initial prediction of drug toxicity by in silico methods followed by in vitro assessment of predicted toxicities on cell linings, and finally, confirmation and actual data collection of toxicity by in vivo models (Buschmann, 2012).

Drug toxicity can never be intentionally studied in humans. Instead, it is performed on animals, and obtained data is extrapolated to predict human toxicity, if any. Various government bodies and societies worldwide work for the welfare of animals. However, this creates controversy about using animals to extrapolate the data for humans. This animal toxicity-based prediction in humans may be very close to the actual clinical toxicity; high genetic variations and outbred lead to high chances of unpredictable drug toxicity too. The higher cost of animal-based drug toxicity studies, complex drug toxicological study protocols, extrapolation of animal data to humans, and extrapolation of effects from high drug dose to low drug dose suggest the development of in silico and in vitro methods for drug toxicological studies (Dumont et al., 2015).

In silico toxicological predictions are the interdisciplinary science that applies information technology to drug toxicology. It reduces the traditional randomized approach and makes the studies more economical and practicable. These in silico methods are based on the computational quantitative structure and activity relationships. In vitro method of drug toxicity assessment uses cell lines (especially human cell lines) to further assess the probability of toxicity and to reduce the time and cost of these assessments (Raunio, 2011).

Drug toxicity assessment essentially deals with various analytical and bioassay methods and includes applied mathematics. However, it must answer some critical questions.

i. Is the drug likely to be toxic?
ii. How can this toxicity be quantitatively measured?
iii. At what minimum dose can this drug show toxic effects?

Drug toxicity assessment combines analytical toxicology, genomics, proteomics, metabolomics, genotoxicity, toxicologic pathology, structure-activity studies, biomathematics and statistics, epidemiology, and more. Most of these can be predicted by in silico methods, identified by in vitro models, and confirmed by in vivo models. The process is briefly summarized in Fig. 2.2.

2.4.1 In silico drug toxicity prediction

Important information regarding the underline system can be determined by in silico methods. This information suggests the need for testing and determining the test priorities. As per the scientific aspects, toxicity studies and data must be available for all the drugs, excipients, and chemicals involved in the synthesis (Pandey et al., 2022; Rajani et al., 2022; Sengupta et al., 2022). Therefore, high accuracy requires chemicals are tested for toxicity. Furthermore, rapid assays can be used for handling significant chemicals together. However, various in vivo toxicity tests, along with guidelines, are suggested by OECD (Myatt et al., 2018). The process is rapidly evolving, which will be majorly dependent on such computational processes. More and more methods are getting included in regulatory guidelines,

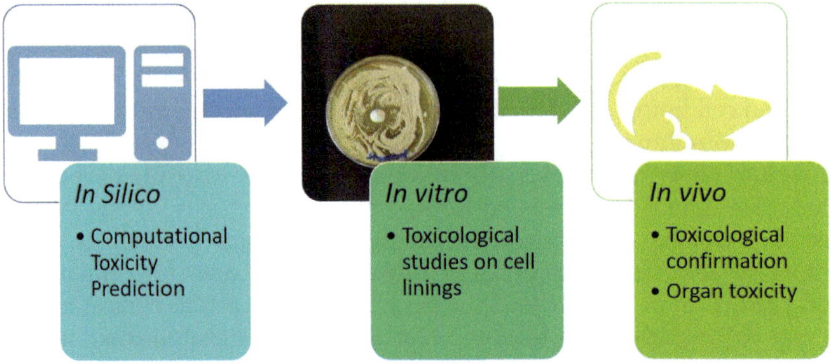

FIGURE 2.2 Scientific sequence of drug toxicity determination.

and data from these studies are being included in drug toxicity assessment documents (Hemmerich and Ecker, 2020).

In combination with in vitro and in vivo data, regulatory authorities are now also accepting in silico data. However, complete acceptance of these methods is yet to be adapted, and in vivo safety documents are required. These in silico data provide the basis of initial dose calculation for in vivo studies, help to protect the scientists working with new drugs, and develop handling, hazard classification, labeling, transportation, and disposal procedures for this drug. Moreover, developments for in silico models for system biology, genomics, proteomics, and metabolomics are still ongoing. Fig. 2.3 represents the flow diagram of in silico drug mutagenicity and carcinogenicity studies (Dearden, 2003).

A challenging situation for in silico models to be used is technological tools and their proprietorship. Although some of the tools are made available by OECD on their website and

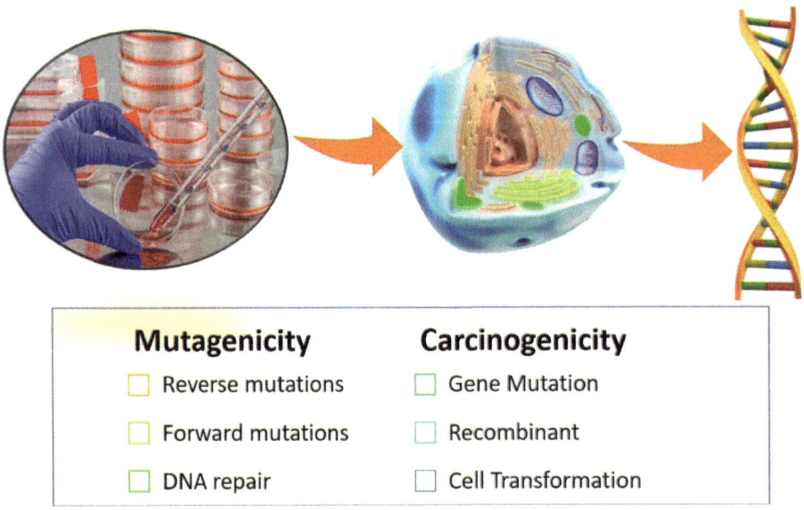

FIGURE 2.3 Flow diagram of in silico drug mutagenicity and carcinogenicity studies.

some more are under development. Proper documentation and scientific presentation of in silico models are also evolving. For proper documentation, in silico toxicology protocols (ISTP) are under development by considering some essential factors like sources of data, nature of studies, nature of protocols, and Good Laboratory Practices (GLPs) status of the laboratory. ISTP can help in validating in silico protocols and predicting the endpoint of the protocol. These ISTP provides the process which leads to the prediction of toxicity (Idakwo et al., 2018).

2.4.2 In vitro drug toxicology study

As per regulatory bodies, safety screening of novel drugs, excipients, chemicals, or other substances of concern (i.e., contaminants) must be conducted using in vitro and in vivo tests where a compound is administered in different doses, and then their effects are observed. As in vitro tests are primarily based on ethical requirements, unnecessary animal testing can be avoided. The toxicity tests on isolated cell systems are alternative cum sequential steps toward studying drug toxicity to in silico tests. These tests gained attention as they predicted the endpoint comparatively faster. In contrast to in silico methods, in vitro tests are well accepted by regulatory bodies as they are similar in approaches and mechanisms. These tests are often used to analyze the effects on cell transformation and gene-based studies, including mutagenicity and oncogenicity. These tests help in the study of the mechanism of drug toxicity (Sung and Shuler, 2010).

Mutagenicity of the drugs is an expression of toxicity that may be expressed in subsequent generations. The theory of somatic mutation as initiating step of chemical oncogenicity is well accepted. Experiments performed by various scientists proved the correlation between mutagenicity and oncogenicity. Therefore these in vitro cell line tests could help to predict the oncogenic potentials of drugs in less time compared to lifetime chronic studies on laboratory animals. However, all the drugs mutagens are not always carcinogens, and vice-versa; for instance, diethyl stilbestrol (a nonsteroidal estrogen) is a carcinogen but not a mutagen (Turkez et al., 2017). Tests involved in the in vitro toxicity analysis can be broadly classified as tests performed on prokaryotic cells or eucaryotic cells. Prokaryotic cells are used as the test objects as they show high mutagenicity. Some of these tests are summarized in Table 2.1.

2.4.2.1 *Eukaryote mutagenicity and mammalian cell mutation*

Due to structural similarities with human cells, in vitro tests are also performed in various eukaryotic cells. Recent developments in cell culture technologies allow both survival and replication of cells, which is the basic principles of mutagenicity tests in these cell linings. Most preferred cells to study such drug toxicity must be isolated from mammals. However, primary cells resembling actual tissues are difficult to culture and have poor cloning abilities. Therefore, some already established mammillary cells, like ovary cells from Chinese hamsters and lymphoma cells from the mouse, are generally used for drug toxicity studies. They also have fewer drug metabolic activities, so they cannot activate metabolic toxicants. Table 2.2 highlights various in vitro mutagenicity and DNA-based tests performed on eukaryotic cells (Sale, 2013; Ouedraogo et al., 2012; OECD, 2022b).

Recent guidelines by OECD also suggest using two cell lines through C3h/10T1/2, Balb/3T3, and mouse embryos. Syrian hamster embryo cells have a different challenge

TABLE 2.1 Various in vitro tests performed in prokaryotic cells.

Test name	Study basis	Microorganism used	Target enzyme(s)
Prokaryote mutagenicity (Ames test)	Reverse mutations	*Salmonella typhimurium*	Liver S9 enzymes
Related tests	Reverse mutations	*Escherichia coli*	Tryptophane mutants
	Reverse mutations	*E. coli*	Utilize nicotinic acid and arginine mutants
	Forward mutations	*S. typhimurium*	Azaguanine in a histidine revertant strain
	Forward mutations	*E. coli*	Galactose non–fermenting one
	Forward mutations	*E. coli*	5-methyltryptophane to 5-methyltryptophane resistance
DNA repair	-	*E. coli*/*Bacillus subtilis*	Polymerase-deficient (DNA repair-deficient)

to score evenly. Some of these in vitro tests have also been performed on cells obtained from cancer patients. On the other hand, some studies also observed cell transformation studies after treatment and exposure to chemotherapeutic drugs and smoking (Vasseur and Lasne, 2012).

2.4.3 In vivo drug toxicity studies

As per the requirements of regulatory authorities, the basis for determining drug toxicity is entirely based on in vivo administration or exposure of the drug to one or more species of the tested animal. These animals are then examined for mortality or sign of toxicities. Detailed pathological examinations of various tissues must be studied if the drug is exposed chronically. Finally, human drug toxicity is predicted using these data and various extrapolation techniques. Some of these in vivo drug toxicity tests are summarized here. To understand the basics, in vivo drug toxicity tests can be divided into general and mechanistic toxicity testing. General toxicity testing without focusing on mechanisms usually wastes time, animal, human, and financial resources. On the other hand, toxicity testing based on mechanisms provides the basis for selecting animal species, doses, and their intervals and methods to extrapolate animal data to predict human drug toxicity.

Another method is based on a targeted organ or system, such as toxicity studies on the skin, eyes, nervous systems, respiratory systems, cardiovascular systems, and others like oncogenicity. Some authors have included this elaborative method in the literature. Here we have presented a more straightforward way of classifying toxicity studies,

TABLE 2.2 Various mutagenicity and DNA based in vitro tests performed in eukaryotic cells.

Test name	Type of study	Cells used	Target enzymes or endpoints
Mutagenicity in simple eukaryotic cells	Gene mutations	Yeasts, or saccharomyces cerevisiae	Purine biosynthetic pathway
Mutagenicity in mammalian cells	Gene mutations	Mouse lymphoma cells or Chinese hamster ovary cells	–
DNA damage and repair	Recombinant test	Yeasts	Gene mutation, oncogenicity, and chromosome damage
DNA synthesis in mammalian cells	–	Primary hepatocytes from adult male rats	Carcinogen aflatoxin B_1 or B_2 – acetylaminofluorene
Chromosome aberrations tests	–	Hepatocytes from rat or Chinese hamster ovary cell line	Chromosome gaps, fragments, breaks, translocations, deletions, ploidy
Related tests	–	Bone marrow cells collected through treated animals	Chromosome gaps, fragments, breaks, translocations, deletions, ploidy
Cell transformation in mammalian cells	–	Embryonic tissue based fibroblast cultures	Carcinogenesis described by transplanting cells inside the host animal as well as monitored the growth of tumor

i.e., classifications based on the duration of drug exposers. In this classification, toxicological studies are divided into four types of tests:

i. Acute toxicity test—a single large dose
ii. Sub-acute toxicity—dose administered for 28 days
iii. Sub-chronic toxicity test—dose administered for 90 days
iv. Chronic toxicity test in combination with oncogenicity test—dose administered for 52 weeks

All these sets of in vivo tests require time, economy, and many animals. Therefore, to make these in vivo drug toxicity studies manageable, all the details related to the drug must be provided to the laboratory performing the test. Details to be provided include chemical structure and identification of the drug, physicochemical properties, pharmacological class, mechanism of action, results of other toxicity studies like in silico, in vitro, and cytotoxicity data, and toxicity data of structurally similar and the drugs of the same pharmacological class.

2.4.3.1 *Acute drug toxicity studies*

Measurement of toxic behavior of drug after short time exposure (i.e., a single dose) is evaluated in acute toxicity studies. This test is performed for all drugs and excipients in their early development stages. This test is primarily performed on rodents and provides initial information on the drug's lethality and potential toxicity. It helps to recognize the mode, i.e., the highest level of the drug's toxic action. Data obtained in this study provides a base for selecting the drug dose for organ-targeted toxicity studies and repeated dose studies. Acute toxicity studies provide information to compare the toxicity of drugs of the same pharmacological class to select the safer treatment for the disease. These results are also essential to selecting the need for childproof packaging, protective equipment, and clothing for the person handling the drug. Acute toxicity tests can be further subdivided as per the administration routes, i.e., acute oral testing, acute skin sensitivity, acute eye contact tests, acute neurotoxicity tests, and others. These tests are briefly discussed here (Program, 2018).

2.4.3.1.1 Acute oral drug toxicity

One of the most effective and well-accepted methods to study acute oral drug toxicity is the determination of the median lethal dose (LD_{50}), which can be defined as the dose of a drug capable of killing half of the test animals. Other methods also include the study of the onset, nature, severity, and reversibility of toxicity following an acute oral dose of the drug. Trevan projected the perception of LD_{50} in 1927. Here, his pioneer study involves administering drugs in different doses to the animal groups, each containing several animals of both genders. The tests were performed for at least three dose levels to determine the dose-response curve. This protocol is still practiced with some modifications as per the requirements. The estimated dose in mg/kg body wt. is denoted as the LD_{50} value. These results also have some statistical confidence limits. This experiment assumes—normal distribution of result data and all or no responses. Findings revealed that various factors like species, age, weight, gender, strain, route of drug administration, time of drug administration, nutrition, gut contents, health, temperature, season, and human error affected the LD_{50} value of drugs. LD_{50} values also promptly vary from laboratory to laboratory. Its reproducibility depends on how closely these variables are controlled (Trevan, 1997).

LD_{50} test is under consideration by regulatory authorities due to its lethal nature. An attempt is to obtain more data and reduce the number of animals. This LD_{50} test is criticized due to:

- **i.** The lethal nature of the test does not give any other acute effects; therefore, it is considered uncritical to obtain a statistically significant value. In addition, it requires large numbers of experimental animals.
- **ii.** Results vary with species, strain, age, gender, etc. The results also differ from laboratory to laboratory.
- **iii.** Regulatory bodies also demand information from chronic toxicity studies
- **iv.** Extrapolation to humans is difficult. Still, this test is conducted to fulfill because of the following recommendations.
- **v.** Properly conducted, it also provides information on the cause, time of death, acute nonlethal effects, affected organs, or reversibility of nonlethal toxic responses.
- **vi.** The slope of the mortality curve provides information on the drug's mode of action, drug metabolism, and detoxication.
- **vii.** The basis of the subchronic test is based on the results of the LD_{50} test.

Despite LD_{50} test having various disadvantages, it is still considered the most important for predicting the toxicity of new drugs. However, regulating agencies mandate the determination of acute toxicity not only by LD_{50} but also by other tests (Zbinden and Flury-Roversi, 1981). A well-planned computer program was developed to simplify experiments and calculate LD_{50}. It was developed by the United States Environmental Protection Agency (USEPA) and works statistically on confidence intervals. Consideration of an initial dose close to the actual LD_{50} must reduce the quantity of tested animals, decrease evaluation time, and minimize the number of evaluating substances required (EPA, 2003). Regulatory bodies provided some alternative tests to LD_{50} for observing acute oral toxicity.

- **i.** The use of the limit test to identify substances having minimum toxicity
- **ii.** Use of a fixed-dose approach
- **iii.** Use of an acute toxic class procedure
- **iv.** The use of an up-and-down method (OECD, 2022a)

The fixed-dose method as well as the acute toxic class approach, are used for the hazardous classification and labeling of drugs. A fixed-dose procedure involves the administration of a single bolus dose, below its LD_{50}, to rodents by oral gavage and detecting the signs of toxicity for 14 successive days. This study ends up with the necropsy on termination day. Acute test other than oral test includes eye irritation and dermal tests is, summarized in Table 2.3. Even on conducting various acute drug toxicity testing, it cannot be predicted which type of tissue or other toxicity can be seen if the drug is repeatedly administered for a long time. The regulatory agencies are also additionally required to accomplish chronic feeding tests. However, these chronic test helps to identify the drugs with higher potential toxicity, which helps to limit the chronic toxicity test to a manageable quantity.

2.4.3.2 *Subacute or repeated drug toxicity studies*

In these repeated dose drug toxicity studies, the drug is administered to animals for 28 days. These studies are performed on rodents to identify organ, inhalation (OECD, 2018b), or dermal toxicities (OECD, 2008, 1981a). These tests are used to find a dose for nontoxicity and the dose of lowest toxicity, which help to decide the first dose for clinical trials.

2.4.3.3 *Subchronic drug toxicity studies*

These tests are performed preferably on rodents and include two types of tests, i.e., oral feeding for 90 days or 28–90 days exposure via dermal or inhalation route (Table 2.4).

Results are described in two parts, i.e., obtained from living animals and obtained from animals after being sacrificed. Further, tests to be performed during subchronic drug toxicity studies are (a) In-life tests and (b) Termination tests.

- **a. In-life tests.** There are different tests that can be performed and including appearance, body weight, behavioral abnormalities, food consumption, eyes, electrocardiogram (ECG), electroencephalogram (EEG), respiration rate, complete hematology, complete blood chemistry, urinalysis, and fecal analysis. Drug and metabolite levels should all be assessed in blood, urine, and fecal samples.

TABLE 2.3 Acute drug toxicity tests other than oral.

Name of test	Experimental animal	Procedure	Endpoint
Eye irritation is not required for materials less than pH 2 and higher than pH 10 (considered to be eye irritants)			
Draize test (no rinse)	Albino rabbit previously n = 6; (now n = 3)	Material left in the eye for 24 h	Graded after 1, 2, and 3 days
Draize test (rinse)	Albino rabbit previously n = 6 (now n = 3)	Influence of rinsing eye just after 1 min exposure	Graded for up to 21 days
Substitute tests	Cultured cells/eyes through slaughtered food animals	Cells are studied for alteration	Not yet acceptable
Modifications	Albino rabbit single animal	Both rinsing and no–rinsing	Severely irritating; no need for further studies
Dermal irritation and sensitization			
Primary irritation	Albino rabbits	Dorsal side in the area of 5 cm^2 was treated with either 0.5 mL or gm	After 4, 24, & 48 h, erythematous and edematous scores
Cutaneous sensitization Buchler (dermal inductions)	Guinea pig	Treated for every 3 days with evenly spaced for 2 weeks, after a 2 week rest	After 4, 24, & 48 h, erythematous and edematous scores
Magnesson and Kligman (intradermal inductions)	Guinea pig	Treated for every 3 days with evenly spaced for 2 weeks, after a 2 week rest	After 4, 24, & 48 h, erythematous and edematous scores
Another test	Guinea pig	Intradermal injection together with Freund's adjuvant[a] and the challenge by dermal application	After 4, 24, & 48 h, erythematous and edematous scores
Another test	Guinea pig	Both induction and challenge are applied topically after intradermal injection of Freund's adjuvant	After 4, 24, & 48 h, erythematous and edematous scores
Phototoxicity and photo-allergy	Guinea pig	U.V. light produces a reactive free-radical intermediate from drugs	Organic radicals act directly with photo-allergy while radicals attach to body proteins, where these modified proteins trigger immune system
Photosensitization	Guinea pig	UV exposer post application	After 4, 24, & 48 h, erythematous and edematous scores

[a]*Substance/chemical mixture which increases the antigenic effect.*

TABLE 2.4 Subchronic drug toxicity tests.

Name of test	Living organism	Procedure	Endpoint	Reference
Subchronic oral tests	Sprague Dawley rat or dog	Three dose levels of oral doses for 28 or 90 days	(a) The highest dose produces toxicity but not a death while (b) the lowest dose causes no toxicity (c) In-life tests and tests on the animal after sacrificed	OECD (2018a)
Subchronic dermal tests	Rat or dog	Three concentrations are applied for 28 or 90 days in suitable solvent corn oil, ethanol, or carboxymethyl cellulose	In-life tests and tests on the animal after sacrificed	OECD (1981b)
Subchronic inhalation tests	Rat or dog	Treated for six to 8 h every day, 5 days each week for 28 or 90 days	In-life tests and tests on the animal after sacrificed	OECD (2018c)

b. **Termination tests.** This test includes microscopic methods, pathological examination, clinical tests, blood chemistry analyses, and detailed target organ studies. High-dose group animals are examined in detail and followed by a lower-dose group until a no-effect group is reached. Organ slides must be observed for necropsy and histology.

2.4.3.4 *Chronic/reproduction drug toxicity studies*

These tests require chronic feeding for the animal's life span or 1 year to a group of rodents in different doses. This test also includes oncogenicity, teratogenicity, and mutagenicity studies. These studies are planned to define the margin of safety and determine various toxic effects. After feeding for 1 year, data is collected for another year. Therefore, the test duration lasts up to 2 years. Three drug doses are selected and given to the groups containing many animals to generate sufficient data. One group is administered with a maximum tolerable dose, calculated in acute and subchronic studies, and two lower doses. Endpoints are similar to those specified in subchronic studies and divided into live tests and testes after sacrifice. On the other hand, chronic drug oncogenicity studies are conducted on rats and mice of both genders, and tumor generation is considered the endpoint (OECD, 2018d,e).

Teratogenicity and reproductive toxicity tests are also required by regulatory authorities and are conducted with chronic drug toxicity studies. These studies must be performed not only during development but also on matured animals. Various teratogenicity tests are summarized in Table 2.5. Even in adult animals, the effect of drug treatment in the premating period, during pregnancy, and lactation is studied. Endpoints in the developmental phase include embryonic development, major organ formation, fetal development, and growth. After the animal's birth, growth, behavior, and development of reproductive physiology are observed. The endpoint of studies in adult animals includes observations of mature eggs & sperm, fertilization, implantation, parturition, and lactation. Probable results are no-effect levels of lower dose groups.

A drug is considered to be teratogenic if it produces adverse effects in the next generation but does not show adverse effects in the mother at the same concentration. Weight change,

TABLE 2.5 Chronic drug teratogenic toxicity tests.

Name of test	Experimental animal	Procedure	Endpoint	References
Single and multiple-generation tests	Rat	25 males/dose group for 70 days premating 25 females/dose group for 14 days premating	• Fertility index • Number of live births • Preimplantation death • Postimplantation death • Time of gestation • Influences on male/female reproductive systems • Survival of pups • Weight gain • Litter size and condition • Time of happen of developmental landmarks • Morphological abnormalities in weanlings	Rorije et al. (2011), Isbrucker et al. (2006), Saghir and Dorato (2016)
Teratology	Rat and rabbit	20 pregnant females/ dosage group	• Structural alterations as well as malformations • Embryo-fetal mortality	Butcher et al. (1980), Khera (1985)
Effect of chemicals in late pregnancy and lactation	Rats, 20 pregnant females/ dosage group	The drug is administered from day 15 of pregnancy to day 21 postpartum	Parturition problems, time of gestation, number as well as size of pups behavioral, physiological testing of the pups	Buhimschi and Weiner (2009a,b), Mehta et al. (2006)

change in regular activities or eating patterns, change in organ weight, and neurotoxicity are symptoms of toxicity in the mother.

2.4.3.4.1 Special tests

Some special tests are conducted to analyze a drug's toxic potential on the central nervous system (CNS)—behavior, motor activity, functional observations, neuropathology, and neurotoxicity. Some major related tests are discussed below.

2.4.3.4.1.1 Drug toxicity in CNS CNS works in a very complex manner; therefore, even if the drug shows toxicity in a particular part of the CNS, the overall function may not be disturbed until the effect is extensive. Moreover, neurotoxicity is analyzed at each level of drug exposure (i.e., acute, subacute, subchronic, and chronic). Neurotoxicity is supplementary to routinely required tests. However, developmental neurotoxicity studies are also performed on drugs. The endpoints and parameters to be studied are presented in Table 2.6. The examined nervous tissues are the spinal cord, brain, and some specific nerves like the sural, optic, tibial, and sciatic nerves. While various tests to be performed in the functional observation battery (FOB) are classified and presented in Table 2.6.

TABLE 2.6 Drug neurotoxicity tests.

Name of test	Experimental animal	Procedure	Endpoint	References
Acute neurotoxicity tests	Rat or mouse 10 −15 animals per sex per dose group	Three dose groups and a control group	Behavioral motor activity FOB, analysis at a particular day of dosing, as well as at 1 and 2 weeks, and neuropathology and histology on a sacrifice	Saunders et al. (2001), Moser (1996)
Subchronic neurotoxicity tests	Rat or mouse dosing for 90 days via diet	Three dose groups and a control group	Behavioral, motor activity, FOB, analysis on selected intervals like weeks 5, 9, and 13 neuropathology and histology on a sacrifice	Moser et al. (1992), Christoph et al. (2003)
Developmental neurotoxicity testing	Rat 20 pregnant female	Three dose groups and a control group	Home cage and open field, motor activity, learning, and memory	Wise et al. (1995), Vorhees et al. (1994)
Delayed neuropathy	Hen	Performed for organophosphates	Ability to inhibit cholinesterase; neurotoxic esterase	Masoud et al. (2009), Henschler et al. (1992)
In vitro BBB model	Rat glial cells	To assess the rate of permeability across the BBB of the drugs	Treated cells have a higher lucifer yellow value than control groups	Stanness et al. (1999), Scism et al. (1999)

BBB, Blood-brain barrier; FOB, functional observation battery.

2.4.3.4.2 Drug metabolic toxicity studies

These studies provide data on probable reactive intermediates and induction/inhibition of the enzymes causing xenobiotic metabolism for possible interaction. This study is performed with radiolabeled isotopes, which facilitate the total recovery of the drug in the body. All the metabolites formed in vivo must be chemically analyzed in blood, lungs, kidneys, liver, and other tissues. Tissue homogenates, fractions of the cells, and purified enzymes are studied to find out events happening through metabolism in the formation of end products. The study of the order of a drug's metabolic reaction is also critical, which is performed by administering various doses to different groups to study in vivo metabolism (Hvastkovs and Rusling, 2016).

2.4.3.4.3 Toxicity due to covalent binding

Some drugs or their metabolites are known to show organ or tissue-specific toxicity. Many carcinogens and anticancer drugs are known to form covalent binding with DNA and form an adduct. Their mechanism of action can predict the toxicity of such drugs. These DNA adducts are an indication of genotoxicity. Some drugs form covalent bonds with protein and again form adducts (Stornetta et al., 2017). These adducts may show lifetime accumulation and indicate possible organ toxicity. Sometimes drugs show covalent binding to tissues when activated by microsomal preparations in vitro, but these are not developed into routine tests. However, they help in predicting the toxicity. Radiolabeled chemicals or dialysis against detergents and separation of adducted antibodies assay of chemically modified DNA or RNA are methods to study such bindings.

2.4.3.4.4 Immunotoxicity and immunotoxicology

These comprise two different types of drug toxicity. Immunotoxicity refers to the contribution of the immune system to the toxic responses of the drug, for instance, as seen in the study for cutaneous sensitization (Bou Zerdan et al., 2021). Immunotoxicology refers to the drug's toxic effect on the immune system, like, in loss of capability to prevent infection (Bussiere, 2010). Examinations for immunotoxicity are normally not mandatory by regulatory bodies.

(a) Potentiation and synergism: It must be studied with combination dosage forms.
(b) Micronucleus test: It is an in vivo examination conducted in mice (in vivo), and the erythrocyte stem cells obtained through bone marrow are generally stained as well as analyzed for micronuclei.

2.5 Computational toxicity in drug development

The drug development process is long and sequential. It includes various steps for toxicity determination by using a computational method. These computational studies are performed to provide:

i. Quantitative structure toxicity relationship
ii. Grouping drugs in toxic categories
iii. Expert systems

These computational methods work on the similarity hypothesis (i.e., drugs with similar structures will have similar toxicity). These computational studies are generally performed in two types (i.e., comprehensive and specific). Here comprehensive type studies are termed expert systems. Based on existing data, these expert systems perform reasoning like a human and represent the properties of the drug based on knowledge rules. While specific type computational systems work based on quantitative structure-activity relationship (QSAR), targeting specific receptors or enzymes (OECD, 2014).

Previously specific computational methods were designed on ligand or target-based. However, it now shifted to a combination of both. These computational toxicity approaches comprise categorizing drugs based on their structure, physicochemical properties, chemical reactivity, and metabolism (Tambe et al., 2021e). However, the missing toxicology data for such categories can be collected from them. Collecting these missing data from the chemical categories is considered a common-sense application of QSAR. Considering physicochemical properties help to find out in vivo bioavailability and pharmaco-toxicokinetics by computational approach (Anup et al., 2021a).

2.5.1 Pharmaco-toxicokinetic, drug metabolic structural alerts

In drug toxicity studies, pharmacokinetics is referred to as toxicokinetics or sometimes biokinetics. Collectively absorption, distribution, metabolism, excretion, and toxicity (ADMET) is the term drug toxicity scientists use for comprehensive profiling of drug toxicokinetics. Computational systems predict and differentiate between the toxicity of a drug and its metabolites based on physicochemical and structurally predicted absorption, distribution, metabolism, and excretion (ADME) (Anup et al., 2021a). The role of drug metabolism in pharmacological and toxicological is well known and can be predicted through computational systems. These reactive metabolites mostly fall into the category of carcinogenic and idiosyncratic and show predicted adverse drug reactions (OECD, 2002).

The ligands binding to cytochrome P450 (CYP), which can be a drug or its metabolites, can be predicted by computational systems, which may act as inhibitors of the enzymes altering the metabolism of drug molecules and other endogenous substances, leading to the prediction of drug-drug or drug-body components toxic interactions (Li et al., 2008). Genotoxicity is a collective term used for mutagenicity and carcinogenicity. These genotoxicity studies involving drug metabolites are a mandatory requirement of drug regulatory agencies. As discussed earlier, complete in vivo determination of genotoxicity is a complex, costly, and time taking method. Therefore, it is high time to predict the same by computational methods. Fifty-seven chemical structures with genotoxicity were grouped by Enoch and Cronin. At the same time, 22 chemical structures were grouped into an idiosyncratic category. Computational drug metabolism prediction, producing such groups, shows a prediction of genotoxicity and idiosyncrasy (Enoch and Cronin, 2010). *In silico* methods judging ADMET forecasts drugs' physicochemical properties, permeability through the gastrointestinal, blood-brain barrier, and other physiological barriers, plasma protein binding, transporter protein's affinity, metabolic clearance, alteration of drug-metabolizing CYP enzymes, and probability of production of reactive metabolites.

2.6 Use of zebrafish in drug discovery toxicology

Evaluating the safety and use of potential drug candidates is the primary objective of toxicology studies in the drug development process. The relevant animal models and vigorously validated procedures fulfill the accomplishment is the vital goal during drug discovery. Hence, to understand the emerging risk for human subjects, the utmost need is to translate the animal model responses, which can be attributed to exploring possible associated risks of the drug candidate. Thus, the toxicologist must be aware of the ethical guidelines and use of toxicology models for safety and evaluation (OECD, 2019).

Zebrafish (*Danio rerio*) is an ideal model organism for drug discovery and toxicology study. Moreover, because of its fecundity and similarity to the morphological and physiological characteristics of mammals, it has become an extremely employed model organism. Further, the amalgamating the scale as well as the throughput of in vitro screens with the physiological intricacy of in vivo analysis, the zebrafish exhibits great contribution to various aspects of the drug development process and toxicology.

Interestingly, the application of zebrafish in pharmacology, as well as toxicology, opens novel avenues to examine and produce novel drug products and identify related disease mechanisms. The use of zebrafish also addresses the 3 R's principle. They do undeniably participate in substituting, decreasing, and refining animal studies and establish it as a "multiorgan culture model." As zebrafish is a valuable technique for performing toxicity analysis, it is an important approach for solving problems as well as determining way to enhance the translation of toxicology findings. In addition, robust estimation of embryonic medium uptake and an efficient understanding of zebrafish structural endpoints might assist in refining biological assays. Moreover, zebrafish have offered new avenues and empathies with various diseases as well as toxic pathways, adverse effect pathways, bioavailability, proteomics, endocrine disturbances, transcriptomics, and metabolism.

2.7 Use of drosophila in drug discovery toxicology

Similar to zebrafish, other animals like drosophila are also getting the attention of drug toxicologists, as these animals have a shorter lifespan and can be developed faster and more economically. The drosophila tests exhibit some advantages. They are generally simple to carry out, do not need mammals as test subjects, and involve an entire eukaryotic animal, including all of its interconnected organ systems as well as activation mechanisms. However, they also have evident drawbacks, such as immunological and hormonal systems that are very unlike those of mammals and the rest of nature (OECD, 1984). Heritable translocations can be identified by precisely studying cells of either male or female progeny at different points of development or by comparing the reproduction of treated or untreated animals and testing for translocations in males with lower fertility.

2.8 Organs-on-a-chip for toxicological assessment in drug development

The drug toxicity profile is the leading reason for the very premature end of clinical trials and further leads to the pulling out of drugs during post-marketing, which may result in human demises as well as financial resources. Moreover, the failure of animal models to predict therapeutic responses in humans is also a problem that brings into question their use for basic research. The predicted reason for this can be the unavailability of effective drug toxicity envisaging models and inadequate understanding of the toxic procedure for preclinical results (Materne et al., 2013; An et al., 2016). The organ-on-a-chip (organ chip) technology bridges the gap between preclinical and clinical outcomes. Microfluidic devices lined with live cells cultivated in fluid flow can accurately reproduce the physiology and pathology of organs at the molecular level. It frequently results in highly effective and durable systems and makes it possible for a more precise model for drug toxicity assessment (Atac et al., 2013; Tambe et al., 2021a).

To accurately simulate organ physiology, including disease conditions, certain technologies reconstruct organ-level structures (such as tissue-tissue interfaces) as well as offer pertinent mechanical signals (such as breathing and peristalsis-like movements). Human "body-on-chips" multiorgan systems that imitate whole-body physiology, drug distribution, as well as disposal may be made by fluidically linking two or more organ chips. Hence, this is an intriguing scientific and technological development in which biology is coupled with microtechnology to mimic critical aspects of human physiology (Miller and Shuler, 2016; Bhatia and Ingber, 2014; Low et al., 2021).

2.9 Toxicogenomics in predictive toxicology in drug development

The evolution of recent ingenious technologies aligned with dramatic increases in genomic knowledge is anticipated to revolutionize toxicological studies by stipulating practical approaches within the understanding and anticipation of the toxicity and efficacy of the latest drugs. Thus, toxicogenomics provides a roadmap for extrapolating findings across species and increases predictability. Toxicogenomics, however, will hasten preclinical safety evaluations and enhance the prognosis of toxic risks, as well as possible risk accumulating for drug-drug or drug-disease interactions. The formulation of a drug depends on understanding the molecular pathways of drug action in addition to conventional characteristics (Vasdev et al., 2021). Mechanistic data is now valued more by various regulatory organizations, which will help the risk analysis (Bandara and Kennedy, 2002; Castle et al., 2002).

In comparison to traditional toxicology methodologies, "toxicogenomics" offers the potential to deliver a more thorough knowledge of molecular pharmacology as well as toxicity. It has been demonstrated to be an effective method for classifying compounds, performing mechanistic research, and finding toxicity biomarkers. Additionally, several biomarkers are helpful in analyzing and grading drugs at much earlier stages of research, leading to improved clinical candidate selection. It is an emerging tool increasingly used for mechanistic or exploratory studies in preclinical and clinical studies, with the overall purpose of generating hypotheses to assist in decision-making (Boorman et al., 2002; Tiwari et al., 2022). Target organs and bodily fluids are specifically sampled, and results from toxicogenomics are combined with data from traditional endpoint measures (clinical chemistry, biochemistry, and histopathology). To confirm the applicability of animal findings to humans as well as determine species-specific effects, it is essential to have a better knowledge of the molecular processes of drug response. As a result, this source of ambiguity in the risk analysis will be significantly reduced. Enhanced knowledge of the toxicity displayed in experimental animal models will increase the prediction performance of extrapolating across experimental animals to humans (Ulrich and Friend, 2002).

2.10 The role of animal models in predicting human toxicology and drug safety

In vivo, preclinical safety models remain the gold standard for assessing human risk. Animal models are ingrained to assess whether a compound proves toxic or non-toxic in humans. Similar to other diagnostic assays and parameters, just by conducting experiments wherein the chemical is administered to both animals and humans. The existence or lack of toxicity can be noticed, and their validity and repeatability may be evaluated (Hudson and Bhogal, 2006). Animal testing is now believed to assist in maintaining human security, the effectiveness of novel medications, and the pharmacodynamic and pharmacokinetic properties of such medications (Tambe et al., 2021b,c,d; Anup et al., 2021b).

Such preclinical testing is required by regulatory agencies worldwide. For the estimation of toxicity, as well as pharmacokinetics, it requires at least two species, often one rodent or one non-rodent species. But for these objectives, a substantial number of animals are utilized in drug evaluation. Interestingly, a fundamental understanding of the most recent method of preclinical safety evaluation establishes the context for three prospective toxicology issues that should be resolved: (a) enhancing various safety assumptions for humans, (b) tackling the "pipeline problem" occurred by high dropout in preclinical toxicology; as well as (c) identifying possible processes of toxicity (Greaves et al., 2004; Heywood, 1981).

Toxicology is well suited to provide patients with efficient and safer medications at a cheaper cost, but to achieve this goal, both technical and nontechnical hurdles must be overcome. Recent developments in the knowledge of the primary mechanism of cell killing as well as the metabolic stimulation of medication to reactive species, provide fresh insights (Kalyane et al., 2022; Polaka et al., 2022; Achanta et al., 2021). However, to enhance mechanism-based safety evaluation for both new and current medications, attention must also be paid to a better understanding of the fundamental processes of drug-induced destination organ cytotoxicity in preclinical models and patients. To advance, basic research must be effectively applied in authentic settings, and the correct technical issues relating to toxicology and drug safety assessment must be prioritized (Schein et al., 1970; Olson et al., 2000; Altman and Bland, 1994).

2.11 Toxicology in preclinical drug development

Drug discovery is a laborious and protracted process that begins with identifying biological targets pertinent to human illness conditions. The main goal of toxicology studies is to assess the safety of possible drug candidates in developing drugs. Validated techniques and pertinent animal models are used to achieve this. The ultimate objective is to translate the responses shown in animal models into a comprehension of the risk for human patients. Toxicology is crucial in finding new drugs and developing new ones.

Toxicologists use quick, quantitative screening techniques during early discovery, concentrating on small endpoints. Early recruitment of medications with the best safety profiles is the goal. These exploratory screenings, which also include in vitro experiments using surrogate markers, GLPs, which are strictly adhered to for all toxicological studies performed in the sustenance of a novel drug application, regulate several aspects of study methods. Medical professionals require a toxicity assessment of the new chemical entity in pertinent animal models. Before the start of the clinical studies. Before the first human dose, in vitro analyses employing proper tissue preparations were the only sources of comparative information regarding human and animal metabolism. The data was acquired to give a preliminary grasp of the applicability of the animal model to human applications. Clinical trials must consider both the response as well as no-effect levels from nonclinical investigations, the onset and period of toxic reactions, the evolution of toxic reactions with dosage time, reversibility, the target organ(s), and the importance of the toxic reactions. The toxicological profile accompanying the initial and ongoing clinical trials are built on the responses to these and other questions. While solving this, the toxicologist must not get caught up in the debate about toxicologic as well as pharmacologic responses (Bass et al., 2009).

During primitive and later research phases of the drug examination and development process, the primary goals of the toxicological profile alter. Thus, screening is the primary emphasis of early drug development. Preclinical safety studies, in the broadest sense, should suitably assess the toxicity of a novel drug candidate in several species, when appropriate, to allow the clinician to be informed of probable side effects during the earliest clinical trials (Mayne et al., 2006). The International Conference on Harmonization (ICH) has made significant progress toward removing significant disparities in the length of toxicity studies required to support clinical trials. Safety pharmacology was acknowledged as a crucial component of the toxicological profile by the ICH Topic M3(M). Investigations should be carried out prior to human exposure with the aim of evaluating impacts on key systems such as the cardiovascular, central nervous, respiratory, or renal systems. Assessments may be carried out independently or as supplements to intended toxicological investigations. Safety pharmacology investigations that are carried out correctly offer valuable data that support more conventional toxicological assessments (Hughes et al., 2011).

The capacity of a chemical to harm DNA or change the DNA sequence in a manner that results in mutation is known as genotoxicity. Neoplasms, inheritable neoplasms, and congenital impairments are the most severe consequences of these mutations. Prior to the first human dosage, in vitro testing for the assessment of mutations, including chromosomal harm must typically be carried out, and the whole test battery must be finished before phase II. Most medications undergo testing as part of their toxicity review. Subchronic examinations are multiple investigations ranging from 2 weeks to 6 months, while acute toxicity testing typically comprises single-dose examinations with a 14-day monitoring period. Multiple-dose trials lasting around 6 months are used in chronic toxicity. In general, a toxicological profile is made up of a number of building blocks that may be added to or eliminated from a study protocol based on information from prior research, data from drugs in the identical therapeutic class, or evidence from drugs with comparable chemical structures.

Biological Toxicology: To complement the populations selected for a clinical study, research on potential negative effects on fertility, fetal development and behavior, and fetal toxicity must be carried out. Draft guideline that outlines an integrated method for evaluating concerns regarding human reproductive, as well as developmental toxicity, was issued by the USFDA (Faqi, 2013).

2.12 Conclusions

Drug toxicity can be measured qualitatively and quantitatively depending on the different laboratory's technical strengths. Different methods are applied for the study of drug-target interactions. Laboratories with chemistry and biochemistry backgrounds prefer to use biochemical methods for drug-target identification. In contrast, genetic laboratories favor genetic methods and people with computational biology fields mainly depend on databases results. Thereby, all these methods are favorable and supportive for therapeutic target identification. Various factors are involved that affect the safety of drugs, such as patient characteristics, environmental conditions, prescribers or health profession-related factors, pharmaceutical factors, animal factors, administration routes, omics, nanotechnology, robotics, and others. The drugs can be toxic or therapeutic depending upon their concentrations or doses. Alternative methods such as in vitro, in vivo, and in silico are adopted to reduce animal testing. Still, researchers cannot avoid animal models for drug toxicity testing due to their limitations. Animal testing delivers knowledge of the functioning organ system, so it is impossible to avoid animal models in the research area. Alternative methods cannot evaluate biochemical and molecular variations of the drug's toxic effects, so these methods need to be improved to accurately detect acute, subchronic, and chronic effects of the compounds. Hence, because of their benefits, much importance will be given to the future development, upgrading, measurement, and authentication of alternative methods.

2.13 List of abbreviations

ADME absorption, distribution, metabolism, and excretion
ADMET absorption, distribution, metabolism, excretion, and toxicity
BBB blood-brain barrier
CNS central nervous system
CYP cytochrome P450
ECG electrocardiogram
EEG electroencephalogram
FOB functional observation battery
GLPs Good Laboratory Practices
IAEC Institute Animal Ethics Committee
ICH International Conference on Harmonization
ISTP in silico toxicology protocols
LD_{50} median lethal dose
OCED Organization for Economic Cooperation and Development
QSAR quantitative structure-activity relationship
USEPA United States Environmental Protection Agency
USFDA United States Food and Drug Administration

References

Achanta, N.S.K., Rajpoot, K., Tekade, R.K., 2021. Drug metabolic kinetics. In: Tekade, R.K. (Ed.), Biopharmaceutics and Pharmacokinetics Considerations. Elsevier, Academic Press, pp. 335–353.

Alshammari, T.M., 2016. Drug safety: the concept, inception and its importance in patients' health. Saudi Pharmaceut. J. 24 (4), 405–412. https://www.ncbi.nlm.nih.gov/pubmed/27330371.

Altman, D.G., Bland, J.M., 1994. Diagnostic tests 2: predictive values. BMJ 309 (6947), 102. https://www.ncbi.nlm.nih.gov/pubmed/8038641.

An, F., Qu, Y., Luo, Y., Fang, N., Liu, Y., Gao, Z., Zhao, W., Lin, B., 2016. A laminated microfluidic device for comprehensive preclinical testing in the drug ADME process. Sci. Rep. 6, 25022. https://www.ncbi.nlm.nih.gov/pubmed/27122192.

Anup, N., Gadeval, A., Rajpoot, K., Tekade, R.K., 2021a. Software used in ADME computation. In: Tekade, R.K. (Ed.), Biopharmaceutics and Pharmacokinetics Considerations. Elsevier, Academic Press, pp. 699–708.

Anup, N., Rajpoot, K., Tekade, R.K., 2021b. Overview of biopharmaceutics and pharmacokinetics. In: Tekade, R.K. (Ed.), Biopharmaceutics and Pharmacokinetics Considerations, vol. 1. Elsevier, Academic Press, pp. 1–16.

Asati, S., Pandey, V., Gour, V., Tiwari, R., Soni, V., Rajpoot, K., Tekade, M., Sharma, M.C., Tekade, R.K., 2022. Toxicity and toxicokinetic considerations in product development and drug research. In: Pharmacokinetics and Toxicokinetic Considerations, vol. 2. Elsevier. https://doi.org/10.1016/b978-0-323-98367-9.00001-9.

Atac, B., Wagner, I., Horland, R., Lauster, R., Marx, U., Tonevitsky, A.G., Azar, R.P., Lindner, G., 2013. Skin and hair on-a-chip: in vitro skin models versus ex vivo tissue maintenance with dynamic perfusion. Lab Chip 13 (18), 3555–3561. https://www.ncbi.nlm.nih.gov/pubmed/23674126.

Bandara, L.R., Kennedy, S., 2002. Toxicoproteomics – a new preclinical tool. Drug Discov. Today 7 (7), 411–418. https://www.ncbi.nlm.nih.gov/pubmed/11916571.

Bass, A.S., Cartwright, M.E., Mahon, C., Morrison, R., Snyder, R., McNamara, P., Bradley, P., Zhou, Y.Y., Hunter, J., 2009. Exploratory drug safety: a discovery strategy to reduce attrition in development. J. Pharmacol. Toxicol. Methods 60 (1), 69–78. https://www.ncbi.nlm.nih.gov/pubmed/19422924.

Bhatia, S.N., Ingber, D.E., 2014. Microfluidic organs-on-chips. Nat. Biotechnol. 32 (8), 760–772. https://www.ncbi.nlm.nih.gov/pubmed/25093883.

Boorman, G.A., Anderson, S.P., Casey, W.M., Brown, R.H., Crosby, L.M., Gottschalk, K., Easton, M., Ni, H., Morgan, K.T., 2002. Toxicogenomics, drug discovery, and the pathologist. Toxicol. Pathol. 30 (1), 15–27. https://www.ncbi.nlm.nih.gov/pubmed/11890469.

Bou Zerdan, M., Moussa, S., Atoui, A., Assi, H.I., 2021. Mechanisms of immunotoxicity: stressors and evaluators. Int. J. Mol. Sci. 22 (15).

Buhimschi, C.S., Weiner, C.P., 2009a. Medications in pregnancy and lactation: part 1. Teratology. Obstet. Gynecol. 113 (1), 166–188. https://www.ncbi.nlm.nih.gov/pubmed/19104374.

Buhimschi, C.S., Weiner, C.P., 2009b. Medications in pregnancy and lactation: Part 2. Drugs with minimal or unknown human teratogenic effect. Obstet. Gynecol. 113 (2 Pt 1), 417–432. https://www.ncbi.nlm.nih.gov/pubmed/19155916.

Buschmann, J., 2012. The OECD guidelines for the testing of chemicals and pesticides. In: Methods in Molecular Biology. Humana Press. https://doi.org/10.1007/978-1-62703-131-8_4.

Bussiere, J.L., 2010. 5.27 - Immunotoxicology of biological response modifiers. In: McQueen, C.A. (Ed.), Comprehensive Toxicology, second ed. Elsevier, Oxford, pp. 521–529 https://www.sciencedirect.com/science/article/pii/B9780080468846006308.

Butcher, R.E., Wootten, V., Vorhees, C.V., 1980. Standards in behavioral teratology testing: test variability and sensitivity. Teratog. Carcinog. Mutagen. 1 (1), 49–61. https://www.ncbi.nlm.nih.gov/pubmed/6119800.

Castle, A.L., Carver, M.P., Mendrick, D.L., 2002. Toxicogenomics: a new revolution in drug safety. Drug Discov. Today 7 (13), 728–736. https://www.ncbi.nlm.nih.gov/pubmed/12110229.

Christoph, G.R., Hansen, J.F., Leung, H.W., 2003. Subchronic inhalation neurotoxicity studies of ethyl acetate in rats. Neurotoxicology 24 (6), 861–874. https://www.ncbi.nlm.nih.gov/pubmed/14637381.

Dearden, J.C., 2003. In silico prediction of drug toxicity. J. Comput. Aided Mol. Des. 17 (2–4), 119–127. https://www.ncbi.nlm.nih.gov/pubmed/13677480.

Dumont, C., Prieto, P., Asturiol, D., Worth, A., 2015. Review of the availability of in vitro and in silico methods for assessing dermal bioavailability. Appl. In Vitro Toxicol. 1 (2), 147–164. https://doi.org/10.1089/aivt.2015.0003.

Enoch, S.J., Cronin, M.T., 2010. A review of the electrophilic reaction chemistry involved in covalent DNA binding. Crit. Rev. Toxicol. 40 (8), 728–748. https://www.ncbi.nlm.nih.gov/pubmed/20722585.

EPA, 2003. The EPA quality assurance project plan table of contents. In: Sampling and Analysis of Environmental Chemical Pollutants. Elsevier.

Faqi, A.S., 2013. Introduction. A Comprehensive Guide to Toxicology in Preclinical Drug Development. Elsevier. https://doi.org/10.1016/b978-0-12-387815-1.00001-0.

Greaves, P., Williams, A., Eve, M., 2004. First dose of potential new medicines to humans: how animals help. Nat. Rev. Drug Discov. 3 (3), 226–236. https://www.ncbi.nlm.nih.gov/pubmed/15031736.

Gupta, R., Polaka, S., Rajpoot, K., Tekade, M., Sharma, M.C., Tekade, R.K., 2022a. Importance of toxicity testing in drug discovery and research. In: Pharmacokinetics and Toxicokinetic Considerations, vol. 2. Elsevier. https://doi.org/10.1016/b978-0-323-98367-9.00016-0.

Gupta, R., Rajpoot, K., Tekade, M., Sharma, M.C., Safavi, M., Tekade, R.K., 2022b. Factors influencing drug toxicity. In: Pharmacokinetics and Toxicokinetic Considerations, vol. 2. Elsevier. https://doi.org/10.1016/b978-0-323-98367-9.00014-7.

Gupta, R., Rajpoot, K., Tekade, M., Sharma, M.C., Tekade, R.K., 2022c. Methods and models for in vitro toxicity. In: Pharmacokinetics and Toxicokinetic Considerations, vol. 2. Elsevier. https://doi.org/10.1016/b978-0-323-98367-9.00006-8.

Hemmerich, J., Ecker, G.F., 2020. In silico toxicology: from structure-activity relationships towards deep learning and adverse outcome pathways. Wiley Interdiscip. Rev. Comput. Mol. Sci. 10 (4), e1475. https://www.ncbi.nlm.nih.gov/pubmed/35866138.

Henschler, D., Schmuck, G., van Aerssen, M., Schiffmann, D., 1992. The inhibitory effect of neuropathic organophosphate esters on neurite outgrowth in cell cultures: a basis for screening for delayed neurotoxicity. Toxicol. Vitro 6 (4), 327–335. https://www.ncbi.nlm.nih.gov/pubmed/20732129.

Heywood, R., 1981. Target organ toxicity. Toxicol. Lett. 8 (6), 349–358. https://www.ncbi.nlm.nih.gov/pubmed/7302965.

Huang, G., Yan, F., Tan, D., 2018. A review of computational methods for predicting drug targets. Curr. Protein Pept. Sci. 19 (6), 562–572. https://www.ncbi.nlm.nih.gov/pubmed/27842478.

Hudson, M., Bhogal, N., 2006. An analysis of the home office statistics of scientific procedures on living animals, great Britain 2004. Altern. Lab Anim. 34 (1), 85–103. https://www.ncbi.nlm.nih.gov/pubmed/16522151.

Hughes, J.P., Rees, S., Kalindjian, S.B., Philpott, K.L., 2011. Principles of early drug discovery. Br. J. Pharmacol. 162 (6), 1239–1249. https://www.ncbi.nlm.nih.gov/pubmed/21091654.

Hunter, P., 2008. A toxic brew we cannot live without. Micronutrients give insights into the interplay between geochemistry and evolutionary biology. EMBO Rep. 9 (1), 15–18. https://www.ncbi.nlm.nih.gov/pubmed/18174893.

Hvastkovs, E.G., Rusling, J.F., 2016. State-of-the-Art metabolic toxicity screening and pathway evaluation. Anal. Chem. 88 (9), 4584–4599.

Idakwo, G., Luttrell, J., Chen, M., Hong, H., Zhou, Z., Gong, P., Zhang, C., 2018. A review on machine learning methods for in silico toxicity prediction. J. Environ. Sci. Health C Environ. Carcinog. Ecotoxicol. Rev. 36 (4), 169–191. https://www.ncbi.nlm.nih.gov/pubmed/30628866.

Isbrucker, R.A., Edwards, J.A., Wolz, E., Davidovich, A., Bausch, J., 2006. Safety studies on epigallocatechin gallate (EGCG) preparations. Part 3: teratogenicity and reproductive toxicity studies in rats. Food Chem. Toxicol. 44 (5), 651–661. https://www.ncbi.nlm.nih.gov/pubmed/16410036.

Kalyane, D., Choudhary, D., Polaka, S., Goykar, H., Karanwad, T., Rajpoot, K., Kumar Tekade, R., 2022. Reactive oxygen nano-generators for cancer therapy. Prog. Mater. Sci. 130, 100974. https://www.sciencedirect.com/science/article/pii/S007964252200055X.

Keiser, M.J., Roth, B.L., Armbruster, B.N., Ernsberger, P., Irwin, J.J., Shoichet, B.K., 2007. Relating protein pharmacology by ligand chemistry. Nat. Biotechnol. 25 (2), 197–206. https://www.ncbi.nlm.nih.gov/pubmed/17287757.

Khera, K.S., 1985. Maternal toxicity: a possible etiological factor in embryo-fetal deaths and fetal malformations of rodent-rabbit species. Teratology 31 (1), 129–153. https://www.ncbi.nlm.nih.gov/pubmed/3983854.

Knight, Z.A., Shokat, K.M., 2007. Chemical genetics: where genetics and pharmacology meet. Cell 128 (3), 425–430. https://www.ncbi.nlm.nih.gov/pubmed/17289560.

Lamb, J., Crawford, E.D., Peck, D., Modell, J.W., Blat, I.C., Wrobel, M.J., Lerner, J., Brunet, J.P., Subramanian, A., Ross, K.N., Reich, M., Hieronymus, H., Wei, G., Armstrong, S.A., Haggarty, S.J., Clemons, P.A., Wei, R., Carr, S.A., Lander, E.S., Golub, T.R., 2006. The Connectivity Map: using gene-expression signatures to connect small molecules, genes, and disease. Science 313 (5795), 1929–1935. https://www.ncbi.nlm.nih.gov/pubmed/17008526.

Li, L., Yin, J., 2019. Drug safety evaluation in China. Curr. Allergy Asthma Rep. 19 (9), 39. https://www.ncbi.nlm.nih.gov/pubmed/31321555.

Li, H., Sun, J., Fan, X., Sui, X., Zhang, L., Wang, Y., He, Z., 2008. Considerations and recent advances in QSAR models for cytochrome P450-mediated drug metabolism prediction. J. Comput. Aided Mol. Des. 22 (11), 843–855. https://www.ncbi.nlm.nih.gov/pubmed/18574695.

Low, L.A., Mummery, C., Berridge, B.R., Austin, C.P., Tagle, D.A., 2021. Organs-on-chips: into the next decade. Nat. Rev. Drug Discov. 20 (5), 345–361. https://www.ncbi.nlm.nih.gov/pubmed/32913334.

Masoud, A., Kiran, R., Sandhir, R., 2009. Impaired mitochondrial functions in organophosphate induced delayed neuropathy in rats. Cell. Mol. Neurobiol. 29 (8), 1245–1255. https://www.ncbi.nlm.nih.gov/pubmed/19517227.

Materne, E.M., Tonevitsky, A.G., Marx, U., 2013. Chip-based liver equivalents for toxicity testing–organotypicalness versus cost-efficient high throughput. Lab Chip 13 (18), 3481–3495. https://www.ncbi.nlm.nih.gov/pubmed/23722971.

Mayne, J.T., Ku, W.W., Kennedy, S.P., 2006. Informed toxicity assessment in drug discovery: systems-based toxicology. Curr. Opin. Drug Discov. Dev 9 (1), 75–83. https://www.ncbi.nlm.nih.gov/pubmed/16445119.

Mehta, A., Pant, S.C., Flora, S.J., 2006. Monoisoamyl dimercaptosuccinic acid induced changes in pregnant female rats during late gestation and lactation. Reprod. Toxicol. 21 (1), 94–103. https://www.ncbi.nlm.nih.gov/pubmed/16040228.

Miller, P.G., Shuler, M.L., 2016. Design and demonstration of a pumpless 14 compartment microphysiological system. Biotechnol. Bioeng. 113 (10), 2213–2227. https://www.ncbi.nlm.nih.gov/pubmed/27070809.

Moser, V.C., 1996. Rat strain- and gender-related differences in neurobehavioral screening: acute trimethyltin neurotoxicity. J. Toxicol. Environ. Health 47 (6), 567–586. https://www.ncbi.nlm.nih.gov/pubmed/8614024.

Moser, V.C., Anthony, D.C., Sette, W.F., Macphail, R.C., 1992. Comparison of subchronic neurotoxicity of 2-hydroxyethyl acrylate and acrylamide in rats. Toxicol. Sci. 18 (3), 343–352. https://doi.org/10.1093/toxsci/18.3.343.

Myatt, G.J., Ahlberg, E., Akahori, Y., Allen, D., Amberg, A., Anger, L.T., Aptula, A., Auerbach, S., Beilke, L., Bellion, P., Benigni, R., Bercu, J., Booth, E.D., Bower, D., Brigo, A., Burden, N., Cammerer, Z., Cronin, M.T.D., Cross, K.P., Custer, L., Dettwiler, M., Dobo, K., Ford, K.A., Fortin, M.C., Gad-McDonald, S.E., Gellatly, N., Gervais, V., Glover, K.P., Glowienke, S., Van Gompel, J., Gutsell, S., Hardy, B., Harvey, J.S., Hillegass, J., Honma, M., Hsieh, J.H., Hsu, C.W., Hughes, K., Johnson, C., Jolly, R., Jones, D., Kemper, R., Kenyon, M.O., Kim, M.T., Kruhlak, N.L., Kulkarni, S.A., Kummerer, K., Leavitt, P., Majer, B., Masten, S., Miller, S., Moser, J., Mumtaz, M., Muster, W., Neilson, L., Oprea, T.I., Patlewicz, G., Paulino, A., Lo Piparo, E., Powley, M., Quigley, D.P., Reddy, M.V., Richarz, A.N., Ruiz, P., Schilter, B., Serafimova, R., Simpson, W., Stavitskaya, L., Stidl, R., Suarez-Rodriguez, D., Szabo, D.T., Teasdale, A., Trejo-Martin, A., Valentin, J.P., Vuorinen, A., Wall, B.A., Watts, P., White, A.T., Wichard, J., Witt, K.L., Woolley, A., Woolley, D., Zwickl, C., Hasselgren, C., 2018. In silico toxicology protocols. Regul. Toxicol. Pharmacol. 96, 1–17. https://www.ncbi.nlm.nih.gov/pubmed/29678766.

OECD, 1981a. Test No. 410: Repeated Dose Dermal Toxicity: 21/28-Day Study. OECD Guidelines for the Testing of Chemicals, Section 4. OECD. https://doi.org/10.1787/9789264070745-en.

OECD, 1981b. Test No. 411: Subchronic Dermal Toxicity: 90-Day Study. OECD Guidelines for the Testing of Chemicals, Section 4. OECD. https://doi.org/10.1787/9789264070769-en.

OECD, 1984. Test No. 477: Genetic Toxicology: Sex-Linked Recessive Lethal Test in *Drosophila melanogaster*. OECD Guidelines for the Testing of Chemicals, Section 4. OECD. https://doi.org/10.1787/9789264071346-en.

OECD, 2002. Report of the OECD Workshop on Environmental Hazard/Risk Assessment. OECD Series on Testing and Assessment. OECD. https://doi.org/10.1787/9789264077935-en.

OECD, 2008. Test No. 407: Repeated Dose 28-Day Oral Toxicity Study in Rodents. OECD Guidelines for the Testing of Chemicals, Section 4. OECD. https://doi.org/10.1787/9789264070684-en.

OECD, 2014. Guidance Document on the Validation of (Quantitative) Structure-Activity Relationship [(Q)SAR] Models. OECD Series on Testing and Assessment. OECD. https://doi.org/10.1787/9789264085442-en.

OECD, 2018a. Test No. 408: Repeated Dose 90-Day Oral Toxicity Study in Rodents. OECD Guidelines for the Testing of Chemicals, Section 4. OECD. https://doi.org/10.1787/9789264070707-en.

OECD, 2018b. Test No. 412: Subacute Inhalation Toxicity: 28-Day Study. OECD Guidelines for the Testing of Chemicals, Section 4. OECD. https://doi.org/10.1787/9789264070783-en.

OECD, 2018c. Test No. 413: Subchronic Inhalation Toxicity: 90-Day Study. OECD Guidelines for the Testing of Chemicals, Section 4. OECD. https://doi.org/10.1787/9789264070806-en.

OECD, 2018d. Test No. 452: Chronic Toxicity Studies. OECD Guidelines for the Testing of Chemicals, Section 4. OECD. https://doi.org/10.1787/9789264071209-en.

OECD, 2018e. Test No. 453: Combined Chronic Toxicity/Carcinogenicity Studies. OECD Guidelines for the Testing of Chemicals, Section 4. OECD. https://doi.org/10.1787/9789264071223-en.

OECD, 2019. Test No. 203: Fish, Acute Toxicity Test. OECD Guidelines for the Testing of Chemicals, Section 2. OECD. https://doi.org/10.1787/9789264069961-en

OECD, 2022a. Test No. 425: Acute Oral Toxicity: Up-and-Down Procedure. OECD Guidelines for the Testing of Chemicals, Section 4. OECD. https://doi.org/10.1787/9789264071049-en.

OECD, 2022b. Test No. 470: Mammalian Erythrocyte Pig-a Gene Mutation Assay. OECD Guidelines for the Testing of Chemicals, Section 4. OECD. https://doi.org/10.1787/4faea90e-en.

Olson, H., Betton, G., Robinson, D., Thomas, K., Monro, A., Kolaja, G., Lilly, P., Sanders, J., Sipes, G., Bracken, W., Dorato, M., Van Deun, K., Smith, P., Berger, B., Heller, A., 2000. Concordance of the toxicity of pharmaceuticals in humans and in animals. Regul. Toxicol. Pharmacol. 32 (1), 56–67. https://doi.org/10.1006/rtph.2000.1399.

Ouedraogo, M., Baudoux, T., Stevigny, C., Nortier, J., Colet, J.M., Efferth, T., Qu, F., Zhou, J., Chan, K., Shaw, D., Pelkonen, O., Duez, P., 2012. Review of current and "omics" methods for assessing the toxicity (genotoxicity, teratogenicity and nephrotoxicity) of herbal medicines and mushrooms. J. Ethnopharmacol. 140 (3), 492–512. https://www.ncbi.nlm.nih.gov/pubmed/22386524.

Pandey, V., Polaka, S., Nalla, L.V., Tekade, M., Sharma, M.C., Tekade, R.K., 2022. Excipient toxicity and safety. In: Tekade, R.K. (Ed.), Pharmacokinetics and Toxicokinetic Considerations, vol. 2. Academic Press, pp. 487–511. https://www.sciencedirect.com/science/article/pii/B9780323983679000251.

Parikh, K.J., Christian, J.R., Rajpoot, K., Tekade, R.K., 2022. Environmental and Safety Aspects of Bionanotechnology. Pharmacokinetics and Toxicokinetic Considerations, vol. 2. Elsevier. https://doi.org/10.1016/b978-0-323-98367-9.00022-6.

Polaka, S., Swetha, K.L., Dittakavi, S., Rajpoot, K., Tekade, R.K., 2021. Bioanalytical method development and validation for establishing bioavailability and bioequivalence. In: Tekade, R.K. (Ed.), Biopharmaceutics and Pharmacokinetics Considerations. Elsevier, pp. 487–516. https://doi.org/10.1016/B978-0-12-814425-1.00001-2.

Polaka, S., Katare, P., Pawar, B., Vasdev, N., Gupta, T., Rajpoot, K., Sengupta, P., Tekade, R.K., 2022. Emerging ROS-modulating technologies for augmentation of the wound healing process. ACS Omega 7 (35), 30657–30672. https://doi.org/10.1021/acsomega.2c02675.

Program, N.T., 2018. The ICCVAM Acute Systemic Toxicity Reference List. Chemical Effects in Biological Systems (CEBS). NIEHS. https://doi.org/10.22427/ntp-data-022-00001-0002-000-7.

Rajani, C., Borisa, P., Bagul, S., Shukla, K., Tambe, V., Desai, N., Tekade, R.K., 2022. Developmental toxicity of nanomaterials used in drug delivery: understanding molecular biomechanics and potential remedial measures. In: Tekade, R.K. (Ed.), Pharmacokinetics and Toxicokinetic Considerations, vol. 2. Academic Press, pp. 685–725. https://www.sciencedirect.com/science/article/pii/B9780323983679000172.

Rajpoot, K., Tekade, R.K., Sharma, M.C., Safavi, M., Tekade, M., 2021a. Pharmacokinetics modeling in drug delivery. In: Tekade, R.K. (Ed.), Biopharmaceutics and Pharmacokinetics Considerations. Elsevier, Academic Press, pp. 279–334.

Rajpoot, K., Tekade, R.K., Sharma, M.C., Tekade, M., 2021b. Pharmacokinetics and biopharmaceutics: "a leader or attendant". In: Tekade, R.K. (Ed.), Biopharmaceutics and Pharmacokinetics Considerations. Elsevier, Academic Press, pp. 17–27.

Rajpoot, K., Desai, N., Koppisetti, H., Tekade, M., Sharma, M.C., Behera, S.K., Tekade, R.K., 2022a. In silico methods for the prediction of drug toxicity. In: Pharmacokinetics and Toxicokinetic Considerations, vol. 2. Elsevier. https://doi.org/10.1016/b978-0-323-98367-9.00012-3.

Rajpoot, K., Tekade, M., Sharma, M.C., Arafat, B., Tekade, R.K., 2022b. Principles and concepts in toxicokinetic. In: Pharmacokinetics and Toxicokinetic Considerations, vol. 2. Elsevier. https://doi.org/10.1016/b978-0-323-98367-9.00023-8.

Raunio, H., 2011. In silico toxicology - non-testing methods. Front. Pharmacol. 2, 33. https://www.ncbi.nlm.nih.gov/pubmed/21772821.

Rim, K.T., 2020. In silico prediction of toxicity and its applications for chemicals at work. Toxicol. Environ. Health Sci. 12 (3), 191–202. https://www.ncbi.nlm.nih.gov/pubmed/32421081.

Rorije, E., Muller, A., Beekhuijzen, M.E., Hass, U., Heinrich-Hirsch, B., Paparella, M., Schenk, E., Ulbrich, B., Hakkert, B.C., Piersma, A.H., 2011. On the impact of second generation mating and offspring in multi-generation reproductive toxicity studies on classification and labelling of substances in Europe. Regul. Toxicol. Pharmacol. 61 (2), 251–260. https://www.ncbi.nlm.nih.gov/pubmed/21878359.

Saghir, S.A., Dorato, M.A., 2016. Reproductive and developmental toxicity testing: examination of the extended one-generation reproductive toxicity study guideline. Regul. Toxicol. Pharmacol. 79, 110–117. https://www.ncbi.nlm.nih.gov/pubmed/27074386.

Sale, J.E., 2013. Translesion DNA synthesis and mutagenesis in eukaryotes. Cold Spring Harbor Perspect. Biol. 5 (3), a012708. https://www.ncbi.nlm.nih.gov/pubmed/23457261.

Saunders, C.R., Shockley, D.C., Knuckles, M.E., 2001. Behavioral effects induced by acute exposure to benzo(a)pyrene in F-344 rats. Neurotox. Res. 3 (6), 557–579. https://www.ncbi.nlm.nih.gov/pubmed/15111245.

Schein, P.S., Davis, R.D., Carter, S., Newman, J., Schein, D.R., Rall, D.P., 1970. The evaluation of anticancer drugs in dogs and monkeys for the prediction of qualitative toxicities in man. Clin. Pharmacol. Ther. 11 (1), 3–40. https://www.ncbi.nlm.nih.gov/pubmed/4983384.

Schneider, P.J., 2018. The impact of technology on safe medicines use and pharmacy practice in the US. Front. Pharmacol. 9, 1361. https://www.ncbi.nlm.nih.gov/pubmed/30524289.

Scism, J.L., Laska, D.A., Horn, J.W., Gimple, J.L., Pratt, S.E., Shepard, R.L., Dantzig, A.H., Wrighton, S.A., 1999. Evaluation of an in vitro coculture model for the blood-brain barrier: comparison of human umbilical vein endothelial cells (ECV304) and rat glioma cells (C6) from two commercial sources. In Vitro Cell. Dev. Biol. Anim. 35 (10), 580–592. https://www.ncbi.nlm.nih.gov/pubmed/10614867.

Sengupta, P., Chatterjee, B., Tekade, R.K., 2022. Drug toxicity and forensic pharmacokinetics. In: Tekade, R.K. (Ed.), Pharmacokinetics and Toxicokinetic Considerations, vol. 2. Academic Press, pp. 425–486. https://www.sciencedirect.com/science/article/pii/B9780323983679000214.

Shete, M.B., Patil, T.S., Deshpande, A.S., Saraogi, G., Vasdev, N., Deshpande, M., Rajpoot, K., Tekade, R.K., 2022. Current trends in theranostic nanomedicines. J. Drug Deliv. Sci. Technol. 71, 103280. https://www.sciencedirect.com/science/article/pii/S1773224722001903.

Slikker Jr., W., de Souza Lima, T.A., Archella, D., de Silva JBJ, Barton-Maclaren, T., Bo, L., Buvinich, D., Chaudhry, Q., Chuan, P., Deluyker, H., Domselaar, G., Freitas, M., Hardy, B., Eichler, H.G., Hugas, M., Lee, K., Liao, C.D., Loo, L.H., Okuda, H., Orisakwe, O.E., Patri, A., Sactitono, C., Shi, L., Silva, P., Sistare, F., Thakkar, S., Tong, W., Valdez, M.L., Whelan, M., Zhao-Wong, A., 2018. Emerging technologies for food and drug safety. Regul. Toxicol. Pharmacol. 98, 115–128. https://www.ncbi.nlm.nih.gov/pubmed/30048704.

Stanness, K.A., Neumaier, J.F., Sexton, T.J., Grant, G.A., Emmi, A., Maris, D.O., Janigro, D., 1999. A new model of the blood–brain barrier: co-culture of neuronal, endothelial and glial cells under dynamic conditions. Neuroreport 10 (18), 3725–3731. https://www.ncbi.nlm.nih.gov/pubmed/10716199.

Stornetta, A., Zimmermann, M., Cimino, G.D., Henderson, P.T., Sturla, S.J., 2017. DNA adducts from anticancer drugs as candidate predictive markers for precision medicine. Chem. Res. Toxicol. 30 (1), 388–409.

Sung, J.H., Shuler, M.L., 2010. In vitro microscale systems for systematic drug toxicity study. Bioproc. Biosyst. Eng. 33 (1), 5–19. https://www.ncbi.nlm.nih.gov/pubmed/19701779.

Tambe, V., Desai, N., Rajpoot, K., Tekade, R.K., 2021a. "Organ-on-a-chip"-based physiologically relevant pharmacokinetic models. In: Tekade, R.K. (Ed.), Biopharmaceutics and Pharmacokinetics Considerations, first ed. Elsevier, pp. 643–673. https://doi.org/10.1016/B978-0-12-814425-1.00024-3.

Tambe, V., Ditani, A., Rajpoot, K., Tekade, R.K., 2021b. Pharmacokinetics aspects of structural modifications in drug design and therapy. In: Tekade, R.K. (Ed.), Biopharmaceutics and Pharmacokinetics Considerations, vol. 1. Elsevier, Academic Press, pp. 83–108.

Tambe, V., Pande, S., Gadeval, A., Rajpoot, K., Raval, N., Tekade, R.K., 2021c. Microdialysis: an emerging technique for pharmacokinetic–pharmacodynamic profiling. In: Tekade, R.K. (Ed.), Biopharmaceutics and Pharmacokinetics Considerations, first ed. Elsevier, pp. 601–616. https://doi.org/10.1016/B978-0-12-814425-1.00018-8.

Tambe, V., Shukla, H., Rajpoot, K., Pandey, M.M., Tekade, R.K., 2021d. Pharmacokinetics aspects of biotechnological products. In: Tekade, R.K. (Ed.), Biopharmaceutics and Pharmacokinetics Considerations. Elsevier, Academic Press, pp. 539–565.

Tambe, V., Sirsat, B., Rajpoot, K., Gadeval, A., Tekade, R.K., 2021e. Pharmacogenomics and drug metabolism. In: Tekade, R.K. (Ed.), Biopharmaceutics and Pharmacokinetics Considerations, vol. 1. Elsevier, Academic Press, pp. 355–385.

Tariq, R.A., Vashisht, R., Sinha, A., Scherbak, Y., 2022. Medication Dispensing Errors and Prevention. StatPearls. https://www.ncbi.nlm.nih.gov/books/NBK519065/.

Tekade, M., Koppisetti, H., Sharma, M.C., Rajpoot, K., Sengupta, P., Kumar, M., Tekade, R.K., 2022. Understanding the concept of signal toxicity and its implications on human health. In: Pharmacokinetics and Toxicokinetic Considerations, vol. 2. Elsevier. https://doi.org/10.1016/b978-0-323-98367-9.00020-2.

Tiwari, A., Joshi, M., Salvi, N., Gupta, D., Gandhi, S., Rajpoot, K., Tekade, R.K., 2022. Toxicity of pharmaceutical azo dyes. In: Pharmacokinetics and Toxicokinetic Considerations, vol. 2. Elsevier. https://doi.org/10.1016/b978-0-323-98367-9.00004-4.

Tolani, P., Gupta, S., Yadav, K., Aggarwal, S., Yadav, A.K., 2021. Big data, integrative omics and network biology. In: Proteomics and Systems Biology. Elsevier. https://doi.org/10.1016/bs.apcsb.2021.03.006.

Trevan, J.W., 1997. The error of determination of toxicity. In: Proceedings of the Royal Society of London Series B, Containing Papers of a Biological Character, vol. 101, pp. 483–514. https://doi.org/10.1098/rspb.1927.0030.

Turkez, H., Arslan, M.E., Ozdemir, O., 2017. Genotoxicity testing: progress and prospects for the next decade. Expert Opin. Drug Metabol. Toxicol. 13 (10), 1089–1098. https://doi.org/10.1080/17425255.2017.1375097.

Ulrich, R., Friend, S.H., 2002. Toxicogenomics and drug discovery: will new technologies help us produce better drugs? Nat. Rev. Drug Discov. 1 (1), 84–88. https://www.ncbi.nlm.nih.gov/pubmed/12119613.

Vasdev, N., Rajpoot, K., Tekade, R.K., 2021. Molecular mechanisms of circadian rhythm and its influence on the pharmacokinetics of drugs. In: Tekade, R.K. (Ed.), Biopharmaceutics and Pharmacokinetics Considerations. Elsevier, Academic Press, pp. 415–449.

Vasseur, P., Lasne, C., 2012. OECD Detailed Review Paper (DRP) number 31 on "cell transformation assays for detection of chemical carcinogens": main results and conclusions. Mutat. Res. 744 (1), 8–11. https://www.ncbi.nlm.nih.gov/pubmed/22120692.

Vorhees, C.V., Acuff-Smith, K.D., Schilling, M.A., Fisher, J.E., Moran, M.S., Buelke-Sam, J., 1994. A developmental neurotoxicity evaluation of the effects of prenatal exposure to fluoxetine in rats. Fund. Appl. Toxicol. 23 (2), 194–205. https://www.ncbi.nlm.nih.gov/pubmed/7982528.

Wacker, S.A., Houghtaling, B.R., Elemento, O., Kapoor, T.M., 2012. Using transcriptome sequencing to identify mechanisms of drug action and resistance. Nat. Chem. Biol. 8 (3), 235–237. https://www.ncbi.nlm.nih.gov/pubmed/22327403.

Wise, L.D., Gordon, L.R., Soper, K.A., Duchai, D.M., Morrissey, R.E., 1995. Developmental neurotoxicity evaluation of acrylamide in Sprague-Dawley rats. Neurotoxicol. Teratol. 17 (2), 189–198. https://www.ncbi.nlm.nih.gov/pubmed/7760778.

Yildirim, M.A., Goh, K.I., Cusick, M.E., Barabasi, A.L., Vidal, M., 2007. Drug-target network. Nat. Biotechnol. 25 (10), 1119–1126. https://www.ncbi.nlm.nih.gov/pubmed/17921997.

Zbinden, G., Flury-Roversi, M., 1981. Significance of the LD50-test for the toxicological evaluation of chemical substances. Arch. Toxicol. 47 (2), 77–99. https://www.ncbi.nlm.nih.gov/pubmed/7271444.

Zhang, Y., Yang, W., Schauberger, G., Wang, J., Geng, J., Wang, G., Meng, J., 2021. Determination of dose–response relationship to derive odor impact criteria for a wastewater treatment plant. Atmosphere 12 (3), 371. https://doi.org/10.3390/atmos12030371.

CHAPTER

3

Role of microRNAs in toxicology

Nupur Vasdev[1], *Muktika Tekade*[2], *Adil Ali Sayyed*[3], *Piyush Gondaliya*[3] *and Rakesh Kumar Tekade*[1]

[1]National Institute of Pharmaceutical Education and Research (NIPER)- Ahmedabad, An Institute of National Importance, Government of India, Department of Pharmaceuticals, Ministry of Chemicals and Fertilizers, Palaj, Gandhinagar, Gujarat, India; [2]School of Pharmacy, Devi Ahilya Vishwavidyalaya, Indore, Madhya Pradesh, India; [3]Department of Transplantation, Mayo Clinic, Jacksonville, FL, United States

3.1 Introduction

Toxicological studies play a vital role in drug development, as most drug candidates fail in human trials due to adverse drug reactions and toxicity issues. In addition, many drugs have been withdrawn from the market with toxicity concerns. Therefore, toxicity assessment in the early phases of drug development can save time as well as expenses in drug development processes. Although various conventional biomarkers are being utilized for toxicity evaluation, they can only be detected at later stages. In the recent decade, miRNAs have emerged as potential biomarkers for assessing toxicities, even at the initial stages.

MicroRNAs (miRNAs) are 21–23 nucleotide long, small non-coding RNA interacting with the 3′-untranslated regions (3′-UTR) of the mature mRNA to control its expression at post transcriptional levels (Gondaliya et al., 2022). Each miRNA can have multiple targets, and a single gene can be targeted by various miRNAs (Sayyed et al., 2021, 2022; Koturbash et al., 2015).

Recent studies have revealed the interaction of different drugs, environmental contaminants, toxins, metals, and nanoparticles with miRNAs, ultimately leading to modulation in miRNAs expression (Tumolo et al., 2022). Even miRNAs expression profiles are altered due to the drug's induced toxicities and perform as a potential biomarker to assess toxicity at the early stages. It was also observed that if drugs or toxicants are causing an adverse effect on various organ systems like the cardiovascular system, hepatic system, respiratory system, and central nervous system, then those toxicants can also vary the expression profile of miRNAs in the targeted organs. The miRNA expression profile was assessed using various tools

Essentials of Pharmatoxicology in Drug Research, Volume 1
https://doi.org/10.1016/B978-0-443-15840-7.00002-6

like quantitative reverse transcription polymerase chain reaction (qRT-PCR), next-generation sequencing, microarrays, and bead-based methods. Computational methods were also used to evaluate the miRNAs and environmental pollutant's interactions. MiRNAs are also crucial for biological processes like cell differentiation, cell growth, cell cycle control, and cell death or apoptosis. As a result, the miRNA's expression will also impact all biological processes (Wang and Cui, 2012; Qiu et al., 2012).

This chapter discussed the biogenesis pathway for the miRNA, its biological function, association with various diseases, tools to assess miRNA expression profile, and the relationship of miRNAs with various toxicities like cardiotoxicity, hepatotoxicity, neurotoxicity, dermatotoxicity, and nephrotoxicity. Here, several interactions of miRNAs with different environmental pollutants such as air toxicants, metals, nanoparticles, and drugs are also covered.

3.2 Understanding miRNA

MiRNAs are small (21–23 nucleotide) noncoding endogenous RNA that help in gene expression regulation by working on their respective mRNA targets. Canonical and noncanonical pathways can be helpful in miRNA biogenesis. miRNA expression profiling has a direct relationship with the pathogenesis of various diseases. Therefore, they are considered potential biomarkers for drug toxicity evaluation. The association of miRNA profile and disease occurrence can be evaluated by several methods.

3.2.1 Biogenesis of miRNAs

Several complex proteins are involved in the biogenesis of the miRNAs. MiRNA biogenesis can be processed by canonical and noncanonical pathways, but the canonical pathway is the dominant one. In the canonical pathway, biogenesis starts from the gene transcription with the help of RNA polymerase II/III to form a stem-loop structure of primary miRNA that generally holds hundreds of base pairs. Then a microprocessor complex of ribonuclease III enzyme (Drosha) and RNA binding protein DiGeorge Syndrome Critical Region 8 (DGCR8) further processes the pri-miRNA or hairpin structure to form premature or precursor miRNA, also known as pre-miRNAs. Pre-miRNAs generally contain 70 nucleotide sequences, and pre-miRNAs are exported to the cytoplasm from the nucleus with the help of a complex of RAS-related nuclear protein-guanosine-5′-triphosphate-ase (Ran-GTPase) and exportin 5. After the export of premature miRNAs into the cytoplasm, the terminal loop of pre-miRNAs is cleaved by RNA endonuclease III Dicer, which is linked with TAR RNA binding protein (TRBP) and processes the pre-miRNA to form a miRNA duplex. Then the miRNA duplex forms an RNA-induced silencing complex (RISC) with the help of the Argonaute (Ago) protein family. This RISC complex unwinds the miRNA duplex to finally form a mature miRNA that can suppress the translation or degrade the mRNA for other processes (O'Brien et al., 2018; Yao, 2016; Yang and Mattes, 2008) (Fig. 3.1).

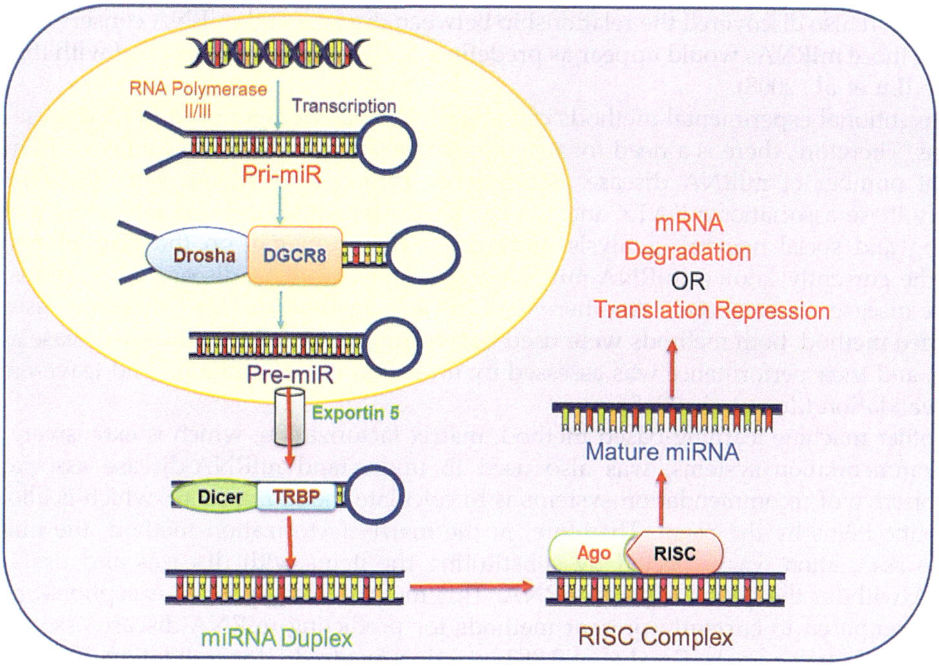

FIGURE 3.1 Biogenesis pathway of miRNA.

3.2.2 Biological functions and association with diseases

Normal and tumor cells showed differential miRNA expression, indicating a link between cancer pathogenesis and dysregulated miRNA. MiRNA expression can be dysregulated due to epigenetic alterations, genetic alteration, single nucleotide polymorphism (SNPs) in genes that code for miRNAs, and defective miRNA. These miRNAs control tumor suppressor genes and oncogenes, and dysregulated miRNAs can lead to various kinds of cancer. Various miRNAs related to cancer were reported that can help explain the pathogenesis of various cancers and help as prognostic and diagnostic markers of cancer.

For example, Grb2-associated binding protein 2 (Gab2) can be utilized as a diagnostic marker for ovarian cancer as it will overexpress in the tumor. Invasion, migration, and epithelial-to-mesenchymal transition of ovarian cancer cells are accelerated using Gab2 by activating PI3K/mTOR. Gab2 also causes the downregulation of miR-200c expression via P13K pathway activation, leading to enhanced CD44 expression and causing ovarian cancer metastasis. Various miRNA cited at the fragile chromosomal location is susceptible to amplification, deletion, and rearrangement that expedite the dysregulation of miRNA, leading to several types of cancer (Khan et al., 2019).

One study was performed to analyze the association of human miRNA with various diseases comprehensively. A network was built for the miRNA-associated diseases, and related or diverse dysfunctional evidence was observed for analogous or diverse disease clusters. This study revealed a negative association between various diseases and miRNA tissue specificity. It also discovered the relationship between diseases and miRNA conservation and showed those miRNAs would appear as predefined miRNA groups associated with the same disease (Lu et al., 2008).

Conventional experimental methods can identify a small number of miRNA disease associations. Therefore, there is a need for new approaches that will help to confirm a more significant number of miRNA disease associations. Two new methods were introduced to identify these associations: KATZ and CATAPULT. The KATZ method integrates machine learning and social network analysis methods. It mainly works on the derived network from the currently known miRNA-miRNA associations, miRNA-disease associations, and disease-disease associations. Another CATAPULT method is the machine learning-governed method. Both methods were used to confirm 242 identified miRNA-disease associations, and their performance was assessed by three-fold cross-validation and leave-one-out cross-validation (Zou et al., 2015).

Another machine learning-based method, matrix factorization, which is extensively used in recommendation systems, was also used to understand miRNA-disease associations. The objective of recommendation systems is to calculate the rating score, which is allocated to specific items by the users. Therefore, in the matrix factorization method, the miRNA-disease association was expected by substituting the items with diseases and users with miRNA without the need for seed miRNA. This method accomplished exceptional performance compared to currently present methods for predicting miRNA-disease associations. This method attains an AUC value of 0.882 by using five-fold cross-validation. This method conquered the main limitation-seed-miRNA problem of currently existing computational methods (Ha et al., 2019).

3.3 Tools for miRNA expression profiling

Tools for miRNA expression profiling are essential to understand the therapeutic function of miRNA and the use of miRNA expression for diagnostic purposes. Several methods, such as quantitative RT-PCR, next-generation sequencing, microarrays, single-molecule measurements, and bead-based methods, are used to quantify miRNA precisely. MiRNA possess unique challenges for expression profiling. Therefore, miRNA expression profiling needs cautious designing of experiments and data analysis. Main cellular processes for the formation of tumor-like cell differentiation, apoptosis, and proliferation are changing with the alteration of miRNA expression. Therefore, a detailed assessment of the alteration in miRNA expression of tumors can be used to understand the critical mechanism of tumorigenesis (Roden et al., 2015).

The small RNA sequence of miRNA makes it challenging to use the conventional reverse transcription method and limits the detection of miRNA expression more accurately and precisely. Currently, two approaches are used to overcome this limitation of detecting the mature miRNA. The first approach works on the extension of miRNA length to further assess easy reverse transcription. Extension of miRNA can be done by 3′ tailing of additional nucleotides or by adaptor ligation method. Adaptor ligation is the most extensively used method for organizing the libraries of small RNA for next-generation sequencing, bead-based detection, or microarray. This method needs ligation of adaptors to both 3′ and 5′ ends of the miRNA, and RNA ligase will help in the adaptor ligation method. These ligated adaptors on the 3′ and 5′ end of the miRNA offer molecular handles for efficient priming of reverse transcription reactions and polymerase chain reactions.

Another miRNA extension technique works on the tailing of miRNA 3′ end with an additional nucleotide. Terminal nucleotidyl transferase catalyses the tailing of miRNA. For example, a poly-A tail that is artificially added permits poly-dT primer binding, which is required for reverse transcription. Lower specificity due to the lower hybridization temperature is the main limitation of the miRNA detection method based on conventional hybridization. Therefore, the extension approaches use several techniques of direct hybridization to overcome the existing problems. Other methods to overcome these limitations are (a) hybridizing the two short oligonucleotides to the miRNA to generate a stacking effect that enhances the specificity; (b) using chemically modified oligonucleotides having high annealing temperatures (Lu et al., 2005; Baker, 2010; Roden et al., 2015).

3.3.1 Microarray

Oligonucleotide miRNA microarrays represent the most extensively used high throughput method for the genome-wide estimation of miRNA expression profiling for numerous samples. Microarray is a powerful method that can monitor thousands of sncRNAs expressions at a time when tens of samples are treated in parallel during a solo experiment. During the last few years, various diverse technical miRNA microarray variants have been developed. Key differences among these variants are the probe immobilization chemistry, oligo probe design, labeling of samples, and detection methods of microarray chip signals. On the CodeLink platform, an exceptional miRNA microarray assay was established to perform the genome-wide assessment of miRNA expression of healthy and diseased samples and to evaluate the difference in expression signatures related to therapeutic intervention, prognosis, and diagnosis. This miRNA microarray incorporates 4104 probes that are printed in duplicate. This microarray can concurrently assess the miRNA profiles of more than 1500 mature miRNA and their analogous precursors from 373 mouse and 474 human miRNA genes (Liu et al., 2008).

Even though the northern blot can concurrently evaluate the miRNA expression profile in diverse conditions, it cannot assess hundreds of miRNA expression profiles. Immobilizing miRNA mixtures on the membrane and hybridizing them with one specific probe limits the assessment by northern blots. These attributes also contribute to its inefficiency in assessing hundreds of miRNAs' molecular amounts. As compared to this northern blot method, miRNA microarray profiling involves the immobilization of known probes in addressable spots. Then these probes are hybridized with the consequent miRNAs of the samples, thus presenting a parallel and high throughput technique for evaluating thousands of miRNA profiles concurrently. Fluorescence intensities are linearly dependent on the miRNA concentration. Sensitivity to identifying target miRNA is a crucial constraint for profiling miRNA microarrays. It was observed that just 0.4 fmol of miRNA was required for QD detection by microarrays, while a 633 nm laser was used as excitation light (Liang et al., 2005).

In yet another study, microarray analysis (Agilent platform) was used for the miRNA profiling of 15 responders and 16 nonresponders. A highly similar miRNA profile was observed within and between responders and nonresponders. The cohort study of 53 squamous cell carcinoma cases was amplified to check the differentially expressed miRNA. Nonresponders showed 12 differentially expressed miRNAs; eight miRNAs were upregulated, and four were downregulated. The qRT-PCR method complied with the microarray findings for differentially expressed miRNAs (Slotta-Huspenina et al., 2018).

3.3.2 Real-time PCR

Quantitative real-time PCR (qRT-PCR) is a consistent technique to examine and verify the miRNA expression profiles in diverse cells, tissue samples, and organisms. Even though several distinguished techniques are used to perform qRT-PCR for determining miRNA expression, two steps are common for all the methods: the first is to obtain cDNA from mature miRNA sequence by reverse transcription, and the second is an amplification of cDNA by standard real-time PCR (Pan et al., 2017).

Due to more sensitivity and reproducibility of this method, qRT-PCR is most widely recognized as the method of choice for quantifying relative gene expression. Still, appropriate data normalization decides the accuracy and precision of the qRT-PCR results. Nonbiological sample-to-sample variations commenced during all the phases, from the preparation of samples to amplification, are corrected necessarily by using reference genes. Incorrect conclusions can also be observed due to unstably expressed reference genes for data normalization.

Usually, it was detected that the universal reference gene that can be appropriate for all tissue variants does not exist. Therefore, selecting the most stably expressed reference gene for definite testing based on the tissue of interest is the most exact and precise approach (Arya et al., 2005; Peltier and Latham, 2008). Various advantages of qRT-PCR over microarrays are: (a) larger dynamic range in comparison to microarray, (b) speed and sensitivity of qRT-PCR assays, and (c) requirement of less amount of starting material, i.e., nanogram range of total RNA (Benes and Castoldi, 2010).

One study was performed to detect the stably expressed miRNAs of rectal cancer tissues that can be used as normalizers or reference genes for future assessment of the miRNA expression profile. Laser micro-dissected tumor tissue and its nearby stromal tissues of rectal cancer patients were used for miRNA expression profiling. Firstly, this high-throughput technique-based miRNAs expression analysis was done to detect the most stably expressed miRNAs from 10 patient specimens. Then qRT-PCR was used to evaluate the stability of these miRNAs in the tissues of 25 rectal cancer patients. Again, the stability of these miRNAs was assessed in normal rectal mucosa and rectal cancer tissues of 28 comparable patients (Eriksen et al., 2016).

Another study identified the most stable miRNAs as reference genes or normalizers in colorectal cancer tissues using qRT-PCR. Ten pairs of normal and colorectal cancer tissues were used for high throughput miRNA expression profiling. The stability of these reference genes was then assessed in 39 normal and 35 tumor tissues. The impact of these reference genes on the relative quantity of recognized tumor suppressors and oncogenic target miRNAs was also made. Two miRNAs were detected as reference genes for two small nucleolar RNA genes and six miRNAs. These reference genes were required for data normalization to facilitate the evaluation of target miRNAs dysregulation among normal and colorectal tumor tissues (Chang et al., 2010).

The qPCR method was used to examine miRNA, and three primers were used to investigate pri- and pre-miRNA. One reverse primer bind to the region inside the hairpin, and two forward primers bind to a region inside the pre-miRNA and outside the hairpin. One primer set amplifies both pri- and pre-miRNA regions, while the other only amplifies pre-miRNA. SYBR green was used to quantify fluorescence (Schmittgen et al., 2004).

The Stem-loop qPCR method was used for the first time for mature miRNA analysis. A mature miRNA-binding stem-loop RT primer was used for the study. A general reverse primer and a miRNA-specific forward primer were used for PCR amplification of cDNA. A Taqman probe specific to mature miRNA was used, and quantification was done by measuring fluorescence (Chen et al., 2005).

Poly(T) adapter was employed for generating cDNA by polyadenylate mature miRNAs using poly(A) polymerase. Forward and reverse primer specific to miRNA binds to poly(T) adapter region for PCR amplification, and SYBR green was used to quantify fluorescence (Forero et al., 2019).

3.3.3 Next-generation sequencing

Second-generation sequencing is next-generation sequencing related to Sanger sequencing, known as first-generation sequencing. 100% accuracy can be achieved by the traditional Sanger sequencing method. This was a revolutionary work as a result of which an individual could discover all creature's genes, including humans. It was a cost-bearing and low-throughput method. The Human Genome Project used approximately three billion US dollars to support the human genome draught map. Still, everyone has a unique genome. The differences can be present in single nucleotide point mutations, also known as single nucleotide polymorphisms (SNP) or allele combinations. Hence, there was a need for a new sequencing method, and NGS came at that time to overcome these limitations. Next-generation sequencing or second-generation sequencing is the most widely used method due to its low cost and high throughput. Replication of the DNA obtained from the reverse transcription of RNA or the original sample was done many times in parallel. Signals were also amplified after multiple times simultaneous sequencing of the amplified DNA. The accuracy of the results was ensured by these amplified signals alone. Dinucleotides or different nucleotides could be added to sequences to provide characteristic signals. Ion torrent, Illumina, 454, and SOLiD are some of the most widely used next-generation sequencing systems (Shendure and Ji, 2008; Hu et al., 2017).

NGS is also recognized as massively parallel sequencing because it enables the profiling of thousands of genes during a single experiment and conquers the cross-hybridization and background signal concerns of microarrays. Concurrent authentication of recognized miRNAs and detection of new miRNAs can also be done using NGS. Getting information on billions of nucleotides in a single experiment decreases the experimental cost. Determining accurate information about nucleotides from a considerable amount of sequence data obtained through high-throughput sequencing is some other advantages of NGS (Liu, 2018).

3.3.4 Bead-based technology for miRNA expression profiling

Various methods like northern blots, cloning approaches, qRT-PCR, bead-based flow cytometric approaches, and microarray assays based on direct hybridization or enzymatic extension coupled with hybridization-based microarray assays were used for miRNA identification and quantification. But there are some technical limitations to these current methods, like the requirement of a massive number of samples or decreasing cross-hybridization from mRNA by enriching the small RNA species. However, variations occur in measurement due to the enrichment procedure. A bead array-based assay involving 735 human miRNAs was introduced to allow high throughput expression profiling for numerous samples. This bead array-based assay was used for profiling miRNAs in peripheral blood. MiRNAs expression was evaluated in the whole blood or the peripheral blood mononuclear cells (PBMCs) of healthy subjects. The influence of different normalization methods, various features of technical reproducibility of results, and the effect of the amount of total RNA input on miRNAs expression pattern were studied to evaluate the performance of this bead array-based assay. The expression profile of miRNAs was validated by the qRT-PCR method (Gaarz et al., 2010).

An extremely specific and sensitive miRNA assay was introduced to overcome the limitations of present miRNA assays. This method has the advantage of high specificity compared to other expression profiling methods based on sequence hybridization. This method has some advantages, such as the requirement of very little, i.e., approximately 2 ng total RNA sample, 3.5–4 log dynamic range, and easy detection of a 1.2–1.3-fold difference between samples. Moreover, it was revealed that formalin-fixed, paraffin-embedded tissues could isolate miRNAs and generate their expression profiles, demonstrating new opportunities for small RNA analysis from archival human tissues. This assay is a modification of the DASL Assay (cDNA mediated selection, annealing, extension, and ligation) that was previously developed for high throughput gene expression profiling (Chen et al., 2008).

The Illumina technology (bead array approach) was utilized to evaluate the multi-parallel expression of all human miRNAs. Total RNA as a template was processed in this method, allowing the opportunity to profile mRNA gene expression in advance experiments. Individual miRNA amplification via multi-parallel polymerase chain reaction was permitted after combining enzymatic polyadenylation with miRNA-specific primer annealing. Traditional confocal laser scanning was used to quantify the signals using fluorescently labeled primers in the PCR amplification (Siegrist et al., 2009).

3.4 Role of miRNA in preclinical and clinical drug safety evaluation

MiRNAs are essential tool for studying drug-induced toxicity as they are the early toxicity marker. Incorporating miRNA profiling into the drug safety testing procedure will harmonize the existing testing approaches and may significantly improve medication safety. Various approaches were used to evaluate drug safety, involving toxicity testing, genotoxicity determination, and clinical pharmacology. The main goal of safety pharmacology studies is to analyze the influence of the drug substance on the various organ system like the central nervous system, cardiovascular system, or respiratory system to further detect the drug's pathophysiological effects and adverse pharmacodynamics substance. Variations in the metabolic processes of animals and humans make it difficult to predict drug toxicity for humans using animal testing. It can cause a problem in detecting the human-specific toxic metabolite in an animal model.

Moreover, enhanced sensitivity due to inconsistent genetic and environmental factors among populations may not be possible to identify in clinical trials. Therefore, the post-marketing phase helps in establishing the complete safety profile of the drug substances. This all signifies the critical requirement of a reliable, fast, and economical substitute for the safety testing of drug substances to detect the toxic potential of the substance (Marrone et al., 2015).

Several studies verified that a wide variety of toxicants that impact organs like the heart, brain, liver, kidney, muscles, and pancreas could also affect the miRNA profile in the target organs. These miRNAs are potential toxicity or tissue injury markers due to their early detection in biological fluids, including urine and blood. There are several proof studies available that show the relationship between miRNA alterations and drug-induced toxicity. All these points indicate the importance of miRNA as a potential translational biomarker and genotype-independent indicator for detecting adverse medication responses in people. Still, relying on a single miRNA as a toxicity biomarker is impossible. Compared to a single miRNA evaluation, a group of miRNA that includes target-specific miRNA should be chosen as an indication of toxicity to increase specificity and provide great diagnostic value (Koturbash et al., 2015).

3.5 MiRNA and drug toxicology

Conventional methods are used to detect drug-induced various toxicities like cardiotoxicity, hepatotoxicity, neurotoxicity, nephrotoxicity, and dermal toxicity. But most of the conventional methods detect the toxicity at the later stages when toxicity is difficult to treat. Even some conventional methods of toxicity detection are invasive and less sensitive. Therefore, miRNA biomarkers for toxicity evaluation became a better alternative to conventional methods of toxicity evaluation. Several miRNAs show upregulation, and several miRNAs show downregulation in different organs due to drug-inducedtoxicity (Fig. 3.2).

3.5.1 MiRNAs and cardiovascular toxicity

Cardiotoxicity can be detected using various methods, including endomyocardial biopsies, echocardiographic cardiac function evaluation (typically by quantifying left ventricular ejection fraction, LVEF), and imaging. However, these methods have significant drawbacks, such as high invasiveness, limited sensitivity, high costs, and late detection of cardiac disease. The circulating biomarkers for DOX-induced cardiotoxicities, such as cardiac troponins (cTn) and brain natriuretic peptide (BNP), have proven to be highly accurate and have been embraced as robust circulating biomarkers. Elevated concentrations of plasma BNP are related to the occurrence of congestive heart failure in the clinical situation. In contrast, cTn is released into the circulatory system during cardiac necrosis and works as the gold standard indicator

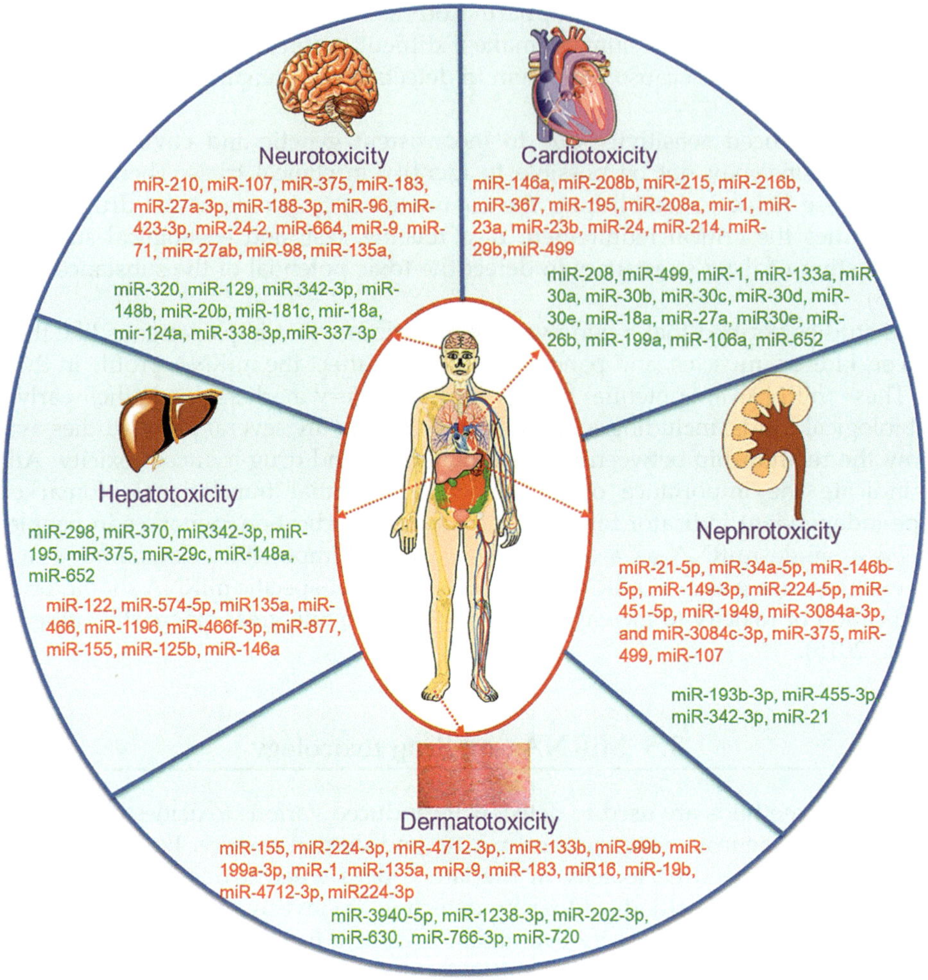

FIGURE 3.2 MiRNAs involved in various toxicities (upregulated (red color) and downregulated (green color) miRNAs).

of heart injury. As a result, troponin levels in the blood only rise after tissue injury, limiting their use as early diagnostic indicators for the onset of heart dysfunction (Lipshultz et al., 2012; Calzetta et al., 2016).

DOX (Doxorubicin) treatment and overexpression of miR-146a enhanced cell death, which was reversed by ectopic ErbB4 expression. MiR-208b was found to be overexpressed in the hearts of all animals given a mid- (2 mg/kg) and high- (3 mg/kg) dose of DOX for 2 weeks. The concentrations of all five miRNAs had dramatically risen after 4 weeks, and dosage dependence was seen. The expression of numerous miRNAs like miR-208b, miR-215, miR-216b, and miR-367 was considerably higher after 6 weeks (Ruggeri et al., 2018). Myocardial damage linked with open-heart surgeries also raised serum and urine-related miR-1 levels, which might indicate future cardiac issues (Zhou et al., 2013).

Adult, postnatal, and embryonic hearts express various miRNAs; their improper expression or genetic deletion has been linked to heart development disturbance, abnormal differentiation of cardiac cells, and cardiac dysfunction. Imbalanced expressions of miRNAs in developing cardiac progenitor cells can lead to congenital or structural abnormalities, such as poor cell migration, proliferation, and differentiation into unsuitable cell types. MiR-195 overexpression in the heart increases hypertrophic development of dilated cardiomyopathy (DCM) in mice by targeting F-box/WD repeat-containing protein 7 (FBXW7) and mitofusin-2 (MFN2) (Wang et al., 2019; Kalayinia et al., 2021).

Furthermore, miR-135b and miR-21-5p, which are linked to the Hippo and Wnt signaling pathways, have been linked not only to the molecular pathogenesis of arrhythmic cardiomyopathy (ARVC) but also to cardiac fibrosis (Naga Prasad and Karnik, 2010). MiR-17−92, which are required for smooth muscle cell proliferation, differentiation, and fibrous matrix formation, controlled BMPR2 expression (Chen and Li, 2017). MiR-1 and miR-208a are abundantly expressed in the heart and are significantly linked to cardiac hypertrophy. Furthermore, the overexpressed miR-23a, miR-24, miR-23b, and miR-214 in cardiac hypertrophy can induce hypertrophic development in cardiomyocytes (Rigaud et al., 2012).

MiR-15 family members were elevated in heart failure and myocardial ischemia, and they also targeted the antiapoptotic factor B-cell lymphoma 2 (Bcl2) to induce apoptosis. MiR-29 family members, whose expression is reduced in the region next to the infarct, promote collagen expression by targeting fibrillin, collagen, and elastin genes (Kalayinia et al., 2021). The expression of 1, 1, 2, 8, and 21 miRNAs were altered in the hearts of mice treated with 6, 9, 12, 18, and 24 mg/kg DOX, respectively. The sole miRNA overexpressed in all DOX-treated animals was a pro-apoptotic miR34a, which showed a substantial dose-related response (Desai et al., 2014). DOX and L-DOX administration reduced let-7g expression in the left atrium and miR-208a expression in the left ventricle. Plasma miR-29b and miR-499 were overexpressed following anthracycline therapy in patients (Skála et al., 2019). After one high DAU (Daunorubicin) dosage, miR-1, miR-208, miR-133a, and miR-499 levels in rats were decreased, but six lower DAU doses had no impact on the miR expression (Doka et al., 2017). Both before and after DOX treatment, the expression of miR-15b, miR-34a, miR-34b, miR-130a, miR-146a, miR-187, miR-199a, miR-199b, miR-214, and miR-424 was different (Holmgren et al., 2016).

3.5.2 MiRNAs and hepatotoxicity

Hepatotoxicity is a prominent cause of clinical trial failure and withdrawal of drugs from the market across the world. New evaluation methods for hepatotoxicity, like miRNA biomarkers, are intended to aid in identifying hazardous compounds early in the research and marketing process, therefore protecting the healthcare of consumers and clinical trial participants and redirecting financial resources to safer molecules (Lin et al., 2017).

Serum alanine aminotransferase (ALT), aspartate aminotransferase (AST), alkaline phosphatase (ALP), and bilirubin are well-established indicators of liver damage. ALT and AST values can be very inconstant in nonclinical species, insensitive to mild to moderate liver injury or chronic liver toxicity, and raised by causes other than liver toxicity. When raised together, bilirubin and ALP are highly specific to liver disease. However, they increase in the blood when a considerable liver injury has occurred.

Another problem is that aminotransferases, particularly ALT, are often poor interpreters of patient mortality for drug-induced liver injury (DILI). Moreover, AST and ALT are elevated in all liver injuries; they cannot be used to distinguish etiology, excluding a few circumstances when the AST/ALT ratio is relevant. These difficulties in interpreting and predicting clinical courses have sparked interest in developing more sensitive and precise indicators of liver injury. In animal models and human clinical settings, urinary and blood miR-122 expression have been linked to acetaminophen (APAP)-induced liver damage. Compared to ALT, miR-122 overexpression in circulation occurs faster and shows less inter-individual variation in response to toxicants like alcohol, APAP, and inflammatory agents. As a result, miRNAs may be more suitable for therapeutic usage in the future than currently recognized biomarkers (Ward et al., 2014; Starckx et al., 2013; Li et al., 2014).

When rats are exposed to hepatotoxins like carbon tetrachloride or acetaminophen, their miRNA expression changes, including downregulation of miR-370 and miR-298, which are considered to control an oxidative stress-related gene. Exposure to tamoxifen, a strong hepatocarcinogen, resulted in the overexpression of numerous oncogenic miRNAs, including the 17–92 cluster, miR-34, and miR-106a (Fukushima et al., 2007; Pogribny et al., 2007).

The alterations in miR-122 were significant and occurred before those in ALT. Substantial elevations in miR-122 levels were discovered earlier than evident histopathologic alterations in the liver, revealing that miR-122 might be employed for early disease diagnostic and surveillance (Zhang et al., 2010). MiR-135a, miR-466g, miR-466f-3p, miR-574-5p, miR-877, and miR-1196 were elevated in the context of fatal hepatotoxicity, while miR-29c, miR-148a, miR-195, miR-342-3p, miR-375, and miR-652 were significantly downregulated (Ward et al., 2012).

3.5.3 MiRNAs and neurotoxicity

New technical breakthroughs and approaches in microarray analysis and genomics have made it feasible to outline the biochemical pathways and miRNAs functions and determine which miRNAs are probable targets of anesthetics. Notch1 has been shown to help developmental processes by influencing cell fate, whereas miR-665 has binding sites in the 3′-untranslated region of Bcl-2-like protein 1 (Bcl-xl) mRNA, which plays a vital role in brain development. Following the administration of various anesthetics, BDNF was discovered to be directly controlled by the elevation of miR-107, miR-210, and miR-375, and BDNF was recognized as a downstream modulator of these miRNAs (Bahmad et al., 2020).

Propofol and sevoflurane are among the most commonly used anesthetics. Furthermore, increasing the dose exposure of sevoflurane administered to new-born rats resulted in a disease of hippocampus neural stem cell (NSCs) proliferation and differentiation. This impact was linked to a rise in miRNA-183 expression and a reduction in NR4A2 expression. MiRNA-183 was previously reported to be linked to an NSCs negative regulation following anesthesia by lowering Sox2 expression levels. The tumor suppressor miRNA-27a-3p was upregulated in newly born mice after exposure to sevoflurane (Liu et al., 2014; Shao and Xia, 2019).

Mice exposed to sevoflurane in early life stages had long-lasting changes in miRNAs of the hippocampus (miR-15a, miR-20b, miR-99a, miR-129-3p, miR-382, and miR-532) and whole brain miRNAs (miR-29a, miR-19a, and miR-145) (Lin et al., 2018). Sevoflurane dramatically increases miRNA-188-3p expression while adversely regulating MDM2-p53 expression (Wang et al., 2018). Additionally, employing miR-96 mimics without anesthetics, Xu et al. associated an elevation in miRNA-96 levels following exposure to sevoflurane with decreased learning and memory function (Xu et al., 2018).

Due to military and manufacturing activity, hexahydro-1,3,5-trinitro-1,3,5-triazine (RDX) is a well-identified pollutant of soil, land, and groundwater. Several investigations have shown that RDX can induce neurotoxicity in humans and animals, including seizures. Stimulating miR-27ab, miR-71, miR-98, and miR-135a expression by RDX can potentially diminish the expression of the genes SULF1, C5ORF13, POLE4, and ROCK2 and hence cause neurotoxicity. Upregulation of miR-27ab or RDX-induced decrease of unknown miRNA expression might increase HMGCR expression and lead to neurotoxicity. RDX-regulated immunological and inflammatory response miRNAs and genes may have a role in RDX-induced neurotoxicity, other side effects, and animal defense responses to RDX (Deng et al., 2014).

MiR-7, primarily expressed in neurons, has been shown to protect cells from oxidative stress by inhibiting α-synuclein translation. 1-methyl-4-phenyl-1,2,3,6-tetrahydropyridine (MPTP) has been shown to protect the cell from oxidative stress in both cultured cells and Parkinson's disease animal models (Junn et al., 2009). MiR-64 and miR-65 may target the ptc-1 and mdl-1 genes, which were shown to be overexpressed in diseased animal models compared to healthy animals and miR-64/miR-65 knockout mice (Asikainen et al., 2010).

3.5.4 MiRNAs and nephrotoxicity

Elevated serum creatinine and blood urea nitrogen (BUN) values are used as indicators of renal damage. Yet, these indicators have limitations in clinical and nonclinical situations, as well as in kidney damage specificity and sensitivity. In addition, miR-34c-3p, a potential miRNA biomarker of renal damage, specifically glomerular cell damage, has been found in blood and urine as a primary indicator of doxorubicin-induced glomerular cell injury (Church et al., 2014).

The 12-week Cd therapy strategy caused kidney impairment, as evidenced by proteinuria and polyuria, as well as a substantial rise in the urine biomarkers β2 microglobulin, Kim-1, and cystatin C. Microarray analysis verified that the expression profiles of 44 miRNAs were considerably elevated. The expression of 54 miRNAs was dramatically reduced in the Cd treatment group compared to the saline control. Compared to the saline control group, miR-21-5p, miR-146b-5p, miR-224-5p, miR-34a-5p, miR-149-3p, miR-3084a-3p, miR-451-5p, miR-1949, and miR-3084c-3p revealed a substantial two-fold or higher over-expression in the treated group. The Cd-treatment group, as compared to the saline control group, displayed substantial downregulation of miR-193b-3p, miR-342-3p, and miR-455-3p (Fay et al., 2018).

MiR-375 was known to be upregulated after inducing nephrotoxicity in in-vitro and in-vivo models by cisplatin. Following cisplatin therapy, 67 miRNAs exhibited substantial and persistent alterations in expression profile: 20 miRNAs were downregulated and 47 were upregulated. TaqMan real-time PCR was used to confirm the elevation of miR-31, miR-212, and mir-375 among the significantly upregulated miRNAs. 3.5-fold upregulation of miR-375 expression in wild-type cells by cisplatin treatment was observed, but it caused only a two-fold downregulation in DN-P53 cells. We discovered a consistent putative miR-375 targeting region in the 3′-UTR of HNF-1 mRNA was discovered by utilizing online databases (Target Scan and MiRanda). They initially looked at how overexpressing miR-375 in rat proximal tubular cells (RPTC) influenced HNF-1 expression. Their findings suggested that NF-κB and P53 are involved in the induction of miR-375 in cisplatin nephrotoxicity. MiR-375 can directly target or suppress HNF-1β (Hao et al., 2017).

Thirty-three miRNAs were known to be differentially expressed with a fold regulation between the nephrotoxicity and non-nephrotoxicity groups. miR-4718, miR-3168, and miR-6125 were the most differentially expressed miRNAs in the nephrotoxicity group. Downregulated miR-17-5p, miR-151b, miR-151a-5p, miR-485-3p, miR-766-3p, and miR-1185-1-3p were among the downregulated differentially expressed miRNAs (Quintanilha et al., 2021).

MiR-107 levels in circulating endothelial cells were shown to be increased in individuals with sepsis-caused AKI. MiR-125b has been identified as a possible biomarker in assessing ischemic kidney damage in patients with AKI. Several miRNAs have been found to be changed in serum samples of individuals with AKI, including miR-26b-5p, miR-10a-5p, miR-27a-3p, miR-29a-3p, miR-93-3p, miR-101-3p, miR-126-3p, miR-127-3p, miR-146a-5p, and miR-210-3p. MiR-21 (overexpressed) and miR-499 (suppressed) appear to be changed in individuals with renal replacement therapy and terminal kidney failure (Brandenburger and Lorenzen, 2020). Cyclosporine A treatment altered the expression of 76 miRNAs. Among those 76 miRNAs, 47 miRNAs were downregulated, and 30 miRNAs were upregulated (Gooch et al., 2017).

3.5.5 MiRNAs and dermatologic toxicity

Because of the strong overexpression of miR-155 in various immune cell lineages, including fibroblasts, lymphocytes, macrophages, mast cells, and dendritic cells, contributes to the pathogenesis of chronic skin inflammation. MiR-155 is associated with immunity and inflammation. Atopic dermatitis (AD) patients have a variable expression of miR-155 in their lesional skin and peripheral circulation. The results revealed that miR-155 was overexpressed in both AD skin tissues and peripheral CD4T cells. A link between the miR-155 expression level in AD peripheral CD4T cells and the severity of the illness was discovered (Mannucci et al., 2017).

MiRNAs regulate cellular differentiation, proliferation, and death, as well as the formation and functioning of melanocytes and immune cells. A study revealed that miR-133b, which was shown to be positioned exactly upstream of the IL17A or IL17F gene, is upregulated in lesional skin from nonsegmental vitiligo (NSV). Furthermore, the immune modulator thymosin 1 (T1) caused the downregulation of miR-3940-5p and overexpression of miR-224-3p and miR-4712-3p in NSV patients. Melanomagenesis and stress response are linked to the loss of miRNA-211. Moreover, miR-99b and miR-199a-3p expression were upregulated in the skin of vitiligo patients. The expression of miR-1, miR-9, miR-135a, and miR-183 was significantly higher in NSV skin than in healthy skin. In the peripheral blood of vitiligo patients, miR-630, miR-202-3p, miR-766-3p, and miR-1238-3p were considerably downregulated. In the NSV patients' serum, miR-16 and miR-19b expressions were elevated, whereas miR-720 was downregulated. In the PBMCs of NSV patients, miR-3940-5p was suppressed, whereas miR-224-3p and miR-4712-3p were considerably elevated (Li, 2020).

3.6 MiRNAs and environmental contaminants

Various environmental contaminants like particulate matter, smoke, air toxicants, metals, nanoparticles, and carcinogens can also cause alteration in miRNA expression profiling. These alterations are helpful in the risk assessment of several diseases caused by environmental contaminants. Various studies were performed to evaluate the interactions of environmental contaminants with the miRNA expression profile (Table 3.1). MiRNAs are early biomarkers that can only detect the disease at the initiation stage. Various toxicants can induce disease via miRNA dysregulation (Fig. 3.3).

3.6.1 Carcinogens

Environmental carcinogen-induced miRNA alterations are helpful in the prediction of future cancer only if the miRNA alteration is irreversible. On the other hand, reversible miRNA alterations are significant for adaptive mechanisms as compared to pathogenic mechanisms. The inability of the cells to re-establish the expression level of miRNAs even after the termination of environmental carcinogen exposure reflects the irreversibility of the miRNA alteration. The duration of exposure to a carcinogen determines the switching of reversibility of miRNA alteration to irreversibility. The miRNA alterations are also affected by the exposure dose of the carcinogen. It was observed in one study that low-dose exposure to cigarette smoke (CS) was not efficient in altering lung miRNA expression significantly, but high-dose exposure altered its expression (Izzotti et al., 2011).

Benzo[a]pyrene-7,8-diol-9,10-epoxide (BPDE) is a Benzo(a) pyrene-activated metabolite. BDPE upregulates miR-22, miR-494, and miR-106a and downregulates miR-10a and miR-506 in transformed malignant human bronchial epithelial cells (16HBE-T). MiR-506 is useful as an anti-oncogene miRNA that suppresses the proliferation of cells and reduces the degree of malignancy. This indicates that the N-Ras oncogene and miR-506 expression levels are inversely correlated, indicating that the N-Ras targets miR-506. This correlation determines the mechanistic basis of the function of miR-506 as an inhibitor of cell growth and tumorigenesis (Izzotti and Pulliero, 2014; Zhao et al., 2011).

Tobacco smoking is found to be a common risk factor for head and neck as well as lung cancer. Tobacco smoking is linked to molecular alterations like miRNA expression dysregulation in both types of cancer. Tobacco-specific nitrosamine 4-(methyl nitrosamino)-1-(3-pyridyl)-1-butanone (NNK) was hypothesized to alter MSH2 and MLH1 expression key Mismatch DNA repair MMR components by endorsing specific miRNA dysregulation in lung and head and neck squamous cancer cells (NCI and FaDu, respectively). In comparison to controls, a low (1 M) or high (2 M) dosage of NNK caused substantial downregulation of "tumor suppressor" miR-422a and overexpression of "oncomirs" miR-21 and miR-155, as

TABLE 3.1 Effect of various toxicants on the expression profile of miRNAs and their targets.

Toxicant	Altered miRNA	Expression	Expression site	Target	Method used for expression	Inference/Effect	Dose of toxicant	Model	Reference
Microcystin-LR	miR-181a	Down-regulated	Brain	Glucose-regulated protein, 78kDa/binding immunoglobulin protein (Grp78/BIP)	miRNA microarray assay, qRT-PCR	Endoplasmic reticulum (ER) stress and neuronal apoptosis in hippocampal CA1 regions of mice	3 μg/kg S.C	C57bl/6 mice	Liu et al. (2020)
2,5-Hexanedione (HD)	105 miRNAs	56 up-regulated, 49 down-regulated	Axons	GSK3β, Map3k1, BDNF and MAP1B	miRNA microarray assay, qRT-PCR, Western blot	Axon-related miRNAs mediate 2,5-hexanedione toxicity	400 mg/kg/day (5 times/wk for 5 weeks)	Sprague–Dawley (SD) rats	Piao et al. (2020)
Arsenic	miR-155, -338, -210. 34a, 124	Up-regulated	Peripheral blood mononuclear cells	DAPK1, EGR2, APP	RNA sequencing, qRT-PCR	Arsenic exposure induces a large number of differentially expressed genes	0.5–4600 μg/L	Bangladeshi female participants	Chen et al. (2020)
Microcystin-LR	319 (mainly miR-16, miR-181a-3p, miR-451, and miR-223)	227 up-regulated, 29 down-regulated (for the highest dose)	Liver	Target gene related to cellular, metabolic, and single-organism processes	High-throughput sequencing, qRT-PCR	4 miRNAs (miR-181a-3p, miR-16, miR-451, miR-223) are intricate in MC-LR toxicity in multiple organs	50 and 200 μg/kg	Silver carp (hypophthalmichthys molitrix)	Feng et al. (2020)
Fructus Meliae Toosendan (FMT)	miR-222	Down-regulated	Serum exosomes & liver	PTEN and PPP2R2A	miRNA microarray analysis, qRT-PCR, biological pathway analysis	miRNA profiles present insights into hepatotoxicity mechanisms of FMT and reveal the protective role of autophagy	20 and 40 g/kg	Male BALB/c mice	Yu et al. (2020)

Alpha-naphthyliso thiocyanate (ANIT) and FP004BA	miR-122-5p, miR-182-5p, miR-192-5p	Up-regulated	Plasma & liver	–	Microarrays & qRT-PCR	Several miRNAs were identified as markers for different stages of liver injury.	50 mg/kg & 100 mg/kg	Male Sprague –Dawley rats	Church et al. (2015)
Isoproterenol (ISO) or allylamine (AAM)	miR-208a-3p	Up-regulated	Plasma	–	Firefly™ circulating miRNA assay	Plasma miR-208a-3p was identified as a strong cardiac injury biomarker	ISO 1.5 mg/kg (i.p.) & AAM 100 mg/kg (per os)	Male hanover Wistar rats	Glineur et al. (2015)
Isoproterenol (ISO), metaproterenol (MET), allylamine (AAM), mitoxantrone (MIT), acetaminophen (APAP)	miR-133a/b, miR-208	Up-regulated	Serum	MyL3 and skeletal muscle troponin (sTnl)	qRT-PCR	miR-133a/b are specific and sensitive markers of skeletal muscle toxicity, and in combination with miR-208, help in differentiating muscle toxicity from cardiotoxicity	APAP (1500 mg/kg), ISO (0.05 mg/kg), AAM (100 mg/kg), MET (5.0 mg/kg), and MIT (10 mg/kg)	Male Sprague –Dawley rats	Calvano et al. (2016)
Silver, gold, and iron oxide nanoparticles	9 miRNAs	5 downregulated, 4 up-regulated	Cells	–	qRT-PCR, miRNA PCR array	Most of the altered miRNAs inhibit cell proliferation and tumorigenesis	AgNP (10 μg/mL), AuNP (10 μg/mL), and SPIONs (10 μg/mL)	HepG2 cells	Brzóska et al. (2019)
Mycotoxin zearalenone (ZEN)	14 miRNAs	–	Porcine uterus, jejunum, and serum	Estrogen receptor α & β	RNA sequencing, qRT-PCR	ZEN significantly altered uterine miRNAs but not miRNAs of the jejunum.	0.17, 1.46, and 4.58 mg/kg	Piglets	Grenier et al. (2019)
Bisphenol A (BPA)		Up-regulated	Liver		Methylated DNA immunoprecipitation-	Hepatic lipid content was increased	25 μg/kg/day	Pregnant CD-1 mice	

(*Continued*)

TABLE 3.1 Effect of various toxicants on the expression profile of miRNAs and their targets.—cont'd

Toxicant	Altered miRNA	Expression	Expression site	Target	Method used for expression	Inference/Effect	Dose of toxicant	Model	Reference
	mi34a and mi122			Nuclear factor E2-related factor 2 (Nrf2)	PCR and pyrosequencing	concomitantly with Nrf2 and pro-lipogenic enzyme expression			Shimpi et al. (2017)
Microcystin-LR (MC-LR)	99 miRNAs	62 downregulated, 37 up-regulated	Human normal liver cell line HL7702	mTOR, Rap1, HIF-1 signaling pathway	High-throughput sequencing, qRT-PCR	Hepatotoxicity induced by MC-LR was linked with variations in miRNAs.	1, 2.5, 5 or 10 μM	Human normal liver cell line HL7702	Yang et al. (2018)
Bisphenol A (BPA)	miR-146a	Overexpressed	Placenta	Aryl hydrocarbon receptors (AhR) and retinoic acid (RA) receptors (RAR and RXR)	Microarray technology & qPCR	miR-146a became a potential biomarker for BPA accumulation in the placenta and to clarify the environmental disease mechanism.	–	Pregnant women	De Felice et al. (2015)
Lead and mercury	74 miRNAs	17 miRNAs downregulated	Cervix	AHR signaling pathway	NanoString nCounter assay	Human cervix miRNA act as novel responders to maternal chemical exposure in pregnancy	–	Pregnant women	Sanders et al. (2015)
Fusarium mycotoxins, zearalenone (ZEN) and deoxynivalenol (DON)	7 miRs	–	Liver and colon	E2F1	qRT-PCR	Disorder in cell proliferation and survival pathway was studied by alteration in miRNA.	DON (12 μg/kg/d), ZEN (40 μg/kg/d), ZEN + DON (40 + 12 μg/kg/d)	Immature gilts	Brzuzan et al. (2015)
Ricin	21 miRNAs	9 downregulated, 12 up-regulated	Lungs and peripheral blood mononuclear cells (PBMCs)	IL-1 and NF-kB pathway	NanoString nCounter miRNA expression assay, qRT-PCR	Activation of several immune regulation pathways was analyzed by transcriptome analysis	7 μg/kg	Mice	Pillar et al. (2019)
Silica nanoparticles	miR-451a	Down-regulated	Human umbilical vein	IL6R signaling pathway		miR-451a can be used as a potential target to		Male Sprague –Dawley (SD) rats	Feng et al. (2019)

			endothelial cells (HUVECs)		Microarray analysis, qRT-PCR, western blot	counter the side effect of nanoparticles.	1.8, 5.4 and 16.2 mg/kg·bw		
Zinc oxide nanoparticles	miR-375, miR-24, miR-29a, miR-34a, miR-103, miR-107, and miR-122	Down-regulated	Liver and pancreas	–	qRT-PCR	Zn nanoparticles altered miRNA expression in pancreatic β cells and liver tissues.	5 mg/kg	Wistar albino rats	Othman et al. (2020)
Toosendan Fructus	81 miRNAs	29 miRNAs up-regulated and 52 miRNA down-regulated	Serum	–	miRNAs chip analysis and qRT-PCR	miRNAs are sensitive biomarkers for hepatotoxicant-induced hepatotoxicity.	10 mg/kg	C57BL/6 mice	Yang et al. (2019)
Nanopolystyrene	7 miRNAs	4 downregulated, 3 up-regulated	*Caenorhabditis elegans*	Wnt signaling pathway	SOLiD sequencing, qRT-PCR	Various biological processes and signaling pathways were associated with altered miRNA by nanopolystyrene exposure	1 μg/L	*Caenorhabditis elegans*	Qu et al. (2019)
Phthalate mixture	miR-141-3p, miR-30d-5p, and miR-184	Up-regulated	Prostate	–	FastQC v0.11.5 sequencing analysis	Alteration in reproductive biometric parameters was detected by miRNA and transcriptome profiling.	20, 200 μg/kg/day, and 200 mg/kg/day	Pregnant female Sprague–Dawley rats	Scarano et al. (2019)
Cadmium	miR-33-5q	Downregulated	Spleen	BNIP3, AKT/mTOR signaling, NF-κB, p-JNK/JNK	qPCR and Western blot	Autophagy was induced by triggering miR-33-5q deregulation through cadmium exposure.	10 mg/kg	Hy-line Brown laying hens	Menghao (2018)
1-Methyl-3-octylimidazolium	miR-125b,	miR-125b downregulated,	Spleen	p38MAPK/NF-κB signaling	qPCR	Lysozyme activity, complement 3 (C3),	1.095 and 4.380 mg/L	Silver carp	Ma et al. (2019)

(Continued)

TABLE 3.1 Effect of various toxicants on the expression profile of miRNAs and their targets.—cont'd

Toxicant	Altered miRNA	Expression	Expression site	Target	Method used for expression	Inference/Effect	Dose of toxicant	Model	Reference
bromide ([C_8mim] Br)	miR-143, miR-155 and miR-21	miR-155 and miR-21 up-regulated				and immunoglobulin M (IgM) content alteration showed the immunotoxic effect of ([C_8mim]Br)			
Metals and polycyclic aromatic hydrocarbons (PAHs)	Ten miRNAs		Urine & blood		qPCR	Expression profile of miRNAs was negatively associated with titanium, antimony, aluminum, & lead and positively associated with tin and molybdenum	Variable exposure	Male coke oven workers	Deng et al. (2019)

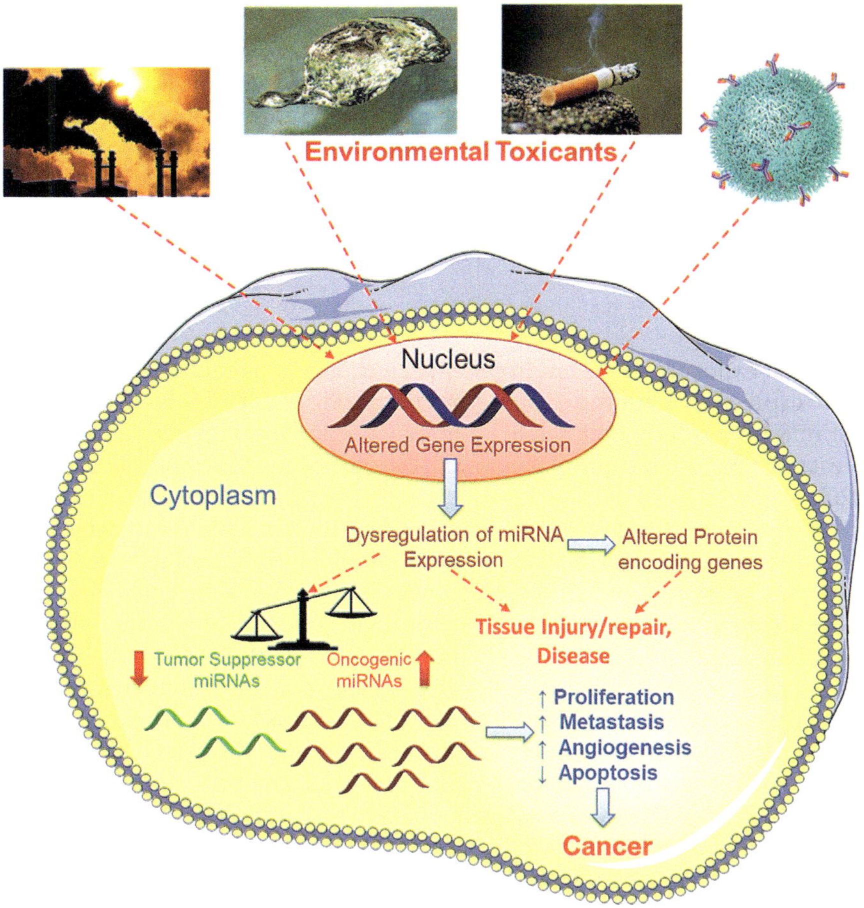

FIGURE 3.3 Effect of various toxicants on disease induction (cancer) via miRNAs dysregulation.

well as reductions in mRNA and MMR protein expression in NCI and FaDu. MiR-21 inhibition in NCI and FaDu restored the NNK-induced decreased MSH2 phenotype, suggesting that miR-21 is involved in MSH2 regulation. Finally, NNK exposure promotes cancer cell growth by increasing NCI and FaDu survival (Doukas et al., 2020).

In comparison to a control diet (corn oil plus cellulose (CCA)), Shah et al. observed that the unique combination of pectin (fermented to butyrate in the colon) plus dietary fish oil (containing three fatty acids) following carcinogen exposure overexpressed a subgroup of putative tumor suppressor miRNAs in the intestinal mucosa and suppressed their predicted target genes (Shah et al., 2016).

One dosage of N-methyl-N-nitrosourea (MNU) and 7,12-dimethylbenz(α)anthracene (DMBA) was administered intraperitoneally to mice. QRT-PCR was used to evaluate the miRNAs expression after 3 and 6 h of therapy. After 3 and 6 h of MNU therapy, reduced expression of miR-34a and miR-155 was observed in the spleen, liver, and kidneys. MiR-21 expression was substantially increased in the kidneys and lungs after 6 h of DMBA treatment, but MNU elevated miR-21 expression levels in the liver after 3 and 6 h compared to DMBA therapy. The fact that miRNAs react differently to carcinogens highlights their potential as epidemiological indicators in the early phases of environmental carcinogenesis (Juhász et al., 2013).

2-acetylaminofluorene (2-AAF) is a mutagenic and carcinogenic fluorene derivative. It's often exploited in carcinogenesis studies. An investigation employing a rodent animal model (rat) revealed that the miR-18, miR-17-5p, miR-20, and miR-93 were overexpressed after dietary exposure to 2-AAF, as measured by qPCR (Pogribny et al., 2011).

3.6.2 Metals/metalloids

Toxic heavy metal exposure in the environment can change epigenetic regulatory markers such as miRNA expression patterns, histone modification, and DNA methylation. Developing changed miRNA profiles as possible biomarkers following metal exposure would be equivalent to establishing a valid profile of miRNA modifications for risk assessment (Wallace et al., 2020).

Human exposure to high levels of Arsenic (As), a hazardous metalloid extensively disseminated in the environment, is linked to various health problems, most notably cancer and cardiovascular diseases. Various epidemiological investigations have revealed evidence that inorganic As exposure can disturb the CVS of humans, including cardiac arrhythmias, ischemic heart failure, and endothelial dysfunction (Tumolo et al., 2022). MiR-126-3p is the abundantly found miRNA in endothelial cells, which contributes to vascular integrity regulation and angiogenesis and is implicated in a no. of cardiovascular pathways; this makes miR-126-3p down-regulation an early indicator for cardiovascular disorders (Wei et al., 2013).

Various levels of As were exposed to the subjects, and urine analysis was done to check the miRNA expression. It was observed that miR-205-5p and miR-200c-3p expression were inversely linked with the exposure of as compared to the control group. Furthermore, the authors compared the expression of these miRNAs in healthy controls and urothelial carcinoma patients. The results showed that miR-205-5p expression was low, suggesting that it may be used as a diagnostic marker for bladder cancer. Both miR-205-5p and miR-200c-3p have antitumor properties. MiR-200c-3p regulates zinc finger E-box-binding homeobox 1 (ZEB1) and ZEB2 to reverse epithelial-mesenchymal transition. As a result, these miRNAs might be involved in tumor genesis and progression (Michailidi et al., 2015).

Lead (Pb) is a hazardous metal that disturbs several physiological systems and is connected to various harmful events, including cardiovascular illness and chronic kidney disease. Using the Nanostring nCounter assay, Sanders et al. explored the connection between metal concentrations and the expression profile of 74 miRNAs. Pregnant women were included in this cohort analysis. Throughout the second trimester of pregnancy, maternal mercury (Hg) and Pb exposure resulted in the downregulation of miR-575 and miR-4286 expression in cervix cells in proportion to tibial bone Pb levels, whereas 17 miRNAs were shown to be adversely linked with toenail Hg levels. According to functional analysis, Hg-associated miRNAs were involved in developing the reproductive system and morphology. At the same time, gene targets associated with Pb were found to be augmented for preeclampsia. Additionally, these miRNAs have been linked to various cell cycles and proliferation pathways, which may influence parturition and the reproductive system. Three genes in the aryl-hydrocarbon receptor (AHR) signaling pathway are expected to be targeted by miR-4286 (Sanders et al., 2015).

Li et al. observed that some miRNAs were affected in placenta samples upon Pb exposure. For example, let-7f-5p, miR-146a-5p, miR-10a-5p, miR-190b, and miR-431-5p were down-regulated, but miR-651 was found to be overexpressed, suggesting that miRNAs may serve as indicators of prenatal environmental exposures (Li et al., 2015).

Mining and pollution can expose workers to Hg, harming their cardiovascular, neurological, and immunological systems. miRNA microarray analysis revealed that the groups exposed to Hg poisoning had four miRNAs downregulated (let-7e-5p, miR-30c-3p, miR-16-5p, and miR-181a-5p) and four miRNAs upregulated (miR-451a, miR-122-5p, miR-92a-3p, and miR-486-5p). QRT-PCR confirmed the higher miR-486-5p and miR-92a-3p levels in mercury-poisoned cells (Ding et al., 2016).

Chromium (Cr), found in soil and rocks, can be gas, liquid, or solid and has many oxidation states. Epidemiological studies have associated exposure to Cr with metabolic and cardiovascular diseases. Dioni et al. investigated 90 obese patients' leukocyte miRNA expression. Forty-three miRNAs were adversely linked with Cr levels during screening, but only 10 were selected for validation. MiR-15b, miR-21-5p, miR-26a-5p, miR-182, miR-183-5p, miR-301, miR-362-3p, miR-451a, and miR-486-3p supported the first phase's pattern. The Functional study found these miRNAs' top canonical pathways to be: axonal guidance signaling, molecular cancer processes, NFAT (nuclear factor of activated T cells) role in cardiac hypertrophy, protein kinase A (PKA) signaling and PTEN signaling. According to bioinformatics, miR-486-3p was positively associated with blood pressure and may be a risk factor in cardiovascular disease due to miRNA communication with the PTEN pathway; miR-451a is negatively associated with glycated hemoglobin (HbA1c) (Dioni et al., 2017).

In a case-control study comprising 360 healthy male coke oven workers, the relationship between various metals and PAHs (polycyclic aromatic hydrocarbons) and miRNA expression was investigated. Many plasma miRNAs have been reported to be adversely linked with Pb, antimony, aluminum, and titanium while positively related to tin and molybdenum. This investigation found a link between some miRNAs and indicators of oxidative stress and genetic damage, like micronuclei and 8-OH-dG (Deng et al., 2019).

3.6.3 Nanoparticles

Nanomaterial exposure may trigger epigenetic modifications that affect gene expression. Variations in miRNA expression have been linked to pathologies. Responses were observed after titanium dioxide (TiO2) NP exposure at maximum concentration. Most deregulated miRNAs, such as miR-25, miR-23a, miR-210, miR-199b, miR-505, and miR-1271, were overexpressed compared to time-matched controls. MiR-96 was highly overexpressed at week 6. There is adequate information to show that NMs can cause various negative consequences, including inflammation, oxidative stress, DNA damage, altered gene expression, lipid peroxidation, reproductive toxicity, apoptosis, immunotoxicity, and carcinogenesis. Most research generated this knowledge has used in in-vitro procedures as appropriate strategies for in vivo-induced effects. But, as they employ short-term exposures and maximum concentrations, most of this research is far from mimicking genuine human exposure scenarios. As a result, in vitro chronic-exposure systems must be implemented in the field and used to test low and non-cytotoxic amounts of the NMs under investigation. BEAS-2B cells demonstrated expression variations in 33 miRNAs associated with cellular stress, inflammation, and carcinogenesis pathways after long-term exposure to MWCNT and TiO2NP (Ballesteros et al., 2021).

One investigation was done to evaluate the influence of silver nanoparticles (AgNPs) on endothelial cell's EA.hy926 epigenome, involving global DNA methylation patterns and miRNA expression levels. There were no alterations in the expression of inflammatory genes, and the reduced expression of the studied miRNAs like miR-126, miR-155, and miR-146 was observed. Ultimately, direct interaction between AgNPs and endothelial cells caused dysregulation of highly functional and highly enriched miRNAs as well as DNA hypermethylation, which might have numerous impacts on endothelial function and integrity (González-Palomo et al., 2021).

One study investigated the effects of low cytotoxic doses of gold nanoparticles (AuNPs), superparamagnetic iron oxide nanoparticles (SPIONs), and silver nanoparticles (AgNPs) on the DNA methylation status of genes involved in inflammation and apoptosis, as well as the miRNAs expression involved in these processes. There were no substantial alterations in the DNA methylation status of control and treated cells. The expression of nine miRNAs was found to be substantially affected by nanoparticle treatment. AgNPs provoked alterations in six miRNAs, AuNPs altered four miRNAs and SPIONs altered two miRNAs. Most miRNAs altered by NP therapy have already decreased cell proliferation and tumorigenesis (Brzóska et al., 2019).

Another study was performed to evaluate the impact of an extensively recognized nanomaterial for medical application, i.e., SPIONs on PC12 cells, a model neuronal cell line. Their findings imply that the cellular miRNAs expression pattern of PC12 cells altered drastically after treatment with SPIONs. NMDAR, one of several candidate mRNAs that were chosen using GO and KEGG pathway enrichment as prospective miRNA targets, was dramatically downregulated by SPIONs therapy. According to this study, SPIONs have a neurotoxic effect on NMDARs, and the thorough annotation of miRNA profiling provides a credible method to analyze the neuro-cytotoxic effects of nanomaterials (Sun et al., 2015).

3.6.4 Air toxicants

Particulate matter (PM) is a complex combination of tiny particles and liquid droplets. Acids, metals, organic compounds, and dust particles or soil are among the significant constituents of particle pollution. In both in-vitro and clinical investigations, miR-10b and miR-128 are the only miRNAs associated with exposure to air pollution. Moreover, two separate investigations were found for the correlation between air pollution and various miRNAs like miR-9, miR-155, miR-21, miR-223, miR-143, miR-222, and miR-338 (Vrijens et al., 2015).

The levels of miRNAs are affected by PM exposure at various stages of pregnancy. In recent research, Tsamou and colleagues used qRT-PCR to examine miRNA expression in 210 placental tissues of mother-new-born couples. During the second trimester of pregnancy, miR-21-5p, miR-146a-5p, and miR-222-3p were negatively related to PM exposure, but miR-21-5p and miR-20a-5p expression in placental tissues was found to be positively related to first-trimester exposure. In silico prediction methods revealed that the tumor suppressor

PTEN is a common potential target of these miRNAs, which was verified by qRT-PCR in a subgroup of the same cohort. PTEN was negatively linked with miR-20a-5p, miR-222-3p, and miR-21-5p, supporting the co-expression of miRNA-PTEN in placental tissue (Tsamou et al., 2018).

Bollati et al. conducted a cohort study on the miRNA profile of blood from steel mill workers; samples were obtained at the start and end of the work week. A qRT-PCR study revealed that miR-222-3p and miR-21-5p levels in leukocytes were considerably higher following three workdays of high metal-rich PM exposure. Furthermore, the level of miR-21-5p was positively linked with 8-hydroxy-guanine (8-OH-dG), demonstrating a link with oxidative stress. Furthermore, bioinformatics analysis confirmed the involvement of these specific miRNAs in inflammation and oxidative stress pathways such as chemokine signaling, TGF, mitogen-activated protein kinase (MAPK) signaling, TLR, and other general function signaling pathways (focal adhesion, apoptosis, etc.) (Bollati et al., 2010).

In multi-centric research involving 143 healthy subjects from the Netherlands, The United Kingdom, Switzerland, and Italy, the effects of black carbon, PM2.5, UFP, and soot on miRNA expression levels were studied. The researchers employed microarray analysis to evaluate the effect of PM2.5 exposure on the expression of seven miRNAs (miR-24-3p, let-7d-5p, miR-502-5p, miR-425-5p, miR-505-3p, miR-4454, miR-4763-3p) isolated from whole blood. Surprisingly, the influence of other contaminants was negligible (Mancini et al., 2020).

Another study employed NGS technology to connect miRNA presence in blood plasma with exposure to PM2.5, PM10, CO, CO_2, NO, NO_2, UFP, and BC in 24 healthy people exposed to air pollutants while resting phase and physical activity. Despite the fact that exposure to a combination of pollutants altered the expression of nine miRNAs (miR-28-3p, miR-30b-5p/30c-5p, miR-146-5p, miR-222-3p, and miR-320a-3p/320b/320c/320d/320e were favorably related; miR-144-3p, miR-192-5p/215-5p, miR-425-5p, and miR-532-5p were negatively linked), no significant influence of PM2.5 and PM10 was detected. But the consequences of CO, CO2, NO, NO2, UFP, and BC were identified (Krauskopf et al., 2019).

Another study examined the long-term impact of PM2.5 revelation on the expression profile of miRNA in serum extracellular vesicles implicated in cardiovascular disease pathways. Elevated concentrations of miR-19b-3p, let-7a-5p, miR-93-5p, miR-15a-5p, miR-23a-3p, miR-126-3p, miR-142-3p, miR-150-5p, and miR-191-5p, and miR-223-3p are associated with inflammation, oxidative stress, and atherosclerosis (Rodosthenous et al., 2016).

After short-term exposure to PM10, expression of miR-99b-5p, let-7c-5p, miR-106a-5p, miR-218-5p, miR-143-3p, miR-642-5p, miR-185-5p, miR-331-3p, and miR-652-3p in extracellular vesicles was found to be suppressed. These miRNAs may have a role in cardiovascular disease and modulate alterations in fibrinogen levels in response to PM10 exposure, indicating that PM may contribute to enhanced coagulation (Pergoli et al., 2017).

After 3 days of PM exposure, upregulation of miR-128 and miR-302c was found in samples of 63 employees. According to pathway analysis, miR-128 was concerned with the pathways of coronary artery disease, whereas miR-302c was implicated in cardiac hypertrophy, coronary artery disease, and heart failure pathways. Both findings emphasize the deleterious impact of exposure to PM on the cardiovascular system (Bollati et al., 2015).

The influence of carcinogenic persistent organic pollutants (POPs) exposure on miRNA and transcriptome profiles in healthy people's buffy coats was examined. A linear model was used to link a cumulative Z-Score of 6 PCB congeners, DDE (a DDT breakdown product), and HCB to the miRNA expression profile, which was then combined with the transcriptome profile. A total of 93 miRNAs (53 favorably and 40 negatively) were found to be significantly linked with the level of exposure (Z-Score) (Krauskopf et al., 2017).

3.7 MiRNA interactions with environmental factors

Several studies have shown that the miRNAs interact functionally with various environmental factors such as drugs, bacteria and virus pathogens, cigarette smoking, industry material, alcohol, stress, exercise, radiation, and sleep. The distinctive roles of miRNAs and the dysregulation of miRNAs due to interaction with environmental factors demonstrate their role in discovering the mechanism of drug response and disease that further helps in the diagnosis, prognosis of disease, and novel pharmacological approaches (Wang and Cui, 2012).

Additionally, miRNAs play a critical role in several vital biological processes like cell growth, cell proliferation, cell control, cell apoptosis, and many more. Hence, abnormality or dysregulation of the miRNA due to miRNA-EF interactions can cause several diseases. For example, has-let-7b was downregulated in pancreatic cancer cells due to gemcitabine. Several studies have revealed the direct connection between diseases, genetic and environmental factors. MiRNAs participate in various diseases as critical genetic factors, and their interaction with EF helps to explain the disease pathogenesis. The computational framework used diverse biological data to quantify miRNA-miRNA and EF-EF similarity and to imagine their interactions (Luo et al., 2018).

The mechanism of EF interactions and new GF-EF interactions were explored using the modeling and computational analysis of the GF-EF interactions. For example, new drug target interactions were identified by revealing several essential insights after modeling and analyzing a particular type of drug, environmental factors, and EF interactions with their targets. Additionally, EF-miRNAs interactions significantly influence and verify phenotypes. It was observed that the EF-miRNAs interactions are extensively related to the characteristics of miRNAs, including the miRNA expression levels, conservation, tissue specificity, and disease spectrum width. The result of this study indicates that the EF-miRNAs interactions are not arbitrary but have a considerable regular pattern. It was also found that the outcome of cancer treatment can be predicted by the miRNA signatures of radiation and cancer treatment drugs (Qiu et al., 2012).

Numerous computational approaches have been proposed to envisage the EF-miRNA interactions. MiREFScan, a computational method based on Laplacian regularised least squares was proposed to predict the EF-miRNA interactions (Chen et al., 2012). Jiang et al. used hypergeometric tests to identify the miRNA-EF interactions by constructing a network of small molecule-miRNA interactions in 23 cancers (Jiang et al., 2012).

Various anticancer drug treatments include hydroxy camptothecin, 5-fluorouracil, all-trans retinoic acid, imatinib, cisplatin, lithium, gemcitabine, curcumin, fludarabine, and epigallocatechin gallate altered the miRNAs profile and cellular sensitivity to these anticancer drugs was modulated by the miRNAs (Wang and Cui, 2012). Epigenetic mechanisms alter many cellular processes and developmental pathways due to the toxicities of various industrial materials.

An industrial plasticizer, Bisphenol A, is extensively used for plastic water bottles and food cans. Recently exposure to BPA has tremendously enhanced the alteration of miRNA expression. A miRNA microarray and a qRT-PCR method were used to explore the impact of BPA exposure on miRNA of human placental cell lines. Validation was done by qRT-PCR, and it was observed that MiR146a was overexpressed in both HTR-8 and 3A cell lines after BPA exposure (Avissar-Whiting et al., 2010).

One study investigated the miRNA alterations by pollutants in the airway epithelial cells. The Diesel exhaust particles (DEP) that are the primary cause of emitted airborne particulate matter (PM) were used as a pollutant in the study. It was observed that the miRNA expression profile was tremendously modulated by DEP exposure in the human airway epithelial cell line. 1.5-folds of alteration in miRNA, either downregulation or upregulation, was observed in 62.9%, i.e., 197 out of 313 detectable miRNAs. The Presumed targets of the 12 mainly altered miRNAs were selected for the molecular network analysis. They showed that the exposure to DEP was related to the strong tumorigenic disease signature and the inflammatory responsive pathway. Results of this study revealed that cellular processes were modified due to the miRNA expression alteration after DEP exposure by gene expression regulation, leading to disease pathogenesis (Jardim Melanie et al., 2009).

Differential miRNA expression in the placenta was investigated to evaluate the influence of maternal cigarette smoking in pregnancy on miRNA expression. It was revealed that miR-16, 21, and 146a were downregulated by maternal cigarette smoking in pregnancy (Maccani and Marsit, 2011).

In another study, lung cancer cells and normal human respiratory epithelial cells were used to evaluate the alteration in miRNA expression and function by cigarette smoke condensate (CSC). It was revealed that miR-31 expression was induced by CSC exposure in both normal and cancer cells. Further, cell proliferation and tumorigenicity were enhanced by miR-31 overexpression, and cell proliferation in lung cancer was decreased by the knockdown of miR-31 expression (Xi et al., 2010). Regular smokers and nonsmokers were tested for the whole genome miRNA expression from the bronchial airway epithelium. It was found that most of the differentially expressed miRNA, including miR-218 in the bronchial airway epithelium, were downregulated in regular smokers (Schembri et al., 2009).

Sathyan et al. observed that ethanol shows teratogenic effects mediated by the miRNAs. They concluded that the ethanol altered a small number of expressed miRNAs, and for a given stage of differentiation, it affects only miRNAs that are typical components of the cellular repertoire. It was also observed that during the developmental stage, ethanol influences more miRNAs. Ethanol-targeted miRNAs demonstrate sensitivity specific to the developmental stage. Various miRNAs that are ethanol sensitive demonstrate their function at several developmental stages. For example, ethanol sensitivity for miR-9 exists for multiple development stages, escalating from embryo through fetus to adulthood (Sathyan et al., 2007).

It was observed that alcohol exposure significantly altered more than 165 mRNA and 41 rat miRNAs in the medial prefrontal cortex (mPFC). Groupings of gene ontology differential expression signified that miRNAs involved in various functional processes related to neuroadaptation, neurotransmission, and synaptic plasticity were altered (Tapocik et al., 2013).

Various conditions are well-known stressors for cells, such as hypoxia, oxidative stress, hyperthermia, and ATP depletion. It was revealed that hyperthermia altered miRNA expression in cells. Some miRNAs like miR-7, 138, and 196b were downregulated, and some miRNAs like miR-125b, 382, and 452 were upregulated after cell exposure to hyperthermia. Cells also showed differentially expressed miRNAs like miR-378, 382, and 452 expressed only in hyperthermia-exposed cells (Wilmink et al., 2010). The miR-130 family was involved in hypoxia-inducible factor 1α (HIF-1α) induced by hypoxia. DDX6 mRNA, an element of the P-bodies, was targeted by the miR-130 family and this mRNA also assists the HIF-1α translation during hypoxia (Saito et al., 2011).

Shin et al. discovered a two-fold increase in miRNA expression after IR exposure to human lung cancer cell line A549. Microarray analysis discovered that cells exposed to 20 and 40 Gy had changes in 12 and 18 miRNA expression, respectively. Target prediction of these miRNAs recommended that genes related to that cell cycle regulation, apoptosis, DNA damage, and repair be targeted by the miRNAs. These results demonstrate that radiation can affect the miRNAs expression levels, and regulation of radiation responses may also involve these miRNAs (Shin et al., 2009).

In an alternative study, the expression profile of miRNAs was investigated after IR exposure to six malignant cell lines. IR exposure showed a 2–3-fold alteration in miR-24–1, let-7i, 151-5p, and 1285 expression levels. These miRNAs are involved in processes like cell proliferation, apoptosis, local immune response, invasion, and radio-resistance. MiR-144 was found as a radiation-responsive miRNA that was expressed after radiation exposure. Tumor formation could be promoted by DNA damage due to high-dose radiation exposure that leads to ionization in the molecule of living cells (Niemoeller et al., 2011).

3.8 Upcoming avenues of miRNA in toxicology

MiRNAs can be used as a potential biomarker for toxicology studies. But the preprocessing and extraction procedures require expertise and specific instrumentations. Therefore, different techniques are in need for future to conquer these limitations. The stability of miRNAs should also be considered while designing new methods for extraction and processing of the miRNAs.

3.8.1 MiRNA-related toxicogenomics

MiRNAs target enormous protein-coding genes; therefore, it is anticipated that miRNAs regulate all biological processes. MiRNAs expression and their targets also get affected by various mechanisms such as mature miRNA mutations or mutations in their mRNA target sequence, epigenetic alterations, and deletions in the miRNAs. These processes alter miRNA expression, which may affect disease development. Various toxicants, oxidative and other types of cellular stress altered the miRNAs expression, demonstrating the crucial role of miRNAs in toxicology that can anticipate a connection between environmental factors and gene expression (Koturbash et al., 2015).

Relationships between exposure to toxicants and genome-wide gene expression pattern alteration were studied in toxicogenomics. Mechanisms of toxicity were identified by new tools provided by the analysis of the resulting molecular signatures, and this analysis also categorizes the compounds based on their biological responses. This analysis also made the identification of a cluster of genes that detect specific toxic responses, and further, this gene cluster works as a biomarker of toxicity. Still, epigenetic factors should also be considered for the complete understanding of the interaction of environmental factors with the genome. Histone modification, DNA methylation, and non-coding RNAs are mainly responsible for the epigenetic regulation of gene expression (Gatzidou et al., 2007; Reamon-Buettner et al., 2008).

Identification of protein targets and in silico screening of chemical compounds using virtual screening small molecule databases was made by Chemogenomics. It can be anticipated that novel leads for the future drug discovery program can be generated using this approach. As the miRNAs profile regulates protein expression, it could also become a crucial tool for predicting efficient drug-target interaction. This effective drug-target interaction due to high protein target expression was favored by the low miRNAs expression profile that regulates the drug's protein target. On the other hand, there are few chances for drug interaction with the target due to the high miRNAs expression profile. Similar to miRNAs role in the prediction of drug-target interactions, it also plays an imperative role in the prediction of toxicant-target interaction and in describing individual susceptibility to toxicants (Lema and Cunningham, 2010).

3.8.2 Circulating miRNAs as toxicity biomarkers

Active secretion, cell death, or cellular injuries can result in the leakage of miRNAs in the biofluids. The dynamic existence of miRNAs in the biofluids appears in various cases for tracking cellular injury and identifying recovery of the cells or tissues. For example, the miRNAs profile can be altered by blood hemolysis, specifically in cases where target tissue-released miRNAs overlap with the erythrocyte-sourced miRNAs (Harrill et al., 2016).

Cell specificity is the primary advantage of miRNAs as biomarkers over conventional biomarkers. Various miRNAs can be transcribed only in specific cell types, and this specificity can be assessed using available database tools. Another potential feature of the miRNAs as a biomarker is the early detection or response to toxicant exposure. miRNA alterations can happen in nontoxic responses to detect the early response to external stimuli before other conventional biomarker changes. Therefore, miRNAs have the potential for risk assessment after slight exposure to external stimuli. Apoptosis or necrosis-like stress conditions shows cellular responses that lead to miRNA alterations followed by infection or toxicity. MiRNAs are sensitive indicators for any change as they can alter by acute and chronic exposure to external factors. Thus, they are an appropriate tool to act as biomarkers for drug-induced toxicity or tissue damage (Marrone et al., 2015; Vrijens et al., 2015).

Even though miRNAs are generally stable in the biofluids that support their use as a suitable biomarker. Still, many observations show the differential stability between circulating miRNAs and their release state. The half-life of miRNAs also plays a critical role in the biomarker potential, as half-life determines the reversal of miRNAs level to baseline and prediction of progression and resolution of any injury (Starkey Lewis et al., 2011b; Schofield et al., 2021). Despite the stability of miRNAs in serum or plasma, various studies demonstrate the degradation of miRNAs in serum after a solo freeze/thaw cycle daily for 10 days or by increasing the incubation at room temperature for 10 days. Another study shows the stability of human plasma miRNAs for 24 h at room temperature, but miRNAs in rat plasma are not constant at room temperature for 24 h (Oda and Yokoi, 2021).

Many challenges should be conquered first before using miRNAs as a regular biomarker. Extraction and pre-processing of the miRNAs are critical to evaluate the miRNAs profile by measuring their level. The chemical extraction method is used to isolate miRNAs from the sample, and commercial kits are used to purify isolated miRNAs. One extra step of verifying the retrieval of oligos spiked-in at extraction should be incorporated for plasma and serum samples with a meager yield of miRNAs. The quality of miRNA samples should be evaluated using a spectrophotometer after the extraction of miRNAs. A proper normalization strategy should be used to evaluate miRNAs (Becker et al., 2010).

Developing new techniques for miRNA detection that do not need specific equipment, training, and time becomes a thrust area of research. Conventional techniques of miRNA detection, such as qRT-PCR, are not suitable for early diagnosis on a large scale. Therefore, better miRNA expression profiling for diagnostic purposes requires the development of a more efficient technique (Ouyang et al., 2019).

Protein assays by commercial kits or automated analyzers are used to standardize the enzymatic assays. Still, variations occur in miRNA methods from researcher to researcher, starting from RNA isolation from the sample to the qRT-PCR and normalizing the data. Therefore, these analytical variations become limitations to comparing the data across independent studies and show the requirement of a consistent and standardized method of miRNAs measurement (Bailey and Glaab, 2018).

MiR-216a, 216b, and 217 are very efficient circulatory biomarkers for pancreatic injury. Various studies and clinical trials showed the importance of these blood-based biomarkers in the detection of pancreatic injury. MiR-375 was not expressed in rat pancreas but was highly expressed in humans. On the other hand, both miR-216a and miR-216b are expressed in human and rat pancreas precisely (Endo et al., 2013). A combination of atorvastatin and ciprofloxacin, gemfibrozil and lovastatin, and pioglitazone-induced skeletal muscle injury were observed by the increased plasma level miR-133b-3p and miR-206-3p (Akai et al., 2017; Watanabe et al., 2019).

Moderate photoreceptor cell death was experienced in rats after administering 50 mg/kg N-methyl-N-nitrosourea (MNU) on the second day. But early upregulation in serum miRNAs, such as a 37-fold increase in miR-183e5p, a 271-fold increase in miR-124e3p, and a 43-fold increase in miR-96e5p was observed after 6 h of administration as compared to time-matched vehicle-treated rats (Kakiuchi et al., 2019). MiR-144 showed promising results as a blood-based biomarker for oxidative stress after exposure to diesel exhaust in asthmatic patients. Antioxidant transcription factor (NRF2) gene expression in the lung was inversely associated with the miR-144 (Yamamoto et al., 2013).

Liver injury induced by acetaminophen was also identified by the elevated miR-122 and miR-192 plasma levels in patients (Starkey Lewis et al., 2011a). Treatment of a low dose of acetaminophen to human blood cells also showed upregulation of miR-19b and miR-29c, but the ALT level was unchanged (Jetten et al., 2012). Liver functions of the human exposed to paraquat were compared with the healthy subject by comparing the miR-122 serum levels. Paraquat-exposed humans showed elevated levels of miR-122 compared to healthy subjects (Ding et al., 2012).

3.9 Conclusion

MiRNAs perform as a potential biomarker for drug toxicity evaluation. Different biological processes are also influenced by the miRNAs, and alteration in the miRNAs profile directly tells about any defect in the biological process. Several methods are used for miRNA expression profiles. Every method has some limitations as compared to other methods. Simultaneously two methods can be used to thoroughly conquer these challenges and evaluate the miRNAs profile. Toxicity induced by different toxicants or contaminants alters the miRNAs profile. Variation in miRNA profile was also observed between normal and diseased groups. There are many advantages of miRNAs as an early biomarker for toxicity evaluation. Still, many challenges should be conquered before using miRNAs as a biomarker. Isolation or extraction of miRNAs from the samples is the first step for miRNA profiling which requires expertise and sufficient time. Although miRNAs are stable in biofluids, circulating miRNAs still show differential stability. In the future new methods should be explored that can reduce the requirements of expertise for isolation or helps in the easy isolation of miRNAs without any sophisticated instruments.

3.10 List of abbreviations

16HBE-T- transformed malignant human bronchial epithelial cells
2-AAF- 2-acetylaminofluorene
8-OH-Dg- 8-hydroxy-guanine
AAM- allylamine
AD- Atopic dermatitis
AgNPs- silver nanoparticles
Ago- Argonaute
AHR- aryl-hydrocarbon receptor
ALP- alkaline phosphatase
ALT- alanine aminotransferase
ANIT- Alpha-naphthylisothiocyanate
APAP- acetaminophen
ARVC- arrhythmic cardiomyopathy
As- arsenic
AST- aspartate aminotransferase
AuNPs- gold nanoparticles
Bcl2- B-cell lymphoma 2
BNP- brain natriuretic peptide
BPA- Bisphenol A
BPDE- Benzo[a]pyrene-7,8-diol-9,10-epoxide
BUN- blood urea nitrogen
CCA- corn oil plus cellulose
Cr- Chromium
CS- cigarette smoke
CSC- cigarette smoke condensate
cTn- cardiac troponins
DAU- Daunorubicin
DCM- Dilated cardiomyopathy
DEP- Diesel exhaust particles
DGCR8- DiGeorge Syndrome Critical Region 8
DILI- drug induced liver injury
DMBA- 7,12-dimethylbenz(α)anthracene

DOX- Doxorubicin
ER- Endoplasmic reticulum
FMT- Fructus Meliae Toosendan
FVXW7- F-box/WD repeat-containing protein 7
Gab2- Grb2 associated binding protein 2
HD- 2,5-hexanedione
Hg- mercury
ISO- isoproterenol
LVEF- left ventricular ejection fraction
MAPK- mitogen-activated protein kinase
MET- metaproterenol
MFN2- mitofusin-2
miRNA- microRNA
MIT- mitoxantrone
MNU- N-methyl-N-nitrosourea
mPFC- medial prefrontal cortex
MPTP- 1-methyl-4-phenyl-1,2,3,6-tetrahydropyridine
NFAT- nuclear factor of activated T cells
NGS- Next-Generation Sequencing
NNK- nitrosamine 4-(methylnitrosamino)-1-(3-pyridyl)-1-butanone
NSCs- neural stem cells
NSV- nonsegmental vitiligo
PAHs- polycyclic aromatic hydrocarbons
PBMCs- peripheral blood mononuclear cells
PKA- protein kinase A
PM- particulate matter
POPs- persistent organic pollutants
qRT-PCR- quantitative real time Polymerase Chain Reaction
Ran-GTPase- RAS-related nuclear protein-guanosine-5′-triphosphate-ase
RDX- hexahydro-1,3,5-trinitro-1,3,5-triazine
RISC- RNA-induced silencing complex
RPTC- rat proximal tubular cells
sncRNAs- small noncoding RNAs
SNP- single nucleotide polymorphism
SPIONs- superparamagnetic iron oxide nanoparticles
TGF- transforming growth factor
TRBP- TAR RNA binding protein
UTR- untranslated regions
ZEB1- zinc finger E-box-binding homeobox 1
ZEN- Mycotoxin zearalenone

References

Akai, S., Oda, S., Yokoi, T., 2017. Establishment of a novel mouse model for pioglitazone-induced skeletal muscle injury. Toxicology 382, 1–9.

Arya, M., Shergill, I.S., Williamson, M., Gommersall, L., Arya, N., Patel, H.R.H., 2005. Basic principles of real-time quantitative PCR. Expert Rev. Mol. Diagn. 5, 209–219.

Asikainen, S., Heikkinen, L., Louhiranta, K., Lakso, M., Wong, G., Nass, R., 2010. Global microRNA expression profiling of *Caenorhabditis elegans* Parkinson's disease models. J. Mol. Neurosci. 41, 210–218.

Avissar-Whiting, M., Veiga, K.R., Uhl, K.M., Maccani, M.A., Gagne, L.A., Moen, E.L., Marsit, C.J., 2010. Bisphenol A exposure leads to specific microRNA alterations in placental cells. Reprod. Toxicol. 29, 401–406.

Bahmad, H., Darwish, B., Dargham, K., Machmouchi, R., Dargham, B., Osman, M., Khechen, Z., Housheimi, N., Abou-Kheir, W., Chamaa, F., 2020. Role of MicroRNAs in anesthesia-induced neurotoxicity in animal models and neuronal cultures: a systematic review. Neurotox. Res. 37.

Bailey, W.J., Glaab, W.E., 2018. Accessible miRNAs as novel toxicity biomarkers. Int. J. Toxicol. 37, 116–120.

Baker, M., 2010. MicroRNA profiling: separating signal from noise. Nat. Methods 7, 687–692.

Ballesteros, S., Vales, G., Velázquez, A., Pastor, S., Alaraby, M., Marcos, R., Hernández, A., 2021. MicroRNAs as a suitable biomarker to detect the effects of long-term exposures to nanomaterials. Studies on TiO(2)NP and MWCNT. Nanomaterials 11, 3458.

Becker, C., Hammerle-Fickinger, A., Riedmaier, I., Pfaffl, M., 2010. mRNA and microRNA quality control for RT-qPCR analysis. Methods 50, 237–243.

Benes, V., Castoldi, M., 2010. Expression profiling of microRNA using real-time quantitative PCR, how to use it and what is available. Methods 50, 244–249.

Bollati, V., Angelici, L., Rizzo, G., Pergoli, L., Rota, F., Hoxha, M., Nordio, F., Bonzini, M., Tarantini, L., Cantone, L., Pesatori, A.C., Apostoli, P., Baccarelli, A.A., Bertazzi, P.A., 2015. Microvesicle-associated microRNA expression is altered upon particulate matter exposure in healthy workers and in A549 cells. J. Appl. Toxicol. 35, 59–67.

Bollati, V., Marinelli, B., Apostoli, P., Bonzini, M., Nordio, F., Hoxha, M., Pegoraro, V., Motta, V., Tarantini, L., Cantone, L., Schwartz, J., Bertazzi, P.A., Baccarelli, A., 2010. Exposure to metal-rich particulate matter modifies the expression of candidate microRNAs in peripheral blood leukocytes. Environ. Health Perspect. 118, 763–768.

Brandenburger, T., Lorenzen, J.M., 2020. Diagnostic and therapeutic potential of microRNAs in acute kidney injury. Front. Pharmacol. 11.

Brzóska, K., Gradzka, I., Kruszewski, M., 2019. Silver, gold, and iron oxide nanoparticles alter miRNA expression but do not affect DNA methylation in HepG2 cells. Materials 12, 1038.

Brzuzan, P., Woźny, M., Wolińska, L., Piasecka, A., Florczyk, M., Jakimiuk, E., Góra, M., Łuczyński, M., Gajecki, M., 2015. MicroRNA expression profiles in liver and colon of sexually immature gilts after exposure to Fusarium mycotoxins. Pol. J. Vet. Sci. 18, 29–38.

Calvano, J., Achanzar, W., Murphy, B., Dipiero, J., Hixson, C., Parrula, C., Burr, H., Mangipudy, R., Tirmenstein, M., 2016. Evaluation of microRNAs–208 and 133a/b as differential biomarkers of acute cardiac and skeletal muscle toxicity in rats. Toxicol. Appl. Pharmacol. 312, 53–60.

Calzetta, L., Orlandi, A., Page, C., Rogliani, P., Rinaldi, B., Rosano, G., Cazzola, M., Matera, M.G., 2016. Brain natriuretic peptide: much more than a biomarker. Int. J. Cardiol. 221, 1031–1038.

Chang, K.H., Mestdagh, P., Vandesompele, J., Kerin, M.J., Miller, N., 2010. MicroRNA expression profiling to identify and validate reference genes for relative quantification in colorectal cancer. BMC Cancer 10, 173.

Chen, C., Ridzon, D.A., Broomer, A.J., Zhou, Z., Lee, D.H., Nguyen, J.T., Barbisin, M., Xu, N.L., Mahuvakar, V.R., Andersen, M.R., 2005. Real-time quantification of microRNAs by stem–loop RT–PCR. Nucleic Acids Res. 33, e179.

Chen, J., Lozach, J., Garcia, E.W., Barnes, B., Luo, S., Mikoulitch, I., Zhou, L., Schroth, G., Fan, J.-B., 2008. Highly sensitive and specific microRNA expression profiling using BeadArray technology. Nucleic Acids Res. 36, e87.

Chen, Q.Y., Shen, S., Sun, H., Wu, F., Kluz, T., Kibriya, M.G., Chen, Y., Ahsan, H., Costa, M., 2020. PBMC gene expression profiles of female Bangladeshi adults chronically exposed to arsenic-contaminated drinking water. Environ. Pollut. 259, 113672.

Chen, W., Li, S., 2017. Circulating microRNA as a novel biomarker for pulmonary arterial hypertension due to congenital heart disease. Pediatr. Cardiol. 38.

Chen, X., Liu, M.-X., Cui, Q.-H., Yan, G.-Y., 2012. Prediction of disease-related interactions between MicroRNAs and environmental factors based on a semi-supervised classifier. PLoS One 7, e43425.

Church, R.J., Mcduffie, J.E., Sonee, M., Otieno, M., Ma, J.Y., Liu, X., Watkins, P.B., Harrill, A.H., 2014. MicroRNA-34c-3p is an early predictive biomarker for doxorubicin-induced glomerular injury progression in male Sprague-Dawley rats. Toxicol. Res. 3, 384–394.

Church, R.J., Otieno, M., Mcduffie, J.E., Singh, B., Sonee, M., Hall, L., Watkins, P.B., Ellinger Ziegelbauer, H., Harrill, A.H., 2015. Beyond miR-122: identification of MicroRNA alterations in blood during a time course of hepatobiliary injury and biliary hyperplasia in rats. Toxicol. Sci. 150, 3–14.

DE Felice, B., Manfellotto, F., Palumbo, A., Troisi, J., Zullo, F., DI Carlo, C., Sardo, A.D.S., DE Stefano, N., Ferbo, U., Guida, M., Guida, M., 2015. Genome–wide microRNA expression profiling in placentas from pregnant women exposed to BPA. BMC Med. Genom. 8, 56.

Deng, Q., Dai, X., Feng, W., Huang, S., Yuan, Y., Xiao, Y., Zhang, Z., Deng, N., Deng, H., Zhang, X., Kuang, D., Li, X., Zhang, W., Zhang, X., Guo, H., Wu, T., 2019. Co-exposure to metals and polycyclic aromatic hydrocarbons, microRNA expression, and early health damage in coke oven workers. Environ. Int. 122, 369–380.

Deng, Y., Ai, J., Guan, X., Wang, Z., Yan, B., Zhang, D., Liu, C., Wilbanks, M., Escalon, B., Meyer, S., Yang, M., Perkins, E., 2014. MicroRNA and messenger RNA profiling reveals new biomarkers and mechanisms for RDX induced neurotoxicity. BMC Genom. 15 (Suppl. 11), S1.

Desai, V.G., Kwekel, C., Vijay, V., Moland, C.L., Herman, E.H., Lee, T., Han, T., Lewis, S.M., Davis, K.J., Muskhelishvili, L., Kerr, S., Fuscoe, J.C., 2014. Early biomarkers of doxorubicin-induced heart injury in a mouse model. Toxicol. Appl. Pharmacol. 281, 221–229.

Ding, E., Zhao, Q., Bai, Y., Xu, M., Pan, L., Liu, Q., Wang, B., Song, X., Wang, J., Chen, L., Zhu, B., 2016. Plasma microRNAs expression profile in female workers occupationally exposed to mercury. J. Thorac. Dis. 8, 833–841.

Ding, X., Ding, J., Ning, J., Yi, F., Chen, J., Zhao, D., Zheng, J., Liang, Z., Hu, Z., Du, Q., 2012. Circulating microRNA-122 as a potential biomarker for liver injury. Mol. Med. Rep. 5, 1428–1432.

Dioni, L., Sucato, S., Motta, V., Iodice, S., Angelici, L., Favero, C., Cavalleri, T., Vigna, L., Albetti, B., Fustinoni, S., Bertazzi, P., Pesatori, A., Bollati, V., 2017. Urinary chromium is associated with changes in leukocyte miRNA expression in obese subjects. Eur. J. Clin. Nutr. 71, 142–148.

Doka, G., Malikova, E., Galková, K., LA Rocca, G., Kruzliak, P., Adamek, M., Rodrigo, L., Krenek, P., Klimas, J., 2017. Downregulation of myogenic microRNAs in sub-chronic but not in sub-acute model of daunorubicin-induced cardiomyopathy. Mol. Cell. Biochem. 432.

Doukas, S., Vageli, D., Lazopoulos, G., Spandidos, D., Sasaki, C., Tsatsakis, A., 2020. The effect of Nnk, A Tobacco smoke carcinogen, on the miRNA and Mismatch DNA repair expression profiles in lung and head and neck squamous cancer cells. Cells 9, 1031.

Endo, K., Weng, H., Kito, N., Fukushima, Y., Iwai, N., 2013. MiR-216a and miR-216b as markers for acute phased pancreatic injury. Biomed. Res. 34, 179–188.

Eriksen, A.H.M., Andersen, R.F., Pallisgaard, N., Sørensen, F.B., Jakobsen, A., Hansen, T.F., 2016. MicroRNA expression profiling to identify and validate reference genes for the relative quantification of microRNA in rectal cancer. PLoS One 11, e0150593.

Fay, M.J., Alt, L.A.C., Ryba, D., Salamah, R., Peach, R., Papaeliou, A., Zawadzka, S., Weiss, A., Patel, N., Rahman, A., Stubbs-Russell, Z., Lamar, P.C., Edwards, J.R., Prozialeck, W.C., 2018. Cadmium nephrotoxicity is associated with altered MicroRNA expression in the rat renal cortex. Toxics 6, 16.

Feng, L., Yang, X., Liang, S., Xu, Q., Miller, M.R., Duan, J., Sun, Z., 2019. Silica nanoparticles trigger the vascular endothelial dysfunction and prethrombotic state via miR-451 directly regulating the IL6R signaling pathway. Part. Fibre Toxicol. 16, 16.

Feng, Y., Chen, X., Ma, J., Zhang, B., Li, X., 2020. Aberrant expressional profiling of known MicroRNAs in the liver of silver carp (*Hypophthalmichthys molitrix*) following microcystin-LR exposure based on samllRNA sequencing. Toxins 12, 41.

Forero, D.A., González-Giraldo, Y., Castro-Vega, L.J., Barreto, G.E., 2019. qPCR-based methods for expression analysis of miRNAs. Biotechniques 67, 192–199.

Fukushima, T., Hamada, Y., Yamada, H., Horii, I., 2007. Changes of micro-RNA expression in rat liver treated by acetaminophen or carbon tetrachloride – regulating role of micro-RNA for RNA expression & minus. J. Toxicol. Sci. 32, 401–409.

Gaarz, A., Debey-Pascher, S., Classen, S., Eggle, D., Gathof, B., Chen, J., Fan, J.-B., Voss, T., Schultze, J.L., Staratschek-Jox, A., 2010. Bead array-based microRNA expression profiling of peripheral blood and the impact of different RNA isolation approaches. J. Mol. Diagn. 12, 335–344.

Gatzidou, E.T., Zira, A.N., Theocharis, S.E., 2007. Toxicogenomics: a pivotal piece in the puzzle of toxicological research. J. Appl. Toxicol. 27, 302–309.

Glineur, S.F., DE Ron, P., Hanon, E., Valentin, J.-P., Dremier, S., DA Costa, A.N., 2015. Paving the Route to plasma miR-208a-3p as an acute cardiac injury biomarker: preclinical rat data supports its use in drug safety assessment. Toxicol. Sci. 149, 89–97.

Gondaliya, P., Sayyed, A.A., Bhat, P., Mali, M., Arya, N., Khairnar, A., Kalia, K., 2022. Mesenchymal stem cell-derived exosomes loaded with miR-155 inhibitor ameliorate diabetic wound healing. Mol. Pharm. 19, 1294–1308.

González-Palomo, A.K., Saldaña-Villanueva, K., Cortés-García, J.D., Fernández-Macias, J.C., Méndez-Rodríguez, K.B., Pérez Maldonado, I.N., 2021. Effect of silver nanoparticles (AgNPs) exposure on microRNA expression and global DNA methylation in endothelial cells EA.hy926. Environ. Toxicol. Pharmacol. 81, 103543.

Gooch, J., King, C., Francis, C., Garcia, P., Bai, Y., 2017. Cyclosporine A alters expression of renal microRNAs: new insights into calcineurin inhibitor nephrotoxicity. PLoS One 12, e0175242.

Grenier, B., Hackl, M., Skalicky, S., Thamhesl, M., Moll, W.-D., Berrios, R., Schatzmayr, G., Nagl, V., 2019. MicroRNAs in porcine uterus and serum are affected by zearalenone and represent a new target for mycotoxin biomarker discovery. Sci. Rep. 9, 9408.

Ha, J., Park, C., Park, S., 2019. PMAMCA: prediction of microRNA-disease association utilizing a matrix completion approach. BMC Syst. Biol. 13, 33.

Hao, J., Lou, Q., Wei, Q., Mei, S., Li, L., Wu, G., Mi, Q.-S., Mei, C., Dong, Z., 2017. MicroRNA-375 is induced in cisplatin nephrotoxicity to repress hepatocyte nuclear factor 1-β. J. Biol. Chem. 292, 4571–4582.

Harrill, A.H., Mccullough, S.D., Wood, C.E., Kahle, J.J., Chorley, B.N., 2016. MicroRNA biomarkers of toxicity in biological matrices. Toxicol. Sci. 152, 264–272.

Holmgren, G., Synnergren, J., Andersson, C.X., Lindahl, A., Sartipy, P., 2016. MicroRNAs as potential biomarkers for doxorubicin-induced cardiotoxicity. Toxicol. Vitro 34, 26–34.

Hu, Y., Lan, W., Miller, D., 2017. Next-generation sequencing for MicroRNA expression profile. In: Huang, J., Borchert, G.M., Dou, D., Huan, J., Lan, W., Tan, M., Wu, B. (Eds.), Bioinformatics in MicroRNA Research. Springer New York, New York, NY.

Izzotti, A., Larghero, P., Longobardi, M., Cartiglia, C., Camoirano, A., Steele, V.E., DE Flora, S., 2011. Dose-responsiveness and persistence of microRNA expression alterations induced by cigarette smoke in mouse lung. Mutat. Res. Fund Mol. Mech. Mutagen 717, 9–16.

Izzotti, A., Pulliero, A., 2014. The effects of environmental chemical carcinogens on the microRNA machinery. Int. J. Hyg. Environ. Health 217, 601–627.

Jardim Melanie, J., Fry Rebecca, C., Jaspers, I., Dailey, L., Diaz-Sanchez, D., 2009. Disruption of microRNA expression in human airway cells by diesel exhaust particles is linked to tumorigenesis-associated pathways. Environ. Health Perspect. 117, 1745–1751.

Jetten, M., Gaj, S., Ruiz Aracama, A., DE Kok, T., Delft, J., Lommen, A., VAN Someren, E., Jennen, D., Claessen, S., Peijnenburg, A., Stierum, R., Kleinjans, J., 2012. 'Omics analysis of low dose acetaminophen intake demonstrates novel response pathways in humans. Toxicol. Appl. Pharmacol. 259, 320–328.

Jiang, W., Chen, X., Liao, M., Li, W., Lian, B., Wang, L., Meng, F., Liu, X., Chen, X., Jin, Y., Li, X., 2012. Identification of links between small molecules and miRNAs in human cancers based on transcriptional responses. Sci. Rep. 2, 282.

Juhász, K., Gombos, K., Szirmai, M., Gőcze, K., Wolher, V., Révész, P., Magda, I., Sebestyén, A., Németh, Á., Ember, I., 2013. Very early effect of DMBA and MNU on MicroRNA expression. In Vivo 27, 113–117.

Junn, E., Lee, K.-W., Jeong, B.S., Chan, T.W., Im, J.-Y., Mouradian, M.M., 2009. Repression of alpha-synuclein expression and toxicity by microRNA-7. Proc. Natl. Acad. Sci. U. S. A. 106, 13052–13057.

Kakiuchi, D., Taketa, Y., Ohta, E., Fujikawa, Y., Nakano-Ito, K., Asakura, S., Hosokawa, S., 2019. Combination of circulating microRNAs as indicators of specific targets of retinal toxicity in rats. Toxicology 411, 163–171.

Kalayinia, S., Arjmand, F., Maleki, M., Malakootian, M., Singh, C.P., 2021. MicroRNAs: roles in cardiovascular development and disease. Cardiovasc. Pathol. 50, 107296.

Khan, S., Ayub, H., Khan, T., Wahid, F., 2019. MicroRNA biogenesis, gene silencing mechanisms and role in breast, ovarian and prostate cancer. Biochimie 167, 12–24.

Koturbash, I., Tolleson, W.H., Guo, L., Yu, D., Chen, S., Hong, H., Mattes, W., Ning, B., 2015. MicroRNAs as pharmacogenomic biomarkers for drug efficacy and drug safety assessment. Biomarkers Med. 9, 1153–1176.

Krauskopf, J., DE Kok, T.M., Hebels, D.G., Bergdahl, I.A., Johansson, A., Spaeth, F., Kiviranta, H., Rantakokko, P., Kyrtopoulos, S.A., Kleinjans, J.C., 2017. MicroRNA profile for health risk assessment: environmental exposure to persistent organic pollutants strongly affects the human blood microRNA machinery. Sci. Rep. 7, 9262.

Krauskopf, J., Van Veldhoven, K., Chadeau-Hyam, M., Vermeulen, R., Carrasco-Turigas, G., Nieuwenhuijsen, M., Vineis, P., DE Kok, T.M., Kleinjans, J.C., 2019. Short-term exposure to traffic-related air pollution reveals a compound-specific circulating miRNA profile indicating multiple disease risks. Environ. Int. 128, 193–200.

Lema, C., Cunningham, M.J., 2010. MicroRNAs and their implications in toxicological research. Toxicol. Lett. 198, 100–105.

Li, L.-M., Wang, D., Zen, K., 2014. MicroRNAs in drug-induced liver injury. J. Clin. Transl. Hepatol. 2, 162–169.

Li, L., 2020. The role of MicroRNAs in vitiligo: regulators and therapeutic targets. Ann. Dermatol. 32, 441.

Li, Q., Kappil, M.A., Li, A., Dassanayake, P.S., Darrah, T.H., Friedman, A.E., Friedman, M., Lambertini, L., Landrigan, P., Stodgell, C.J., Xia, Y., Nanes, J.A., Aagaard, K.M., Schadt, E.E., Murray, J.C., Clark, E.B., Dole, N., Culhane, J., Swanson, J., Varner, M., Moye, J., Kasten, C., Miller, R.K., Chen, J., 2015. Exploring the associations between microRNA expression profiles and environmental pollutants in human placenta from the National Children's Study (NCS). Epigenetics 10, 793–802.

Liang, R.-Q., Li, W., Li, Y., Tan, C.-Y., Li, J.-X., Jin, Y.-X., Ruan, K.-C., 2005. An oligonucleotide microarray for microRNA expression analysis based on labeling RNA with quantum dot and nanogold probe. Nucleic Acids Res. 33, e17.

Lin, D., Liu, J., Hu, Z., Cottrell, J., Kass, I., 2018. Neonatal anesthesia exposure impacts brain microRNAs and their associated neurodevelopmental processes. Sci. Rep. 8.

Lin, H., Ewing, L., Koturbash, I., Gurley, B., Miousse, I., 2017. MicroRNAs as biomarkers for liver injury: current knowledge, challenges and future prospects. Food Chem. Toxicol. 110.

Lipshultz, S.E., Miller, T.L., Scully, R.E., Lipsitz, S.R., Rifai, N., Silverman, L.B., Colan, S.D., Neuberg, D.S., Dahlberg, S.E., Henkel, J.M., Asselin, B.L., Athale, U.H., Clavell, L.A., Laverdière, C., Michon, B., Schorin, M.A., Sallan, S.E., 2012. Changes in cardiac biomarkers during doxorubicin treatment of pediatric patients with high-risk acute lymphoblastic leukemia: associations with long-term echocardiographic outcomes. J. Clin. Oncol. 30, 1042–1049.

Liu, C.-G., Calin, G.A., Volinia, S., Croce, C.M., 2008. MicroRNA expression profiling using microarrays. Nat. Protoc. 3, 563–578.

Liu, J., Huang, Y., Cai, F., Dang, Y., Liu, C., Wang, J., 2020. MicroRNA-181a regulates endoplasmic reticulum stress in offspring of mice following prenatal microcystin-LR exposure. Chemosphere 240, 124905.

Liu, P., 2018. MicroRNA expression analysis: next-generation sequencing. In: Raghavachari, N., Garcia-Reyero, N. (Eds.), Gene Expression Analysis: Methods and Protocols. Springer New York, New York, NY.

Liu, Y.-R., Laghari, Z., Novoa, C., Hughes, J., Webster, J., Goodwin, P.E., Wheatley, S., Scotting, P., 2014. Sox2 acts as a transcriptional repressor in neural stem cells. BMC Biol. 15.

Lu, J., Getz, G., Miska, E.A., Alvarez-Saavedra, E., Lamb, J., Peck, D., Sweet-Cordero, A., Ebert, B.L., Mak, R.H., Ferrando, A.A., Downing, J.R., Jacks, T., Horvitz, H.R., Golub, T.R., 2005. MicroRNA expression profiles classify human cancers. Nature 435, 834–838.

Lu, M., Zhang, Q., Deng, M., Miao, J., Guo, Y., Gao, W., Cui, Q., 2008. An analysis of human MicroRNA and disease associations. PLoS One 3, e3420.

Luo, H., Lan, W., Chen, Q., Wang, Z., Liu, Z., Yue, X., Zhu, L., 2018. Inferring microRNA-environmental factor interactions based on multiple biological information fusion. Molecules 23, 2439.

Ma, J., Chen, X., Xin, G., Li, X., 2019. Chronic exposure to the ionic liquid [C8mim]Br induces inflammation in silver carp spleen: involvement of oxidative stress-mediated p38MAPK/NF-κB signalling and microRNAs. Fish Shellfish Immunol. 84, 627–638.

Maccani, M.A., Marsit, C.J., 2011. Exposure and fetal growth-associated miRNA alterations in the human placenta. Clin. Epigenet. 2, 401–404.

Mancini, F.R., Laine, J.E., Tarallo, S., Vlaanderen, J., Vermeulen, R., Van Nunen, E., Hoek, G., Probst-Hensch, N., Imboden, M., Jeong, A., Gulliver, J., Chadeau-Hyam, M., Nieuwenhuijsen, M., DE Kok, T.M., Piepers, J., Krauskopf, J., Kleinjans, J.C.S., Vineis, P., Naccarati, A., 2020. microRNA expression profiles and personal monitoring of exposure to particulate matter. Environ. Pollut. 263, 114392.

Mannucci, C., Casciaro, M., Minciullo, P., Calapai, G., Navarra, M., Gangemi, S., 2017. Involvement of microRNAs in skin disorders: a literature review. Allergy Asthma Proc. 38, 9–15.

Marrone, A.K., Beland, F.A., Pogribny, I.P., 2015. The role for microRNAs in drug toxicity and in safety assessment. Expert Opin. Drug Metabol. Toxicol. 11, 601–611.

Menghao, C., 2018. Cadmium induces BNIP3-dependent autophagy in chicken spleen by modulating miR-33-AMPK axis. Chemosphere 194, 396–402, 2018 v.194.

Michailidi, C., Hayashi, M., Datta, S., Sen, T., Zenner, K., Oladeru, O., Brait, M., Izumchenko, E., Baras, A., Vandenbussche, C., Argos, M., Bivalacqua, T.J., Ahsan, H., Hahn, N.M., Netto, G.J., Sidransky, D., Hoque, M.O., 2015. Involvement of epigenetics and EMT-related miRNA in arsenic-induced neoplastic transformation and their potential clinical use. Cancer Prev. Res. 8, 208–221.

Naga Prasad, S.V., Karnik, S.S., 2010. MicroRNA regulators of signaling networks in dilated cardiomyopathy. J. Cardiovasc. Transl. Res. 3, 225–234.

Niemoeller, O.M., Niyazi, M., Corradini, S., Zehentmayr, F., Li, M., Lauber, K., Belka, C., 2011. MicroRNA expression profiles in human cancer cells after ionizing radiation. Radiat. Oncol. 6, 29.

O'brien, J., Hayder, H., Zayed, Y., Peng, C., 2018. Overview of microRNA biogenesis, mechanisms of actions, and circulation. Front. Endocrinol. 9, 402.

Oda, S., Yokoi, T., 2021. Recent progress in the use of microRNAs as biomarkers for drug-induced toxicities in contrast to traditional biomarkers: a comparative review. Drug Metabol. Pharmacokinet. 37, 100372.

Othman, M.S., Hafez, M.M., Abdel Moneim, A.E., 2020. The potential role of zinc oxide nanoparticles in microRNAs dysregulation in STZ-induced type 2 diabetes in rats. Biol. Trace Elem. Res. 197, 606–618.

Ouyang, T., Liu, Z., Han, Z., Ge, Q., 2019. MicroRNA detection specificity: recent advances and future perspective. Anal. Chem. 91, 3179–3186.

Pan, X., Murashov, A.K., Stellwag, E.J., Zhang, B., 2017. Using quantitative real-time PCR to detect microRNA expression profile during embryonic stem cell differentiation. In: Zhang, B. (Ed.), RNAi and Small Regulatory RNAs in Stem Cells: Methods and Protocols. Springer New York, New York, NY.

Peltier, H.J., Latham, G.J., 2008. Normalization of microRNA expression levels in quantitative RT-PCR assays: identification of suitable reference RNA targets in normal and cancerous human solid tissues. RNA (New York, N.Y.) 14, 844–852.

Pergoli, L., Cantone, L., Favero, C., Angelici, L., Iodice, S., Pinatel, E., Hoxha, M., Dioni, L., Letizia, M., Albetti, B., Tarantini, L., Rota, F., Bertazzi, P.A., Tirelli, A.S., Dolo, V., Cattaneo, A., Vigna, L., Battaglia, C., Carugno, M., Bonzini, M., Pesatori, A.C., Bollati, V., 2017. Extracellular vesicle-packaged miRNA release after short-term exposure to particulate matter is associated with increased coagulation. Part. Fibre Toxicol. 14, 32.

Piao, F., Chen, Y., Yu, L., Shi, X., Liu, X., Jiang, L., Yang, G., Wang, N., Gao, B., Zhang, C., 2020. 2,5-hexanedione-induced deregulation of axon-related microRNA expression in rat nerve tissues. Toxicol. Lett. 320, 95–102.

Pillar, N., Haguel, D., Grad, M., Shapira, G., Yoffe, L., Shomron, N., 2019. Characterization of microRNA and gene expression profiles following Ricin intoxication. Toxins 11, 250.

Pogribny, I., Tryndyak, V., Boyko, A., Rodriguez-Juarez, R., Beland, F., Kovalchuk, O., 2007. Induction of microRNAome deregulation in rat liver by long-term tamoxifen exposure. Mutat. Res. 619, 30–37.

Pogribny, I.P., Muskhelishvili, L., Tryndyak, V.P., Beland, F.A., 2011. The role of epigenetic events in genotoxic hepatocarcinogenesis induced by 2-acetylaminofluorene. Mutat. Res. Genet. Toxicol. Environ. Mutagen 722, 106–113.

Qiu, C., Chen, G., Cui, Q., 2012. Towards the understanding of microRNA and environmental factor interactions and their relationships to human diseases. Sci. Rep. 2, 318.

Qu, M., Luo, L., Yang, Y., Kong, Y., Wang, D., 2019. Nanopolystyrene-induced microRNAs response in *Caenorhabditis elegans* after long-term and lose-dose exposure. Sci. Total Environ. 697, 134131.

Quintanilha, J.C.F., Cursino, M.A., Borges, J.B., Torso, N.G., Bastos, L.B., Oliveira, J.M., Cobaxo, T.S., Pincinato, E.C., Hirata, M.H., Geraldo, M.V., Lima, C.S.P., Moriel, P., 2021. MiR-3168, miR-6125, and miR-4718 as potential predictors of cisplatin-induced nephrotoxicity in patients with head and neck cancer. BMC Cancer 21, 575.

Reamon-Buettner, S.M., Mutschler, V., Borlak, J., 2008. The next innovation cycle in toxicogenomics: environmental epigenetics. Mutat. Res. Rev. Mutat. Res. 659, 158–165.

Rigaud, V., Fernandes-Silva, M., Guimaraes, G., Bacal, F., Bocchi, E., 2012. MicroRNAs: new players in heart failure. Mol. Biol. Rep. 40.

Roden, C., Mastriano, S., Wang, N., Lu, J., 2015. microRNA expression profiling: technologies, insights, and prospects. In: Santulli, G. (Ed.), MicroRNA: Medical Evidence: From Molecular Biology to Clinical Practice. Springer International Publishing, Cham.

Rodosthenous, R.S., Coull, B.A., Lu, Q., Vokonas, P.S., Schwartz, J.D., Baccarelli, A.A., 2016. Ambient particulate matter and microRNAs in extracellular vesicles: a pilot study of older individuals. Part. Fibre Toxicol. 13, 13.

Ruggeri, C., Gioffré, S., Achilli, F., Colombo, G., D'alessandra, Y., 2018. Role of microRNAs in doxorubicin-induced cardiotoxicity: an overview of preclinical models and cancer patients. Heart Fail. Rev. 23, 1–14.

Saito, K., Kondo, E., Matsushita, M., 2011. MicroRNA 130 family regulates the hypoxia response signal through the P-body protein DDX6. Nucleic Acids Res. 39, 6086–6099.

Sanders, A.P., Burris, H.H., Just, A.C., Motta, V., Amarasiriwardena, C., Svensson, K., Oken, E., Solano-Gonzalez, M., Mercado-Garcia, A., Pantic, I., Schwartz, J., Tellez-Rojo, M.M., Baccarelli, A.A., Wright, R.O., 2015. Altered miRNA expression in the cervix during pregnancy associated with lead and mercury exposure. Epigenomics 7, 885–896.

Sathyan, P., Golden, H.B., Miranda, R.C., 2007. Competing interactions between micro-RNAs determine neural progenitor survival and proliferation after ethanol exposure: evidence from an ex vivo model of the fetal cerebral cortical neuroepithelium. J. Neurosci. 27, 8546–8557.

Sayyed, A.A., Gondaliya, P., Bhat, P., Mali, M., Arya, N., Khairnar, A., Kalia, K., 2022. Role of miRNAs in cancer diagnostics and therapy: a recent update. Curr. Pharmaceut. Des. 28, 471–487.

Sayyed, A.A., Gondaliya, P., Mali, M., Pawar, A., Bhat, P., Khairnar, A., Arya, N., Kalia, K., 2021. MiR-155 inhibitor-laden exosomes reverse resistance to cisplatin in a 3D tumor spheroid and xenograft model of oral cancer. Mol. Pharm. 18, 3010–3025.

Scarano, W.R., Bedrat, A., Alonso-Costa, L.G., Aquino, A.M., Fantinatti, B.E.A., Justulin, L.A., Barbisan, L.F., Freire, P.P., Flaws, J.A., Lemos, B., 2019. Exposure to an environmentally relevant phthalate mixture during prostate development induces microRNA upregulation and transcriptome modulation in rats. Toxicol. Sci. 171, 84–97.

Schembri, F., Sridhar, S., Perdomo, C., Gustafson, A.M., Zhang, X., Ergun, A., Lu, J., Liu, G., Zhang, X., Bowers, J., Vaziri, C., Ott, K., Sensinger, K., Collins, J.J., Brody, J.S., Getts, R., Lenburg, M.E., Spira, A., 2009. MicroRNAs as modulators of smoking-induced gene expression changes in human airway epithelium. Proc. Natl. Acad. Sci. U. S. A. 106, 2319–2324.

Schmittgen, T.D., Jiang, J., Liu, Q., Yang, L., 2004. A high-throughput method to monitor the expression of microRNA precursors. Nucleic Acids Res. 32, e43.

Schofield, A.L., Brown, J.P., Brown, J., Wilczynska, A., Bell, C., Glaab, W.E., Hackl, M., Howell, L., Lee, S., Dear, J.W., 2021. Systems analysis of miRNA biomarkers to inform drug safety. Arch. Toxicol. 95, 3475–3495.

Shah, M.S., Kim, E., Davidson, L.A., Knight, J.M., Zoh, R.S., Goldsby, J.S., Callaway, E.S., Zhou, B., Ivanov, I., Chapkin, R.S., 2016. Comparative effects of diet and carcinogen on microRNA expression in the stem cell niche of the mouse colonic crypt. Biochim. Biophys. Acta 1862, 121–134.

Shao, C.-Z., Xia, K.-P., 2019. Sevoflurane anesthesia represses neurogenesis of hippocampus neural stem cells via regulating microRNA-183-mediated NR4A2 in newborn rats. J. Cell. Physiol. 234, 3864–3873.

Shendure, J., Ji, H., 2008. Next-generation DNA sequencing. Nat. Biotechnol. 26, 1135–1145.

Shimpi, P.C., More, V.R., Paranjpe, M., Donepudi, A.C., Goodrich, J.M., Dolinoy, D.C., Rubin, B., Slitt, A.L., 2017. Hepatic lipid accumulation and Nrf2 expression following perinatal and peripubertal exposure to Bisphenol A in a mouse model of nonalcoholic liver disease. Environ. Health Perspect. 125, 087005.

Shin, S., Cha, H.J., Lee, E.-M., Lee, S.-J., Seo, S.-K., Jin, H.-O., Park, I.-C., Jin, Y.-W., An, S., 2009. Alteration of miRNA profiles by ionizing radiation in A549 human non-small cell lung cancer cells. Int. J. Oncol. 35, 81–86.

Siegrist, F., Singer, T., Certa, U., 2009. MicroRNA expression profiling by bead array technology in human tumor cell lines treated with interferon-alpha-2a. Biol. Proced. Online 11, 113.

Skála, M., Hanousková, B., Skálová, L., Matouskova, P., 2019. MicroRNAs in the diagnosis and prevention of drug-induced cardiotoxicity. Arch. Toxicol. 93.

Slotta-Huspenina, J., Drecoll, E., Feith, M., Habermehl, D., Combs, S., Weichert, W., Bettstetter, M., Becker, K., Langer, R., 2018. MicroRNA expression profiling for the prediction of resistance to neoadjuvant radiochemotherapy in squamous cell carcinoma of the esophagus. J. Transl. Med. 16, 109.

Starckx, S., Batheja, A., Verheyen, G.R., Jonghe, S.D., Steemans, K., Dijck, B.V., Singer, M., Bogdan, N., Snoeys, J., Vinken, P., 2013. Evaluation of miR-122 and other biomarkers in distinct acute liver injury in rats. Toxicol. Pathol. 41, 795–804.

Starkey Lewis, P., Dear, J., Platt, V., Simpson, K., Craig, D., Antoine, D., French, N., Dhaun, N., Webb, D., Costello, E., Neoptolemos, J., Moggs, J., Goldring, C., Park, B., 2011a. Circulating microRNAs as potential markers of human drug-induced liver injury. Hepatology 54, 1767–1776.

Starkey Lewis, P.J., Dear, J., Platt, V., Simpson, K.J., Craig, D.G., Antoine, D.J., French, N.S., Dhaun, N., Webb, D.J., Costello, E.M., 2011b. Circulating microRNAs as potential markers of human drug-induced liver injury. Hepatology 54, 1767–1776.

Sun, B., Liu, R., Ye, N., Xiao, Z.-D., 2015. Comprehensive evaluation of microRNA expression profiling reveals the neural signaling specific cytotoxicity of superparamagnetic iron oxide nanoparticles (SPIONs) through N-Methyl-D-Aspartate receptor. PLoS One 10, e0121671.

Tapocik, J.D., Solomon, M., Flanigan, M., Meinhardt, M., Barbier, E., Schank, J.R., Schwandt, M., Sommer, W.H., Heilig, M., 2013. Coordinated dysregulation of mRNAs and microRNAs in the rat medial prefrontal cortex following a history of alcohol dependence. Pharmacogenomics J. 13, 286–296.

Tsamou, M., Vrijens, K., Madhloum, N., Lefebvre, W., Vanpoucke, C., Nawrot, T.S., 2018. Air pollution-induced placental epigenetic alterations in early life: a candidate miRNA approach. Epigenetics 13, 135–146.

Tumolo, M.R., Panico, A., DE Donno, A., Mincarone, P., Leo, C.G., Guarino, R., Bagordo, F., Serio, F., Idolo, A., Grassi, T., Sabina, S., 2022. The expression of microRNAs and exposure to environmental contaminants related to human health: a review. Int. J. Environ. Health Res. 32, 332–354.

Vrijens, K., Bollati, V., Nawrot, T.S., 2015. MicroRNAs as potential signatures of environmental exposure or effect: a systematic review. Environ. Health Perspect. 123, 399–411.

Wallace, D.R., Taalab, Y.M., Heinze, S., Tariba Lovaković, B., Pizent, A., Renieri, E., Tsatsakis, A., Farooqi, A.A., Javorac, D., Andjelkovic, M., Bulat, Z., Antonijević, B., Buha Djordjevic, A., 2020. Toxic-metal-induced alteration in miRNA expression profile as a proposed mechanism for disease development. Cells 9, 901.

Wang, J., Cui, Q., 2012. Specific roles of MicroRNAs in their interactions with environmental factors. J. Nucleic Acids 978384.

Wang, L., Qin, D., Shi, H., Zhang, Y., Li, H., Han, Q., 2019. MiR-195-5p promotes cardiomyocyte hypertrophy by targeting MFN2 and FBXW7. BioMed Res. Int. 2019, 1580982.

Wang, L., Zheng, M., Wu, S., Niu, Z., 2018. MicroRNA-188-3p is involved in sevoflurane anesthesia-induced neuroapoptosis by targeting MDM2. Mol. Med. Rep. 17.

Ward, J., Bala, S., Petrasek, J., Szabo, G., 2012. Plasma microRNA profiles distinguish lethal injury in acetaminophen toxicity: a research study. World J. Gastroenterol. 18, 2798–2804.

Ward, J., Kanchagar, C., Veksler-Lublinsky, I., Lee, R.C., Mcgill, M.R., Jaeschke, H., Curry, S.C., Ambros, V.R., 2014. Circulating microRNA profiles in human patients with acetaminophen hepatotoxicity or ischemic hepatitis. Proc. Natl. Acad. Sci. U. S. A. 111, 12169–12174.

Watanabe, K., Oda, S., Matsubara, A., Akai, S., Yokoi, T., 2019. Establishment and characterization of a mouse model of rhabdomyolysis by coadministration of statin and fibrate. Toxicol. Lett. 307, 49–58.

Wei, Y., Nazari-Jahantigh, M., Neth, P., Weber, C., Schober, A., 2013. MicroRNA-126, -145, and -155. Arterioscler. Thromb. Vasc. Biol. 33, 449–454.

Wilmink, G.J., Roth, C.L., Ibey, B.L., Ketchum, N., Bernhard, J., Cerna, C.Z., Roach, W.P., 2010. Identification of microRNAs associated with hyperthermia-induced cellular stress response. Cell Stress Chaperones 15, 1027–1038.

Xi, S., Yang, M., Tao, Y., Xu, H., Shan, J., Inchauste, S., Zhang, M., Mercedes, L., Hong, J.A., Rao, M., Schrump, D.S., 2010. Cigarette smoke induces C/EBP-β-mediated activation of miR-31 in normal human respiratory epithelia and lung cancer cells. PLoS One 5, e13764.

Xu, C., Niu, J.-J., Zhou, J.-F., Wei, Y.-S., 2018. MicroRNA-96 is responsible for sevoflurane-induced cognitive dysfunction in neonatal rats via inhibiting IGF1R. Brain Res. Bull. 144.

Yamamoto, M., Singh, A., Sava, F., Pui, M., Tebbutt, S.J., Carlsten, C., 2013. MicroRNA expression in response to controlled exposure to diesel exhaust: attenuation by the antioxidant N-acetylcysteine in a randomized crossover study. Environ. Health Perspect. 121, 670–675.

Yang, F., Li, L., Yang, R., Wei, M., Sheng, Y., Ji, L., 2019. Identification of serum microRNAs as potential toxicological biomarkers for toosendanin-induced liver injury in mice. Phytomedicine 58, 152867.

Yang, M., Mattes, J., 2008. Discovery, biology and therapeutic potential of RNA interference, microRNA and antagomirs. Pharmacol. Therapeut. 117, 94–104.

Yang, S., Chen, L., Wen, C., Zhang, X., Feng, X., Yang, F., 2018. MicroRNA expression profiling involved in MC-LR-induced hepatotoxicity using high-throughput sequencing analysis. J. Toxicol. Environ. Health Part A 81, 89–97.

Yao, S., 2016. MicroRNA biogenesis and their functions in regulating stem cell potency and differentiation. Biol. Proced. Online 18, 8.

Yu, L., Zheng, J., Li, J., Wang, Y., Lu, X., Fan, X., 2020. Integrating serum exosomal microRNA and liver microRNA profiles disclose the function role of autophagy and mechanisms of Fructus Meliae Toosendan-induced hepatotoxicity in mice. Biomed. Pharmacother. 123, 109709.

Zhang, Y., Jia, Y., Zheng, R., Guo, Y., Wang, Y., Guo, H., Fei, M., Sun, S., 2010. Plasma microRNA-122 as a biomarker for viral-, alcohol-, and chemical-related hepatic diseases. Clin. Chem. 56, 1830–1838.

Zhao, Y., Liu, H., Li, Y., Wu, J., Greenlee, A.R., Yang, C., Jiang, Y., 2011. The role of miR-506 in transformed 16HBE cells induced by anti-benzo[a]pyrene-trans-7,8-dihydrodiol-9,10-epoxide. Toxicol. Lett. 205, 320–326.

Zhou, X., Mao, A., Wang, X., Duan, X., Yao, Y., Zhang, C., 2013. Urine and serum microRNA-1 as novel biomarkers for myocardial injury in open-heart surgeries with cardiopulmonary bypass. PLoS One 8, e62245.

Zou, Q., Li, J., Hong, Q., Lin, Z., Wu, Y., Shi, H., Ju, Y., 2015. Prediction of microRNA-disease associations based on social network analysis methods. BioMed Res. Int. 2015, 810514.

CHAPTER

4

Exosomes as mediators of chemical-induced toxicity

Suryanarayana Polaka[1], *Muktika Tekade*[2], *Nupur Vasdev*[1], *Tanisha Gupta*[1], *Bhakti Pawar*[1], *Maliheh Safavi*[3] *and Rakesh Kumar Tekade*[1]

[1]National Institute of Pharmaceutical Education and Research (NIPER)- Ahmedabad, An Institute of National Importance, Government of India, Department of Pharmaceuticals, Ministry of Chemicals and Fertilizers, Palaj, Gandhinagar, Gujarat, India; [2]School of Pharmacy, Devi Ahilya Vishwavidyalaya, Indore, Madhya Pradesh, India; [3]Department of Biotechnology, Iranian Research Organization for Science and Technology, Tehran, Iran

4.1 Introduction

Intracellular and intercellular communication are essential for regulating the tissue's biological functions. Cells communicate with each other through various stimuli, including genetic and environmental. This stimulus helps in passing information from one cell to another cell in the form of signaling molecules and transcription factors. It is widely accepted that the signals passing from one cell to another are through cytokines, neurotransmitters, hormones, and growth factors via their specific receptor expression on the receptor cell surface. However, recent research has demonstrated a novel intercellular communication mechanism via extracellular vesicles (EVs) (Bang and Thum, 2012). EVs play a vital part in cell-to-cell contact, thereby expressing their consequences both locally and on multiple distant organs (Guay and Regazzi, 2017). EVs have attained a substantial reputation in various disease progression and targeting certain diseases therapeutically. EVs are classified into three major classes: apoptotic bodies, macro-vesicles, and exosomes. Apoptotic bodies are the largest EVs, containing a size range from 500 to 4000 nm, which are released especially during apoptosis of the cells through plasma membrane outward budding (Revenfeld et al., 2014). Macrovesicles are small in size (50–1000 nm) compared to the apoptotic bodies but larger than exosomes (50–150 nm). A budding process in the endo-lysosomal pathway causes the release of macrovesicles from the plasma membrane (Samanta et al., 2018).

Essentials of Pharmatoxicology in Drug Research, Volume 1
https://doi.org/10.1016/B978-0-443-15840-7.00007-5

To date, the research focus on exosomes has been explored majorly in cancer, immunology, and biomarker identification. Exosomes have been studied extensively for their role in immune system modulation, tumor progression, metastatic tumor development, and as an alternative therapeutic delivery system (Théry et al., 2009). Exosomes can also produce a toxic response as they are involved in intercellular communication. However, the toxicological aspects of exosomes are not explicitly mentioned in the publications, and the research on exosome-mediated toxicity is still in its infancy stage. This chapter emphasizes the discussion on exosome biogenesis, composition, and biological functions. Furthermore, we also enlisted the impact of chemical toxins on the exosome composition and disease progression. It also provides brief insights into the importance of exosomes in toxicology and the future direction of exosome research.

4.2 Generation and composition of exosomes

4.2.1 Generation of exosomes

Cells produce different compositions of extracellular vesicles under normal and stress conditions. Recent research shows that under pathological conditions, the synthesis and composition of exosomes alter due to various signaling mechanisms. The release of the exosomes from the plasma membrane occurs through the fusion of the multivesicular bodies (MVBs) (Booth et al., 2006). Essentially, exosomes are produced from the late endosomes. Intraluminal vesicles (ILVs) are produced from the invagination of the late endosomes inside the MVBs (Minciacchi et al., 2015). During the process of invagination, some proteins and cytosolic components are incorporated into the ILVs. The released ILVs in the extracellular space are called exosomes (Sahu et al., 2011; Record, 2014). On the other hand, these ILVs undergo degradation by lysosomes (Fig. 4.1). Canonical exosomes contain biconcave shapes when synthesized by artificial methods and during drying. However, the shape of the exosomes appears as spheroids in solution under the transmission electron microscope (TEM) (Yellon and Davidson, 2014). The typical characteristics for exosomes like density are approximately 1.13–1.19 g/mL upon sucrose gradient isolation (Zakharova et al., 2007; Bobrie et al., 2011).

ILVs formation requires ESCRT complex (ESCRT 0 to III). These proteins work collectively to fasten the MVBs formation, protein cargo sorting, and vesicle budding process (Hurley, 2015). The ESCRT pathway begins with protein identification and then involves the ubiquitin subunit of ESCRT-0 in protein sequestration to the exact location on the endosomes. Then the ESCRT-0 interacts with the ESCRT-I and II to form a complex, and finally, the resultant complex will associate with the ESCRT-III. This ESCRT complex helps the budding process. During the breakage of the buds to generate ILVs from MVBs, the ESCRT-III dissociates from the MVBs with the help of the sorting protein Vsp4 (Henne et al., 2011). Despite the fact that the arguments regarding the involvement of the ESCRT complex in the biogenesis of the exosomes, ESCRT complex components and some specific proteins were determined in the exosomes isolated from different cell types (Villarroya-Beltri et al., 2014). These observations provide strong evidence of ESCRT's involvement in the exosome's biogenesis. However, there are other possible mechanisms involved in the biogenesis of the exosomes, like non-ESCRT-dependent exosome biogenesis.

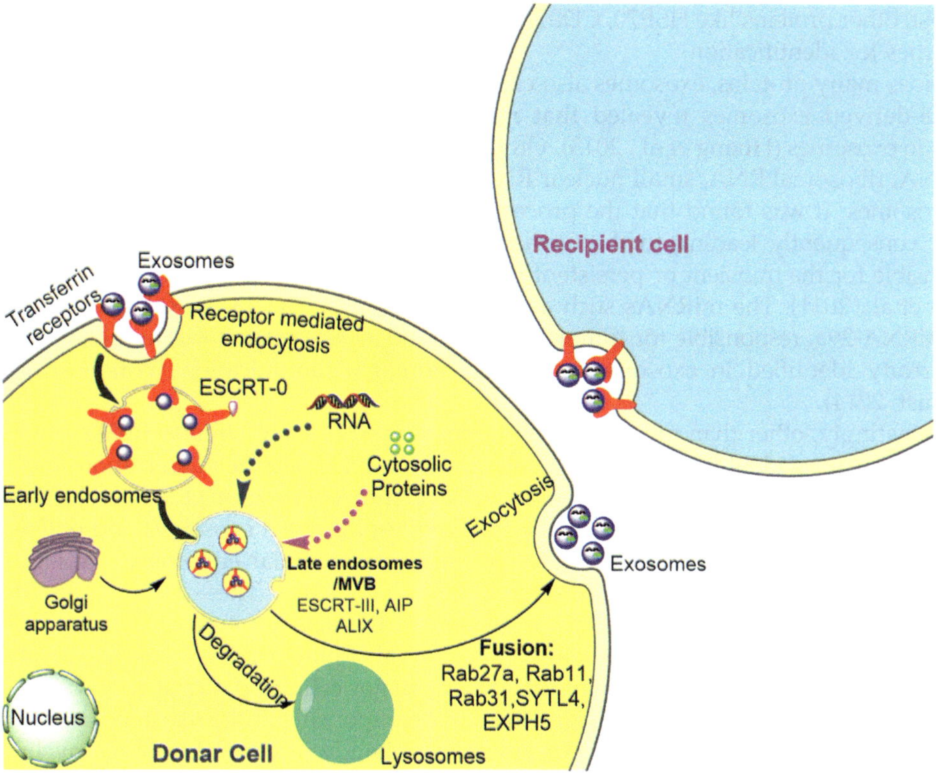

FIGURE 4.1 **Biogenesis and release of the exosomes via endocytosis and exocytosis pathways.** *AIP*, ALIX: ALG-2-interacting protein; *ESCORT*, Endosomal-sorting complexes required for transport; *EXPH5*, Exophilin 5; *MVB*, Multivesicular bodies; *RNA*, Ribonucleic acid; *SYTL4*, Synaptotagmin like 4.

4.2.2 Detailed components of exosomes

The composition of the exosomes is purely dependent on the cell type from which they originate. Exosomes are considered mini kinds of parental cells. Exosomes contain various essential types of machinery like nucleic acids, sorted proteins, and lipids. A large variety of proteins (4400), lipids (194), mRNAs (1639), and miRNAs (764) are identified in the exosome's origin from diverse cell types. Owing to their complex architecture, exosomes possess potential functional diversity for many applications (Mathivanan et al., 2012; Kim et al., 2013). A typical exosome enriched with various functional proteins possesses different functions, like tetraspanins (CD9, CD63, and CD81) help in cell penetration, fusion, and invasion; heat shock proteins such as HSP70 and HSP90 participate in the process of antigen binding and presentation as a response to stress. Furthermore, exosomes also consist of proteins that help in MVB formation, such as Alix and TSG101, and contain proteins involved in the process of membrane transportation and fusion (annexin, Rab) (Vlassov et al., 2012). Among the various proteins present in the exosomes, Alix, fotillin, and TSG101 are involved in exosome biogenesis and make them discrete from the ectosomes after plasma membrane shedding. In contrast, other proteins like HSP70, CD81, CD63, and CD9 are widely known for the marker's properties for identification.

Besides many proteins, exosomes also contain different RNAs. RNA sequencing of human plasma-derived exosomes revealed that microRNAs (miRNAs) are the highly abundant RNAs in exosomes (Huang et al., 2013). Other RNAs like small nucleolar RNA, piwi interacting RNA, ribosomal RNA, small nuclear RNA, and long noncoding RNA are also present in the exosomes. It was found that the process of miRNAs delivery via exosomes is unidirectional, consequently leading to the formation of an intercellular network, which may be responsible for the transient or persistent phenotypic variations in the recipient cells (Mittelbrunn et al., 2011). The miRNAs such as miRNA-320, miRNA-214, miRNA-126, miRNA-1, and miRNA-29a, responsible for tumorigenesis, angiogenesis, exocytosis, and hematopoiesis are already identified in exosome-based intercellular communication (Waldenström and Ronquist, 2014).

Fascinatingly, other than miRNAs, long noncoding RNAs and circular RNAs (circRNAs) have recently been identified in the exosomes and found they are the main responsible agents for many biological reactions, including cancer development (Hewson et al., 2016). Alice et al. described that lncRNA H19 packed inside the Huh7 cell-derived exosomes and delivered to the endothelial cells (ECs), leading to the metastasis via vascular endothelial growth factor (VEGF) mediated exosomes increase (Conigliaro et al., 2015). These studies demonstrate the importance of lncRNA transfer via exosomes in the development of tumors. lncRNAs are not only involved in tumor development, they also play a critical role in maintaining the tumor microenvironment by manipulating the major cellular pathways.

Apart from the nucleic acids and proteins, lipid components of the exosomes also play an essential role in the bioactivity of the exosomes. Phosphatidylserine (PS), sphingomyelin (SM), cholesterol, arachidonic acid, phosphatidic acid and, prostaglandins, and fatty acids are also enriched in the exosomes, and they are the main responsible factors for the stability and structural integrity of the exosomes. The exosomes are equipped with some functional lipolytic enzymes, which makes them autonomous bodies able to synthesize different bioactive lipids.

Evidence suggests that the accumulation of fatty acids and prostaglandins can stimulate prostaglandin-mediated biological functions in the body (Subra et al., 2010). The endosomal arachidonic acid delivered by the exosomes can be transported to the prostaglandin E synthase and cyclooxygenase located in the endoplasmic reticulum to synthesize more PGE_2. Similarly, the endoplasmic reticulum of the recipient cell can inhibit the cholesterol epoxide hydrolase enzyme upon fatty acid binding, which is the main responsible enzyme for the cleavage of cholesterol 5,6 epoxide into the cholestanetriol (Kedjouar et al., 2004; de Medina et al., 2011). Exosomes can be released and taken up by the target cells. Hence, since exosomes can modulate lipid metabolism, they should be considered for atherosclerosis pathogenesis (Zakharova et al., 2007). The findings show that the lipid composition of the exosomes can act as alternative biomarkers for disease diagnosis and prognosis other than proteins and RNAs. A more detailed composition of the exosomes is demonstrated in Fig. 4.2.

4.2.3 The biological role of exosomes

Exosomes are essential for controlling common biological processes like immune surveillance, repair of tissue, blood clotting, and stem cell maintenance (Samanta et al., 2018).

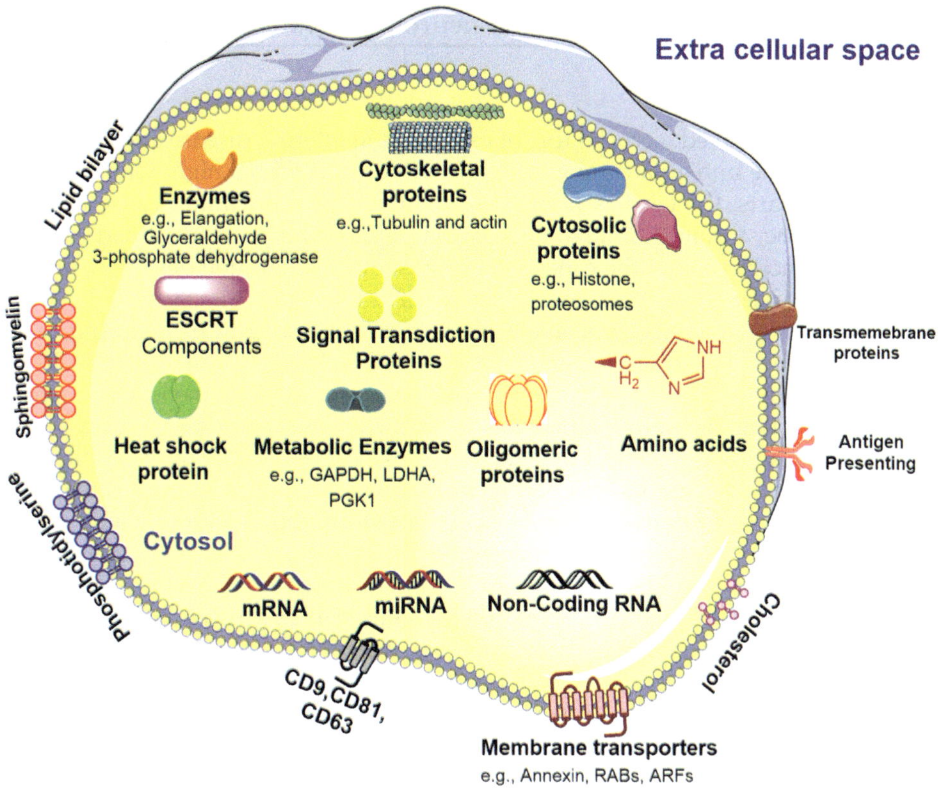

FIGURE 4.2 **Biomolecular composition of exosomes.** *ARFs*, ADP ribosylation factors; *CD*, Cluster of differentiation; *GAPDH*, Glyceraldehyde 3-phosphate dehydrogenase; *LDHA*, Lactate dehydrogenase A; *miRNA*, MicroRNA; *PGK1*, Phosphoglycerate kinase 1; *RNA*, Ribonucleic acid.

Dendritic cells derived exosomes may be involved in generating immune responses. Exosomes derived from dendritic cells may trigger the major histocompatibility complex (MHC) I and II molecules and then be involved in activating T cells such as CD4+ and CD8+ (Zitvogel et al., 1998). The regulatory mechanism of the cell response is owned by exosomes due to their property to transport cargo from one cell to another, including mRNAs, transcription factors, miRNAs, oncogenes, and infectious particles. Transmission of exosome signals occurs either by stimulating the receptors in the neighboring cells or by merging with the recipient cells plasma membrane (Gonda et al., 2019). Exosomes can either stimulate or inhibit the expression of natural killer cells and CD8+ cells based on their source of origin (Gonda et al., 2019). Intercellular communication by the exosomes in in vivo was first reported by Dr. Raposo in 1996. Dr. Raposo proved that the exosomes released by the B lymphoblastoid cells with MHC II particles could be used to constrain the T cell response (Raposo et al., 1996). This finding led other researchers to work on the important role of the exosomes in other diseases' pathogenesis and progression, such as neurodegenerative diseases, carcinogenesis, cardiovascular diseases, and infectious diseases (Rajendran et al., 2006; Hoshino et al., 2015; Harischandra et al., 2017).

4.3 Exosome's role in cancer and neurodegenerative disease progress

4.3.1 Cancer

Cancer biology has paved a crucial role of exosomes in altering disease and health. Cancer is characterized by the unregulated abnormal growth of cells with a high potential to spread to different body parts. Cancer has now been identified as the leading cause of mortality throughout the globe, around 1.8 million newly diagnosed cases were identified in 2020. Major questions of cancer are how the cancer cell grows, evades immune detection, and metastasize? Cancer cells release various signaling particles or molecules that eventually reduce the immune cell activity to the uncontrollable growth of cells and recruit neighboring cells. This cell-to-cell communication occurs through the exosomes released by the cancer cells, which contain numerous biomolecules that can bind to the receptor and then either activate or silence the downstream signaling pathways.

Benedikter et al. studied the effect of cigarette smoke extract on the airway epithelial cell-mediated exosome release and its effect on pathological roles. It is well known that cigarette smoke extract produces oxidative stress. Hence, the authors further investigated the role of oxidative stress on the release of exosomes and found that any thiol antioxidants, such as glutathione (GSH) or N-acetyl-L-cysteine (NAC), can be able to stop the release of exosomes. The authors exposed human bronchial epithelial cells (BEAS-2B) to the cigarette smoke extract, acrolein, hydrogen peroxide, bacitracin, 5,5′-dithiobis-(2-nitrobenzoic acid) (DTNB), Rutin or antibody clone RL_{90} with and without the presence of GSH and NAC. The flow cytometer was used to measure the exosomes released into the media using the CD63+ and CD81+ markers. Exosomes are isolated by ultracentrifugation techniques for characterization. Glutathione and glutathione disulfide presence in the cells were measured using a glutathione reductase cycling assay and a flow cytometer using exofacial thiols. The results demonstrated the release of exosomes upon exposure to cigarette smoke extract and their prevention upon exposure to GSH or NAC. Acrolein was found to be able to limit the NAC reversible exosome induction, and hydrogen peroxide possessed no effect on the exosome release. Membrane impermeable and nonspecific thiol inhibitors are found to stimulate exosome release. The authors concluded that endogenous compounds like acrolein released during inflammation might influence the release of exosomes in smokers and ex-smokers with chronic obstructive pulmonary disease complications. Antioxidants like GSH and NAC can reversibly inhibit cigarette smoke extract and acrolein-stimulated exosome release. Hence, they can be used as a clinical candidate to achieve the clinical benefits of antioxidants (Benedikter et al., 2017).

$PM_{2.5}$ particles are fine particle air pollutants with a particle size of less than or equal to 2.5 microns (Huang et al., 2015). Exposure to these particles, either long-term or short-term, may cause health problems (Honda et al., 2017). Exposure to particle sizes less than 2.5 microns increases the risk of respiratory diseases (Chen et al., 2016). Xu et al. investigated the effect of $PM_{2.5}$ on the release of Wnt3a-enriched exosomes from A549 human epithelial lung cancer cells. The results demonstrated a high level of Wnt3a-enriched exosomes released upon exposure to $PM_{2.5.}$ Exosomes enriched in Wnt3a activate the β-catenin signaling in the A549 human epithelial lung cancer cells. However, the released exosomes do not show any effect on the invasion and migration of cancer cells but have a positive effect on the A549 cancer cells by the Wnt3a/β-catenin pathway in in vitro.

Furthermore, these results were validated in vivo by findings that exosomes also promoted tumor growth in in vivo. These results show the direct effect of $PM_{2.5}$ on lung cancer progression. Inhibiting the Wnt3a/β-catenin signaling pathway could be a promising approach to slowing the progression of $PM_{2.5}$-induced lung cancer (Xu et al., 2019).

Xu et al. studied the effect of 1.0 μM arsenite-treated human bronchial epithelial cells (HBE) on the transfer of exosomal miRNA-21 to the untreated HBE cells by a noncontact, coculture method. Furthermore, the authors evaluated the effect of transferred miRNA-21 on the recipient cells. The results demonstrated that miRNA-21 is actively involved in the intercellular communication between cancerous and normal HBE cells. It was found that exosomes released from the arsenite-treated HBE cells induced proliferation of the normal HBE cells, whereas in the case of exosomes released from miRNA-21 depleted cells did not show any effect on cell proliferation. The authors concluded that the transformed HBE cells secrete exosomes containing miRNA-21 and subsequently induce the proliferation of the normal HBE cells. These findings support the concept of exosomal communication between the cells to transfer the miRNAs during carcinogenesis induced by environmental toxins (Xu et al., 2015).

Chronic use of platinum drugs, such as carboplatin, cisplatin, and paclitaxel, for treating ovarian cancer leads to acquired drug resistance and causes an 80% cancer recurrence. Drug-resistant cancer cells own higher drug efflux potential, antioxidant properties, and enhanced damage repair properties of DNA, making them immune to chemotherapeutic drugs (Stewart, 2007). Crow et al. studied how platinum-containing drug-resistant cancer cells affect cancer cell progression and found that platinum-resistant cancer cells secrete exosomes enriched with the miRNA-21, which is responsible for promoting the epithelial-mesenchymal transition. Epithelial to mesenchymal transition is a crucial step in cancer development (Crow et al., 2017). Cancer cells resistant to platinum had mutations in the SMAD4. SMAD4 is a transcription factor that is majorly engaged in the communication pathway intracellularly and epithelial to mesenchymal transition. Authors proposed that platinum contain drugs increase the release of exosome miRNA-21, stimulating SMAD4 mutations, thereby enhancing cancer cell survival and progression (Pohl et al., 2010). Yang et al. proposed that exosomes released by the tumor stem cells significantly regulate the Wnt, β-catenin, and Hedgehog to maintain cancer cell proliferation (Yang et al., 2016). Different components in the cargo of exosomes help deregulation of immune surveillance and encourage cancer cell growth, leading to resistant and malignant cancers.

4.3.2 Neurological diseases

Exosomes act as one vital mediator for intercellular communication. Hence, it increases the progression of some neurological diseases such as Parkinson's, Amyotrophic lateral sclerosis, Alzheimer's disease, Prion disease, and Huntington's diseases via transferring the proteins, mRNAs, or other molecules associated with the pathology (Tsilioni et al., 2014). Exosomes transport toxic proteins, mutated or misfolded, to the healthy neuronal cells, which are a template for the disease's progression by oligomer formation. Prominently, many environmental and genetic factors can induce the secretion of exosomes. Environmental factors like pesticides, metals, and brain traumatic injury play a predominant part in the inception of neurological diseases (Berry et al., 2010; Gardner et al., 2015). Here in this section, we mainly focused on the critical role of environmental factors in exosome release and their impact on neurological disease progression.

Neurological disorders share similar pathological features like misfolding and aggregation of the disease-specific toxic protein species (Sweeney et al., 2017). These diseases generally arise due to the continuous stream of protein misfolding, mainly due to errors in biogenesis, mutations, and pathological stressors. The proteins like β-amyloid (Aβ), α-synuclein (αSyn), tau, and prion proteins acquire abnormal β-sheet structures in their proteins, which are generally absent in normal cells (Hipp et al., 2014). A wealth of information is now available to support the theory of exosome involvement in the cell-to-cell transmission of misfolded toxic proteins. This has been supported by the reports in which authors reported that Aβ and αSyn have been identified in the exosomes and can act as a potential mediator to spread them intercellularly with the healthy cells and spread the disease progression (Rajendran et al., 2006; Emmanouilidou et al., 2010).

The exosome distribution of toxic proteins like αSyn grabbed interest when the pathogenic aggregated αSyn was identified in the cerebrospinal fluid-derived exosomes from the patient with Parkinson's disease and dementia along with Lewy bodies. Both these diseases are very complex disorders whose etiology is not identified correctly. Furthermore, evidence for the genetic interaction stimulated neurodegenerative disorders was found when the juvenile onset of Parkinsons was associated with genes such as ATP13A2 and PARK9 (Gitler et al., 2009; Santoro et al., 2011). ATP13A2 is mainly involved in transporting cations such as zinc, selenium, manganese, and selenium from the cytosol to the lysosomes (Schmidt et al., 2009). It was found that overexpression of these ATP13A2/PARK9 genes enhances the αSyn release via exosomes in the primary cortical cells of mice and H4 cells (Tsunemi et al., 2014). However, complete proof for the sole reason of exosome cargo-mediated delivery of the toxic proteins and their involvement in the pathology of Parkinson's and other diseases has yet to be defined.

Some pesticides are toxic to neurons, and chronic exposure to these toxins can lead to the development of neurological diseases (Kanthasamy et al., 2005; Rokad et al., 2016). Rotenone is among such neurotoxic pesticides utilized in agriculture and the management of water, enhancing the expression of αSyn and its deposition in the brain cells, where it majorly contributes to the degeneration of nigral neurons (Betarbet et al., 2000). In in vivo wild-type mice, Pan-Montojo et al. demonstrated the delivery of synthesized pathological αSyn upon rotenone exposure in the enteric neuronal system to the substantia nigra and vagus nerve (Pan-Montojo et al., 2010). Later, in another study, the same authors demonstrated that rotenone stimulates the exosome secretion of αSyn from the enteric neurons and their delivery to the presynaptic sympathetic neurons. This study provided evidence of the involvement of environmental toxins in αSyn exosome release (Pan-Montojo et al., 2012). Much interest is being created in the environmental factors' effects on the microbiome-gut-brain axis in neurological diseases pathogenesis (Ghaisas et al., 2016).

Recent research evidence suggests that the toxic Aβ aggregated proteins can increase the pathology of Alzheimer's disease brain. However, the mechanism by which these proteins spread into healthy neurons has not yet been established. Numerous reports have shown the pathogenic characteristics of soluble Aβ protein on the cellular functions and synaptic membrane of neurons (Walsh et al., 2002; Selkoe and Disease, 2008). It has been hypothesized that exosomes might be involved in the delivery of toxic Aβ protein to the affected part of the brain (Guo and Lee, 2014).

Few researchers tried to identify the exosome presence in the cerebrospinal fluid and blood and some tried to prove that the exosomes were enriched with the monomeric Aβ protein and tau protein delivery from diseased cells to healthy cells (Rajendran et al., 2006; Fiandaca et al., 2015; Eitan et al., 2013). However, no study has proved the soluble Aβ protein presence in the exosomes of Alzheimer's disease patients.

For the first time, Sinha et al. identified exosomes from Alzheimer's patients' brains and found a higher level of Aβ oligomer in the exosomes. After extraction and culture, the authors found that these exosomes act as a delivery vehicle for transferring toxic proteins from one cell to another. These results were validated by blocking the exosomes' biogenesis, release, and uptake, which were found to decrease the toxic proteins spreading and their related toxicity. Authors proposed that exosomes are centrally involved in the disease progression of Alzheimer's disease. Thus, they can be used as alternative diagnostic agents or develop new therapeutics to treat Alzheimer's disease (Sinha et al., 2018).

Prion disease is one of the deadliest neurodegenerative diseases caused by protein aggregation, prion replication, and spongiform degeneration in significant parts of the brain (Harischandra et al., 2014). Numerous metals are known for their binding efficiency toward prion protein (PrP), and the PrP metal-ion tendency plays an essential role in prion disease pathogenesis (Choi et al., 2006). Recent studies have demonstrated that metal ions like Mn, Cu, and Cd promote structural changes in the PrP protein, resulting in its aggregation and toxicity (Kanthasamy et al., 2012; Yen et al., 2016). In addition, PrP protein was found in the exosome cargo, leading to the delivery of pathological prion protein (Liu et al., 2016).

Recent investigations demonstrated that inducing the exosome release enhances the cell-to-cell transfer of prion proteins (Guo et al., 2016). Furthermore, exosomes are known for their delivery of miRNAs, such as miRNA-146a, from donor to recipient cells, thereby regulating prion expression. The miRNA-146a level rises during metal toxicity and oxidative stress and has been identified as a responsible factor for rare human prion disease (Lukiw et al., 2011). Table 4.1 summarizes the research carried out to investigate the role of toxins and their effects on exosome-mediated cancer and neurodegenerative disease progression.

4.4 The importance of exosome in toxicology: a biomarker perspective

Chemical exposure and cellular stress can affect the biogenesis, release, and uptake of exosomes (de Jong et al., 2012; Harischandra et al., 2018). Exosome cargo is sensitive to these responses, which may help the toxicology in various aspects. Exosome cargo component analysis can be carried out to identify the biomarkers of exposure, exposure-associated disease, and exposure-mediated effects. To date, preclinical and clinical studies have been carried out to identify novel exosome biomarkers for kidney and liver injury. Current diagnostics are based on the protein levels and their expressions to grade the disease stage. However, these clinical readouts cannot differentiate between the type and extent of or severity of the diseases (Szabo and Momen-Heravi, 2017). Recent research has identified exosome miRNAs as a biomarker from blood and urine that can be used to overcome the current diagnostic limitations. Researchers find a unique nature of exosomes during alcoholic liver damage, hepatitis-ischemic injury, inflammatory liver injury, and various types of acute kidney injuries (Zhou et al., 2006; Bala et al., 2012; Cho et al., 2017).

TABLE 4.1 Chemical-induced toxicities for developing pathological conditions of diseases.

Toxicants	Disease	Exosomes cargo involved in the pathogenesis	Mechanism	References
Manganese	Parkinson's disease, neurodegenerative diseases	α-synuclein and ASC	Transfer of αSynuclein and ASC-enriched exosomes to the other cells	Harischandra et al. (2019)
Rotenone	Parkinson's disease, neurodegenerative diseases	α-synuclein	Transfer of αSynuclein toxic protein enriched exosomes to the other cells	Pan-Montojo et al. (2012)
Paraquat	Amylotropic lateral sclerosis	TDP-43	Transfer of TDP-43 toxic proteins enriched exosomes to the other cells	Nonaka et al. (2013)
Cigarette smoke extract	Lung cancer	miRNAs	miRNAs enriched exosomes transfer to the healthy cells	Goldkorn and Filosto (2010)
Radiation	Tracheal cancer	miRNAs, chemokines, and integrins	miRNAs, chemokines, and integrins enriched exosomes transfer to the healthy cells	Mutschelknaus et al. (2016)
Arsenite	Lung and liver cancer	miRNA-21 and miRNA-155	miRNA-21 and miRNA-155 enriched exosomes transfer to the healthy cells	Xu et al. (2015), Chen et al. (2017)

ASC, apoptosis-associated speck-like protein containing a CARD; *TDP*, TAR DNA-binding protein.

Interestingly, in a few cases, exosomes were identified earlier than the onset of clinical diseases, creating tremendous opportunities for immediate interventions (Beltrami et al., 2012). Upon radiation exposure for exosome profiling, organ-specific damage can be detected (Kulkarni et al., 2016). miRNAs present in the exosomes are also identified as novel multi-organ drug toxicity markers, including cardiotoxicity (Nishimura et al., 2015). In conclusion, exosome biomarkers can differentiate the type and severity of the diseases and can also identify the exposure associated with the diseases. Furthermore, we can also identify the acute damage type of the diseases. Furthermore, exosomes can be identified before the disease's onset, allowing for early interventions.

4.5 Future directions of the exosome research

Many researchers are interested in exosomes because of their ability to transport cargo containing miRNAs, proteins, and various lipids and peptides to distant cells. The current focus of exosome research is to identify novel biomarkers for the early detection of various diseases and their progression, as well as to deliver therapeutics via exosomes to create cell-based delivery systems for effective targeted delivery of the loaded therapeutics. Exosomes show great potential to revolutionize the field of nanomedicine (Gadekar et al., 2021; Gorain et al., 2016; Muniswamy et al., 2019; Prajapati et al., 2009).

The advantages of using exosomes as a nanomedicine include exosomes can cross the blood-brain barrier easily. Exosomes are highly stable due to the membrane composition, such as cholesterol, sphingomyelin saturated fatty acids, glycerophospholipid, and phosphatidylserine. The composition of the exosomes also favors the permeation of the therapeutically loaded exosomes through the target cell membrane. Furthermore, exosomes derived from similar species possess very little or no immunogenicity, which thus decreases the risk of immune reactions. However, despite the rich literature on the potential of these nanovesicles as diagnostics and therapeutics, it is too early to relate the changes in the exosome cargo with different diseases due to a lack of clinical studies for validating the results perceived in the preclinical investigations. Therefore, it is vital to appreciate the fundamental differences between the types of cell and exosomal content, which is disease-specific.

Another direction of exosome research that grabbed attention is understanding the exosome's involvement in various disease pathogenesis and progression. As briefed in this recent research chapter, chronic exposure to environmental toxins can induce exosome biogenesis and consequently be involved in disease pathogenesis. It has been observed in many cases that the composition of the exosomes is altered in the targeted patient compared to the healthy subject. However, the underlying mechanisms behind the altered composition of exosomes upon exposure to the chemicals and disease progression are not crystal clear yet. Therefore, future investigations into the exosomes need to focus on molecular-level mechanistic studies to understand how the toxins affect the biochemical composition of the exosome and how these secreted exosomes alter the microenvironment of the disease target area. These kinds of investigations will provide an alternative target for therapeutics.

4.6 Conclusion

After a thorough review of the above-listed reports, it is evident that environmental toxins can stimulate exosomes, thereby triggering disease pathogenesis. Exosomes play an essential role in the pathogenesis and progression of disease due to their inherent capability to deliver biologically active molecules like miRNA, proteins, mRNA, and lipids from one cell to another. Due to technological advancement, very sensitive assays are now available to identify the exosomes in various biofluids, including blood, saliva, urine, and cerebrospinal fluid, making them an alternative biomarker for identifying disease progression. Future studies on the exosomes should be devoted to understanding the molecular mechanism behind the altered cargo of the exosomes and their release pattern. Furthermore, efforts need to be devoted to understanding how the released exosomes impact the microenvironment of the recipient cell to support the pathogenesis of the disease.

4.7 List of abbreviations

ATP13A2 ATPase cation transporting 13A2
Cd cadmium
Cu copper
DNA deoxyribonucleic acid

GSH glutathione
MHC major histocompatibility complex
MiRNA MicroRNA
Mn manganese
mRNAs messenger RNAs
NAC N-acetyl-L-cysteine (NAC)
RNAs ribonucleic acid
αSyn Alpha-synuclein

References

Bala, S., Petrasek, J., Mundkur, S., Catalano, D., Levin, I., Ward, J., Alao, H., Kodys, K., Szabo, G., 2012. Circulating microRNAs in exosomes indicate hepatocyte injury and inflammation in alcoholic, drug-induced, and inflammatory liver diseases. Hepatology 56, 1946–1957.

Bang, C., Thum, T., 2012. Exosomes: new players in cell–cell communication. Inter. J. Biochem. & Cell Biol. 44, 2060–2064.

Beltrami, C., Clayton, A., Phillips, A.O., Fraser, D.J., Bowen, T., 2012. Analysis of urinary microRNAs in chronic kidney disease. Biochem. Soc. Transac. 40, 875–879.

Benedikter, B.J., Volgers, C., Van Eijck, P.H., Wouters, E.F., Savelkoul, P.H., Reynaert, N.L., Haenen, G.R., Rohde, G.G., Weseler, A.R., Stassen, F.R., 2017. Cigarette smoke extract induced exosome release is mediated by depletion of exofacial thiols and can be inhibited by thiol-antioxidants. Free Rad. Biol. Med. 108, 334–344.

Berry, C., LA Vecchia, C., Nicotera, P.J.C.D., 2010. Paraquat and Parkinson's disease. Differentiation 17, 1115–1125.

Betarbet, R., Sherer, T.B., Mackenzie, G., Garcia-Osuna, M., Panov, A.V., Greenamyre, J.T., 2000. Chronic systemic pesticide exposure reproduces features of Parkinson's disease. Nature Neurosci. 3, 1301–1306.

Bobrie, A., Colombo, M., Raposo, G., Théry, C., 2011. Exosome secretion: molecular mechanisms and roles in immune responses. Traffic 12, 1659–1668.

Booth, A.M., Fang, Y., Fallon, J.K., Yang, J.-M., Hildreth, J.E., Gould, S., 2006. Exosomes and HIV Gag bud from endosome-like domains of the T cell plasma membrane. J. Cell Biol. 172, 923–935.

Chen, C., Luo, F., Liu, X., Lu, L., Xu, H., Yang, Q., Xue, J., Shi, L., Li, J., Zhang, A., 2017. NF-kB-regulated exosomal miR-155 promotes the inflammation associated with arsenite carcinogenesis. Cancer Lett. 388, 21–33.

Chen, Z.-H., Wu, Y.-F., Wang, P.-L., Wu, Y.-P., Li, Z.-Y., Zhao, Y., Zhou, J.-S., Zhu, C., Cao, C., Mao, Y.-Y., 2016. Autophagy is essential for ultrafine particle-induced inflammation and mucus hyperproduction in airway epithelium. Autophagy 12, 297–311.

Cho, Y.E., Mezey, E., Hardwick, J.P., Salem Jr., N., Clemens, D.L., Song, B.J., 2017. Increased ethanol-inducible cytochrome P450-2E1 and cytochrome P450 isoforms in exosomes of alcohol-exposed rodents and patients with alcoholism through oxidative and endoplasmic reticulum stress. Hepatol. Commun. 1, 675–690.

Choi, C.J., Kanthasamy, A., Anantharam, V., Kanthasamy, A.G., 2006. Interaction of metals with prion protein: possible role of divalent cations in the pathogenesis of prion diseases. Neurotoxicology 27, 777–787.

Conigliaro, A., Costa, V., Dico, A.L., Saieva, L., Buccheri, S., Dieli, F., Manno, M., Raccosta, S., Mancone, C., Tripodi, M., 2015. CD90+ liver cancer cells modulate endothelial cell phenotype through the release of exosomes containing H19 lncRNA. Mol. Cancer 14, 1–11.

Crow, J., Atay, S., Banskota, S., Artale, B., Schmitt, S., Godwin, A.K., 2017. Exosomes as mediators of platinum resistance in ovarian cancer. Oncotarget 8, 11917.

De Jong, O.G., Verhaar, M.C., Chen, Y., Vader, P., Gremmels, H., Posthuma, G., Schiffelers, R.M., Gucek, M., VAN Balkom, B.W., 2012. Cellular stress conditions are reflected in the protein and RNA content of endothelial cell-derived exosomes. J. Extracell. Vesic. 1, 18396.

De Medina, P., Paillasse, M.R., Ségala, G., Khallouki, F., Brillouet, S., Dalenc, F., Courbon, F., Record, M., Poirot, M., Silvente-Poirot, S., 2011. Importance of cholesterol and oxysterols metabolism in the pharmacology of tamoxifen and other AEBS ligands. Chem. Phys. Lipids 164, 432–437.

Eitan, E., Hutchison, E., Marosi, K., Comotto, J., Mustapic, M., Nigam, S.J.A.M., 2013. Extracellular vesicle-associated abeta mediates trans-neuronal bioenergetic and Ca (2+)-handling deficits in Alzheimer's disease models. NPJ Aging Mech. of Dis. 2 (25), 3780–3801, 2016.

Emmanouilidou, E., Melachroinou, K., Roumeliotis, T., Garbis, S.D., Ntzouni, M., Margaritis, L.H., Stefanis, L., Vekrellis, K., 2010. Cell-produced α-synuclein is secreted in a calcium-dependent manner by exosomes and impacts neuronal survival. J. Neurosc. 30, 6838–6851.

Fiandaca, M.S., Kapogiannis, D., Mapstone, M., Boxer, A., Eitan, E., Schwartz, J.B., Abner, E.L., Petersen, R.C., Federoff, H.J., Miller, B.L., 2015. Identification of preclinical Alzheimer's disease by a profile of pathogenic proteins in neurally derived blood exosomes: a case-control study. Alzheimer's & Dementia 11, 600–607.e1.

Gadekar, V., Borade, Y., Kannaujia, S., Rajpoot, K., Anup, N., Tambe, V., Kalia, K., Tekade, R.K., 2021. Nanomedicines accessible in the market for clinical interventions. J. Contr. Release 330, 372–397.

Gardner, R.C., Burke, J.F., Nettiksimmons, J., Goldman, S., Tanner, C.M., Yaffe, K., 2015. Traumatic brain injury in later life increases risk for Parkinson disease. Ann. Neurolog. 77, 987–995.

Ghaisas, S., Maher, J., Kanthasamy, A., 2016. Gut microbiome in health and disease: linking the microbiome–gut–brain axis and environmental factors in the pathogenesis of systemic and neurodegenerative diseases. Pharmacol. & Ther. 158, 52–62.

Gitler, A.D., Chesi, A., Geddie, M.L., Strathearn, K.E., Hamamichi, S., Hill, K.J., Caldwell, K.A., Caldwell, G.A., Cooper, A.A., Rochet, J.-C., 2009. α-Synuclein is part of a diverse and highly conserved interaction network that includes PARK9 and manganese toxicity. Nature Genet. 41, 308–315.

Goldkorn, T., Filosto, S., 2010. Lung injury and cancer: mechanistic insights into ceramide and EGFR signaling under cigarette smoke. Am. J. Respir. Cell Mol. Biol. 43, 259–268.

Gonda, A., Kabagwira, J., Senthil, G.N., Wall, N.R., 2019. Internalization of exosomes through receptor-mediated endocytosis. Mol. Cancer Res. 17, 337–347.

Gorain, B., Choudhury, H., Tekade, R.K., Karan, S., Jaisankar, P., Pal, T.K., 2016. Comparative biodistribution and safety profiling of olmesartan medoxomil oil-in-water oral nanoemulsion. Regul. Toxicol. Pharmacol. 82, 20–31.

Guay, C., Regazzi, R., 2017. Exosomes as new players in metabolic organ cross-talk. Obesity & Metabol. 19, 137–146.

Guo, B.B., Bellingham, S.A., Hill, A.F., 2016. Stimulating the release of exosomes increases the intercellular transfer of prions. J. Biol. Chem. 291, 5128–5137.

Guo, J.L., Lee, V.M., 2014. Cell-to-cell transmission of pathogenic proteins in neurodegenerative diseases. Nature Med. 20, 130–138.

Harischandra, D.S., Ghaisas, S., Rokad, D., Kanthasamy, A.G., 2017. Exosomes in toxicology: relevance to chemical exposure and pathogenesis of environmentally linked diseases. Toxicol. Sci. 158, 3–13.

Harischandra, D.S., Ghaisas, S., Rokad, D., Zamanian, M., Jin, H., Anantharam, V., Kimber, M., Kanthasamy, A., Kanthasamy, A.G., 2018. Environmental neurotoxicant manganese regulates exosome-mediated extracellular miRNAs in cell culture model of Parkinson's disease: relevance to α-synuclein misfolding in metal neurotoxicity. Neurotoxicology 64, 267–277.

Harischandra, D.S., Kondru, N., Martin, D.P., Kanthasamy, A., Jin, H., Anantharam, V., Kanthasamy, A.G., 2014. Role of proteolytic activation of protein kinase Cδ in the pathogenesis of prion disease. Prion 8, 143–153.

Harischandra, D.S., Rokad, D., Neal, M.L., Ghaisas, S., Manne, S., Sarkar, S., Panicker, N., Zenitsky, G., Jin, H., Lewis, M., 2019. Manganese promotes the aggregation and prion-like cell-to-cell exosomal transmission of α-synuclein. Sci. Signal. 12.

Henne, W.M., Buchkovich, N.J., Emr, S.D., 2011. The ESCRT pathway. Develop. Cell 21, 77–91.

Hewson, C., Capraro, D., Burdach, J., Whitaker, N., Morris, K.V., 2016. Extracellular vesicle associated long non-coding RNAs functionally enhance cell viability. Non-coding RNA Res. 1, 3–11.

Hipp, M.S., Park, S.-H., Hartl, F.U., 2014. Proteostasis impairment in protein-misfolding and-aggregation diseases. Trends Cell Biol. 24, 506–514.

Honda, T., Pun, V.C., Manjourides, J., Suh, H., 2017. Anemia prevalence and hemoglobin levels are associated with long-term exposure to air pollution in an older population. Environ. int. 101, 125–132.

Hoshino, A., COSTA-Silva, B., Shen, T.-L., Rodrigues, G., Hashimoto, A., Mark, M.T., Molina, H., Kohsaka, S., DI Giannatale, A., Ceder, S., 2015. Tumour exosome integrins determine organotropic metastasis. Nature 527, 329–335.

Huang, L., Pu, Z., Li, M., Sundell, J., 2015. Characterizing the indoor-outdoor relationship of fine particulate matter in non-heating season for urban residences in Beijing. PloS one 10, e0138559.

Huang, X., Yuan, T., Tschannen, M., Sun, Z., Jacob, H., Du, M., Liang, M., Dittmar, R.L., Liu, Y., Liang, M., 2013. Characterization of human plasma-derived exosomal RNAs by deep sequencing. BMC genomics 14, 1–14.

Hurley, J.H., 2015. ESCRT s are everywhere. The EMBO J. 34, 2398–2407.

Kanthasamy, A., Choi, C., Jin, H., Harischandra, D., Anantharam, V., Kanthasamy, A., 2012. Effect of divalent metals on the neuronal proteasomal system, prion protein ubiquitination and aggregation. Toxicol. Lett. 214, 288–295.

Kanthasamy, A.G., Kitazawa, M., Kanthasamy, A., Anantharam, V., 2005. Dieldrin-induced neurotoxicity: relevance to Parkinson's disease pathogenesis. Neurotoxicology 26, 701–719.

Kedjouar, B., DE Médina, P., Oulad-Abdelghani, M., Payré, B., Silvente-Poirot, S., Favre, G., Faye, J.-C., Poirot, M., 2004. Molecular characterization of the microsomal tamoxifen binding site. J. Biol. Chem. 279, 34048–34061.

Kim, D.K., Kang, B., Kim, O.Y., Choi, D.S., Lee, J., Kim, S.R., Go, G., Yoon, Y.J., Kim, J.H., Jang, S.C., 2013. EVpedia: an integrated database of high-throughput data for systemic analyses of extracellular vesicles. J. Extracell. Vesic. 2, 20384.

Kulkarni, S., Koller, A., Mani, K.M., Wen, R., Alfieri, A., Saha, S., Wang, J., Patel, P., Bandeira, N., Guha, C., 2016. Identifying urinary and serum exosome biomarkers for radiation exposure using a data dependent acquisition and SWATH-MS combined workflow. Int. J. Rad. Oncol. Biol. Phys. 96, 566–577.

Liu, S., Hossinger, A., Hofmann, J.P., Denner, P., Vorberg, I.M., 2016. Horizontal transmission of cytosolic Sup35 prions by extracellular vesicles. MBio 7.

Lukiw, W., Dua, P., Pogue, A., Eicken, C., Hill, J., 2011. Upregulation of micro RNA-146a (miRNA-146a), a marker for inflammatory neurodegeneration, in sporadic Creutzfeldt–Jakob disease (sCJD) and Gerstmann–Straussler–Scheinker (GSS) syndrome. J. Toxicol. & Environ. Health 74, 1460–1468.

Mathivanan, S., Fahner, C.J., Reid, G.E., Simpson, R., 2012. ExoCarta 2012: database of exosomal proteins. RNA Lipids 40, D1241–D1244.

Minciacchi, V.R., Freeman, M.R., DI Vizio, D., 2015. Extracellular vesicles in cancer: exosomes, microvesicles and the emerging role of large oncosomes. Semin. Cell Dev. Biol. 41–51. Elsevier.

Mittelbrunn, M., Gutiérrez-Vázquez, C., Villarroya-Beltri, C., González, S., Sánchez-Cabo, F., González, M.Á., Bernad, A., Sánchez-Madrid, F., 2011. Unidirectional transfer of microRNA-loaded exosomes from T cells to antigen-presenting cells. Nature Commun. 2, 1–10.

Muniswamy, V.J., Raval, N., Gondaliya, P., Tambe, V., Kalia, K., Tekade, R.K., 2019. 'Dendrimer-Cationized-Albumin' encrusted polymeric nanoparticle improves BBB penetration and anticancer activity of doxorubicin. Int. J. Pharm. 555, 77–99.

Mutschelknaus, L., Peters, C., Winkler, K., Yentrapalli, R., Heider, T., Atkinson, M.J., Moertl, S., 2016. Exosomes derived from squamous head and neck cancer promote cell survival after ionizing radiation. PloS one 11, e0152213.

Nishimura, Y., Kondo, C., Morikawa, Y., Tonomura, Y., Torii, M., Yamate, J., Uehara, T., 2015. Plasma miR-208 as a useful biomarker for drug-induced cardiotoxicity in rats. J. Appl. Toxicol. 35, 173–180.

Nonaka, T., Masuda-Suzukake, M., Arai, T., Hasegawa, Y., Akatsu, H., Obi, T., Yoshida, M., Murayama, S., Mann, D.M., Akiyama, H., 2013. Prion-like properties of pathological TDP-43 aggregates from diseased brains. Cell Rep. 4, 124–134.

Pan-Montojo, F., Anichtchik, O., Dening, Y., Knells, L., Pursche, S., Jung, R., Jackson, S., Gille, G., Spillantini, M.G., Reichmann, H., 2010. Progression of Parkinson's disease pathology is reproduced by intragastric administration of rotenone in mice. PloS one, 1–1.

PAN-Montojo, F., Schwarz, M., Winkler, C., Arnhold, M., O'sullivan, G.A., Pal, A., Said, J., Marsico, G., Verbavatz, J.-M., Rodrigo-Angulo, M., 2012. Environmental toxins trigger PD-like progression via increased alpha-synuclein release from enteric neurons in mice. Sci. Rep. 2, 1–12.

Pohl, M., Radacz, Y., Pawlik, N., Schoeneck, A., Baldus, S.E., Munding, J., Schmiegel, W., Schwarte-Waldhoff, I., Reinacher-Schick, A., 2010. SMAD4 mediates mesenchymal–epithelial reversion in SW480 colon carcinoma cells. Anticancer Res. 30, 2603–2613.

Prajapati, R.N., Tekade, R.K., Gupta, U., Gajbhiye, V., Jain, N.K., 2009. Dendimer-mediated solubilization, formulation development and in vitro-in vivo assessment of piroxicam. Mol. Pharm. 6, 940–950.

Rajendran, L., Honsho, M., Zahn, T.R., Keller, P., Geiger, K.D., Verkade, P., Simons, K., 2006. Alzheimer's disease β-amyloid peptides are released in association with exosomes. Proceed. Nat. Acad. Sci. 103, 11172–11177.

Raposo, G., Nijman, H.W., Stoorvogel, W., Liejendekker, R., Harding, C.V., Melief, C., Geuze, H., 1996. B lymphocytes secrete antigen-presenting vesicles. J. Exper. Med. 183, 1161–1172.

Record, M., 2014. Intercellular communication by exosomes in placenta: a possible role in cell fusion? Placenta 35, 297–302.

Revenfeld, A.L.S., Bæk, R., Nielsen, M.H., Stensballe, A., Varming, K., Jørgensen, M., 2014. Diagnostic and prognostic potential of extracellular vesicles in peripheral blood. Clin. Ther. 36, 830–846.

Rokad, D., Ghaisas, S., Harischandra, D.S., Jin, H., Anantharam, V., Kanthasamy, A., Kanthasamy, A.G., 2016. Role of neurotoxicants and traumatic brain injury in-synuclein protein misfolding and aggregation. Brain Res. Bull.

Sahu, R., Kaushik, S., Clement, C.C., Cannizzo, E.S., Scharf, B., Follenzi, A., Potolicchio, I., Nieves, E., Cuervo, A.M., Santambrogio, L., 2011. Microautophagy of cytosolic proteins by late endosomes. Development. Cell 20, 131–139.

Samanta, S., Rajasingh, S., Drosos, N., Zhou, Z., Dawn, B., Rajasingh, J., 2018. Exosomes: new molecular targets of diseases. Acta Pharmacologica Sinica 39, 501–513.

Santoro, L., Breedveld, G.J., Manganelli, F., Iodice, R., Pisciotta, C., Nolano, M., Punzo, F., Quarantelli, M., Pappatà, S., DI Fonzo, A., 2011. Novel ATP13A2 (PARK9) homozygous mutation in a family with marked phenotype variability. Neurogenetics 12, 33–39.

Schmidt, K., Wolfe, D.M., Stiller, B., Pearce, D.A., 2009. Cd^{2+}, Mn^{2+}, Ni^{2+} and Se^{2+} toxicity to *Saccharomyces cerevisiae* lacking YPK9p the orthologue of human ATP13A2. Biochem. and Biophys. Res. Commun. 383, 198–202.

Selkoe, D.J., 2008. Soluble oligomers of the amyloid β-protein: impair synaptic plasticity and behavior. Synaptic Plast. Mech. Alzheimer's Dis. 89–102.

Sinha, M.S., Ansell-Schultz, A., Civitelli, L., Hildesjö, C., Larsson, M., Lannfelt, L., Ingelsson, M., Hallbeck, M., 2018. Alzheimer's disease pathology propagation by exosomes containing toxic amyloid-beta oligomers. Acta Neuropathologica 136, 41–56.

Stewart, D., 2007. Mechanisms of resistance to cisplatin and carboplatin. Crit. Rev. Oncol./Hemat. 63, 12–31.

Subra, C., Grand, D., Laulagnier, K., Stella, A., Lambeau, G., Paillasse, M., DE Medina, P., Monsarrat, B., Perret, B., Silvente-Poirot, S., 2010. Exosomes account for vesicle-mediated transcellular transport of activatable phospholipases and prostaglandins. J. Lipid Res. 51, 2105–2120.

Sweeney, P., Park, H., Baumann, M., Dunlop, J., Frydman, J., Kopito, R., Mccampbell, A., Leblanc, G., Venkateswaran, A., Nurmi, A., 2017. Protein misfolding in neurodegenerative diseases: implications and strategies. Transl. Neurodegen. 6, 1–13.

Szabo, G., Momen-Heravi, F., 2017. Extracellular vesicles in liver disease and potential as biomarkers and therapeutic targets. Nature Rev. Gastroenterol. & Hepatol. 14, 455.

Théry, C., Ostrowski, M., Segura, E., 2009. Membrane vesicles as conveyors of immune responses. Nature Rev. Immunol. 9, 581–593.

Tsilioni, I., Panagiotidou, S., Theoharides, T.C., 2014. Exosomes in neurologic and psychiatric disorders. Clin. Ther. 36, 882–888.

Tsunemi, T., Hamada, K., Krainc, D., 2014. ATP13A2/PARK9 regulates secretion of exosomes and α-synuclein. J. Neurosci. 34, 15281–15287.

Villarroya-Beltri, C., Baixauli, F., Gutiérrez-Vázquez, C., Sánchez-Madrid, F., Mittelbrunn, M., 2014. Sorting it out: regulation of exosome loading. Semin. Cancer Biol. 3–13. Elsevier.

Vlassov, A.V., Magdaleno, S., Setterquist, R., Conrad, R., 2012. Exosomes: current knowledge of their composition, biological functions, and diagnostic and therapeutic potentials. Biochimica et Biophysica Acta (BBA)-Gen. Subject 1820, 940–948.

Waldenström, A., Ronquist, G., 2014. Role of exosomes in myocardial remodeling. Circ. Res. 114, 315–324.

Walsh, D.M., Klyubin, I., Fadeeva, J.V., Cullen, W.K., Anwyl, R., Wolfe, M.S., Rowan, M.J., Selkoe, D., 2002. Naturally secreted oligomers of amyloid β protein potently inhibit hippocampal long-term potentiation in vivo. Nature 416, 535–539.

Xu, H., Jiao, X., Wu, Y., Li, S., Cao, L., Dong, L., 2019. Exosomes derived from PM2. 5-treated lung cancer cells promote the growth of lung cancer via the Wnt3a/β-catenin pathway. Oncol. Rep. 41, 1180–1188.

Xu, Y., Luo, F., Liu, Y., Shi, L., Lu, X., Xu, W., Liu, Q., 2015. Exosomal miR-21 derived from arsenite-transformed human bronchial epithelial cells promotes cell proliferation associated with arsenite carcinogenesis. Archiv. Toxicol. 89, 1071–1082.

Yang, Q., Diamond, M.P., AL-Hendy, A., 2016. Early life adverse environmental exposures increase the risk of uterine fibroid development: role of epigenetic regulation. Front. pharm. 7, 40.

Yellon, D.M., Davidson, S.M., 2014. Exosomes: nanoparticles involved in cardioprotection? Circ. Res. 114, 325–332.

Yen, C.-F., Harischandra, D.S., Kanthasamy, A., Sivasankar, S., 2016. Copper-induced structural conversion templates prion protein oligomerization and neurotoxicity. Sci. Adv. 2, e1600014.

Zakharova, L., Svetlova, M., Fomina, A.F., 2007. T cell exosomes induce cholesterol accumulation in human monocytes via phosphatidylserine receptor. J. Cell. Phys. 212, 174–181.

Zhou, H., Pisitkun, T., Aponte, A., Yuen, P.S., Hoffert, J.D., Yasuda, H., Hu, X., Chawla, L., Shen, R.-F., Knepper, M.A., 2006. Exosomal Fetuin-A identified by proteomics: a novel urinary biomarker for detecting acute kidney injury. Kid. Inter. 70, 1847–1857.

Zitvogel, L., Regnault, A., Lozier, A., Wolfers, J., Flament, C., Tenza, D., Ricciardi-Castagnoli, P., Raposo, G., Amigorena, S., 1998. Eradication of established murine tumors using a novel cell-free vaccine: dendritic cell derived exosomes. Nature Med. 4, 594–600.

CHAPTER

5

Drug-induced oxidative stress as a mechanism of toxicity

Tanisha Gupta[1], Shyam Gomte[1], Bhakti Pawar[1], Muktika Tekade[2], Kuldeep Rajpoot[1], Nidhi Raval[3] and Rakesh Kumar Tekade[1]

[1]National Institute of Pharmaceutical Education and Research (NIPER)-Ahmedabad, An Institute of National Importance, Government of India, Department of Pharmaceuticals, Ministry of Chemicals and Fertilizers, Palaj, Gandhinagar, Gujarat, India; [2]School of Pharmacy, Devi Ahilya Vishwavidyalaya, Indore, Madhya Pradesh, India; [3]University of British Columbia, Pharmaceutical Sciences Building, Vancouver, BC, Canada

5.1 Introduction

Oxidative stress (OS) is the situation that turns out due to an imbalance between the generation and deposition of reactive oxygen species (ROS) in distinctive tissues and cells and the capacity of the physiological system to detoxify these metabolic reactive products (Pizzino et al., 2017; Kalyane et al., 2022). OS is concerned with various disorders like cardiovascular disorders, neurodegenerative disorders, diabetes mellitus, and several other abnormalities (Hayes et al., 2020; Sies, 2015). Cells can produce ROS and reactive nitrogen species (RNS) as a product of the biotransformation process (Hayes et al., 2020).

ROS is widely identified as a detrimental molecule to cells since it harms nucleic acid, lipids, and protein inside the cells (Nathan and Cunningham-Bussel, 2013). ROS can produce in high-energy environments where strong metabolism is required and should not be neglected. In certain conditions, increased ROS production results in oxidative damage to the body and pathogens. ROS species disrupt normal cells and tissues by oxidative damage and have a significant role in growth, development, immunity, and homeostasis processes (Shadel and Horvath, 2015; Polaka et al., 2022a). ROS are generally chemically reactive species containing oxygen atoms. The reactivity may arise due to non-paired electrons and non-radical species, including hydrogen peroxide (H_2O_2). Some ROS example includes peroxide

Essentials of Pharmatoxicology in Drug Research, Volume 1
https://doi.org/10.1016/B978-0-443-15840-7.00014-2

ion, hydroxyl ion, superoxide radicals, hydroxyl radical, oxygen, and hydrogen peroxides. These are the additional products of biotransformation reactions and have a significant role in homeostasis and cellular signaling pathways. Endogenous, as well as exogenous mechanisms, can produce ROS. One of the essential precursors for ROS generation in the cell is the powerhouse of the cell, i.e., mitochondria.

Mitochondria generate superoxide radicals as the additional product of oxidative phosphorylation reaction, producing ROS species (Devasagayam et al., 2004). Interestingly, cells have their mechanism, such as an antioxidant-based mechanism involving various elements like superoxide dismutase (SOD), catalase, and glutathione peroxidase, which has a role in preserving cells from ROS-generated oxidative damage (Deponte, 2013). Another well-known example includes mitochondrial manganese SOD, which changes the superoxide radical into peroxides. Later, it was reduced to water with the help of enzyme peroxidases (Harrison et al., 2005). This chapter overviews the generalized concept of OS with its role in toxicity. Finally, we can go through various detection techniques available for OS determination (Deavall et al., 2012).

In recent times, scientists have concentrated on the safe delivery of pharmaceuticals. However, several factors, such as medical conditions, may significantly impact the results of the medication in respect of toxicity (Gupta et al., 2022b; Kumawat et al., 2020), body warmness (Desai et al., 2021), age (Rajpoot et al., 2021a), stomach food composition (Polaka et al., 2022b), enzyme secretions (Achanta et al., 2021; Tambe et al., 2021e; Rajpoot et al., 2020a), sleeping pattern (Choudhary et al., 2021; Vasdev et al., 2021), and sex of patients (Anup et al., 2021a; Polaka et al., 2022a).

By adjusting various pharmacokinetic characteristics of chemotherapeutic drugs, such as absorption, distribution, metabolism, and excretion across the body, the harmful impact of any pharmaceutical agents can be reduced (Anup et al., 2021c; Padiyar et al., 2020; Polaka et al., 2021a; Rajpoot et al., 2020b, 2021c). The nanoformulation has the capability to improve the pharmaceutical properties of the drug (Gadekar et al., 2021; Gorain et al., 2016; Muniswamy et al., 2019; Prajapati et al., 2009). Several innovative strategies were reported for developing fitting classes of the dosage form (Youngren et al., 2013; Tekade and Chougule, 2013). In this connection, many techniques, models, as well as software are used to calculate the ideal dosage of active ingredients to achieve the intended result while minimizing hazardous consequences (Anup et al., 2021b; Polaka et al., 2021b; Rajpoot et al., 2021b; Tambe et al., 2021a, 2021c, 2021d).

Additionally, to confirm medication toxicity, a variety of methods are utilized, including in silico (Rajpoot et al., 2022a); in vitro toxicity studies (Gupta et al., 2022c); in vivo animal models, toxicokinetic, and toxicodynamic considerations (Rajpoot et al., 2022b); the toxic effects of ingredients (Tiwari et al., 2022; Gupta et al., 2022a); and distinct biomarkers (Tekade et al., 2022).

5.2 Oxidative stress

As mentioned earlier, OS generates ROS, which damages the cells through various mechanisms. In other words, it indicates the misbalance between antioxidants and oxidants in the body system. The concept of OS was used first time in 1985 (Sies, 2019). Moreover, the review

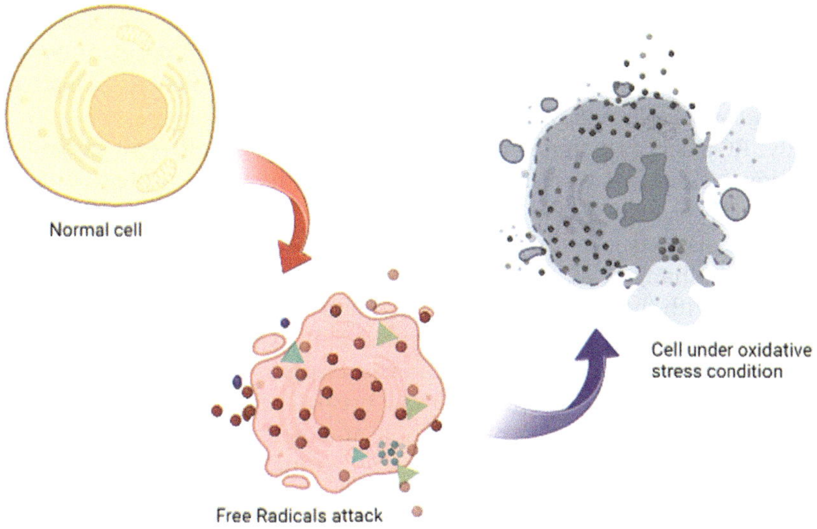

FIGURE 5.1 Oxidative stress condition of cells due to the attack of free radicals.

published on the biochemistry of OS gives more details about prooxidants' exogenous and endogenous precursors and a comprehensive understanding of antioxidants and prooxidants (Sies, 1986). Finally, a more concise definition of OS was given by Sies et al., stating that OS is the condition of misbalance between antioxidants and oxidants on the side of oxidants, resulting in disturbance of redox signaling pathway and prevent and/or molecular harm (Fig. 5.1) (Sies, 2019).

5.2.1 ROS and its role in OS

ROS indicates the ROS generated after the biotransformation reaction. In a normal physiological state, the ROS generation is well balanced by the corresponding amount of their depletion by antioxidants (Finkel and Holbrook, 2000). ROS extensively produced in the cell organelles such as peroxisomes, endoplasmic reticulum, and mostly in mitochondria (Murphy, 2009). The controlled ROS generation is required to maintain the process of homeostasis. An enhanced oxidant level has harmful effects on cells, like provoking and initiating several signaling pathways and oxidation of different components of cells such as lipids, proteins, and carbohydrates. These effects are associated with diseases like aging and diabetes (Forbes et al., 2008; Finkel and Holbrook, 2000; Kumawat et al., 2020). As mentioned earlier, ROS consists of a family of molecules like H_2O_2, hydroxyl radical, peroxynitrite, nitric acid, superoxide anion hydrochloric acid, and other radicals. The radicals like superoxide and hydroxyl radicals are highly unstable.

Furthermore, hydrogen peroxide and other radicals freely circulate and have a longer life (Sies, 1991). Interestingly, distinctive exogenous sources like ionizing radiation, ultraviolet light, toxins found in the environment, chemotherapeutic agents, and inflammatory mediators such as cytokines can initiate ROS generation (Finkel and Holbrook, 2000). Several investigations confirmed that many intracellular ROS production is developed from mitochondria.

However, only about 4% of oxygen is transformed into radical formation (Lenaz et al., 2002). Besides catalase, glutathione peroxidase, and superoxide dismutase, other antioxidants consist of vitamin E, flavonoids, vitamin C, glutathione, and carotenoids construct other antioxidants (Finkel and Holbrook, 2000).

Additionally, ROS acts as a signaling molecule by activating different signaling pathways and transcription factors like tyrosine kinases, mitogen-activated protein kinases, activator protein-1, specificity protein-1, and nuclear factor-kB, which results in the modulation of inflammation, fibrosis, cell growth and differentiation, and angiogenesis (Ha et al., 2008). In context with OS, Zhang et al. studied the anticancer drugs effects on the progression of OS, which is linked with the repair of DNA and alteration in biotransformation. With the utilization of the cellular model, it has been revealed that ROS generation starts with a single dose of anticancer drugs such as doxorubicin and cisplatin. The levels of ROS correspond to the construction of double-stranded DNA breaks. Interestingly, the knockdown of BRCA1 is related to homologous recombination and aggregation of ROS. The generation of ROS associated with inflammatory mediators levels includes interlukin-6, tumor necrosis factor, and interleukin-1β. It can be concluded from the study DNA construction is associated with biotransformation alteration, and several side effects were observed due to the production of OS (Zhang et al., 2022).

5.2.2 The antioxidant guardians of cells

The cellular defense mechanism involves an antioxidant system that helps to arrest, interfere with, and restore oxidative damage. This kind of defense system involves quenchers and non-enzymatic scavengers called antioxidants. Additionally, the enzymes like hydroxy-peroxidases, superoxide dismutase, and catalases are also involved (Koch et al., 2004; Koehler et al., 2006). The glutathione is widely present as intracellular nonprotein thiol, which is responsible for reducing disulfide bonds generated inside cytoplasmic proteins via acting as an electron donor. Glutathione-based complexes like thioredoxin GSH and GSH-S transferase contribute to most of the redox buffer in the cytosol. Mitochondrial GSH constitutes about 10%–15% of total GSH in the liver and renal proximal tubule. Apart from this, glutathione peroxidase (GPx) is present in two different types in the mitochondria, which are mainly phospholipid hydroperoxide (PHGPx) and GPx1. The PHGPx is inducible and catalyzes phospholipid hydroperoxide regeneration by utilizing the GSH-reducing potential, which is available in the cytosol. On the other hand, GPx1 is present in the mitochondrial matrix.

Moreover, superoxide dismutase (SOD) is available in three forms, mainly SOD1, SOD2, and SOD3. SOD1 is Cu/Zn SOD present in intermembrane space and cytoplasm. Whereas SOD2 is manganese SOD present in the mitochondrial matrix, and SOD3 is extracellular localization of Cu/Zn SOD. SOD promotes superoxide eradication by enhancing the spontaneous dismutation rate constant (Pereira et al., 2012).

5.3 Activation of ROS via signaling pathways in drug-induced OS

The production of ROS in cellular organelles such as chloroplast or mitochondria results in nuclear transcriptome alteration, showing that necessary information must be passed from these cellular compartments to the nucleus; however, the signal identity that transmits information remains unclear. ROS affects gene expression through its three-principal mode of action like catalase activity, SOD activity, and glutathione peroxidase activity. Some ROS sensors may be generated to promote signaling cascades that are ultimately responsible for gene expression. Consequently, the signaling pathway components may be oxidized by ROS. Additionally, ROS can alter the expression of a gene by changing and targeting the transcription factors activity (Apel and Hirt, 2004).

5.3.1 ROS in mitogen-activated protein kinase (MAPK) signaling pathways

MAPK signaling components in rice and Arabidopsis genomes are extraordinarily complicated, with over 100 MAPK, MAPKK, and MAPKKK genes in both plants, according to sequence analysis. Signaling modules of MAPK are involved in eliciting stress, hormone, and cytokinesis responses. H_2O_2 stimulates the MAPKs, MPK3, and MPK6 in Arabidopsis via MAPKKK ANP1. Freezing, heat shock, and salt stress tolerance were all improved when ANP1 was overexpressed in transgenic plants (Kovtun et al., 2000). Similarly, H_2O_2 is also responsible for enhancing the Arabidopsis nucleoside diphosphate kinase 2 expression (Moon et al., 2003). Because NDPK2 can interact with and activate the MAPKs, MPK3, and MPK6, the impact of nucleoside-diphosphate kinase-2 (NDPK2) may be mediated by them. It concludes that different stress conditions can promote ROS generation, which activates MAPK signaling pathways.

5.3.2 ROS generation of transcription factors

The ROS-induced gene expression mechanism in prokaryotes was compared. Plants and fungi may have similar processes (Georgiou, 2002). In the case of *E. coli.*, the factor OxyR has vital importance in oxidative-induced signaling (Zheng et al., 1998). Similarly, Yap1 plays the same role in budding yeast. Yap1 and OxyR are the transcription factors that regulate gene expression due to OS conditions. ROS controls the activity of various transcription factors like Yap1 and OxyR by covalent modifications of cysteine thiol groups in Yap1 and OxyR. However, the distinct difference between Yap1 and OxyR is that budding yeast transcription factors cannot sense ROS directly. Still, it can be possible via the activity of Gpx3, which act as peroxiredoxin and hydroperoxides.

Moreover, the gene expression based on OS may be regulated through transcription factors interactions with distinct OS-sensitive cis-elements in the promoters of these genes. It has been seen that OS-sensitive elements are found in animals, yeast, and plants. Gene expression induced with H_2O_2 in Arabidopsis microarray study reveals putative H_2O_2-responsive cis-elements in genes regulated by H_2O_2 (Desikan et al., 2001).

5.4 Drug-induced organ-increased cellular OS

Toxicity induced by chemical moiety is a vital concern; however, this can be significantly influenced by many factors (Gupta et al., 2022b). To overcome these toxicity effects, a deep understanding of the signal toxicity concept and its consequences on human health is highly

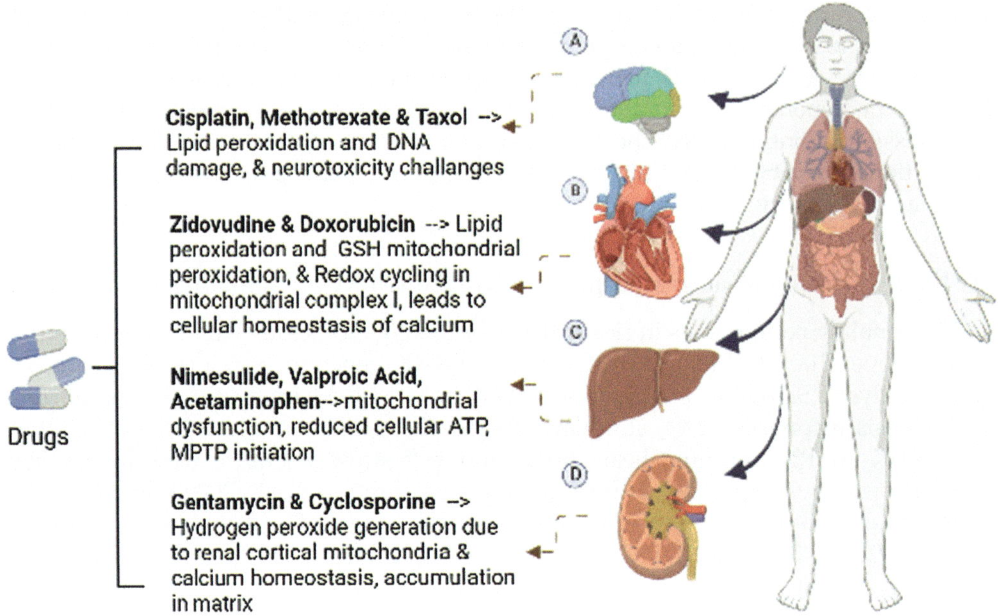

FIGURE 5.2 Drug-induced organ-specific OS.

needed (Tiwari et al., 2022; Tekade et al., 2022; Gupta et al., 2022a). In recent times, several methods and models have been utilized to identify the toxicity effect of drugs (Rajpoot et al., 2022a; Gupta et al., 2022c; Asati et al., 2022). Some therapeutics can exhibit significant cellular OS to different organs (e.g., liver, heart, kidney, etc.). Few significant toxicity effects caused by therapeutic agents are discussed in this section (Fig. 5.2).

5.4.1 Liver

Most therapeutic agent produces hepatic toxicity, which is a significant challenge for the pharmaceutical industry. In addition, the pharmacokinetics (Tambe et al., 2021b) and toxicokinetic (Rajpoot et al., 2022b, 2022c) properties of therapeutic molecules also have a significant effect on inducing toxicity in the body. However, it was revealed from various studies that idiosyncratic liver toxicity induced by the drug may be initiated in parts by OS (Boelsterli, 2002; Tafazoli et al., 2005). Various drugs, namely acetaminophen, valproic acid, nimesulide, are concerned with drug-initiated hepatic injury via mitochondrial dysfunction, reduced cellular ATP, and initiation of MPTP (Stirnimann et al., 2010). The drug acetaminophen toxicity produces by the reactive metabolite generation (NAPQI), which reduces GSH and attaches to mitochondrial protein. Consequently, it starts mitochondrial OS with peroxynitrite production via the amplification of c-Jun-N-terminal kinase initiation, resulting in damage of DNA in mitochondria leading to injury of cells or death (Jaeschke and Bajt, 2006; Jaeschke et al., 2011). Initially, GSH first catches NAPQI, and the GSH adduct is eliminated. Moreover, after GSH reduces, NAPQI reacts with proteins to produce acetaminophen adduct.

Furthermore, valproic acid, a widely used antiepileptic drug, is concerned with hepatotoxicity issues because of microvesicular steatosis. The OS mechanism in the hepatotoxicity pathogenesis produced by valproic acid was reported. Various reports show distinct modifications in OS markers. Additionally, when combined with valproic acid, hepatocyte imaging exhibits enhanced ROS production (Chang and Abbott, 2006).

The effects of rifampicin-isoniazid (INH-RIF)-induced liver damage on liver OS and inflammatory reaction were examined in research on the polyphenolic-rich extract of Crocus sativus L. petals (CSP). In contrast to silymarin, which was given in a recommended dose for 14 days, the INH-RIF was given in a range of doses to Wistar rats. Histological examinations have revealed that group II compared to group I exhibits prominent hepatocellular necrosis and inflammation as well as a modification in the normal architecture of the liver. In group III, silymarin therapy stopped all histological aberrations produced by INH-RIF. Group III has the most remarkable rate of hepatocyte development, demonstrating strong hepatoprotective action. Similar to group III, group V also experienced substantial recovery; however, it was less pronounced and more notable than group III (Fig. 5.3) (Wali et al., 2020).

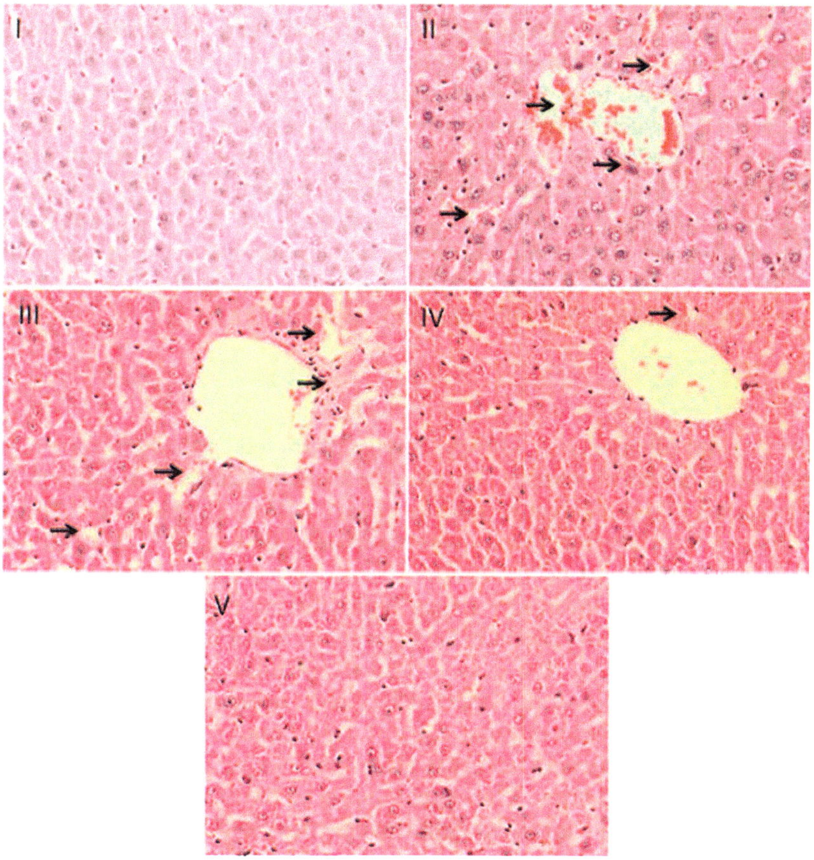

FIGURE 5.3 Effect of various CSP dosages on the histoarchitecture of the liver in INH-RIF-induced liver damage. Several test groups are shown in micrographs of colon histopathological sections staining; group I showed the typical integrated cellular architecture. The characteristic cellular disintegration of INH-RIF poisoning is seen in group II. CSP therapy provided a defense against INH-RIF-induced histopathological damage in groups III, IV, and V. *Reproduced with permission from Wali, A. F., Pillai, J. R., AL Dhaheri, Y., Rehman, M. U., Shoaib, A., Sarheed, O., et al., 2020. Crocus sativus L. Extract containing polyphenols modulates oxidative stress and inflammatory response against anti-tuberculosis drugs-induced liver injury. Plants, 9, 167. under Creative Commons Attribution (CC BY) license Copyright © 2020.*

5.4.2 Heart

The free radicals agglomeration in the peripheral blood has an adverse impact on the heart system, as in pathophysiological states and aging (D'Alessandro et al., 2011). An antiretroviral drug-like zidovudine is used widely in the therapy of acquired immunodeficiency syndrome (AIDs), an inhibitor of replication of human immunodeficiency virus (HIV). However, a limitation associated with zidovudine is cardiotoxicity. Zidovudine therapy also results in the peroxidation of lipids and GSH mitochondrial peroxidation (de la Asunción et al., 1998). Dilatory supplements like vitamin E and vitamin C prevent mitochondrial OS conditions. Moreover, therapeutic agents like doxorubicin are widely employed as anticancer agents in various cancer therapies. However, it is concerned with dose-related myocardial damage, potentiating congestive heart failure (Lefrak et al., 1973). Doxorubicin may cause OS via the mechanism of redox cycling in mitochondrial complex I, resulting in harm to mitochondria and destruction of cellular and mitochondrial homeostasis of calcium (Sardão et al., 2009; Oliveira et al., 2004).

In a study, rats having type 1 diabetes mellitus (T1DM) were examined by researchers for cardioprotective impacts of curcumin nanoparticle (NC) therapy compared to that of conventional curcumin (CC) on acute myocardial infarction (AMI). Histological analyses indicated healthy myocardial architecture in the control group rats (Fig. 5.4A). In contrast, the AMI group animals had multifocal necrosis along with diffuse infiltration of leukocytes (Fig. 5.4B). The T1DM group of rats solely exhibited blood stasis (Fig. 5.4C). The T1DM-AMI group showed multifocal necrosis along with widespread leukocyte infiltration and stasis (Fig. 5.4D). Rats given traditional curcumin had multifocal necrosis and inflammatory leukocyte infiltration, whereas rats given NC displayed localized subendocardial necrosis and leukocyte infiltration (Fig. 5.4G,H) (Boarescu et al., 2021).

5.4.3 Kidney

In comparison with other organs, kidneys have a restricted capacity to repair. Kidneys are highly vulnerable to chemical toxicity. Various therapeutic agents cause about 20% of individuals and hospitals to receive events of acute kidney failure. On the other hand, in geriatric individuals, drug-induced nephrotoxicity was about 66% (Betton et al., 2005; Naughton, 2008; Kumawat et al., 2020; Rajpoot et al., 2021a). The classes of various drugs like anticancer agents, nonsteroidal anti-inflammatory drugs (NSAIDs), immunosuppressants, and antibiotics are potentiating renal injury, and OS is the primary factor in producing toxicity. The antibiotics like gentamycin belong to a class of aminoglycosides and generate kidney toxicity (Cuzzocrea et al., 2002; Walker et al., 1999). It has been revealed that gentamycin produces hydrogen peroxide with the help of renal cortical mitochondria (Walker and Shah, 1987). It has been indicated from studies as iron was released from renal cortical mitochondria and proven with in vivo investigations. The outcomes show that the radicals such as hydroxyl radicals or other oxidants have a role in gentamycin-provoked kidney failure.

Similarly, cyclosporine is an immunosuppressant used in immunosuppression, transplantation of organs, and increasing patient survival (Holzmacher et al., 2005; Tariq et al., 1999). Since it has limitations like it produces nephrotoxicity proven from many reports. Kidney toxicity may be associated with decreased blood flow to the kidney, which results in

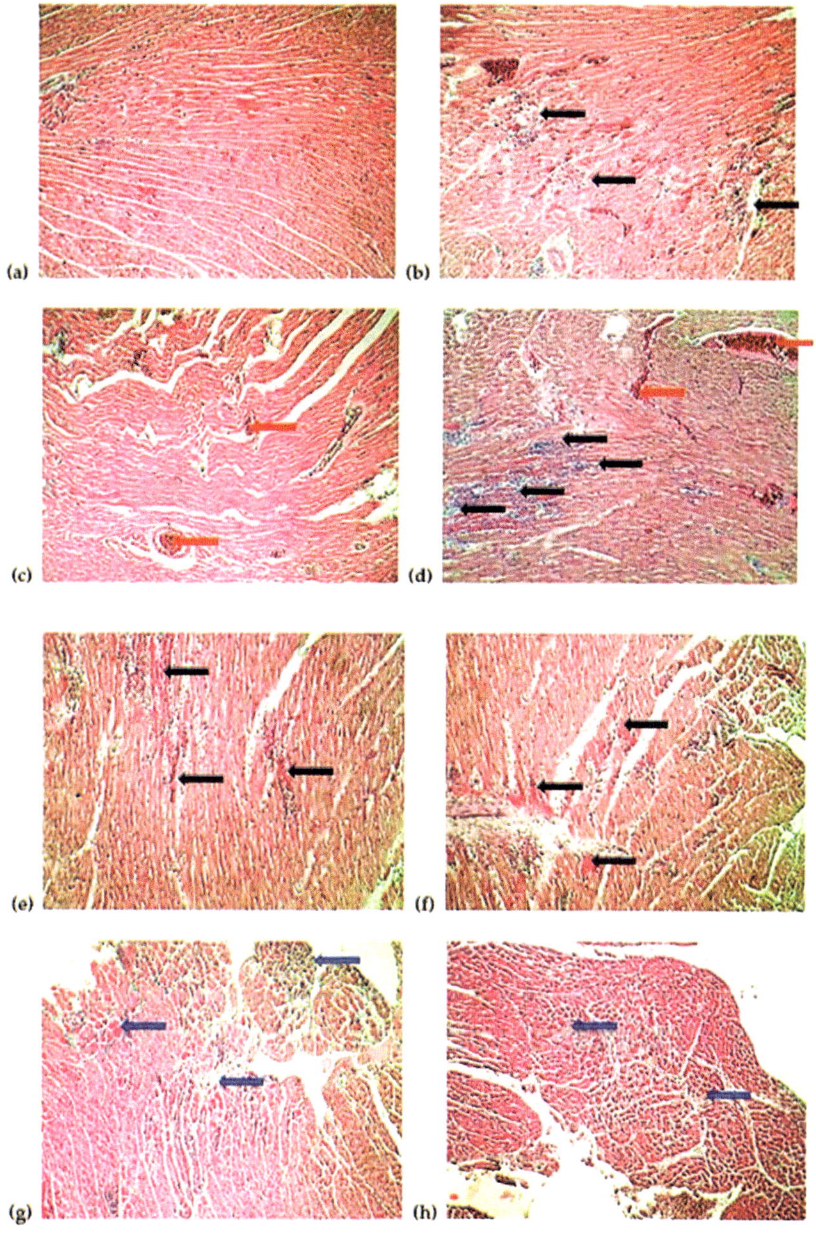

FIGURE 5.4 Heart tissue histopathological investigations. (A) Normal myocardium architecture; (B) AMI (multifocal necrosis with widespread leukocyte infiltration; black arrow); (C) T1DM (blood stasis in a constricted blood vessel containing readily identifiable integral RBCs; red arrow); (D) T1DM-AMI (multifocal necrosis with widespread, leukocyte infiltration; black arrow); E S-T. *Adapted with permission from reference Boarescu, P.-M., Boarescu, I., Bulboacă, A. E., Bocşan, I. C., Pop, R. M., Gheban, D., 2021. Multi-organ protective effects of curcumin nanoparticles on drug-induced acute myocardial infarction in rats with type 1 diabetes mellitus. Appl. Sci., 11, 5497. under Creative Commons Attribution (CC BY) license. Copyright: © 2021.*

hypoxia-based injury encouraged by enhanced production of ROS (Tariq et al., 1999). It has been revealed from previous studies that cyclosporine provoked renal toxicity through modifications of calcium homeostasis, enhanced calcium accumulation in the matrix, and enhanced ROS generation (Simon et al., 2001).

In a study, rats with T1DM were used by researchers for the investigation to confirm the nephroprotective influence of NC therapy in comparison to the traditional CC on AMI. The kidneys' typical architecture was visible during a histopathological analysis of the control group's kidneys (Fig. 5.5A). Blood stasis was detected in rats having AMI (Fig. 5.5B). On the other hand, the rats in the T1DM as well as T1DM and AMI groups both developed glomerular collapse and blood stasis (Fig. 5.5C and D). Delivery of turmeric lessened kidney histology stasis (Fig. 5.5E and F). Similar outcomes were seen in the group that provided NC following the delivery of STZ (Fig. 5.5G), but the group that got NC earlier had healthy kidneys (Fig. 5.5H) (Boarescu et al., 2021).

5.4.4 Brain

The brain is an organ that is exceptionally susceptible to damage by free radicals as it has a greater oxygen consumption rate, a wide supply of transition metals, large content of unsaturated lipids, and lesser regeneration power compared to other types of tissues (Jovanović and Jovanović, 2011). Many anticancer agents such as cisplatin, methotrexate, and taxol produce neurotoxicity and may be involved in minor modifications in neuropathy, consciousness, paralysis, cerebral infarctions, and other significant complications.

Cisplatin, a platinum-derived anticancer agent, has restrictions in application because of the peripheral nervous system genesis dysfunction, which may complicate and continue over the long term. It has been illustrated that lignin, an antioxidant used with cisplatin, and cisplatin has detrimental effects on the brain, such as peroxidation of lipids and DNA damage were inhibited (Giridharan et al., 2012). Moreover, it has been seen from histological investigations of the peripheral nervous system that antioxidant alpha-tocopherol plays a crucial role in protecting mice from various neurologic damage initiated by cisplatin treatment. Other anticancer agents, such as methotrexate and folic acid antagonists, are used in various cancer therapies. Since methotrexate is also concerned with neurotoxicity challenges. In this context, Uzar et al. illustrated that caffeic acid phenyl ether arrested the peroxidation of lipids promoted by methotrexate in rats. Similarly, in another study, it has been observed that chlorogenic acid helps to prevent higher peroxidation of lipids after the methotrexate treatment (Vardi et al., 2012; Uzar et al., 2006).

5.5 Various techniques to study OS-induced drug toxicity

The ROS has been generated during the OS conditions. However, due to their short duration, relatively low steady-state concentrations, and highly reactive nature, the lack of accurate and repeatable methods to assess ROS is a difficulty in the research of OS. Apart from this, to characterize each ROS molecule's biological activity, its concentration must be explicitly measured in the presence of other oxygen metabolites. OS can be determined by various

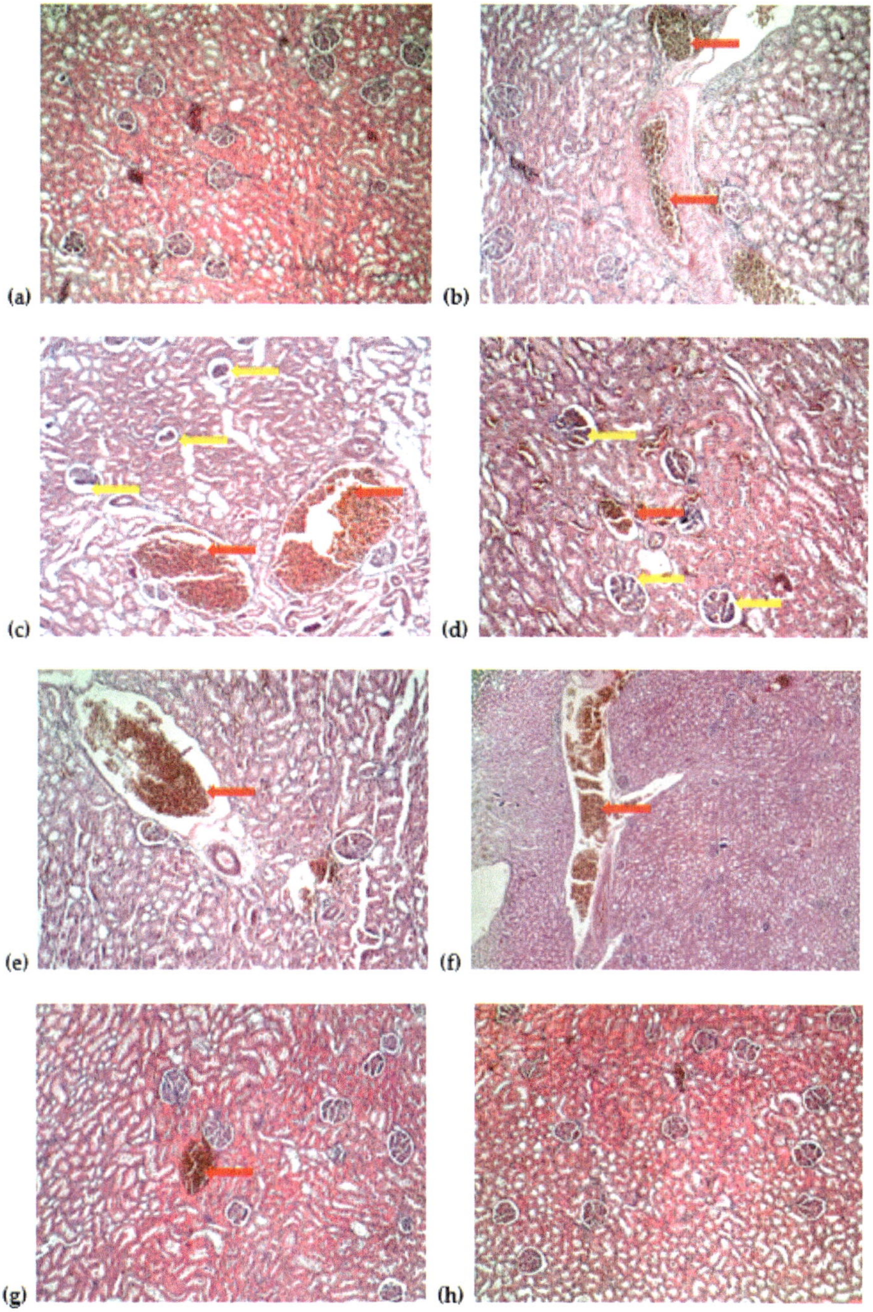

FIGURE 5.5 Histopathology of the renal tissue. (A) The kidneys' typical structure, (B) AMI (blood stasis in a constricted blood vessel containing readily visible integrated RBCs (*red arrow*)), (C) T1DM (glomerular collapse (*yellow arrow*) and blood stasis in a constricted blood vessel having visible integral RBCs (*red arrow*)), (D) T1DM-AMI (glomerular collapse (*yellow arrow*) and blood stasis in a constricted blood vessel containing readily identifiable integrated RBCs (*red arrow*)), (E) S-T1DM-CC-AMI (blood stasis (*red arrow*)), (F) CC-T1DM-CC-AMI (blood stasis (*red arrow*)), (G) S-T1DM-NC-AMI (blood stasis (*red arrow*)), (H) NC-T1DM-NC-AMI (*the kidneys' typical structure*). *Adapted with permission from reference Boarescu, P.-M., Boarescu, I., Bulboacă, A. E., Bocşan, I. C., Pop, R. M., Gheban, D., et al., 2021. Multi-organ protective effects of curcumin nanoparticles on drug-induced acute myocardial infarction in rats with type 1 diabetes mellitus. Appl. Sci. 11, 5497. under Creative Commons Attribution (CC BY) license. Copyright: © 2021.*

techniques, which mainly involve in vitro as well as in vivo techniques. They are detailed as follows (Noh and Ha, 2011).

5.5.1 ROS in vitro detection techniques

The ideal OS marker should possess two prime requirements the marker should be increased when exposed to enhanced inducers of OS, and the marker should remain stable in the absence of OS. Interestingly, the fluorometric assays are carried out with maximum sensitivity for detecting OS in living cells (Chen et al., 2011; Kuznetsov et al., 2011).

In the fluorometric assays, cells are primarily treated with a nano-fluorescent compound which becomes fluorescent on reacting with ROS. Many kinds of classical and novel dyes can be used for the detection of ROS. The 2′,7′-dichlorodihydrofluorescein diacetate (H_2 DCF) is a hydrophobic compound transformed into a hydrophilic nonfluorescent derivative by the enzyme esterase which eliminates acetate groups. In the presence of intracellular ROS, the membrane-impermeable H_2DCF is quickly oxidized to highly fluorescent 2′,7′-dichloro-fluorescein (DCF). Moreover, the DCF method of ROS detection can be used for mitochondrial as well as non-mitochondrial ROS detection (Kuznetsov et al., 2011). However, the DCF distinct disadvantage is that when it is oxidized to its fluorescent form, the substance begins to leak out of the cells. In addition, the DCF intracellular half-life is only minutes. Hence, it restricts its application to fluorescence-activated cell sorting or confocal microscopy and microplate reader assay methods in intact cells (Keller et al., 2004). Interestingly, the metals such as Fe^{2+} initiate the oxidation of DCFH in oxygen and hydrogen peroxide presence (Kalyanaraman et al., 2012).

Similarly, a dye like dihydrocalcein-AM is easily permeated to cell membranes. It results in oxidized green fluorescence calcein that has excellent retaining characteristics in cells which intact with the membranes. Compared with DCFDA dye, calcein exhibits are less prone to photo-oxidation, which may be useful while using microscopy. Moreover, MitoSox is a fluorogenic HE derivative dye that emits red fluorescence when oxidized directly by superoxide anion. Its phosphonium is positively charged, which enables it to be targeted to mitochondria (Vardi et al., 2012; Zielonka and Kalyanaraman, 2010). MitoSox aggregates in the mitochondria as a function of mitochondrial membrane potential and fluorescence when oxidized and then binds to mitochondrial DNA. From the number of studies, MitoSox has been authenticated by flow cytometry and confocal microscopy for specific detection of mitochondrial superoxide generation in endothelial cells. Fibroblasts, keratinocytes, cardiomyocytes, isolated blood vessels, and neuronal cells (Mukhopadhyay and Fox, 1998).

Interestingly, in recent years, a Coumarin-Neutral Red nanoprobe was developed and appears to be helpful in detecting hydroxyl radicals. However, it shows very weak sensitivity to other ROS like, hydrogen peroxide, superoxide anion, hypochlorite, and singlet O_2 (Ganea et al., 2011). In addition, various approaches are available for detecting ROS, such as electron spin resonance spectroscopy, redox proteomics, and imaging techniques (Shete et al., 2022).

5.5.2 ROS in vivo detection techniques

Compared to in vitro detection of ROS techniques, the approaches to detecting in vivo ROS are still deficient. Samples from treated animals can be taken and evaluated for markers like antioxidant enzymes and the status of GSH, as well as downstream processes like protein and lipid oxidation and oxidation of DNA. Additionally, samples can be investigated by available kits and plate reader techniques. Long back in 2005, ROS could be measured noninvasive by quantifying the OS damage in humans via exhaled aldehydes breath analysis which is the free radical damage indicators in the human body (Smith et al., 2007). This is the individual device in use in humans, and it's utilized to track how efficient antioxidant pills and exercise are at lowering free radical levels. Interestingly, scientists have designed precisely sensitive and specific nanoparticles based on peroxalate. These synthesized nanoparticles are useful for in vivo detection due to their wavelength emission (460–630 nm), and show specificity and high sensitivity (Lee et al., 2007).

5.6 Approaches to investigate antioxidant status

The status of cellular antioxidants produced can be easily determined by determining the activity of GSH peroxidase, catalase, GSH reductase, SOD as well as decreased GSH levels (Lautraite et al., 2003). The conventional techniques to assess GSH determination consists of a biochemical assay based on the compound reaction like o-phthalaldehyde or 5,5′-dithio-bis-2-nitrobenzoic acid, which directly produced fluorescent or chromophoric compounds determined by fluorescent or Ultraviolet/visible spectroscopy, respectively. Since these studies are more time-consuming and do not go for high throughput experimental studies. On the other hand, GSH can be easily determined by well-known analytical techniques like high-performance liquid chromatography (HPLC). However, it is time-consuming and has a higher cost (Redegeld et al., 1988).

Besides, fluorescent-activated cell sorting (FACS) and labeling the intracellular thiols with fluorescent compounds are accepted alternative techniques. Recently, a combination of microchip electrophoresis with laser-promoted fluorescence was employed to determine mitochondria's hydrogen peroxide and GSH levels. Moreover, the catalase activity can be assessed by utilizing assays depending on changes in the H_2O_2 absorbance at 240 nm. Additionally, various commercial kits are accessible for GSH reductase, catalase, SOD, and GSH peroxidase (Outten and Culotta, 2004; Oyanagui, 1984; Kowaltowski et al., 2000). Table 5.1 explains various kinds of oxidative damage and markers used to determine OS (Pereira et al., 2012).

5.7 Animal models suitable to study OS

The animal models are developed to quantify OS toxicity via the knockout of vital antioxidant enzymes. Research can be conducted utilizing exogenously delivered toxicants to elicit OS, examining and characterizing the animal model's reaction to the exogenous insult. Another option is using genetic models with the persistently pro-oxidative environment inside specific tissues or cells to produce pathology; as an outcome, e.g., heterozygous SOD2 knockout mouse ($SOD2^{+/-}$). These animals had a half decrease in SOD activity and a phenotype that indicates impaired mitochondrial function and enhanced oxidative damage, such as

TABLE 5.1 Ex vivo and in vitro determination of OS.

Category of damage	Markers	References
Peroxidation of lipids	8-Isoprostane, malondialdehyde, 4-hydroxynoneal	Mas-Bargues et al. (2021)
Oxidation/ nitration of proteins	3-Nitrotyrosine, advanced oxidation protein products, advanced glycation products, protein carbonyl content	Rabbani and Thornalley (2009)
RNA/DNA damage	UV DNA damage, 8-hydroxy guanosine, 8-hydroxy deoxyguanosine, double-strand DNA breaks	Figueroa-González and Pérez-Plasencia (2017)
Antioxidants	Superoxide dismutase, catalase, glutathione, total antioxidant capacity	Birben et al. (2012)
ROS	In vivo and in vitro ROS	Rabbani et al. (2018), More and Makola (2020)

a 30%–80% enhancement in mitochondrial and nuclear oxidation of DNA (8-oxo-dG). It can be used to investigate liver toxicity and toxicity that occurred due to zidovudine (Boelsterli and Hsiao, 2008).

Similarly, the λ-glutamyl-transpeptidase (GGT)-deficient mice eliminate a lot of GSH in their urine and have tissue-specific GSH depletion (Will et al., 2000). Consequently, it results in cataract development, growth suppression, variation in coat color, and early death of mice. Interestingly, incorporating N-acetylcysteine into GGT-deficient mice drinking water results in a phenotype alteration. These kinds of mice can be used to investigate cisplatin toxicity in the kidney, and oxidative damage can be quantified. Moreover, the homozygous Trx2 mouse is lethal, and a reduction in the Trx2 levels results in mitochondrial activity reduction by reduced levels of ATP, enhanced H_2O_2 formation, and a decline in OXPHOS activity (Perez et al., 2008). These mice have more significant oxidative damage to lipids, proteins, and DNA. Interestingly, they had high sensitivity to apoptosis and oxidative damage induced with diquat. Table 5.2 explains the different kinds of mouse models used to study OS (Pereira et al., 2012).

5.8 Antioxidative therapy in clinical trials

Clinical studies are significant to the progression of antioxidative therapy. The information regarding various clinical trials on antioxidant therapy is present at the http://www.ClinicalTrials.gov Website. The vitamins such as vitamin E, which has antioxidant activity, are frequently investigated for their antioxidant property as a dietary supplement in clinical trials for hepatic disease in phase 2/3. Besides that, the antioxidants like Coenzyme Q10 and zinc were also studied in phase 2. Some of the compounds which act as partial antioxidants, such as metadoxime, silymarin, and N-acetylcysteine, are investigated for nonalcoholic steatohepatitis (NASH) or adrenoleukodystrophy (ALD) in phase four clinical study (Li et al., 2015).

TABLE 5.2 Various mouse models used to investigate drug-induced OS.

Animal models	Type of dysregulation	Examples
Glutathione peroxidase $^{(+/-)}$ mouse model	Greatly sensitive to ROS producers, No increase in the oxidative damage basal levels Not exhibit any balancing antioxidant mechanisms	Ethanol, doxorubicin Acetaminophen
Thioredoxin 2 $^{(+/-)}$ mouse model	Reduction in mitochondrial activity by reduced ATP levels and enhanced H_2O_2 production with declining OXPHOS activity	Diquat
	Apoptosis, embryonic lethality	-
Manganese superoxide dismutase 2 $^{(+/-)}$ model	Enhanced oxidative damage and reduced mitochondrial activity	Methamphetamine, zidovudine
Catalase model $^{(+/-)}$	Slows the decomposing rate of extracellular H_2O_2	Ethanol
	Significant enhancement in oxidative damage due to photochemical reaction	
λ-Glutamyl-transpeptidase (GGT)-deficient mice	Excretion of glutathione in urine Glutathione depletion in specific tissues	Cisplatin, Bleomycin

Moreover, chocolate, green tea extract, and ginger have been employed as antioxidants for hepatic disease. Interestingly, resveratrol and quercetin have been isolated from plants and show antioxidant activity, used in hepatic disease in phase 3. Despite some encouraging findings from clinical trials, antioxidant therapy still has a long way to go. In contrast, many antioxidants are highly efficient for disease prevention or treatment in animal models. Still, they do not appear beneficial in humans for treating established diseases. Anti-TNF, for example, which has shown to be effective in animal models, does not appear to be helpful in humans with acute alcoholic hepatitis. Hence, translational research is of prime importance in the case of antioxidant therapy in the clinic (Li et al., 2015).

5.9 Opportunities for the future: personalized healthcare

In recent years, it has been indicated that it can be possible to employ ROS determination to anticipate potential phototoxicity produced by various chemicals (Onoue et al., 2008). Since there may be a distinct difference in susceptibility and severity of toxicity produced. Cisplatin-produced ototoxicity shows that it depends on dose as well as distinct interindividual differences in toxicity in individuals taking the same amount of cisplatin dose (Bokemeyer et al., 1998).

Besides that, it has been hypothesized that genetic factors play a crucial role in determining the vulnerability to the cisplatin effects. In a clinical study involving 173 individuals with testicular cancer, the glutathione-S-transferase (GST), genetic variants play a vital role in cisplatin-produced ototoxicity. It has been confirmed from the study that Val-GSTP1 proved to have a protective nature, while GSTM1 was found to be detrimental (Oldenburg et al., 2007). However, studies are ongoing to discover key genetic components responsible for cisplatin-produced ototoxicity (Mukherjea and Rybak, 2011). It may be helpful in the future to predict vulnerability to cisplatin-produced ototoxicity based on genetic mechanisms and applications to control the risk of ototoxicity in various individuals.

Similarly, it has been found that different protein variants are concerned with the metabolism and transport of doxorubicin, like SOD2 and SLC22A16 transporter (Bray et al., 2010; Glynn et al., 2009; Tambe et al., 2021e). Hence, the doxorubicin promoted redox imbalance, and genetic variation based on its cellular accumulation can be associated with its therapeutic activity as well as toxicity. Interestingly, the relationship between vulnerability to doxorubicin-promoted cardiac damage and BRCA2 status has been demonstrated (Singh et al., 2012). BRCA2 is a gene that encodes a protein entangled in the repair of chromosomal damage, and it is a signal of increased harm to ovarian and breast cancer. In the knockout mice depleting BRCA2 distinctively in cardiomyocytes, doxorubicin exposure was found in enhanced cardiotoxicity due to the higher levels of cytochrome *c* release, accumulation of *p*53, and apoptosis in cardiomyocytes (Singh et al., 2012). The above examples, such as cisplatin and doxorubicin, demonstrate the ability of genetic variations to evaluate vulnerability to the toxicity of two drugs for which OS can be a vital contributor to adverse drug events.

5.10 Conclusion

The described drugs in this chapter show the potential for oxidative damage and have a substantial role in human toxicity. Still, it is unclear how OS affects the developing safety profile of newer medications. Therefore, additional research is needed to shed light on a person's sensitivity to particular ROS-dependent mechanisms of toxicity. Recognizing these individual variations and the toxicity potential of oxidants is becoming more critical, not just for current medicines but also for personalizing clinical drug research.

5.11 List of abbreviations

AIDs acquired immunodeficiency syndrome
ALD adrenoleukodystrophy
AMI acute myocardial infarction
CC curcumin
CSP Crocus sativus L. petals
DCF 2′,7′-dichlorofluorescein
FACS fluorescent-activated cell sorting
GGT λ-glutamyl-transpeptidase
GPx glutathione peroxidase
GST glutathione-S-transferase
H_2 DCF 2′,7′-dichlorodihydrofluorescein diacetate
H_2O_2 hydrogen peroxide
HIV human immunodeficiency virus
HPLC high-performance liquid chromatography
INH-RIF rifampicin-isoniazid
MAPK mitogen-activated protein kinase

NASH nonalcoholic steatohepatitis
NC curcumin nanoparticle
NDPK2 nucleoside-diphosphate kinase-2
NSAIDs nonsteroidal anti-inflammatory drugs
OS oxidative stress
PHGPx phospholipid hydroperoxide
RNS reactive nitrogen species
ROS reactive oxygen species
SOD superoxide dismutase
T1DM type 1 diabetes mellitus

References

Achanta, N.S.K., Rajpoot, K., Tekade, R.K., 2021. Drug metabolic kinetics. In: Tekade, R.K. (Ed.), Biopharmaceutics and Pharmacokinetics Considerations, 1. Elsevier, Academic Press, pp. 335–353.

Anup, N., Desai, N., Rajpoot, K., Tekade, R.K., 2021a. Kinetics of maternal–fetal drug transfer. In: Tekade, R.K. (Ed.), Biopharmaceutics and Pharmacokinetics Considerations.

Anup, N., Gadeval, A., Rajpoot, K., Tekade, R.K., 2021b. Software used in ADME computation. In: Tekade, R.K. (Ed.), Biopharmaceutics and Pharmacokinetics Considerations. Elsevier, Academic Press.

Anup, N., Rajpoot, K., Tekade, R.K., 2021c. Overview of biopharmaceutics and pharmacokinetics. In: Tekade, R.K. (Ed.), Biopharmaceutics and Pharmacokinetics Considerations. Elsevier, Academic Press.

Apel, K., Hirt, H., 2004. Reactive oxygen species: metabolism, oxidative stress, and signal transduction. Annu. Rev. Plant Biol. 55, 373–399.

Asati, S., Pandey, V., Gour, V., Tiwari, R., Soni, V., Rajpoot, K., Tekade, M., Sharma, M.C., Tekade, R.K., 2022. Toxicity and toxicokinetic considerations in product development and drug research. Pharmacokinetics and Toxicokinetic Considerations, 2. Elsevier, pp. 401–424.

Betton, G.R., Kenne, K., Somers, R., Marr, A., 2005. Protein biomarkers of nephrotoxicity; a review and findings with cyclosporin A, a signal transduction kinase inhibitor and N-phenylanthranilic acid. Cancer. Biomarkers. 1, 59–67.

Birben, E., Sahiner, U.M., Sackesen, C., Erzurum, S., Kalayci, O., 2012. Oxidative stress and antioxidant defense. World Allergy Organ. J. 5, 9–19.

Boarescu, P.-M., Boarescu, I., Bulboacă, A.E., Bocşan, I.C., Pop, R.M., Gheban, D., Râjnoveanu, R.-M., Râjnoveanu, A., Rosian, S.H., Buzoianu, A.D., Bolboacă, S.D., 2021. Multi-organ protective effects of curcumin nanoparticles on drug-induced acute myocardial infarction in rats with type 1 diabetes mellitus. Appl. Sci. 11, 5497.

Boelsterli, U.A., 2002. Mechanisms of NSAID-induced hepatotoxicity: focus on nimesulide. Drug Saf. 25, 633–648.

Boelsterli, U.A., Hsiao, C.-J.J., 2008. The heterozygous Sod2+/− mouse: modeling the mitochondrial role in drug toxicity. Drug Discov. Today 13, 982–988.

Bokemeyer, C., Berger, C.C., Hartmann, J.T., Kollmannsberger, C., Schmoll, H.J., Kuczyk, M.A., Kanz, L., 1998. Analysis of risk factors for cisplatin-induced ototoxicity in patients with testicular cancer. Br. J. Cancer 77, 1355–1362.

Bray, J., Sludden, J., Griffin, M., Cole, M., Verrill, M., Jamieson, D., Boddy, A., 2010. Influence of pharmacogenetics on response and toxicity in breast cancer patients treated with doxorubicin and cyclophosphamide. Br. J. Cancer 102, 1003–1009.

Chang, T.K., Abbott, F.S., 2006. Oxidative stress as a mechanism of valproic acid-associated hepatotoxicity. Drug Metab. Rev. 38, 627–639.

Chen, X., Tian, X., Shin, I., Yoon, J., 2011. Fluorescent and luminescent probes for detection of reactive oxygen and nitrogen species. Chem. Soc. Rev. 40, 4783–4804.

Choudhary, D., Goykar, H., Rajpoot, K., Tekade, R.K., 2021. Chronopharmacokinetics. In: Tekade, R.K. (Ed.), Biopharmaceutics and Pharmacokinetics Considerations, 2. Elsevier, Academic Press, pp. 1–26.

Cuzzocrea, S., Mazzon, E., Dugo, L., Serraino, I., DI Paola, R., Britti, D., DE Sarro, A., Pierpaoli, S., Caputi, A., Masini, E., Salvemini, D., 2002. A role for superoxide in gentamicin-mediated nephropathy in rats. Eur. J. Pharmacol. 450, 67–76.

D'alessandro, A., Rinalducci, S., Zolla, L., 2011. Redox proteomics and drug development. J. Proteonomics 74, 2575–2595.

DE LA Asunción, J.G., DEL Olmo, M.L., Sastre, J., Millán, A., Pellín, A., Pallardó, F.V., Viña, J., 1998. AZT treatment induces molecular and ultrastructural oxidative damage to muscle mitochondria. Prevention by antioxidant vitamins. J. Clin. Invest. 102, 4–9.

Deavall, D.G., Martin, E.A., Horner, J.M., Roberts, R., 2012. Drug-induced oxidative stress and toxicity. J. Toxicol. 2012, 645460.

Deponte, M., 2013. Glutathione catalysis and the reaction mechanisms of glutathione-dependent enzymes. Biochim. Biophys. Acta 1830, 3217–3266.

Desai, N., Koppisetti, H., Rajpoot, K., Tekade, M., Sharma, M.C., Tekade, R.K., 2021. Influence of fever on pharmacokinetics of drugs. In: Tekade, R.K. (Ed.), Biopharmaceutics and Pharmacokinetics Considerations, , I ed.1. Elsevier, pp. 451–463.

Desikan, R., S, A.H.-M., Hancock, J.T., Neill, S.J., 2001. Regulation of the Arabidopsis transcriptome by oxidative stress. Plant Physiol. 127, 159–172.

Devasagayam, T.P., Tilak, J.C., Boloor, K.K., Sane, K.S., Ghaskadbi, S.S., Lele, R.D., 2004. Free radicals and antioxidants in human health: current status and future prospects. J. Assoc. Phys. India 52, 794–804.

Figueroa-González, G., Pérez-Plasencia, C., 2017. Strategies for the evaluation of DNA damage and repair mechanisms in cancer. Oncol. Lett. 13, 3982–3988.

Finkel, T., Holbrook, N.J., 2000. Oxidants, oxidative stress and the biology of ageing. Nature 408, 239–247.

Forbes, J.M., Coughlan, M.T., Cooper, M.E., 2008. Oxidative stress as a major culprit in kidney disease in diabetes. Diabetes 57, 1446–1454.

Gadekar, V., Borade, Y., Kannaujia, S., Rajpoot, K., Anup, N., Tambe, V., Kalia, K., Tekade, R.K., 2021. Nanomedicines accessible in the market for clinical interventions. J. Controlled Release 330, 372–397.

Ganea, G.M., Kolic, P.E., EL-Zahab, B., Warner, I.M., 2011. Ratiometric coumarin-neutral red (CONER) nanoprobe for detection of hydroxyl radicals. Anal. Chem. 83, 2576–2581.

Georgiou, G., 2002. How to flip the (redox) switch. Cell 111, 607–610.

Giridharan, V.V., Thandavarayan, R.A., Bhilwade, H.N., Ko, K.M., Watanabe, K., Konishi, T., 2012. Schisandrin B, attenuates cisplatin-induced oxidative stress, genotoxicity and neurotoxicity through modulating NF-κB pathway in mice. Free Radic. Res. 46, 50–60.

Glynn, S.A., Boersma, B.J., Howe, T.M., Edvardsen, H., Geisler, S.B., Goodman, J.E., Ridnour, L.A., Lonning, P.E., Borresen-Dale, A.L., Naume, B., Kristensen, V.N., Chanock, S.J., Wink, D.A., Ambs, S., 2009. A mitochondrial target sequence polymorphism in manganese superoxide dismutase predicts inferior survival in breast cancer patients treated with cyclophosphamide. Clin. Cancer Res. 15, 4165–4173.

Gorain, B., Choudhury, H., Tekade, R.K., Karan, S., Jaisankar, P., Pal, T.K., 2016. Comparative biodistribution and safety profiling of olmesartan medoxomil oil-in-water oral nanoemulsion. Regul. Toxicol. Pharmacol. 82, 20–31.

Gupta, R., Polaka, S., Rajpoot, K., Tekade, M., Sharma, M.C., Tekade, R.K., 2022a. Importance of toxicity testing in drug discovery and research. In: Pharmacokinetics and Toxicokinetic Considerations. Academic Press, pp. 117–144.

Gupta, R., Rajpoot, K., Tekade, M., Sharma, M.C., Safavi, M., Tekade, R.K., 2022b. Factors influencing drug toxicity. In: Pharmacokinetics and Toxicokinetic Considerations. Academic Press, pp. 27–50.

Gupta, R., Rajpoot, K., Tekade, M., Sharma, M.C., Tekade, R.K., 2022c. Methods and models for in vitro toxicity. In: Pharmacokinetics and Toxicokinetic Considerations. Academic Press, pp. 145–174.

Ha, H., Hwang, I.A., Park, J.H., Lee, H.B., 2008. Role of reactive oxygen species in the pathogenesis of diabetic nephropathy. Diabetes Res. Clin. Pract. 82 (Suppl. 1), S42–S45.

Harrison, J.F., Hollensworth, S.B., Spitz, D.R., Copeland, W.C., Wilson, G.L., Ledoux, S.P., 2005. Oxidative stress-induced apoptosis in neurons correlates with mitochondrial DNA base excision repair pathway imbalance. Nucleic Acids Res. 33, 4660–4671.

Hayes, J.D., Dinkova-Kostova, A.T., Tew, K.D., 2020. Oxidative stress in cancer. Cancer Cell 38, 167–197.

Holzmacher, R., Kendziorski, C., Michael Hofman, R., Jaffery, J., Becker, B., Djamali, A., 2005. Low serum magnesium is associated with decreased graft survival in patients with chronic cyclosporin nephrotoxicity. Nephrol. Dial. Transplant. 20, 1456–1462.

Jaeschke, H., Bajt, M.L., 2006. Intracellular signaling mechanisms of acetaminophen-induced liver cell death. Toxicol. Sci. 89, 31–41.

Jaeschke, H., Mcgill, M.R., Williams, C.D., Ramachandran, A., 2011. Current issues with acetaminophen hepatotoxicity–a clinically relevant model to test the efficacy of natural products. Life Sci. 88, 737–745.

Jovanović, Z., Jovanović, S., 2011. Resistance of nerve cells to oxidative injury. Med. Pregl. 64, 386–391.

Kalyanaraman, B., Darley-Usmar, V., Davies, K.J., Dennery, P.A., Forman, H.J., Grisham, M.B., Mann, G.E., Moore, K., Roberts 2ND, L.J., Ischiropoulos, H., 2012. Measuring reactive oxygen and nitrogen species with fluorescent probes: challenges and limitations. Free Radic. Biol. Med. 52, 1–6.

Kalyane, D., Choudhary, D., Polaka, S., Goykar, H., Karanwad, T., Rajpoot, K., Kumar Tekade, R., 2022. Reactive oxygen nano-generators for cancer therapy. Prog. Mater. Sci. 130, 100974.

Keller, A., Mohamed, A., Dröse, S., Brandt, U., Fleming, I., Brandes, R.P., 2004. Analysis of dichlorodihydrofluorescein and dihydrocalcein as probes for the detection of intracellular reactive oxygen species. Free Radic. Res. 38, 1257–1267.

Koch, O.R., Pani, G., Borrello, S., Colavitti, R., Cravero, A., Farre, S., Galeotti, T., 2004. Oxidative stress and antioxidant defenses in ethanol-induced cell injury. Mol. Aspect. Med. 25, 191–198.

Koehler, C.M., Beverly, K.N., Leverich, E.P., 2006. Redox pathways of the mitochondrion. Antioxidants Redox Signal. 8, 813–822.

Kovtun, Y., Chiu, W.L., Tena, G., Sheen, J., 2000. Functional analysis of oxidative stress-activated mitogen-activated protein kinase cascade in plants. Proc. Natl. Acad. Sci. U. S. A. 97, 2940–2945.

Kowaltowski, A.J., Vercesi, A.E., Rhee, S.G., Netto, L.E., 2000. Catalases and thioredoxin peroxidase protect *Saccharomyces cerevisiae* against Ca2+-induced mitochondrial membrane permeabilization and cell death. FEBS Lett. 473, 177–182.

Kumawat, A., Raval, N., Reddy, G., Rajpoot, K., Tekade, R.K., 2020. Gene delivery to tackle diabetic nephropathy. In: Tekade, R.K. (Ed.), The Future of Pharmaceutical Product Development and Research. Academic Press, pp. 515–537.

Kuznetsov, A.V., Kehrer, I., Kozlov, A.V., Haller, M., Redl, H., Hermann, M., Grimm, M., Troppmair, J., 2011. Mitochondrial ROS production under cellular stress: comparison of different detection methods. Anal. Bioanal. Chem. 400, 2383–2390.

Lautraite, S., Bigot-Lasserre, D., Bars, R., Carmichael, N., 2003. Optimisation of cell-based assays for medium throughput screening of oxidative stress. Toxicol. Vitro 17, 207–220.

Lee, D., Khaja, S., Velasquez-Castano, J.C., Dasari, M., Sun, C., Petros, J., Taylor, W.R., Murthy, N., 2007. In vivo imaging of hydrogen peroxide with chemiluminescent nanoparticles. Nat. Mater. 6, 765–769.

Lefrak, E.A., Pitha, J., Rosenheim, S., Gottlieb, J.A., 1973. A clinicopathologic analysis of adriamycin cardiotoxicity. Cancer 32, 302–314.

Lenaz, G., Bovina, C., D'aurelio, M., Fato, R., Formiggini, G., Genova, M.L., Giuliano, G., MERLO Pich, M., Paolucci, U., Parenti Castelli, G., Ventura, B., 2002. Role of mitochondria in oxidative stress and aging. Ann. N. Y. Acad. Sci. 959, 199–213.

Li, S., Tan, H.Y., Wang, N., Zhang, Z.J., Lao, L., Wong, C.W., Feng, Y., 2015. The role of oxidative stress and antioxidants in liver diseases. Int. J. Mol. Sci. 16, 26087–26124.

Mas-Bargues, C., Escrivá, C., Dromant, M., Borrás, C., Viña, J., 2021. Lipid peroxidation as measured by chromatographic determination of malondialdehyde. Human plasma reference values in health and disease. Arch. Biochem. Biophys. 709, 108941.

Moon, H., Lee, B., Choi, G., Shin, D., Prasad, D.T., Lee, O., Kwak, S.S., Kim, D.H., Nam, J., Bahk, J., Hong, J.C., Lee, S.Y., Cho, M.J., Lim, C.O., Yun, D.J., 2003. NDP kinase 2 interacts with two oxidative stress-activated MAPKs to regulate cellular redox state and enhances multiple stress tolerance in transgenic plants. Proc. Natl. Acad. Sci. U. S. A. 100, 358–363.

More, G.K., Makola, R.T., 2020. In-vitro analysis of free radical scavenging activities and suppression of LPS-induced ROS production in macrophage cells by Solanum sisymbriifolium extracts. Sci. Rep. 10, 6493.

Mukherjea, D., Rybak, L.P., 2011. Pharmacogenomics of cisplatin-induced ototoxicity. Pharmacogenomics 12, 1039–1050.

Mukhopadhyay, C.K., Fox, P.L., 1998. Ceruloplasmin copper induces oxidant damage by a redox process utilizing cell-derived superoxide as reductant. Biochemistry 37, 14222–14229.

Muniswamy, V.J., Raval, N., Gondaliya, P., Tambe, V., Kalia, K., Tekade, R.K., 2019. Dendrimer-Cationized-Albumin' encrusted polymeric nanoparticle improves BBB penetration and anticancer activity of doxorubicin. Int. J. Pharmaceut. 555, 77–99.

Murphy, M.P., 2009. How mitochondria produce reactive oxygen species. Biochem. J. 417, 1–13.

Nathan, C., Cunningham-Bussel, A., 2013. Beyond oxidative stress: an immunologist's guide to reactive oxygen species. Nat. Rev. Immunol. 13, 349–361.

Naughton, C.A., 2008. Drug-induced nephrotoxicity. Am. Fam. Physician 78, 743–750.

Noh, H., Ha, H., 2011. Reactive oxygen species and oxidative stress. Diabetes and the Kidney, 170. Karger Publishers, pp. 102–112.

Oldenburg, J., Kraggerud, S.M., Cvancarova, M., Lothe, R.A., Fossa, S.D., 2007. Cisplatin-induced long-term hearing impairment is associated with specific glutathione s-transferase genotypes in testicular cancer survivors. J. Clin. Oncol. 25, 708–714.

Oliveira, P.J., Bjork, J.A., Santos, M.S., Leino, R.L., Froberg, M.K., Moreno, A.J., Wallace, K.B., 2004. Carvedilol-mediated antioxidant protection against doxorubicin-induced cardiac mitochondrial toxicity. Toxicol. Appl. Pharmacol. 200, 159–168.

Onoue, S., Kawamura, K., Igarashi, N., Zhou, Y., Fujikawa, M., Yamada, H., Tsuda, Y., Seto, Y., Yamada, S., 2008. Reactive oxygen species assay-based risk assessment of drug-induced phototoxicity: classification criteria and application to drug candidates. J. Pharm. Biomed. Anal. 47, 967–972.

Outten, C.E., Culotta, V.C., 2004. Alternative start sites in the *Saccharomyces cerevisiae* GLR1 gene are responsible for mitochondrial and cytosolic isoforms of glutathione reductase. J. Biol. Chem. 279, 7785–7791.

Oyanagui, Y., 1984. Reevaluation of assay methods and establishment of kit for superoxide dismutase activity. Anal. Biochem. 142, 290–296.

Padiyar, A., Agrawal, O.P., Rajpoot, K., Tekade, R.K., 2020. Hydrotropy, mixed hydrotropy, and mixed solvency as trending concept for solubilization of lipophilic drugs. In: Tekade, R.K. (Ed.), The Future of Pharmaceutical Product Development and Research. Academic Press, pp. 145–178.

Pereira, C.V., Nadanaciva, S., Oliveira, P.J., Will, Y., 2012. The contribution of oxidative stress to drug-induced organ toxicity and its detection in vitro and in vivo. Expet Opin. Drug Metabol. Toxicol. 8, 219–237.

Perez, V.I., Lew, C.M., Cortez, L.A., Webb, C.R., Rodriguez, M., Liu, Y., Qi, W., Li, Y., Chaudhuri, A., van Remmen, H., Richardson, A., Ikeno, Y., 2008. Thioredoxin 2 haploinsufficiency in mice results in impaired mitochondrial function and increased oxidative stress. Free Radic. Biol. Med. 44, 882–892.

Pizzino, G., Irrera, N., Cucinotta, M., Pallio, G., Mannino, F., Arcoraci, V., Squadrito, F., Altavilla, D., Bitto, A., 2017. Oxidative stress: harms and benefits for human health. Oxid. Med. Cell. Longev. 2017, 8416763.

Polaka, S., Desai, N., Kshirsagar, B., Rajpoot, K., Tekade, R.K., 2021a. Revamping the pharmacokinetics of poorly soluble drugs using different formulations. In: Biopharmaceutics and Pharmacokinetics Considerations. Academic Press, pp. 387–413.

Polaka, S., Swetha, K.L., Dittakavi, S., Rajpoot, K., Tekade, R.K., 2021b. Bioanalytical method development and validation for establishing bioavailability and bioequivalence. In: Biopharmaceutics and Pharmacokinetics Considerations. Academic Press, pp. 487–516.

Polaka, S., Makwana, V., Vasdev, N., Sheth, A., Rajpoot, K., Sengupta, P., Tekade, R.K., 2022a. Engineering immunity via skin-directed drug delivery devices. J. Contr. Release 345, 385–404.

Polaka, S., Rajpoot, K., Tekade, M., Sharma, M.C., Tekade, R.K., 2022b. Food–drug interactions and their implications on oral drug bioavailability. In: Pharmacokinetics and Toxicokinetic Considerations. Academic Press, pp. 263–289.

Prajapati, R.N., Tekade, R.K., Gupta, U., Gajbhiye, V., Jain, N.K., 2009. Dendimer-mediated solubilization, formulation development and in vitro–in vivo assessment of Piroxicam. Mol. Pharmaceut. 6, 940–950.

Rabbani, N., Thornalley, P.J., 2009. Quantitation of markers of protein damage by glycation, oxidation, and nitration in peritoneal dialysis. Perit. Dial. Int. 29, 51–56.

Rabbani, P.S., Abdou, S.A., Sultan, D.L., Kwong, J., Duckworth, A., Ceradini, D.J., 2018. In vivo imaging of reactive oxygen species in a murine wound model. JoVE 141, 58450.

Rajpoot, K., Desai, N., Koppisetti, H., Tekade, M., Sharma, M.C., Behera, S.K., Tekade, R.K., 2022a. In silico methods for the prediction of drug toxicity. In: Pharmacokinetics and Toxicokinetic Considerations. Academic Press, pp. 357–383.

Rajpoot, K., Katare, P., Tekade, M., Sharma, M.C., Polaka, S., Sengupta, P., Tekade, R.K., 2022b. Toxicokinetic and toxicodynamic considerations in drug research. In: Pharmacokinetics and Toxicokinetic Considerations. Academic Press, pp. 751–776.

Rajpoot, K., Tekade, M., Sharma, M.C., Arafat, B., Tekade, R.K., 2022c. Principles and concepts in toxicokinetic. In: Pharmacokinetics and Toxicokinetic Considerations, pp. 1–26.

Rajpoot, K., Tekade, M., Sharma, M.C., Sreeharsha, N., Sharma, A., Tekade, R.K., 2020a. Recombinant blood products and therapeutic enzymes: an update. In: The Future of Pharmaceutical Product Development and Research. Academic Press, pp. 447–482.

Rajpoot, K., Tekade, M., Sreeharsha, N., Sharma, M.C., Tekade, R.K., 2020b. Recent advancements in solubilization of hydrophobic drugs. In: The Future of Pharmaceutical Product Development and Research. Academic Press, pp. 109–144.

Rajpoot, K., Tekade, R.K., Chatterjee, B., Sharma, M.C., Tekade, M., 2021a. Biopharmaceutical considerations in the pediatric and geriatric formulation development. In: Biopharmaceutics and Pharmacokinetics Considerations. Academic Press, pp. 109–144.

Rajpoot, K., Tekade, R.K., Sharma, M.C., Safavi, M., Tekade, M., 2021b. Pharmacokinetics modeling in drug delivery. In: Biopharmaceutics and Pharmacokinetics Considerations. Academic Press, pp. 279–334.

Rajpoot, K., Tekade, R.K., Sharma, M.C., Tekade, M., 2021c. Pharmacokinetics and biopharmaceutics: a leader or attendant. In: Biopharmaceutics and Pharmacokinetics Considerations. Academic Press, pp. 17–27.

Redegeld, F., van Opstal, M., Houdkamp, E., van Bennekom, W., 1988. Determination of glutathione in biological material by flow-injection analysis using an enzymatic recycling reaction. Anal. Biochem. 174, 489–495.

Sardão, V.A., Oliveira, P.J., Holy, J., Oliveira, C.R., Wallace, K.B., 2009. Morphological alterations induced by doxorubicin on H9c2 myoblasts: nuclear, mitochondrial, and cytoskeletal targets. Cell Biol. Toxicol. 25, 227–243.

Shadel, G.S., Horvath, T.L., 2015. Mitochondrial ROS signaling in organismal homeostasis. Cell 163, 560–569.

Shete, M.B., Patil, T.S., Deshpande, A.S., Saraogi, G., Vasdev, N., Deshpande, M., Rajpoot, K., Tekade, R.K., 2022. Current trends in theranostic nanomedicines. J. Drug Deliv. Sci. Technol. 71, 103280.

Sies, H., 1986. Biochemistry of oxidative stress. Angew Chem. Int. Ed. Engl. 25, 1058–1071.

Sies, H., 1991. Oxidative stress: from basic research to clinical application. Am. J. Med. 91, 31S–38S.

Sies, H., 2015. Oxidative stress: a concept in redox biology and medicine. Redox Biol. 4, 180–183.

Sies, H., 2019. Oxidative stress: eustress and distress in redox homeostasis. Stress: Physiol., Biochem. Pathol. 3, 153–163 (Elsevier).

Simon, N., Morin, C., Bruguerolle, B., Tillement, J.P., 2001. Effects of trimetazidine on altered functions of rat kidney induced by cyclosporine. Therapie 56, 583–587.

Singh, K.K., Shukla, P.C., Quan, A., Desjardins, J.F., Lovren, F., Pan, Y., Garg, V., Gosal, S., Garg, A., Szmitko, P.E., Schneider, M.D., Parker, T.G., Stanford, W.L., Leong-Poi, H., Teoh, H., AL-Omran, M., Verma, S., 2012. BRCA2 protein deficiency exaggerates doxorubicin-induced cardiomyocyte apoptosis and cardiac failure. J. Biol. Chem. 287, 6604–6614.

Smith, D., Turner, C., Španěl, P., 2007. Volatile metabolites in the exhaled breath of healthy volunteers: their levels and distributions. J. Breath Res. 1, 014004.

Stirnimann, G., Kessebohm, K., Lauterburg, B., 2010. Liver injury caused by drugs: an update. Swiss Med. Wkly. 140, w13080.

Tafazoli, S., Spehar, D.D., O'brien, P.J., 2005. Oxidative stress mediated idiosyncratic drug toxicity. Drug Metab. Rev. 37, 311–325.

Tambe, V., Desai, N., Rajpoot, K., Tekade, R.K., 2021a. Organ-on-a-chip"-based physiologically relevant pharmacokinetic models. In: Biopharmaceutics and Pharmacokinetics Considerations. Academic Press, pp. 643–673.

Tambe, V., Ditani, A., Rajpoot, K., Tekade, R.K., 2021b. Pharmacokinetics aspects of structural modifications in drug design and therapy. In: Biopharmaceutics and Pharmacokinetics Considerations. Academic Press, pp. 83–108.

Tambe, V., Kathar, U., Raval, N., Rajpoot, K., Shilpi, S., Khatri, K., Tekade, R.K., 2021c. Positron emission tomography as a noninvasive tool in pharmacokinetic studies. In: Biopharmaceutics and Pharmacokinetics Considerations. Academic Press, pp. 617–641.

Tambe, V., Pande, S., Gadeval, A., Rajpoot, K., Raval, N., Tekade, R.K., 2021d. Microdialysis: an emerging technique for pharmacokinetic–pharmacodynamic profiling. In: Biopharmaceutics and Pharmacokinetics Considerations. Academic Press, pp. 601–616.

Tambe, V., Sirsat, B., Rajpoot, K., Gadeval, A., Tekade, R.K., 2021e. Pharmacogenomics and drug metabolism. In: Biopharmaceutics and Pharmacokinetics Considerations. Academic Press, pp. 355–385.

Tariq, M., Morais, C., Sobki, S., AL Sulaiman, M., AL Khader, A., 1999. N-acetylcysteine attenuates cyclosporin-induced nephrotoxicity in rats. Nephrol. Dial. Transplant. 14, 923–929.

Tekade, R.K., Chougule, M.B. 2013. Formulation development and evaluation of hybrid nanocarrier for cancer therapy: Taguchi orthogonal array based design. BioMed Res. Int. 2013, 712678.

Tekade, M., Koppisetti, H., Sharma, M.C., Rajpoot, K., Sengupta, P., Kumar, M., Tekade, R.K., 2022. Understanding the concept of signal toxicity and its implications on human health. Pharmacokinetics and Toxicokinetic Considerations, 2. Elsevier, pp. 99–116.

Tiwari, A., Joshi, M., Salvi, N., Gupta, D., Gandhi, S., Rajpoot, K., Tekade, R.K., 2022. Toxicity of pharmaceutical azo dyes. Pharmacokinetics and Toxicokinetic Considerations, 2. Elsevier, pp. 569–603.

Uzar, E., Koyuncuoglu, H.R., Uz, E., Yilmaz, H.R., Kutluhan, S., Kilbas, S., Gultekin, F., 2006. The activities of antioxidant enzymes and the level of malondialdehyde in cerebellum of rats subjected to methotrexate: protective effect of caffeic acid phenethyl ester. Mol. Cell. Biochem. 291, 63–68.

Vardi, N., Parlakpinar, H., Ates, B., 2012. Beneficial effects of chlorogenic acid on methotrexate-induced cerebellar Purkinje cell damage in rats. J. Chem. Neuroanat. 43, 43–47.

Vasdev, N., Rajpoot, K., Tekade, R.K., 2021. Molecular mechanisms of circadian rhythm and its influence on the pharmacokinetics of drugs. In: Tekade, R.K. (Ed.), Biopharmaceutics and Pharmacokinetics Considerations, 1. Elsevier, Academic Press, pp. 415–449.

Wali, A.F., Pillai, J.R., AL Dhaheri, Y., Rehman, M.U., Shoaib, A., Sarheed, O., Jabnoun, S., Razmpoor, M., Rasool, S., Paray, B.A., Ahmad, P., 2020. Crocus sativus L. Extract containing polyphenols modulates oxidative stress and inflammatory response against anti-tuberculosis drugs-induced liver injury. Plants 9, 167.

Walker, P.D., Barri, Y., Shah, S.V., 1999. Oxidant mechanisms in gentamicin nephrotoxicity. Ren. Fail. 21, 433–442.

Walker, P.D., Shah, S.V., 1987. Gentamicin enhanced production of hydrogen peroxide by renal cortical mitochondria. Am. J. Physiol. 253, C495–C499.

Will, Y., Fischer, K.A., Horton, R.A., Kaetzel, R.S., Brown, M.K., Hedstrom, O., Lieberman, M.W., Reed, D., 2000. γ-Glutamyltranspeptidase–Deficient knockout mice as a model to study the relationship between glutathione status, mitochondrial function, and cellular function. Hepatology 32, 740–749.

Youngren, S.R., Tekade, R.K., Gustilo, B., Hoffmann, P.R., Chougule, M.B. 2013. Stat6 sirna matrix-loaded gelatin nanocarriers: formulation, characterization, and *ex vivo* proof of concept using adenocarcinoma cells. BioMed Res. Int. 2013, 858946.

Zhang, Y., Ding, C., Zhu, W., Li, X., Chen, T., Liu, Q., Zhou, S., Zhang, T.C., Ma, W., 2022. Chemotherapeutic drugs induce oxidative stress associated with DNA repair and metabolism modulation. Life Sci. 289, 120242.

Zheng, M., Aslund, F., Storz, G., 1998. Activation of the OxyR transcription factor by reversible disulfide bond formation. Science 279, 1718–1721.

Zielonka, J., Kalyanaraman, B., 2010. Hydroethidine- and MitoSOX-derived red fluorescence is not a reliable indicator of intracellular superoxide formation: another inconvenient truth. Free Radic. Biol. Med. 48, 983–1001.

CHAPTER

6

Role of "toxicant-induced loss of tolerance" in the emergence of disease

Anand More[1], *Muktika Tekade*[2], *Nagaraja Sreeharsha*[3,4] *and Rakesh Kumar Tekade*[1]

[1]National Institute of Pharmaceutical Education and Research (NIPER)- Ahmedabad, An Institute of National Importance, Government of India, Department of Pharmaceuticals, Ministry of Chemicals and Fertilizers, Palaj, Gandhinagar, Gujarat, India; [2]School of Pharmacy, Devi Ahilya Vishwavidyalaya, Indore, Madhya Pradesh, India; [3]Department of Pharmaceutics, Vidya Siri College of Pharmacy, Bengaluru, Karnataka, India; [4]Department of Pharmaceutical Sciences, College of Clinical Pharmacy, King Faisal University, Al-Ahsa, Saudi Arabia

6.1 Introduction

The first description of the two-step disease mechanism for TILT was published in the 1990s and is characterized by the development of new intolerances and multisystem symptoms subclass of people after significant chemical exposure. It can occur as a single event or as repeated exposure to low levels (Ashford and Miller, 1998; Miller, 1997; Masri et al., 2021). The global observations of the TILT mechanism do not fall under the purview of traditional toxicology or allergy, in contrast to established known processes for damage that involves several steps known to be the reason for endocrine and cancer-like problems. Initiation in Stage I of TILT starts after exposure to a specific material or combination of such materials (chemicals) that usually affects the nervous system with or without the immune system. To initiate the process, this chemical exposure has to react with at least a few of such systems in a manner that makes people resistant to later triggering events. After the initiation stage, Stage II, i.e., Triggering, comes into the picture, where the impacted cannot tolerate routine exposures to various substances with different structural properties

Essentials of Pharmatoxicology in Drug Research, Volume 1
https://doi.org/10.1016/B978-0-443-15840-7.00010-5

at levels that have never bothered them before and are not bothersome to the majority of people (Masri et al., 2021).

Chemically different substances may trigger, such as inhalants, ingestants, chemical vapors from solvents, fragrances, smoke, and specific medicine, or food. After initiation, exposure to these "triggers" led to symptoms like fatigue, rash, mood swipe, headache, weakness, memory impairment, concentration-related issues (called "brain fog"), and lungs problem. After the onset of symptoms from previous exposure, many foods and medications that were previously tolerated can cause symptoms. Initiation is neither observed nor reported frequently, but the masking phenomenon can disguise the triggering, thereby preventing their observation (Masri et al., 2021). Fig. 6.1 gives the overall idea about the role development of illness.

As described above, it develops in two stages. Stage I initiation, where exposure to even low or high events like solvent hazards, pesticides, chemical entities, or pesticides, can lead to loss of natural or prior tolerance, followed by stage II, i.e., triggering where even small amounts of earlier tolerated chemicals (exhaust from traffic, medicines, or combination of it) can trigger symptoms. Usually, these two stages are hidden from the medical practitioner as he diagnoses the patient based on symptoms. The connection between symptoms and triggers is concealed by masking. It is also possible for the initial exposure event that breaks down tolerance to go unnoticed (Masri et al., 2021; Miller, 2001a).

Nowadays, multiple chemical sensitivity, environmental illness, and idiopathic environmental intolerance are no longer commonly used terms. Instead, "Chemical Intolerance" and "TILT" are used more frequently. However, these should not be viewed as distinct illnesses but as somewhat different ways of describing the same cluster of allergy-like symptoms that do not fall under the traditional definition of allergies but still affect vast numbers of people domestically and internationally. Since TILT, unlike other theories, which only describe symptoms, does more than that, so the terminology has evolved, making it a

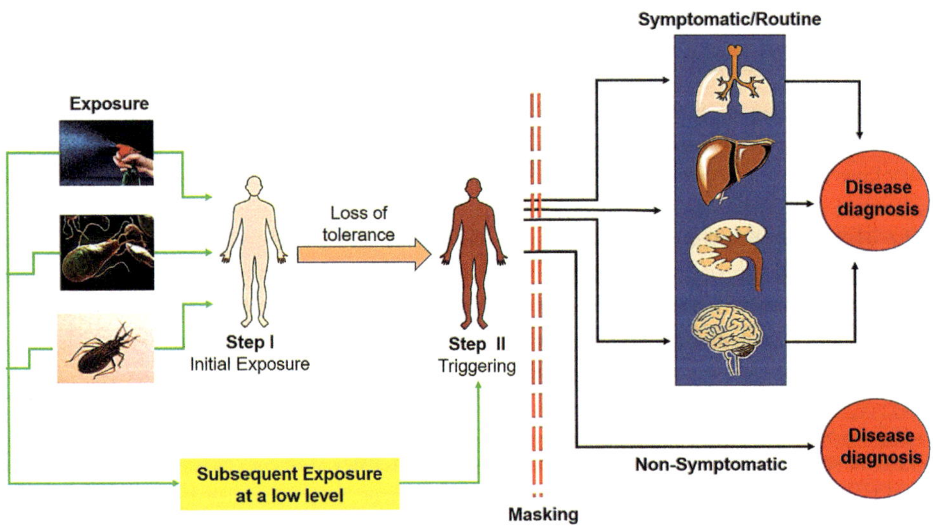

FIGURE 6.1 Toxicity-induced loss of tolerance.

preferred term. An overall disease mechanism known as TILT encompasses this entire class of diseases, similar to other contemporary disease mechanisms that science has learned to comprehend, such as immunological disorders or infectious conditions (Masri et al., 2021; Rossi et al., 2018).

Multiple chemical sensitivity is still a contentious topic in the health sector with a wildly varying presentation with negative physical responses to low concentrations of numerous common chemicals, like preservatives, paints, disinfectants, pesticides, etc., so when such chemicals react physically, it leads to acute to chronic level symptoms. Symptoms may vary from system to system, like GIT reactions, respiratory tract problems, memory loss, headache, depression, immunological dysfunction, muscle pain, etc. Unlike an allergy, MCS is not consistently associated with immunological dysfunction. Even numerous findings revealed that repeated exposure to such chemicals might affect brain physiology too. This is because an elevated level of peroxynitrite, nitric oxide, and other immunological disturbances hampers glutamate receptor (NMDA) functionality (Drexler and Greiner, 2020; Rossi et al., 2018).

Earlier, two theories were proposed for diseases, namely the immune theory and germ theory. Germ theory is the oldest, while TILT theory is the latest theory. In germ theory, responses are triggered by numerous germs/antigens; the involvement of different organs has been seen. In the case of immune theory, an antigen triggers the development of antibodies, and further invasion of antigen can result in an antigen-antibody complex (response) (Masri et al., 2021; Miller, 2001). Due to a masking condition, most patients may even be unaware they have intolerances. The connection between a person's symptoms and triggering exposures is frequently hidden by masking. It helps to understand why there is a change in symptoms from individual to individual and even from day to day in the same person. It has several interactive components: apposition, addiction, and habituation (Miller, 2001a).

Despite the relative newness of the term "TILT," reports of illnesses with similar symptoms go back much further in time (Tabershaw and Cooper, 1966; Randolph, 1961). At first glance, it seemed like the condition was confined to North America. However, in 1995, researchers from nine European countries funded by the European Commission found that they shared similar observations (Ashford et al., 1995; Miller and Ashford, 1995). Intriguingly, this cross-national study compared distinct manifestations of "chemical sensitivity" and uncovered distinct chemical sensitivity triggers. They presented proof for the two-stage disease process described by Miller as TILT (Miller, 2001a). This chapter mainly focuses on toxicity causing loss of tolerance in the emergence of the disease, its features like anomaly, causality, generalizability, novelty, and the evaluation and consequences of TILT (Miller, 1999).

The exact mechanism for the disease is yet to be established, but Fig. 6.2 gives an idea about the general mechanism for the disease. In the case of germ theory, a germ or pathogen is the causative agent for disease emergence. Specific causes, specific diseases, or sometimes a group of pathogens may contribute to the pathology of the disease. Germs like bacteria or viruses may enter the body by wounded skin or respiratory channels. Then they start to reproduce there and start their colonization in the host body. During their lifecycle, they produce toxins or metabolites like endotoxin or exotoxin, which cause disease. Even this reproduces germs and starts infecting the other host. All this led to acute to chronic levels hampering the body system. For example, HIV causes AIDS. In the case of immune theory,

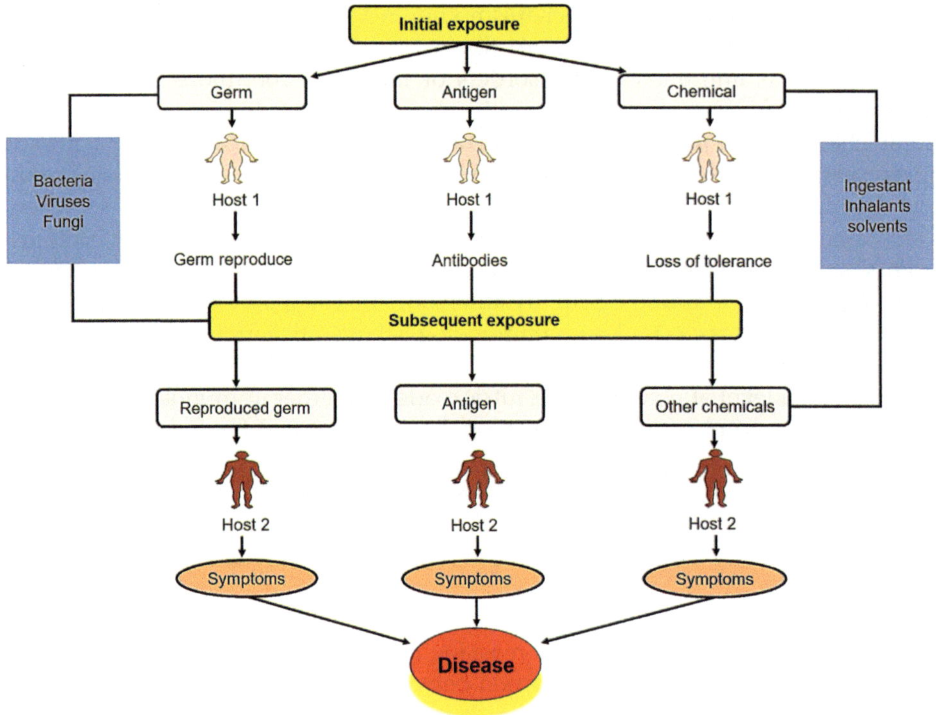

FIGURE 6.2 Brief overview of germ theory, immune theory, and TILT theory.

like germ theory, germs and antigens are the culprit for disease emergence. Different responses vary from the GI tract to the skin, respiratory system, and brain; an example, Allergic rhinitis (Miller, 2001; Cabrera-Perez et al., 2017).

6.2 Toxicant-induced loss of tolerance

Toxicant-provoked loss of tolerance (or TILT) is the name given to the two-step disease process by which some people who are sensitive to toxins (such as those found in air pollutants, spillages, or pesticide implementations) lose their normal tolerance for these substances. This leads to a situation where previously tolerated exposures now cause adverse reactions. Reactions can take the form of either compulsive or avoidant behaviors. Some affected people may react to specific triggers hidden (masked) by their reactions to other, more common chemicals, foods, and drugs. Nevertheless, when it comes to planning human challenge studies in this field, a few key clinical observations need to be considered (Masri et al., 2021). Before performing meaningful test challenges on these patients, it is necessary to have a solid understanding of the commonly reported biphasic, commonly observed withdrawal pattern of the patient's symptoms. This is especially true for the symptoms that involve the CNS and its related phenomenon like masking (Miller, 1999; Miller, 2001) (Table 6.1).

TABLE 6.1 A brief overview of features and characteristics of the new theory of disease.

Feature	Characteristic	Example	Reference
Anomaly	Not fit to the existing disease pattern	Genetic abnormalities	Miller (1999), Miller (2001b)
Causality	Relation between cause and exposure agent	Diarrhea is caused by bacteria and parasite	Miller (1999)
Generalizability	The general relation between a disease class and a drug class	Nephrotoxicity and ototoxicity by aminoglycosides	Miller (1999)
Novelty	New disease mechanisms established	In Alzheimer's disease	Miller (1999)

6.2.1 Features of a new theory of disease

6.2.1.1 Anomaly

An anomaly is a condition that is reported by reliable people but doesn't fit into any of the known disease models (Bartkowiak and Applications, 2011; Zhu et al., 2020). Some abnormality in the patient's clinical presentation or response is required before a novel disease theory is advanced. Over the last century, the immune theory of disease grew out of the fact that some people who get sick don't get sick again after they get better. The emergence of a novel theory requires the presence of an anomaly.

Investigators observed that "generally, there is a period of some extended professional insecurity produced as a result of standard scientific puzzles failing to resolve as expected repeatedly. When the old rules don't work, it's time to start looking for something better. The meeting of the ACS on chemical sensitivity and four other federally sponsored meetings on the same topic in the last few years are all lead up to the search for new anomalies. Clinicians increasingly see patients who report multiple chemical intolerances after single, recognizable chemical exposure. Because of the wide range of backgrounds these people represent, it is safe to say that workers, goat keepers, office workers, etc., who have few commonalities beyond a common trigger event and the subsequent emergence of shared intolerances stand out as a curious outliers (Miller, 2001b; Miller, 1999).

6.2.1.2 Causality

Causality is the causal evidence linking an exposure or agent to the ailment. Second, the exposure or agent being studied, whether an antigen, germ, or chemical, must be the causative factor in the observed illnesses for the new theory of disease to be accepted. The relationship between a cause and its effect, or between two phenomena that tend to occur together, is meant by the term "causality" in this context (Vaishampayan et al., 2019; Zhu et al., 2020). Researchers may find only hints of a causal link at the outset of investigating a phenomenon. As time passes and knowledge expands, certain conditions must be met before a cancer diagnosis can be scientifically confirmed. As an illustration, consider the afterthoughts of Robert Koch's germ theory of disease. Causality has been established using various scientific criteria for different diseases, including those caused by bacteria, immunological disorders, viruses,

CNS infections, and long-term illnesses. All nine of Hill's (1965) criteria (consistency, association capability, association strength, biological gradient, temporality, plausibility, experiment, coherence, and analogy) aid in the establishment of causality for environmental-induced diseases (Grant and Boucher, 2010). Hill warns that it takes more than one of his criteria to establish causation and that the absence of any of them does not rule out the possibility of such a connection. These criteria help to validate causation when taken as a whole. TILT appears to involve two sequential steps (initiation and triggering). Each stage may call for a slightly different strategy for establishing a causal connection.

Further proof from animal studies and epidemiological inquiries will likely be necessary to validate the reason for disease initiation (first step). However, Hill argued that there was one criterion that gives valid proof or evidence for causality, and that might be a direct experiment (human studies and animal studies). As a result, a causal hypothesis is provided by the TILT triggering phase that can be tested in humans (Miller, 1999).

6.2.1.3 Generalizability

Third, a new theory of disease needs to be generalizable or applicable to a broad category of etiological factors like a wide variety of pathogens or antigens. Also, a reasonable explanation for a group of diseases is required. To be generalizable means that the results can be applied to all instances of a given class or group (Webb and Shavelson, 2005; Zhu et al., 2020). Max Boehr, who wrote about the transferability of the germ theory in 1868, said, "The theory of infection has the characteristic of all good pathological theories. It gives a clear and intelligible definition to a wide range of anatomical and clinical causes, as well as related experiences and findings of credible observers" (Carter, 1985).

In a study where background chemical exposures in this hospital ward had reduced to the minimum levels possible so that patients can be monitored to see if they improve when triggers are removed. Also, we want to see if patients' symptoms improve after receiving placebo-controlled, double-blind tests will help us figure out whether environmental factors play a role in the development of these and other diseases. Charles Darwin once said that incorporating taxonomy into his research, "Facts are grouped in science to derive general laws from them." Similarly, TILT provides a theory because it is the culmination of thousands of cases observed by doctors. Therefore, TILT satisfies the requirement of generalizability. Because of this generalizability, we can anticipate illness after various chemical exposures, such as a chemical spill, use of pesticides, or war (Miller, 1999).

6.2.1.4 Novelty

Besides being anomalous, causal, and applicable to a wide range of cases, a novel theory of disease must also offer a compellingly different way of thinking about the illness at hand that is a novelty. The term "novel" indicates that the theory has not been previously described. If the proposed mechanism turns out to be similar to one already known, then the proposed explanation is not novel (Zhu et al., 2020). While TILT does have some similarities to both allergens and toxins, it does not strictly follow either set of guidelines. Even though both TILT and toxicity involve adverse effects on the environmental agent, in most cases, the doses associated with TILT are many times lower than what is considered toxic. However, TILT is also similar to allergies in other ways. Both processes require two steps and result in heightened sensitivity. Chemically intolerant people have historically been "allergic" to various

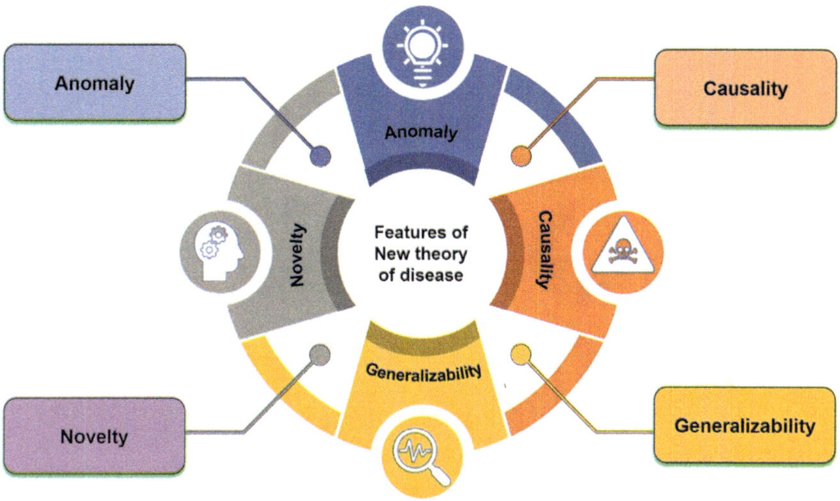

FIGURE 6.3 Features of a new theory of diseases.

substances like food, drug, dust, etc. Nonetheless, research has not linked chemical intolerances to IgE or other antibodies but involved a specific antigen-antibody interaction in the case of allergy (Miller, 1999) (Fig. 6.3).

6.2.2 Features of TILT relevant to its testing

The TILT phenomenon seems to involve a two-stage process, as described by several researchers who have looked into it. Regarding humans, it is more challenging to model the first stage (initiation) due to ethical concerns than it is to model the second stage (triggering). In the end, animal models and epidemiologic studies might be able to explore the first stage. Patients' biphasic, stimulatory-and-withdrawal-like symptoms, especially CNS, need to be understood before testing such patients. Another critical factor called masking need to be minimized; else, it would mask the responses from low-level chemical exposure. Randolph compared the symptoms associated with alcohol and drug addiction. The critical difference between TILT and addiction is dose dependency. TILT is a dose-dependent phenomenon, whereas addiction is not. Chemicals or biologicals can induce TILT, but in the case of addiction, it is not the case (Miller, 2001) (Fig. 6.4).

6.2.3 Common symptoms of TILT

TILT-related symptoms can affect any organ in the human body. Many neurological symptoms, such as memory loss, mood swings, and brain fog, can be debilitating. It is possible to develop intolerances that cause various symptoms depending on the specific event (like exposure to Gulf War chemicals or sick building). Symptoms that are frequently reported include:

i. Inability to focus, memory loss
ii. Mood swings

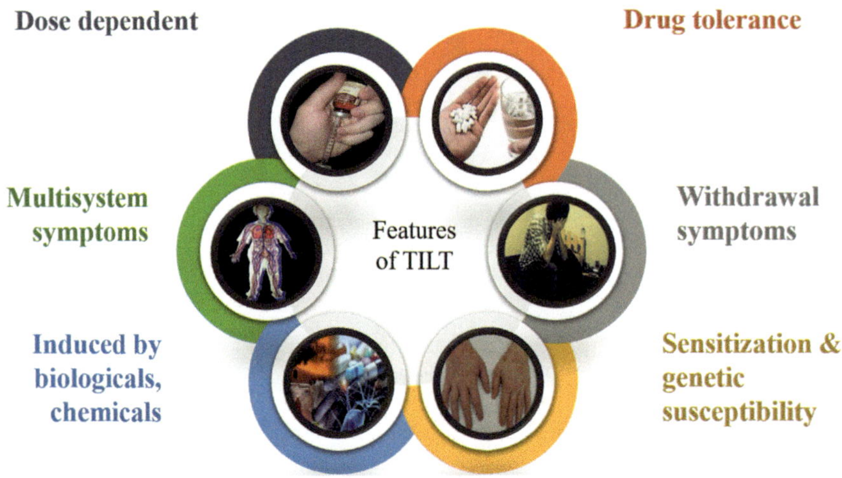

FIGURE 6.4 Commonly observed TILT feature.

iii. GIT symptoms
iv. Headache and confusion
v. Myalgia and respiratory symptoms
vi. Allergic symptoms
vii. Depression and dizziness

6.2.4 Common triggers for TILT

Numerous triggers can lead to TILT, but some of them, like certain drugs, chemicals, and food, are frequently involved in the emergence of the disease. Initial low or high-level exposure led to the loss of tolerance, and subsequent exposure to such an agent gave rise to a multisystem symptom. A few such triggers for TILT are discussed here.

i. **Drugs:** Many known antibiotics cause allergic reactions. Ampicillin and tetracycline antibiotics commonly cause an allergic reaction. Drug intolerance can be natural, like aspirin can be naturally seen in teas, nuts, vegetables, etc. Histamine is a well-known allergic agent present in dried fruits, vinegar, fermented food, and meats, and consumption of such food led to TILT. Diarrhea, rashes, difficulties in breathing, and headache are commonly associated with salicylate sensitivity.
ii. **Chemicals:** Most of the time, people's lives are contaminated by chemical exposures in their homes and workplaces. Moving to or renovating a new house can accompany exposure to new furniture, paint, and carpet that may act as a trigger source. Even sometimes, fragranced or laundry cloth may become problematic to someone intolerant of them. With industrialization, this problem is increasing day by day.
iii. **Food:** Food intolerances should not be confused with food allergies, even though some symptoms may be the same. The most significant distinction is that, unlike food

intolerances, allergies always involve immunoglobulins, or "IgE." Eggs, tree nuts, wheat, and cow's milk, are among the common foods that cause severe immune system reactions that affect the body's organs. Unlike an allergy, food intolerance symptoms are not that much severe. Food intolerances are more common than food allergies. Instead of allergies, food intolerances are more common in people with chemical sensitivities than allergies.

6.2.5 Common conditions that trigger TILT

Like common triggers, particular conditions have been attributed to toxicity-induced loss of tolerance. The simultaneous presence of such conditions and exposure to chemicals can affect the multisystem, which could be challenging to treat.

i. Skin conditions like eczema, eruption
ii. Neurological conditions like MCS, attention related disorders, seizures
iii. CVS events like high blood pressure, arrhythmias
iv. Respiratory problems like asthma, airway dysfunction
v. Fibromyalgia, lupus, arthritis
vi. Gulf war syndrome, implant syndrome
vii. Sinusitis, tinnitus, polyps

6.2.6 Empirical approaches for the investigation of toxicant-induced loss of tolerance

To understand the toxicant-induced loss of tolerance, it is necessary to investigate both the onset of symptoms and the beginning of chemical sensitivity in individuals who have been affected. Chemical sensitivity can cause a wide range of symptoms and may even represent a group of symptoms. It is unlikely that conventional population-based epidemiologic methods will help describe the triggering stages. Tests or studies should be such in which subjects can serve as their control, like in placebo-controlled studies, double-blind studies, etc. Parallel research should also be conducted on a control group, which is crucial for determining how the EMU (Environmentally controlled medical unit) affects responses. Masking is another aspect that needs to be considered because it could play a crucial role.

On the other hand, traditional research methods focusing on populations could prove beneficial when investigating the beginning stages of chemical sensitivity. The likelihood of success for such studies increases when confounding variables are kept to a minimum. Selecting study participants who experienced the same or similar exposures before their ailments may be an effective strategy (Miller et al., 1997).

6.3 Stages of TILT

It is a disease process with two stages initially discovered in the 1990s (Masri et al., 2021; Miller, 1997). Multi-system signs and innovative start aversions occur in a subgroup of people after a severe event of chemical exposure or constant contact at a low level. The global observations of the TILT mechanism do not fall under either conventional toxicological or classical allergies, unlike the well-known multistep damage mechanisms described in the development of various malignancies and endocrine disruptions. Although toxicant-induced loss of tolerance (TILT) is a two-step illness process proposed to describe chemical intolerance, nothing is known about the exposures that induce the disease.

6.3.1 Initiation (stage 1)

Initiation, the first stage of TILT, starts when a person is exposed to a chemical or a combination of substances that usually impact the immune system and/or neurological system. For commencement to occur, chemicals must interact with one (or both) of these systems so that humans grow intolerant to subsequent triggering events. The first step (initiation) is more challenging to simulate in people due to ethical problems compared to the second stage (triggering). Animal models and epidemiologic research may finally show the first stage (Miller, 2000).

6.3.2 Triggering (stage 2)

Following commencement, afflicted persons cannot tolerate extensive exposure every day to a variety of structurally diverse compounds at levels that previously did not causes the effect. Ingestants, inhalants, implants, and skin contacts, such as scents, solvents used for cleaning, cigarette, specific meals, medicine, and other exposures, may cause a reaction. Exposure to such "triggers" causes symptoms such as fatigue, pain, dimmer vision, hastiness, temper swings, concentration and related problems (often referred to as "brain fog"), and breathing problems after it starts.

6.4 Characteristics affecting TILT

What we do know is that any process purporting to explain TILT must explain the traits most closely linked with this condition, as observed by patients and physicians all across the world: (a) Stimulatory and withdrawal symptoms, (b) Masking, (c) Acclimatization, (d) Apposition, and (e) Addiction (Table 6.2).

6.4.1 Symptoms of stimulation and withdrawal

Randolph began by describing the progression of these people's reactions to chemicals and diets through time (Randolph, 1962). Their symptoms, he noted, were strikingly similar to those associated with alcohol and drug abuse (Siegel, 2005). According to Randolph, food and caffeine addictions were the lowest rungs on an addiction ladder, which progressed from food, and a combination of food with medicines; on the lower rungs are chemicals like caffeine and alcohol, and on the higher rungs are substances like nicotine and other naturally occurring and synthetically manufactured compounds (Moss and Randolph, 1980).

TABLE 6.2 Common traits associated with TILT.

Traits	Characteristics	References
Stimulatory and withdrawal symptoms	Symptoms similar to alcohol and drug abuse	Miller (2001b), Masri et al. (2021)
Masking	Hides the relationship between symptoms and triggers	Masri et al. (2021)
Acclimatization	Symptom severity decreases with repeated closely timed exposures	Miller (2001), Miller (1997)
Apposition	It tends to mask the effect of interest	Miller (2001), Miller (1997)
Addiction.	Deliberately take caffeine, alcohol, nicotine, or other substances	Miller (2001), Miller (1997)

Chemically sensitive people are similar to drug addicts because they both have tremendous desires and terrible withdrawal symptoms. Chemically sensitive individuals' stimulatory and withdrawal symptoms are generally comparable to individuals experienced by normal people exposed to far higher doses of identical medications. According to Gulf War veterans with unexplained ailments, intoxication can be caused by consuming just one alcoholic beverage and a bad hangover (National Academies of Sciences and Medicine, 2016; Cory-Slechta and Wedge, 2016). Finally, there are many similarities between drug addiction and TILT. It also displays toxicity and allergy-like characteristics. On the other hand, its likeness to addiction is arguably most evident and has missed the notice of numerous clinicians and investigators.

6.4.2 Masking

Assume that TILT is a process that underpins chronic tiredness, migraines, asthma, and depression. It's understandable to question why people who experience these symptoms don't similarly describe chemical sensitivities. In actuality, some, but not all, patients do report them (Fiedler et al., 1996). Various chemically sensitive individuals with these diseases say that they didn't start feeling better until they avoided enough of their issue irritants, either unintentionally or consciously. Most say they wouldn't have known what was making them sick if they hadn't avoided so many chemicals and foods at once or hadn't unmasked themselves.

Masking and unmasking are nonscientific phrases with no scientific counterpart. Nonetheless, the outcome of studies in this field may be determined by investigators' capacity to comprehend masking and unmasking and alter these factors intelligently. Masking appears to have at least three connected components: acclimatization, apposition, and addiction, altogether restricted by the result of low-level pharmacological trials in these individuals. These three components are likely to work together in real life, although they are treated separately here. Assume that researchers wanted to put a putatively sensitive person to the test by exposing him to a modest dose of xylene. Molhave's mixture contains xylene, a prevalent indoor air pollutant (Mølhave et al., 1986). Earlier in the trial, how did researchers confirm that their subjects were unmasked (at absolute baseline)? So, the masking component needs to be examined and managed.

6.4.3 Acclimatization

Adaption happens in the majority of people after prolonged or recurrent exposure to a variety of environmental stresses. As a result, as the exposure continues, the symptoms will lessen. When chemically sensitive patients are exposed to more chemicals, their symptoms improve; nevertheless, when the exposure is discontinued, these persons generally experience significant withdrawal symptoms. As a result, what they're describing is more comparable to habit than adaptability. Assume that the xylene-sensitive patient works at a hospital and is regularly exposed to low amounts of xylene. Exposure to xylene at levels below the smell threshold (0.62 ppm) may have little or no effect on a person who has worked in the same building for the previous week (Association, 1989). Hence, depending on how freshly a sensitive subject has been exposed to the test drug or a chemically similar agent, their response to a challenge might range from none to maximum. Due to habituation, if not enough time has passed, such as less than 04 days, the challenge may result in a deceptive adverse reaction. Sensitivity may have decreased if too much time has gone by, such as weeks or months.

6.4.4 Apposition

Assume that the study subject is hypersensitive to a variety of chemicals. The subject got up early on the day of his challenge testing, put on perfumed soap or hair spray, did breakfast made on a gas burner, and reached the laboratory after driving through heavy traffic. He takes an elevator into the laboratory building and is exposed to people wearing various colognes. His responses might overlap in time if he was susceptible to multiple exposures. These kinds of reactions are believed to last for hours or even days. If this is the case, they may persist in a placebo challenge, resulting in a false positive. As a result, the second feature of masking that must be handled before and throughout challenge trials is the apposition or juxtaposition of the effects of carefully scheduled exposures (Miller, 1997).

6.4.5 Addiction

The addiction stage starts with initiation, maintenance, and withdrawal; later, it may lead to abstinence or even relapse (Ashford and Miller, 1998). Many symptoms that chemically sensitive individuals experience are similar to those usually linked with addiction. Addiction might be a factor in disguising. Alcohol, cigarette, and caffeine addicts knowingly or unknowingly period their next "hit" to avoid removal symptoms, a condition that happens in all three addictions. Chemically sensitive patients, on the other hand, have been found to develop a food addiction. The most common addictive substances in Randolph's patients were wheat, eggs, milk, and corn. Bioactive components such as tyramine, monosodium glutamate, and opiates may be found in foods (Winsky-Sommerer et al., 2004).

People who regularly use cigarettes, alcohol, caffeine, and foods containing active substances may need to avoid testing since the pharmacological qualities of these drugs may mask or overcome the effects of an experimental challenge. Failure to remove addictions before testing may result in false positive challenges due to lingering effects from an addiction taken hours or days before the dummy trial or unfair negative trials due to addictions masking (Vandaele and Ahmed, 2021).

6.5 Toxicant-induced loss of tolerance-induced conditions

Today, we are keen-sighted of a consistent pattern of illness in people exposed to chemicals in more than a dozen countries. Anomalies in science reveal the flaws in present models and motivate the quest for innovative ones (Miller, 1994). The fact that intolerances develop in a wide range of demographic groups with little in common other than an initial chemical exposure event is a significant anomaly that points to TILT as a possible new disease explanation. Asthma, migraine headaches, melancholy, chronic weariness, fibromyalgia, and "Gulf War syndrome" could all be explained by it (Miller, 1994). Approximately partial persons who are chemically prejudiced claim that their sickness originated from a specific exposure event, such as an oil spill, long-lasting solvent exposure, insect killer application, indoor air pollution, and combustion products. A small percentage of people exposed to settings such as these seem to progress chronic illnesses that last for years, if not decades, after they were first exposed and suffer from the different disease conditions that may be originated in TILT (Miller and Prihoda, 1999) (Fig. 6.5).

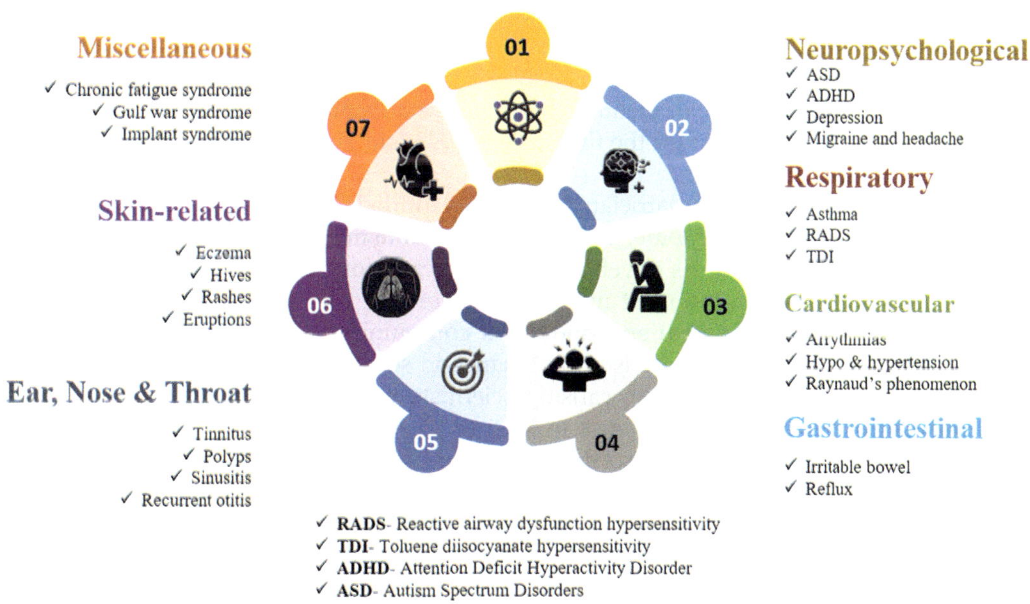

FIGURE 6.5 Commonly observed TILT-induced conditions.

6.5.1 Neuropsychological-related condition

Neurotoxicity is a term that defines the neurophysiological changes that occur as a result of toxic substance exposure, which can include cognitive alterations, memory problems, mood swings, and the beginning of dementia or psychiatric problems. Toxic substances commonly used in heavy metals, medicines, organophosphates, bacterial and animal neurotoxins are examples of agents. Following exposure, acute versus chronic hazardous neurophysiological changes may occur. The type of neurotoxic exposure may lead to central nervous system injury, emotional disorders, and/or cognition impairments, etc.

Heavy metal neurotoxicity, such as lead, mercury, and arsenic, is most typically investigated in chronic and acute exposure. Common acute exposure symptoms include nausea, headaches, cognitive difficulties, and emotional disruptions. Heavy metal exposure is more common in industrial workplace situations, where chronic, long-term exposure is more prevalent. Neurodegeneration and mental symptoms are more common due to such long-term exposure. Increased depression, anxiety, and irritability are examples of psychiatric signs. Chronic exposure can cause various symptoms, including exhaustion, slowed processing speed, fine and gross motor impairments, and generalized cognitive impairment. The cognitive impairments that underpin the exposures are outlined here, with particular attention devoted to the individual chemicals and/or chemical groups that were most frequent throughout each exposure episode (Molot et al., 2021; Liu et al., 2019; Huff et al., 2019).

6.5.1.1 Autism spectrum disorders (ASD)

Autism spectrum disorder (ASD) is a social development condition that impairs a person's brain development and, as a result, their behavior. These symptoms should be present from early childhood and have a significant impact on everyday life for a diagnosis of autism to be made. Autistic individuals exist in their world. Differences in behavior, social communication, interaction, specific interests, and sensory processing describe it. These characteristics might make it difficult for persons on the autism spectrum to interact with their surroundings. This is a widespread developmental disease on the autism spectrum that American psychiatrist Leo Kanner discovered for the first time in 1943 (eid ziad Al-Adwan and Al-Naimat, 2019).

Like Kanner, the Austrian pediatrician Asperger identified the clinical indicators of autism that underlie the Asperger syndrome, a disorder on the autism spectrum, in 1944 (eid ziad Al-Adwan and Al-Naimat, 2019). As of yet, no definitive cause or treatment for autism has been identified, making it one of the most mysterious disorders. The pattern of its expansion is rather unusual. Because of verbal and nonverbal communication issues and the repetition of certain behavioral patterns, there is an imbalance in social interaction. Its occurrence has skyrocketed in the last few decades, causing scientists worldwide to examine the disease from every angle possible, from its cause to its cure.

The origins of autism spectrum disorder (ASD) are still poorly understood, and recent evidence suggests that environmental and genetic factors significantly influence the condition's development. However, to investigate the environmental elements linked to this condition, it is necessary first to define the term "environment." In medicine, the environment refers to everything that exists outside of a person's body, like air, water, and food, that has the potential to affect their health. Also, the environment is everything that surrounds us within our mother's uterus when we are in her womb. Some researchers focused on environmental variables like parents' age, medical history, and pregnancy-related drug exposure, which contributed to the high risk of autism.

The prevalence of autism is believed to be between 2% and 6% in children. The incidence rate is 3 to times higher in males than in females. According to data, the number of cases identified with autism in the United States is increasing. This increase is due to increased autism sensitivity in public and improved diagnostic criteria - the fact is that other diseases like hyperactivity and schizophrenia are being diagnosed at the cost of autism. 75%–50% of autistic kids are also mentally retarded, and 30% have seizures, confirming the concerns that autism is caused by an organic or hereditary factor (eid ziad Al-Adwan and Al-Naimat, 2019).

6.5.1.2 Attention deficit hyperactivity disorder (ADHD)

One of the most common childhood diseases, attention deficit hyperactivity disorder (ADHD), can last throughout adolescence and adulthood. About 11% of children aged 4–17 have attention deficit hyperactivity disorder (ADHD). Children with ADHD typically begin displaying symptoms between the ages of three and six. In most cases, a diagnosis of ADHD is made in a kid when they are 7 years old. Young boys are three times more likely than young girls to develop this condition. ADHD isn't just a problem for kids. Daily, about 4% of American people over the age of 18 struggle with ADHD tendencies. It is diagnosed equally in males and females in maturity. Symptoms include the inability to stay focused and pay attention, problems managing behavior, and hyperactivity (over-activity).

It is common for all children to be inattentive, hyperactive, or impulsive, but these behaviors are more severe and occur more frequently in children with ADHD. A child must experience symptoms for at least 6 months and to a more considerable extent than other children of the same age to be diagnosed with the disease. Although several studies imply that genes influence ADHD, scientists are unsure what causes it. ADHD, like many other illnesses, is most likely caused by a mix of circumstances. In addition to heredity, researchers are investigating potential environmental factors, such as brain injury, nutrition, and social environment, which may all play a role in ADHD.

Studies show a link between cigarette smoking and alcohol consumption during pregnancy and the development of ADHD in children. Furthermore, children who are exposed to high levels of lead, which can be found in plumbing fixtures or paint in ancient houses, may be at an increased risk of developing ADHD. According to recent British research, there may be a link between ingesting certain food additives, such as artificial colors or preservatives, and increased activity. The findings are being confirmed, and more research is being conducted to learn more about how food chemicals affect hyperactivity.

Other illnesses or ailments are present in some children with ADHD. They could, for example, have one or more of the following:

a. **A learning disability:** A preschooler with a learning disability could have trouble understanding specific sounds or words or expressing them verbally. Reading, spelling, writing, and math may be difficult for a school-aged child.
b. **Oppositional defiant disorder:** Children with this disorder, which causes them to be stubborn or rebellious, frequently dispute with adults and refuse to follow regulations.

c. **Conduct disorder:** This condition includes activities such as lying, stealing, fighting, or bullying others. They can destroy property, break into residences, and possess or use firearms. These children and teenagers are also more likely to use illegal substances. Children with conduct disorders are more likely to have problems at school or with the police.
d. **Bipolar disorder:** It is a mental illness that can be chronic or periodic. It can induce a wide range of odd, frequently dramatic, changing mood, energy, activity, and attention or focus changes. Bipolar disorder is also known as manic depression. Extreme mood swings from mania (an exceptionally high elevated mood) to depression in short periods may be present in some children with ADHD.
e. **Tourette syndrome:** Although just a small percentage of children have this neurological abnormality, many of those who do also have ADHD. Nervous tics and repetitive behaviors, such as eye blinks, facial twitches, or grimacing, are common in patients with Tourette syndrome. Others regularly clear their throats, snort or sniff, or bark out unpleasant phrases. Medication can be used to control these habits (Faraone et al., 2005).

6.5.1.3 Depression

Depression is linked to hypoactivation of prefrontal cortical (PFC) areas (including lateral and anterior cingulate cortex) and over-reactivity of the amygdala, a critical signaling site for neural threat response to unpleasant emotion and anxiety on a system level. It is a significant cause of global impairment. Environmental exposures are common in everyday life, adjustable, and may affect human neurobiology.

Air pollution, toxic compounds, heavy metals, noise, and radiation are examples of detrimental exposures. Natural environments, disasters, urbanization, and climate change are among the physical features of a few contextual contexts that we have explored. Sustained symptoms of sorrow, sleep difficulties, poor energy, worry, and emotions of insignificance characterize the disorder. Depression is a lethal illness, with suicide being the most severe complication. Depression risk varies by age, education, income, sex, and the frequency and scope of its occurrence in different countries show different patterns and trends.

According to recent studies, noise and chemical pollution are two examples of environmental factors that may have a neurological impact and alter the likelihood of depression, particularly in genetically predisposed people. A direct impact on a particular structure of the brain, which can lead to cell damage or functional alterations in the CNS systems. Heavy metals such as cadmium, lead, and arsenic can be acquired through various sources, including traffic, diet, and industrial emissions, such as dust in urban and industrial regions. It's possible that they'll cause neurotoxicity, and, through epigenetic mechanisms, increase the likelihood of neurodevelopmental disorders and depression.

Some studies have also found that exposure to chemicals, pesticides, and solvents like toluene can cause psychological disorders like depression. These chemical-related disorders place a significant financial and healthcare burden on the economy and healthcare system (Grandjean and Bellanger, 2017). Many workers are exposed to chemical hazards in their regular tasks due to many countries' industrialization. Solvents such as ethyl, benzene, toluene, and xylenes are commonly used in industrial and commercial processes. According to WHO studies, the clinical picture solvent solvents damage to the neurological system includes subjective symptoms such as memory and attentional problems, depressed mood, irritability, sleep disturbances, and exhaustion. On the other hand, long-term occupational exposure to organic solvents is usually associated with depressive and anxiety symptoms (Bast-Pettersen, 2009).

6.5.1.4 Migraine and headaches

Migraine is a widespread ailment that causes significant morbidity and economic costs worldwide. Migraineurs frequently mention barometric pressure changes, intense sunlight, flickering lights, air quality, and scents as triggers for their headaches. Migraine sufferers are also affected by the environment of their homes and workplaces. However, few controlled research studies confirm the impact of chemical and environmental exposure on migraine and headaches. Migraine's direct costs are proportional to the severity of the pain and incapacity it causes, and they skyrocket with prescription medications. However, indirect expenses exceed medical expenditures, and work-related incapacity is the most crucial factor in migraine's economic burden (Lee et al., 2018).

Headaches are a typical symptom following exposures at work or in the environment. It's noted as a complaint after being exposed to metal fumes as well as solvent vapors, which are utilized in industries and as fuels to dissolve other chemicals. The acuteness and intensity of the symptoms are determined by the source of the intoxicant, its molecular form, the route of entry, and the dose of exposure. Symptoms may not show for years or develop over time due to increased exposure. Pain can be caused by brain swelling (tin, lead) and temporary hypoxia or vasodilation (zinc, manganese, nickel).

Despite the lack of published data on chemical exposure headaches, a computer listing from the Hazardous Substance Data Bank indicates a database of over 700 compounds of various types that can induce headaches. The headaches reported in the low-exposure group lasted an average of 4.9 h. The majority of people experienced single daily headaches as a result of their daily exposures. Overexposure to chemicals may begin to experience severe headaches within minutes. All these people had a headache that was unlike anything they had ever felt, lasting several days. These people had never had frequent periodic headaches before, but after the actual headache went away, they developed a periodic headache syndrome, with recurrent headaches many times a month. The headaches were described as episodic, with recurrences lasting anywhere from 8 months to more than 3 years, with no substantial improvement in frequency or intensity.

Even though the absence of controlled human studies on the neurotoxic consequences of chemical exposure at work, case reports and cross-sectional epidemiological studies of acute nervous system symptoms such as headache, dizziness, and seizures can be found in the literature. In occupational exposure to chemicals and solvents in the pharmaceutical and chemical sectors, confusion, memory and concentration problems, irritability, sudden wrath, and exhaustion might occur (Lipton and Bigal, 2005).

6.5.2 Respiratory system-related conditions

Respiratory disease is the leading cause of death for most people and is one of the top 10 causes worldwide. According to the World Health Organization, 65 million individuals suffer from respiratory ailments ranging from mild to severe. Respiratory sickness is responsible for about 90% of deaths in low- and middle-income nations. Occupational respiratory disease is a lung disease or ailment caused by inhaling particles, fog, vapor, or hazardous gas at the workplace. The amount of material accumulated in the respiratory system and the sort of lung illness that the magnitude and type of inhalation determine the results. Organic and inorganic particles cause lung illness, vapors, and gases from hydrocarbons, insecticidal chemicals, plastics, and plastic burners.

According to the World Health Organization, 41 million people died from noncommunicable diseases (NCDs) in 2016, accounting for 71% of all deaths globally (Lindström et al., 2021). The respiratory tract is one of the most commonly affected organs. Asthma and chronic obstructive pulmonary disease (COPD), in particular, had a significant impact on the 4.2 million deaths globally due to respiratory disorders in 2008. Also, chemical pneumonitis, bronchitis, respiratory hypersensitivity reaction, acute chemical pneumonitis, Reactive Airways Dysfunction Syndrome (RADS), and Toluene Diisocyanate (TDI) Hypersensitivity reactions are common disorders due to exposure to environmental toxins, like heavy metals, persistent organic pollutants and tobacco smoke in the workplace (Faria et al., 2021).

Exposure to toxic agents at the workplace and inhalation of gases, chemicals, vapors, and fumes are defined in the Iowa Administrative Code as they are occupationally related to asthma, respiratory hypersensitivity reaction, bronchitis, and acute chemical pneumonitis. An increase in the size of the lung tissue (Swelling), fluid flow into the air gaps in the lung, and a diminished capacity to take in oxygen and release carbon dioxide are all symptoms of acute chemical pneumonitis. Death may occur in difficult situations due to a shortage of oxygen supply to the tissues (hypoxia). Chronic chemical pneumonitis can develop after prolonged exposure to a lung irritant at low levels. This creates inflammation, which can lead to fibrosis (scarring), a reduction in oxygen exchange, as well as stiffness of the lungs. If left untreated, this illness can lead to respiratory collapse and death.

Air hunger (a feeling of not being able to obtain enough air), strange lung sounds (wet or gurgling), difficulty breathing, an unpleasant feeling, and cough, or maybe a burning sensation in the chest are all acute exposure. Cough (not always present), growing impairment related to dyspnoea, fast breathing, and dyspnoea with little exercise are all symptoms of chronic exposure. Many typical home and industrial pollutants can cause acute and chronic lung irritation. Chlorine is one of the most irritating compounds that may be ingested. Dangerous exposure can occur at home (when using bleach-containing cleaning products), workplace, or during unforeseen incidents like spills and swimming pools. Other hazardous compounds can be inhaled in a variety of circumstances, including factories (particularly during welding, smelting, and other metal operations), solvent or pesticide manufacturing or use, fires (house fires, wildfires), and grain and fertilizer dust (Lux et al., 2020).

Workers in all jobs may regularly be exposed to chemicals and disinfectants, particularly in essential critical services like health care, transportation, grocery stores, emergency personnel, and other workforce sectors (ILO, 2020b). Due to an anticipated increase in global demand for several disinfectants, chemical industry workers may be dealing with larger quantities of these chemicals (ILO, 2020b). Quaternary ammonium, peroxyacetic acid, hydrogen peroxide, peroxyacetic acid, sodium hypochlorite, isopropanol, octanoic acid, ethanol, phenolic, trimethylene glycol, glycolic acid, L-lactic acid, are some of the chemicals that are widely used to disinfect against COVID-19 (Suarez-Lopez et al., 2021). In particular, quaternary ammonium and sodium hypochlorite have been linked to an increased risk of COPD, may affect fertility, and can aggravate asthma symptoms (Emanuel et al., 2020).

In addition, the occupational population is exposed to unique asthma and COPD hazards. Airborne pollutants that cause asthma and COPD include diisocyanates, formaldehyde, anhydrides, and metal salts. COPD is also triggered by inorganic or organic dust or gases, such as mine and cement dust. Asthma is brought on or aggravated by exposure to chemicals at work. These drugs can cause asthma in one of three ways: first allergic reactivity, an irritating response, and a reaction that causes an accumulation of naturally occurring substances in the lungs, such as histamines, leading to an asthma attack.

Occupational asthma is a disease characterized by fluctuating airflow limitation or airway hyperresponsiveness, both of which are produced by causes or situations specific to a particular occupational environment rather than stimuli received in environments other than the job. Coughing, chest stiffness, wheezing, dyspnoea, and breathing difficulty are asthma symptoms. Also, nasal congestion, eye irritation, and runny nose could be there. This may be an allergic reaction, but it might also be an irritating reaction from being exposed to asthma triggers at work. More than 300 workplace chemicals have been identified as potential asthma triggers. Animal proteins, like those found in scales, dander, fur, hair, bodily wastes, and saliva, are among these compounds. Paints, varnishes, adhesives, laminates, and soldering resin are made with chemicals like acids, diisocyanates, and anhydrides. The chemicals are utilized in insulation, packaging, foam mattresses, and upholstery. Proteins observed in flour, natural rubber latex, hemp, cereals, cotton, rye, flax, papain, and wheat, a digestive enzyme collected from papaya, are among the plant substances. Platinum, chromium, and nickel sulfate are metals.

The World Trade Center (WTC) disaster in New York in 2001 blasted smoke clouds, gasoline, and debris throughout the surrounding neighborhood, devouring streets and moving into homes and other structures as well as surrounding them. Airborne particles and their resuspension caused heavy and protracted exposures for first responders and adjacent neighbors during clean-up procedures. Many people had respiratory symptoms, including "WTC cough," a novel illness characterized by a persistent cough and severe breathing difficulties. As per US Government Accountability Office, practically answering firemen experienced severe respiratory ailments, which put hundreds of firefighters' careers on hold (Andarini et al., 2019).

Reactive airway dysfunction syndrome (RADS) is an extreme kind of work-related asthma brought on by irritants that develop quickly and without a latency period after a single encounter with a very irritating concentration of a respiratory irritant. The pathogenesis of RADS is unknown; however, airway damage, hyperresponsiveness, chronic airway inflammation, and remodeling are all thought to result from exposure to high concentrations of an irritating agent. A 27-year-old male suffered from cough, dyspnoea, and chemical burns 6 h after inhaling and splashing an industrial disinfectant containing a mixture of acetic acid, hydrogen peroxide, and peracetic acid. He was a nonsmoker who had never had atopy, asthma, or lung illness. He was diagnosed with RADS and began treatment for asthma. At the age of 4 months, his diffusion capacity returned to normal. He was still symptomatic 18 months later, with severe and chronic airway blockage on spirometry, requiring a mix of asthma medications, including high-dose inhaled corticosteroids, long-acting beta-2 agonist, and long-acting muscarinic antagonist (Chew and Tan, 2017).

In both animals and humans, exposure to toluene diisocyanate (2, 4- and 2,6-TDI) has been shown to have adverse effects on the respiratory system. Sudden acute bronchospasm attacks, pulmonary edema, and respiratory distress may be life-threatening and may occur days, or even months, after the first exposure. Acute effects include sensory irritation and respiratory inflammation in non-sensitized asthmatic subjects, asthmatic episodes in non-sensitized subjects, sensitization and induction of asthma with repeated exposures, and lung function declines due to chronic exposure without evidence of sensitization. Once TDI-sensitized individuals have developed asthma, even low diisocyanate doses (one to 10 parts per billion) might trigger attacks. Three clerical workers exposed to TDI fumes from a nearby polyurethane manufacturing developed asthma, according to a British case study. Exhaust from the factory was inhaled into the ventilation system of the building next door, causing delayed or late-type asthmatic symptoms in the clerical staff. Painting a TDI-containing varnish onto a surface in a chamber exposed the workers to an estimated concentration of 1 part per billion TDI was used to confirm TDI-induced asthma. Only when exposed to TDI-containing varnish did asthmatic symptoms occur.

A critical evaluation of the case histories and clinical data of 621 isocyanate workers was presented in clinical studies. Of these, 247 had bronchial asthma diagnosed, which was followed by chronic bronchitis, rhinitis, conjunctivitis, and several other less common conditions like allergic alveolitis hypersensitivity reactions. A faster loss in lung function with prolonged TDI exposure in the absence of occupational asthma is another pulmonary endpoint that many studies look into (Baur et al., 1994).

6.5.3 Cardiovascular system-related conditions

Cardiovascular disease (CVD) is the world's leading morbidity and mortality cause for men and women. In 2017, roughly 18 million people died from CVD, resulting in a loss of life expectancy of 330 million years, with 35.6 million years lost due to incapacity. The illness has risen to become the primary cause of death (approximately 40% of all fatalities) in emerging countries like the United States, China, and Brazil. As a result, identifying new preventive risk factors is critical, especially for people in low and middle-income nations. Environmental deterioration and heavy metal exposure in the workplace may directly impact the development of CVD. It is now recognized as a significant risk to global health on a personal and societal level.

Recent studies have provided offensive evidence concerning the rising prevalence of diabetes and high blood pressure relating to environmental exposure to heavy metals cadmium (Cd), like arsenic (As), mercury (Hg), and lead (Pb), and a few essential trace metals such as cobalt (Co), chromium (Cr), copper (Cu), molybdenum (Mo), magnesium (Mg), nickel (Ni), manganese (Mn), selenium (Se), zinc (Zn) tungsten (W), and vanadium (V). Over the last two decades, evidence of the involvement of heavy metal exposure in CVD risk has significantly expanded. A recent meta-analysis of almost 350,000 people from 37 countries found that exposure to As, Pb, Cd, and Cu was directly linked to an increased risk of CVD incidence and mortality, with a dose-response curve linear in form. In the same meta-analysis, no significant link between Hg exposure and CVD risk was discovered. Prospective cohort data on Zn and CVD risk were also mixed, with the greatest category of Se consumption associated with decreased cardiovascular disease risk (Yang et al., 2020).

Analyses of cross-sectional data from 7404 participants in a Hispanic Community Health Study in the USA, aged 18 to 74. Participants had clinical examinations, including ECGs, filled out questionnaires, and they came from four different US regions. At least one of the following conditions was considered CVD: coronary heart disease, heart failure, atrial fibrillation, or cerebrovascular illness. Rates of occurrence were calculated using Poisson regression models representing the connection between occupational exposure and CVD and CVD subtypes. Organic solvents (6.5%), pesticides (4.7%), and metals (8.5%), were all reported as being present in current occupations by Hispanic/Latino workers. Overall, 6.1% of participants had some CVD, with coronary heart disease (4.3%) being the most frequent (1.0%), heart failure (0.8%), cerebrovascular disease (1.0%), and atrial fibrillation (0.8%) being the next most prevalent (0.7%). After adjusting for sociodemographic, lifestyle, acculturation, and occupational characteristics, the prevalence ratios for any CVD were 2.18 (95% CI 1.34−3.55), coronary heart disease 2.20 (95% CI 1.31−3.71), cerebrovascular disease 1.38 (95% CI 0.62 3.03), heart failure 0.91 (95% CI 0.23−3.54), and atrial fibrillation 5.92 (95% CI 1.89−18.61). Exposure to metals was linked to a nearly fourfold increase in the risk of atrial fibrillation (Bulka et al., 2019b).

The relationship between hazardous chemical exposure and cardiovascular disease in those employed in the chemical product industry was investigated by researchers. The findings indicate that reactive oxygen species and oxidative stress, both of which are caused by exposure to dangerous substances, work as mediators, changing the physiological levels of EP and NEP to increase blood pressure. Lipid peroxidation causes an increase in triglyceride, blood glucose levels, and cholesterol, which contributes to the development of cardiovascular disease. Several studies have found that exposure to hazardous chemicals increases the physiological levels of leptin, brain-derived neurotrophic factor (BDNF), and neurotransmitters such as serotonin, dopamine, and catecholamines, all of which are linked to food intake desire, as well as that exposure to SO_2, CO_2, NO_2, and PM10 from pollution influences CVD development (Kim et al., 2012).

Workers in a petrochemical factory were shown to have a higher prevalence of hypertension. Heart disease was more common among workers who were exposed to high amounts of styrene than those exposed to moderate levels or the general population. The workers repeatedly exposed to high levels of styrene in plastic unit manufacturing sites had higher cholesterol, systolic blood pressure, and fasting glucose than non-exposed controls. Overall, the results show that ROS and oxidative stress caused by exposure to dangerous chemicals act as mediators, changing physiological levels of epinephrine and norepinephrine to raise BP and eventually increase chances of CVD development through lipid peroxidation-induced increases in cholesterol, triglycerides, and blood glucose (Nsanzabera, 2022; Bulka et al., 2019a).

6.5.4 GIT-related conditions

Researchers studied the relationship between workplace features and circumstances and the occurrence of GIT disorders. A group of 891 people had routine colonoscopies and gastroscopies and interviews about their work settings and exposures. Data were then statistically evaluated to see if any correlations could be found. Certain gastrointestinal illnesses, such as ulcers and gastritis, are common among shift workers. Still, a few studies have looked into the relationship with other kinds of GIT diseases, like inflammatory bowel disease. The Greek Statistical classification of jobs says that (STEP-92) the study included a representative sample of individuals from all professional groupings. During the study period, 809 people were diagnosed with one of the eight gastrointestinal disorders: peptic ulcer 155 (19.2%), gastritis 102 (12.6%), Crohn's disease 106 (13.1%), ulcerative colitis 46 (5.7%), colon cancer 119 (14.7%) and stomach cancer. Polyps 126 (15.6%), constipation 127 (15.7%), and diarrhea 7.2% (Chiu et al., 2020).

Exposure to toluene has been linked to an increased risk of different gastrointestinal malignancies, and working as a painter has regularly been linked to a 40% greater risk of lung cancer. There is evidence that trichloroethylene exposure increases the risk of liver cancer and non-lymphoma, Hodgkin's tetrachloroethylene exposure increases the risk of esophageal and cervical cancer, and carbon tetrachloride exposure increases the risk of lymph hematopoietic malignancies. The cohort with the highest methylene chloride exposure was linked to increased liver and biliary tract malignancies.

Long-term occupational exposure to high levels of inorganic arsenic develops gastrointestinal effects, including nausea, vomiting, abdominal pain, and diarrhea. Mercury and methylmercury are toxic to the gastrointestinal tract and may induce kidney toxicity if ingested (Baker et al., 2018).

Benzene and trichloroethylene (TCE) have been classed by International Agency for Research on Cancer (IARC) as carcinogenic to humans (group 1). In contrast, some solvents, such as methylene chloride and tetrachloroethylene, have been categorized as possibly carcinogenic (group 2A). Exposure to toluene has been linked to an increased risk of different gastrointestinal malignancies, and working as a painter has regularly been linked to a 40% greater risk of lung cancer. There is evidence that trichloroethylene exposure increases the risk of liver cancer and non-lymphoma, Hodgkin's tetrachloroethylene exposure increases the risk of esophageal and cervical cancer, and carbon tetrachloride exposure increases the risk of lymph hematopoietic malignancies. The cohort with the highest methylene chloride exposure was linked to an increased incidence of liver and biliary tract malignancies (Ore et al., 2022; Park and work, 2021).

Bisphenols, phthalates, POPs, heavy metals, and pesticides were the main chemicals studied to determine how ambient exposure affected the gut flora. These chemical classes were taken into consideration for the study since they are frequently present in human environments, and there is mounting proof that they impact the composition of the gut microbiota (Chiu et al., 2020).

The available evidence of the study suggests that exposure to environmental toxins like heavy metals, pesticides, nanoparticles, polycyclic aromatic hydrocarbons, dioxins, furans, polychlorinated biphenyls, and noncaloric artificial sweeteners has been linked to the development of metabolic, neoplastic, inflammatory, and immunological illnesses (Gadekar et al., 2021; Gorain et al., 2016; Muniswamy et al., 2019; Prajapati et al., 2009).

Moreover, the effects of the environmental chemicals on gut microbiota highly depend on sex and age (Martínez-Castillo et al., 2021; Youngren et al., 2013; Tekade and Chougule, 2013).

6.5.5 Ear, nose and throat (ENT) related conditions

Many industrial hazards, such as chemicals, noise, atmospheric pressure changes, allergens, carcinogens, and trauma, are likely to damage components of the human body, like the ear, nose, and throat. Allergens or carcinogens can travel through these parts to other body regions, including the lungs, gastrointestinal tract, and brain. General hazardous airborne pollutants are the risks in a chemical environment.

Gaseous and particulate substances find their way to the lungs by inhalation. Insecticides like phenol, cresol, and organophosphates like Parathion are absorbed via the skin. Insecticides like phenol, cresol, and organophosphates like Parathion are absorbed via the skin. Metals, aromatic carbons, aliphatic chemicals, toxic fumes, and dust are all dangerous substances in the chemical environment. Mist, fog, vapors, and dust are examples of these. When in the air, they all behave the same manner. Due to the issue of personal vulnerability and individual behaviors, assimilation and subsequent hazardous manifestations vary from work to work in the same sort of activity. Following are some occupational diseases caused by these chemical hazards (Asher and Guilford, 2016).

- **Pneumoconiosis and Occupational Asthma:** Cotton dust in textile and flour dust in food industries induce pneumoconiosis and occupational asthma. To transit these hazardous chemicals, the nose and throat serve as conduit linking the lower respiratory tract to the atmosphere.
- **Extrinsic Allergic Alveolitis:** Allergic rhinitis precedes extrinsic allergic alveolitis, which is caused by fungal spores.
- **Cement Dermatitis:** Primary irritant dermatitis is induced by handling cement. Ulcerations of the oral and nasal mucous membranes occur from inhaling cement dust.
- **Nasal cavity malignancy** is caused by organic pollutants such as isopropyl oil. Furniture workers are exposed to wood dust as a result of their work. Leather dust is also a factor.
- **Carcinoma of the Paranasal Sinuses:** The leading cause is inorganic pollutants such as nickel in refinery workers.
- **Nasopharyngeal Cancer:** Formaldehyde dust, smoke particulates, and some aromatic hydrocarbons are known to cause nasopharyngeal cancer. Tobacco and alcohol users are more prone to this cancer (Concha-Barrientos et al., 2004).

6.5.6 Skin-related conditions

The National Institute for Occupational Safety and Health (NIOSH) and the Centres for Disease Control and Prevention (CDC) estimated that over 13.2 million workers in the United States are exposed to toxins that can be absorbed via the skin, across a wide range of occupational industries and sectors. Workers in the following industries and sectors are at risk of potentially dangerous skin exposures: agriculture, cosmetology, manufacturing, health care, painting, mechanics, printing/lithography, cleaning, and building, to name a few. There are over 82,000 chemicals in industrial usage, with an estimated 700 new chemicals being launched each year, resulting in a substantial risk of chemical exposure to the skin.

Skin exposures in the workplace can cause several diseases, which can have a detrimental influence on an individual's health, capacity to work, medical bills, and lost work due to illness, with annual costs estimated to surpass $1 billion in the United States alone. According to the Bureau of Labour Statistics (BLS), about 34,400 cases were due to skin disorders in 2012, or 3.4 per 10,000 employees, outnumbering occupational respiratory illnesses.

The three types of chemical-skin interactions are direct skin effects, systemic consequences, and immune-mediated skin effects. Hundreds of chemicals (acrylic resins, metals rubber additives, chemicals) found in almost all industries have been identified as causing direct effects such as irritation, necrosis, corrosion, and immunological responses such as contact dermatitis or urticaria. Still, the amount and types of molecules that contribute to systemic effects are mostly unknown (Anderson and Meade, 2014).

Contact dermatitis is the most frequent type of occupational illness in the United States, accounting for 90%–95% of all occupational skin disorders and having a sizable socioeconomic impact. Itching, soreness, swelling, redness, and the creation of a rash are common signs of acute dermatitis, which can lead to chronic alterations such as pigmentation changes, skin thickness, and cracking after repeated or protracted exposure. It can be caused by the chemical's direct effects on the skin, irritant contact dermatitis (ICD), or immune-mediated effects, such as urticaria and allergic contact dermatitis (ACD). Acute exposures to extremely irritating compounds like acids, bases, and oxidizing agents, as well as a high frequency of wet labor and chronic cumulative exposures to moderate irritants like detergents and light cleaning agents, can all lead to ICD (Anderson and Meade, 2014).

Allergic contact dermatitis is a common and chronic skin condition that is frequently linked to environmental variables, primarily those related to the workplace. In the human environment, more than 3700 chemicals have been identified as contact allergens. 12.5% to 40.6% of the population in North America and Western Europe has been diagnosed as allergic to at least one chemical. Metals are one of the most common contact allergies. Common metals that cause contact allergic dermatitis after prolonged consumption include nickel, cobalt, and chromium, while other metal ions may produce hypersensitivity reactions. Many recent studies have reported the link between heavy metal load (lead, cadmium, platinum) and allergy responses.

In several studies, metal implants used in many medical applications, like intravascular stents, cardiac pacemakers, dental implants, and implanted gynecologic devices, are considered vital sources of metal sensitization. Although metal hypersensitivity reactions differ by patient, they include, urticarial, eczematous bullous, inflammation, and vasculitis eruptions comparable to AD symptoms (Nicolopoulou-Stamati et al., 2016).

Atopic dermatitis is a chronic inflammatory skin illness that primarily affects children and causes severe itching, xerosis, and apparent eczematous skin lesions. Atopic dermatitis significantly influences patients and their family's quality of life. Atopic dermatitis has seen a rise in its expected lifetime prevalence by a factor of two in the last 30 years, particularly in metropolitan areas in developed countries, highlighting the role of lifestyle and environment in the etiology of atopic disorders. We may come into contact with millions of chemical molecules throughout our lives. Chemical allergies have been increasingly exposed to a range of sources in recent decades, particularly in industrialized countries. Some of these end up in our surroundings as automobile exhaust fumes, pesticides, industrial dust, fertilizers, cigarette smoke, and insecticides. Preservatives, pigments, perfumes, surfactants, chelating agents favor, and flavor enhancers are also found in most personal hygiene products, cosmetics, processed foods, and pharmaceuticals. Amalgam fillings, dental implants, prosthetic jewelry, and jewelry could all discharge heavy metals (Kim, 2015).

Several cross-sectional studies have found a link between air pollution exposure and eczema symptoms. A study found that eczema symptoms were strongly linked to benzene,

PM10, nitrogen oxide chemicals, and carbon monoxide exposure in 9- to 11-year-old children. In Taiwan, a nationwide assessment of nearly 30,000 children found that flexural eczema was linked to exposure to traffic-related air pollution. In an urban area, a birth cohort study discovered strong positive connections between eczema and distance to the nearest major road and a positive relationship between NO_2 exposure and eczema. Several studies have found that outdoor air pollution impacts the prevalence of Alzheimer's disease. The lifetime frequency of AD eczema was substantially linked with 3-year mean amounts of PM10, nitrogen oxide chemicals, and carbon monoxide in a study involving 4907 French children (Kim, 2015). In an urban US birth cohort study, exposure to butyl benzyl phthalate during pregnancy was linked to the development of eczema at 2 years of age. Outdoor air pollution appears to be one of the most potent risk factors for the development of Alzheimer's disease, according to these studies (Nakamura et al., 2013).

6.5.7 Miscellaneous conditions

i. **Chronic fatigue syndrome:** chronic fatigue syndrome (CFS) is a common ailment. More than 2 million Americans are thought to have CFS, many of whom go undiagnosed. CFS affects twice as many women as it does men, and it is more common in people over 40. Several doctors have reported multisystem symptoms similar to chronic fatigue syndrome and chemical intolerance in some patients after surgical implant procedures. Importantly, silicone can seep out of intact breast implant membranes over time, causing inflammatory and immune reactions. The chemical nature of implants may contain metals that migrate into neighboring tissue. Processing aids and peroxides have also helped cure implant gels (Bjørklund et al., 2020). A causal association between breast implant illness (BII) and symptoms is supported by reports that implant removal can relieve symptoms in 40%–60% of people. "These patients had no adverse reactions to perfumes, room fresheners, deodorants, hairsprays, cleaning agents, cigarette smoke, exhaust fumes, carpeting, fabric dyes, adhesives, caulking, glues, stain removers, detergents, dry cleaning products, paints, lacquers, insecticides, pesticides, and printing resins before implantation," Brawer summarized his observations of over 500 breast implant recipients. Following the onset of their systemic sickness, they began to experience nausea, dizziness, and headaches when exposed to practically all of the above. He also saw a "deep parallelism" between TILT and his findings spanning four decades (Masri et al., 2021).

ii. **Gulf War syndrome** is a multi-symptomatic chronic condition affecting military personnel from both sides of the Persian Gulf War, which lasted from 1990 to 1991. It has been related to many acute and chronic symptoms, including muscle discomfort, fatigue, cognitive issues, insomnia, rashes, and diarrhea. Approximately 250,000 of the 697,000 United States soldiers who served in the 1991 Gulf War suffer from chronic multi-symptom sickness, a dangerous condition.

During the Gulf War, chemical weapons were a known risk factor due to their use or proximity to military troops. Ten thousand US troops were subjected to the organophosphate (OP) nerve agents like sarin and cycloserine, which inhibit the enzyme acetylcholinesterase, when US forces blew up an Iraqi munitions store at Khamisiyah (AChE). Even low doses of OP can cause acute symptoms, which may signal the initiation of

TILT. OP insecticides were also routinely used in the Gulf to prevent vector-borne disease among US troops. At least 40,000 service members may have been overexposed to OPs, according to the US Department of Defense.

Pyridostigmine bromide (PB) pills were given to an estimated 250,000 US soldiers as a pre-treatment medicine to protect them from nerve agent exposure. PB is a carbamate chemical that acts on the central nervous system similarly to OP insecticides. Except for battle, PB was exclusively approved in the United States for treating myasthenia gravis, a chronic muscle illness in which patients have antibodies to their cholinergic receptors. PB was never approved for those with normal nervous system function, let alone those chemically vulnerable. It's possible that they were overexposed to OPs. Combustion products from burn pits and oil well fires were two other primary Gulf exposures.

One study found that consuming PB tablets, being within one mile of an exploding Scud missile, putting insecticides on the skin, and being exposed to oil and smoke were all linked to Gulf War Illness. The central and peripheral cholinergic nerve systems (which require the neurotransmitter acetylcholinesterase) were the most prominent symptoms described by Gulf War veterans. Excess sickness in Gulf War veterans was linked, in part, to exposure to acetylcholinesterase inhibitors, such as PB, pesticides, and nerve agents, according to Golomb (Wessely, 2001).

iii. **World Trade Centre disaster:** The WTC disaster in New York City in 2001 blasted clouds of smoke, gasoline, and debris throughout the neighborhood, engulfing streets and entering homes and other structures. Airborne particles and their re-suspension caused heavy and protracted exposures for first responders and adjacent neighbors during clean-up procedures. Many people had respiratory symptoms, including "WTC cough," a novel illness characterized by a persistent cough and severe breathing difficulties. Many people had respiratory symptoms, including "WTC cough," a novel illness characterized by a persistent cough and severe breathing difficulties.

iv. As per the US Government Accountability Office, every responding fireman experienced severe respiratory ailments, putting hundreds of firefighters' careers on hold. Combustion products and chemicals used in furnishings, construction materials, and upkeep are among the pollutants linked to the WTC disaster. Polycyclic aromatic hydrocarbons (PAHs), asbestos, pesticides, dioxins, polychlorinated biphenyls, phthalates, and brominated fire retardants (BFR) were found in dust samples from the wreckage (Landrigan et al., 2004; Jordan et al., 2011).

v. **Tunnel workers**

Chemical intolerances were developed among construction workers developing a subway tunnel under an old fuel station (Davidoff et al., 1998). As the tunnel was being dug, they were exposed to dirt contaminated with gasoline vapors (60 ppm benzene) for 2 months. Following the closure of the tunnel due to elevated benzene levels, the authors randomly interviewed 30 of the remaining 70 employees, examined their health and chemical intolerances, and then did so again 10–13 months later. They were compared to a control group of 24 people drawn at random from the general community. Approximately one-fourth of the exposed workers (26.7%) reported new chemical intolerances and other TILT-like traits. Other potentially significant exposures in such a restricted tunnel area include particles, soil microorganisms, diesel exhaust, and carbon monoxide, in addition to benzene from gasoline. In addition to benzene from gasoline, other potentially significant exposures in such a constrained tunnel region would include particulates, soil microorganisms, diesel exhaust, and carbon monoxide. According to the authors, Workers in this group were low-income males who did not have a history of reporting CI-related symptoms and were not litigious (Ulvestad et al., 2000; You et al., 2014).

vi. Oil Spill

Oil spills often happen because of our daily reliance on oil and petroleum products. Every day, Canada consumes about 450,000 tons of oil and petroleum products. The United States (US) uses nearly 10 times this amount, and about 20 million tons are used daily worldwide. The self-reported oil spill exposure and birth outcomes growth study of southern Louisiana women at the time of the Gulf oil spill estimates that between 2012 and 2016, 1375 women reported at least one live birth due to the oil leak. A total of 573 babies were born before and after the oil leak. Self-reported financial repercussions, direct contact with oil, traumatic experiences, loss of coast use, and engagement in litigation were all indicators of oil spill exposure. Low birth weight (LBW; birth weight 2500 g) and preterm birth (PTB; birth $>$ 3 weeks early) were the two most common birth outcomes.

The United States Coast Guard (USCG) conducted the clean-up effort following the Deepwater Horizon (DWH) oil leak in 2010. Few human studies investigate acute and long-term cardiovascular problems linked to oil spill exposure. There was a modestly elevated incidence of chronic respiratory problems among active duty Coast Guard employees who had been exposed to oil during spill clean-up (Krishnamurthy et al., 2019; Alexander et al., 2018).

6.6 Evaluation of exposures causing toxicant-induced loss of tolerance

Chemical intolerance has mainly been ignored in the medical and public health fields. Even though between 15 and 36% of the population of the United States reports being intolerant to a few chemicals and around 5% reporting of MCS the physician (Miller and Prihoda, 1999). Currently, there is no well-established standard treatment for MCS. Sometimes it is difficult to know the actual exposure because of such sensitivity or tolerance, and multi-system involvement arises. So, it is always advised to keep yourself away from such exposures. That's why MCS treatment is not simple and demands active participation from the patient. It becomes more complex, especially in patients with neurological conditions. Even biomarkers and combinations of the drug are more and less used for the disease management of the patient.

6.6.1 Biomarkers

Biomarkers can distinguish specific viruses and bacteria that cause infectious diseases, as well as the specific antigens and antibodies associated with immunological reactions that came into existence (Savvateeva et al., 2019). After a few years, germ and immune theories of the disease have been proposed. Similarly, the discovery of disease-specific biomarkers for conditions associated with TILT may not come for some time. It would appear that TILT has some similarities to addiction. Even though the problem has been identified previously and research has been going on for decades, there is still no test that can diagnose addiction. Addiction can only be accurately diagnosed through abstaining from the substance in question and observing how the body reacts. The same seems to be the case with abdication. After a few times, it is possible that with the help of more sophisticated tools and techniques, one can evaluate TILT on a more ground level (Miller, 1999).

6.6.2 Diagnosis and treatment

If chemically intolerant people also have intolerances to chemicals, drugs, and food, then eliminating all potential/primary triggers at the same time should improve their symptoms. Drug therapy may also include if TILT causes abdiction or addiction. Consider that above 50 different drugs have been investigated for their potential in treating cocaine addiction. Still, none of them have been proven to be efficient as of yet.

Cocaine has been referred to as a "dirty drug" because it affects a wide variety of brain cells (Butini et al., 2016). It also includes those involved in the neurotransmitter systems of noradrenaline, serotonin, and dopamine. Dopamine is linked with five different types of receptors that are already known. If the treatment of cocaine addiction is so complex, imagine how difficult it would be to treat the health effects that result from complex chemical environments that involve dozens or even hundreds of different substances. In the meantime, the approach that is most likely to produce the desired outcomes is the one that involves the elimination of all potentially offensive substances, also known as unmasking. This is the simplest method. It would not make much sense for someone addicted to cocaine to try to counteract the numerous symptoms they are experiencing with other nonaddictive drugs while still engaging in cocaine use (Miller, 1999).

6.7 Consequences of toxicant-induced loss of tolerance

TILT is a novel disease theory, so its advantages and consequences/limitations come. It is impossible to encompass all of the varied conditions that have been ascribed to TILT, just as it is impossible to encompass all of the conditions that have been ascribed to any other theory of disease, like immune theory and germ theory, explains an overarching mechanism that underlies a group of diseases. The germ theory and the immune theory both involve multiple syndromes and various symptoms involving any organ system. It would be equivalent to creating a case definition for the TILT class of diseases. It would be impossible to try and find a single case definition that would fit all infectious diseases or all diseases in general. As a potential substitute to case definition for investigation, the subject can rate the intensity of their symptoms and their reaction to food, chemical inhalant, drugs, and masking indexes from 0 to 100 scale (Miller and Prihoda, 1999; Miller, 1999).

6.8 Conclusion

Toxicant-induced loss of tolerance is a two-step process, namely initiation followed by triggering. Exposure to inhalants, ingestants, chemical vapors from solvents, fragrances, smoke, pesticides, specific medicine or food, etc., may serve as triggers that lead to symptoms like fatigue, rash, mood swipe, headache, weakness, memory impairment, concentration-related issues (called "brain fog"), and lungs problem. Germ theory and immune theory cannot provide an approachable mechanism for the disease or chemical sensitivity. Though it explains the causality factor of disease Anomaly, novelty, generalizability, and causality can be explained by TILT. This theory explains disease mechanism in two steps, i.e., initiation and subsequent triggering at low levels, considering a phenomenon called masking. It is like an iceberg where we can only see a small portion of ice (in this case, it is symptoms) above the seawater. Still, the actual depth of the iceberg below the seawater (i.e., initiation and triggering) is unknown. TILT is a novel theory and provides a robust and mechanistic approach to the etiology of the disease. However, still, it needs human challenge studies to provide evidence/proof for the same.

6.9 List of abbreviations

ACD Allergic contact dermatitis
AChE Acetylcholinesterase
ACS American chemical society
ADHD Attention deficit hypersensitive disorder
AIDS Acquired immunodeficiency syndrome
ASD Autism spectrum disorder
BDNF Brain-derived neurotrophic factor
BLS Bureau of labour statistics
CDC Disease control and prevention
CFS Chronic fatigue syndrome
CI Chemical intolerance
CNS Central nervous system
COPD Chronic obstructive pulmonary disease
COVID-19 Coronavirus disease of 2019
CVD Cardio vascular disease
GIT Gastro-intestinal tract
HIV Human immunodeficiency virus
IgE Immunoglobulin-E
MCS Multiple chemical sensitivity
NCD Noncommunicable disease
NIOSH National institute for occupational safety and health
NMDA N-methyl-D-aspartic acid
OP Organophosphates
PB Pyridostigmine bromide
RADS Reactive airway dysfunction hypersensitivity
TDI Toluene diisocyanate hypersensitivity
TILT Toxicant-induced loss of tolerance
WHO World health organization
WTC World trade centre

References

Alexander, M., Engel, L.S., Olaiya, N., Wang, L., Barrett, J., Weems, L., Schwartz, E.G., Rusiecki, J.A.J.E.R., 2018. The deepwater horizon oil spill coast guard cohort study: a cross-sectional study of acute respiratory health symptoms. Environ. Res. 162, 196–202.

Andarini, D., Camelia, A., Listianti, A.N., 2019. Occupational respiratory symptoms caused by chemical hazard on hairdresser workers in Palembang. J. Kesehat. Masy. 15, 6–14.

Anderson, S.E., Meade, B.J., 2014. Potential health effects associated with dermal exposure to occupational chemicals. EHI 8, S15258.

Asher, B.F., Guilford, F.T., 2016. Oxidative stress and low glutathione in common ear, nose, and throat conditions: a systematic review. Altern. Ther. Health Med. 22, 44–50.

Ashford, N., Heinzow, B., Lutjen, K., Marouli, C., Molhave, L., Monah, B., Papadopoulos, S., Rest, K., Rosdahl, D., Siskos, P.J., 1995. Chemical sensitivity in selected European countries: an exploratory study. A Report to the European Commission. Ergonomia.

Ashford, N.A., Miller, C.S., 1998. Low-level chemical exposures: a challenge for science and policy. Environ. Sci. Technol. 32, 508–509.

Association, A.I.H., 1989. Odor thresholds for chemicals with established occupational health standards, Aiha.

Baker, M., Bergstresser, D., Serafeim, G., Wurgler, J., 2018. Financing the Response to Climate Change: The Pricing and Ownership of US Green Bonds. National Bureau of Economic Research.

Bartkowiak, A.M., Applications, I.M., 2011. Anomaly, novelty, one-class classification: a comprehensive introduction. Int. J. Comput. Inf. Syst. Ind. Manag. Appl. 3, 61–71.

Bast-Pettersen, R.J.N., 2009. The neuropsychological diagnosis of chronic solvent induced encephalopathy (CSE)—a reanalysis of neuropsychological test results in a group of CSE patients diagnosed 20 years ago, based on comparisons with matched controls. Neurotoxicology 30, 1195–1201.

Baur, X., Marek, W., Ammon, J., Czuppon, A., Marczynski, B., Raulf-Heimsoth, M., Roemmelt, H., Fruhmann, G.J., 1994. Respiratory and other hazards of isocyanates. Int. Arch. Occup. Environ. Health 66, 141–152.

Bjørklund, G., Dadar, M., Pivina, L., Dosa, M.D., Semenova, Y., Maes, M.J., 2020. Environmental, neuro-immune, and neuro-oxidative stress interactions in chronic fatigue syndrome. Mol. Neurobiol. 57, 4598–4607.

Bulka, C.M., Daviglus, M.L., Persky, V.W., Durazo-Arvizu, R.A., Lash, J.P., Elfassy, T., Lee, D.J., Ramos, A.R., Tarraf, W., Argos, M.J.H., 2019a. Association of occupational exposures with cardiovascular disease among US Hispanics/Latinos. Heart 105, 439–448.

Bulka, C.M., Persky, V.W., Daviglus, M.L., Durazo-Arvizu, R.A., Argos, M.J., 2019b. Multiple metal exposures and metabolic syndrome: a cross-sectional analysis of the National Health and Nutrition Examination Survey 2011–2014. Environ. Res. 168, 397–405.

Butini, S., Nikolic, K., Kassel, S., Brückmann, H., Filipic, S., Agbaba, D., Gemma, S., Brogi, S., Brindisi, M., Campiani, G.J., 2016. Polypharmacology of dopamine receptor ligands. Prog. Neurobiol. 142, 68–103.

Cabrera-Perez, J., Badovinac, V.P., Griffith, T.S., 2017. Enteric immunity, the gut microbiome, and sepsis: rethinking the germ theory of disease. Exp. Biol. Med. 242, 127–139.

Carter, K.C., 1985. Ignaz semmelweis, carl mayrhofer, and the rise of germ theory. Med. Hist. 29, 33–53.

Chew, S., Tan, K.J., 2017. P136 Pneumonitis and reactive airways dysfunction syndrome with persistent airway obstruction due to inhalation of industrial disinfectant: a case report. Chest 151, A33.

Chiu, K., Warner, G., Nowak, R.A., Flaws, J.A., Mei, W.J., 2020. The impact of environmental chemicals on the gut microbiome. Toxicol. Sci. 176, 253–284.

Concha-Barrientos, M., Nelson, D.I., Driscoll, T., Steenland, N.K., Punnett, L., Fingerhut, M., PRÜSS-Üstün, A., Leigh, J., Tak, S.W., Corvalan, C.J., 2004. Selected Occupational Risk Factors, pp. 1651–1801.

Cory-Slechta, D., Wedge, R., 2016. Gulf War and Health: Volume 10: Update of Health Effects of Serving in the Gulf War, 2016. National Academies Press.

Davidoff, A.L., Keyl, P.M., Meggs, W.J., 1998. Development of multiple chemical sensitivities in laborers after acute gasoline fume exposure in an underground tunneling operation. Arch. Environ. Health 53, 183–189.

Drexler, H., Greiner, A., 2020. Multiple Chemical Sensitivity, pp. 2539–2546.

Eid Ziad AL-Adwan, F., AL-Naimat, Y.M.J., 2019. Autism spectrum disorder (ASD); symptoms, causes, diagnosis, intervention, and counseling needs of the families in Jordan. Mod. Appl. Sci. 13, 1–48.

Emanuel, E.J., Persad, G., Upshur, R., Thome, B., Parker, M., Glickman, A., Zhang, C., Boyle, C., Smith, M., Phillips, J.P., 2020. Fair allocation of scarce medical resources in the time of Covid-19. N. Engl. J. Med. 382 (21), 2049–2055.

Faraone, S.V., Perlis, R.H., Doyle, A.E., Smoller, J.W., Goralnick, J.J., Holmgren, M.A., Sklar, P., 2005. Molecular genetics of attention-deficit/hyperactivity disorder. Psychiatr. Clin. 57, 1313–1323.

Faria, V.S., Silva, S.A., Marchini, J.F., 2021. Reactive airways dysfunction syndrome following inhalation of hydrogen chloride vapor. Autops. Case Rep. 11.

Fiedler, N., Kipen, H.M., Deluca, J., Kelly-Mcneil, K., Natelson, B.J., 1996. A controlled comparison of multiple chemical sensitivities and chronic fatigue syndrome. Psychosom. Med. 58, 38–49.

Gadekar, V., Borade, Y., Kannaujia, S., Rajpoot, K., Anup, N., Tambe, V., Kalia, K., Tekade, R.K., 2021. Nanomedicines accessible in the market for clinical interventions. J. Contr. Release 330, 372–397.

Gorain, B., Choudhury, H., Tekade, R.K., Karan, S., Jaisankar, P., Pal, T.K., 2016. Comparative biodistribution and safety profiling of olmesartan medoxomil oil-in-water oral nanoemulsion. Regul. Toxicol. Pharmacol. 82, 20–31.

Grandjean, P., Bellanger, M.J., 2017. Calculation of the disease burden associated with environmental chemical exposures: application of toxicological information in health economic estimation. Environ. Health 16, 1–13.

Grant, W.B., Boucher, B.J., 2010. Are Hill's criteria for causality satisfied for vitamin D and periodontal disease?. Dermato-endocrinology, 2 (1), 30–36.

Huff, R.D., Carlsten, C., Hirota, J.A., 2019. An update on immunologic mechanisms in the respiratory mucosa in response to air pollutants. J. Allergy Clin. Immunol. 143, 1989–2001.

Jordan, H.T., Miller-Archie, S.A., Cone, J.E., Morabia, A., Stellman, S.D., 2011. Heart disease among adults exposed to the September 11, 2001 world trade center disaster: results from the world trade center health registry. Prev. Med. 53, 370–376.

Kim, K.-W., Won, Y.L., Ko, K.S., Heo, K.-H., Chung, Y.H., 2012. The effects of hazardous chemical exposure on cardiovascular disease in chemical products manufacturing workers. Toxicol. Res. 28, 269–277.

Kim, K., 2015. Influences of environmental chemicals on atopic dermatitis. Toxicol. Res. 31, 89–96.

Krishnamurthy, J., Engel, L.S., Wang, L., Schwartz, E.G., Christenbury, K., Kondrup, B., Barrett, J., Rusiecki, J.A., 2019. Neurological symptoms associated with oil spill response exposures: results from the deepwater horizon oil spill coast guard cohort study. Environ. Int. 131, 104963.

Landrigan, P.J., Lioy, P.J., Thurston, G., Berkowitz, G., Chen, L., Chillrud, S.N., Gavett, S.H., Georgopoulos, P.G., Geyh, A.S., Levin, S., 2004. Health and environmental consequences of the world trade center disaster. Environ. Health Prospect. 112, 731–739.

Lee, H., Myung, W., Cheong, H.-K., Yi, S.-M., Hong, Y.-C., Cho, S.-I., Kim, H., 2018. Ambient air pollution exposure and risk of migraine: synergistic effect with high temperature. Environ. Int. 121, 383–391.

Lindström, I., Lantto, J., Karvala, K., Soini, S., Ylinen, K., Suojalehto, H., Suuronen, K.J.O., Medicine, E., 2021. Occupations and exposure events in acute and subacute irritant-induced asthma. Occup. Environ. Med. 78, 793–800.

Lipton, R.B., Bigal, M.E., 2005. Migraine: epidemiology, impact, and risk factors for progression. Headache 45, S3–S13.

Liu, X., Ouyang, W., Shu, Y., Tian, Y., Feng, Y., Zhang, T., Chen, W., 2019. Incorporating bioaccessibility into health risk assessment of heavy metals in particulate matter originated from different sources of atmospheric pollution. Environ. Pollut. 254, 113113.

Lux, H., Baur, X., Budnik, L.T., Heutelbeck, A., Teixeira, J.P., Neumann, E., Adliene, D., Puišo, J., Lucas, D., Löndahl, J., 2020. Outdoor air pollution from industrial chemicals causing new onset of asthma or COPD: a systematic review protocol. J. Occup. Med. Toxicol. 15, 1–10.

Martínez-Castillo, M., García-Montalvo, E.A., Arellano-Mendoza, M.G., Sánchez-Peña, L.D.C., Soria Jasso, L.E., Izquierdo-Vega, J.A., Valenzuela, O.L., Hernández-Zavala, A.J.H., Toxicology, E., 2021. Arsenic exposure and non-carcinogenic health effects. Hum. Exp. Toxicol. 40, S826–S850.

Masri, S., Miller, C.S., Palmer, R.F., Ashford, N., 2021. Toxicant-induced loss of tolerance for chemicals, foods, and drugs: assessing patterns of exposure behind a global phenomenon. Environ. Sci. Eur 33, 1–19.

Miller, C., Ashford, N., Doty, R., Lamielle, M., Otto, D., Rahill, A., Wallace, L., 1997. Empirical approaches for the investigation of toxicant-induced loss of tolerance. Environ. Health Perspect. 105, 515–519.

Miller, C., Prihoda, T., 1999. A controlled comparative study of chemical intolerances among MCS patients, implant recipients and Gulf War veterans. Tox. Ind. Health 386–398.

Miller, C.S., 2000. Mechanisms of action of addictive stimuli toxicant-induced loss of tolerance.

Miller, C.S., Ashford, N.A., 1995. Chemical sensitivity: perspectives from North America and Europe.

Miller, C.S., 2001a. Toxicant-induced loss of tolerance. Addiction 96, 115–137.

Miller, C.S., 2001b. The compelling anomaly of chemical intolerance. Ann. N. Y. Acad. Sci. 933, 1–23.

Miller, C.S., 1997. Toxicant-induced loss of tolerance–an emerging theory of disease? Environ. Health Prospect. 105, 445–453.

Miller, C.S., 1994. White paper: chemical sensitivity: history and phenomenology. Toxicol. Ind. Health 10, 253–276.

Miller, C.S., 1999. Are we on the threshold of a new theory of disease? Toxicant-induced loss of tolerance and its relationship to addiction and abdiction. Toxicol. Ind. Health 15, 284–294.

Miller, C.S., 2001. Toxicant-induced loss of tolerance–an emerging theory of disease? Townsend Lett. Dr. (212) 76-76.

Mølhave, L., Bach, B., Pedersen, O.F.J.E.I., 1986. Human reactions to low concentrations of volatile organic compounds, 12, 167–175.

Molot, J., Sears, M., Marshall, L.M., Bray, R.I.J.R.O.E.H., 2021. Neurological susceptibility to environmental exposures: pathophysiological mechanisms in neurodegeneration and multiple chemical sensitivity. Environ. Health Rev. 37, 509–530.

Moss, R.W., Randolph, T.G., 1980. An Alternative Approach to Allergies: The New Field of Clinical Ecology Unravels the Environmental Causes of Mental and Physical Ills. Lippincott & Crowell, New York.

Muniswamy, V.J., Raval, N., Gondaliya, P., Tambe, V., Kalia, K., Tekade, R.K., 2019. 'Dendrimer-Cationized-Albumin' encrusted polymeric nanoparticle improves BBB penetration and anticancer activity of doxorubicin. Int. J. Pharm. 555, 77–99.

Nakamura, Y., Oscherwitz, J., Cease, K.B., Chan, S.M., Muñoz-Planillo, R., Hasegawa, M., Villaruz, A.E., Cheung, G.Y., Mcgavin, M.J., Travers, J.B.J.N., 2013. Staphylococcus δ-toxin induces allergic skin disease by activating mast cells. Nature 503, 397–401.

National academies of Sciences, E., 2016. Gulf War and Health: Volume 10: Update of Health Effects of Serving in the Gulf War.

Nicolopoulou-Stamati, P., Maipas, S., Kotampasi, C., Stamatis, P., Hens, L., 2016. Chemical pesticides and human health: the urgent need for a new concept in agriculture. Public Health Front. 4, 148.

Nsanzabera, C., 2022. Risk prediction and factors associated with cardiovascular diseases among workers and their spouses in two beverage processing industries in Rwanda. JKUAT-COHES.

Ore, A., Adewale, A.A., Kehinde, S.A., Faniyi, T.O., Oladeji, A.D., Rufus, P.C., Akande, A.A., Chukwuemeka, I.E., 2022. Potential roles of oxidative stress and insulin resistance in diisononyl phthalate induced dyslipidemia and hepatosteatosis in BALB/c mice. Adv. Redox Res. 5, 100038.

Park, R.M.J.S., Work, H.A., 2021. Risk assessment for toluene diisocyanate and respiratory disease human studies. Saf. Health Work 12, 174–183.

Prajapati, R.N., Tekade, R.K., Gupta, U., Gajbhiye, V., Jain, N.K., 2009. Dendimer-mediated solubilization, formulation development and in vitro-in vivo assessment of piroxicam. Mol. Pharm. 6, 940–950.

Randolph, T.G., 1961. Human ecology and susceptibility to the chemical environment. Ann. Allergy 19, 908.

Randolph, T.G., 1962. Human Ecology and Susceptibility to the Chemical Environment.

Rossi, S., Pitidis, A.J.J.O.O., Medicine, E., 2018. Multiple chemical sensitivity: review of the state of the art in epidemiology, diagnosis, and future perspectives. J. Occup. Environ. Med. 60, 138.

Savvateeva, E.N., Rubina, A.Y., Gryadunov, D.A., 2019. Biomarkers of community-acquired pneumonia: a key to disease diagnosis and management. BioMed Res. Int. 2019.

Siegel, S., 2005. Drug tolerance, drug addiction, and drug anticipation. Curr. Dir. Psychol. Sci. 14, 296–300.

Suarez-Lopez, J.R., Cairns, M.R., Sripada, K., Quiros-Alcala, L., Mielke, H.W., Eskenazi, B., Etzel, R.A., Kordas, K., 2021. COVID-19 and children's health in the United States: consideration of physical and social environments during the pandemic. Environ. Res. 197, 111160.

Tabershaw, I., Cooper, W.C., 1966. Sequelae of acute organic phosphate poisoning. J. Occup. Health 8, 5–20.

Tekade, R.K., Chougule, M.B., 2013. Formulation development and evaluation of hybrid nanocarrier for cancer therapy: taguchi orthogonal array based design. BioMed Res. Int. 2013, 712678.

Ulvestad, B., Bakke, B., Melbostad, E., Fuglerud, P., Kongerud, J., Lund, M.B., 2000. Increased risk of obstructive pulmonary disease in tunnel workers. Thorax 55, 277–282.

Vaishampayan, S., Palshikar, G.K., Apte, M., Attar, V.Z., 2019. Causality: an overlooked aspect in anomaly detection. In: TENCON 2019–2019 IEEE Region 10 Conference (TENCON). IEEE, pp. 2413–2417.

Vandaele, Y., Ahmed, S., 2021. Habit, choice, and addiction. Neuropsychopharmacology 46, 689–698.

Webb, N.M., Shavelson, R.J., 2005. Generalizability theory: overview. Am. Psychol.

Wessely, S., 2001. Ten years on: what do we know about the Gulf War syndrome? Clin. Med. 1, 28.

Winsky-Sommerer, R., Yamanaka, A., Diano, S., Borok, E., Roberts, A.J., Sakurai, T., Kilduff, T.S., Horvath, T.L., DE Lecea, L., 2004. Interaction between the corticotropin-releasing factor system and hypocretins (orexins): a novel circuit mediating stress response. J. Neurosci. Res. 24, 11439–11448.

Yang, A.-M., Lo, K., Zheng, T.-Z., Yang, J.-L., Bai, Y.-N., Feng, Y.-Q., Cheng, N., Liu, S.-M., 2020. Environmental heavy metals and cardiovascular diseases: status and future direction. Chronic Dis. Transl. Med. 6, 251–259.

You, D., Smith, A.H., Rempel, D., 2014. Meta-analysis: association between wrist posture and carpal tunnel syndrome among workers. Saf. Health Work 5, 27–31.

Youngren, S.R., Tekade, R.K., Gustilo, B., Hoffmann, P.R., Chougule, M.B., 2013. STAT6 siRNA matrix-loaded gelatin nanocarriers: formulation, characterization, and ex vivo proof of concept using adenocarcinoma cells. BioMed Res. Int. 2013, 858946.

Zhu, S., Chen, C., Sultani, W., 2020. Video anomaly detection for smart surveillance. Computer Vision: A Reference Guide. Springer.

CHAPTER

7

Types of cellular responses to chemical toxicants

Deepak Kumar Gupta[1], *Akhilesh Tiwari*[1], *Megha Joshi*[2], *Muktika Tekade*[3], *Kuldeep Rajpoot*[4], *Nupur Vasdev*[4], *Omar Husham Ahmed Al-Attraqchi*[5] *and Rakesh Kumar Tekade*[4]

[1]Indira Gandhi National Tribal University, Amarkantak, Madhya Pradesh, India; [2]Vikram University, Ujjain, Madhya Pradesh, India; [3]School of Pharmacy, Devi Ahilya Vishwavidyalaya, Indore, Madhya Pradesh, India; [4]National Institute of Pharmaceutical Education and Research (NIPER)- Ahmedabad, An Institute of National Importance, Government of India, Department of Pharmaceuticals, Ministry of Chemicals and Fertilizers, Palaj, Gandhinagar, Gujarat, India; [5]Centre for Drug Research, Universiti Sains Malaysia, George Town, Penang, Malaysia

7.1 Introduction

Scientists have paved their interest in the safe delivery of drugs; however, many factors may significantly influence the outcomes of the drug in terms of toxicity like disease conditions (Kumawat et al., 2020; Gupta et al., 2022b, 2022c), body temperature (Desai et al., 2021), age (Rajpoot et al., 2021a, 2021b, 2021c), diet (Polaka et al., 2022b), enzyme levels (Rajpoot et al., 2020a, 2020b; Achanta et al., 2021; Tambe et al., 2021d), sleeping pattern (Choudhary et al., 2021; Vasdev et al., 2021), sex (Anup et al., 2021a; Polaka et al., 2022a), etc. The toxic effect of any chemical agents can be minimized by modifying different pharmacokinetic parameters of drug agents like absorption, distribution, metabolism, and elimination through the body (Padiyar et al., 2020; Rajpoot et al., 2020a, 2020b, 2021a, 2021b, 2021c; Anup et al., 2021c; Polaka et al., 2021a).

In this regard, different methods and models, along with software, are employed, which can determine the optimum dose of chemical agents to elicit the desired effect by reducing

Essentials of Pharmatoxicology in Drug Research, Volume 1
https://doi.org/10.1016/B978-0-443-15840-7.00026-9

toxic effects (Anup et al., 2021b; Polaka et al., 2021b; Rajpoot et al., 2021a, 2021b, 2021c; Tambe et al., 2021a, 2021b, 2021c). Additionally, several approaches are used to confirm drug toxicity, such as in silico (Rajpoot et al., 2022a), in vitro toxicity studies (Gupta et al., 2022b, 2022c), in vivo animal models, toxicokinetic and toxicodynamic considerations (Rajpoot et al., 2022b), the toxicity of ingredients (Gupta et al., 2022a; Tiwari et al., 2022), and different biomarkers evaluation (Tekade et al., 2022).

7.1.1 What is "cellular dysfunction"?

Cellular dysfunction is a state in which there is total loss or impairment in the functioning of the cells. It becomes a cause of many physical and chemical abnormities like cancer (Rajani et al., 2020; Ditani et al., 2021), diabetes (Kumawat et al., 2020), Huntington's disease, and acute brain injury. Eventually, cell dysfunction leads to organ dysfunction. The main cause of cellular dysfunction is the impairment of energy production, which leads to metabolic shutdown in the cell (Achanta et al., 2021; Tambe et al., 2021d). Cellular dysfunction is a common complication of sepsis, other systemic inflammations, or a combination of the two. Cellular dysfunction is thought to be caused by a decrease in mitochondrial energy generation and protein synthesis (Seo et al., 2000; Chow et al., 2017; Madreiter-Sokolowski et al., 2018).

7.1.2 Mechanism of cellular dysfunction

Cellular dysfunction can be caused by systemic inflammation or endogenous toxic exposure, ranging from reversible cellular dysfunction to permanent cellular damage and cell death (West, 2017). The immune system ability to deal with the disease determines the fate of the afflicted cell, tissue, or organ. Reversible cellular dysfunctions are usually nonlethal and may be treated with medications or surgery, but irreversible cellular dysfunction occurs when the disease develops to the point that the cell damage is permanent (Fig. 7.1) (Kubben and Misteli, 2017; Kumari and Jat, 2021). There are four types of hypotheses for DNA adducts (Seo et al., 2000; Miller and Zachary, 2017);

i. **Hypothesis 1:** According to this hypothesis, a single adduct in conformation can affect DNA polymerase properties/behaviors and their impact on dNTP selection as it affects

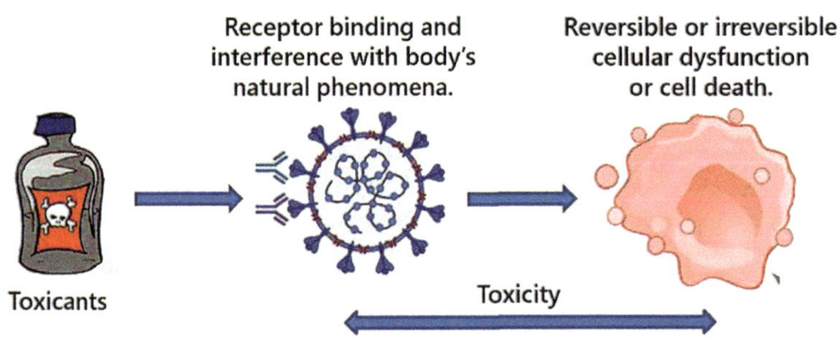

FIGURE 7.1 General mechanism of cellular dysfunction.

all surrounding components; that's why it induces different biological endpoints. Hypothesis 1 can only rationalize structure factors, but it is unknown how this hypothesis rationalizes biological factors.

ii. **Hypothesis 2:** This hypothesis explains how biological factors can cause mutagenesis.

iii. **Hypothesis 3:** As per this hypothesis, adducts may take on numerous conformations, each of which might result in a different set of biological consequences (e.g., mutagenic patterns of varying severity).

iv. **Hypothesis 4:** According to this hypothesis, different biological systems (e.g., a variety of DNA polymerases) handle the same adduct in various ways (for example, in distinct sequence contexts).

7.2 Chemical factors causing cellular dysfunction

Many factors directly or indirectly affect cellular functioning, impairing the body's organ function and resulting in physiological diseases (Asati et al., 2022; Gupta et al., 2022a, 2022b, 2022c). These factors are different, and effects include an imbalanced diet, heredity, chemical exposure, and different internal chemical reactions (redox, oxidative stress). Above all, factors trigger particular organs and may lead to cellular dysfunction, and this dysfunction may affect one or more physiological organs (Kumawat et al., 2020; Gupta et al., 2022b, 2022c; Rajpoot et al., 2022a; Tiwari et al., 2022). Park et al. presented evidence supporting mitochondrial dysfunction's role in sporadic Parkinson's disease (PD) (Park et al., 2015, 2018a, 2018b).

7.2.1 Chemicals causing DNA adducts

Chemical compounds resulting in DNA adduct formation may lead to DNA mutations, which can further trigger apoptosis pathways (Quezada-Maldonado et al., 2021). These mutations may trigger oncogenes and/or deactivate tumor suppressors. This condition leads to uncontrolled cell multiplication and induction of malignant or benign tumors (e.g., benzopyrene) (Du et al., 2021; Myers et al., 2021).

DNA adduct formation is the process of fragmentation of DNA which forms covalent connections with specific carcinogenic chemicals like acetaldehyde, benzopyrene-diol epoxide, safrole, etc. This might start a cancerous cell formation (Heymann et al., 2018; Sanchez et al., 2018; Yang et al., 2020). When a chemical bind to DNA, it becomes a nucleotide. This complex damages DNA, causing it to replicate abnormally. This could be the beginning of a mutation, leading to cancer if DNA repair doesn't occur properly. The chemical that attaches to DNA is our primary source of worry. Instead of doing a whole-body examination to diagnose cancer, a test to find the DNA adducts might be used to identify cancer in its early stages. The DNA findings can be acquired sooner when a scanning tunneling microscope is utilized. In scientific investigations, DNA adducts are employed as biomarkers (Rajalakshmi et al., 2015; Shete et al., 2022).

Acetaldehyde, a significant component of tobacco smoke, is one of the chemicals that forms DNA adducts (Sanchez et al., 2018). Cisplatin attaches to DNA and induces cross-linking, resulting in cell death (Yimit et al., 2019). The binding of DNA molecules to mutagenic and carcinogenic chemicals results from their exposure to specific genotoxic agents and their respective metabolites. The adoption of DNA adductomic techniques has resulted in the development of several methods for identifying DNA adducts. The ability to identify numerous polycyclic aromatic hydrocarbons (PAH)-derived DNA adducts simultaneously enhances exposure assessment and provides a systematic and sophisticated insight into the carcinogenic process following PAH combination exposure (Gao et al., 2018; Stading et al., 2021). Lung cancer acquires a significant portion of the cancer mortality rate graph concerning other cancers worldwide. The fundamental question is what in DNA adducts is responsible for cancer. DNA adducts act as biomarkers for carcinogen exposure, like tobacco smoke. However, numerous meta-analytic investigations have revealed the co-relationship between DNA adducts and malignancy (Mohideen et al., 2021).

One of the meta-analyses used 22 studies on bronchial adducts on 1091 people, out of which 887 had lung cancer, and 204 were healthy persons with no indication of lung cancer. The findings demonstrated that these adducts were responsible for a higher risk of lung cancer. The random effects model observed a mean ratio $(MR)_{lung\ cancer}$ value for bronchial adducts was 2.64, 95% confidence interval (CI) of 2.00–3.50. After filtering the persons having smoking behaviors, a substantial difference was observed in lung cancer patients with substantially higher levels of bronchial adduct than healthy people. The formation of bronchial adducts was later found to be highly connected to the inhalation of carcinogens found in tobacco smoke, confirming its relationship to volatile carcinogens. Finally, using meta-regression, the $MR_{smoking}$ estimate of bronchial adducts was 2.28, with a 95%CI of 1.10–4.73. The study discovered evidence of bronchial adducts as a cause of lung cancer induced by chemicals, not merely related to exposure (Ewa and Danuta, 2017; Ceppi et al., 2017).

7.2.2 Chemicals causing protein adducts

Protein adducts are covalent changes caused by electrophiles reacting with nucleophilic sites in proteins, such as the N-terminus or amino acid side chains with sulfhydryl or amine functionalities (Zanon et al., 2021). Protein adducts can cause one or more of the following abnormalities in the body (a) protein malfunction followed by activation of cell death pathways and (b) autoimmunity (Khan and Wang, 2018; Hwa Yun et al., 2020). Protein adducts stimulate oncogenes or inactivate tumor suppressors, resulting in uncontrollable cell proliferation and malignancy (e.g., diclofenac glucuronidation metabolite). Chemicals that interact with protein targets and form protein adducts lead to abnormal activation and inactivation of ion channels responsible for cellular dysfunctions and cell death (Jarabek et al., 2009). Acrylamide and 2,5-hexanedione are two examples of neurotoxicants that are thought to work by forming protein adducts (Hoet and Lauwerys, 2020).

Protein adducts play a crucial part in the start of toxicity, although their importance is not well understood. Adduct formation alters the structures and/or functions of essential proteins, including catalysis, ion translocation, protein-protein interactions, and so on, resulting in toxicity. For example, acute organophosphate toxicity is mediated by the covalent binding of organophosphate to serine residues in nerve cells, resulting in persistent inactivation of acetylcholinesterase (AChE) (Naughton and Terry, 2018; Ranjan and Jindal, 2022). Fig. 7.2 illustrates the protein adduct process.

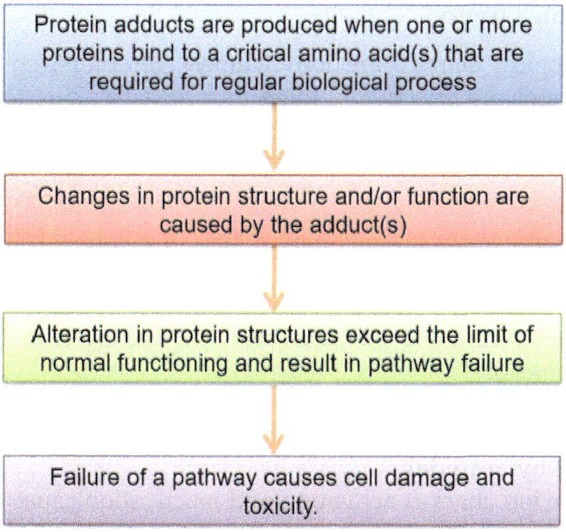

FIGURE 7.2 Protein adducts process.

Protein adducts have promising possibilities as biomarkers in the diagnosis of chemical poisoning, the investigation of toxicant exposure, the clinical monitoring of medicines, as well as the assessment of pharmacological reactions to treatment. Serum albumin and hemoglobin are the most commonly used indicators because of their multiple benefits, such as presence in large quantities in the blood, including a variety of variable amino acids, and so on (LoPachin and DeCaprio, 2005). According to current evidence, there are correlations between the creation of adducts by certain drugs and different sorts of damage, including mutation, malignancy, and developmental repercussions. The clinical manifestation of a toxic impact is generally tissue-specific and might be delayed.

7.2.3 Chemicals causing oxidative stress

A chemical alteration of DNA occurs due to exposure to genotoxic agents and their reactive metabolites. Oxidative stress is caused by a mismatch between the creation and buildup of reactive oxygen species (ROS) in cells and tissues and the biological system's ability to detoxify these reactive products (Yang and Bartlett, 2016). Chemicals responsible for oxidative protein stress oxidize the DNA or protein molecules, resulting in either DNA mutation, protein dysfunction, or both (e.g., benzene, CCl4). A high amount of oxygen concentration in these compounds can potentially play a role in their reactive oxidative activity. Oxidative stress is typically induced by substances containing more oxygen (phenol, ketone, etc.), such as tertiary butyl hydroquinone. The SO_3 species in oil sands process-affected water (OSPW) has recently been found to be responsible for yeast cytotoxicity, which is caused by oxidative stress and has deleterious effects on cellular membranes (Sun et al., 2017; Gault, 2019; Pizzino et al., 2017). Oxidative stress arises when the production of free radicals and the ability of cells to eliminate them are out of balance. For example, excess hydroxyl radicals and peroxynitrite can increase lipid peroxidation, deteriorating cell membranes and lipoproteins (Sun et al., 2017).

7.2.4 Chemicals interacting with protein targets

The four primary targets for pharmacological activity are ion channels, receptors, enzymes, and carrier molecules. Most medications are effective in these four scenarios due to their binding to specific target proteins. Following are the chemicals that interact with target proteins in specific ways (Jarabek et al., 2009):

i. Chemicals that prohibit the production of cellular building components like nucleotides, lipids, and amino acids (for example, Amanita phalloides, a kind of death cap mushroom).
ii. Chemicals change ion channels and metabolism by blocking bioactive metabolic enzymatic processes (for example, sarin inhibits AChE and increases acetylcholine levels to activate signaling pathways and ion channels).
iii. Chemicals that block proteins or enzymes involved in oxygen absorption, fuel use, and ATP production eventually deplete energy and cause cell death (for example, the enzyme cytochrome *c* oxidase is inhibited by cyanide).
iv. Chemicals that cause aberrant or irregular ion channel activation and inactivation cause widespread cellular malfunction, cell death, and various other undesirable physiological effects (tetrodotoxin, for example, shuts voltage-gated $Na+$ channels).

7.3 Types of cellular responses to toxicants

Cells produce different responses after exposure to toxicants. These cellular responses can be of different types like inflammation, carcinogenesis, genotoxicity (Tambe et al., 2021d), disruption of cell signaling (Tekade et al., 2022), altered development and reproduction, microbiome alterations and modulation of toxicity, nanotoxicology, neuroinflammation, neurodegeneration, etc. All these cellular responses are discussed in detail in the next section.

7.3.1 Inflammation

The immune system is a host defense system comprising many biological structures and processes within an organism that protects against diseases, and inflammation is one of those processes. Inflammation is an autoimmune process that occurs when any pathogen tries to invade body tissue (Polaka et al., 2022a). Inflammation is categorized as acute inflammation and chronic inflammation. Acute inflammation starts immediately, becomes severe in a short time, and lasts for less time up to 2 weeks. Chronic inflammation is slow, long-term, and lasts for months to years (Pahwa et al., 2020).

Diseases involving chronic inflammation are diabetes, CVS disorders, arthritis, COPD, rheumatoid arthritis, and allergies. When acute inflammation continues for a long time, it becomes chronic. Events such as vasodilation, increased blood flow, capillary permeability, and movement of neutrophils to the infected tissue occur in inflammation. In response to foreign stimuli, macrophages release inflammatory mediator cytokines, namely IL-1 and TNF-α. These mediators induce the endothelial cells at the injury site to release selectins and integrins. When reaching the injury site, leukocytes get activated by other cytokines and chemokines, which release the inflammatory mediators. Neutrophils consist of lysozymes that lead to the destruction of foreign matter. Neutrophils also tend to phagocytosis (Kuprash and Nedospasov, 2016).

The immune system's response is inflammation to damaging stimuli, including infections, damaged cells, toxic substances, or irradiation. It works by removing unwanted stimuli and initiating the healing process. As a result, inflammation is an important defense mechanism for maintaining a healthy life. During acute inflammatory responses, cellular and molecular mechanisms and interactions limit the risk of damage or infection. This mitigation mechanism aids in the re-establishment of tissue homeostasis as well as the disappearance of acute inflammation. On the other hand, uncontrolled acute inflammation can become chronic, leading to various chronic inflammatory illnesses (Chen et al., 2017; Hirano et al., 2021).

Acute and/or chronic inflammatory responses in the brain, heart, liver, pancreas, kidneys, lungs, intestines, and reproductive system can result in tissue damage or sickness (Fig. 7.3). Inflammatory cells are activated by infectious and noninfectious stimuli, as well as cell damage, through inflammatory signaling pathways, the most common of which are NF-B, MAPK, and JAK-STAT (Yokoyama et al., 2017).

In vivo cell death triggers an inflammatory reaction. The resulting hyperemia, plasma protein leakage, and leukocyte recruitment play a major role in tissue defense and host defense healing phenomena. This response can also cause tissue damage, which can lead to the onset of several diseases. Because inflammation plays an integral part in these processes, it's crucial to comprehend the mechanisms governing this response. This path's basic shape is well recognized. Injured cells send out "danger signals," which warn the host that the cell is about to die. Some of these compounds bind to cellular receptors, triggering the production of pre-inflammatory cytokines. Other chemicals produced by dead cells promote the production of extracellular mediators. The inflammatory response is then orchestrated by the mediators, which trigger the various vascular and cellular components, followed by activation of

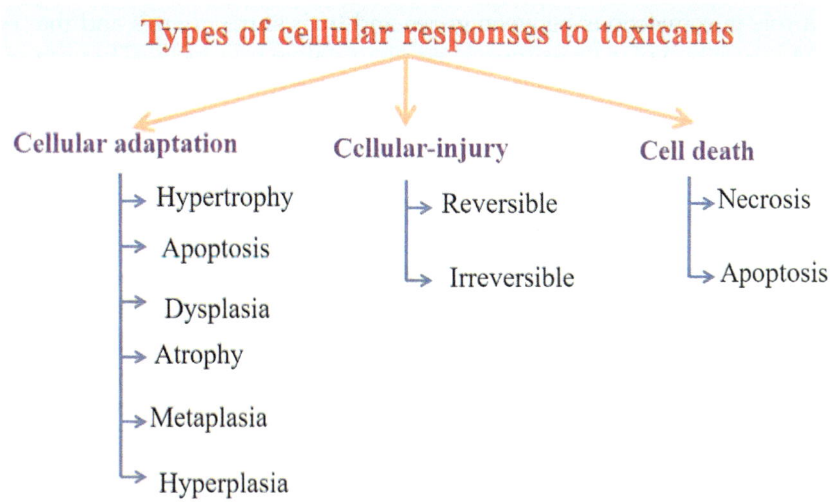

FIGURE 7.3 Types of cellular responses to toxicants.

respective responses. In addition to causing inflammation, dendritic cells are activated when dead cells give out dangerous signals. It drives the formation of immune responses to antigens in and around the dying cells. Many of the chemicals and mechanisms that play a role in these processes are yet to be known (Pizzino et al., 2017).

7.3.2 Genotoxicity and epigenetics

Genotoxicity is the ability of xenobiotics to damage genetic information in the cells. Exposure to chemical and biological agents can result in epigenetic alterations, which may lead to various diseases, including cancer. The chemicals that induce epigenetic alterations are referred to as epimutagens which include ions such as chromium, arsenic, nickel, lead, copper, mercury, and cadmium (Jennifer and Maciej, 2013; Zhou and Xi, 2018). It is observed that these ions impact the epigenome by inducing changes in DNA methylation and modification of histone proteins, affecting chromatin structure and miRNA expression (Dusinska et al., 2017).

Mechanism of nanomaterials-induced genotoxicity is carried out by the biomolecules involved in normal genome function or causing injury to DNA/chromosomal malformations. Oxidative stress is the critical mechanism for nanomaterial-induced genotoxicity. The generation of ROS causes DNA injury and damage to lipids and proteins. The secondary mechanism causing genotoxicity induced by nanomaterials includes extracellular ROS via inflammatory responses of macrophages and neutrophils (Dusinska et al., 2017; Kalyane et al., 2022).

Genetic diversity is widely acknowledged to substantially influence susceptibility to common diseases, medicine and toxicant responses, and disease outcomes. With more data from human and model organism research becoming available, the understanding that epigenetic marks differ throughout the population is emerging (Burggren, 2016; Hu and Barrett, 2017). Furthermore, the link between genetic diversity, toxicological consequences, and epigenetics is being researched. Recent research suggests that chromatin states and transcriptional regulation play a role in connections between genes and their surroundings and that epigenetics can aid in the association of expression-related quantitative trait loci (QTL) with disease outcomes (Schmidt et al., 2016; Yu et al., 2016). However, investigations of Epigenetics and Gene-environment add to the difficulty of experimental designs, making it difficult to choose the most useful epigenetic readouts that can be conducted efficiently across different persons, poisoning signs and symptoms, as well as exposures and tissue types. We believe assessing chromatin accessibility in conjunction with total RNA levels, is the most cost-effective, comprehensive, and feasible way to characterize the interindividual heterogeneity to toxicant responses and the intricacy of epigenetic and regulatory activities, among many epigenetic experimental methodologies available (Lewis et al., 2017; Lauschke et al., 2019).

Epigenetic reprogramming has been considered a component of cancer cells' "genome instability" enabling feature, and it is also widely known that carcinogens can alter the epigenetic state of cells. The most often documented toxicant-induced epigenome modifications include DNA methylation, histone/chromatin remodeling, and altered miRNA expression. Because of the potential influence of gene expression patterns and, as a result, toxicity phenotypes are influenced by epigenotoxic effects. Furthermore, epigenetic modifications have been proposed as an essential biomarker of carcinogen exposure and its effect (Gupta, 2018).

There has been evidence of epigenetic changes in various tissues of mice when 1,3 butadiene was administered by inhalation. Loss of histone proteins and reduced DNA repair activity were observed in those mice. Increased histone markers in the liver suggest genomic instability, and these epigenetic alterations may lead to a carcinogenic process. MiRNA and DNA damage: miRNA regulates gene expression by directly binding to RNA. Induction of processing and nuclear export of miRNA is suggested during the damage of DNA. Formaldehyde, as a toxicant, is known to damage the DNA and cause the induction of miRNA expression (Chappell and Rager, 2017).

7.3.3 Carcinogenesis

Carcinogenesis, also known as oncogenesis or tumorigenesis, is the process through which healthy cells become cancerous (Fig. 7.4). Cellular, genetic, and epigenetic alterations, as well as aberrant cell division, characterize the process. Cell division is a physiological phenomenon occurring in nearly all tissues under various conditions. A balance between proliferation and programmed cell death (apoptosis) is typically maintained to protect the integrity of tissues and organs. The carcinogenic factors are divided into three types, namely (i) primary factors, (ii) secondary factors, and (iii) favoring factors. Primary factors comprise chemical substances and viruses. The primary factors act at the molecular level mainly on nucleic acids (RNA and DNA). A secondary factor involves genetic inheritance, which can be due to the inactivation of tumor suppressor genes. Uni or bilateral retinoblastoma is known to occur in children due to genetic inheritance. Favoring factors are the risk factors which include nutrition, age, environment, etc. (D'Arcy, 2019).

7.3.3.1 *Physical factors*

Ionizing and nonionizing radiations play a significant role in carcinogenesis. Ionizing radiations impact the cell nucleus, chromosomes, and DNA level (rupturing phosphorylated bond occurs with the breakage of one or two filaments). These biological actions either result in cell death or act as a carrier of the mutated cell.

7.3.3.2 *Genetic instability*

For normal somatic cells, their ability to multiply is limited and is controlled by the enzyme telomerase. As telomere length diminishes, chromosome fusion and other abnormalities trigger apoptosis or mutation in daughter cells. Tumor cells reactivate the telomerase activity and overcome the potential replication block. The G_1S is the critical phase for controlling the proliferation of cells undergoing genetic abnormalities. Signals from growth factors allow cells to move from inactive G_1 to the G_0 stage, ultimately leading to the S stage, where the DNA synthesis is initiated. Receptor tyrosine kinase activates (RTKs) several signaling pathways that promote the cycle entry upon binding to growth factors. These RTKs are targets for mutations and result in benign and malignant tumors (Peters and Gonzalez, 2018).

According to the most widely accepted hypothesis of carcinogenesis, somatic mutations, changes in DNA, and epimutations occur because cancer disturbs these ordered processes by interfering with the programming that controls them, causing the usual balance between

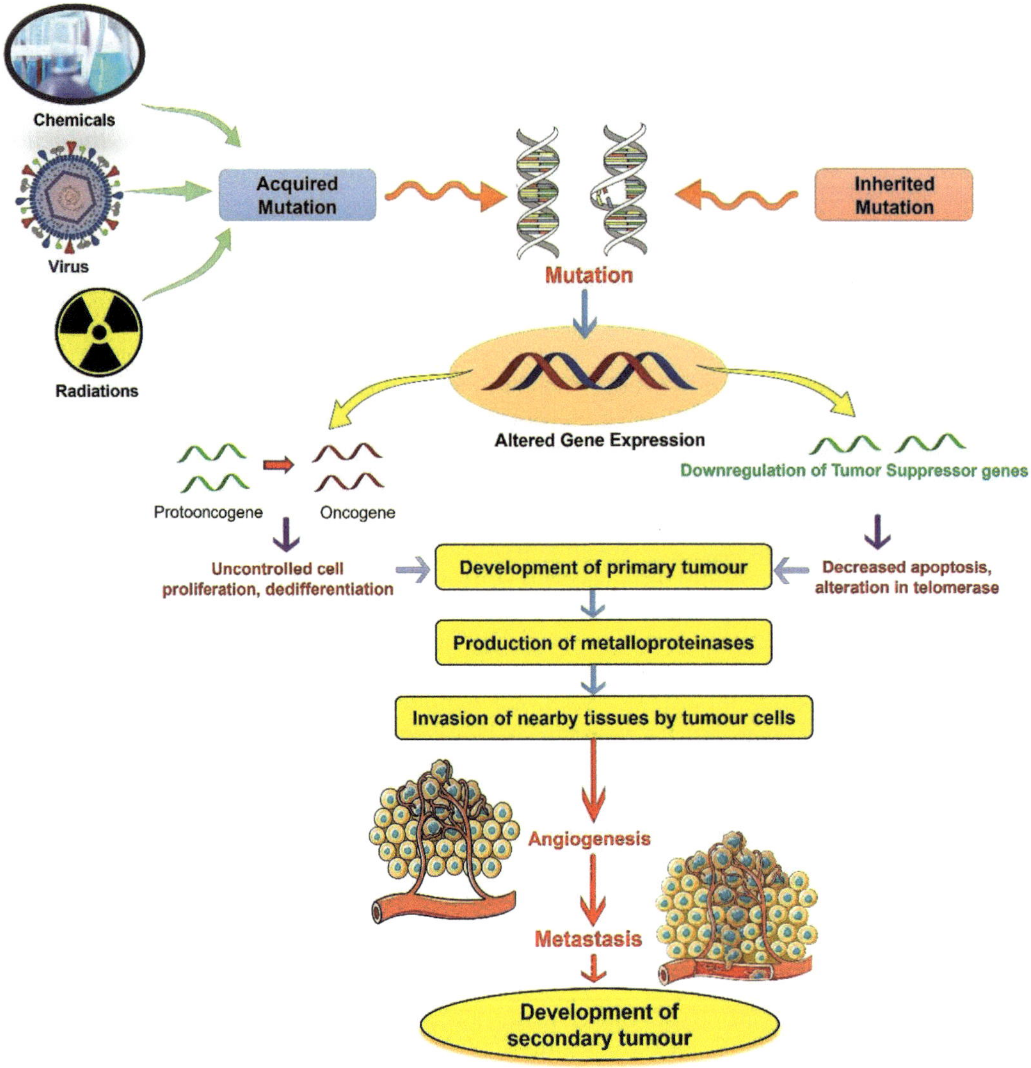

FIGURE 7.4 Simplified outline of the genesis of cancer.

proliferation and cell death to be disrupted. This causes unregulated cell division and natural selection to evolve those cells in the body. Only a small percentage of mutations cause cancer, while most do not (Compton, 2020). Mutagens create DNA mutations, whereas carcinogens cause cancer due to those mutations. Mutagens are not all carcinogens, and carcinogens are not all mutagens (Basu, 2018). Nitrogen mustards (developed from mustard gas used by the military in 1917) were identified in 1946 to produce mutations in fruit flies and inhibit tumor formation in mice (Worek et al., 2016). Methods for assessing the mutagenesis potential of chemical and physical agents were developed by genetic toxicology (Turkez et al., 2017).

In the 1970s, a cellular-based assay for genetic alterations was developed by Bruce Ames and colleagues. This assay was named as Ames assay. Many government regulatory bodies now demand sophisticated versions of these procedures to evaluate substances for mutagenicity. Often, cancer is caused by a chemical's metabolite (breakdown product), not the original molecule. When a foreign substance is digested, it should be made less hazardous, but this does not always happen. This hazardous compound can then interact with cellular DNA or proteins, posing a severe health risk, and resulting in the formation of cancerous cells and this process is known as bioactivation. It's also possible that a chemical might enhance bioactivation or speed cancer growth. The study of cancer's fundamental biology is continuing. The genetic sciences assist in understanding why some people are more cancer-prone than others (Yokoyama et al., 2017).

7.3.4 Disruption of cell signaling

Cell signaling, in simple words, can be defined as communication between cells. There are four major kinds of signaling, namely paracrine signaling, autocrine signaling, endocrine signaling, and signaling by direct contact. Disruption in cell signaling may lead to severe consequences like cancer as there is constant activation of signaling pathways instructing the cell to multiply. Cell signaling disruption may be due to mutation of receptors, protein kinases, or transcription factors that keep the proteins in an active state (Fig. 7.5). The free radical theory

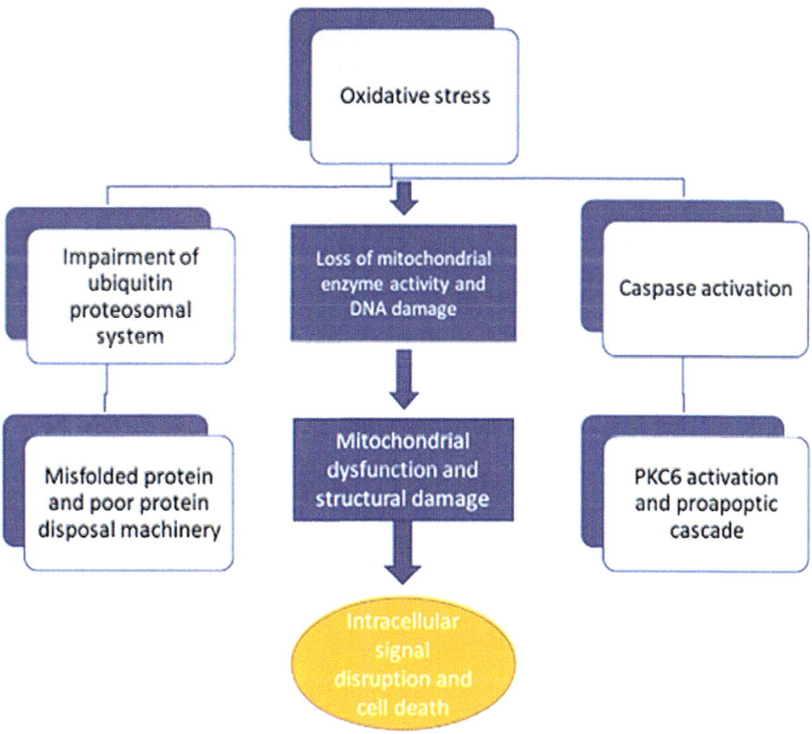

FIGURE 7.5 A flowchart summary of crucial downstream signaling targets of oxidative stress during environmental exposure to neurotoxic pesticides and metals leading to disruption of intracellular signaling.

of aging can also be one factor that serves disruption of cell signaling. Interleukin-6 (IL-6) trans-signaling via soluble IL-6 receptor (sIL-6R) has emerged as a prominent regulator of inflammation in endothelial cells. One hypothesis was carried out considering that selective inhibition of the IL-6 trans-signaling pathway will attenuate inflammation and subsequently leads to barrier disruption in retinal endothelial cells (Valle et al., 2019).

7.3.4.1 Disruption of extracellular signaling

Extracellular signaling pathways can be classified according to the type of receptors involved. Multiple receptor subtypes are ionotropic receptors, GPCRs, enzyme-coupled receptors, and nuclear receptors. There are three possibilities for disruption of cell signaling: (i) modulation of the signal, (ii) blocking signal at the receptor, and (iii) mimicking the signal (Pope and Hester, 2020).

7.3.4.2 Disruption of intracellular signaling

Intracellular signaling begins with the binding of an extracellular signaling molecule with a specific receptor protein leading to cellular responses such as cell growth, immune regulation, tissue repair, homeostatic regulation, neurotransmission, and apoptosis (Pope and Liu, 2020).

Signal transduction pathways convert ligand signals into target cells' biological activity changes, and they are becoming a more popular target for drug development. In cellular systems, signal transduction is a critical biological activity. It affects various biological activities in the cell, and its disruption can result in various illnesses, phenotypes, and medication treatment results. The molecules link and interact in a predetermined manner in signaling pathways through dynamic and refined signal transduction, allowing living creatures to fulfill an overall function in a harmonic manner (McCarthy et al., 2017; Espinosa-Riquer et al., 2020). The following are some instances of disease-related cell signaling disruption (Pizzino et al., 2017):

i. Signaling mechanisms guiding cancer cells to grow and divide constantly activated in cancer cells. Changes (mutations) in receptors, protein kinases, or transcription factors maintaining the proteins are common causes.
ii. Protein kinases, phosphorylated proteins, and other chemical molecules are becoming more significant therapeutic targets. Inhibiting these enzymes can impair signal-transduction pathways, which are essential in cancer and inflammatory disorders.

7.3.4.3 Changes in the cancer genome cause intracellular signaling to be disrupted

A simplified signaling pathway highlights known examples of true oncogenes that are dysregulated in various ways. A signaling pathway can be disturbed in numerous places, and a range of genetic and epigenomic changes can contribute to this, eventually leading to cancer (Fig. 7.6).

7.3.5 Altered development and reproduction

Oxidative stress significantly impacts the pathophysiology of the body's functions. Many severe disorders originated from it, including neurodegeneration and adverse reproductive

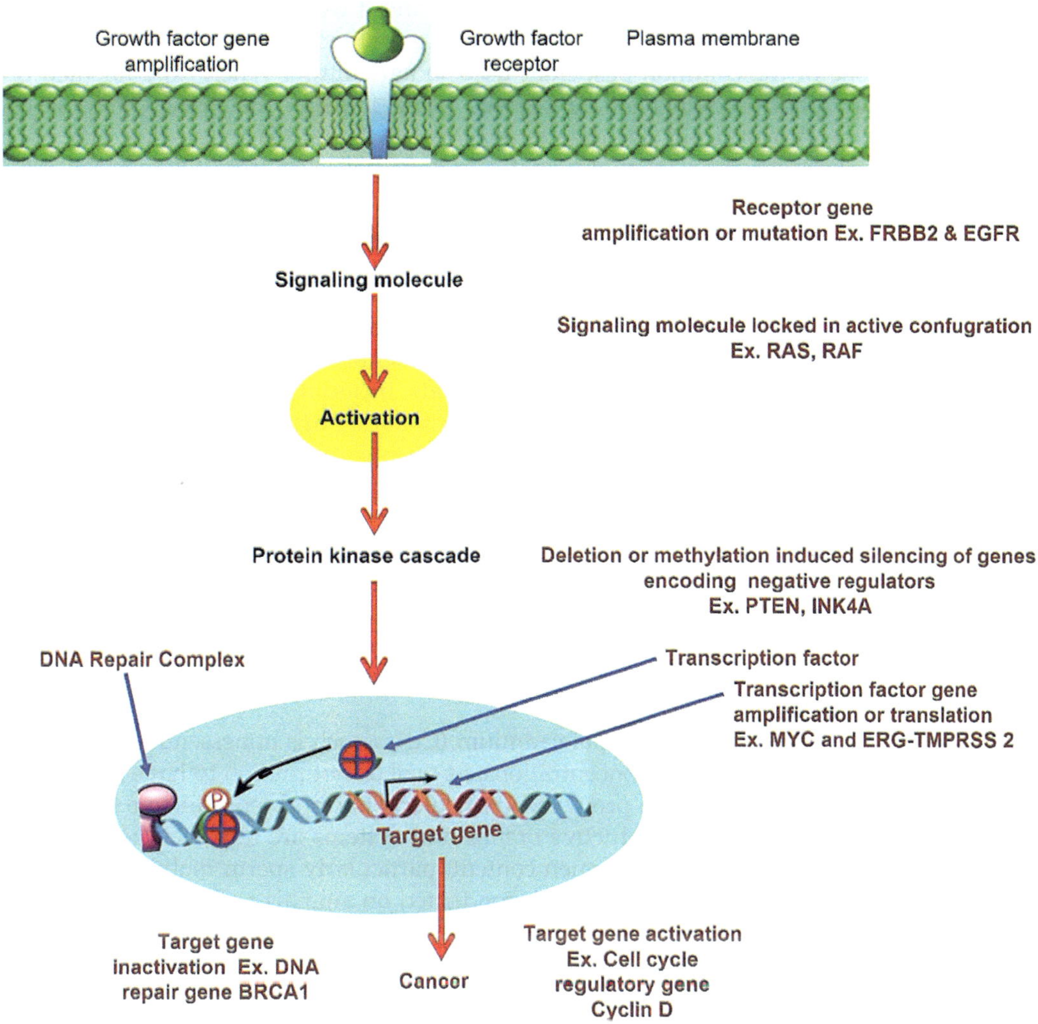

FIGURE 7.6 Changes in the cancer genome disrupt intracellular signaling.

outcomes. ROS has been found to play a role in every stage of pregnancy, i.e., ovarian steroid biosynthesis, oocyte maturation, fertilization, and luteal maintenance. Prooxidants and antioxidants are associated with polycystic ovarian syndrome and infertility. Prooxidative shifting may lead to adverse consequences like miscarriages, embryopathy, preeclampsia, fetal growth restriction (FGR), and preterm premature rupture of membranes (PPROM) (Steller et al., 2018).

Dyslipidemia is a term that can be used to refer to lipid imbalances, namely hypercholesterolemia and hypertriglyceridemia. Dyslipidemia is associated with many pathophysiological conditions, such as obesity and cardiovascular diseases. In one of the animal studies, male Wistar rats were fed hydrogenated vegetable fat, and it was observed that sperm concentration, sperm head morphology, and motility were improved (Collodel et al., 2020). Quinalphos (QP) is one of the common pesticides used in agriculture. When experimented on Swiss albino mice, pharmacokinetic data showed three folds of increased QP in testes compared to serum. A significant decrease in fertilization, lower blastocyst rate, and poor blastocyst quality was observed when spermatozoa were collected from QP-exposed mice and were subjected to in vitro fertilization. Fertilizing ability was decreased, which appeared to be mediated through elevated oxidative stress and altered steroidogenesis in testes due to exposure to quinalphos (Kumari et al., 2021).

According to published research, chemical exposures could affect reproductive behavior and lead to congenital disabilities, subfecundity, fertility problems, spontaneous abortion, stunted growth, and intrauterine fetal death in experimental animals as well as wildlife. The environment contains many exogenous compounds, including pharmaceuticals, industrial and agricultural chemicals, food additives, and cosmetics. Important considerations concerning the effects on health are raised by people being exposed to these substances continuously. One of the primary toxicity endpoints for environmental toxins has now been identified in the male reproductive system. Adolescent infertility brought on by exposure to environmental toxins has become a severe issue in developed nations (Pineau, 2020). There are also worries that the methodologies used to detect, describe, and prioritize these compounds for vulnerability analysis, and safety management objectives are inadequate, given the growing evidence linking various environmental contaminants, including disturbances to breast health in human societies (Matouskova et al., 2022; Parikh et al., 2022; Polaka et al., 2022b).

Considering the poisonous heavy metal cadmium (Cd), which is nonessential, harmful to the environment, dangerous at low concentrations, as well as not proven to have any potential health benefits. Numerous health problems, particularly harmful reproductive health, are caused by its exposure. Male's reproductive organs and systems are impacted by Cd exposure, which impairs spermatogenesis, semen content, particularly sperm mobility, hormone production, and release. According to research conducted on animals and people, it also impacts menstrual periods and female fertility, including the hormone levels of the reproductive system (Kumar and Sharma, 2019). Furthermore, research showed that irrespective of the species, age group, or amount of exposure, atrazine was linked to damage to the male fertility system in rats. In atrazine-administered rats, the testicular injury could be caused by oxidative stress and apoptosis-related pathways (Zhu et al., 2021).

7.3.6 Microbiome alterations and modulation of toxicity

Toxicant modulation of the microbiome is the replacement in the microbiota that occurs due to chemical exposure. Alterations in the gut microbiome may be caused due to obesity, inflammatory bowel disease, and diabetes. Various research found that when the gut microbiome was incubated with arsenic, the gut bacteria could adsorb or take up arsenic and reduce the free arsenic levels in the culture medium. The exposure to arsenic altered the expression of genes of the p53 signaling pathway and the genes associated with hepatocellular carcinoma. Gut microbiome disruption enhances the toxic effect of arsenic and may lead to arsenic-induced hepatocellular carcinoma (Chi et al., 2019).

Many researchers have concluded that Bisphenol A (BPA), which is a common chemical found in plastics and epoxy resins, exerts a toxic effect on different organs and systems through various mechanisms, including epigenetic modifications and effects on cell signaling pathways, microbiome, and metabolome in different species (McDonough et al., 2021). Various studies show that alteration in the gut microbiome contributes to pancreatic ductal adenocarcinoma (PDAC). The use of proton pump inhibitors is known to cause gut dysbiosis, which increases the risk of pancreatic cancer (Kohi et al., 2022).

The gut microbiome, sometimes called the super organ, contains up to 100 trillion bacteria, with individual species biodiversity. They play a crucial part in various biochemical functions associated with metabolic, immunity, and neurological reactions (Arun et al., 2021). Exposure to heavy metals stunts the development and modifies the phyla that make up the gut microbiome. As this goes, the gut microbiota works to eliminate the heavy metals via changing the biophysical environment, intestinal absorption, and boosting the enzymes that help heavy metals be metabolized (Arun et al., 2021).

The human gut microbiota is susceptible to disruption when exposed to various harmful environmental chemicals. Human illness risk is closely linked to perturbations in the gut microbiota caused by the surrounding. Functional gut microbiota changes are an extensively recognized method by which environmental toxins impose harmful implications on humans (Tu et al., 2020). Radiation enteropathy is a result of altered gut flora after radiation dose. Using two processes, namely translocation and dysbiosis, the gut microbiota may affect radiation-induced gastrointestinal mucositis (Liu et al., 2021). Chemotherapeutic causes gastrointestinal toxicity by harming the intestinal mucosa and significantly upsetting the gut ecology. Gastrointestinal dysbiosis has been linked to anxiety, stress, pain, poor brain ability, as well as cardiovascular disorders, according to animal models and human research. Lately, a potential connection has been made between chemotherapy-induced disturbance of the gut microbiota as well as long-term consequences in people with cancer (Ciernikova et al., 2021).

Different strategies for gut microbiota modulation are used, like probiotics, prebiotics, and postbiotics. Probiotics restore microbial dysbiosis and exert immunomodulation. Prebiotics are nondigestible food ingredient that selectively stimulates the growth of specific bacteria. Postbiotics refer to the soluble byproducts and metabolites secreted by gut microbiota that exerts biological activities on the host (Fong et al., 2020).

7.3.7 Nanotoxicology

Nanotoxicology studies how manufactured nanoparticles interact with biological systems and the environment, focusing on the relationship between nanomaterial physicochemical qualities and the generation of toxic or hostile biological responses. Additionally, it is a subbranch of toxicology that deals with the potentially toxic effects of nanoscale structures or particles with diameters less than 100 nm. Having an advantage of nano size, nanomaterials are hypothesized to penetrate cellular membranes, biological barriers, and tissues more quickly compared to heavy bulk-sized materials (Fig. 7.7) (Singh et al., 2019). The importance of studying and understanding the toxicity of nanoparticles arises from the ever-increasing usage and application of nanomaterials in different areas and disciplines (Krug and Wick, 2011).

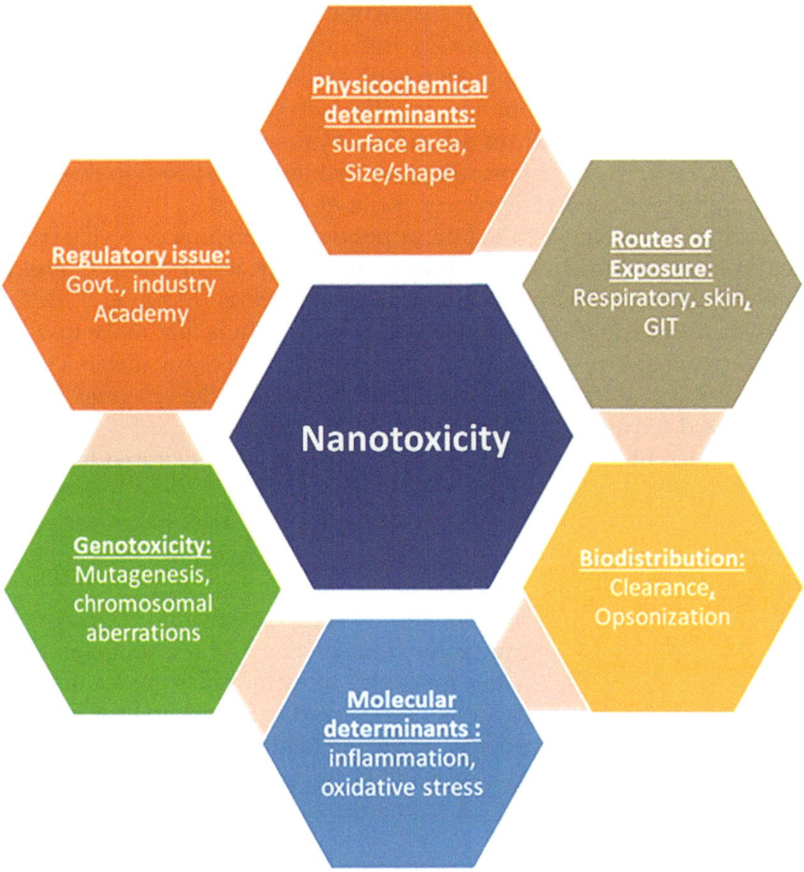

FIGURE 7.7 Nanotoxicity and related issues.

In both industrial and medical applications of nanoparticles, indirect and direct exposure of the cells to the nanoparticles may occur. Therefore, proper understanding of how the cell responds and handles the nanoparticles is essential for developing safe nanoparticle-based materials and medications (Oberdörster, 2010; Akçan et al., 2020).

7.3.7.1 Factors of nanoparticles toxicity

There are various factors that affect the strength of the toxicity of nanoparticles (Akçan et al., 2020). In particular, the size of the particles has been shown to be a relatively important determining factor of the overall toxicity of the nanoparticles (Chen et al., 2015). Specifically, nanoparticles with smaller particle sizes tend to exhibit higher toxicity, mainly due to the larger overall surface areas of the particles. This high surface area causes a greater number of molecules to bind to the surface leading to an increased toxic effect (Browning et al., 2013). The chemical composition and charge of the surface are also considered to be important toxicity factors, as the charge of the surface determines the adsorption of charged biomolecules and ions to the nanoparticles (Li et al., 2015). The positively charged nanoparticles are more toxic as they are easily attracted to the negatively charged membrane and interact with enzymes, proteins, and DNA. There is evidence in biological assays that silver nanoparticles continuously release silver ions during their transport until their final location (Singh et al., 2019). A study found that charged NPs induced cell death through apoptosis, and neutrally charged NPs lead to necrosis in HaCat cells (Gupta, 2018).

7.3.7.2 Mechanism of nanoparticles cellular toxicity

The primary mechanism of cellular toxicity caused by nanoparticles is ROS induction leading to oxidative stress (Fu et al., 2014). Although ROS production in the cell is typically required to carry out specific roles, such as in cell signaling cascades or as a defense mechanism by the immune system's cells, but imbalanced and excessive production of ROS can lead to detrimental effects on the cell. Because of the high reactivity of the ROS, it can react with DNA, proteins, and other vital biomolecules leading to cellular dysfunction (Qi et al., 2017).

The ROS induction by nanoparticles seems to be caused by the reactive prooxidant functional groups on the surface of the particles (Knaapen et al., 2004). Other possible mechanisms of toxicity have also been investigated; for instance, in an in vitro study conducted on silver-based nanoparticles, glutathione depletion and superoxide dismutase (SOD) activity were assessed, in addition to ROS production. The results showed that the levels of glutathione, which is a substance required for a balanced antioxidant status in the cell, were reduced. Also, a very slight reduction in the activity of SOD was observed (Avalos et al., 2014).

Concerning the levels of ROS production induced by nanoparticles, particle size seems to be the primary determining factor (Fu et al., 2014). In a study using gold nanoparticles, the ROS production caused by nanoparticles with different diameters was measured. The study covered nanoparticles with a diameters range of 5–250 nm. The results showed that nanoparticles with smaller diameters exhibited higher toxicity, confirming the inverse relationship between toxicity and particle size (Misawa and Takahashi, 2011). The higher toxicity was mainly attributed to the larger surface area of the nanoparticles with smaller diameters.

The oxidative stress in the cell caused by the nanoparticles eventually causes DNA damage and apoptosis. Various forms of DNA damage have been observed, such as strand breakage and chromosomal fragmentation (Singh et al., 2009; Al Gurabi et al., 2015). Also, induction of gene mutation can occur, which leads to genotoxicity (Dusinska et al., 2019). The typical cellular response to this DNA damage is usually the initiation of the DNA repair mechanisms. However, in cases where the DNA damage cannot be repaired, cell cycle arrest may occur, with apoptosis occurring subsequently (Khanna et al., 2015). In an in vivo study, the toxicity of silver-based nanoparticles was assessed in a *Drosophila melanogaster* fruit fly model. The effects of the nanoparticles included the induction of heat shock stress and oxidative stress. Also, DNA damage occurred and high apoptosis rates were observed in cells of the fruit fly model (Ahamed et al., 2010).

Given that oxidative stress is the leading cause of nanoparticle toxicity, various solutions have been attempted to circumvent their adverse effects (Khanna et al., 2015). For instance, coating the surface of the nanoparticles with a free radicals-scavenger substance can reduce toxicity. The free radicals-scavenger is usually encapsulated inside a suitable polymer (Stevanović et al., 2014). An in vitro study showed that iron-oxide nanoparticles coated with chitosan oligosaccharide exhibited reduced ROS induction and cytotoxic effects compared to uncoated iron-oxide nanoparticles (Shukla et al., 2015).

7.3.8 Neuroinflammation

The cell types that are responsible for inflammation are leukocytes and endothelial cells. Signaling molecules comprise nitric oxide (NO), prostaglandins, cytokines, and proteins. Innate immunity comprises generic, nonspecific responses of the immune system, usually triggered by specific pathogen-derived molecules known as pathogen-associated molecular patterns (PAMPs). Inflammatory responses associated with the brain and spinal cord are termed neuroinflammation. Manifestations vary from disease, infection, injury, and stress (DiSabato et al., 2016; Polaka et al., 2022a). Microglia, innate immune cells of the CNS, play a vital role in controlling neuroinflammatory responses. Cells convert from inactivated to an activated phagocytic state during chronic neuroinflammation. It has the potential to produce cytokines and neurotoxic molecules that cause neurodegeneration. Astrocytes belong to a different class of glial cells that contributes to the release of the proinflammatory mediator TNF-α (Lyman et al., 2014).

Neuroinflammation results from a complex interaction between cells in the central nervous system (CNS), including neurons, macroglia, microglia, and invading leukocytes. The beginning of injury, environmental circumstances, genetic history, and age/past experiences alter this complex neuroinflammatory circuit's integrated response. The inflammatory response involves a complicated network of several cell types. Activated macrophages, monocytes, and other cells regulate local responses to tissue injury and infection. At the site of tissue injury, damaged epithelium and endothelial cells generate chemicals that initiate the inflammatory cascade, as well as chemokines and growth factors that recruit neutrophils and monocytes. Neutrophils, monocytes, lymphocytes, i.e., natural killer cells (NK cells), T cells, and B cells, and mast cells are the first cells to arrive at an injury site. They are considered the first line of the defense mechanism of the human body (Chen et al., 2017). Depending on the etiology, neuroinflammation manifests itself in a variety of ways. These forms of neuroinflammation are outlined below, along with their unique routes (Rock and Kono, 2008).

(a) **Injury**: The onset of apoptosis in response to damage and the demyelination of neuronal cells results in inflammation at the injury site. The second phase, which involves reactive gliosis, edema, and cavitation of the spinal parenchyma, begins after this, as well as the possibility of irreversible spinal cord function loss.

(b) **Immune responses in the periphery**: The blood-brain barrier protects the brain from toxins in the bloodstream. It comprises endothelial and astrocyte cells and serves as a physical barrier between the circulatory system and the brain. Astrocyte junctions govern what gets through the barrier. Still, they can be disrupted after an injury, resulting in an influx of T lymphocytes, B cells, and macrophages invading the brain, increasing inflammation.

(c) **Infection**: Encephalitis (brain inflammation) and meningitis can be caused by bacteria, viruses, fungus, and, on rare occasions, by parasites or protozoa (The meninges—the tissue layers that envelop the brain and spinal cord—are inflamed). Infections of all kinds stimulate a unique mechanism that leads to neuroinflammation.

(d) **Aging**: Further study has discovered that an increase in activated microglia, a hallmark of active immune system response, has been seen in the brains of the elderly, suggesting another link between aging and neuroinflammation.

(e) **Neurodegenerative disease**: Neuroinflammation and neurodegenerative illness are inextricably related. Neuroinflammation is linked to Parkinson's disease (PD), Alzheimer's disease (AD), and multiple sclerosis (MS) diseases that affect people. To begin with, it is assumed that neuroinflammation is a significant contributor to AD-related neurodegeneration.

7.3.9 Neurodegeneration

Neurodegenerative disease is characterized by progressive loss of the population of neurons. The most common neurodegenerative disorders are PD and AD. Others include Huntington's disease and spinal muscular atrophy (SMP). Amyloid-beta, tau, alpha-synuclein, TDP-43, or the prion protein are a few of the proteins that can aggregate and are associated with the pathogenesis of neurodegenerative diseases. The pathophysiological hypothesis of neurodegenerative diseases relies on the fact that some proteins change their conformations, thereby gaining toxicity or losing their physiological functions and generating small oligomeric or large fibrillary aggregates, resulting in neurotoxicity and neurodegeneration (Fig. 7.8).

Degenerative nerve diseases impact various physiological processes, including balance, mobility, speech, breathing, and heart function. Many of these diseases are passed on from generation to generation. A medical condition such as alcoholism, a tumor, or a stroke may be to blame. Other probable causes include toxins, chemicals, and infections. The term neurodegeneration comes from the prefix "neuro-," which refers to nerve cells (i.e., neurons), and the word "degeneration," which refers to the loss of structure or function in tissues or organs (Kawachi and Lassmann, 2017; Rajpoot, 2020).

7.3.9.1 Causes of neurodegeneration

Genetic mutations are responsible for a tiny percentage of neurological illnesses (less than 5%). Toxic protein build-up and the formation of neurotoxic chemicals as a result of lack of

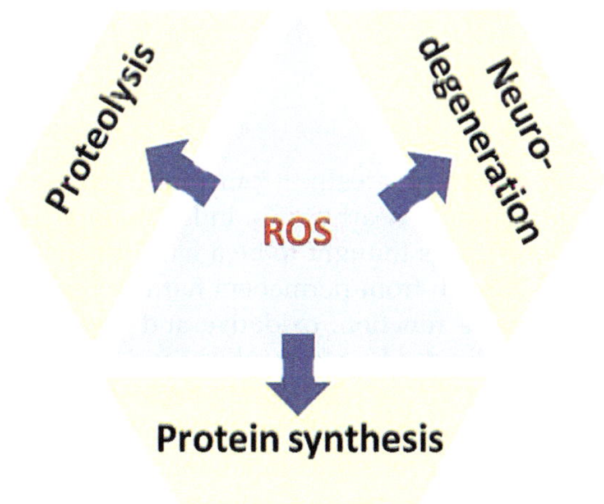

FIGURE 7.8 Role of ROS in neurodegeneration.

mitochondrial activity in the brain is one of the major causes of neurodegeneration. Experts concur that the effect is the encouragement of Apoptosis (programmed cell death), a type of cell death that occurs when a cell is programmed to die, which is the purposeful suicide of a cell to shield other adjacent neurons from hazardous chemicals (Lewis et al., 2017). The origin of the complicated and lethal neurodegenerative condition known as amyotrophic lateral sclerosis (ALS) is still unknown. Human-induced pluripotent stem cell (hiPSC) models have recently made advancements that make it possible to research the genetic causes of ALS in patient-derived neural cell types such as motor neurons and glia. Whereas astrocyte failure has historically been assumed to aggravate the development of illness, astrocytic dysfunction could have a more substantial direct impact on the onset and development of illness. However, just a small number of ALS risk-associated genes are being studied for their effect on astrocyte dysfunction and neurodegeneration (Halpern et al., 2019).

Endotoxin is a lipopolysaccharide (LPS) that makes up a large portion of gram-negative bacteria's exterior membrane and is found in significant amounts in the stomach, mouth, skin, as well as other tissues when bacteria are invaded. Endotoxin concentrations in the bloodstream are typically modest, but they rise with gastrointestinal inflammation, periodontal illness, and neurological disorders. Endotoxin at these concentrations activates brain microglia and causes inflammatory processes in normal healthy blood. Elevated endotoxin concentrations cause memory impairments, destruction of brain synapses and neurons, microglial stimulation, priming, and/or tolerance in animals. Endotoxin may interact with many agreeable proteins to produce a variety of neurodegenerative disorders by promoting amyloid as well as tau accumulation and neuropathology (Brown, 2019).

7.4 Forms of cell death

The two basic types of cell death that have been identified are apoptosis and necrosis (Fig. 7.9). Necrosis occurs when cells are irreversibly damaged by external stimulation. On the other hand, apoptosis is a process in which cells die and is thought to be a type of spontaneous cell death in which a cell kills itself in response to a signal (Table 7.1).

7.4.1 Necrosis

The term "necrosis" refers to uncontrolled and abrupt cell death. It causes the cell membrane to rupture, allowing the cell contents to spill out into nearby cells. Inflammatory cells are also activated as a result of this. As a result, necrosis is thought to be a harmful and infectious disease process (Tomasetti et al., 2017). Cell death from permanent harm is referred to as necrosis. Swelling of organelles, loss of organelle function, oxidative and hydrolytic breakdown of intracellular membranes and macromolecules by electrophiles and free radicals. Eventually, lysis is all degenerative processes necrotizing cells during necrosis (loss of cellular constituents to surrounding tissues due to cell membrane rupture). As cellular components and free radicals released into the extracellular matrix attract inflammatory cells, necrosis usually results in the formation of an inflammatory response (Zhao and Xia, 2019).

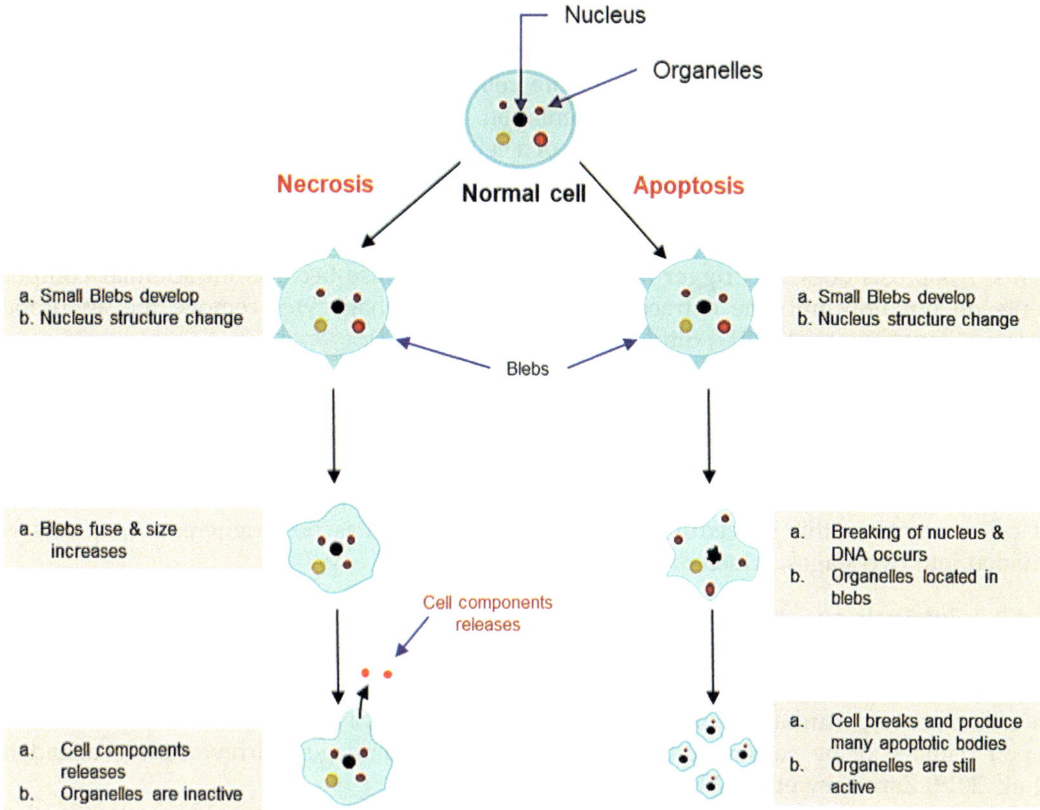

FIGURE 7.9 Phenomenon of cell death in necrosis and apoptosis.

TABLE 7.1 Forms of cell death.

Necrosis	Apoptosis
Cell death in a submissive state. It does not entail any cellular activity activation.	A powerful kind of cell destruction. It induces phagocytosis or suicide in cells but is less hazardous than necrosis.
Early loss of plasma membrane activity followed by cell swelling and bursting.	Caspase-dependent, which is a protein involved in programmed cell death
Inflammation is caused when a cell explodes. As a result, cells are activated in reaction to tissue injury.	Dying cells shrink, releasing membrane apoptotic bodies that are immunological cells phagocytose such as mast cells.

7.4.2 Apoptosis: programmed cell death

Apoptosis, on the other hand, is a more organized kind of cell death (sometimes known as "cell suicide" or "planned cell death"). Apoptosis is a process in which particular enzymes are activated, causing the systematic fragmentation of cell contents into blebs of the cell membrane that pinch off from the primary cell to create apoptotic bodies. Unlike necrosis, when organelle and energy synthesis ceases before cellular fragmentation, the cell continues to create energy and proteins during fragmentation. Apoptosis produces a large number of apoptotic bodies, each of which is made up of a cellular membrane encasing intact and functioning cellular components. Apoptosis can be caused by several types of oxidative stress, including the presence of too many oxygen-derived free radicals, which can occur as a result of the excessive free radical formation and/or a lack of or depletion of endogenous antioxidants. Apoptosis does not trigger an inflammatory response because intracellular components do not flow into the extracellular matrix; local phagocytes remove the apoptotic corpses (Ikwegbue et al., 2017; Sifuentes-Franco et al., 2018).

Apoptosis is characterized by cell shrinkage with or without a minimal effect on organelles. Apoptosis, unlike necrosis, is a particular cell death procedure that can occur in both healthy as well as pathological conditions (Carneiro and El-Deiry, 2020). Small apoptotic bodies appear on the wounded cell's surface, including 'phagocytic' signals. In vivo, phagocytes identify these signals and consume the bodies (Medina et al., 2020). There is no leaking of cell contents in this procedure; therefore, inflammation is not triggered. Apoptosis is divided into two stages, which are as follows.

7.4.2.1 *Intrinsic apoptosis*

Intrinsic apoptosis (also known as mitochondrial apoptosis) happens when a cell dies due to various factors, including intracellular damage and oncogenic stress. Intracellular sensors in cells react to perturbations by activating signaling pathways to restore homeostasis and repair damage or by causing intrinsic apoptosis if the damage is irreversible (Valizadeh et al., 2019; Zamaraev et al., 2020; Li et al., 2021).

The intrinsic apoptotic pathway can be triggered by chemotherapy and/or radiation. For example, external and endogenous stimuli that activate it include DNA damage, ischemia, and oxidative stress. It also helps in the production of new cells and the clearance of damaged ones. The intrinsic process causes mitochondrial membrane breakdown and cytochrome *c* release into the cytoplasm, where it forms an apoptosome with the inactive form of caspase-9 and apoptotic protease activating factor 1 (APAF1). This complex hydrolyzes adenosine triphosphate to cleave and activate caspase 9. The initiator caspase-9 then cleaves and activates caspases-3/6/7, resulting in cell death. Extracellular signals generally generated by immune system cytotoxic cells and primarily induce apoptosis via the extrinsic pathway are fundamentally different (Han et al., 2020; Lan et al., 2021; Peterson et al., 2022).

The intrinsic apoptosis route activates caspase-3 or cleaves bid (BH3 interacting domain death agonist), resulting in mitochondrial dysfunction, cytochrome *c* release, and caspase-9 and caspase-3 activation. Caspase-3 triggers apoptosis in various organs, causing DNA damage and cell death (Jayaram and Krishnamurthy, 2021).

7.4.2.2 *Extrinsic apoptosis*

In molecular biology, the term "extrinsic pathway" refers to both the extrinsic apoptotic and extrinsic coagulation pathways. The first sort of extrinsic route, the extrinsic apoptotic pathway, will be the subject of this article. One of the signaling pathways that might trigger cell apoptosis is the extrinsic apoptosis pathway (programmed cell death) (Bedoui et al., 2020).

Apoptosis is a phenomenon of organized structure alterations and DNA fragmentation that leads to cell death. Cellular events from the outside or inside stimulate it. Extrinsic pathway mediated by death receptors is one of them. Death receptors include Fas receptors, tumor necrosis factor (TNF) receptors, and TNF-related apoptosis-inducing ligand (TRAIL) receptors. TNF-R1 interacts with TNF to cause the recruitment of adaptor proteins such as Fas-associated protein with death domain (FADD) and TNF-R1-associated death domain protein (TRADD). These adaptor proteins further recruit a series of downstream factors, including Caspase-8, a critical mediator of the extrinsic pathway, resulting in cell apoptosis (Holbrook et al., 2019; Li et al., 2020).

The extrinsic route of apoptosis is triggered when a death ligand binds to a death receptor, such as TNF- to TNFR1. The 29 transmembrane receptor proteins in the TNFR family are organized in homo trimers and are activated by ligand contact(s). They all share cysteine-rich extracellular domains and an 80-amino-acid-long cytoplasmic domain known as the death domain (DD). The death domain is required to transmit death signals from the cell surface to intracellular signaling pathways (Przedborski et al., 2003).

7.5 Repair mechanisms

Nonhomologous recombination and homologous recombination end joining are the two fundamental processes for healing double-strand breaks. Homologous recombination entails the exchange of nucleotide sequences to repair damaged bases on both strands of DNA using a sister chromatid (Wagener-Ryczek et al., 2021).

7.5.1 DNA repair

DNA repair is a collection of processes that identify and repair DNA damage. Direct reversal of damage, repair of excision, and repairing double-strand breaks in DNA are three different forms of repair processes. The damage is targeted for direct reversal repair. Photo reactivation, for instance, is a process in which pyrimidine bases are separated by the photolyase enzyme in DNA—fused by ultraviolet (UV) radiation (a light-driven enzyme) (Galluzzi et al., 2017; Gu et al., 2021; Huang and Zhou, 2021).

i. A DNA methyl transferase or DNA glycosylase identifies and removes the alkyl group for direct alkylation reversal. Excision repair can be either particular or general. DNA glycosylases selectively recognize and remove the mismatched nucleotide in base excision repair. The repair machinery identifies a wide range of deformities in the double helix induced by mismatched bases. Nucleotide excision repair is a process that involves the removal of one or more nucleotides. Because replication is stopped at the actual site of damage, post-replication repair occurs downstream of the lesion. Okazaki fragments are short segments of DNA that are created so that replication can occur.
ii. Recombination repair, which takes the sequence from an intact sister chromosome to fix the damaged ones, or error-prone repair, which uses the broken strand as a

sequence template, fills in the gap left by the damaged site. Repairs that are prone to errors are inefficient and prone to mutation.

iii. When the DNA of a cell is damaged, it causes the cell to die, and it often chooses to duplicate it rather than waiting for it to be repaired (translation synthesis). While this may result in mutations, it is preferable to a complete stoppage of DNA replication, resulting in cell death. When DNA repair fails, on the other hand, the need for good DNA repair is emphasized. Free radicals oxidize guanine, resulting in G-T transversion, among the human cancer mutations that are most common.

7.5.1.1 The direct reversal DNA repair mechanism

A way of repair is DNA reversal in direct manner damage that does not require the usage of a template. UV exposure promotes the formation of pyrimidine dimers, which can change the structure of the DNA chain and impede outside of the devastated area transcription. Using light energy to break down a covalent connection between nearby pyrimidine nucleotides that is abnormal, this dimerization reaction may be inverted by using photoreactivation as a direct reversal. Humans do not experience this photoreactivation (Li et al., 2018; Kay et al., 2019). The damage induced by alkylating agents interaction with DNA can also be reversed by direct reversal. Guanine methylation changes DNA structure by producing a thymine-complementing product rather than a cytosine-complementing product. The methylation product is transported to the active site; methylguanine methyltransferase (MGMT) is a protein that can return guanine to its natural state (Cortez, 2019; Ganesa et al., 2022).

7.5.1.2 DNA repair by excision

When one of the two strands of the double helix is damaged, excision is the general method of repair. The strand that isn't faulty acts as a blueprint for the rest of the strands. On the other strand, damaged DNA is eliminated, and new nucleotides are produced in its stead (Mao and Wyrick, 2019; Caldecott, 2020). Excision repair may be divided into three categories:

1. Base-excision repair

A single base that has been damaged is discovered and removed during base-excision repair. The process is dependent on a group of enzymes called glycosylases. Before the nucleotide gap on the DNA strand is filled by DNA polymerase, the enzymes remove the damaged base, forming an apurinic (AP) site that is repaired by AP endonuclease (Caldecott, 2020).

2. Excision repair of nucleotides

Excision repair of nucleotides is a popular method for repairing DNA damage that identifies multiple damaged basest nucleotides. This technique is utilized in humans to repair the damage produced by UV radiation, i.e., the production of pyrimidine dimers. The procedure starts with the identification of damage, and then endonucleases break the DNA polymerase on both sides before it can recombine (Kumar et al., 2020; Liebelt et al., 2020).

3. Mismatch repair

It is the third excision method, which happens when the bases are misaligned and integrated, inserted during replication of the DNA strand, and not removed by DNA polymerase during proofreading. Missed faults are eventually fixed by enzymes that detect and remove mismatched bases, allowing the original sequence to be restored in mismatch repair (Baretti and Le, 2018).

7.5.1.3 Repairing double-strand breaks in DNA

Repairing both damaged DNA strands is required to maintain genomic integrity. The two basic mechanisms are homologous recombination and nonhomologous end joining for healing double-strand breaks. Homologous recombination, which uses a sister chromatid to repair damaged nucleotides on both DNA strands, involves the exchange of nucleotide sequences. Classical nonhomologous end joining uses small DNA sequences termed microhomologies to rejoin the break ends in the absence of a uniform template (Portt et al., 2011; Loreto et al., 2014; Galluzzi et al., 2020).

According to studies, double-strand fractures can also be healed through alternate processes, i.e., annealing with single strands and alternate joining under specific circumstances. These procedures are carcinogenic and can potentially cause mutations and the loss of genetic information. In the genome, end joining is used to link scattered nucleotide repeats. It is achieved by single-stranded annealing; this causes the repeat to be duplicated and the intervening section to be deleted. The procedure for repairing double-strand breakage in alternative joining is unclear, although it has been shown to jeopardize. End breaks on different chromosomes are merged to maintain genomic integrity (Galluzzi et al., 2020).

7.5.2 Protein repair

Different intrinsic and extrinsic variables have an ongoing impact on proteins. Damaged proteins have an impact on a variety of intracellular processes, leading to a variety of illnesses and diseases. Only a few methods for protein repair have been identified, such as the methionine sulfoxide reductases reducing methionine sulfoxide residues, L-isoaspartate methyl transferase converting isoaspartyl residues to L-aspartate, while fructosamine-3-kinase deglycates protein-bound fructosamine (Elmore, 2007).

Lysosomes and proteasomes are two different types of lysosomes. They are the main proteolytic enzymes responsible for protein breakdown. Because protein repair and breakdown are so necessary, researchers have increasingly focused on modulating these systems in various physiological circumstances, including aging and illness. In the field of protein repair enzymes, genetic manipulation has shown encouraging results. Still, no potent inhibitors have yet been found, and just one activating chemical has been reported to the best of the author's knowledge. On the other hand, different medications and natural chemicals that interfere with proteolysis have been discovered and/or manufactured, leading to the maintenance of homeostasis and/or a delay in disease development (Elmore, 2007).

7.5.2.1 Protein damage can be reversible or irreversible

Chemical instability causes protein, like other biomolecules, to alter over time or be assaulted by substances such as reactive oxygen and nitrogen species that are highly reactive with specific amino acid side chains, aldehydes, and di-carbonyls. Reactive oxygen species can bind to proteins directly or indirectly through other molecules. The formation of oxidized by-products from their contact with lipids and carbohydrates has an irreversible reaction with proteins. We'll talk about specific reversible and irreversible protein damage in the following section, focusing on the enzyme systems in charge of reversing harm when possible (Krisko and Radman, 2019; Kiely-Collins et al., 2021).

7.5.2.1.1 Lipid peroxidation products and protein conjugation

Under oxidative stress, unconstrained radicals produced in the cell can assault cellular membranes directly. Free radicals oxidize polyunsaturated fatty acids due to a chain reaction that disintegrates into a slew of oxidized substances such as acrolein, 4-hydroxy-2-nonenal, and malondialdehyde. The final products of Lipid peroxidation have progressed to an advanced level, which can interact with proteins and build up over time. Some problems caused by old age are natural precursors of carbonyl-reactive chemicals produced by lipid peroxidation in biomembranes. PUFAs, including arachidonic acid, linoleic acid, and linolenic acid, are oxidized through a series of nonenzymatic phases 4-hydroxy-2-nonenal is an unsaturated aldehyde with four hydroxyl groups (Vingerhoets, 2001).

7.5.2.1.2 Oxidation and carbonylation of proteins processes

Reactive oxygen species, as previously noted, may react with proteins directly. Free radicals oxidize proteins in a site-specific manner, and cations of redox metals (e.g., copper and iron) are commonly involved. Protein oxidative modifications can be divided into two types: the first oxidize and break the peptide bond, while the second alters the side chains. Phenylalanine is converted into tyrosine during oxidation and then tyrosine to di-tyrosine. Furthermore, tyrosine is preferred as a nitrification goal, resulting in the creation of nitrotyrosine (Topkaya et al., 2018).

7.5.2.1.3 Glycation and glycoxidation of proteins

Through a Schiff base formation, sugar ketones or aldehydes can react quickly and nonenzymatically, involving the amino groups on the side chains of proteins. Even though it is possible to reverse this response, the base of the Schiff can be gradually rearranged to produce the product of Amadori, fructosamine when glucose is the reactive sugar. Early-stage glycation adducts result from these reactions, which characterize early-stage processes. It's been proposed that specialized enzymes like amadoriase and fructosamine-3-kinase target these adducts for repair. However, additional glycation adduct modification by cyclization, oxidation, fragmentation, dehydration, and/or rearrangement of early-stage glycation adducts is possible (Eker et al., 2009).

7.5.2.1.4 Deamidation of proteins and isomerization of amino acids

Proteins may spontaneously change their aspartyl and asparaginyl residues, such as isomerization, racemization, and deamidation, in addition to lipid peroxidation products that cause glycoxidation, oxidation, glycation, and the production of protein adducts. Proline, which is generally found trans-configured, cis-proline, an abnormal isomeric form of the amino acid, can also be found. Despite this, deamidation and isomerization hotspots exist for asparagine and aspartic acid. Both types of residues can form a succinimide ring intermediate when the nucleophilic attack on the peptide bond nitrogen atom of the following carbonyl group residue on the side chain happens. This succinimide is unstable and can disintegrate into a combination of aspartyl and isoaspartyl residues when hydrolyzed. Racemization of the succinimide results in the formation of residues containing D-aspartyl, D-succinimidyl, and D-isoaspartyl. Deamidation can cause spontaneous asparagine hydrolysis, resulting in an aspartyl residue (Delmar et al., 2019; Lawson et al., 2022).

7.5.2.1.5 Modification of proteins by oxidation that is reversible

Cysteine and methionine residues are the most popular sensitive amino acids to oxidation by almost all forms of reactive oxygen species. Although certain oxidation products of methionine and cysteine can be converted to methionine and cysteine again inside proteins, this is not the case for other amino acids. Cysteine is an amino acid containing a thiol side chain that is significant due to the thiol group's strong reactivity. Many proteins have both structural and functional elements. The sulfur atom in cysteine can take on a variety of oxidation states in physiological settings. When cysteine is oxidized, a sulfenic acid or a disulfide bridge, which can be transformed into bridges of disulfide or sulfonic acid, is formed as a result of subsequent oxidation in two very unstable and reactive tautomeric forms. Enzymatic systems may reverse both oxidation products. However, sulfonic acid reduction by the presence of oxidized cysteines in the active regions of peroxiredoxin has been demonstrated using sulfiredoxin (Portt et al., 2011).

7.5.2.2 Protection mechanisms for protein maintenance and repair

Unlike DNA, which has a large number of repair enzymes and routes to combat oxidative and other types of damage, proteins have a limited number of enzymes and mechanisms that help to repair this damage. Most changed proteins are degraded, and just a few repair mechanisms have been found related to protein damage. Within proteins, cysteine and methionine's oxidation products can be reduced to their reduced forms when it comes to oxidative damage to proteins having amino acids with sulfur (Portt et al., 2011).

Small proteins like thioredoxin and glutaredoxin have reduced versions. Glutathione/glutathione reductase and thioredoxin reductase oxidize these compounds and then recycle them back to their reduced forms, and they are two of the most critical systems in the reversal of disulfide bridge oxidation and sulfenic acid oxidation, respectively (Portt et al., 2011).

7.5.2.2.1 Activities of the enzyme methionine sulfoxide reductase

The action of methionine sulfoxide reductases was initially discovered in yeast in 1960 and then in larger species shortly after. Thioredoxin and thioredoxin reductase were discovered with nicotinamide adenine dinucleotide phosphate (NADPH), representing two out of three elements that make up the methionine sulfoxide reduction. Initially, it is based on the ability of a methionine auxotrophic *E. coli* strain to flourish in the presence of solely L-methionine sulfoxide as a source of methionine in the growing medium. Later, in *E. coli*, a third protein component required for the enzymatic reduction of sulfoxide of methionine was found (Galluzzi et al., 2020).

Ultimately, scientists partly isolated an *E. coli* enzyme capable of facilitating the reduction of carbon dioxide of methionine sulfoxides in proteins, as well as showing that the ribosomal protein L12 activity in *E. coli* was restored simultaneously. Methionine sulfoxide reductase (Msr)-A, the whole first Msr enzyme identified practically. It's found in the majority of higher eukaryotic cell types and tissues, and it's found in all living things. Furthermore, MsrA is one of 300 proteins essential for aerobic living and can be present in all bacteria's genomes (Galluzzi et al., 2020).

7.5.2.2.2 Distribution and localization of methionine sulfoxide reductases

Msr genes may be found in various organisms, including practically all creatures from microbes to *Homo sapiens*, *Staphylococcus aureus*, and *Arabidopsis thaliana*, except parasites and hyperthermophilic microorganisms. They contain multiple copies of either msrA, msrB, or both msrA and msrB. In contrast, Drosophila Melanogaster, *E. coli*, and *C. elegans* (*D. melanogaster*) have single msrA and msrB genes. MsrA and MsrB have little in common in terms of sequence and structure, despite catalyzing the same chemical process. In Neisseria gonorrhoeae, a single gene, pilB, encodes both msrA and msrB, resulting in a fused (Reductases of methionine sulfoxide) MsrA and MsrB polypeptide (Loreto et al., 2014).

7.5.2.2.3 Gene control by methionine sulfoxide reductases

The calcium phospholipid-binding protein (CPBP), a homolog of elongation factor 1c that cooperates with other proteins to bind the msrA promoter, was discovered in yeast and is necessary for the transcriptional regulation of the msrA gene. It was discovered that CPBP regulates the expression of the msrA gene favorably, and deletion of CPBP led to lower MsrA RNA and protein expression. Furthermore, cytosolic thioredoxin (Trx1) was discovered to be required for yeast activity of the msrA transcription factor during normal growth circumstances. Following persistent oxidative stress, CPBP binds to the msrA promoter. Subsequently, through transcriptional regulation, the heme oxygenase-1's yeast homolog has been related to antioxidants inside the cell defense via modulating antioxidant enzymes such as methionine sulfoxide reductases, c-glutamylcysteine synthetase, glutathione peroxidase, catalase, and glutathione peroxidase (Chondrogianni et al., 2014).

7.5.2.2.3.1 Other potential protein repair mechanisms Two more methods for repairing proteins have been described, in addition to methionine sulfoxide reductases. Protein L-isoaspartate methyl transferase (PIMT) transforms isoaspartyl residues in proteins to L-aspartate, converting them from aspartate and asparagine, while fructosamine-3-kinase phosphorylates protein-bound fructosamine. Protein maintenance systems such as chaperone, heat-shock proteins, peptidyl-prolyl cis-trans isomerases, and protein disulfide isomerases play a crucial part in protein homeostasis. Still, they're not discussed in this chapter since they're more concerned with the folding and refolding of proteins than with protein damage repair (Portt et al., 2011).

7.5.2.2.4 L-isoaspartate methyl transferase, a protein, methylates proteins

As previously established, asparagine deamidation occurs spontaneously, like aspartyl residue isomerization and racemization. Asparagine or aspartate residues are replaced by isoaspartate residues, resulting in a kinked polypeptide chain. The ubiquitous enzyme PIMT, which can catalyze the conversion of such isoaspartate residues to the regular L-aspartyl form, is found in all species, from bacteria to humans. On the other hand, the L-asparaginyl form does not appear to be regenerable. The PIMT's capacity to identify damaged aspartyl residues was originally discovered in an enzyme of mammals (Portt et al., 2011).

7.5.2.2.5 Protein deglycation occurs when fructosamine-3-kinase phosphorylates protein-bound fructosamine

It has been considered that glycation-induced protein damage is irreversible. Certain enzymes, known as deglycase and amadoriases, have been discovered in bacteria and fungi that catalyze the transformation/fructosamine oxidation and related ketoamine oxidation. A Schiff base is generated from these reactions, which can subsequently be hydrolyzed to release the sugar moiety from the lysine attached to the protein (aldose or ketoaldose). However, it's unclear if these enzymes may function on proteins and whether Fructosamine and other low-molecular-weight ketoamines react readily (Portt et al., 2011).

7.5.3 Lipid repair

The first sort of oxidative damage to be researched was lipid peroxidation. Membrane phospholipids are constantly exposed to oxidative stress. A multitude of chain reactions is involved in the lipid peroxidation process that starts when a hydrogen atom (from carbon) is removed from a sequence of unsaturated fatty acyls. A lipid peroxyl radical (LOO$^{\cdot}$) is formed when oxygen combines with a fatty acid in an aerobic environment. LOO may boost the initiated peroxidation chain reaction by removing nearby hydrogen atoms of an unsaturated fatty acid (Eisenberg et al., 2009). Cholesterol has also been oxidized, producing several epoxides and alcohols (Chondrogianni et al., 2014).

Lipid replacement therapy, or functional oral supplements containing phospholipids and antioxidants found in cell membranes, has been utilized to restore cellular function. It works by replacing Membrane glycerophospholipids that have been degraded, generally by oxidation, and have accumulated with age and in various clinical circumstances. This method is distinct from previous dietary and intravenous phospholipid intervention methods because of phospholipid composition and oxidation defense during storage, ingestion, digesting, and absorption. Protective compounds that noncovalently bind to phospholipid micelles and inhibit enzymatic and biliary disruption are also used (Chondrogianni et al., 2014).

Phospholipids are made to safeguard you in a variety of natural ways. Lipoprotein receptors, transport, carrier molecules, circulating cells, and lipoproteins are all involved in this process. Until they are delivered to cells and tissues, they can be transported to intracellular membranes by both selective and nonspecific transport mechanisms. They spontaneously replenish and encourage the clearance of damaged membrane lipids once given to membrane locations. Membrane damage, usually oxidative but sometimes enzymatic, leads to cellular dysfunction in many chronic clinical illnesses. Clinical investigations recently have shown the effectiveness of restoring mitochondrial activity, lipid replacement therapy used, and lowering tiredness in elderly individuals and patients with a range of clinical illnesses defined by mitochondrial dysfunction and fatigue as prominent symptoms (Chondrogianni et al., 2014).

7.6 Conclusion

Reversible cellular malfunction, irreversible cellular damage, and cell death can all be caused by toxins. Cellular atrophy and substrate deposition are two possible cellular reactions to toxic damage. Various chemicals affect cellular dysfunction by forming DNA and protein adducts, causing oxidative stress, and by interacting with protein targets. Cell membrane breakdown, impairment of cellular repair processes, and reduction of cellular power generation are some of the primary causes of cell death. Cell death can be occurred by necrosis or apoptosis. Toxicants showed diverse cellular responses like carcinogenicity, genotoxicity, inflammation, neuroinflammation, neurodegeneration, cell signaling disruption, and many more. These cellular responses alter the organs functioning and lead to impairment in normal physiology. Oxidative stress brought on by oxygen-derived free radicals may induce apoptosis. Typically, apoptosis does not result in an inflammatory reaction. DNA repair, protein repair, and lipid repair mainly help as repair mechanisms for the cellular responses to toxicants.

7.7 List of abbreviations

AChE Acetylcholinesterase
AD Alzheimer's disease
ALS Amyotrophic lateral sclerosis
AP Apurinic
APAF1 Apoptotic protease activating factor 1
Cd Cadmium
CNS Central nervous system
CPBP Calcium phospholipid-binding protein
DD Death domain
FADD Fas-associated protein with death domain
hiPSC Human induced pluripotent stem cell
LOO Lipid peroxyl radical
LPS Lipopolysaccharide
MGMT Methylguanine methyltransferase
MR Mean ratio
MS Multiple sclerosis
Msr Methionine sulfoxide reductase
NK Cells natural killer cells
nm Nanometer
OSPW Oil sands process affected water
PAH Polycyclic aromatic hydrocarbons
PD Parkinson's disease
PIMT Protein L-isoaspartate methyl transferase
QTL Quantitative trait loci
ROS Reactive oxygen species
SOD Superoxide dismutase
TNF Tumor necrosis factor
TRADD TNF-R1-associated death domain protein
TRAIL TNF-related apoptosis-inducing ligand
Trx1 Thioredoxin
UV Ultraviolet
XP Xeroderma pigmentosum

References

Achanta, N.S.K., Rajpoot, K., Tekade, R.K., 2021. Drug metabolic kinetics. In: Tekade, R.K. (Ed.), Biopharmaceutics and Pharmacokinetics Considerations. Elsevier, Academic Press, pp. 335–353.

Ahamed, M., Posgai, R., Gorey, T.J., Nielsen, M., Hussain, S.M., Rowe, J.J., 2010. Silver nanoparticles induced heat shock protein 70, oxidative stress and apoptosis in *Drosophila melanogaster*. Toxicol. Appl. Pharmacol. 242 (3), 263–269.

Akçan, R., Aydogan, H.C., Yildirim, M.S., Tastekin, B., Sağlam, N., 2020. Nanotoxicity: a challenge for future medicine. Turk. J. Med. Sci. 50 (4), 1180–1196.

Al Gurabi, M.A., Ali, D., Alkahtani, S., Alarifi, S., 2015. In vivo DNA damaging and apoptotic potential of silver nanoparticles in Swiss albino mice. OncoTargets Ther. 8, 295.

Anup, N., Desai, N., Rajpoot, K., Tekade, R.K., 2021a. Kinetics of maternal–fetal drug transfer. In: Tekade, R.K. (Ed.), Biopharmaceutics and Pharmacokinetics Considerations, pp. 145–162.

Anup, N., Gadeval, A., Rajpoot, K., Tekade, R.K., 2021b. Software used in ADME computation. In: Tekade, R.K. (Ed.), Biopharmaceutics and Pharmacokinetics Considerations. Elsevier, Academic Press, pp. 699–708.

Anup, N., Rajpoot, K., Tekade, R.K., 2021c. Overview of biopharmaceutics and pharmacokinetics. In: Tekade, R.K. (Ed.), Biopharmaceutics and Pharmacokinetics Considerations, vol. 1. Elsevier, Academic Press, pp. 1–16.

Arun, K.B., Madhavan, A., Sindhu, R., Emmanual, S., Binod, P., Pugazhendhi, A., et al., 2021. Probiotics and gut microbiome—prospects and challenges in remediating heavy metal toxicity. J. Hazard Mater. 420, 126676.

Asati, S., Pandey, V., Gour, V., Tiwari, R., Soni, V., Rajpoot, K., et al., 2022. Toxicity and toxicokinetic considerations in product development and drug research. In: Pharmacokinetics and Toxicokinetic Considerations, vol. 2. Elsevier, pp. 401–424.

Avalos, A., Haza, A.I., Mateo, D., Morales, P., 2014. Cytotoxicity and ROS production of manufactured silver nanoparticles of different sizes in hepatoma and leukemia cells. J. Appl. Toxicol. 34 (4), 413–423.

Baretti, M., Le, D.T., 2018. DNA mismatch repair in cancer. Pharmacol. Therapeut. 189, 45–62.

Basu, A.K., 2018. DNA damage, mutagenesis and cancer. Int. J. Mol. Sci. 19 (4), 970.

Bedoui, S., Herold, M.J., Strasser, A., 2020. Emerging connectivity of programmed cell death pathways and its physiological implications. Nat. Rev. Mol. Cell Biol. 21 (11), 678–695.

Brown, G.C., 2019. The endotoxin hypothesis of neurodegeneration. J. Neuroinflammation 16 (1), 180.

Browning, L.M., Lee, K.J., Nallathamby, P.D., Xu, X.-H.N., 2013. Silver nanoparticles incite size-and dose-dependent developmental phenotypes and nanotoxicity in zebrafish embryos. Chem. Res. Toxicol. 26 (10), 1503–1513.

Burggren, W., 2016. Epigenetic inheritance and its role in evolutionary biology: re-evaluation and new perspectives. Biology 5 (2), 24.

Caldecott, K.W., 2020. Mammalian DNA base excision repair: dancing in the moonlight. DNA Repair 93, 102921.

Carneiro, B.A., El-Deiry, W.S., 2020. Targeting apoptosis in cancer therapy. Nat. Rev. Clin. Oncol. 17 (7), 395–417.

Ceppi, M., Munnia, A., Cellai, F., Bruzzone, M., Peluso, M.E.M., 2017. Linking the generation of DNA adducts to lung cancer. Toxicology 390, 160–166.

Chappell, G.A., Rager, J.E., 2017. Epigenetics in chemical-induced genotoxic carcinogenesis. Curr. Opin. Toxicol. 6, 10–17.

Chen, L., Deng, H., Cui, H., Fang, J., Zuo, Z., Deng, J., et al., 2017. Inflammatory responses and inflammation-associated diseases in organs. Oncotarget 9 (6), 7204–7218.

Chen, L.Q., Fang, L., Ling, J., Ding, C.Z., Kang, B., Huang, C.Z., 2015. Nanotoxicity of silver nanoparticles to red blood cells: size dependent adsorption, uptake, and hemolytic activity. Chem. Res. Toxicol. 28 (3), 501–509.

Chi, L., Xue, J., Tu, P., Lai, Y., Ru, H., Lu, K., 2019. Gut microbiome disruption altered the biotransformation and liver toxicity of arsenic in mice. Arch. Toxicol. 93 (1), 25–35.

Chondrogianni, N., Petropoulos, I., Grimm, S., Georgila, K., Catalgol, B., Friguet, B., et al., 2014. Protein damage, repair and proteolysis. Mol. Aspects Med. 35, 1–71.

Choudhary, D., Goykar, H., Rajpoot, K., Tekade, R.K., 2021. Chronopharmacokinetics. In: Tekade, R.K. (Ed.), Biopharmaceutics and Pharmacokinetics Considerations. Elsevier, Academic Press, pp. 163–194.

Chow, J., Rahman, J., Achermann, J.C., Dattani, M.T., Rahman, S., 2017. Mitochondrial disease and endocrine dysfunction. Nat. Rev. Endocrinol. 13 (2), 92–104.

Ciernikova, S., Mego, M., Chovanec, M., 2021. Exploring the potential role of the gut microbiome in chemotherapy-induced neurocognitive disorders and cardiovascular toxicity. Cancers 13 (4).

Collodel, G., Castellini, C., Lee, J.C., Signorini, C., 2020. Relevance of fatty acids to sperm maturation and quality. Oxid. Med. Cell. Longev. 2020, 7038124.

Compton, C., 2020. Cancer initiation, promotion, and progression and the acquisition of key behavioral traits. In: Cancer: The Enemy from Within. Springer, pp. 25–48.

Cortez, D., 2019. Replication-coupled DNA repair. Mol. Cell 74 (5), 866–876.

D'Arcy, M.S., 2019. Cell death: a review of the major forms of apoptosis, necrosis and autophagy. Cell Biol. Int. 43 (6), 582–592.

Delmar, J.A., Wang, J., Choi, S.W., Martins, J.A., Mikhail, J.P., 2019. Machine learning enables accurate prediction of asparagine deamidation probability and rate. Mol. Ther. Methods Clin. Dev. 15, 264–274.

Desai, N., Koppisetti, H., Rajpoot, K., Tekade, M., Sharma, M.C., Tekade, R.K., 2021. Influence of fever on pharmacokinetics of drugs. In: Tekade, R.K. (Ed.), Biopharmaceutics and Pharmacokinetics Considerations. Elsevier, pp. 451–463.

DiSabato, D.J., Quan, N., Godbout, J.P., 2016. Neuroinflammation: the devil is in the details. J. Neurochem. 139, 136–153.

Ditani, A.S., Mallick, P.P., Anup, N., Tambe, V., Polaka, S., Sengupta, P., et al., 2021. Biosimilars accessible in the market for the treatment of cancer. J. Control. Release 336, 112–129.

Du, X., Li, D., Wang, G., Fan, Y., Li, N., Chai, L., et al., 2021. Chemoprotective effect of atorvastatin against benzo(a) pyrene-induced lung cancer via the inhibition of oxidative stress and inflammatory parameters. Ann. Transl. Med. 9 (4), 355.

Dusinska, M., Mariussen, E., Rundén-Pran, E., Hudecova, A.M., Elje, E., Kazimirova, A., et al., 2019. In vitro approaches for assessing the genotoxicity of nanomaterials. In: Nanotoxicity. Springer, pp. 83–122.

Dusinska, M., Tulinska, J., El Yamani, N., Kuricova, M., Liskova, A., Rollerova, E., et al., 2017. Immunotoxicity, genotoxicity and epigenetic toxicity of nanomaterials: new strategies for toxicity testing? Food Chem. Toxicol. 109 (Pt 1), 797–811.

Eisenberg, T., Knauer, H., Schauer, A., Büttner, S., Ruckenstuhl, C., Carmona-Gutierrez, D., et al., 2009. Induction of autophagy by spermidine promotes longevity. Nat. Cell Biol. 11 (11), 1305–1314.

Eker, A.P.M., Quayle, C., Chaves, I., van der Horst, G.T.J., 2009. DNA repair in mammalian cells. Cell. Mol. Life Sci. 66 (6), 968–980.

Elmore, S., 2007. Apoptosis: a review of programmed cell death. Toxicol. Pathol. 35 (4), 495–516.

Espinosa-Riquer, Z.P., Segura-Villalobos, D., Ramírez-Moreno, I.G., Pérez Rodríguez, M.J., Lamas, M., Gonzalez-Espinosa, C., 2020. Signal Transduction pathways activated by innate immunity in mast cells: translating sensing of changes into specific responses. Cells 9 (11), 2411.

Ewa, B., Danuta, M.-Š., 2017. Polycyclic aromatic hydrocarbons and PAH-related DNA adducts. J. Appl. Genet. 58 (3), 321–330.

Fong, W., Li, Q., Yu, J., 2020. Gut microbiota modulation: a novel strategy for prevention and treatment of colorectal cancer. Oncogene 39 (26), 4925–4943.

Fu, P.P., Xia, Q., Hwang, H.-M., Ray, P.C., Yu, H., 2014. Mechanisms of nanotoxicity: generation of reactive oxygen species. J. Food Drug Anal. 22 (1), 64–75.

Galluzzi, L., Kepp, O., Chan, F.K.-M., Kroemer, G., 2017. Necroptosis: mechanisms and relevance to disease. Annu. Rev. Pathol. 12, 103–130.

Galluzzi, L., Linkermann, A., Kepp, O., Kroemer, G., 2020. Pathophysiology of cancer cell death. In: Abeloff's Clinical Oncology. Elsevier, pp. 74–83.e74.

Ganesa, S., Sule, A., Sundaram, R.K., Bindra, R.S., 2022. Mismatch repair proteins play a role in ATR activation upon temozolomide treatment in MGMT-methylated glioblastoma. Sci. Rep. 12 (1), 1–15.

Gao, P., da Silva, E., Hou, L., Denslow, N.D., Xiang, P., Ma, L.Q., 2018. Human exposure to polycyclic aromatic hydrocarbons: metabolomics perspective. Environ. Int. 119, 466–477.

Gault, I.G.M., 2019. Oil Sands Process-Affected Water Toxicity Attribution and Evaluating Ageing as a Remediation Strategy.

Gu, S., Bodai, Z., Cowan, Q.T., Komor, A.C., 2021. Base editors: expanding the types of DNA damage products harnessed for genome editing. Gene Genome Editing 1, 100005.

Gupta, P.K., 2018. Illustrated Toxicology. Elsevier.

Gupta, R., Polaka, S., Rajpoot, K., Tekade, M., Sharma, M.C., Tekade, R.K., 2022a. Importance of toxicity testing in drug discovery and research. In: Pharmacokinetics and Toxicokinetic Considerations, vol. 2. Elsevier, pp. 117–144.

Gupta, R., Rajpoot, K., Tekade, M., Sharma, M.C., Safavi, M., Tekade, R.K., 2022b. Factors influencing drug toxicity. In: Pharmacokinetics and Toxicokinetic Considerations, vol. 2. Elsevier, pp. 27–50.

Gupta, R., Rajpoot, K., Tekade, M., Sharma, M.C., Tekade, R.K., 2022c. Methods and models for in vitro toxicity. In: Pharmacokinetics and Toxicokinetic Considerations, vol. 2. Elsevier, pp. 145–174.

Halpern, M., Brennand, K.J., Gregory, J., 2019. Examining the relationship between astrocyte dysfunction and neurodegeneration in ALS using hiPSCs. Neurobiol. Dis. 132, 104562.

Han, C., Liu, Z., Zhang, Y., Shen, A., Dong, C., Zhang, A., et al., 2020. Tumor cells suppress radiation-induced immunity by hijacking caspase 9 signaling. Nat. Immunol. 21 (5), 546–554.

Heymann, H.M., Gardner, A.M., Gross, E.R., 2018. Aldehyde-induced DNA and protein adducts as biomarker tools for alcohol use disorder. Trends Mol. Med. 24 (2), 144–155.

Hirano, S.-i., Ichikawa, Y., Sato, B., Yamamoto, H., Takefuji, Y., Satoh, F., 2021. Potential therapeutic applications of hydrogen in chronic inflammatory diseases: possible inhibiting role on mitochondrial stress. Int. J. Mol. Sci. 22 (5), 2549.

Hoet, P., Lauwerys, R., 2020. Biological monitoring of occupational neurotoxicants. In: Occupatinal Neurotoxicology. CRC Press, pp. 49–74.

Holbrook, J., Lara-Reyna, S., Jarosz-Griffiths, H., McDermott, M., 2019. Tumour necrosis factor signalling in health and disease. F1000Research 8, F1000. Faculty Rev-1111.

Hu, J., Barrett, R.D.H., 2017. Epigenetics in natural animal populations. J. Evol. Biol. 30 (9), 1612–1632.

Huang, R., Zhou, P.-K., 2021. DNA damage repair: historical perspectives, mechanistic pathways and clinical translation for targeted cancer therapy. Signal Transduct. Target. Ther. 6 (1), 1–35.

Hwa Yun, B., Guo, J., Bellamri, M., Turesky, R.J., 2020. DNA adducts: formation, biological effects, and new biospecimens for mass spectrometric measurements in humans. Mass Spectrom. Rev. 39 (1–2), 55–82.

Ikwegbue, P.C., Masamba, P., Oyinloye, B.E., Kappo, A.P., 2017. Roles of heat shock proteins in apoptosis, oxidative stress, human inflammatory diseases, and cancer. Pharmaceuticals 11 (1), 2.

Jarabek, A.M., Pottenger, L.H., Andrews, L.S., Casciano, D., Embry, M.R., Kim, J.H., et al., 2009. Creating context for the use of DNA adduct data in cancer risk assessment: I. Data organization. Crit. Rev. Toxicol. 39 (8), 659–678.

Jayaram, S., Krishnamurthy, P.T., 2021. Role of microgliosis, oxidative stress and associated neuroinflammation in the pathogenesis of Parkinson's disease: the therapeutic role of Nrf2 activators. Neurochem. Int. 145, 105014.

Jennifer, M., Maciej, W., 2013. Nanoparticle technology as a double-edged sword: cytotoxic, genotoxic and epigenetic effects on living cells. J. Biomater. Nanobiotechnol. 4 (1), 53–63.

Kalyane, D., Choudhary, D., Polaka, S., Goykar, H., Karanwad, T., Rajpoot, K., Kumar Tekade, R., 2022. Reactive oxygen nano-generators for cancer therapy. Prog. Mater. Sci. 130, 100974.

Kawachi, I., Lassmann, H., 2017. Neurodegeneration in multiple sclerosis and neuromyelitis optica. J. Neurol. Neurosurg. Psychiatr. 88 (2), 137–145.

Kay, J., Thadhani, E., Samson, L., Engelward, B., 2019. Inflammation-induced DNA damage, mutations and cancer. DNA Repair 83, 102673.

Khan, M.F., Wang, G., 2018. Environmental agents, oxidative stress and autoimmunity. Curr. Opin. Toxicol. 7, 22–27.

Khanna, P., Ong, C., Bay, B.H., Baeg, G.H., 2015. Nanotoxicity: an interplay of oxidative stress, inflammation and cell death. Nanomaterials 5 (3), 1163–1180.

Kiely-Collins, H., Winter, G.E., Bernardes, G.J.L., 2021. The role of reversible and irreversible covalent chemistry in targeted protein degradation. Cell Chem. Biol. 28 (7), 952–968.

Knaapen, A.M., Borm, P.J., Albrecht, C., Schins, R.P., 2004. Inhaled particles and lung cancer. Part A: mechanisms. Int. J. Cancer 109 (6), 799–809.

Kohi, S., Macgregor-Das, A., Dbouk, M., Yoshida, T., Chuidian, M., Abe, T., et al., 2022. Alterations in the duodenal fluid microbiome of patients with pancreatic cancer. Clin. Gastroenterol. Hepatol. 20 (2), e196–e227.

Krisko, A., Radman, M., 2019. Protein damage, ageing and age-related diseases. Open Biol. 9 (3), 180249.

Krug, H.F., Wick, P., 2011. Nanotoxicology: an interdisciplinary challenge. Angew. Chem. Int. Ed. 50 (6), 1260–1278.

Kubben, N., Misteli, T., 2017. Shared molecular and cellular mechanisms of premature ageing and ageing-associated diseases. Nat. Rev. Mol. Cell Biol. 18 (10), 595–609.

Kumar, N., Raja, S., Van Houten, B., 2020. The involvement of nucleotide excision repair proteins in the removal of oxidative DNA damage. Nucleic Acids Res. 48 (20), 11227–11243.

Kumar, S., Sharma, A., 2019. Cadmium toxicity: effects on human reproduction and fertility. Rev. Environ. Health 34 (4), 327–338.

Kumari, R., Jat, P., 2021. Mechanisms of cellular senescence: cell cycle arrest and senescence associated secretory phenotype. Front. Cell Dev. Biol. 9, 645593.

Kumari, S., Dcunha, R., Sanghvi, S.P., Nayak, G., Kalthur, S.G., Raut, S.Y., et al., 2021. Organophosphorus pesticide quinalphos (Ekalux 25 EC) reduces sperm functional competence and decreases the fertilisation potential in Swiss albino mice. Andrologia e14115.

Kumawat, A., Raval, N., Reddy, G., Rajpoot, K., Tekade, R.K., 2020. Gene delivery to tackle diabetic nephropathy. In: Tekade, R.K. (Ed.), The Future of Pharmaceutical Product Development and Research, vol. 1. Academic Press, pp. 515–537.

Kuprash, D., Nedospasov, S.J.B., 2016. Molecular and cellular mechanisms of inflammation. Biochemistry (Moscow) 81 (11), 1237–1239.

Lan, Y.-Y., Chen, Y.-H., Liu, C., Tung, K.-L., Wu, Y.-T., Lin, S.-C., et al., 2021. Role of JNK activation in paclitaxel-induced apoptosis in human head and neck squamous cell carcinoma. Oncol. Lett. 22 (4), 1–11.

Lauschke, V.M., Zhou, Y., Ingelman-Sundberg, M., 2019. Novel genetic and epigenetic factors of importance for inter-individual differences in drug disposition, response and toxicity. Pharmacol. Therapeut. 197, 122–152.

Lawson, K.E., Dekle, J.K., Evans, M.N., Adamczyk, A.J., 2022. Deamidation reaction network mapping of pharmacologic and related proteins: impact of solvation dielectric on the degradation energetics of asparagine dipeptides. React. Chem. Eng. 7, 1525–1543.

Lewis, L., Crawford, G.E., Furey, T.S., Rusyn, I., 2017. Genetic and epigenetic determinants of inter-individual variability in responses to toxicants. Curr. Opin. Toxicol. 6, 50–59.

Li, K., van Delft, M.F., Dewson, G., 2021. Too much death can kill you: inhibiting intrinsic apoptosis to treat disease. EMBO J. 40 (14), e107341.

Li, P., Stetler, R.A., Leak, R.K., Shi, Y., Li, Y., Yu, W., et al., 2018. Oxidative stress and DNA damage after cerebral ischemia: potential therapeutic targets to repair the genome and improve stroke recovery. Neuropharmacology 134, 208–217.

Li, X., Liu, W., Sun, L., Aifantis, K.E., Yu, B., Fan, Y., et al., 2015. Effects of physicochemical properties of nanomaterials on their toxicity. J. Biomed. Mater. Res. Part A 103 (7), 2499–2507.

Li, Z., Yuan, W., Lin, Z., 2020. Functional roles in cell signaling of adaptor protein TRADD from a structural perspective. Comput. Struct. Biotechnol. J. 18, 2867–2876.

Liebelt, F., Schimmel, J., Verlaan–de Vries, M., Klemann, E., van Royen, M.E., van der Weegen, Y., et al., 2020. Transcription-coupled nucleotide excision repair is coordinated by ubiquitin and SUMO in response to ultraviolet irradiation. Nucleic Acids Res. 48 (1), 231–248.

Liu, J., Liu, C., Yue, J., 2021. Radiotherapy and the gut microbiome: facts and fiction. Radiat. Oncol. 16 (1), 9.

LoPachin, R.M., DeCaprio, A.P., 2005. Protein adduct formation as a molecular mechanism in neurotoxicity. Toxicol. Sci. 86 (2), 214–225.

Loreto, C., La Rocca, G., Anzalone, R., Caltabiano, R., Vespasiani, G., Castorina, S., et al., 2014. The role of intrinsic pathway in apoptosis activation and progression in Peyronie's disease. BioMed Res. Int. 2014, 616149.

Lyman, M., Lloyd, D.G., Ji, X., Vizcaychipi, M.P., Ma, D., 2014. Neuroinflammation: the role and consequences. Neurosci. Res. 79, 1–12.

Madreiter-Sokolowski, C.T., Sokolowski, A.A., Waldeck-Weiermair, M., Malli, R., Graier, W.F., 2018. Targeting mitochondria to counteract age-related cellular dysfunction. Genes 9 (3), 165.

Mao, P., Wyrick, J.J., 2019. Organization of DNA damage, excision repair, and mutagenesis in chromatin: a genomic perspective. DNA Repair 81, 102645.

Matouskova, K., Szabo, G.K., Daum, J., Fenton, S.E., Christiansen, S., Soto, A.M., et al., 2022. Best practices to quantify the impact of reproductive toxicants on development, function, and diseases of the rodent mammary gland. Reprod. Toxicol. 112, 51–67.

McCarthy, A.J., Coleman-Vaughan, C., McCarthy, J.V., 2017. Regulated intramembrane proteolysis: emergent role in cell signalling pathways. Biochem. Soc. Trans. 45 (6), 1185–1202.

McDonough, C.M., Xu, H.S., Guo, T.L., 2021. Toxicity of bisphenol analogues on the reproductive, nervous, and immune systems, and their relationships to gut microbiome and metabolism: insights from a multi-species comparison. Crit. Rev. Toxicol. 1–18.

Medina, C.B., Mehrotra, P., Arandjelovic, S., Perry, J.S.A., Guo, Y., Morioka, S., et al., 2020. Metabolites released from apoptotic cells act as tissue messengers. Nature 580 (7801), 130–135.

Miller, M.A., Zachary, J.F., 2017. Mechanisms and morphology of cellular injury, adaptation, and death. In: Pathologic Basis of Veterinary Disease. Elsevier, pp. 2–43.e19.

Misawa, M., Takahashi, J., 2011. Generation of reactive oxygen species induced by gold nanoparticles under X-ray and UV irradiations. Nanomed. Nanotechnol. Biol. Med. 7 (5), 604–614.

Mohideen, K., Sudhakar, U., Balakrishnan, T., Almasri, M.A., Al-Ahmari, M.M., Al Dira, H.S., et al., 2021. Malondialdehyde, an oxidative stress marker in oral squamous cell carcinoma—a systematic review and meta-analysis. Curr. Issues Mol. Biol. 43 (2), 1019–1035.

Myers, J.N., Harris, K.L., Rekhadevi, P.V., Pratap, S., Ramesh, A., 2021. Benzo (a) pyrene-induced cytotoxicity, cell proliferation, DNA damage, and altered gene expression profiles in HT-29 human colon cancer cells. Cell Biol. Toxicol. 37 (6), 891–913.

Naughton, S.X., Terry Jr., A.V., 2018. Neurotoxicity in acute and repeated organophosphate exposure. Toxicology 408, 101–112.

Oberdörster, G., 2010. Safety assessment for nanotechnology and nanomedicine: concepts of nanotoxicology. J. Intern. Med. 267 (1), 89–105.

Padiyar, A., Agrawal, O.P., Rajpoot, K., Tekade, R.K., 2020. Hydrotropy, mixed hydrotropy, and mixed solvency as trending concept for solubilization of lipophilic drugs. In: Tekade, R.K. (Ed.), The Future of Pharmaceutical Product Development and Research. Academic Press, pp. 145–178.

Pahwa, R., Goyal, A., Bansal, P., Jialal, I., 2020. Chronic Inflammation. StatPearls.

Parikh, K.J., Christian, J.R., Rajpoot, K., Tekade, R.K., 2022. Environmental and safety aspects of bionanotechnology. In: Pharmacokinetics and Toxicokinetic Considerations, vol. 2. Elsevier, pp. 605–650.

Park, J.-S., Davis, R.L., Sue, C.M., 2018a. Mitochondrial dysfunction in Parkinson's disease: new mechanistic insights and therapeutic perspectives. Curr. Neurol. Neurosci. Rep. 18 (5), 21.

Park, J.-S., Davis, R.L., Sue, C.M., 2018b. Mitochondrial dysfunction in Parkinson's disease: new mechanistic insights and therapeutic perspectives. Curr. Neurol. Neurosci. Rep. 18 (5), 1–11.

Park, J.S., Blair, N.F., Sue, C.M., 2015. The role of ATP13A2 in Parkinson's disease: clinical phenotypes and molecular mechanisms. Mov. Disord. 30 (6), 770–779.

Peters, J.M., Gonzalez, F.J., 2018. The evolution of carcinogenesis. Toxicol. Sci. 165 (2), 272–276.

Peterson, K., Palmer, B., Christensen, C., Bailey, S., Mizrachi, D., 2022. Constitutively active death receptor induces apoptosis in mammalian cells. Arch. Mol. Biol. Genet. 1 (1), 20–28.

Pineau, C., 2020. An Overview of Male Reproductive Toxicants: Facts and Opinions. Toxic Chemical and Biological Agents. Springer Netherlands, Dordrecht.

Pizzino, G., Irrera, N., Cucinotta, M., Pallio, G., Mannino, F., Arcoraci, V., et al., 2017. Oxidative stress: harms and benefits for human health. In: Oxidative Medicine and Cellular Longevity, vol 2017, p. 8416763.

Polaka, S., Desai, N., Kshirsagar, B., Rajpoot, K., Tekade, R.K., 2021a. Revamping the pharmacokinetics of poorly soluble drugs using different formulations. In: Tekade, R.K. (Ed.), Biopharmaceutics and Pharmacokinetics Considerations. Elsevier, pp. 387–413.

Polaka, S., Makwana, V., Vasdev, N., Sheth, A., Rajpoot, K., Sengupta, P., Tekade, R.K., 2022a. Engineering immunity via skin-directed drug delivery devices. J. Control. Release 345, 385–404.

Polaka, S., Rajpoot, K., Tekade, M., Sharma, M.C., Tekade, R.K., 2022b. Food–drug interactions and their implications on oral drug bioavailability. In: Pharmacokinetics and Toxicokinetic Considerations, vol. 2. Elsevier, pp. 263–289.

Polaka, S., Swetha, K.L., Dittakavi, S., Rajpoot, K., Tekade, R.K., 2021b. Bioanalytical method development and validation for establishing bioavailability and bioequivalence. In: Tekade, R.K. (Ed.), Biopharmaceutics and Pharmacokinetics Considerations. Elsevier, pp. 487–516.

Pope, C.N., Hester, K., 2020. Disruption of Extracellular Signaling. An Introduction to Interdisciplinary Toxicology. Elsevier, pp. 69–80.

Pope, C.N., Liu, J., 2020. An Introduction to Interdisciplinary Toxicology: From Molecules to Man. Academic Press.

Portt, L., Norman, G., Clapp, C., Greenwood, M., Greenwood, M.T., 2011. Anti-apoptosis and cell survival: a review. Biochim. Biophys. Acta Mol. Cell Res. 1813 (1), 238–259.

Przedborski, S., Vila, M., Jackson-Lewis, V., 2003. Series introduction: neurodegeneration: what is it and where are we? J. Clin. Invest. 111 (1), 3–10.

Qi, J., Wang, J., Gong, Z., Zhou, J.-M., 2017. Apoplastic ROS signaling in plant immunity. Curr. Opin. Plant Biol. 38, 92–100.

Quezada-Maldonado, E.M., Sánchez-Pérez, Y., Chirino, Y.I., García-Cuellar, C.M., 2021. Airborne particulate matter induces oxidative damage, DNA adduct formation and alterations in DNA repair pathways. Environ. Pollut. 287, 117313.

Rajalakshmi, T.R., AravindhaBabu, N., Shanmugam, K.T., Masthan, K.M.K., 2015. DNA adducts-chemical addons. J. Pharm. BioAllied Sci. 7 (Suppl. 1), S197–S199.

Rajani, C., Borisa, P., Karanwad, T., Borade, Y., Patel, V., Rajpoot, K., Tekade, R.K., 2020. Cancer-targeted chemotherapy: emerging role of the folate anchored dendrimer as drug delivery nanocarrier. In: Chauhan, A., Kulhari, H. (Eds.), Pharmaceutical Applications of Dendrimers. Elsevier, pp. 151–198.

Rajpoot, K., 2020. Nanotechnology-based targeting of neurodegenerative disorders: a promising tool for efficient delivery of neuromedicines. Curr. Drug Targets 21 (8), 819–836.

Rajpoot, K., Desai, N., Koppisetti, H., Tekade, M., Sharma, M.C., Behera, S.K., Tekade, R.K., 2022a. In silico methods for the prediction of drug toxicity. In: Pharmacokinetics and Toxicokinetic Considerations, vol. 2. Elsevier, pp. 357–383.

Rajpoot, K., Katare, P., Tekade, M., Sharma, M.C., Polaka, S., Sengupta, P., Tekade, R.K., 2022b. Toxicokinetic and toxicodynamic considerations in drug research. In: Pharmacokinetics and Toxicokinetic Considerations, vol. 2. Elsevier, pp. 751–776.

Rajpoot, K., Tekade, M., Sharma, M.C., Sreeharsha, N., Sharma, A., Tekade, R.K., 2020a. Recombinant blood products and therapeutic enzymes: an update. In: Tekade, R.K. (Ed.), The Future of Pharmaceutical Product Development and Research. Academic Press, pp. 447–482.

Rajpoot, K., Tekade, M., Sreeharsha, N., Sharma, M.C., Tekade, R.K., 2020b. Recent advancements in solubilization of hydrophobic drugs. In: Tekade, R.K. (Ed.), The Future of Pharmaceutical Product Development and Research. Academic Press, pp. 109–144.

Rajpoot, K., Tekade, R.K., Chatterjee, B., Sharma, M.C., Tekade, M., 2021a. Biopharmaceutical considerations in the pediatric and geriatric formulation development. In: Tekade, R.K. (Ed.), Biopharmaceutics and Pharmacokinetics Considerations, vol. 1. Elsevier, Academic Press, pp. 109–144.

Rajpoot, K., Tekade, R.K., Sharma, M.C., Safavi, M., Tekade, M., 2021b. Pharmacokinetics modeling in drug delivery. In: Tekade, R.K. (Ed.), Biopharmaceutics and Pharmacokinetics Considerations. Elsevier, Academic Press, pp. 279–334.

Rajpoot, K., Tekade, R.K., Sharma, M.C., Tekade, M., 2021c. Pharmacokinetics and biopharmaceutics: "a leader or attendant". In: Tekade, R.K. (Ed.), Biopharmaceutics and Pharmacokinetics Considerations. Elsevier, Academic Press, pp. 17–27.

Ranjan, A., Jindal, T., 2022. Enzymatic Targets of Organophosphates. Toxicology of Organophosphate Poisoning. Springer, pp. 45–66.

Rock, K.L., Kono, H., 2008. The inflammatory response to cell death. Annu. Rev. Pathol. 3, 99–126.

Sanchez, A.B., Garcia, C.C.M., Freitas, F.P., Batista, G.L., Lopes, F.S., Carvalho, V.H., et al., 2018. DNA adduct formation in the lungs and brain of rats exposed to low concentrations of [$^{13}C_2$]-acetaldehyde. Chem. Res. Toxicol. 31 (5), 332–339.

Schmidt, S.V., Krebs, W., Ulas, T., Xue, J., Baßler, K., Günther, P., et al., 2016. The transcriptional regulator network of human inflammatory macrophages is defined by open chromatin. Cell Res. 26 (2), 151–170.

Seo, K.-Y., Jelinsky, S.A., Loechler, E.L., 2000. Factors that influence the mutagenic patterns of DNA adducts from chemical carcinogens. Mutat. Res. Rev. Mutat. Res. 463 (3), 215–246.

Shete, M.B., Patil, T.S., Deshpande, A.S., Saraogi, G., Vasdev, N., Deshpande, M., et al., 2022. Current trends in theranostic nanomedicines. J. Drug Deliv. Sci. Technol. 71, 103280.

Shukla, S., Jadaun, A., Arora, V., Sinha, R.K., Biyani, N., Jain, V., 2015. In vitro toxicity assessment of chitosan oligosaccharide coated iron oxide nanoparticles. Toxicol. Rep. 2, 27–39.

Sifuentes-Franco, S., Padilla-Tejeda, D.E., Carrillo-Ibarra, S., Miranda-Diaz, A.G., 2018. Oxidative stress, apoptosis, and mitochondrial function in diabetic nephropathy. Internet J. Endocrinol. 2018, 1875870.

Singh, A.V., Laux, P., Luch, A., Sudrik, C., Wiehr, S., Wild, A.M., et al., 2019. Review of emerging concepts in nanotoxicology: opportunities and challenges for safer nanomaterial design. Toxicol. Mech. Methods 29 (5), 378–387.

Singh, N., Manshian, B., Jenkins, G.J., Griffiths, S.M., Williams, P.M., Maffeis, T.G., et al., 2009. NanoGenotoxicology: the DNA damaging potential of engineered nanomaterials. Biomaterials 30 (23–24), 3891–3914.

Stading, R., Gastelum, G., Chu, C., Jiang, W., Moorthy, B., 2021. Molecular mechanisms of pulmonary carcinogenesis by polycyclic aromatic hydrocarbons (PAHs): implications for human lung cancer. Semin. Cancer Biol. 76, 3–16.

Steller, J.G., Alberts, J.R., Ronca, A.E., 2018. Oxidative stress as cause, consequence, or biomarker of altered female reproduction and development in the space environment. Int. J. Mol. Sci. 19 (12), 3729.

Stevanović, M., Bračko, I., Milenković, M., Filipović, N., Nunić, J., Filipič, M., Uskoković, D.P., 2014. Multifunctional PLGA particles containing poly (l-glutamic acid)-capped silver nanoparticles and ascorbic acid with simultaneous antioxidative and prolonged antimicrobial activity. Acta Biomater. 10 (1), 151–162.

Sun, J., Peng, H., Alharbi, H.A., Jones, P.D., Giesy, J.P., Wiseman, S.B., 2017. Identification of chemicals that cause oxidative stress in oil sands process-affected water. Environ. Sci. Technol. 51 (15), 8773–8781.

Tambe, V., Desai, N., Rajpoot, K., Tekade, R.K., 2021a. "Organ-on-a-chip"-based physiologically relevant pharmacokinetic models. In: Tekade, R.K. (Ed.), Biopharmaceutics and Pharmacokinetics Considerations. Elsevier, pp. 643–673.

Tambe, V., Kathar, U., Raval, N., Rajpoot, K., Shilpi, S., Khatri, K., Tekade, R.K., 2021b. Positron emission tomography as a noninvasive tool in pharmacokinetic studies. In: Tekade, R.K. (Ed.), Biopharmaceutics and Pharmacokinetics Considerations. Elsevier, Academic Press, pp. 617–641.

Tambe, V., Pande, S., Gadeval, A., Rajpoot, K., Raval, N., Tekade, R.K., 2021c. Microdialysis: an emerging technique for pharmacokinetic–pharmacodynamic profiling. In: Tekade, R.K. (Ed.), Biopharmaceutics and Pharmacokinetics Considerations. Elsevier, pp. 601–616.

Tambe, V., Sirsat, B., Rajpoot, K., Gadeval, A., Tekade, R.K., 2021d. Pharmacogenomics and drug metabolism. In: Tekade, R.K. (Ed.), Biopharmaceutics and Pharmacokinetics Considerations, vol. 1. Elsevier, Academic Press, pp. 355–385.

Tekade, M., Koppisetti, H., Sharma, M.C., Rajpoot, K., Sengupta, P., Kumar, M., Tekade, R.K., 2022. Understanding the concept of signal toxicity and its implications on human health. In: Pharmacokinetics and Toxicokinetic Considerations, vol. 2. Elsevier, pp. 99–116.

Tiwari, A., Joshi, M., Salvi, N., Gupta, D., Gandhi, S., Rajpoot, K., Tekade, R.K., 2022. Toxicity of pharmaceutical azo dyes. In: Pharmacokinetics and Toxicokinetic Considerations, vol. 2. Elsevier, pp. 569–603.

Tomasetti, C., Li, L., Vogelstein, B., 2017. Stem cell divisions, somatic mutations, cancer etiology, and cancer prevention. Science (New York, N.Y.) 355 (6331), 1330–1334.

Topkaya, S.N., Ozyurt, V.H., Cetin, A.E., Otles, S., 2018. Nitration of tyrosine and its effect on DNA hybridization. Biosens. Bioelectron. 102, 464–469.

Tu, P., Chi, L., Bodnar, W., Zhang, Z., Gao, B., Bian, X., et al., 2020. Gut microbiome toxicity: connecting the environment and gut microbiome-associated diseases. Toxics 8 (1).

Turkez, H., Arslan, M.E., Ozdemir, O., 2017. Genotoxicity testing: progress and prospects for the next decade. Expert Opin. Drug Metabol. Toxicol. 13 (10), 1089–1098.

Valizadeh, A., Majidinia, M., Samadi-Kafil, H., Yousefi, M., Yousefi, B., 2019. The roles of signaling pathways in liver repair and regeneration. J. Cell. Physiol. 234 (9), 14966–14974.

Valle, M.L., Dworshak, J., Sharma, A., Ibrahim, A.S., Al-Shabrawey, M., Sharma, S., 2019. Inhibition of interleukin-6 trans-signaling prevents inflammation and endothelial barrier disruption in retinal endothelial cells. Exp. Eye Res. 178, 27–36.

Vasdev, N., Rajpoot, K., Tekade, R.K., 2021. Molecular mechanisms of circadian rhythm and its influence on the pharmacokinetics of drugs. In: Tekade, R.K. (Ed.), Biopharmaceutics and Pharmacokinetics Considerations. Elsevier, Academic Press, pp. 415–449.

Vingerhoets, A., 2001. An introduction to behavioral endocrinology (2nd ed.), Edited by R.J. Nelson, Sinauer Associates, Sunderland MA, 2000. ISBN: 0-87893-616-5 (pkb.). 724 pp. Biol. Psychol. 56 (2), 171–172.

Wagener-Ryczek, S., Merkelbach-Bruse, S., Siemanowski, J., 2021. Biomarkers for homologous recombination deficiency in cancer. J. Personalized Med. 11 (7), 612.

West, A.P., 2017. Mitochondrial dysfunction as a trigger of innate immune responses and inflammation. Toxicology 391, 54–63.

Worek, F., Jenner, J., Thiermann, H., 2016. Chemical Warfare Toxicology: Volume 1: Fundamental Aspects. Royal Society of Chemistry.

Yang, S., Liu, J.D.H., Diem, M., Wesseling, S., Vervoort, J., Oostenbrink, C., Rietjens, I.M.C.M., 2020. Molecular dynamics and in vitro quantification of safrole DNA adducts reveal DNA adduct persistence due to limited DNA distortion resulting in inefficient repair. Chem. Res. Toxicol. 33 (9), 2298–2309.

Yang, X., Bartlett, M.G., 2016. Identification of protein adduction using mass spectrometry: protein adducts as biomarkers and predictors of toxicity mechanisms. Rapid Commun. Mass Spectrom. 30 (5), 652–664.

Yimit, A., Adebali, O., Sancar, A., Jiang, Y., 2019. Differential damage and repair of DNA-adducts induced by anticancer drug cisplatin across mouse organs. Nat. Commun. 10 (1), 1–11.

Yokoyama, C., Sueyoshi, Y., Ema, M., Mori, Y., Takaishi, K., Hisatomi, H., 2017. Induction of oxidative stress by anticancer drugs in the presence and absence of cells. Oncol. Lett. 14 (5), 6066–6070.

Yu, C.-H., Pal, L.R., Moult, J., 2016. Consensus genome-wide expression quantitative trait loci and their relationship with human complex trait disease. OMICS J. Integr. Biol. 20 (7), 400–414.

Zamaraev, A.V., Zhivotovsky, B., Kopeina, G.S., 2020. Viral infections: negative regulators of apoptosis and oncogenic factors. Biochemistry (Moscow) 85 (10), 1191–1201.

Zanon, P.R.A., Yu, F., Musacchio, P., Lewald, L., Zollo, M., Krauskopf, K., et al., 2021. Profiling the Proteome-Wide Selectivity of Diverse Electrophiles, p. 10.

Zhao, Z., Xia, J., 2019. Computational approaches for modeling signal transduction networks. In: Encyclopedia of Bioinformatics and Computational Biology. Elsevier, pp. 856–863.

Zhou, Q., Xi, S., 2018. A review on arsenic carcinogenesis: epidemiology, metabolism, genotoxicity and epigenetic changes. Regul. Toxicol. Pharmacol. 99, 78–88.

Zhu, S., Zhang, T., Wang, Y., Zhou, X., Wang, S., Wang, Z., 2021. Meta-analysis and experimental validation identified atrazine as a toxicant in the male reproductive system. Environ. Sci. Pollut. Control Ser. 28 (28), 37482–37497.

CHAPTER

8

Toxicant-induced injury and tissue repair

Tanisha Gupta[1], *Shyam Gomte*[1], *Krutika H. Pardeshi*[2], *Prashant L. Pingale*[3], *Muktika Tekade*[4], *Manoj Kumar*[5] *and Rakesh Kumar Tekade*[1]

[1]National Institute of Pharmaceutical Education and Research (NIPER)- Ahmedabad, An Institute of National Importance, Government of India, Department of Pharmaceuticals, Ministry of Chemicals and Fertilizers, Palaj, Gandhinagar, Gujarat, India; [2]Department of Pharmaceutics, School of Pharmaceutical Sciences, Sandip University, Nashik, Maharashtra, India; [3]Department of Pharmaceutics, GES's Sir Dr. M. S. Gosavi College of Pharmaceutical Education and Research, Nashik, Maharashtra, India; [4]School of Pharmacy, Devi Ahilya Vishwavidyalaya, Indore, Madhya Pradesh, India; [5]Department of Radiology, Stanford University, Stanford, CA, United States

8.1 Introduction

Toxicants can exert an adverse effect at cellular and molecular levels triggering significant damage and repair response. These damages or dysfunctions can be reversible or irreversible, causing either a recovery process or cell death. Toxicokinetics and toxicodynamics evaluations are broadly performed to understand the toxic and beneficial effects of a chemical substance or a pharmacological agent within the body. Pharmacological agents could have side effects with toxicity. When a drug is approved as a product, its new chemical entities must comply with safety and regulatory guidelines meeting the defined parameters of absorption, distribution, metabolism, and excretion (ADME) (Mehendale, 2005). When a toxin substance is absorbed and distributed throughout the body, its metabolization produces water-soluble metabolites to be eliminated from the body. These metabolized toxins may further generate reactive metabolites and free radicals that can adversely interact with cellular macromolecules causing tissue and functional damage or inducing injuries at cellular, tissue, and organ levels (Hayes and Kruger, 2014).

Essentials of Pharmatoxicology in Drug Research, Volume 1
https://doi.org/10.1016/B978-0-443-15840-7.00013-0

At the molecular level, toxins can exhibit a wide range of adverse effects with significant health consequences. These toxic injuries could change the normal functioning of entire organs, impacting the body's overall functions and wellness. The production of nanomedicine is growing rapidly and is evident by growing number of clinial and preclinical investigations (Youngren et al., 2013; Tekade and Chougule, 2013). Given this rise, there is a need for new testing standards to assess the toxicological impact and hazards to human health and the environment (Gadekar et al., 2021; Gorain et al., 2016; Muniswamy et al., 2019; Prajapati et al., 2009). Toxicant-induced injuries can be repairable or unrepairable depending on the extent of damage at the cellular, molecular, and organ level. Also, the outcomes of toxic exposure depend upon the individual's health status and the ability of organs, cells, and tissues to resist the toxin effects via adaptation and/or repair mechanisms (van Benthem, 2021).

The liver is the primary site of metabolism. It has a vital functional role in the digestion of food, storing energy, and releasing carbohydrates called glycan. The liver is divided into several separate lobes constructed by parenchyma cells called hepatocytes. These cells play pivotal roles in metabolism, body detoxification, and protein synthesis. Hepatocytes are also the storehouse of cytosolic and microsomal drug-metabolizing enzymes. Therefore, toxicant-induced injuries in liver cells could severely impair liver functions. These damages are believed to be proportional to the metabolism mediated by drug metabolizing enzymes (DME) producing reactive chemical metabolites (Hayes and Kruger, 2014; Mehendale, 2005).

Moreover, some nonlethal cellular damage may result in cellular degeneration and impaired routine maintenance processes. Injured hepatocytes could accumulate lipids, water, glycogen, metabolic waste products, or pigments leading to inflammation and immune reactions. Lipid accumulation in liver cells leads to hepatic lipidosis or steatosis, a harmful disease state of the liver that is often observed in patients overconsuming alcohol. Cell degeneration can often be reversed if the triggering cause is eliminated; however, cell death occurs when the cell's self-repair capacity is severely compromised (van Benthem, 2021).

Tissue repair is a regenerative and systematic recovery process after an injury. All injured tissues undergo the basic repair steps of removing and replacing dead and missing cells with regenerating healthy ones. Regeneration and replacement are two distinct modes of tissue repair. Tissue regeneration revitalizes the injured tissue to its original functional state. The depositing scar tissue fills structural gaps. Alternatively, replacement occurs when regeneration is impossible; it involves depositing connective tissue to replace irreversibly damaged tissues. Sometimes, repair primarily consists of regeneration, and how much regeneration is possible is determined by two factors: (i) the extent of damage to the tissue "scaffolding" and (ii) the tissue type and where the injury occurs. If only the organ parenchymal cells get damaged, but the fundamental scaffolding of the extracellular matrix remains intact, full regeneration is feasible. Complete regeneration is impossible if the scaffolding around which the cells are arranged is damaged (Krafts, 2014).

This chapter discusses toxicant-induced injury, its complication, and its mechanism. Here we cover the factor affecting the tissue repair process, the role of the metabolic and excretory system, and the extracellular matrix and protein's role in tissue repair after toxicant-induced injury.

8.2 Toxicant-induced injuries and complications

Toxicants interact with diverse targets in cells after entering living organisms to exert their inhibitory or activating harmful effects. Such interactions disrupt cellular homeostasis, and cells may adapt, survive, or perish due to a series of molecular and cellular incidents, depending on the time and extent of exposure (Pope, 2020). Numerous interactions between the organism and the invasive toxin result in a toxic effect as part of the cellular processes that lead to the toxicities manifestation. When a toxin interacts with its targets, it interacts with intrinsic target molecules or modifies the environment, causing cell structure and function perturbations that activate repair mechanisms at the cellular, molecular, or tissue levels. Toxicity occurs when the interferences caused by the toxicant surpass the repair capacity and when the repair process has become dysfunctional. Cancer, fibrosis, and tissue necrosis are examples of toxicity induced by chemicals (Gregus, 2010). Some of the symptoms of toxicant-induced injury are teratogenicity, mutagenicity, acute respiratory distress syndrome, carcinogenicity, breath shortness, headache, rashes, vision loss, vomiting, etc. The liver and kidney are especially susceptible to the effects of systemically absorbed toxins because they have prominent role in metabolism and excretion. Based on this, two main kinds of toxicant-induced injury are observed: toxic hepatic injury and toxic renal injury (van Benthem, 2021).

Toxicant-induced injuries have been demonstrated by earlier studies where damage extends and proliferate even after the primary toxicant metabolites are excreted from the body (Chilakapati et al., 2007a, 2007b; Mangipudy et al., 1995). One good example is the hepatotoxicant such as thioacetamide (half-life 2.5 h) which exhibited hepatotoxic properties in rats. Initially, low to moderate doses resulted in hepatic injury and necrosis. While the rats recovered well in 4 days, the experimental group with 12 times increase in the dose showed significant growth in the hepatic injury, and all the rats died due to hepatic toxicity. Further evaluation showed plasma ALT peaked after 24 h, confirming that hepatic injuries may result in extended proliferation after thioacetamide metabolites are excreted from the body (Chilakapati et al., 2007b; Mangipudy et al., 1996; Shankar et al., 2003).

Commonly used analgesics such as acetaminophen, widely known as paracetamol, have antipyretic action. The higher doses of acetaminophen and its metabolites, N-acetyl-para-aminoquinone (NAPQ1), lead to the depletion of glutathione (GSH) levels and could result in liver toxicity, liver necrosis, and ultimately death of an individual. The half-life of acetaminophen in mice is nearly 1 h, and it is believed that after 8 h, no acetaminophen is present in the body. Moreover, the injury initiated by acetaminophen and its metabolites extending is unknown and needs to be addressed (Mangipudy et al., 1995, 1996; Shankar et al., 2003). Hepatotoxicity is more common in diabetic patients taking pharmacological therapy. Its causes and predisposing factors (Wang et al., 2007) are not well understood. Renal injury from toxicants also results in significant morbidity and delays the process of drug development (Pianta et al., 2013).

In other studies, Salama et al. studied the result of L-carnitine on short-term lung injury caused by toxicants like potassium dichromate in rats. The initiation of the Nrf2/HO-1 pathway of signaling maintains antioxidant stress on cells. It exhibits cytoprotective and anti-inflammatory functions toward acute lung injury. The concentration of L-carnitine was measured by the levels of malondialdehyde (MDA) and glutathione (GSH). Additionally, lung contents were evaluated, including protein kinase B (AKT), glutathione cysteine ligase modifier subunit (GCLM), transforming growth factor β1 (TGFβ1), nuclear factor erythroid-2 related factor 2 (Nrf2), heme oxygenase-1 (HO-1), NADPH quinone oxidoreductase 1 enzyme (NQO1), and Kelch-like ECH-associated protein 1 (Keap1). It was observed that L-carnitine-induced rats showed enhanced levels of AKT, Nrf2, GSH, and their ideal genes, along with depletion in the levels of TGFβ1 and MDA. Interestingly, L-carnitine reduces the goblet cells, alveolar walls were destroyed, and blood cells become clogged in the tissue of the lungs initiated by potassium dichromate toxicant. L-carnitine positively reduced acute lung injury caused by toxic potassium dichromate (Salama et al., 2021).

8.3 Mechanisms of toxicant-induced injury

Each toxicant has a specific chemical property that determines its action in interacting with a particular cell receptor or site at the organ level. For the specific pharmacological activity, a drug molecule must be absorbed and distributed efficiently into the bloodstream for its site of action, followed by its biotransformation and excretion from the body (Gupta, 2016). Toxicity-induced injury has been well studied and observed for the dose-response phenomenon (Fig. 8.1). The recovery from toxicant-induced injury mainly through tissue repair mechanisms influenced by various factors such as strain or species, age, caloric restriction, nutrition, and disease condition (Mehendale, 2005). The mechanism and predisposing factors related to toxicant-induced liver toxicity in diabetic individuals are unclear. These mechanisms of toxicant-induced injury mainly include three processes: (a) Inflammatory cells present at the injured site used to mediate the spread of injury, (b) Oxidative stress and damage from free radicals, and (c) Discharge of lysosomal and cytosolic degradative enzymes from dead cells that target and kill the surrounding cell (Kemp et al., 2008; Poli, 1993). These processes are further discussed in detail below.

8.3.1 Inflammation and development of injury

Inflammation is the primary reaction to injuries and infection. Inflammation is a signal for immune cell activation and initiating the tissue repair process. Cytokines and inflammatory cells recruited at the injury site can also damage normal cells (Jaeschke and Smith, 1997). Later, the macrophages recruited at the site of injury secrete several inflammatory mediators like interleukin-8 (IL-8), interleukin-1 (IL-1), and tissue necrosis factor α (TNF-α), initiating and inducing the monocytes, neutrophils at the injury site. These inflammatory cells also release several mediators, such as bioactive lipids, cytokines, reactive oxygen and nitrogen species, and hydrolytic enzymes that contribute to pathogenesis and tissue injury (Blazka et al., 1995). Interestingly, it has been seen that cytokine antagonist helps to stop tissue regeneration and result in tissue injury in the intestines, lungs, liver, heart, kidney, etc. In addition, neutrophils and kupffer cells at the liver injury site damage the neighboring normal cells. However, it was observed that the propagation of tissue injury is not driven by inflammatory cells (Ju et al., 2002).

8.3.2 Free radicals in toxicant-induced tissue injury

Free radicals contribute to the development and pathophysiology of toxic liver injury and have received much attention recently (Poli et al., 1987; Freeman and Crapo, 1982). Free radicals such as hydroxyl radicals, superoxide anion, oxides of N_2, H_2O_2, and peroxynitrites are generated during oxidative stress conditions. Moreover, free radical generation is capable of beginning tissue injury. However, the function of free radicals in the development of tissue

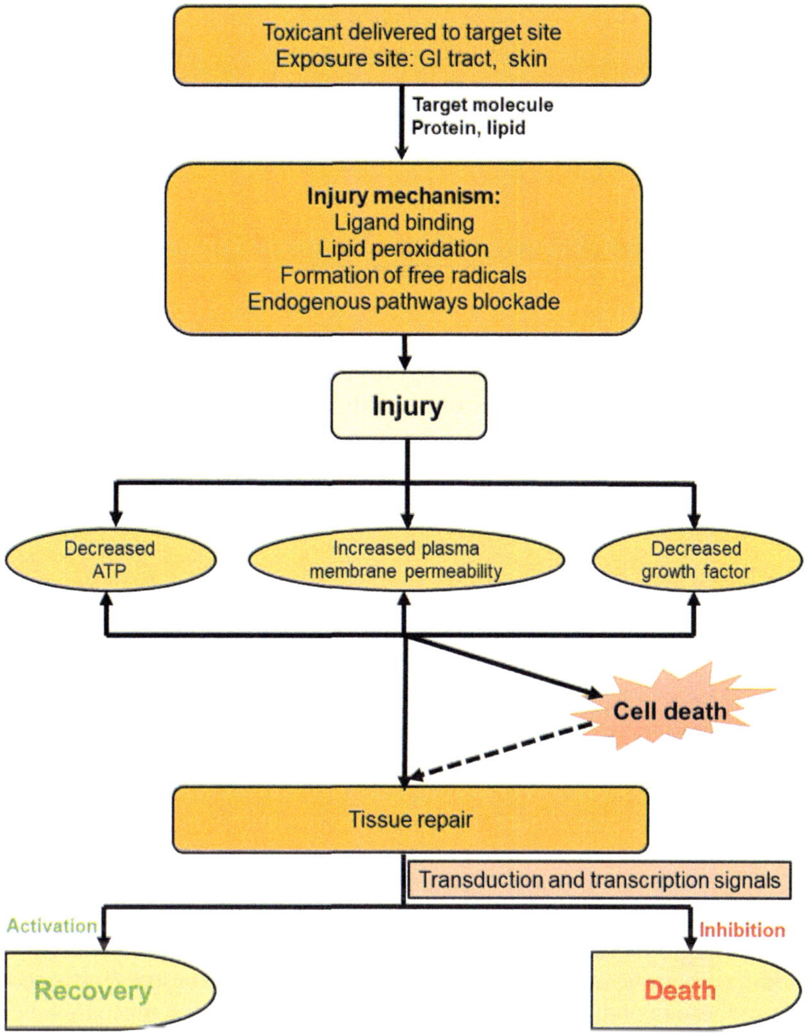

FIGURE 8.1 Mechanism of toxicant-induced injury.

injury is still unknown. The propagation of tissue injuries by lipid peroxidation is related to the free-radical theory (Kellogg and Fridovich, 1975). However, its role in the development of damage is still obscure. Initially, it was seen that free radical generation intensifies the tissue injury; however, the cause of this injury development is not shown yet (Mehendale, 2012).

8.3.3 Death proteins and injury development

Death protein function in injury development and progression is a less studied mechanism. It mainly involves the discharge of hydrolytic enzymes from the dead cells into the ECM of a calcium-rich (Ca+) environment. This mechanism also destroys the surrounding normal cells (Mehendale, 2012). The enzymes such as phospholipases, proteases, lysosomal enzymes, and endonucleases are collectively known as death proteins. Death proteins are usually pathognomic in nature, meaning they may be inidcative of certain disease conditions that may be leading to the death of cells. However, the exact mechanism of death proteins in tissue injury development remains unclear and not well explored.

8.4 Factors influencing tissue repair

The tissue repair process is cyclic and self-propagative based on the molecular signals at the injury sites. The molecular signals and tissue recovery rates could be impacted by age, species, strain, caloric restriction, disease condition, nutrition, etc. When estimating the risk of toxicant exposure in the context of public health, a wide range of responses could be expected based on these factors.

These elements influence recovery and response and could explain the wide range of interindividual variability in drug and toxicant responses. Some of the factors are discussed below:

8.4.1 Aging

Age is a vital factor in tissue repair, and aging is usually stimulated by toxicant-induced tissue injury. The population of people over 60 is expanding quicker than any other age group, and aging is a risk factor for the slow healing of wounds and tissue repair. Moreover, animal investigation and clinical investigations revealed aging delay wound healing process. It is widely accepted that aging slows down the wound healing mechanism in healthy older persons, but not an actual deterioration in healing quality (Guo and Dipietro, 2010). Compared to adults, newborn animals can mount faster and have more efficient tissue regeneration throughout the early stages of development (Mehendale, 2005). This has been well examined in neonates and 2-month-old young adults with CCl_4 and chlordecone + CCl_4-amped hepatic damage in Sprague–Dawley rats (Dalu et al., 1995a, 1995b; Dalu and Mehendale, 1996).

In a rat study using 2-month-old young adult rats, the neonates were resistant to CCl_4 and CD + CCl_4-induced hepatic injury. The research demonstrated that the continued hepatocyte multiplication in these neonatal rats with developing livers was the mechanism causing such resistance. These mechanisms and molecular signals underlying this improved tissue repair in elderly rats are being investigated. Similarly, older mice exhibit delayed angiogenesis, collagen synthesis, and re-epithelialization compared to young mice. Moreover, in the elders, delayed wound healing is linked to a different response of inflammation, such as in the wound area delayed T-cell infiltration, changes in the synthesis of chemokines, and reduction in phagocytic activity of macrophages (Swift et al., 2001). Several treatments have been investigated to minimize the age-related deterioration of healing.

8.4.2 Species or strain

The species or strain also affects the tissue repair mechanism. The LD50 value of carbon tetrachloride (CCL_4) as a toxicant was examined in the Sprague–Dawley rat and Mongolian gerbils. It was seen that the LD50 value was 35 times less in gerbils than in rats. The toxicant CCL_4-induced injury in gerbils was more significant since the tissue repair mechanism was very slow. Gerbils are also exceptionally resistant to CCl_4 toxicity when exacerbated by chlordecone (Cai and Mehendale, 1990, 1991). However, the tissue repair mechanism in rats was quicker than in Mongolian gerbils. Hence, the species or strains could affect tissue repair by slowing or fastening the repair process (Mehendale, 2005).

8.4.3 Nutrition

Nutritional elements like lipids, proteins, and carbohydrates influence the toxicant-induced tissue injury and its repair process. Numerous studies have shown that modifying the tissue repair response by modulating nutritional variables can directly affect the eventual result of toxicity. For example, the CYP450-mediated metabolism of thioacetamide was unaffected by glucose loading, but the compensatory tissue repair response was significantly reduced (Chanda et al., 1995). Moreover, malnutrition or certain dietary deficiencies can substantially affect the healing of wounds during trauma or surgery. Tissue repair is influenced by protein, vitamins, fat, energy, and mineral metabolism.

8.4.3.1 Amino acids, proteins, and carbohydrates

Glucose is the primary fuel source for producing ATP, which gives energy for forming new tissues and angiogenesis (Shepherd, 2003). To avoid the depletion of protein substrates and other amino acids, glucose must be used as a precursor for the synthesis of ATP (Arnold and Barbul, 2006). Similarly, proteins are vital nutritional factors for routine wound healing. Fibroblast proliferation, capillary formation, collagen synthesis, proteoglycan synthesis, and wound remodeling is protein deficit that can be hampered. Collagen is the most widely found protein in connective tissue, and it is made chiefly of hydroxyproline, glycine, and proline.

Moreover, arginine is the semi-essential category of amino acids necessary during rapid growth and extreme stress on the body's defense mechanisms. However, the synthesis of proline requires arginine as a precursor. Enough arginine levels are necessary for collagen deposition, wound contraction, and angiogenesis (Shepherd, 2003). Like arginine, glutamine is the most seen amino acid in plasma and a primary cell source of metabolic energy that proliferate quickly, such as lymphocytes, fibroblasts, epithelial cells, and macrophages. After major surgery, trauma, or sepsis, glutamine levels in the blood drop, and this amino acid supplement improves the balance of nitrogen and reduces immunosuppression (Guo and Dipietro, 2010).

8.4.3.2 Vitamins and trace elements

The various types of vitamins, like vitamins C and E, have antioxidant and anti-inflammatory activity. Ascorbic acid plays multiple functions in the healing of the wound. However, vitamin C deficiency has several consequences for tissue repair. Ascorbic acid deficiency has been associated with reduced collagen production and proliferation of fibroblast, angiogenesis reduction, and enhanced capillary fragility, all of which have been connected to impaired healing. Similarly, vitamin E is anti-inflammatory and has been linked to reducing excessive scar tissue production in chronic wounds. Moreover, the deficiency of vitamin A results in impaired tissue repair and wound healing. The antioxidant activity, enhanced proliferation of fibroblast, alteration of cellular differentiation and proliferation, enhanced hyaluronate and collagen production, and reduced MMP-modified extracellular matrix breakdown are all biological features of vitamin A (Campos et al., 2008).

8.4.3.3 Fatty acids

Lipids are also helpful in the process of tissue repair and wound healing. Lipids are given to postoperative or severely ill patients as a dietary supplement to help them fulfill their energy needs and provide essential structural blocks for wound healing and tissue regeneration. Omega-3 fatty acids such as docosahexaenoic acid and eicosapentaenoic acid found in fish oil have long been recommended for their health advantages. Pro-inflammatory cytokine synthesis, gene expression, metabolism of the cell, and wound site angiogenesis are all affected by omega-3 fatty acids (McDaniel et al., 2008; Shingel et al., 2008; Arnold and Barbul, 2006).

8.4.4 Advancement of wound

Healing wounds is a biological mechanism in the human body and can be attained by four means: hemostasis, inflammation, proliferation, and remodeling. Wounds that do not heal properly, such as delayed chronic and acute wounds, have not progressed through the regular stages of recovery. Due to a delayed, partial, or disorganized healing process, such wounds usually develop pathologic inflammation. Many factors influence the healing process, which includes local and systemic factors. The local factors include infection and oxygenation, and systemic factors include age, stress, gender, disease condition, alcoholism, smoking, medication, and nutrition. Moreover, the wound-healing process involves macrophages, neutrophils, keratinocytes, lymphocytes, endothelial cells, and fibroblasts. In any particular phase of healing, single or several elements may play a role, assisting in the healing process's overall outcome (Gosain and DiPietro, 2004). For example, following a skin injury, the exposed subendothelium, tissue factor, and collagen initiate aggregation of platelets, leading to degranulation and the release of growth factors and chemokines to generate the clot. In total, above procedures will result in successful clot hemostasis. In addition, macrophages are innate immune cells that eat microorganisms through the process called phagocytosis. The hemostasis and inflammatory phases can take up to 72 h to complete. The subsequent proliferative phase is marked by many cell types and a large amount of connective tissue. Keratinocytes, fibroblasts, and endothelial cells are all present in the wound. The ECM matrix, including collagen, elastin, proteoglycans, and hyaluronic acid, creates granulation tissue to restore the initially formed clot. The final stage of wound healing is the remodeling of the wound, which requires a balance of cell death and new cell creation (Lindley et al., 2016; Gauglitz et al., 2011; Berman et al., 2017; Su et al., 2010).

8.4.5 Ailment condition

Usually, it has been observed that an ailment condition affects the normal tissue repair process and delays the tissue repair process. Some diseases include cancer, cardiovascular diseases, diabetes mellitus, stress, and obesity, in which the wound-healing process is compromised. Individuals who have diabetes showed a significant impairment in repairing acute wounds. The secondary issues include kidney and cardiovascular difficulties and poor wound healing. Prolonged hypoxia, driven by both a lack of perfusion and a scarcity of angiogenesis, is harmful to wound healing.

Similarly, obesity increases the threat of various disorders, including diabetes, coronary heart disease, cancer, hypertension, stroke, respiratory issues, sleep apnea, and poor wound healing. The infection of wounds, hematoma, seroma development, dehiscence, venous ulcers, and pressure ulcers are common wound problems in obese people. The treatment of thioacetamide (300 mg/kg) was given in streptozotocin-induced type-I diabetes in rats. Interestingly, it was found that it significantly stops the tissue repair mechanism and results in 100% mortality (Wang et al., 2000a, 2000b). Furthermore, the diabetes-induced rats have more liver damage, partially due to increased thioacetamide-bioactivation enzymes CYP2E1 and CYP2E2 (Wang et al., 2001). However, a specific inhibitor of CYP2E1, diallyl sulfide (DAS), cannot protect diabetic rats from thioacetamide-induced liver damage and mortality. Thus, it can be said that diabetic individuals are significantly vulnerable to toxicant-induced hepatic injury because of the inhibition of the tissue repair mechanism (Mehendale, 2005; Guo and Dipietro, 2010).

8.5 Role of metabolic and excretory systems in toxicant-induced injury and tissue repair

8.5.1 Liver

The liver is the largest organ in the adult human body, weighing about 1.5 kg (2.5% of body weight). Many hazardous chemicals enter the body by circulation and transport to the liver following absorption. As a result, the liver is the first organ to come into contact with ingested chemicals, which are highly available in blood in concentrated form. As a primary site of metabolism, liver consists of various metabolizing enzymes that maintain nutritional homeostasis and promote xenobiotic metabolism and excretion; nuclear receptors that regulate enzyme production are also present in the liver (Kester, 2014). Different hepatic cells act as a reservoir of microsomal and cytosolic drug-metabolizing enzymes; therefore, the liver could become a main target for chemical-induced damage. The amount of liver damage caused by the chemical equals the number of enzyme-mediated metabolites (Boll et al., 2001; Plaa et al., 2014). Since ancient times, the amazing ability of the liver to regenerate after medical surgery or cell damage has been well known (Michalopoulos, 2007). Regeneration of the liver has been studied in various models, like rodents (Fausto et al., 1995). Studies have discovered a complex signaling pathways network regulated by chemokines, cytokines, growth regulators, and hormones that promotes liver regeneration after mechanical ablation of the liver (Fausto et al., 1995). Liver is particularly susceptible to chemical attacks.

Hepatotoxic substances include a variety of metals, vitamins, bacteria, plant, fungal, and animal toxins, as well as hundreds of synthetic medicines and compounds. Most hepatotoxic components selectively harm any liver cell as they are arranged in a distinctive zonal arrangement. Two-stage toxic hepatic damage proceeds, with Stage I representing the toxic damage and Stage II showing the opposing reactions—the balance between the advancement of injury and the healing of damage determines the ultimate result. A cascade of distress signals leads to toxic damage, causing healthy cells in the area to proliferate and replace dead cells. The degree of the damage, as well as the time and dose correlations, determines whether the injury recovers or progresses.

8.5.1.1 Stage I: toxic injury

Toxicity may harm cells in three ways: (1) direct cell damage, (2) mitochondria dysfunction, and (3) activating an autoimmune response. Furthermore, certain drugs and their metabolites directly bind to particular receptors, which triggers and decreases the expression of signal transduction activated due to receptors, which can have either positive or adverse effects. The most common mechanism of hepatotoxicity is harm caused by toxic metabolites generated by the cytochrome P450 system. Strong electrophiles, including nucleic acid, protein, and low-molecular-weight nucleophiles like glutathione, can form covalent bonds with stable and essential nucleophilic macromolecules like nucleic acids and proteins. Glutathione shortage can result in oxidative stress, which can result in protein, nucleotide, and lipoprotein damage, as well as lipid peroxidation.

8.5.1.2 Stage II: Injury repair or injury progression

Tissue healing is a continuous process that keeps an injury from becoming fatal by preventing it from advancing to organ dysfunction. It is impacted by species, breed, age, and other personal characteristics. According to research, the dose-dependent tissue healing process increases until a dosage threshold is achieved. Tissue repair is accelerated at low-to-moderate dosages, but as the dose rises, the start is delayed. As a result, at dosages beyond a specific limit, the tissue repair response is insufficient and too late to prevent further damage (Kester, 2014).

Drug and host factors are the two major players in drug-induced liver injury (DILI), which may communicate in a multidimensional way at various functional pathways, determining person susceptibility, clinical outcome, and phenotype. Mechanisms engaged in the onset of cellular damage are probably drug-specific. They may result from the interaction between drug-specific properties and host-specific actions. Host factors dominate host reactions to the injury insult (i.e., inflammation, immune response, repair, and tissue injury) once it has been established that damage has occurred. Host factors like age, genetics, gender, lifestyles, comedication and disease conditions are likely to influence these responses (Fig. 8.2) (Chen et al., 2015).

8.5.2 Kidney

Acute kidney injury (AKI) is a broad term referring to various medical conditions. This illness spectrum covers all renal problems, from mild dysfunction to dialysis. AKI is caused by ischemia and toxins, affecting 5%–35% of all surgical patients, with a 2-5-fold increase in mortality risk (Kanbay et al., 2010).

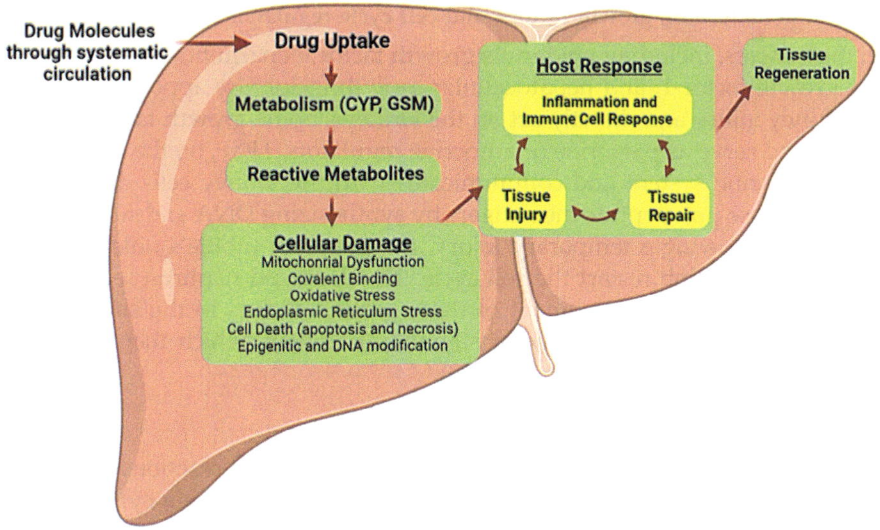

FIGURE 8.2 Role of the liver in toxicant-induced injury and tissue regeneration.

8.5.2.1 Renal tissue injury classification

8.5.2.1.1 Primary injury

Ischemia and cytotoxic damage are the primary causes of renal injury. Numerous causes of kidney injury include spinal Bifida, immune deficiency, obstructive conditions, and contagious conditions (including small vessel vasculitis, which are most influential in kidney biology because of the enormous number of small vessels present, particularly blood vessels of glomerular blood). Proteinuria, hematuria, and glomerulopathy are all symptoms of epithelial cell damage induced by diaphragm rupture. Two infected kidney disorders include pyelonephritis and renal abscess complications.

8.5.2.1.2 Secondary injury

The next cause of kidney damage is a generalized illness, such as trauma, protracted hunger, injury of nonrenal organs, sepsis which may include failure of multiple organs, and AKI, with a 70% mortality rate. Hyperglycemia in diabetes mellitus activates the RAS, which promotes inflammation via the angiotensin-1, i.e., the AT1 receptor (Doi et al., 2009).

8.5.2.1.3 Kidney tissue repair

Several investigations have found a complex and diverse connection between tissue healing and the development or reversal of renal damage. Tissue regeneration appears to be slowed timely by damage, resulting in injury regression and opening the door to healing. The structural re-developing after acute tubule injury is primarily due to the simultaneous proliferation of persisting epithelial cells to adapt to nearby cell loss (Witzgall et al., 1994).

8.5.2.1.4 Adhesion molecules, growth factors, and cell cycle regulators

Several messengers, including epidermis growth factor, heparin-bound epidermis growth, insulin-like growth factor-1, and hepatocellular growth factor, are appeared to be increased after acute kidney injury and directly act on the kidneys. Some growth factors are generated in the kidneys and serve as paracrine or autocrine regulators. HGF, on the other hand, works through the endocrine system and communicates with the kidney cells during circulation. Cells respond to these polypeptide messengers by synthesizing DNA and subsequently going through mitosis. Following a temporary injury, the proximal tubule's quiescent endothelial cells and Henle's loop limb restart the cell cycle. The damaged nephron sections eventually become highly reactive. The attachment of these growth factors to the site-specific surface of cell receptors activates the intracellular signaling pathway, which then commits the cell to a new phase of the cell cycle (Schena, 1998).

8.5.2.1.5 Angiogenesis

Microvascular permeability is caused by endothelial leukocyte reactions with the glycocalyx peeling. Cell-cell contact alteration leads to the collapse of the actin cytoskeleton and the rupture of a matrix of the perivascular system. Because of this, heme concentration and obstruction in the vascular system develop. To maintain artery flow and improve tissue perfusion, the kidney reacts to these hypoxic conditions by secreting a range of vasoactive and angiogenic chemicals. Endogenous RAS activation in the murine proximal tubular epithelium in vitro leads to enhanced external angiotensin II syntheses with self-critical effects to create a vascular endothelial factor for growth (VEGF). In the kidneys of both humans and animals, VEGF stimulates vascular multiplication and repair tissues (Feliers and Kasinath, 2010).

8.5.2.1.6 Renal progenitors

Damaged tissue cells are usually repaired from communities of surviving epithelial cells after an infection. These cells can proliferate, grow and differentiate into new cells or go deeper into the cell cycle. One of the regulators for this divergence and re-differentiation in favor of healing and survivability is the Foxc2 transcription factor. If the uninephrectomized mouse is implanted with epithelial-mesenchymal transitional epithelial cells, the cells have generated immature glomeruli, which shows this technique can transfer the features of the kidney progenitor (Hader et al., 2010).

8.5.2.1.7 Mesenchymal stem cells

Mesenchymal stem cells have been implicated in healing acute tubular damage following injury and restoring performance in chronic kidney disease. Microvesicles released by these cells may contain mRNA that transmits mesenchymal stem cell differentiative characteristics and transcription and proliferation regulatory factors that offer apoptosis tolerance. The cells are also considered to interact with each other and impact the activity and repair of the progenitor cells (Bruno et al., 2009).

8.5.3 Lungs

Improper cell proliferation and diversification may cause many lung diseases, including carcinoma, following a chemical injury to the airway epithelium. The transcription factor of the activator protein 1, which consists mainly of protein dimers Jun fos and Jun, serves as an environmental sensor for different hazardous stimuli and controls gene expression in a range of biological activities. AP-1 families Jun C, Jun B, and fra1 are necessary for embryonic development, while Jun D, Fos C, and Fos B are essential for proper postnatal growth, according to gene interruption studies. This implies their abnormal activation following toxic damage, while necessary for normal cellular functions, may contribute to the genesis of lung diseases. The Jun and Fos expression in in vivo and in vitro lung cells supports this notion of various environments and carcinogens. More significantly, numerous members of the AP-1 group are consistently generated in several carcinogenic lung malignancies (Reddy and Mossman, 2002). Particular toxins stimulate different mitogen-activated protein kinases, activating the AP-1 signaling pathway after contact with the cells. Various contaminants trigger different MACKs, and AP-1 binds its target sites in promoters after activation to control the expression of multiple genes involved in diverse biological processes.

8.5.4 Spleen

It is considered that bone marrow is the most common source of macrophage inflammation. On the other hand, the spleen was discovered to function in studies as a repository of inflammatory monocytes. After tissue damage, spleen monocytes enter the circulation and travel to inflammation sites where they act as macrophages and contribute to proinflammatory and anti-inflammatory reactions (Swirski et al., 2009; Robbins et al., 2012). The macrophages have been connected with acetaminophen-induced hepatic injury pathogenesis. They play a significant role in enhancing inflammation and tissue damage. Evidence suggests that these various measures are at the expense of distinct macrophage subpopulations progressively developing in the liver after acetaminophen overdose.

Research by Mili Mandal has shown that, after acetaminophen poisoning in the spleen, distinct populations of pro- and anti-inflammatory macrophages develop in the Liver. Reducing hepatotoxicity means that interaction is mostly pro-inflammatory/cytotoxic or mediator-controlled cells. The spleen has been shown to serve as a reservoir for inflammatory monocytes, which increase response to tissue injury or infections. The above research results have shown a high, low, and medium level Ly6C marker of pro-inflammatory and anti-inflammatory in the spleen following the administration of Acetaminophen. The hypothesis that the spleen functions as a cellular reservoir are supported by the fact that each of these monocyte subpopulations increased after ingesting acetaminophen. Monocytes from bone marrow travel through the spleen in cell tracking assays before settling in atherosclerotic lesions (Nahrendorf et al., 2007; Swirski et al., 2009; Robbins et al., 2012; Mandal et al., 2016).

8.5.5 Skin

There are several explanations for wounds, including surgical, traumatic, external pressures (pressure, burning, and cutting), and pathological or vascular diseases such as diabetes mellitus. These injuries are categorized as chronic or acute based on the impact of their causes. However, this is not always possible; all aspects of wound therapy attempt to heal the wound entirely and quickly. It is challenging to heal chronic wounds (Chen et al., 2008). Such interactions promote cell migration, commence angiogenesis, and epithelization, encourage matrix creation and restoration in the wounded region, and interact with specific cell surface receptors to control tissue healing. Different growth factor families, including epidermal growth factor (EGF), fibroblast growth factor (FGF), transforming growth factor (TGF), and platelet-derived growth factor (PDGF) were investigated in the field of wound healing. The healing process is the subject of several surveys.

The importance of stromal cell-generated factor 1 is also becoming more evident during the healing process in regulating epidermal cell migration and proliferation. The created EGF is vital for the epithelialization of platelets, macrophages, and fibroblasts. Generated FGF promotes the growth of granulated tissue and epithelization and matrix formation through keratinocytes, mast cells, fibroblasts, endothelial cells, smooth muscle cells, and chondrocytes. The TGF-β, essential for inflammation, tissue development, epithelialization, and matrix forming and restoration, is produced by platelets, keratinocytes, macrophages, lymphocytes, and fibroblasts. All platelets, keratinocytes, and macrophages are produced by PDGF, which are engaged in every stage of the wound healing process.

Pierce et al. found that through various mechanisms, both PDGF and TGF-β enhanced wound healing in vivo. In short, PDGF functions in chemo-attraction for macrophages and fibroblasts and stimulates the production of growth factors such as TGF-β. Some research proved the importance of each wound repair growth factor; in addition, several studies indicated the ability of combined growth factors and carriers to improve wound treatment for their delivery. Although topical administration of growth factors has accelerated wound healing, its therapeutic application still faces barriers. Various research projects are designed to identify the optimum balance of biomaterials and growth factors to produce a conduit suited for maintaining the integrity and stability of the growth factor. Due to the dynamic process of wound repair, whether long-term or short-term growth factors need to be provided and how long thorough healing is uncertain. In addition, the wound healing cascade contains a lot of cell-component interaction. The problem is combining many development components and relating them to a particular harm situation (Pierce et al., 1989).

8.6 Cytokine release and recruitment of phagocytic cells for tissue repair

8.6.1 Macrophages

Tissue-residing inflammatory monocytes control the process of repair, regeneration, and fibrosis of injured tissue. Monocytes and macrophages are crucial to start the tissue healing process maintenance. These cells undergo phenotypic and functional alterations in response to tissue injury. Tissue healing and fibrosis are intricate processes involving monocytes or macrophages. The early cellular reaction to an injury is driven by chemokine, metalloproteinase matrix (MMP), and other proinflammatory cytokines generated by macrophages. When macrophages diminish early after damage, the inflammatory response typically decreases substantially. However, macrophage removal can cause damage to the wound and a less successful rehabilitation and healing process (Wynn and Vannella, 2016).

Macrophages are a diverse and adaptable group of cells that play a pivotal role in wound healing and tissue regeneration. TGF-β, the prototypical profibrogenic cytokine produced by macrophages, acts on myofibroblasts to encourage activation and synthesis of extracellular matrix (ECM). In addition, they can generate high amounts of thrombospondin-1, which is a potent stimulator of transforming growth factor-β in vivo. Macrophages being a significant source of soluble mediators such as TNF- and IL-1 platelet-derived growth factor, IL-1, IL-4, IL-13, TNF-, CCL7, and CCL8, and a wide range of certain chemokines can encourage migration of leukocyte and maintain the inflammatory response (Ramachandran et al., 2015). At the time of infection, neutrophils move to the wound site, obliterate pathogens there, and recruit immune cells. When macrophages encounter and engulf apoptotic neutrophils, they release cytokines that suppress inflammation and repair the tissue (Fig. 8.3) (Bouchery and Harris, 2017).

8.6.1.1 *Macrophages in tissue regeneration*

In the event of infection or injury, the immune system plays an essential role in effectively managing the regeneration and repair of injured or damaged tissues. Molecular patterns associated with pathogens (PAMPs) and molecular patterns related to damage (DAMPs) are released throughout tissue injury via invading pathogens or dying and dead cells, respectively (Zhang et al., 2010). Pattern recognition receptors (PRRs), which are mainly expressed by innate immune cells, identify these molecules and activate inflammation signaling pathways in dendritic cells, TRMs, neutrophils, and other cell populations (e.g., endothelial cells and fibroblasts) (Gong et al., 2020). When these cells are activated, they release various proinflammatory cytokines and chemokines, which cause innate inflammatory cells to migrate to the wound site.

During a successful wound healing, macrophages (primarily moMs) adopt a "classically activated" phenotype (also called M1) wherein they release reactive oxygen species (ROS), antimicrobial peptides, and inflammatory cytokines (e.g., TNFα, IL-12, IL-6) to enhance inflammation (Mosser and Edwards, 2008; Ogle et al., 2016). M1 macrophages are highly phagocytic, which allows them to remove bacteria and debris from the environment of the wound (Hesketh et al., 2017). After the acute phase of inflammation settles, the prominent

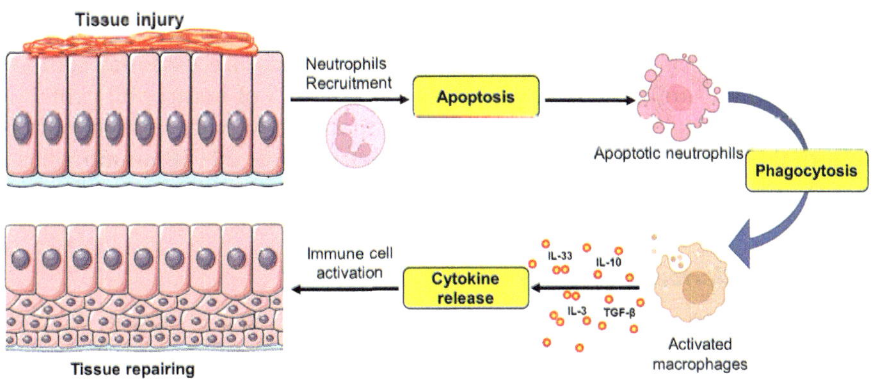

FIGURE 8.3 Role of neutrophils and macrophages in tissue repair.

population of macrophages transformed into an "alternatively activated" phenotype (also called M2). M2 macrophages secrete anti-inflammatory mediators, particularly IL-10, as well as growth factors (e.g., PDGF, TGF-β), which help in the healing of tissue by sustaining angiogenesis, boosting proliferation and ingrowth of progenitor cells, and encouraging remodeling and assembly of ECM (Biswas and Mantovani, 2010; Martin and García, 2021).

8.6.2 Neutrophil

Neutrophils are the most common immune cell in human blood. They protect the host from pathogenic organisms and other potentially toxic reagents. Neutrophils are involved in innate immunity and healthy skin; they are not often visible, but they are produced in abundance during injury. They are the initial inflammatory cells circulating in the wound area, consistent with their initial infection protection activity. Their ability to generate many cytokines and growth factors allows them to decrease the danger of infection. Antimicrobials and proteases help to kill and degrade harmful bacteria and generate neutrophils. Neutrophils cannot be essential for the repair of skin damage. According to animal studies, neutrophils can hinder re-epithelization or improve scar tissue formation in wounds with a low risk of infection (Theilgaard-Mönch et al., 2004). After an infection, neutrophils circulating at the wound place are attracted quickly and execute various activities. They generate several proinflammatory mediators that recruit and stimulate other inflammatory cells and cause inflammation development. In typical wounds, recruited neutrophils will ultimately die and be eaten by macrophages, producing an inflammatory response resolution mechanism (Fig. 8.3).

8.6.2.1 Neutrophil granules: a rich source of proteases

Many antibacterial chemicals, proteases, and neutrophils are equipped to destroy and break down possible infections. Most of these compounds are stored in the cytoplasm of granules. Once phagocytosis has devoured a microbe, it can be released into the phagolysosome or the extracellular environment (Nathan, 2006).

8.6.2.2 Azurophilic granules

Azurophil granules are packed with antimicrobial proteins and acidic hydrolases and were previously thought to be primary lysosomes. Azurophil granules, like lysosomes, have granulysin (CD63) in their membrane. Alpha-defensins are essential components of azurophil granules and are thought to contribute at least 5% of neutrophil protein content. Defensins are small proteins up to 3.5 kDa and are cationic, cytotoxic, and antimicrobial peptides. Neutrophils consist of four closely linked a-defensins of 29–30 amino acids (human neutrophil peptide1–4) preserved in azurophil granules rich with defensin (Faurschou and Borregaard, 2003).

8.6.2.3 Neutrophil-derived proteases

Proteases in neutrophil granules are common in addition to a spectrum of antibacterial compounds. The primary purpose of these proteases is to aid in killing and degrading germs. Still, neutrophils can also be employed to divide the membrane and matrix of the basement.

This helps the neutrophils travel from circulation to the tissue and, after that, to the damaged location. These proteases are essential for clinical practice since they inflict further damage to the host tissues when produced in large numbers in the extracellular area by neutrophils. Serine and metalloproteinases are two protease kinds crucial in wound healing and are produced by neutrophils (Parks et al., 2004).

8.6.2.4 Serine proteases

Cathepsin G, elastase, and protease are all serine proteases produced by neutrophils. All the proteases feature an azurophilated grain pattern of histidine-aspartic acid-serine in their active sites. Most studies were performed with elastase and cathepsin G on neutrophil serine protease. The ECM components protein elastin, fibronectin, laminin and Vitronectin, have same proteolytic activity. According to the current study, the activity of these proteases can be utilized as an early indication for identifying chronic injuries.

8.6.2.5 Matrix metallo-proteinases

Neutrophils maintain many MMPs in their granules and secretory vesicles in addition to serine proteases. MMPs are a group of enzymes preserved for pro-domains and catalytic zinc-binding domains. MMP-2, MMP-8, and MMP-9, utilized for wound healing, are the essential MMPs discovered in neutrophil granulates. Various research projects found that these proteins majorly affect wound healing. MMP-8 is a protein that cleaves fibrillary collagen and is primarily expressed in neutrophils and is usually called collagenase-2 (Witko-Sarsat et al., 2000). While neutrophils are crucial for infection control, the development of chronic wounds can be attributed to the increased neutrophil activity or neutrophil persistence at the site of an injury. Although absolute neutrophil and MMP-based serine proteases are needed to eliminate organisms and restorative wounds efficiently, data from different underlying studies and clinical studies show that overabundance of neutrophil activity may increase site harmful effects, lead to long-term inflammatory response, further tissue destruction, and ultimately to improperly healed injury (Wilgus et al., 2013).

8.7 Re-epithelialization and tissue repair

The skin is composed of an epidermis that works as a barrier to the external environment. The dermis offers mechanical resistance and is securely fixed to the epidermis. The epidermis is composed primarily of keratinocytes. The aged skin gets continually renewed by the proliferation and differentiation of progeny cells (Jung et al., 2007). The process of adolescent recovery includes blood coagulation, inflammation, keratinocyte migration, keratinocyte proliferation, granulated tissue development, and neovascular tissue formation. The development of skin thickness and new epithelia is referred to as re-epithelialization. When the total thickness of the skin is removed, a larger and longer defect is created than an incision. Re-epithelialization occurs in the second and third stages around 16–24 h following its spread during the damage phase. The injured site attracts neutrophils, mono-cell, and macrophages when the membrane of the skin/blood is interrupted.

Keratinocytes and other cutaneous cells, chemical and cytokine proliferation then stimulate keratinocytes, phenotype changes through growth factors, chemical cells, and cytokines. The activated phenotype is characterized by cytoskeleton network alterations and receptor changes in the cell membrane. Keratinocytes enter the curing site and form new adhesion complexes by polymerizing cytoskeleton actin fibers. The structures and signals of intracellular receptors that don't have the enzyme activity interact with integrated and syndecan (Rousselle et al., 2019).

A tissue that formed a wound-healing model comprised of human keratinocytes and fibroblasts was investigated for re-epithelializing pathways. A 6 mm biopsy punch was employed to injure replicated human skin. Three days after the damage, model research revealed two independent and complementary ways to govern wound recurrence. Probably mitotic pressure comes through the push force from the neighboring unwounded epidermis. The second pathway is the migratory language in which keratinocytes travel independently, as with the migratory leapfrog paradigm (Ortonne et al., 2004). Skin conditions therapy now includes wound re-epithelialization technology, such as autographing, allographs, wound dressings, and tissue-engineering alternatives. Epithelization speed and reliability are usually related to ECM synthesis and vascularization features. More profound knowledge of aggregate cell migration is medically essential. Epithelial barrier repair is the goal of epithelial cells in wound cure (Rousselle et al., 2019).

8.7.1 Tissue repair

The tissue repair and regeneration begin once the injury is induced or occurs due to trauma or a particular clinical condition. Reparation of the tissue is a basic linear process that drives cell proliferation employing growth factors, leading to the combination of the changes that occur, including soluble mediators and blood cells. The biological and biochemical events of tissue regeneration are stages of inflammatory reactions, cell proliferation, the production of extracellular matrix components, and the post-repair period, called remodeling (Fig. 8.4) (Gonzalez et al., 2016).

8.7.1.1 Inflammatory stage

Injured blood capillaries constrict, and the blood discharged coagulates during an acute vascular inflammation that contributes to preserving the artery integrity. Coagulation is the aggregation in the fibrin network of thrombus and platelets depending on the activation and aggravation by certain stimuli of these cells (Martin, 1997). The fibrin network organizing the required temporary matrix for cell cycle progression, in addition to re-establishing homeostasis and building a barrier against invasion by microorganisms, restores skin function as a protective barrier while preserving skin integrity. This also enables cell migration into the milieu of the lesion and the stimulation of fibroblast growth. The leukocyte influx in the injury region characterizes the cell response in the inflammatory phase. This reaction is fast and corresponds to the main signs of inflammation at the lesion's location. Inflammatory cells help heal the wound by facilitating the release and removal of various cell debris from lysosomal enzymes and reactive oxygen species (Medrado et al., 2003).

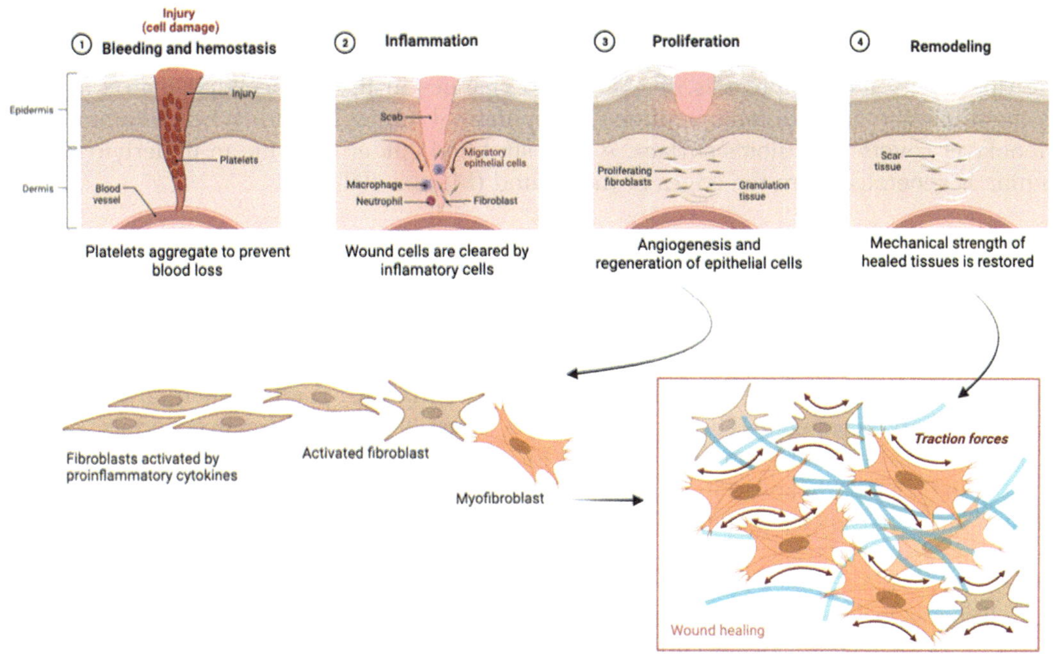

FIGURE 8.4 Steps in tissue repair.

Many neutrophils are transmigrated into the endothelium cells within a few hours after the lesion, caused by proinflammatory cytokines, including interleukin-1, tumor necrosis factor α, and Interferon γ at the site. Monocytes migrate from nearby blood arteries, which enter the lesion region 48 h after lesion formation, and novel gene expression profiles distinguish them into macrophages. These cells can function as antigenic cells and promote neutrophil phagocytosis by signaling chemokines (Eming et al., 2007).

8.7.1.2 Proliferative stage

The proliferative stage minimizes fibroplasia and tissue size by contacting and providing a viable epithelial barrier to activate keratinocytes. The processes begin in the microambience of the lesion. They can persist up to 14 days within the first 48 h of the lesion formation (Li et al., 2007). According to the study, the contraction is initiated by myofibroblast, rich in α-smooth muscle actin, and wound contraction is performed at this stage. The cells that cluster on the wound's edges carry out a contractive activity that leads to the lesion boundaries in the center (Calin et al., 2010).

8.7.1.3 Remodeling stage

Remodeling is the next healing phase that begins 2–3 weeks after the lesion onset and can continue for one or more years. The primary aim of the restructuring step is to maximize tensile strength by reorganizing the extracellular matrix, reducing it, and resynthesizing it. At this stage, an attempt is made in the healing process to resume normal cellular morphology and reconstruct the granulated tissue to reduce the number of cellular and vascular scar tissues and gradually increase the collagen fiber concentration. This stage is characterized by the ripening of the components, the profound changes in the extracellular matrix as well as the resolution of acute inflammation. The epidermal migration ends when a keratinocyte monolayer covers the lesion's surface. A new stratified epidermis with an underlying basal lamina is generated from the edges of the wound (Martin, 1997).

8.8 Proteins and extracellular matrix (ECM) in tissue regeneration

8.8.1 Role of proteins in tissue regeneration

The three main constituents in the extracellular matrix (ECM) are protein, glycosaminoglycan, and glycoconjugate. The connective tissue consists of an ECM matrix and its components, as well as cell adhesion receptors that form a complex network of cells in every tissue and organ (Kusindarta and Wihadmadyatami, 2018). Protein, collagen, fibronectin, vitronectin, and laminins play a significant function in tissue regeneration, as mentioned in Table 8.1.

8.8.1.1 Collagen

Collagen is the readily available structural protein in mammals and the primary constituent of the ECM in nearly all hard and soft tissues. It accounts for about 30% of the body's total protein (Sheehy et al., 2017). Different types of collagen are available in the ECM of various tissues. Collagen type I is the most prevalent collagen type in tendons and bones. In contrast, collagen type II is found in articular cartilage. A set of 29 distinct collagen species have been determined to date. Collagen is necessary for keeping the mechanical stability of the ECM and is engaged in essential biological processes such as repair, morphogenesis, and remodeling (Abou Neel et al., 2013). To create collagen-based biocomposites, purified collagen serves as an essential building block, which can be mixed with proteins and macromolecules and then polymerized to develop applications in tissue engineering scaffolds. There are two types of collagen-based biomaterials. The biomaterials created by decellularizing organs and tissues fall under one category. This method eliminates cells through mechanical, enzymatic, or chemical processes. It leaves an ECM architecture with functional proteins in its place (Lu et al., 2011; Gilbert et al., 2006). The biomaterials from purified collagen extracted and isolated from tissues like skin or tendons fall under the second category (Sheehy et al., 2018). As previously stated, collagen is a highly appealing natural polymer for tissue engineering; it is the major ECM component and thus contains inbuilt biochemical and structural cues to enhance tissue formation. Because collagen is so durable, it is possible to create scaffolds based on porous collagen using electrospinning, lyophilization, and 3D bioprinting processes (Haugh et al., 2011).

8.8.1.2 Glycosaminoglycan (GAGs)

Glycosaminoglycans (GAGs) are negatively charged polysaccharide chains that form proteoglycan molecules and are also recognized as mucopolysaccharides. They are made up of disaccharide units that have been present in all mammalian tissues (Afratis et al., 2012). The molecular structure of these molecules determines their wide range of functions within the

TABLE 8.1 Function of extracellular matrix-associated proteins in tissue regeneration.

Protein	Function	Ref.
Collagens	➢ Promote regeneration of connective tissue. ➢ Provide elasticity and strength to the skin.	Riha et al. (2021)
Glycosaminoglycans	➢ Help in the proliferation and adhesion of cells. ➢ Promote the functioning of immune cells and the signaling of growth factors.	Tayebi and Moharamzadeh (2017)
Fibronectin	➢ Extracellular matrix component that controls the behavior of the cell. ➢ Boosts tissue repair and regulates motility and attachment of cells.	Parisi et al. (2020)
Vitronectin	➢ Binds with plasminogen, collagen, glycosaminoglycans, and urokinase receptor. ➢ Stabilizes the plasminogen activation inhibitor-1 inhibitory conformation.	Schvartz et al. (1999)
Elastin	➢ Helpful in repairing scars and healing wounds. ➢ It gives elasticity, recoil, and stretch to the skin.	Baumann et al. (2021)
Tenascin	➢ Modulates growth, adhesion, and migration of cells. ➢ Helpful in the condensation of the mesenchymal cell.	Chiquet-Ehrismann and Chiquet (2003)
Galectin	➢ Role in immune responses, inflammation, autophagy, signaling, and migration of cells. ➢ Helpful in diseases like cancer, diabetes, wound repair, fibrosis, etc.	Johannes et al. (2018)
Laminin	➢ Promotes homeostasis and tissue morphogenesis via regulation of tissue architecture, matrix-mediated signaling, adhesion, and migration of cells.	Hamill et al. (2009)
SPARC (secreted protein acidic and rich in cysteine)	➢ Regulates growth of cells via interaction with cytokines and extracellular matrix.	Bradshaw (2009)
Osteopontin	➢ Involvement in the pathogenesis of cancer, various chronic inflammatory disease, atherosclerosis, etc. ➢ Regulates biomineralization and inhibits vascular calcification.	Lund et al. (2009)

body. While hydration of cells and scaffolding of structure was previously thought to be the only roles of GAGs, a study showed that GAGs play an essential role in cell signaling, which regulates a wide range of biochemical processes (Raman et al., 2005).

The control of cell proliferation and growth, cell adhesion promotion, wound healing, and anticoagulation are just few examples of the involved GAGs processes (Casale and Crane, 2019). Based on their central disaccharide molecular units, the chondroitin sulfate/dermatan sulfate, heparin/heparan sulfate, hyaluronic acid, and keratan sulfate are the four main GAG groups (Prydz, 2015). Mechanical strength and wound resistance are two of GAGs' primary responsibilities as ECM constituents in the epidermal, dermal, and hypodermal layers. Together with other connective tissue molecules like collagen and elastin, they function in a delicate three-dimensional network (Varkey et al., 2015). Biopolymers can create skin engineering scaffolds and carriers for wound healing because they contain natural macromolecules like GAGs and different proteins (Wartenberg et al., 2021).

8.8.1.3 Fibronectin

Fibronectin (FN) is a multidomain glycoprotein with a molecular weight of around 230–270 kD found in almost all extracellular matrixes (ECM). Another type of such protein is found in blood plasma (Bason et al., 2018). Both cellular and plasma forms are typically made up of two nearly identical subunits that are made up of three different varieties of repetitive modules (Types I-III). This glycoprotein's primary function is to promote cell proliferation, migration, spreading, and adhesion, yet it is also required to grow many organs and tissues during embryogenesis (Hosoyama et al., 2019; Kusindarta and Wihadmadyatami, 2018). It is also involved in the healing of wounds as well as cellular morphology. Due to fibronectin's ability to bind to $\alpha5\beta1$ cell membrane integrin through an RGD sequence, it plays a vital role in enhancing the result of cell adhesion (Klimek and Ginalska, 2020). Changes in fibronectin conformation reveal additional binding sites, which contribute to the formation of fibrils and convert fibrils into an insoluble, stabilized form. Once constructed, the fibronectin matrix contributes to fabricating other extracellular matrix proteins, thereby influencing tissue organization. Fibronectin is essential for matrix assembly initiation, maturation, and progression during fibrillogenesis (Singh and Schwarzbauer, 2012).

8.8.1.4 Elastin

An ECM fibrous protein, elastin comprises a single tropoelastin component to provide durability and flexibility to the connective tissues. Only one human gene encodes the tropoelastin, secreted by many cells, including fibroblasts, smooth muscle, endothelial cells, keratinocytes, and chondrocytes with unglycosylated protein of 60 kDa (Mithieux et al., 2013). Valine, proline, and glycine amino acid sequence is responsible for their elasticity. Elastic fibers, generated by elastin and microfibrils, are essential components of organs and connective and vascular tissues. The RGD sequences in the elastin molecule facilitate cell growth and adhesion (Vindin et al., 2019).

Elastin is an essential structural ECM protein and is not utilized recurrently as other ECM proteins (such as fibronectin, collagen, and laminins) in biomaterials engineering, mainly due to the complex purification process. During this technique, some contaminations may occur. Therefore, their existence might lead to an immunological reaction in the body (Sorushanova et al., 2019). Synthetic tropoelastin, elastin-like polypeptides (ELPs), α-elastin, and elastin-like recombinases (ELRs) are some of the artificial elastin forms that have been created (Spicer, 2019).

8.8.1.5 Laminins

Laminins are cross-shaped glycoproteins with trimeric structures of α, β, and γ chains. There are five, four, and three distinct genetic forms of each isoform, respectively. Laminins are cross- or T-shaped molecules with two or three short arms and one long arm (Domogatskaya et al., 2012). These proteins interact to make adhesion space between various tissues. The ECM basement membrane (MB) contains laminins, nidogens, perlecan, collagen type IV, and agrin. The assembly and structure of MB are mainly dependent on laminins. These glycoproteins are essential for cell adherence, migration, differentiation, and healing of wounds. It is evident that laminins significantly contribute to the normal function of blood vessels, tendons, and other connective soft tissues that have a role in the pathogenesis of soft tissue injury and connective tissue damage (Grounds et al., 2005). They also function in the early development of embryos and organogenesis. Laminins and peptides derived from laminin have been used with surprising efficiency in biodegradable polymer enrichment (Klimek and Ginalska, 2020).

8.8.1.6 Tenascins

The tenascins are polymorphic, molecularly weighted glycoproteins in the ECM between 150 and 380 kDa. Tenascins consist of identical subunits composed of several repeat domains, including type III fibronectin domains, EGF, heptad repeats, and globular domains at the C-terminal. The first isomer found was the C-isomer of tenascin, which is a huge monomer of 300 kDa in hexamer form (Okamoto and Imanaka-Yoshida, 2012). Tenascin-C high levels were observed in patients' blood with rheumatoid arthritis and in synovial fluid after human injury. The role of tenascin-C in ECM injury was shown to be diverse, including the mediation of both fibrotic and inflammatory processes to promote tissue healing. Tenascin-C works in ventricular remodeling by releasing cardiomyocytes from extracellular matrix adhesion and promoting matrix metalloproteinase expression. In calcified aortic valves, tenascin-C and matrix metalloproteinase-12 were shown to have a role in elastic fiber fragmentation (Midwood et al., 2011). It was believed that after an injury, they managed the muscle healing. Tenascins are essential for maintaining the mechanical behavior of weight-bearing ECM and the efficient recovery of ECM upon mechanical damage (Halper and Kjaer, 2014).

8.8.1.7 Thrombospondins

A family of five modular glycoproteins, each expressed by a separate gene, is called TSP (thrombospondins). TSP-1 and TSP-2 are in Group A, while in Group B are TSPs 3–5. TSPs influence cell activity in a range of tissues by connecting components, including heparan sulfate proteoglycans and a variety of cell membrane receptors, to the extracellular matrix. They are called extracellular matrix "adhesion-modulating components." TSP-1 is a protein typically kept in platelets but released by the injury from its granules to the tissue healing. It consists of three subunits of 150 kDa, with each unit having a G-like laminate and N-terminal domain forming a homotrimer. TSP-1 does not interact with and bind with structural components of the blood vessel wall but does so through controlling nitric oxide production. It is well-recognized for the pathophysiology of atherosclerosis and peripheral vascular disease (Halper and Kjaer, 2014).

8.8.1.8 Osteopontin

Osteopontin is a glycosylated phosphoprotein that may be found in the extracellular matrix in mineralized tissues and body fluids. Osteopontin expression rises during cancer and angiogenesis under inflammatory and cellular stimuli. Osteopontin can activate numerous signal pathways and influence cell functions by binding and interacting with specific cell-surface receptors, such as integrin and CD44. Osteopontin can affect endothelial and epithelial cell motility, extracellular invasion, and cell attachment by interacting with surface cell receptors. Osteopontin also plays an essential role in controlling tissue remodeling (Denhardt et al., 2001). Osteopontin activity has been demonstrated to enhance wound healing compared to healthy skin. The osteopontin knock-out mice display wound healing abnormalities, including disruption to the matrix and alterations in collagen fibrillogenesis in its cartilage compared with its counterparts. The above referenced study indicated that osteopontin can regulate MSC migration during the repair of skin injuries through interaction with CD44. Finally, with osteopontin, there was substantial migration of MSC to damaged areas and differentiation of skin cells into various types. It was shown that osteopontin migrations to MSCs in vitro were increased, and endogenous MSCs could be attracted to skin lesions and distinguished between keratinocytes and endothelial (Wang et al., 2017).

8.8.1.9 Secreted protein acidic and rich in cysteine (SPARC)

The extracellular matrix-associated protein SPARC (32 kDa) is known as osteonectin. The term SPARC is not restricted to bones, as its name indicates (osteonectin), but it is present in many tissues, platelets, and muscles, which are not mineralized. SPARC functions are the critical processes for tissue regeneration, widespread dispersion during embryogenesis, tissue reparations, cell turnover, cell differentiation, and remodeling. SPARC performs various functions, including metabolic homeostasis, inflammation reduction, extracellular matrix remodeling, and collagen maturation, that create a favorable tissue regeneration environment. In contrast, in such a homeostatic environment, the capacity of tissues to renew and repair is improved. SPARC's regeneration properties are used in various bioengineering applications including obesity, cancer, sarcopenia, and diabetes (Ghanemi et al., 2022).

8.8.1.10 Vitronectin

Precursor vitronectin is a polypeptide with 478 amino acids. The main product of vitronectin is the single chain 75 kDa polypeptide precursor in the liver released by receptor-mediated endocytosis or exocytosis into a space between ECM. As a pro-inflammatory response, tissues experiencing trauma exhibit high amounts of vitronectin mRNA, with more vitronectin building up in the extravascular area in the affected tissues.

Increased vitronectin expression in the liver is followed by inflammation or acute damage. Vitronectin is a protein of the acute phase injury. The level of vitronectin doubles in plasma and is maintained for up to 5 days following surgery. According to animal models and cell lines studies, an acute phase reactions and chronic inflammation enhance the expression of the vitronectin gene. Vitronectin is also a predeterminent for interleukin 6 (Singh et al., 2010).

8.8.2 Role of ECM in regeneration of tissue

The ECM is the most crucial component in creating new pathways and tissues. ECM participates in various activities, including pathologies, neurodegenerative tissue regeneration, mesenchymal-conditioned media, or brain regeneration. The involvement of fibroblast migration and propagation substantially impacts lesion cure at the injury site. Fibroblasts are the ECM component. The result of wound healing may be affected by fibroblast growth. Fibroblasts create wound-related collagen, which affects the process of re-epithelization in wound healing. During proliferation, fibroblasts create collagen of type III that aids in closing the wound. Since TGF increases fibroblast production of bFGF, the fibroblast growth activity is increased during proliferation. More fibroblast also leads to higher collagen production.

Collagen fiber is a significant extracellular matrix fibroblast protein used to restore the damaged strength and function of the tissue. Collagen fibers have been observed to be substantially deposit 8–10 days following damage, after which the number of fibroblasts increases subsequently. ECM is also involved in various activities, such as using mesenchymal conditions in or without mesenchymal disorders, neurological regeneration, and wound treatment. In addition, in the case of peripheral nerve injuries, a decellularized chemical technique and an acellular nerve allograft can be employed to eliminate antigens that cause program rejections while retaining the bulk of ECM components that can successfully guide and accelerate nerve regeneration. Significant effort has been made to induce the direct axonal development of peripheral nerve injury using an in vivo model in the field of tissue engineering (Klimek and Ginalska, 2020).

Proteins found on extracellular vesicles isolated from a wide range of cell types can preclude the death of cells, enhance vascular integrity and neovascularization, modify the immune system at multiple cellular levels, and stimulate proliferation and migration of cells, the outgrowth of neurite and ECM components secretion. EV proteins protect various cell types from apoptosis and necroptosis. One proposed mechanism is reducing reactive oxygen species (ROS) levels by EV. The proteins on EVs induce polarization of macrophages and T cells toward M2 phenotypes and anti-inflammatory regulatory T cells (Treg) while inhibiting the proliferation of inflammatory CD8+ T cells, CD4+ T cells, and natural killer (NK) cells. TLR4 differentiation of myeloid primary response 88 (MyD88)-NF-B signaling activation is a primary immune modulation mechanism.

Angiogenesis is aided by EV-mediated intracellular pathways upregulation in endothelial cells such as VEGF, sonic hedgehog Shh/RhoA, and Wnt/β-catenin signaling. The Shh/Gli signaling activation and subsequent release of nitric oxide (NO) result in vascular protection. EV-associated proteins stimulate cell migration and proliferation in a variety of cell types. The activation of Wnt/β-catenin signaling can stimulate the proliferation of various skin cell types. Other proteins associated with EV promote neurite outgrowth and ECM secretion (Fig. 8.5) (Roefs et al., 2020).

8.9 Summary and future perspectives

The injury caused by exposure to various toxins leads to toxicant-induced injury. Tissues repair mechanism is followed after the injury leading to an array of cellular and molecular repairing process. Toxicants may harm living organisms by interacting with various cell targets after they enter the body. The toxic effect are exerted through physical, molecualar and cellular pathways when a toxicant and its metabolits are spread within the body. Metabolic and excretory organs such as the liver, lung, spleen, skin, and kidney play a vital role

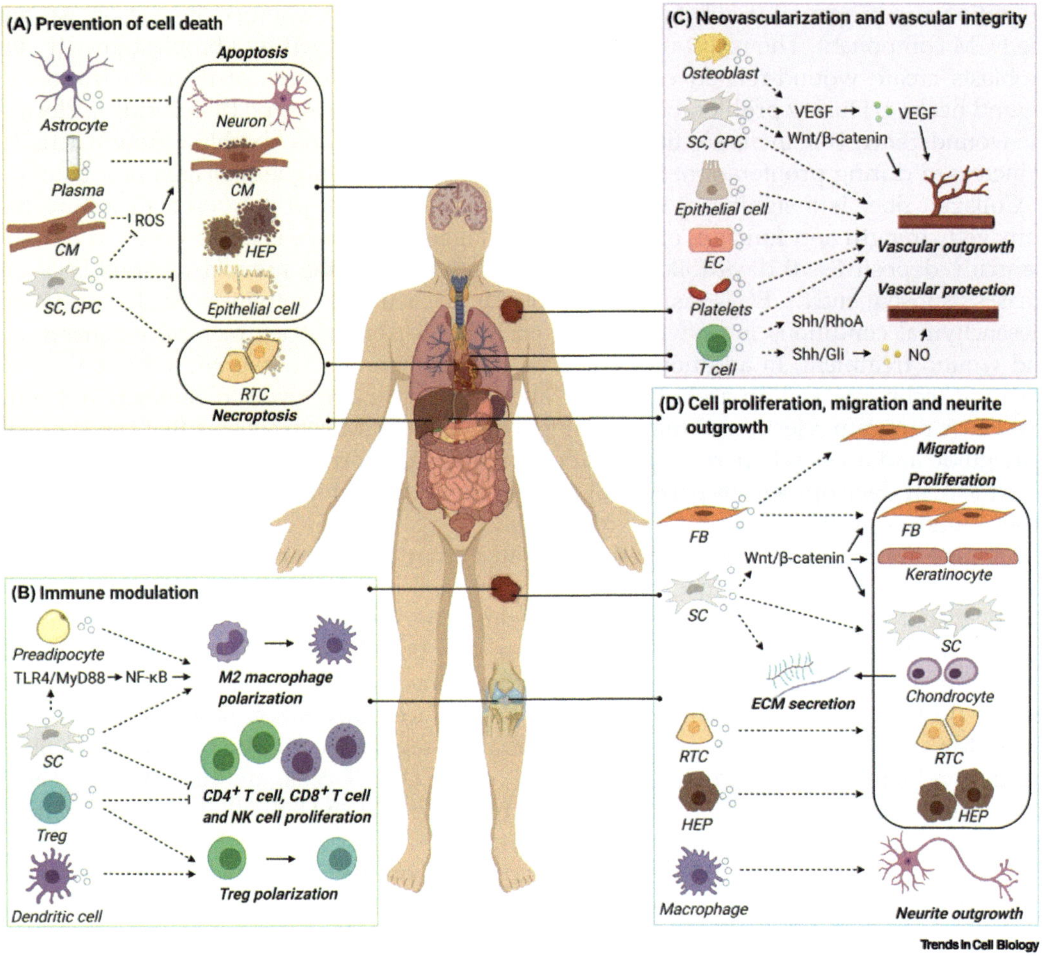

FIGURE 8.5 Process of tissue repair altered by proteins associated with extracellular vesicles. *Adapted from Roefs, M., Sluijter, J. Vader, P., 2020. Extracellular vesicle-associated proteins in tissue repair. Trends Cell Biol. 30, 990–1013.*

elimination of injury causing toxins and the tissue repair process. Immune cells, such as macrophages play a significant part in the beginning, resolution, and maintenance of the tissue healing process. At the same time, neutrophils protect the host cells from microbial conditions. After the injury occurs, the tissue repair and regeneration mechanism start, followed by the inflammatory, proliferative, and remodeling stages. Extracellular matrix and several proteins like collagen, fibronectin, elastin, laminin, etc. play a significant part in repairing or creating new tissues, restoring its structural integrity. The mechanism underlying the toxicant-induced injury and consequent tissue repair process is yet to be explored broadly as new investigations continue in that direction. More novel and systematic approaches are warranted to study the broader consequences of toxicant-induced injuries and their impact on human health.

8.10 List of abbreviation

AKI Acute kidney injury
ALT Alanine transaminase
AT1 Angiotensin-1
ECM Extracellular matrix
EGF Epidermal growth factor
ELPs Elastin-like polypeptides
ELRs Elastin-like recombinamers
FGF Fibroblast growth factor
GAGs Glycosaminoglycan
GCLM Glutathione cysteine ligase modifier subunit
GSH Glutathione
HGF Hepatocyte growth factor
HO-1 Heme oxygenase-1
IFN Interferon
IGF Insulin-like growth factor-1
IL-1 Interleukin-1
IL-8 Interleukin-8
IL10 Interleukin-10
MB Basement membrane
MDA Malondialdehyde
MMP Matrix metalloproteinases
MSCs Mesenchymal stem cells
NAPQ1 N-acetyl-para-amino-quinone
NQO1 NADPH quinone oxidoreductase 1
Nrf2 Nuclear factor erythroid-2 related factor 2
PDGF Platelet-derived growth factor
RAS Renin-angiotensin system
SDF-1 Stromal cell derived factor 1
SPARC Secreted protein acidic and rich in cysteine
TGF-β1 Transforming growth factor β1
TNF-α Tissue necrosis factor α
TSPs Thrombospondins
VEGF Vascular endothelial growth factor

References

Abou Neel, E.A., Bozec, L., Knowles, J.C., Syed, O., Mudera, V., Day, R., Hyun, J.K., 2013. Collagen—emerging collagen based therapies hit the patient. Adv. Drug Deliv. Rev. 65, 429–456.

Afratis, N., Gialeli, C., Nikitovic, D., Tsegenidis, T., Karousou, E., Theocharis, A.D., Pavão, M.S., Tzanakakis, G.N., Karamanos, N.K., 2012. Glycosaminoglycans: key players in cancer cell biology and treatment. FEBS J. 279, 1177–1197.

Arnold, M., Barbul, A., 2006. Nutrition and wound healing. Plast. Reconstr. Surg. 117, 42s–58s.

Bason, C., Gallorini, M., Berardi, A., 2018. The extracellular matrix, growth factors and morphogens in biomaterial design and tissue engineering. Extracellular Matrix for Tissue Engineering and Biomaterials.

Baumann, L., Bernstein, E.F., Weiss, A.S., Bates, D., Humphrey, S., Silberberg, M., Daniels, R., 2021. Clinical relevance of elastin in the structure and function of skin. Aesthet. Surg. J. Open Forum 3, ojab019.

Berman, B., Maderal, A., Raphael, B., 2017. Keloids and hypertrophic scars: pathophysiology, classification, and treatment. Dermatol. Surg. 43 (Suppl. 1), S3–s18.

Biswas, S.K., Mantovani, A., 2010. Macrophage plasticity and interaction with lymphocyte subsets: cancer as a paradigm. Nat. Immunol. 11, 889–896.

Blazka, M.E., Wilmer, J.L., Holladay, S.D., Wilson, R.E., Luster, M.I., 1995. Role of proinflammatory cytokines in acetaminophen hepatotoxicity. Toxicol. Appl. Pharmacol. 133, 43–52.

Boll, M., Weber, L.W., Becker, E., Stampfl, A., 2001. Mechanism of carbon tetrachloride-induced hepatotoxicity. Hepatocellular damage by reactive carbon tetrachloride metabolites. Z. Naturforsch. C J. Biosci. 56, 649–659.

Bouchery, T., Harris, N.L., 2017. Specific repair by discerning macrophages. Science 356, 1014.

Bradshaw, A.D., 2009. The role of SPARC in extracellular matrix assembly. J. Cell Commun. Signal. 3, 239–246.

Bruno, S., Grange, C., Deregibus, M.C., Calogero, R.A., Saviozzi, S., Collino, F., Morando, L., Busca, A., Falda, M., Bussolati, B., Tetta, C., Camussi, G., 2009. Mesenchymal stem cell-derived microvesicles protect against acute tubular injury. J. Am. Soc. Nephrol. 20, 1053–1067.

Cai, Z., Mehendale, H.M., 1991. Hepatotoxicity and lethality of halomethanes in Mongolian gerbils pretreated with chlordecone, phenobarbital or mirex. Arch. Toxicol. 65, 204–212.

Cai, Z.W., Mehendale, H.M., 1990. Lethal effects of CCl4 and its metabolism by Mongolian gerbils pretreated with chlordecone, phenobarbital, or mirex. Toxicol. Appl. Pharmacol. 104, 511–520.

Calin, M.A., Coman, T., Calin, M.R., 2010. The effect of low level laser therapy on surgical wound healing. Rom. Rep. Phys. 62, 617–627.

Campos, A.C., Groth, A.K., Branco, A.B., 2008. Assessment and nutritional aspects of wound healing. Curr. Opin. Clin. Nutr. Metab. Care 11, 281–288.

Casale, J., Crane, J.S., 2019. Biochemistry, Glycosaminoglycans.

Chanda, S., Mangipudy, R.S., Warbritton, A., Bucci, T.J., Mehendale, H.M., 1995. Stimulated hepatic tissue repair underlies heteroprotection by thioacetamide against acetaminophen-induced lethality. Hepatology 21, 477–486.

Chen, L., Tredget, E.E., Wu, P.Y., Wu, Y., 2008. Paracrine factors of mesenchymal stem cells recruit macrophages and endothelial lineage cells and enhance wound healing. PLoS One 3, e1886.

Chen, M., Suzuki, A., Borlak, J., Andrade, R.J., Lucena, M.I., 2015. Drug-induced liver injury: interactions between drug properties and host factors. J. Hepatol. 63, 503–514.

Chilakapati, J., Korrapati, M.C., Hill, R.A., Warbritton, A., Latendresse, J.R., Mehendale, H.M., 2007a. Toxicokinetics and toxicity of thioacetamide sulfoxide: a metabolite of thioacetamide. Toxicology 230, 105–116.

Chilakapati, J., Korrapati, M.C., Shankar, K., Hill, R.A., Warbritton, A., Latendresse, J.R., Mehendale, H.M., 2007b. Role of CYP2E1 and saturation kinetics in the bioactivation of thioacetamide: effects of diet restriction and phenobarbital. Toxicol. Appl. Pharmacol. 219, 72–84.

Chiquet-Ehrismann, R., Chiquet, M., 2003. Tenascins: regulation and putative functions during pathological stress. J. Pathol. 200, 488–499.

Dalu, A., Cronin, G.M., LYN-Cook, B.D., Mehendale, H.M., 1995a. Age-related differences in TGF-alpha and protooncogenes expression in rat liver after a low dose of carbon tetrachloride. J. Biochem. Toxicol. 10, 259–264.

Dalu, A., Mehendale, H.M., 1996. Efficient tissue repair underlies the resiliency of postnatally developing rats to chlordecone + CCl4 hepatotoxicity. Toxicology 111, 29–42.

Dalu, A., Warbritton, A., Bucci, T.J., Mehendale, H.M., 1995b. Age-related susceptibility to chlordecone-potentiated carbon tetrachloride hepatotoxicity and lethality is due to hepatic quiescence. Pediatr. Res. 38, 140–148.

Denhardt, D.T., Burger, E.H., Kazanecki, C., Krishna, S., Semeins, C.M., Klein-Nulend, J., 2001. Osteopontin-deficient bone cells are defective in their ability to produce NO in response to pulsatile fluid flow. Biochem. Biophys. Res. Commun. 288, 448–453.

Doi, K., Leelahavanichkul, A., Yuen, P.S., Star, R.A., 2009. Animal models of sepsis and sepsis-induced kidney injury. J. Clin. Invest. 119, 2868–2878.

Domogatskaya, A., Rodin, S., Tryggvason, K., 2012. Functional diversity of laminins. Annu. Rev. Cell Dev. Biol. 28, 523–553.

Eming, S.A., Krieg, T., Davidson, J.M., 2007. Inflammation in wound repair: molecular and cellular mechanisms. J. Invest. Dermatol. 127, 514–525.

Faurschou, M., Borregaard, N., 2003. Neutrophil granules and secretory vesicles in inflammation. Microb. Infect. 5, 1317–1327.

Fausto, N., Laird, A.D., Webber, E.M., 1995. Liver regeneration. 2. Role of growth factors and cytokines in hepatic regeneration. Faseb. J. 9, 1527–1536.

Feliers, D., Kasinath, B.S., 2010. Mechanism of VEGF expression by high glucose in proximal tubule epithelial cells. Mol. Cell. Endocrinol. 314, 136–142.

Freeman, B.A., Crapo, J.D., 1982. Biology of disease: free radicals and tissue injury. Lab. Invest. 47, 412–426.

Gadekar, V., Borade, Y., Kannaujia, S., Rajpoot, K., Anup, N., Tambe, V., Kalia, K., Tekade, R.K., 2021. Nanomedicines accessible in the market for clinical interventions. J. Contr. Release 330, 372–397.

Gauglitz, G.G., Korting, H.C., Pavicic, T., Ruzicka, T., Jeschke, M.G., 2011. Hypertrophic scarring and keloids: pathomechanisms and current and emerging treatment strategies. Mol. Med. 17, 113–125.

Ghanemi, A., Yoshioka, M., St-Amand, J., 2022. Secreted protein acidic and rich in cysteine as an exercise-induced gene. Towards novel molecular therapies for immobilization-related muscle atrophy in elderly patients. Genes 13, 1014.

Gilbert, T.W., Sellaro, T.L., Badylak, S.F., 2006. Decellularization of tissues and organs. Biomaterials 27, 3675–3683.

Gong, T., Liu, L., Jiang, W., Zhou, R., 2020. DAMP-sensing receptors in sterile inflammation and inflammatory diseases. Nat. Rev. Immunol. 20, 95–112.

Gonzalez, A.C.D.O., Costa, T.F., Andrade, Z.D.A., Medrado, A.R.A.P., 2016. Wound healing-a literature review. An. Bras. Dermatol. 91, 614–620.

Gorain, B., Choudhury, H., Tekade, R.K., Karan, S., Jaisankar, P., Pal, T.K., 2016. Comparative biodistribution and safety profiling of olmesartan medoxomil oil-in-water oral nanoemulsion. Regul. Toxicol. Pharmacol. 82, 20–31.

Gosain, A., Dipietro, L.A., 2004. Aging and wound healing. World J. Surg. 28, 321–326.

Gregus, Z., 2010. Chapter 3. Mechanisms of toxicity. In: Klaassen, C.D., Watkins, J.B. (Eds.), Casarett & Doull's Essentials of Toxicology, 2e. The McGraw-Hill Companies, New York, NY.

Grounds, M.D., Sorokin, L., White, J., 2005. Strength at the extracellular matrix-muscle interface. Scand. J. Med. Sci. Sports 15, 381–391.

Guo, S., Dipietro, L.A., 2010. Factors affecting wound healing. J. Dent. Res. 89, 219–229.

Gupta, P.K., 2016. Absorption, distribution, and excretion of toxicants. Fundamentals of Toxicology.

Hader, C., Marlier, A., Cantley, L., 2010. Mesenchymal-epithelial transition in epithelial response to injury: the role of Foxc2. Oncogene 29, 1031–1040.

Halper, J., Kjaer, M., 2014. Basic components of connective tissues and extracellular matrix: elastin, fibrillin, fibulins, fibrinogen, fibronectin, laminin, tenascins and thrombospondins. Adv. Exp. Med. Biol. 802, 31–47.

Hamill, K.J., Kligys, K., Hopkinson, S.B., Jones, J.C., 2009. Laminin deposition in the extracellular matrix: a complex picture emerges. J. Cell Sci. 122, 4409–4417.

Haugh, M.G., Murphy, C.M., Mckiernan, R.C., Altenbuchner, C., O'brien, F.J., 2011. Crosslinking and mechanical properties significantly influence cell attachment, proliferation, and migration within collagen glycosaminoglycan scaffolds. Tissue Eng. Part A 17, 1201–1208.

Hayes, A.W., Kruger, C.L., 2014. Hayes' Principles and Methods of Toxicology. Crc Press.

Hesketh, M., Sahin, K.B., West, Z.E., Murray, R.Z., 2017. Macrophage phenotypes regulate scar formation and chronic wound healing. Int. J. Mol. Sci. 18.

Hosoyama, K., Lazurko, C., Muñoz, M., Mctiernan, C.D., Alarcon, E.I., 2019. Peptide-based functional biomaterials for soft-tissue repair. Front. Bioeng. Biotechnol. 7, 205.

Jaeschke, H., Smith, C.W., 1997. Mechanisms of neutrophil-induced parenchymal cell injury. J. Leukoc. Biol. 61, 647–653.

Johannes, L., Jacob, R., Leffler, H., 2018. Galectins at a glance. J. Cell Sci. 131.

Ju, C., Reilly, T.P., Bourdi, M., Radonovich, M.F., Brady, J.N., George, J.W., Pohl, L.R., 2002. Protective role of Kupffer cells in acetaminophen-induced hepatic injury in mice. Chem. Res. Toxicol. 15, 1504–1513.

Jung, K., Park, H.-J., Kim, Y.-H., Hong, J.-P., 2007. Expression of tumor necrosis factor-α and cyclooxygenase-2 mRNA in porcine split-thickness wounds treated with epidermal growth factor by quantitative real-time PCR. Res. Vet. Sci. 82, 344–348.

Kanbay, M., Kasapoglu, B., Perazella, M.A., 2010. Acute tubular necrosis and pre-renal acute kidney injury: utility of urine microscopy in their evaluation- a systematic review. Int. Urol. Nephrol. 42, 425–433.

Kellogg 3rd, E.W., Fridovich, I., 1975. Superoxide, hydrogen peroxide, and singlet oxygen in lipid peroxidation by a xanthine oxidase system. J. Biol. Chem. 250, 8812–8817.

Kemp, W.L., Burns, D.K., Brown, T.G., 2008. Chapter 1. Cellular Pathology. Pathology: The Big Picture. The McGraw-Hill Companies, New York, NY.

Kester, J.E., 2014. Liver. In: Wexler, P. (Ed.), Encyclopedia of Toxicology, third ed. Academic Press, Oxford.

Klimek, K., Ginalska, G., 2020. Proteins and peptides as important modifiers of the polymer scaffolds for tissue engineering applications-A review. Polymers 12.

Krafts, K.P., 2014. Tissue Repair. Encyclopedia of Toxicology, third ed. Elsevier.

Kusindarta, D., Wihadmadyatami, H., 2018. The role of extracellular matrix in tissue regeneration. Tissue Regen. 65.
Li, J., Chen, J., Kirsner, R., 2007. Pathophysiology of acute wound healing. Clin. Dermatol. 25, 9–18.
Lindley, L.E., Stojadinovic, O., Pastar, I., Tomic-Canic, M., 2016. Biology and biomarkers for wound healing. Plast. Reconstr. Surg. 138, 18s–28s.
Lu, H., Hoshiba, T., Kawazoe, N., Koda, I., Song, M., Chen, G., 2011. Cultured cell-derived extracellular matrix scaffolds for tissue engineering. Biomaterials 32, 9658–9666.
Lund, S.A., Giachelli, C.M., Scatena, M., 2009. The role of osteopontin in inflammatory processes. J. Cell Commun. Signal. 3, 311–322.
Mandal, M., Gardner, C.R., Sun, R., Choi, H., Lad, S., Mishin, V., Laskin, J.D., Laskin, D.L., 2016. The spleen as an extramedullary source of inflammatory cells responding to acetaminophen-induced liver injury. Toxicol. Appl. Pharmacol. 304, 110–120.
Mangipudy, R.S., Chanda, S., Mehendale, H.M., 1995. Tissue repair response as a function of dose in thioacetamide hepatotoxicity. Environ. Health Perspect. 103, 260–267.
Mangipudy, R.S., Rao, P.S., Mehendale, H.M., 1996. Effect of an antimitotic agent colchicine on thioacetamide hepatotoxicity. Environ. Health Perspect. 104, 744–749.
Martin, K.E., García, A.J., 2021. Macrophage phenotypes in tissue repair and the foreign body response: implications for biomaterial-based regenerative medicine strategies. Acta Biomater. 133, 4–16.
Martin, P., 1997. Wound healing—aiming for perfect skin regeneration. Science 276, 75–81.
Mcdaniel, J.C., Belury, M., Ahijevych, K., Blakely, W., 2008. Omega-3 fatty acids effect on wound healing. Wound Repair Regen. 16, 337–345.
Medrado, A.R., Pugliese, L.S., Reis, S.R.A., Andrade, Z.A., 2003. Influence of low level laser therapy on wound healing and its biological action upon myofibroblasts. Laser Surg. Med. 32, 239–244.
Mehendale, H.M., 2005. Tissue repair: an important determinant of final outcome of toxicant-induced injury. Toxicol. Pathol. 33, 41–51.
Mehendale, H.M., 2012. Once initiated, how does toxic tissue injury expand? Trends Pharmacol. Sci. 33, 200–206.
Michalopoulos, G.K., 2007. Liver regeneration. J. Cell. Physiol. 213, 286–300.
Midwood, K.S., Hussenet, T., Langlois, B., Orend, G., 2011. Advances in tenascin-C biology. Cell. Mol. Life Sci. 68, 3175–3199.
Mithieux, S.M., Wise, S.G., Weiss, A.S., 2013. Tropoelastin–a multifaceted naturally smart material. Adv. Drug Deliv. Rev. 65, 421–428.
Mosser, D.M., Edwards, J.P., 2008. Exploring the full spectrum of macrophage activation. Nat. Rev. Immunol. 8, 958–969.
Muniswamy, V.J., Raval, N., Gondaliya, P., Tambe, V., Kalia, K., Tekade, R.K., 2019. 'Dendrimer-Cationized-Albumin' encrusted polymeric nanoparticle improves BBB penetration and anticancer activity of doxorubicin. Int. J. Pharm. 555, 77–99.
Nahrendorf, M., Swirski, F.K., Aikawa, E., Stangenberg, L., Wurdinger, T., Figueiredo, J.L., Libby, P., Weissleder, R., Pittet, M.J., 2007. The healing myocardium sequentially mobilizes two monocyte subsets with divergent and complementary functions. J. Exp. Med. 204, 3037–3047.
Nathan, C., 2006. Neutrophils and immunity: challenges and opportunities. Nat. Rev. Immunol. 6, 173–182.
Ogle, M.E., Segar, C.E., Sridhar, S., Botchwey, E.A., 2016. Monocytes and macrophages in tissue repair: implications for immunoregenerative biomaterial design. Exp. Biol. Med. 241, 1084–1097.
Okamoto, H., Imanaka-Yoshida, K., 2012. Matricellular proteins: new molecular targets to prevent heart failure. Cardiovasc. Ther. 30, e198–e209.
Ortonne, P.D.J.-P., Löning, T., Schmitt, D., Thivolet, J., 2004. Immunomorphological and ultrastructural aspects of keratinocyte migration in epidermal wound healing. Virchows Arch. 392, 217–230.
Parisi, L., Toffoli, A., Ghezzi, B., Mozzoni, B., Lumetti, S., Macaluso, G.M., 2020. A glance on the role of fibronectin in controlling cell response at biomaterial interface. Jpn. Dent. Sci. Rev. 56, 50–55.
Parks, W.C., Wilson, C.L., López-Boado, Y.S., 2004. Matrix metalloproteinases as modulators of inflammation and innate immunity. Nat. Rev. Immunol. 4, 617–629.
Pianta, T.J., Buckley, N.A., Peake, P.W., Endre, Z.H., 2013. Clinical use of biomarkers for toxicant-induced acute kidney injury. Biomark. Med. 7, 441–456.

Pierce, G.F., Mustoe, T.A., Lingelbach, J., Masakowski, V.R., Griffin, G.L., Senior, R.M., Deuel, T.F., 1989. Platelet-derived growth factor and transforming growth factor-beta enhance tissue repair activities by unique mechanisms. J. Cell Biol. 109, 429–440.

Plaa, G., Charbonneau, M., Plante, I., 2014. Detection and evaluation of chemically induced liver injury. Hayes' Principles and Methods of Toxicology.

Poli, G., 1993. Liver damage due to free radicals. Br. Med. Bull. 49, 604–620.

Poli, G., Albano, E., Dianzani, M.U., 1987. The role of lipid peroxidation in liver damage. Chem. Phys. Lipids 45, 117–142.

Pope, C.N.L.J., 2020. An Introduction to Interdisciplinary Toxicology: From Molecules to Man. Academic Press, London.

Prajapati, R.N., Tekade, R.K., Gupta, U., Gajbhiye, V., Jain, N.K., 2009. Dendimer-mediated solubilization, formulation development and in vitro-in vivo assessment of piroxicam. Mol. Pharm. 6, 940–950.

Prydz, K., 2015. Determinants of glycosaminoglycan (GAG) structure. Biomolecules 5, 2003–2022.

Ramachandran, P., Iredale, J.P., Fallowfield, J.A., 2015. Resolution of liver fibrosis: basic mechanisms and clinical relevance. Semin. Liver Dis. 35, 119–131.

Raman, R., Sasisekharan, V., Sasisekharan, R., 2005. Structural insights into biological roles of protein-glycosaminoglycan interactions. Chem. Biol. 12, 267–277.

Reddy, S.P., Mossman, B.T., 2002. Role and regulation of activator protein-1 in toxicant-induced responses of the lung. Am. J. Physiol. Lung Cell Mol. Physiol. 283, L1161–L1178.

Riha, S.M., Maarof, M., Fauzi, M.B., 2021. Synergistic effect of biomaterial and stem cell for skin tissue engineering in cutaneous wound healing: a concise review. Polymers 13, 1546.

Robbins, C.S., Chudnovskiy, A., Rauch, P.J., Figueiredo, J.L., Iwamoto, Y., Gorbatov, R., Etzrodt, M., Weber, G.F., Ueno, T., VAN Rooijen, N., Mulligan-Kehoe, M.J., Libby, P., Nahrendorf, M., Pittet, M.J., Weissleder, R., Swirski, F.K., 2012. Extramedullary hematopoiesis generates Ly-6C(high) monocytes that infiltrate atherosclerotic lesions. Circulation 125, 364–374.

Roefs, M., Sluijter, J., Vader, P., 2020. Extracellular vesicle-associated proteins in tissue repair. Trends Cell Biol. 30, 990–1013.

Rousselle, P., Braye, F., Dayan, G., 2019. Re-epithelialization of adult skin wounds: cellular mechanisms and therapeutic strategies. Adv. Drug Deliv. Rev. 146, 344–365.

Salama, A., Fayed, H.M., Elgohary, R., 2021. L-carnitine alleviated acute lung injuries induced by potassium dichromate in rats: involvement of Nrf2/HO-1 signaling pathway. Heliyon 7, e07207.

Schena, F.P., 1998. Role of growth factors in acute renal failure. Kidney Int. Suppl. 66, S11–S15.

Schvartz, I., Seger, D., Shaltiel, S., 1999. Vitronectin. Int. J. Biochem. Cell Biol. 31, 539–544.

Shankar, K., Vaidya, V.S., Apte, U.M., Manautou, J.E., Ronis, M.J., Bucci, T.J., Mehendale, H.M., 2003. Type 1 diabetic mice are protected from acetaminophen hepatotoxicity. Toxicol. Sci. 73, 220–234.

Sheehy, E., Cunniffe, G., O'brien, F., 2018. Collagen-based biomaterials for tissue regeneration and repair. Peptides and Proteins as Biomaterials for Tissue Regeneration and Repair. Elsevier.

Sheehy, E., Cunniffe, G., O'brien, F., 2017. Collagen-based biomaterials for tissue regeneration and repair. Peptides and Proteins as Biomaterials for Tissue Regeneration and Repair.

Shepherd, A.A., 2003. Nutrition for optimum wound healing. Nurs. Stand. 18, 55–58.

Shingel, K.I., Faure, M.P., Azoulay, L., Roberge, C., Deckelbaum, R.J., 2008. Solid emulsion gel as a vehicle for delivery of polyunsaturated fatty acids: implications for tissue repair, dermal angiogenesis and wound healing. J. Tissue Eng. Regen. Med. 2, 383–393.

Singh, B., Su, Y.-C., Riesbeck, K., 2010. Vitronectin in bacterial pathogenesis: a host protein used in complement escape and cellular invasion. Mol. Microbiol. 78, 545–560.

Singh, P., Schwarzbauer, J.E., 2012. Fibronectin and stem cell differentiation—lessons from chondrogenesis. J. Cell Sci. 125, 3703–3712.

Sorushanova, A., Delgado, L.M., Wu, Z., Shologu, N., Kshirsagar, A., Raghunath, R., Mullen, A.M., Bayon, Y., Pandit, A., Raghunath, M., Zeugolis, D.I., 2019. The collagen suprafamily: from biosynthesis to advanced biomaterial development. Adv. Mater. 31, e1801651.

Spicer, C., 2019. Hydrogel scaffolds for tissue engineering: the importance of polymer choice. Polym. Chem. 11.

Su, W.H., Cheng, M.H., Lee, W.L., Tsou, T.S., Chang, W.H., Chen, C.S., Wang, P.H., 2010. Nonsteroidal anti-inflammatory drugs for wounds: pain relief or excessive scar formation? Mediat. Inflamm. 2010, 413238.

Swift, M.E., Burns, A.L., Gray, K.L., Dipietro, L.A., 2001. Age-related alterations in the inflammatory response to dermal injury. J. Invest. Dermatol. 117, 1027–1035.

Swirski, F.K., Nahrendorf, M., Etzrodt, M., Wildgruber, M., Cortez-Retamozo, V., Panizzi, P., Figueiredo, J.L., Kohler, R.H., Chudnovskiy, A., Waterman, P., Aikawa, E., Mempel, T.R., Libby, P., Weissleder, R., Pittet, M.J., 2009. Identification of splenic reservoir monocytes and their deployment to inflammatory sites. Science 325, 612–616.

Tayebi, L., Moharamzadeh, K., 2017. Biomaterials for Oral and Dental Tissue Engineering.

Tekade, R.K., Chougule, M.B., 2013. Formulation development and evaluation of hybrid nanocarrier for cancer therapy: taguchi orthogonal array based design. BioMed Res. Int. 2013, 712678.

Theilgaard-Mönch, K., Knudsen, S., Follin, P., Borregaard, N., 2004. The transcriptional activation program of human neutrophils in skin lesions supports their important role in wound healing. J. Immunol. 172, 7684–7693.

van Benthem, P., 2021. Skills development-Toxicology MSDT.

Varkey, M., Ding, J., Tredget, E.E., 2015. Advances in skin substitutes—potential of tissue engineered skin for facilitating anti-fibrotic healing. J. Funct. Biomater. 6, 547–563.

Vindin, H., Mithieux, S.M., Weiss, A.S., 2019. Elastin architecture. Matrix Biol. 84, 4–16.

Wang, T., Fontenot, R.D., Soni, M.G., Bucci, T.J., Mehendale, H.M., 2000a. Enhanced hepatotoxicity and toxic outcome of thioacetamide in streptozotocin-induced diabetic rats. Toxicol. Appl. Pharmacol. 166, 92–100.

Wang, T., Shankar, K., Bucci, T.J., Warbritton, A., Mehendale, H.M., 2001. Diallyl sulfide inhibition of CYP2E1 does not rescue diabetic rats from thioacetamide-induced mortality. Toxicol. Appl. Pharmacol. 173, 27–37.

Wang, T., Shankar, K., Ronis, M.J., Mehendale, H.M., 2000b. Potentiation of thioacetamide liver injury in diabetic rats is due to induced CYP2E1. J. Pharmacol. Exp. Therapeut. 294, 473–479.

Wang, T., Shankar, K., Ronis, M.J., Mehendale, H.M., 2007. Mechanisms and outcomes of drug- and toxicant-induced liver toxicity in diabetes. Crit. Rev. Toxicol. 37, 413–459.

Wang, W., Li, P., Li, W., Jiang, J., Cui, Y., Li, S., Wang, Z., 2017. Osteopontin activates mesenchymal stem cells to repair skin wound. PLoS One 12, e0185346.

Wartenberg, A., Weisser, J., Schnabelrauch, M., 2021. Glycosaminoglycan-based cryogels as scaffolds for cell cultivation and tissue regeneration. Molecules 26, 5597.

Wilgus, T.A., Roy, S., Mcdaniel, J.C., 2013. Neutrophils and wound repair: positive actions and negative reactions. Adv. Wound Care 2, 379–388.

Witko-Sarsat, V., Rieu, P., Descamps-Latscha, B., Lesavre, P., Halbwachs-Mecarelli, L., 2000. Neutrophils: molecules, functions and pathophysiological aspects. Lab. Invest. 80, 617–653.

Witzgall, R., Brown, D., Schwarz, C., Bonventre, J.V., 1994. Localization of proliferating cell nuclear antigen, vimentin, c-Fos, and clusterin in the postischemic kidney. Evidence for a heterogenous genetic response among nephron segments, and a large pool of mitotically active and dedifferentiated cells. J. Clin. Invest. 93, 2175–2188.

Wynn, T.A., Vannella, K.M., 2016. Macrophages in tissue repair, regeneration, and fibrosis. Immunity 44, 450–462.

Youngren, S.R., Tekade, R.K., Gustilo, B., Hoffmann, P.R., Chougule, M.B., 2013. STAT6 siRNA matrix-loaded gelatin nanocarriers: formulation, characterization, and ex vivo proof of concept using adenocarcinoma cells. BioMed Res. Int. 2013, 858946.

Zhang, Q., Raoof, M., Chen, Y., Sumi, Y., Sursal, T., Junger, W., Brohi, K., Itagaki, K., Hauser, C.J., 2010. Circulating mitochondrial DAMPs cause inflammatory responses to injury. Nature 464, 104–107.

CHAPTER

9

Computer-aided technologies in drug discovery and toxicity prediction

Bhakti Pawar[1], *Santosh Kumar Behera*[1], *Muktika Tekade*[2], *Nizar Al-Shar'i*[3] *and Rakesh Kumar Tekade*[1]

[1]National Institute of Pharmaceutical Education and Research (NIPER)- Ahmedabad, An Institute of National Importance, Government of India, Department of Pharmaceuticals, Ministry of Chemicals and Fertilizers, Palaj, Gandhinagar, Gujarat, India; [2]School of Pharmacy, Devi Ahilya Vishwavidyalaya, Indore, Madhya Pradesh, India; [3]Faculty of Pharmacy, Jordan University of Science and Technology, Irbid, Jordan

9.1 Introduction

Drug discovery and development is a lengthy, complex, and cost-intensive process (Gadekar et al., 2021; Gorain et al., 2016; Muniswamy et al., 2019; Prajapati et al., 2009). It is usually associated with a high risk of failure (a drug candidate will not succeed), as high as up to 96% (Hinkson et al., 2020). Data obtained from clinical trials have shown four main reasons for such failures: lack of clinical efficacy, toxicity, poor drug-likeness, and poor strategic planning and commercial value. Toxicity-related issues account for about 30% of these failures (Duxin Sun et al., 2022). Therefore, the utilization of computational methods to accelerate and enrich drug discovery processes is steadily growing in all aspects of product development (Youngren et al., 2013; Tekade and Chougule, 2013). These methods have established milestones in the drug development pipeline, from target identification and mechanism of action to lead and drug candidate identification. A computer model for finding nontoxic medicinal compounds from a pool of small molecules is always appreciated in the pharmaceutical industry (Macalino et al., 2015).

Currently, ample computational tools and techniques have been used to measure drug safety and efficacy. For drug safety assessment, generally, in-vitro and in-vivo tests are implemented. Computational methods are always preferable to these in vitro and in vivo experimental techniques because they are efficient, quick, affordable, accurate, and, majorly, they may be carried out before a chemical is manufactured. Several computer-aided drug design

https://doi.org/10.1016/B978-0-443-15840-7.00004-X

(CADD) techniques are used nowadays to shorten the tenure of drug discovery. It helps scientists to focus mainly on the most promising compounds. Computational power is being used to accelerate the drug research and development process throughout the globe. Scientists use chemical and biological information regarding ligands and/or targets to find and improve novel medicines. There are many computational techniques that are available today for assessing drug safety that is classified into three classes: read-across, qualitative as well as quantitative regression. At the early stages of compound safer evaluation, it is more important to determine if a drug candidate is hazardous or nonhazardous, extremely hazardous or mildly hazardous, instead of the exact toxicity level (Yang et al., 2018).

QSTR models might be developed for a small number of chemical analogs to predict their precise toxicity values. Moreover, read-across is also a viable method for predicting some toxicity endpoints from comparable structures with experimental toxicity values for such a small set of molecules. Such approaches possess excellent accuracy, particularly in the local chemical space, and may occasionally substitute cell culture or animal studies to get specific outcomes. Additionally, structure warnings might be obtained from the models to induce detrimental signs on tissues that scientists could utilize to modify the structure to minimize the risk in early drug discovery (Pizzo et al., 2015).

ADME investigations aim to learn how a chemical (drug compound/medication molecule) is metabolized within the body. This process frequently includes toxicology tests, which result in the acronym ADMET. The reason behind focusing mainly on drug toxicity is, according to (Guengerich, 2011), that factors such as human pharmacokinetics, clinical efficacy, financial, formulation, and preclinical toxicity, and clinical-stage adverse events are majorly related to drug toxicity. Among all the factors, preclinical toxicity constitutes almost 31%. One of the most significant aspects of existing drug development is the prediction of a drug candidate's toxicity. Although in vivo toxicology studies will always be necessary, in silico toxicity studies assist in avoiding the high expense, labor time, and ethical concerns associated with animal research. Acute (one-time) or repeated exposures can determine toxicity at varying dosages and via various ingestion methods. Toxicity Checker, PreADMET, ProTox-II, eMolTox, TOXNET, ToxiM, ToxCast, Tox21, SuperToxic, and Lazar toxicity are some of the currently used web servers/databases for investigating the toxicity of a compound.

Multiple computer models have been created to enhance in silico drug toxicity predictions. There are few computer-based (in silico) methods to study the toxicity of new chemical entities which detect structural alerts (SAs). SAs are necessary substructures that cause toxicity. They are linked to toxicity, so medicinal chemists could use them to improve the structure of drugs to lower the risk. Automatic identification of structural alerts by in silico methods has become a trend with the growth of chemoinformatics and the explosion of accessible information. Many techniques and tools for detecting SAs have been developed, including SARpy, a fragment-based technique (Ferrari et al., 2013), whereas MolFea and MoSS are graph-based techniques (Yang et al., 2017).

SARpy (SAR in python) is a technique that creates a SAR (structure-activity relationship) model using big data without any prior information. SARpy (fragment-based method) considers only complete branches or cycles as SA. It is a free technique that works on the principle of string mining to generate substructures (Ferrari et al., 2013). Drug side effects are among the leading causes of death in developed countries. Toxicology is cited as the second most frequent justification for abandoning the development of innovative pharmaceuticals during future stages of clinical trials and removing drugs from the market. Structure-activity relationships (SARs) can predict ADEs from the earliest phases of drug development since, unlike other methods, they need knowledge of the structural formulas of drug candidates. To meet the requirement of in silico drug adversity investigation, a cost-free ADVERPred was made available to estimate five ADEs related to the chemical structure (Ivanov et al., 2018). MoSS is a graph-based technique that defines a chemical molecule as a mathematical graph. The graph contains a group of vertices and edges, representing atoms and bonds of composites, respectively. The next step is to find substructures by using graphical information.

MolFea, a linear substructure mining program, uses the Levels Version Space algorithm to address the lowest and highest frequency limitations. However, as MolFea only considers linear substructures, its limitations are apparent. This shortcoming was overcome by the MoSS approach, which utilizes depth-first search association rules for mining substructures containing cyclic structures as well as aliphatic chains (Yang et al., 2017).

Another tool for predicting molecule's toxicity is the ToxAlerts, which gathers structural alerts discovered via computational methods or specified by professionals. It can anticipate toxicity based on the presence of structural alerts. Expert techniques rely on experts' skills as well as experience to infer the mechanistic pathway of toxicity (Van Leeuwen et al., 2009). This can be done for individual chemicals or entire chemical classes. Unlike reading across, which is utilized to conclude toxicity from similar chemicals, structural warnings are intended to identify potential risks and aid in understanding the underlying process. Expert methods are designed to assist in evaluating chemicals for which no prior knowledge is available, so they can utilize mechanistic evidence and data from safety screenings to decide their safety profile.

9.1.1 The read-across method

It is a technique for filling in data gaps for new chemical entities. It is based on the generation of chemical groups from structural data. The fundamental principle is that the bioactivities of similar structures will be similar (Johnson and Maggiora, 1990; Escher and Bitsch, 2021). As a result, read-across is carried out by recognizing related compounds and analyzing their bioactivity, inferring the parent compound's nontoxicity.

The TIMES model belongs to the hybrid category that includes the theory of toxicity. It contains a reference library of possible bio-metabolic alterations in addition to abiotic processes and the probability of their occurrence under particular conditions (Arabi, 2021). The harmful effects are measured after alterations in the model that utilizes transformation probabilities or rate data decoded from biotransformation charts. The mutagenicity endpoint was used to assess the TIMES model's capacity to generate activated metabolites. This model takes into account the various biotransformation ways which might be used for the detoxification of compounds following biotransformation. Around 30 biotransformations (reactions such as hydroxylation, tautomerization, acetylation, sulfation, oxidation, hydrolysis, dealkylation, glucuronidation, dehalogenation isomerization, and epoxidation were studied).

Limeng Pu et al. described eToxPred, a novel method for estimating the toxicological pathways for molecules with high accuracy. To assess NCEs, eToxPred uses algorithms of ML trained on molecular fingerprints. Multiple datasets comprising well-known medicines, potentially dangerous substances, natural products, and synthesized bioactive compounds are utilized for the assessment of the outcome. On the other hand, eToxPred predicts accuracy for the ability of synthesis and toxicity with an average square error of just 4% and 72%, respectively (Pu et al., 2019).

Sanguinetti MC et al. noted an extensive set of drugs could cause fatal cardiac arrhythmia by blocking the hERG (human Ether-à-go-go-Related Gene) channels of K^+ ion. As a result, accurate detection of presumed nonblockers, as well as hERG blockers in the compound reference library, is critical for cardiotoxicity prediction. Pred-hERG, a recently developed technique, uses characteristics based on externally predictive QSAR models of hERG blockade to evaluate cardiac toxicity. A binary model, Pred-hERG, uses atomic contribution possibility charts as well as a multiclass model; both are integrated for the final prediction. It gives high prediction accuracy around. Pred-hERG has a highly accurate classification rate of 0.8 and a multiclass accuracy of 0.7, which is encouraging (Sanguinetti and Tristani-Firouzi, 2006).

ChemTox (http://www.cyprotex.com/insilico/physiological modeling/chemtox) can be used to predict essential toxicity characteristics such as Ames mutagenicity and medium lethal dose (LD_{50}) (Mortelmans and Zeiger, 2000). Molecular descriptors are being used to develop QSPR methods, which are usually obtained with a compound structure. Because this technique relies on a collection of specialized descriptors to create QSPR models for specific toxicity, it may not be appropriate for assessing toxicity and medication side effects. Like chemTox, based on the study of toxic fragments found in drugs with established LD_{50} values, ProTox predicts rodent oral toxicity (Drwal et al., 2014). But the advantage of using ProTox is with a collection of protein-ligand pharmacophores, known as toxicophores. ProTox also assesses potential targets linked through undesired drug effects and the primary toxic pathways.

Researchers have designed the models to estimate the toxicity of six different classes utilizing an LLL (local lazy learning) technique for multiple learning (tumorigenicity, acute toxicity, skin and eye irritation, mutagenicity, multiple-dose effects, and reproductive consequences) (Lu et al., 2017). They verified almost 17,120 molecules and added molecular fingerprints (FCFP_4 and ECFP_4), chemical-chemical interaction, as well as descriptors. The working of the model was satisfactory for the above-mentioned toxicities, as well as specific vital structures responsible for toxicity were found (Alqahtani, 2017).

9.2 Toxicity evaluation by in silico methods at an early phase

Twenty to 40% of drug rejections during drug discovery are attributable to safety limits. Even before the drug is synthesized, it is a good idea to check for potential toxicity. For this purpose, many in silico models using various methodologies for toxicity prediction have been developed. In the following section, we have discussed how in silico techniques help to predict different toxicities at early drug discovery.

9.2.1 Carcinogenicity and mutagenicity

The Carcinogenic Potency Database (CPDB) is used for the majority of predictive models in which $\geq$1500 compounds are listed and named as (cancer-causing agents or noncancer-causing agents) based on their TD_{50} values (Gold et al., 2005). Models such as Naïve Bayes, kNN, probabilistic neural network, and SVM are used to predict chemical carcinogenesis (Tanabe et al., 2013; Zhang et al., 2016; Singh et al., 2013; Li et al., 2015). Zhang et al. created CarcinoPred-EL, which allows researchers to estimate the ability of a compound to cause cancer with the help of software.

9.2.2 Hepatotoxicity

Kim et al. employed weighted molecular fingerprints to create a computational algorithm for the estimation of DILI. They have utilized 881 sections of molecular fingerprints as a standard for representing the existence or nonexistence of every substructure of chemicals. Random forest and support vector machine techniques are used to screen the bioactive constituents present in the herbal compounds that cause DILI. According to the prediction results, many herbal substances can potentially produce drug-induced liver impairment (Kim and Nam, 2017).

From 2000 to 2015, Hewitt explored in silico models for drug-induced liver injury prediction. Models like statistics as well as expert-based systems were utilized (Ellison et al., 2022). In these models, hybrid or chemical descriptors were utilized as standard. Several ML approaches, like linear discriminant analysis and ANN, were applied to determine overall hepatotoxicity endpoints (Yang et al., 2018).

Zhu and Kruhlak used pharmacovigilance data from the FDA adverse event reporting system to create a human hepatotoxicity database for QSTR models (Zhu and Kruhlak, 2014). Various approaches (SVM logistic regression, gradient boosting AdaBoost, Xgboost, Catboost Lightgbm, and ExtraTrees) were developed to estimate liver toxicity or DILI. A DILI rank dataset containing 450 compounds was divided into 400:50 for evaluation, as well as five times cross-validation was used. An entire procedure was carried out 100 times. The eight fingerprints among the 12 were chosen using FDA data. The best five among nine base classifiers and seven molecular descriptors were used (Wang et al., 2019).

9.2.3 Acute oral toxicity

Acute toxicity is mainly classified as inhalational, oral, and dermal. From all of this, this toxicity is mainly evaluated for computerized evaluation. Zhu et al. collected 7385 chemicals with LD_{50} values and developed different models for chemical acute oral toxicity prediction. Several machine-learning approaches were created and implemented based on the dataset to generate classifiers and regression models to estimate LD_{50} (Zhu et al., 2009).

9.2.4 Irritation and corrosion

In the pharmaceutical and cosmetics sectors, ocular and dermal corrosion/irritation is a paramount concern. To predict dermal and ocular corrosion, researchers have analyzed the present models in Toxtree, Case Ultra, and Derek Nexus (Verheyen et al., 2017). They found their performance inadequate due to their slight pertinence domain and low accuracy.

9.2.5 Endocrine disruption

Endocrine disruption can be caused by chemicals that interact through receptors located on the nucleus, like androgen (AR) and estrogen receptors (ER), as improper targeting. Or when they are opened to the surrounding. Chen et al. (2014) utilized molecular fingerprints and ML approaches for creating in silico approaches for the estrogen receptor and androgen receptor binding, with the excellent result in the investigation being 0.79 and 0.84, respectively (Chen et al., 2014).

9.3 Risk mitigation in the early drug discovery phase and guiding compound design and selection

It is well known that drug toxicity is a leading cause of drug failure in the late phase and withdrawal of the drug from the market. The primary risk factors related to drug toxicity can be categorized into (1) drug-related (toxic reactive metabolite) and (2) patient-related (genetic and nongenetic processes). The liver is a major target organ for toxicity. Thompson et al. proposed using a Hepatic Liability Panel together with in vitro techniques to detect reactive metabolites for decreasing risk, which therapeutic candidates would lead to liver damage (idiosyncratic and non-idiosyncratic). This will allow researchers to design and select the drug that is less likely to cause liver damage in the discovery stage. The panel is measured utilizing toxicity tests which measure CYP450-dependent and mitochondrial damage, bile salt export pump inhibition, and independent cell toxicity (Thompson et al., 2011).

9.4 Techniques to avoid and minimize reactive metabolites

An optimal risk mitigation plan for RM should give reliable, quantitative data that can be used to support decision-making and reflect the level of clinical hazard. It is the most critical step in late drug discovery when it's time to decide whether or not to pursue certain compounds through the development and clinical phases. To evaluate this problem, it has been suggested that assessing drug and/or metabolite covalent binding on hepatic proteins can give a meaningful, measurable indication of the extent of safety reactive metabolite (Evans et al., 2004).

Notably, the strongest association was seen when covalent binding in human hepatocytes was combined with dose, whereas dose alone can't effectively differentiate among medicines in various classes of safety groups (Nakayama et al., 2009). This will entail using technologies that can identify specific flaws in compounds and be utilized in conjunction with the time intervals and capacities required during the design of the process. (i) SAs, (ii) in vitro Hepatic Liability Panel assays (BSEP, THLE toxicity, and HepG2 mitochondrial toxicity will be used. (iii) in vitro DMPK assays (trapping of electrophilic intermediates, time-dependent CYP inhibition, assessment of acyl glucuronide stability, and metabolite identification), We anticipate that once the Hepatotoxicity Matrix is validated, we can choose molecules for studying important parameters such as ADME, the ability of a compound to cause liver damage, efficacy.

For example, thiazolidinediones, a class of drugs used to treat people with Type 2 diabetes, exemplify how we think our mitigation strategy will offer value. Troglitazone, the first commercial drug in the class, was taken off the market in the United States in the year 2000 because of hepatic injury. Compared to novel molecules such as Pioglitazone and Rosiglitazone, they seem to have a much lesser risk of hepatotoxicity that is commonly utilized for treating diabetes. The exact reason behind the toxicity of Troglitazone is not yet apparent. In contrast, much information about Rosiglitazone and Pioglitazone is available about their relative safety and toxicity in the public domain.

If we consider the key features by reviewing the available data for all the three drugs (Troglitazone, Rosiglitazone, and Pioglitazone), such as daily dose, covalent binding in human hepatocytes (Usui et al., 2009), cell toxicity (Lloyd et al., 2002; Gao et al., 2004), and BSEP inhibition (Masubuchi, 2006; Snow and Moseley, 2007; Roth and Ganey, 2010), it was clear that when the dose is not taken into account, comparing with remaining two drugs, Troglitazone shows stronger covalent binding; however, daily dose and covalent binding places Troglitazone in a separate reactive metabolite class than Pioglitazone and Rosiglitazone as shown in Fig. 9.1. As a result, in the screening stage, researchers can get an idea of whether or not to pursue a particular drug.

Table 9.1 compares the three thiazolidinediones based on their daily dose, covalent binding, covalent binding × dose, hepatotoxicity classification, cell cytotoxicity, bile salt export pump inhibition, and CYP bioactivation. Collecting such quantitative data will help plan the risk mitigation of reactive metabolites.

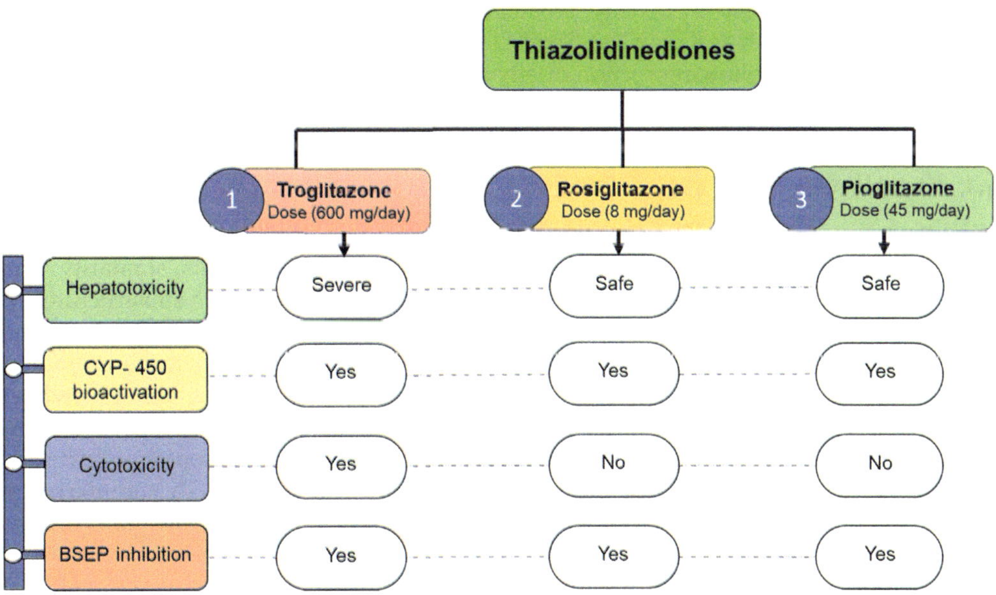

FIGURE 9.1 Brief description of thiazolidinediones.

TABLE 9.1 Comparative study of thiazolidinediones based on different parameters.

Parameters	Troglitazone	Rosiglitazone	Pioglitazone	References
Daily dose (mg/day)	600	8	45	Usui et al. (2009)
Covalent binding (pmol/mg protein) was determined with the help of four-arm assays by using NADPH, UDPGA, $MgCl_2$, and GSH	118	11	11	Usui et al. (2009)
Covalent binding × dose	70,800	88	495	Usui et al. (2009)
Hepatotoxicity classification (based on the in vitro DMPK assay)	Severe (withdrawn)	Safe (no label)	Safe (no label)	Nakayama et al. (2009)
Cell cytotoxicity (determined by performing various in vitro DMPK assays)	Yes	No	No	Masubuchi (2006)
Bile salt export pump inhibition	Yes	Yes	Yes	Snow and Moseley (2007)
CYP bioactivation	Yes	Yes	Yes	–

9.5 Different in silico toxicological approaches and case studies of toxicity prediction

In silico techniques used in toxicity prediction are primarily based on machine learning models. Web servers such as KnowTox, ToxiM, and ProTox-II, are the most widely used tools to predict toxicity. The following section briefly discusses the outline of these webservers and case studies describing how they can help predict the toxicity of a compound.

9.5.1 KnowTox

KnowTox demands an input such as query compound and offers in silico risk assessment support. It encompasses conformal prediction with 88 ToxCast endpoints, similarity search for supporting read-across, and use of structural alert for searching toxic substructures. For example, KnowTox has been applied to study two triazoles among in-house datasets. These have been discontinued for a variety of factors despite being expected to be antifungals. These two structures contain epoxide, triazole attached with thioether, and phenyl with halogen groups. Based on the estimations of all 88 conformal prediction models, both triazoles were active at 15 endpoints concerning DNA binding, nuclear receptor, cytokine, cell cycle, cell adhesion molecules, cell morphology, proteases, and CYP. To summarize, the conformal prediction models produce reasonable predictions for the possible harmful consequences of these molecules.

Furthermore, it was found that with the pursuit of SA, toxicity estimation is aided by evidence from the available data regarding substructures already having toxicity endpoints.

Three structural alerts (acyclic bivalent sulfur moiety, halogenated benzene, and epoxide) were found for Triazoles 1 & 2. Liu et al. have studied a total of 23 therapeutic moieties comprising acyclic bivalent sulfur molecules. Eight have been linked to liver toxicity, while the remaining 14 are probably liver toxic. Although liver toxicity may be ruled out, potential liver toxicity for these moieties should be considered. Another important note is offered in the case of epoxide substructure, which is a highly reactive group; it makes the structure more electrophile.

Generally, nucleophiles will attack electrophile molecules, generating a ring-opening mechanism involved in an S_N2-type reaction, leading to mutagenicity or carcinogenicity. Moreover, risk assessment was performed by taking advantage of the ToxCast database. ToxCast database was used to separate 7912 chemicals for a query compound to find the compounds with the maximum Tanimoto resemblance. The toxicity data of these most comparable molecules are shown. Next, a similarity search was carried out where eight somewhat similar molecules were found to be similar. The resemblances were seen in triazole-substructure and halogenated benzene. The similarity search does not find any additional molecules with an epoxide substructure. Even though ToxCast provides 985 assays, the two most resembled structures for triazoles were studied. Propiconazole, alike triazole 1, was found to be active at various endpoints for nuclear receptors, among others (for example, estrogen, CAR, thyroid receptors, PXR as well as androgen), GPCRs (for example, opioid receptors, muscarinic histamine receptor H2 as well as cholinergic receptors), and cytochromes P450 (1a, 2c, 2b, 2d, 3a, 19).

Similarly, bromuconazole, the most comparable molecule to triazole 2, was mostly limited to receptors present on the nucleus (examples; retinoic acid, PXR estrogen receptors, and androgen), cytochromes P450 (3a, 2a, 19A12b, 2c), and DNA binding (p53, AhR sterol regulatory element-binding protein). Note that the substitution of halogen is a crucial step. For example, bromine in bromuconazole is highly reactive than F- and Cl- substitution. As a result, specific toxic effects in bromuconazole may be more distinct than in compounds lacking Br-functional group, like triazoles 1&2. As a result, certain harmful effects in bromuconazole may be more distinct compared to moieties with no Br, like triazoles (1&2) (Liu et al., 2015).

Briefly, in-house investigations revealed that animals that were previously injected with two triazoles had shown signs of liver enzyme upregulation, liver damage, and aromatase inhibition. In addition to this information about triazoles, Knebel et al. have recently explained the molecular mechanism behind triazole-induced liver toxicity. The KnowTox program reproduces the significant in vivo effects of 1 & 2 triazole drugs that were previously considered for development (Knebel et al., 2019; Morger et al., 2020) (Fig. 9.2).

9.5.2 ToxiM

ToxiM is Machine Learning-based webserver that supports and categorizes molecules into two classes. Generally, the toxicity of a query molecule will be predicted with the assistance of regression models for aqueous solubility and permeability with the Caco-2 cell line.

9.5.2.1 How to use the ToxiM webserver?

The user can submit the query compound via its PubChem CID or insert a structural data file (SDF) file to the toxicity prediction website. For toxicity prediction, the SDF is run through

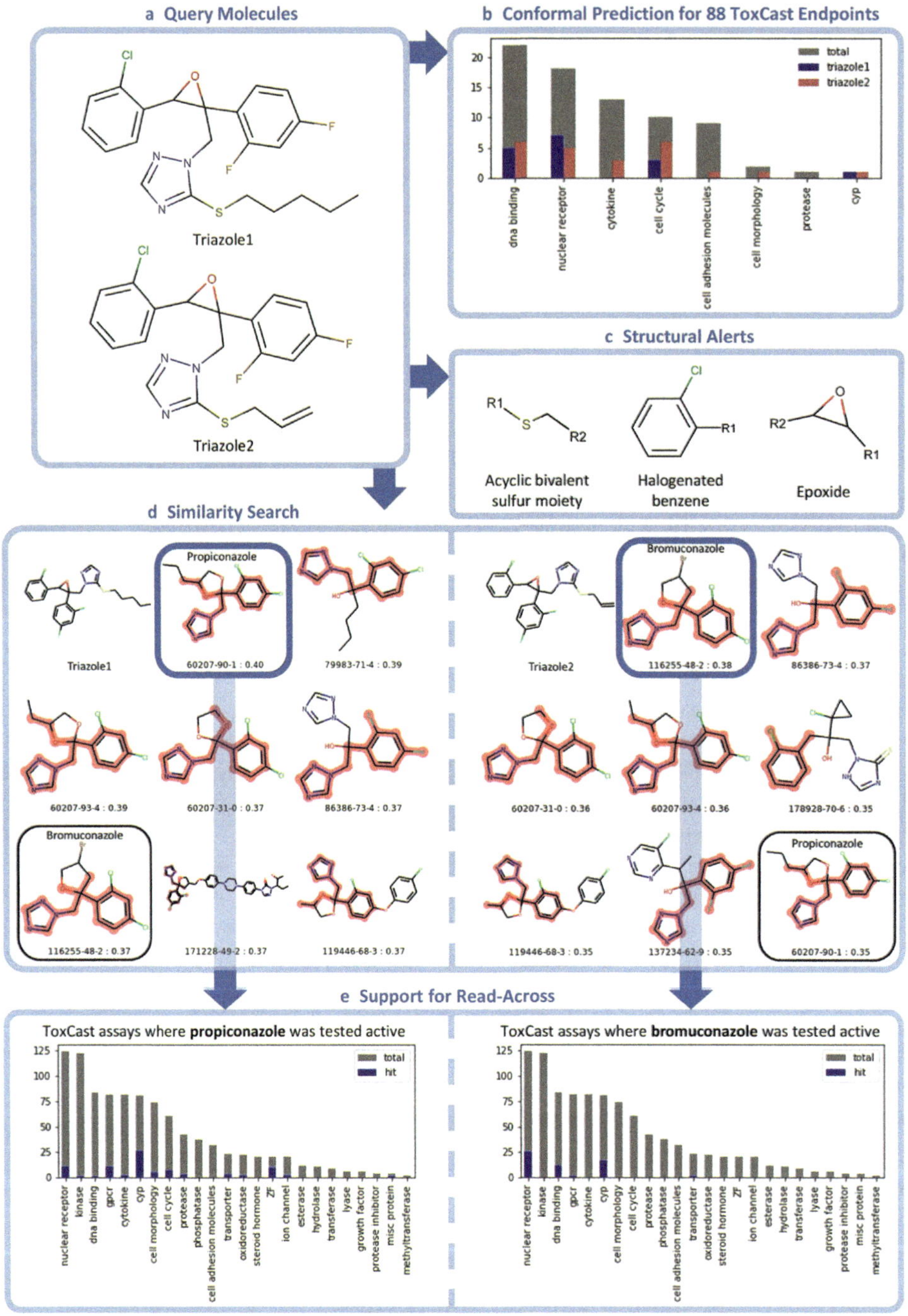

FIGURE 9.2 Stepwise guidance for the user to apply the KnowTox tool. (A) Two different Triazoles (1 and 2) are presented as a query. (B) Conformal prediction for different endpoints (Gray). Red and Blue triazoles 1 and triazole 2 seem to be active (C) Structural alerts for triazoles 1&2. (D) Similarity search found for Triazole 1 and triazole 2 and their most similar molecules in ToxCast with CAS number as well as Tanimoto similarity. Red marked order displays the most common substructure. (E) Experimental information from ToxCast for propiconazole (left) and bromuconazole (right). Gray: assays present in ToxCast. Blue: (active compound). *Adopted from Morger, A., Mathea, M., Achenbach, J. H., Wolf, A., Buesen, R., Schleifer, K. J., Landsiedel, R., Volkamer, A., 2020. KnowTox: pipeline and case study for confident prediction of potential toxic effects of compounds in early phases of development. J. Cheminf. 12, 1–17 under a Creative Commons Attribution 4.0 International License (https://creativecommons.org/licenses/by/4.0/legalcode).*

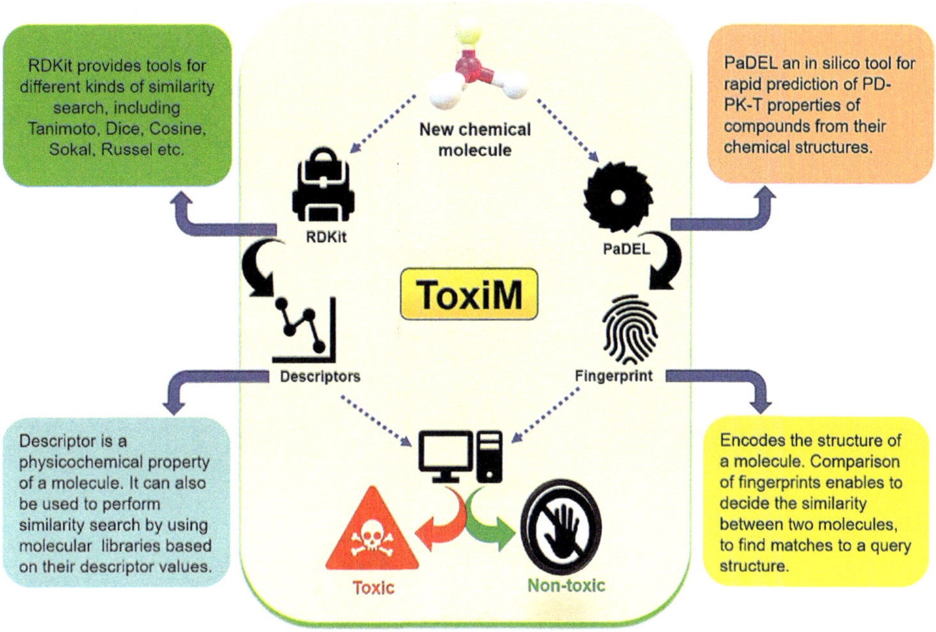

FIGURE 9.3 Schematic presentation of ToxiM webserver.

the web server's algorithm. A total of three models were present in the ToxiM webserver: fingerprint, descriptor, and hybrid. The given SDF file is then run through these models. The input compound is analyzed through the selected models and is then classified into two categories: toxic and nontoxic (Fig. 9.3). The webserver is available at http://metagenomics.iiserb.ac.in/ToxiM/. Detailed information on toxicity prediction by ToxiM is given on the website (Sharma et al., 2017).

9.5.3 ProTox-II

The ProTox-II interface is simple and user-friendly. The user can type the compound's name or insert the Simplified Molecular-Input Line-Entry System (SMILES) series of chemicals to forecast its probable toxicities. There are five main classification steps in the ProTox-II platform: (i) toxicological pathways (12 models), (ii) toxicity targets (15 models), (iii) toxico logical endpoints (four models), (iv) acute toxicity (oral toxicity model with six different toxicity classes), and (v) organ toxicity (one model) as shown in Fig. 9.4. The user gets the option of drawing the chemical structure by using the chemical editor. In the next section, we briefly discussed the toxicity prediction of Etonogestrel and Tolcapone using the ProTox-II webserver as case studies.

9.5.3.1 Etonogestrel

Etonogestrel is approved as a hormonal contraceptive categorized under the fifth level of toxicity for acute oral toxicity with an LD_{50} concentration of 5000 mg/kg with a usual

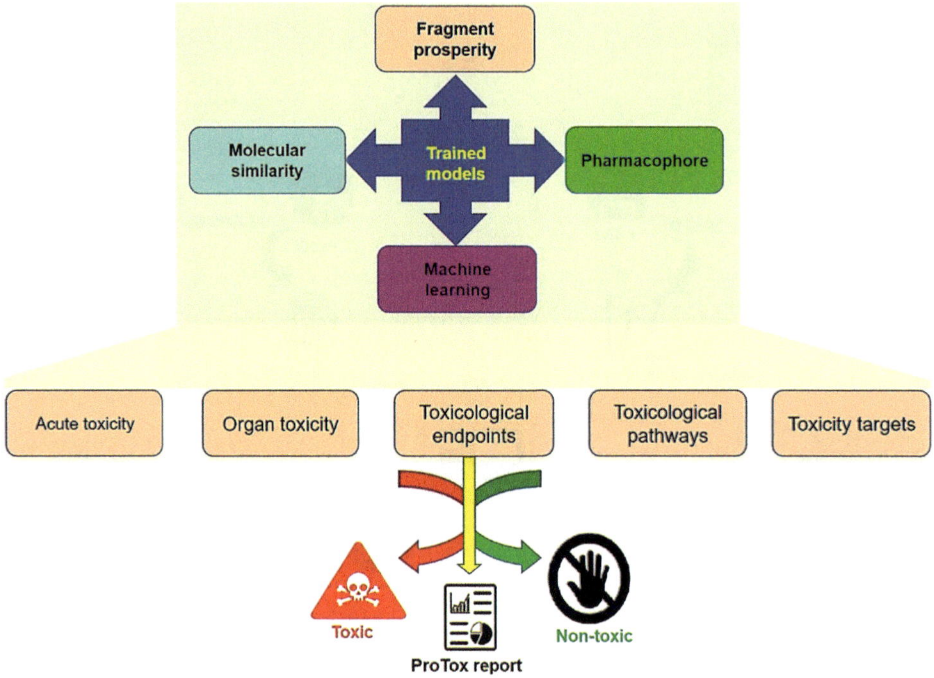

FIGURE 9.4 Flowchart for ProTox-II webserver.

similarity and prediction accuracy of 92.31% and 72.9%, respectively. A confidence score is a number between 0 and 1 that indicates the probability that a Machine Learning model's output is valid and will meet a user's request. The confidence score for organ toxicity (liver toxicity) of etonogestrel was found to be 0.68. It was seen that for five various toxicity pathways (ER, ARLBD, ER-LBD, SR-ARE, and NR-AR), etonogestrel was found to be active along with maximum confidence scores of 0.76, 0.94, 0.73, 0.57, and 0.96, resp. (Banerjee et al., 2018).

Moreover, etonogestrel shows toxicity against three targets, Androgen Receptor, Amine Oxidase A, and Progesterone Receptor A. Though etonogestrel is categorized in the lesser acute toxic class, it was found to cause liver damage and is simultaneously active for three toxicity targets and five toxicity pathways. However, etonogestrel is safe; its interaction with molecular targets might show a toxic effect.

9.5.3.2 *Tolcapone*

Tolcapone is a withdrawn drug (catechol-o-methyl transferase inhibitor). It is an excellent compound that connects different designs under the ProTox-II method (Siramshetty et al., 2016). Tolcapone has an LD_{50} value of 1600 mg/kg, which is described as the fourth toxicity class for acute oral toxicity. An average similarity and prediction toxicity value for Tolcapone was found to be 100%, respectively. Tolcapone was studied for its organ toxicity (hepatotoxicity), and the predicted confidence score was 0.79.

In contrast, the confidence score for the toxicological endpoint (immunotoxicity) was 0.52 (Desbonnet et al., 2012). Furthermore, Tolcapone, with a confidence score of 0.99, was found active for MMP toxicity. It was predicted that Tolcapone has a low binding affinity with Prostaglandin G/H Synthase 1 and Amine Oxidase A. This is an excellent example that shows molecules can be active for more than one type of toxicity, therefore, can exhibit severe toxic effects.

9.6 Conclusion

Using the in silico toxicity prediction technique is an alternative to animal testing. Toxicity determination of any new chemical entity has become the easiest task due to the availability of different toxicity databases, web servers, and software. However, it is imperative to have a model that will perform precisely so we can apply it to the novel compound confidently. This will give an idea about the applicability of the software. Moreover, it is also crucial that the model should suggest reliable and informative predictions. Machine learning-based models involve a popular confidence estimation technique, conformal prediction. Conformal prediction helps to optimize the models with little effort and gives reliable predictions. However, there is a growing need for robust in silico tools which will give both reliability and applicability. The more we use in silico tools, the more knowledge we can gain from them, ultimately leading to better toxicity prediction.

9.7 List of abbreviations

ANN Artificial neural network
Aq. Aqueous
BSEP Bile salt export pump inhibition
CADD Computer-aided drug design
CAR Chimeric antigen receptor
CPDB Carcinogenic Potency Database
DILI Drug-induced liver injury
DMPK Drug metabolism pharmacokinetic
ECFP Extended connectivity fingerprint
FCFP Feature-class fingerprint
GPCRs *G-protein*-coupled receptors
GSH Glutathione
hERG Human Ether-à-go-go-Related Gene
LLL Local lazy learning
MMP Matrix metalloproteinase
NADPH Nicotinamide adenine dinucleotide phosphate
NCEs New chemical entity
PXR Pregnane X receptor
QSAR Quantitative-structure activity relationships
QSPR Quantitative-structure property relationships
QSTR Quantitative structure-toxicity relationship
SAR Structure-activity relationship
SARpy SAR in python
SAs Structural alerts
SDF Structure data file
SMILES Simplified Molecular-Input Line-Entry System
TIMES Tissue metabolism simulator
UDPGA Uridine diphosphate glucuronic acid

References

Alqahtani, S., 2017. In silico ADME-Tox modeling: progress and prospects. Expert Opin. Drug Metabol. Toxicol. 13, 1147–1158.

Arabi, A.A., 2021. Artificial intelligence in drug design: algorithms, applications, challenges and ethics. Fut. Drug Discov. FDD59.

Banerjee, P., Eckert, A.O., Schrey, A.K., Preissner, R., 2018. ProTox-II: a webserver for the prediction of toxicity of chemicals. Nucleic Acids Res. 46, W257–W263.

Chen, Y., Cheng, F., Sun, L., Li, W., Liu, G., Tang, Y., 2014. Computational models to predict endocrine-disrupting chemical binding with androgen or oestrogen receptors. Ecotoxicol. Environ. Saf. 110, 280–287.

Desbonnet, L., Tighe, O., Karayiorgou, M., Gogos, J.A., Waddington, J.L., O'tuathaigh, C.M., 2012. Physiological and behavioural responsivity to stress and anxiogenic stimuli in COMT-deficient mice. Behav. Brain Res. 228, 351–358.

Drwal, M.N., Banerjee, P., Dunkel, M., Wettig, M.R., Preissner, R., 2014. ProTox: a web server for the in silico prediction of rodent oral toxicity. Nucleic Acids Res. 42, W53–W58.

Duxin Sun, W.G., Hongxiang, H., Simon, Z., 2022. Why 90% of clinical drug development fails and how to improve it? Acta Pharm. Sin. B 12, 3049–3062.

Ellison, C., Hewitt, M., Przybylak, K., 2022. In silico models for hepatotoxicity. In: Silico Methods for Predicting Drug Toxicity. Springer.

Escher, S.E., Bitsch, A., 2021. Read-across methodology in toxicological risk assessment. In: Reichl, F.-X., Schwenk, M. (Eds.), Regulatory Toxicology. Springer International Publishing, Cham.

Evans, D.C., Watt, A.P., Nicoll-Griffith, D.A., Baillie, T.A., 2004. Drug– protein adducts: an industry perspective on minimizing the potential for drug bioactivation in drug discovery and development. Chem. Res. Toxicol. 17, 3–16.

Ferrari, T., Cattaneo, D., Gini, G., Golbamaki Bakhtyari, N., Manganaro, A., Benfenati, E., 2013. Automatic knowledge extraction from chemical structures: the case of mutagenicity prediction. SAR QSAR Environ. Res. 24, 365–383.

Gadekar, V., Borade, Y., Kannaujia, S., Rajpoot, K., Anup, N., Tambe, V., Kalia, K., Tekade, R.K., 2021. Nanomedicines accessible in the market for clinical interventions. J. Contr. Release 330, 372–397.

Gao, J., Garulacan, L.A., Storm, S.M., Hefta, S.A., Opiteck, G.J., Lin, J.-H., Moulin, F., Dambach, D.M., 2004. Identification of in vitro protein biomarkers of idiosyncratic liver toxicity. Toxicol. Vitro 18, 533–541.

Gold, L.S., Manley, N.B., Slone, T.H., Rohrbach, L., Garfinkel, G.B., 2005. Supplement to the carcinogenic potency database (CPDB): results of animal bioassays published in the general literature through 1997 and by the National toxicology program in 1997–1998. Toxicol. Sci. 85, 747–808.

Gorain, B., Choudhury, H., Tekade, R.K., Karan, S., Jaisankar, P., Pal, T.K., 2016. Comparative biodistribution and safety profiling of olmesartan medoxomil oil-in-water oral nanoemulsion. Regul. Toxicol. Pharmacol. 82, 20–31.

Guengerich, F.P., 2011. Mechanisms of drug toxicity and relevance to pharmaceutical development. Drug Metabol. Pharmacokinet. 26 (1), 3–14.

Hinkson, I.V., Madej, B., Stahlberg, E.A., 2020. Accelerating therapeutics for opportunities in medicine: a paradigm shift in drug discovery. Front. Pharmacol. 11, 770.

Ivanov, S.M., Lagunin, A.A., Rudik, A.V., Filimonov, D.A., Poroikov, V.V., 2018. ADVERPred–Web service for prediction of adverse effects of drugs. J. Chem. Inf. Model. 58 (1), 8–11.

Johnson, M.A., Maggiora, G.M., 1990. Concepts and Applications of Molecular Similarity. Wiley.

Kim, E., Nam, H., 2017. Prediction models for drug-induced hepatotoxicity by using weighted molecular fingerprints. BMC Bioinf. 18, 25–34.

Knebel, C., Buhrke, T., Süssmuth, R., Lampen, A., MARX-Stoelting, P., Braeuning, A., 2019. Pregnane X receptor mediates steatotic effects of propiconazole and tebuconazole in human liver cell lines. Arch. Toxicol. 93, 1311–1322.

Li, X., Du, Z., Wang, J., Wu, Z., Li, W., Liu, G., Shen, X., Tang, Y., 2015. In silico estimation of chemical carcinogenicity with binary and ternary classification methods. Mol. Inform. 34, 228–235.

Liu, R., Yu, X., Wallqvist, A., 2015. Data-driven identification of structural alerts for mitigating the risk of drug-induced human liver injuries. J. Cheminf. 7, 1–8.

Lloyd, S., Hayden, M.J., Sakai, Y., Fackett, A., Silber, P.M., Hewitt, N.J., Li, A.P., 2002. Differential in vitro hepatotoxicity of troglitazone and rosiglitazone among cryopreserved human hepatocytes from 37 donors. Chem. Biol. Interact. 142, 57–71.

Lu, J., Zhang, P., Zou, X.-W., Zhao, X.-Q., Cheng, K.-G., Zhao, Y.-L., Bi, Y., Zheng, M.-Y., Luo, X.-M., 2017. In silico prediction of chemical toxicity profile using local lazy learning. Comb. Chem. High Throughput Screen. 20, 346–353.

Macalino, S.J.Y., Gosu, V., Hong, S., Choi, S., 2015. Role of computer-aided drug design in modern drug discovery. Arch Pharm. Res. (Seoul) 38, 1686–1701.

Masubuchi, Y., 2006. Metabolic and non-metabolic factors determining troglitazone hepatotoxicity: a review. Drug Metabol. Pharmacokinet. 21, 347–356.

Morger, A., Mathea, M., Achenbach, J.H., Wolf, A., Buesen, R., Schleifer, K.-J., Landsiedel, R., Volkamer, A., 2020. KnowTox: pipeline and case study for confident prediction of potential toxic effects of compounds in early phases of development. J. Cheminf. 12, 1–17.

Mortelmans, K., Zeiger, E., 2000. The Ames Salmonella/microsome mutagenicity assay. Mutat. Res. 455, 29–60.

Muniswamy, V.J., Raval, N., Gondaliya, P., Tambe, V., Kalia, K., Tekade, R.K., 2019. "Dendrimer-Cationized-Albumin" encrusted polymeric nanoparticle improves BBB penetration and anticancer activity of doxorubicin. Int. J. Pharm. 555, 77–99.

Nakayama, S., Atsumi, R., Takakusa, H., Kobayashi, Y., Kurihara, A., Nagai, Y., Nakai, D., Okazaki, O., 2009. A zone classification system for risk assessment of idiosyncratic drug toxicity using daily dose and covalent binding. Drug Metabol. Dispos. 37, 1970–1977.

Pizzo, F., Gadaleta, D., Lombardo, A., Nicolotti, O., Benfenati, E., 2015. Identification of structural alerts for liver and kidney toxicity using repeated dose toxicity data. Chem. Cent. J. 9, 1–11.

Prajapati, R.N., Tekade, R.K., Gupta, U., Gajbhiye, V., Jain, N.K., 2009. Dendimer-mediated solubilization, formulation development and in vitro-in vivo assessment of piroxicam. Mol. Pharm. 6, 940–950.

Pu, L., Naderi, M., Liu, T., Wu, H.-C., Mukhopadhyay, S., Brylinski, M., 2019. e toxpred: a machine learning-based approach to estimate the toxicity of drug candidates. BMC Pharmacol. Toxicol. 20, 1–15.

Roth, R.A., Ganey, P.E., 2010. Intrinsic versus idiosyncratic drug-induced hepatotoxicity—two villains or one? J. Pharmacol. Exp. Therapeut. 332, 692–697.

Sanguinetti, M.C., Tristani-Firouzi, M., 2006. hERG potassium channels and cardiac arrhythmia. Nature 440, 463–469.

Sharma, A.K., Srivastava, G.N., Roy, A., Sharma, V.K., 2017. ToxiM: a toxicity prediction tool for small molecules developed using machine learning and chemoinformatics approaches. Front. Pharmacol. 8, 880.

Singh, K.P., Gupta, S., Rai, P., 2013. Predicting carcinogenicity of diverse chemicals using probabilistic neural network modeling approaches. Toxicol. Appl. Pharmacol. 272, 465–475.

Siramshetty, V.B., Nickel, J., Omieczynski, C., Gohlke, B.-O., Drwal, M.N., Preissner, R., 2016. Withdrawn—a resource for withdrawn and discontinued drugs. Nucleic Acids Res. 44, D1080–D1086.

Snow, K.L., Moseley, R.H., 2007. Effect of thiazolidinediones on bile acid transport in rat liver. Life Sci. 80, 732–740.

Tanabe, K., Kurita, T., Nishida, K., Lučić, B., Amić, D., Suzuki, T., 2013. Improvement of carcinogenicity prediction performances based on sensitivity analysis in variable selection of SVM models. SAR QSAR Environ. Res. 24, 565–580.

Tekade, R.K., Chougule, M.B., 2013. Formulation development and evaluation of hybrid nanocarrier for cancer therapy: Taguchi Orthogonal Array based design. BioMed Res. Int. 712678.

Thompson, R.A., Isin, E.M., Li, Y., Weaver, R., Weidolf, L., Wilson, I., Claesson, A., Page, K., Dolgos, H., Kenna, J.G., 2011. Risk assessment and mitigation strategies for reactive metabolites in drug discovery and development. Chem. Biol. Interact. 192, 65–71.

Usui, T., Mise, M., Hashizume, T., Yabuki, M., Komuro, S., 2009. Evaluation of the potential for drug-induced liver injury based on in vitro covalent binding to human liver proteins. Drug Metabol. Dispos. 37, 2383–2392.

van Leeuwen, K., Schultz, T.W., Henry, T., Diderich, B., Veith, G., 2009. Using chemical categories to fill data gaps in hazard assessment. SAR QSAR Environ. Res. 20, 207–220.

Verheyen, G.R., Braeken, E., VAN Deun, K., VAN Miert, S., 2017. Evaluation of existing (Q) SAR models for skin and eye irritation and corrosion to use for REACH registration. Toxicol. Lett. 265, 47–52.

Wang, Y., Xiao, Q., Chen, P., Wang, B., 2019. In silico prediction of drug-induced liver injury based on ensemble classifier method. Int. J. Mol. Sci. 20, 4106.

Yang, H., Li, J., Wu, Z., Li, W., Liu, G., Tang, Y., 2017. Evaluation of different methods for identification of structural alerts using chemical ames mutagenicity data set as a benchmark. Chem. Res. Toxicol. 30, 1355–1364.

Yang, H., Sun, L., Li, W., Liu, G., Tang, Y., 2018. In silico prediction of chemical toxicity for drug design using machine learning methods and structural alerts. Front. Chem. 6, 30.

Youngren, S.R., Tekade, R.K., Gustilo, B., Hoffmann, P.R., Chougule, M.B., 2013. STAT6 siRNA matrix-loaded gelatin nanocarriers: formulation, characterization, and ex vivo proof of concept using adenocarcinoma cells. BioMed Res. Int. 2013, 858946.

Zhang, H., Cao, Z.-X., Li, M., Li, Y.-Z., Peng, C., 2016. Novel naïve Bayes classification models for predicting the carcinogenicity of chemicals. Food Chem. Toxicol. 97, 141–149.

Zhu, H., Martin, T.M., Ye, L., Sedykh, A., Young, D.M., Tropsha, A., 2009. Quantitative structure– activity relationship modeling of rat acute toxicity by oral exposure. Chem. Res. Toxicol. 22, 1913–1921.

Zhu, X., Kruhlak, N.L., 2014. Construction and analysis of a human hepatotoxicity database suitable for QSAR modeling using post-market safety data. Toxicology 321, 62–72.

CHAPTER

10

Predicting toxicity from chemical structure of a drug compound

Bhakti Pawar[1], Anand More[1], Nagaraja Sreeharsha[2,3], Muktika Tekade[4] and Rakesh Kumar Tekade[1]

[1]National Institute of Pharmaceutical Education and Research (NIPER)- Ahmedabad, An Institute of National Importance, Government of India, Department of Pharmaceuticals, Ministry of Chemicals and Fertilizers, Palaj, Gandhinagar, Gujarat, India; [2]Department of Pharmaceutical Sciences, College of Clinical Pharmacy, King Faisal University, Al-Ahsa, Saudi Arabia; [3]Department of Pharmaceutics, Vidya Siri College of Pharmacy, Bengaluru, Karnataka, India; [4]School of Pharmacy, Devi Ahilya Vishwavidyalaya, Indore, Madhya Pradesh, India

10.1 Introduction

Drug discovery and development is a complex and time-consuming process. Determination of toxicity is of utmost importance concerning public health. Prediction of toxicity with the help of traditional methods takes time, and eventually, it delays the drug development process and causes failure in clinical trials (Gadekar et al., 2021; Gorain et al., 2016; Muniswamy et al., 2019; Prajapati et al., 2009). The utilization of animals for toxicity prediction has some restrictions. Moreover, it is time-consuming and costlier. Because of interspecies variations and distinct disease models, the data provide little insight into human toxicity reactions (Johnson, 2013).

Animal trials, therefore, cannot predict how the human body will react to novel drugs and cannot eliminate risk. As a result, methodologies need to decrease animal testing, prompt risk assessment, and reduce evaluation costs in the pharmaceutical business and regulatory decision-making processes (Raies and Bajic, 2016). To evaluate the toxicity of novel substances, experimental toxicological methods such as in vivo and in vitro procedures can be utilized; however, these methods alone are not thought to be the most productive or sensitive. In silico tox determination should be performed to minimize the expenses and vagueness related to preclinical studies. For drug safety assessment, numerous computer models

https://doi.org/10.1016/B978-0-443-15840-7.00008-7

have been created thus far. These models can be broadly categorized into qualitative classification, quantitative regression, and read-across.

One of the most popular and sophisticated toxicity prediction techniques is known as quantitative structure-activity relationships (QSAR), which is focused mainly on the compound's structural properties (Yang et al., 2018). In the initial stage of risk evaluation, we only need to know the category of the compound, whether it is toxic, nontoxic, or slightly toxic. The exact toxicity value is needed in the initial stage, so these categories are used. Read-across is also a feasible method for determining particular toxicity criteria for those special chemicals from their identical structural features and experimental toxicity levels (Escher and Bitsch, 2021). These models can occasionally take the role of in vitro or in vivo experiments for specific endpoints because of their excellent accuracy, particularly in a limited chemical region. In recent years, the scenario has changed from traditional animal testing of the drug to virtual screening of the drug with the help of in silico technology. In silico techniques are usually based on the different toxicity datasets which are already existing to predict the toxicity with the help of chemical structure. Furthermore, structural alerts (SAs), which serve as the prerequisites for a substance to have harmful effects on organs, can be produced from the algorithms.

The European Union updated its framework for chemical control in 2006 and issued new rules for the registration, evaluation, authorization, and restriction of chemicals (REACH). To control the use of chemicals and prevent unnecessary use European chemical agency (ECHA) was formed. Recently, eTox software was developed to gather all the information regarding the safety of small molecules from pharmaceutical and public toxicological reports (Pu et al., 2019).

Similarly, in the United State, toxicity in the 21st century, i.e., (The tox21) database, was created to reduce animal testing and start using in silico techniques (Mayr et al., 2016). Thus, the creation of web-based toxicity prediction systems significantly impacts conserving resources and time during the drug discovery process. Artificial intelligence (AI), especially machine learning (ML), has been used widely not only for product development (Youngren et al., 2013; Tekade and Chougule, 2013) but also for toxicity prediction. Machine learning involves multiple algorithms to determine different organ-specific toxicity. VenomPred is another machine learning-based web tool to predict the toxicity of compounds (Galati et al., 2022).

This chapter comprehensively expounds on the prediction of toxicity with the help of the chemical structure of the compound and different methods for the determination of structural compounds. A brief overview of how machine learning helps decide toxic compounds has also been elaborated in this chapter.

10.2 Toxicity prediction based on chemical structure

Drug discovery and development is an extensive process with a high risk that can be reduced with the help of in silico toxicity prediction tools. Drug failure in the preclinical trial is often due to its toxic behavior toward different tissues, organs, or systems. A variety of in vitro assays can be used to detect the toxicity of a chemical before preclinical testing;

however, synthesis of the compound itself can be expensive. Utilizing in silico toxicity prediction tools such as data mining and machine learning methods to estimate chemical or drug-induced toxicity offers helpful information on potential liability and facilitates initial phase workflow optimization. As the properties of any chemical depend upon its molecular structure, based on these structures, toxicity can be predicted. A chemical must pass from its administration site to its site of action, where it must then attach to or interact with its receptor or target to exhibit its toxicity. A stepwise flowchart has been provided for the toxicity prediction based on chemical structure in Fig. 10.1.

ChemTox is an in silico technique that predicts the toxicity of a chemical using its molecular structure without synthesizing the compound, its physicochemical, or toxicological data (Pu et al., 2019). It is also reported that this workflow predicts Ames mutagenicity, rat acute dose LD_{50} administered intravenously (IV) or per oral (p.o.). Moreover, it also helps to predict aqueous solubility simply with the help of the molecular structure of the chemical. The input for this workflow is a chemical structure that has to insert as a standard format which can be in the form of SMILES, mol, or SDF. This model work based on quantitative-structure property relationships (QSPRs) that calculate the toxicity with the help of known responses obtained from the chemicals. The output is usually given in the form of a KNIME data table. This table can be saved as a database or file. Currently, there are many software that predict toxicity with the help of available databases such as TOXNET, ToxCast, Tox21, PubChem, etc. The previous chapter of this book also comprehensively describes the software and databases.

Similarly, OpenTox is another toxicity prediction software with inbuilt ToxPredict as an application that uses chemical structure and its name as an input (Lam et al., 2004, https://www.opentox.net/library/toxicity-prediction). This OpenTox software contains pre-calibrated toxicity models; based on such models, the given chemical structure is verified, and toxicity is predicted. ToxPredict has 16 different models which address 14 endpoints that can be used directly in a ready-to-use format. OpenTox possesses different web services such as structure names, characteristics, datasets, algorithms, models, and validation. The following section discusses the different structural alerts and methods to detect structural alerts used to find out the various toxicity-causing structural parts.

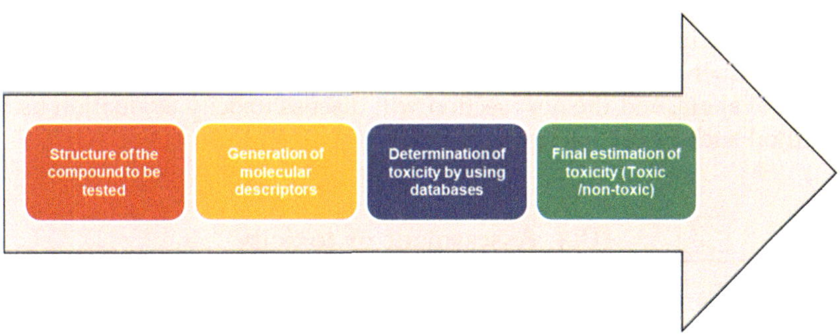

FIGURE 10.1 Stepwise guide for the toxicity prediction based on chemical structure.

10.3 Methods for detecting structural alerts

Structural alerts (SAs) are chemical substructures that can cause toxicity to different organs (Pizzo et al., 2015). Ames mutagenicity is one of the most extensively researched endpoints for structural alerts. At first, researchers used to find substructures by studying the structure-activity relationship of toxic chemical compounds (Benigni and Bossa, 2006). Examples of commercially used toxicity prediction software are Derek Nexus, and Genetox Expert (Ridings et al., 1996) Alerts from LeadScope. Furthermore, the automatic finding of SA becomes part of in silico toxicology (Lepailleur et al., 2013; Floris et al., 2017). Method detection for structural alerts is classified as (i) fragment-based, (ii) graph-based, and (iii) fingerprint-based (Yang et al., 2018).

As we have discussed earlier in the previous chapter, SARpy is one of the fragment-based methods which involve fragmentation of the molecule, which means initially, it cleaves the bond of molecular structure. It then verifies the fragment according to the toxic or nontoxic molecule. For instance, Computer Automated Structure Evaluation (CASE) utilizes Koniocortex-Like Network (KLN) as a code that shows nonlinear expressions for molecules to find structural alerts (Klopman, 1984; Klopman and McGonigal, 1981). This SARpy model allows researchers to evaluate the carcinogenicity of many new drug molecules (Golbamaki and Benfenati, 2016). Similarly, with the help of the hologram quantitative structure-activity relationship (HQSAR) model, CatSAR can generate all the feasible substructures; it is a part of the commercially available product of SYBYL from Tripos Inc (Yang et al., 2019).

According to the graph-based approach, chemical molecules are mathematical graphs with vertices and edges, respectively, that stand in for the atoms and bonds of chemicals. Therefore, the aim of finding substructures is changed to finding subgraphs (Liu et al., 2011). As mentioned in Chapter 9 about MolFea, which is a graph-based linear program that mostly finds the substructure using a stepwise Version space algorithm (Yang et al., 2018). However, the fact that MolFea only mines linear substructures makes this flaw clear. This flaw was overcome by the Moss algorithm that uses in-depth mining of substructures and considers side chains and cycles. One more graph-based program is Gaston, which has three sub-pathways: paths, trees, and cycles. This software allows researchers to use their codes while searching substructures such as [C, O], which means carbon and oxygen.

Another method for detecting structural alerts is fingerprint-based. Molecular fingerprints act as a library of predefined fragments. Various descriptors are being used, such as PaDEL-Calculation of fingerprints of MDL MACCS containing 166 essential substructures was done with the help of a descriptor (Yap, 2011). These substructures can be used to determine SA by calculating their frequencies with the help of a dataset. Till now, we have seen different ways to detect structural alerts, and the next section will discuss toxicity evaluation using a newly developed method such as read-across.

10.4 Assessment of toxicity

Toxicity Assessment: The Guidelines for Carcinogen Risk Assessment provide an outline of the fundamental principles that guide the process of determining a substance's level of toxicity. The National Research Council (NRC) provided standards for evaluating acute toxicity a while back (National Research Council, 1994). The identification of hazards and the evaluation of dose-response relationships are the first two steps in the assessment of toxicity. The process of identifying potential hazards involves describing the different classes of toxicity (like neurotoxicity, carcinogenicity, etc.) that a substance is capable of causing as well as an analysis of the circumstances under which these various forms of toxicity might manifest in human beings who have been exposed to the substance (Stern, 2010). The data used in the identification process are usually obtained from studies conducted on animals and other experimental work. Still, they can also originate from epidemiologic research. Dose-response analysis is a more in-depth assessment of the circumstances in which the toxic properties of a chemical might become apparent in people who have been exposed to that chemical which focuses heavily on the dose-effect relationship (National Research Council, 1994).

10.4.1 Assessment of toxicity using reading across

One of the most challenging obstacles in finding alternatives to animal testing is the safety assessment for repeated dose toxicity (Hartung, 2009). Read across work on the principle of structural resemblance among target molecule and origin. Toxicity assessment by reading can be done by comparing the bioavailability or partition coefficient (relative) parameters of target substances with identical toxicological functionality molecules (Barratt, 2000). Because the molecular structure of a chemical already contains information about its properties, it is possible to deduce whether or not it is toxic based solely on its chemical composition. Various factors must be evaluated when contemplating chemical similarities to implement read-across, like possible metabolites, stability (chemical), exposure route, target tissue concentration, etc., and it also depends on whether toxicity is caused by active moiety or by the metabolite of it. Even similarities in the pharmacodynamics of drugs can lead to toxicity (Berggren et al., 2015).

Four types of possibilities can be possible with the read-across method:

- **i.** Compounds are chemically similar but do not undergo metabolism to elucidate the toxicity
- **ii.** Compounds are chemically similar but undergo metabolism to elucidate the toxicity
- **iii.** Low toxicity chemicals
- **iv.** Different chemicals from the structurally similar group with different toxicities

In the first case, the substance is not undergoing metabolism or may show slow metabolism. In such cases, it is difficult to determine whether the parent drug or metabolite causes toxicity. As there is a similarity in parent compounds, metabolites are excluded from the toxicity argument. In the second case, compounds have less resemblance than that mentioned in the first case but have a similar substructure that can lead to identical metabolites upon biotransformation. But it is challenging to have in vitro evidence for the same as in vitro model could not identify the primary metabolite and its related toxicity or effect upon biotransformation. Simply, these kinds of models do not have metabolic activity. But HepaRG cells predict the toxicity and show metabolic activity (Mueller et al., 2014).

In the third case, the compound has no or less toxicity; in such cases, there is no general mechanism between the target molecule and source. So negative read across demands more data to achieve the same certainty as the positive read method. This case is crucial as cosmetics and other consumable products fit into this category. So, this reading across methods would help conclude whether the use of new, less toxic substances is required or not based on an assessment of toxicity caused by them. In the fourth case, at least one structural analog shows different potency or effect. In such a case, it would be difficult to find a mechanistic relationship explaining why some analogs show desired properties while some have different adverse effects (Berggren et al., 2015).

10.4.1.1 Development of reading across the method

The analog approach (AN), also entitled as one to one approach, and the category approach (CA), also termed many to one approach, are the two approaches that can be used to develop read across the method. The analog approach utilizes one or a few analogs, while the category approach utilizes several analogs in toxicity assessment. Since two analogs could have different toxicity profiles, it's possible that AN is affected by outliers (Venkatapathy and Wang, 2013). It is helpful to use various analogs for CA to identify patterns among a category. Doing so might also enhance confidence in toxicity forecasting (Modi et al., 2012; Jeliazkova et al., 2010).

To determine whether a chemical falls within a category, CA mandates defining the category boundary (Jeliazkova et al., 2010) and executing a technique called "combination of predictions" for such analog, which has conflict in toxicity profiles. This is done using maximum, median, mode, minimum, average, quadratic, linear, or other nonlinear combination methods of toxicity prediction (Dimitrov and Mekenyan, 2010). This method can be qualitative or quantitative. It depends on the toxicity endpoint; if the toxicity endpoint is qualitative, then it is qualitative; else, it is qualitative (Raies and Bajic, 2016). Interpolation and extrapolation approaches to reading across are also crucial in developing the method. The interpolation approach assesses toxicity by interpolating the chemical analog toxicity over a target chemical. This approach is comparatively better than the extrapolation approach, where toxicity is assessed only by extrapolating from a single side.

10.4.1.2 Advantages of the read-across method

i. Easy interpretation and implementation (Worth et al., 2013)
ii. It can be qualitative or quantitative, based on endpoint result (Enoch, 2010)
iii. It helps to assess the similarity between chemicals (Dimitrov and Mekenyan, 2010)

10.4.1.3 Limitations of reading across the method

i. Model interpretation can be complicated by similarity measures (complex) (Raies and Bajic, 2016)
ii. Read-across uses small datasets compared to QSAR (Gajewicz, 2017)
iii. Accuracy of the method can be affected by factors like choice and no of analog, its chemical properties, strength, etc. (Dimitrov and Mekenyan, 2010)

10.4.1.4 Hypothetical example of reading across the method

Think about a similar group of surfactants, such as alkyl betaines, with 8-, 10-, 12-, 14-, and 16-carbon alkyl chains. Interpolation from findings of toxicity tests conducted on the 8-, 12-, and 16-carbon series could be used to generate conservative estimates of the systemic toxicities of the 10- and 14-carbon chemicals (Barratt, 2000).

The further sections aim to overview one of the in silico techniques, such as machine learning, for determining toxicity depending on the molecular structure of a chemical.

10.5 Chemical structure-based toxicity prediction by machine learning

Assessment of toxicity is of the utmost significance in the process of developing and approving new drugs. It is common knowledge that for drugs to be approved for use, they must first be tested in clinical settings (Janodia et al., 2007; Ting, 2006). Clinical trials almost always involve some degree of inherent danger. In late clinical trials involving humans, it was discovered that about half of newly developed medications were either unsafe or ineffective (Hwang et al., 2016). For instance, Sitaxentan was hastily pulled from markets worldwide because it caused specific and irrevocable hepatic damage in humans (Galiè et al., 2011; Erve et al., 2013).

The riskiness of clinical tests draws attention to the significance of preclinical evaluations, which are an absolute prerequisite to forestall the introduction of dangerous drugs into a human clinical trial. The animal trial, a common way of preclinical evaluation, does not provide sufficient information besides being laborious and will cost a lot of money. Due to the differences between species and the different disease models used, the results do not provide much guidance regarding human toxicity reactions (Johnson, 2013; Akhtar, 2015). For example, sitaxentan did not cause any obvious signs of liver damage in animal studies (Owen et al., 2012). Still, hepatotoxicity notably affected human subjects (Galiè et al., 2011; Erve et al., 2013). Because of this, the human body's reaction to new medicines cannot be determined using animal tests, and there is no risk exemption provided (Johnson, 2013; Thomas et al., 2018). It is essential to conduct high-throughput computer toxicity prediction to cut down on the costs and uncertainties that are inherently associated with animal experiments. For example, QSAR methods like the Hansch approach, Free-Wilson method, and QSAR regression analysis method. But with new challenges, these methods are becoming obsolete. A machine learning approach has been used to overcome all problems and address new challenges.

10.5.1 Machine learning

A subfield of AI called "machine learning" employs sophisticated algorithms to enable machines to understand data and predict future outcomes. The principle of machine learning algorithms developed from research on pattern recognition and cluster analysis include decision trees, support vector machines (SVM), artificial neural networks (ANN), and Bayesian classifiers. This algorithm has also been used in data mining. Nowadays, more researchers are using machine learning to predict toxicity due to its benefits, such as speed, cost-effectiveness, and high accuracy. Various machine learning techniques have different findings. Performance can be significantly impacted by variables like computational representations and datasets (Wu and Wang, 2018). Toxicity prediction from machine learning depends on data collection and Performance, discussed in other sections.

10.5.1.1 Data collection

The volume of data being obtained determines how accurate toxicity predictions will be. One of the largest collections of toxicology databases in the world is TOXNET, which was founded in 1985. The first database on acute toxicity can be found in the Hazardous Substances Data Bank (HSDB) (Fonger, 1995; Fonger et al., 2014). One more high-throughput tox database is Toxicity Forecaster (ToxCast). It consists of acute as well as chronic toxicity data. Various commonly used databases for toxicity prediction have been mentioned in Table 10.1.

10.5.1.2 Performance

Combining molecular descriptors and machine learning yielded a prediction model resembling a QSAR, which has been implemented for decades to examine the quantifiable connection between biological activity and compound structure. This includes toxic effects also toxicity toward the surrounding substance, making it a traditional technique for predicting toxicity (Bradbury, 1994; Wu and Wang, 2018). Studies of the QSAR take into account both the two-dimensional structures of chemical molecules and the parameters of biological activity.

In the early days of research, scientists relied on straightforward pattern recognition techniques, like k-NN, to categorize compounds and make predictions about their toxicities. However, it is difficult for simple, straightforward pattern recognition to process asymmetric data, especially when there are considerably fewer positive samples than negative samples or vice versa (Dunn, 1988). Because nontoxic compounds are not expressly identified, uneven information is regularly found in the toxicity database. Luckily, decision tree class ANNs and algorithms, like random forests, can properly classify and predict asymmetric data while

TABLE 10.1 Common databases used for toxicity prediction by machine learning.

Database	Database description	References
ToxCast	Thousands of chemicals toxicity data	Kavlock et al. (2012)
DrugBank	Drug data and targets	Wishart et al. (2018)
TOXNET	Toxicology databases	Fonger et al. (2000)
ToxBank Data Warehouse	Systemic toxicity data	Kohonen et al. (2013)
SuperToxic	Web and literature toxicology data	Schmidt et al. (2009)
PubChem	Overall information on drugs, patent	Kim et al. (2016)
ToxCast	Pathology, survival, and toxicology data. Biochemical effects	Tice et al. (2013)

demonstrating powerful generalization capacity (Kumar and Anitha, 2014; Murphey et al., 2004; Chen et al., 2004).

Using MACCS, FP2, and ECFP6 fingerprints in conjunction with 2D QSAR and ANN model, testing can attain average regression of 0.75 (r test value). Deep learning multi-task neural networks performed so well that they were able to predict toxicity in NIH/3T3 cells with an AUC (Area under curve) value of 0.9, which is marginally more remarkable than the AUC of 0.87 in random forests (RFs), that can be used as molecular fingerprints as an input to the model (Dahl et al., 2014). In addition to ANNs, RFs have also proven to be effective when applied to the prediction of QSAR. RF could pass validation using a molecular fingerprint on the QSAR external test set (Wu and Wang, 2018).

10.6 Conclusion

Since the early assessment of a lead compound's toxicity profile is crucial for its development, the fast and effective evaluation of the potential toxicity of small molecules is a hot topic for the entire scientific community. It constitutes a domain of particular interest in drug discovery. This chapter discusses different in silico techniques for the determination of the toxicity of compounds based on structure. Different webserver tools such as ChemTox, OpenTox, eToxpred, etc., which are readily available to researchers, are also discussed in the above sections. Methods for detecting structural alerts, such as fragment-based, graph-based, and fingerprint-based, are also discussed. These methods utilize algorithms such as SARpy, MoSS, and bio alerts. Another method for the assessment of toxicity is read-across. A read-across method involves extrapolating in vivo animal statistics from one to multiple source compounds to a target substance that has not been evaluated. Now it's the need of the hour to develop better techniques to predict the compound's toxicity and overcome the lack of existing techniques.

10.7 List of abbreviations

AI Artificial intelligence
AN Analogue approach
ANN Artificial neural networks
AUC Area under the curve
CA Category approach
CASE Computer automated structure evaluation
ECHA European chemical agency
HQSAR Hologram quantitative structure-activity relationship
IV Intravenously
KLN Koniocortex-Like Network
KNIME Konstanz Information Miner
ML Machine learning
NRC National Research Council
PO Per oral
QSAR Quantitative structure-activity relationships
QSPRs Quantitative-structure property relationships

SAs Structural alert
SMILES Simplified molecular input line entry system
SVM Support vector machines
ToxCast Toxicity Forecaster

References

Akhtar, A., 2015. The flaws and human harms of animal experimentation. Camb. Q. Healthc. Ethics 24, 407–419.

Barratt, M.D., 2000. Prediction of toxicity from chemical structure. Cell Biol. 16, 1–13.

Benigni, R., Bossa, C., 2006. Structural alerts of mutagens and carcinogens. Curr. Comput. Aided Drug Des. 2, 169–176.

Berggren, E., Amcoff, P., Benigni, R., Blackburn, K., Carney, E., Cronin, M., et al., 2015. Chemical safety assessment using read-across: assessing the use of novel testing methods to strengthen the evidence base for decision making. Environ. Health Perspect. 123, 1232–1240.

Bradbury, S.P., 1994. Predicting modes of toxic action from chemical structure: an overview. SAR QSAR Environ. Res. 2, 89–104.

Chen, C., Liaw, A., Breiman, L., 2004. Using Random Forest to Learn Imbalanced Data, vol. 110. University of California, Berkeley, p. 24.

Dahl, G.E., Jaitly, N., Salakhutdinov, R., 2014. Multi-task neural networks for QSAR predictions. arXiv preprint arXiv:1406.1231.

Dimitrov, S., Mekenyan, O., 2010. An introduction to read-across for the prediction of the effects of chemicals. In: In Silico Toxicology: Principles and Applications, pp. 372–383.

Dunn 3rd, W.J., 1988. QSAR approaches to predicting toxicity. Toxicol. Lett. 43, 277–283.

Enoch, S.J., 2010. Chemical category formation and read-across for the prediction of toxicity. In: Recent Advances in QSAR Studies: Methods and Applications, pp. 209–219.

Erve, J.C., Gauby, S., Maynard Jr., J.W., Svensson, M.A., Tonn, G., Quinn, K.P., 2013. Bioactivation of sitaxentan in liver microsomes, hepatocytes, and expressed human P450s with characterization of the glutathione conjugate by liquid chromatography tandem mass spectrometry. Chem. Res. Toxicol. 26, 926–936.

Escher, S., Bitsch, A., 2021. Read-across methodology in toxicological risk assessment. Regul. Toxicol. 525–538.

Floris, M., Raitano, G., Medda, R., Benfenati, E., 2017. Fragment prioritization on a large mutagenicity dataset. Mol. Inform. 36, 1600133.

Fonger, G.C., 1995. Hazardous substances data bank (HSDB) as a source of environmental fate information on chemicals. Toxicology 103, 137–145.

Fonger, G.C., Hakkinen, P., Jordan, S., Publicker, S., 2014. The National Library of Medicine's (NLM) hazardous substances Data Bank (HSDB): background, recent enhancements and future plans. Toxicology 325, 209–216.

Fonger, G.C., Stroup, D., Thomas, P.L., Wexler, P., 2000. TOXNET: a computerized collection of toxicological and environmental health information. Toxicol. Ind. Health 16, 4–6.

Gadekar, V., Borade, Y., Kannaujia, S., Rajpoot, K., Anup, N., Tambe, V., et al., 2021. Nanomedicines accessible in the market for clinical interventions. J. Control. Release 330, 372–397.

Gajewicz, A., 2017. What if the number of nanotoxicity data is too small for developing predictive Nano-QSAR models? An alternative read-across based approach for filling data gaps. Nanoscale 9 (24), 8435–8448.

Galati, S., DI Stefano, M., Martinelli, E., Macchia, M., Martinelli, A., Poli, G., Tuccinardi, T., 2022. VenomPred: a machine learning based platform for molecular toxicity predictions. Int. J. Mol. Sci. 23, 2105.

Galiè, N., Hoeper, M.M., Gibbs, J.S.R., Simonneau, G., 2011. Liver toxicity of sitaxentan in pulmonary arterial hypertension. Eur. Respir. J. 37, 475–476.

Golbamaki, A., Benfenati, E., 2016. In silico methods for carcinogenicity assessment. In: Silico Methods for Predicting Drug Toxicity. Springer.

Gorain, B., Choudhury, H., Tekade, R.K., Karan, S., Jaisankar, P., Pal, T.K., 2016. Comparative biodistribution and safety profiling of olmesartan medoxomil oil-in-water oral nanoemulsion. Regul. Toxicol. Pharmacol. 82, 20–31.

Hartung, T., 2009. Toxicology for the twenty-first century. Nature 460, 208–212. https://www.opentox.net/library/toxicity-prediction.

Hwang, T.J., Carpenter, D., Lauffenburger, J.C., Wang, B., Franklin, J.M., Kesselheim, A.S., 2016. Failure of investigational drugs in late-stage clinical development and publication of trial results. JAMA Intern. Med. 176, 1826–1833.

Janodia, M.D., Sreedhar, D., Virendra, L., Ajay, P., Udupa, N., 2007. Drug development process: a review. Pharm. Rev. 5, 2214–2221.

Jeliazkova, N., Jaworska, J., Worth, A., 2010. Open source tools for read-across and category formation. In: Silico Toxicology: Principles and Applications, pp. 408–445.

Johnson, D.E., 2013. Fusion of nonclinical and clinical data to predict human drug safety. Expert Rev. Clin. Pharmacol. 6, 185–195.

Kavlock, R., Chandler, K., Houck, K., Hunter, S., Judson, R., Kleinstreuer, N., et al., 2012. Update on EPA's ToxCast program: providing high throughput decision support tools for chemical risk management. Chem. Res. Toxicol. 25, 1287–1302.

Kim, S., Thiessen, P.A., Bolton, E.E., Chen, J., Fu, G., Gindulyte, A., et al., 2016. PubChem substance and compound databases. Nucleic Acids Res. 44, D1202–D1213.

Klopman, G., 1984. Artificial intelligence approach to structure-activity studies. Computer automated structure evaluation of biological activity of organic molecules. J. Am. Chem. Soc. 106, 7315–7321.

Klopman, G., Mcgonigal, M., 1981. Computer simulation of physical-chemical properties of organic molecules. 1. Molecular system identification. J. Chem. Inf. Comput. Sci. 21, 48–52.

Kohonen, P., Benfenati, E., Bower, D., Ceder, R., Crump, M., Cross, K., et al., 2013. The ToxBank data warehouse: supporting the replacement of in vivo repeated dose systemic toxicity testing. Mol. Inform. 32, 47–63.

Kumar, R.S., Anitha, Y., 2014. An efficient approach for asymmetric data classification. Int. J. Innov. Res. Adv. Eng. 1, 157–161.

Lam, C.W., James, J.T., Mccluskey, R., Hunter, R.L., 2004. Pulmonary toxicity of single-wall carbon nanotubes in mice 7 and 90 days after intratracheal instillation. Toxicol. Sci. 77, 126–134.

Lepailleur, A., Poezevara, G., Bureau, R., 2013. Automated detection of structural alerts (chemical fragments) in (eco) toxicology. Comput. Struct. Biotechnol. J. 5, e201302013.

Liu, P., Agrafiotis, D.K., Rassokhin, D.N., 2011. Power Keys: a novel class of topological descriptors based on exhaustive subgraph enumeration and their application in substructure searching. J. Chem. Inf. Model. 51, 2843–2851.

Mayr, A., Klambauer, G., Unterthiner, T., Hochreiter, S., 2016. DeepTox: toxicity prediction using deep learning. Front. Environ. Sci. 3, 80.

Modi, S., Hughes, M., Garrow, A., White, A., 2012. The value of in silico chemistry in the safety assessment of chemicals in the consumer goods and pharmaceutical industries. Drug Discov. Today 17, 135–142.

Mueller, D., Krämer, L., Hoffmann, E., Klein, S., Noor, F., 2014. 3D organotypic HepaRG cultures as in vitro model for acute and repeated dose toxicity studies. Toxicol. In Vitro 28, 104–112.

Muniswamy, V.J., Raval, N., Gondaliya, P., Tambe, V., Kalia, K., Tekade, R.K., 2019. 'Dendrimer-Cationized-Albumin' encrusted polymeric nanoparticle improves BBB penetration and anticancer activity of doxorubicin. Int. J. Pharm. 555, 77–99.

Murphey, Y.L., Guo, H., Feldkamp, L.A., 2004. Neural learning from unbalanced data. Appl. Intell. 21, 117–128.

National Research Council, D. O. E. A. L. S., Board on Environmental Studies and Toxicology, Commission on Life Sciences, Committee on Risk Assessment of Hazardous Air Pollutants, June 1, 1994. Science and Judgment in Risk Assessment, first ed. Routledge, Washington (DC).

Owen, K., Cross, D.M., Derzi, M., Horsley, E., Stavros, F.L., 2012. An overview of the preclinical toxicity and potential carcinogenicity of sitaxentan (Thelin®), a potent endothelin receptor antagonist developed for pulmonary arterial hypertension. Regul. Toxicol. Pharmacol. 64, 95–103.

Pizzo, F., Gadaleta, D., Lombardo, A., Nicolotti, O., Benfenati, E., 2015. Identification of structural alerts for liver and kidney toxicity using repeated dose toxicity data. Chem. Cent. J. 9, 1–11.

Prajapati, R.N., Tekade, R.K., Gupta, U., Gajbhiye, V., Jain, N.K., 2009. Dendimer-mediated solubilization, formulation development and in vitro-in vivo assessment of piroxicam. Mol. Pharm. 6, 940–950.

Pu, L., Naderi, M., Liu, T., Wu, H.-C., Mukhopadhyay, S., Brylinski, M., 2019. eToxPred: a machine learning-based approach to estimate the toxicity of drug candidates. BMC Pharmacol. Toxicol. 20, 1–15.

Raies, A.B., Bajic, V.B., 2016. In silico toxicology: computational methods for the prediction of chemical toxicity. Wiley Interdiscip. Rev. Comput. Mol. Sci. 6, 147–172.

Ridings, J., Barratt, M., Cary, R., Earnshaw, C., Eggington, C., Ellis, M., et al., 1996. Computer prediction of possible toxic action from chemical structure: an update on the DEREK system. Toxicology 106, 267–279.

Schmidt, U., Struck, S., Gruening, B., Hossbach, J., Jaeger, I.S., Parol, R., et al., 2009. SuperToxic: a comprehensive database of toxic compounds. Nucleic Acids Res. 37, D295–D299.

Stern, B.R., 2010. Essentiality and toxicity in copper health risk assessment: overview, update and regulatory considerations. J. Toxicol. Environ. Health Part A 73, 114–127.

Tekade, R.K., Chougule, M.B., 2013. Formulation development and evaluation of hybrid nanocarrier for cancer therapy: taguchi orthogonal array based design. BioMed Res. Int. 2013, 712678.

Thomas, R.S., Paules, R.S., Simeonov, A., Fitzpatrick, S.C., Crofton, K.M., Casey, W.M., Mendrick, D.L., 2018. The US Federal Tox21 Program: a strategic and operational plan for continued leadership. Altex 35, 163.

Tice, R.R., Austin, C.P., Kavlock, R.J., Bucher, J.R., 2013. Improving the human hazard characterization of chemicals: a Tox21 update. Environ. Health Perspect. 121, 756–765.

Ting, N., 2006. Introduction and new drug development process. In: Dose Finding in Drug Development. Springer.

Venkatapathy, R., Wang, N.C.Y., 2013. Developmental toxicity prediction. In: Reisfeld, B., Mayeno, A.N. (Eds.), Computational Toxicology: Volume II. Humana Press, Totowa, NJ.

Wishart, D.S., Feunang, Y.D., Guo, A.C., Lo, E.J., Marcu, A., Grant, J.R., et al., 2018. DrugBank 5.0: a major update to the DrugBank database for 2018. Nucleic Acids Res. 46, D1074–D1082.

Worth, A.P., Lapenna, S., Serafimova, R., 2013. QSAR and metabolic assessment tools in the assessment of genotoxicity. In: Computational Toxicology. Springer.

Wu, Y., Wang, G., 2018. Machine learning based toxicity prediction: from chemical structural description to transcriptome analysis. Int. J. Mol. Sci. 19, 2358.

Yang, H., Sun, L., Li, W., Liu, G., Tang, Y., 2018. In silico prediction of chemical toxicity for drug design using machine learning methods and structural alerts. Front. Chem. 6, 30.

Yang, J., Gu, W., Li, Y., 2019. Biological enrichment prediction of polychlorinated biphenyls and novel molecular design based on 3D-QSAR/HQSAR associated with molecule docking. Biosci. Rep. 39.

Yap, C.W., 2011. PaDEL-descriptor: an open source software to calculate molecular descriptors and fingerprints. J. Comput. Chem. 32, 1466–1474.

Youngren, S.R., Tekade, R.K., Gustilo, B., Hoffmann, P.R., Chougule, M.B., 2013. STAT6 siRNA matrix-loaded gelatin nanocarriers: formulation, characterization, and ex vivo proof of concept using adenocarcinoma cells. BioMed Res. Int. 2013, 858946.

CHAPTER

11

Toxicokinetics and organ-specific toxicity

Pankaj Vinodrao Dixit[1], *Dinesh Kumar Mishra*[1], *Kuldeep Rajpoot*[2], *Muktika Tekade*[3], *Nagendra Sai Kumar Achanta*[4], *Neelima Anup*[2] and *Rakesh Kumar Tekade*[2]

[1]Indore Institute of Pharmacy, Indore, Madhya Pradesh, India; [2]National Institute of Pharmaceutical Education and Research (NIPER)- Ahmedabad, An Institute of National Importance, Government of India, Department of Pharmaceuticals, Ministry of Chemicals and Fertilizers, Palaj, Gandhinagar, Gujarat, India; [3]School of Pharmacy, Devi Ahilya Vishwavidyalaya, Khandwa Road, Indore, Madhya Pradesh, India; [4]University of Campania, Luigi Vanvitelli, Caserta, Italy

11.1 Introduction

Toxicokinetics is the amalgamation of the word's toxin and kinetics. Toxins have been well known to humanity since their evolution as they are the most important weapons of one species against another to defend or capture one another. The development of science and specific pharmacology has helped us understand how these toxins affect body function via the study of pharmacodynamics vis-à-vis the fate of these foreign substances in the body (i.e., pharmacokinetics (PK)) (Tambe et al. 2021d, 2021e). PK deals with the fate of an ingested or administered substance in the body by studying its absorption, distribution, metabolism, and excretion (Boroujerdi, 2015; Rajpoot et al. 2021b, 2021c; Polaka et al., 2021a; Anup et al., 2021c).

Due to the explosion of pharmacologically active chemicals in the late 20th century and the systematization of the drug discovery process after the thalidomide tragedy, the application of PK principles is more clearly being defined in the discipline of toxicology. Thus, in a nutshell, toxicology is significantly aided by understanding how the body handles toxins. The absorption, distribution, metabolism, and excretion of a toxin play a pivotal role in

Essentials of Pharmatoxicology in Drug Research, Volume 1
https://doi.org/10.1016/B978-0-443-15840-7.00016-6

understanding the harmful effects but also helps in designing remedial measures. Additionally, some factors like fever (Desai et al., 2021), patients state like pregnancy (Anup et al., 2021a), and age of patients (Rajpoot et al., 2021a) should also be considered during the designing of dosage forms (Vasdev et al., 2021; Tambe et al., 2021b; Achanta et al., 2021). Paracelsus has rightly said that the "dose" of any chemical can makes it a poison, i.e., all drugs marked as medicines, in essence, may become toxins if inappropriately consumed (Abbott, 1993). This has given a great impetus for the regulatory toxicological screening of all such purported "New Chemical Entities."

Patient related conditions such as existing medical problems, may significantly influence the medication's toxicological effects. Some crucial factors that may influence the ingested medicines performance and may cause toxicity are body temperature (Desai et al., 2021), age (Rajpoot et al., 2021a), diet (Polaka et al., 2022b), enzyme levels (Achanta et al., 2021; Tambe et al., 2021f; Rajpoot et al., 2020b), sleeping pattern (Choudhary et al., 2021; Vasdev et al., 2021), sex (Anup et al., 2021a; Polaka et al., 2022a), etc. Therefore, scientists are constantly focusing on the development and safe administration of medicines (Gupta et al., 2022b; Kumawat et al., 2020).

The detrimental effects of any pharmacological agents could be abated by modifying the PK features of chemotherapeutics that comprehend absorption, distribution, metabolism, and excretion throughout the body (Anup et al., 2021c; Padiyar et al., 2020; Polaka et al., 2021a; Rajpoot et al. 2020c, 2021c). For the establishment of a therapeutic dose of chemical entities and subduing adverse effects, several methodologies, models, and software are utilized (Anup et al., 2021b; Polaka et al., 2021b; Rajpoot et al., 2021b; Tambe et al. 2021a, 2021c, 2021d), for instance, the use of technological and methodological advancements for assessing drug toxicity, like in silico computational modeling studies (Rajpoot et al., 2022a), distinct bioindicators (Tekade et al., 2022), in vitro toxicity analysis (Gupta et al., 2022c), in vivo animal studies, toxicokinetic as well as toxicodynamic studies (Rajpoot et al., 2022b), and the toxic impacts of different formulation components (Tiwari et al., 2022; Gupta et al., 2022a).

Organization for Economic Co-operation and Development (OECD) guideline cites the most relevant internationally agreed testing methods, of which Test no. 417 expounds the in vivo studies which renders information on toxicokinetics (OECD, 2010). The guideline illustrates the potentiality of toxicokinetics in understanding the dose-dependent toxic effects of the parent drug and/or xenobiotics in the plasma of experimental animals. In addition, the role of tissue drug concentration and its metabolism on particular site is also described. The guideline further helps to develop paradigms to understand the risk of toxicities in humans compared to animals. The role of determining the temporal behavior of drugs in tissues from the data is that we correlate plasma levels with either efficacy or toxicity for generalization. In fact, it is the tissue level that ultimately seals fate. There are numerous examples wherein the plasma levels do not explain efficacy or toxicity. For instance, azithromycin exhibits high concentrations in soft tissues (Matzneller et al., 2013), and aminoglycosides show peak concentrations in critical organs, which are decisive in toxicity determination (Peloquin et al., 2004). Nowadays, no observed adverse effect level (NOAEL) to human exposure is a crucial predictor for human safety risk, which is calculated by analyzing drug and metabolite concentrations in animal plasma.

Humans are exposed to various chemicals via the environment, inhalation, skin exposure, and water. Advances in living standards have paved the way for numerous other sources like

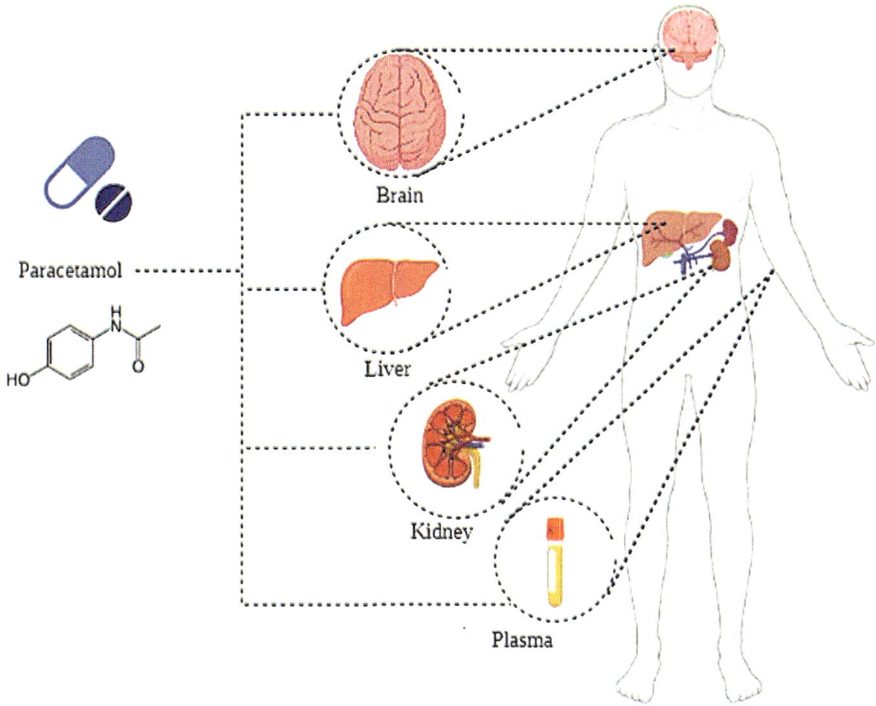

FIGURE 11.1 Influence of route of administration on toxicity.

cosmetics, sanitizers, detergents, bleaches, pesticides, and a wide variety of drugs. The administration route also impacts exposure to various organ systems in addition to temporal variation in the systemic circulation. A scheme is depicted in Fig. 11.1. These observations are highlighted by Ning et al., who focused on investigating the influence of the route of drug administration on the median lethal dose (LD_{50}) values of 527 chemical compounds (Ning et al., 2015). The author concluded that all parenteral routes yielded LD_{50} values that co-related well with intravenous (IV), intramuscular (IM), and intraperitoneal (IP) routes. However, the correlation of these values was very poor when oral data were compared. The importance of differences in PK and organ exposures to varying drug concentrations were discussed to explain the observations. This type of experimental data repeatedly spotlights the need for a thorough understanding of the movement and exposure of drugs in different body compartments. It highlights the importance of radiographic mass balance studies as mandatory regulatory protocols.

Administration of drugs via parenteral or intravenous route encompasses intradermal (into the skin); subcutaneous (beneath the skin into the fatty layer), intramuscular (into muscles), intrathecal (into the cerebrospinal fluid (CSF) of the spinal cord), and a few more that are rarely used which comprehend intraarterially (directly into arteries), intrapleural (into pleural or chest cavity) (Fig. 11.2) and often directly into the tumor site or an organ as in case of cancer therapy.

FIGURE 11.2 Routes of drug administration.

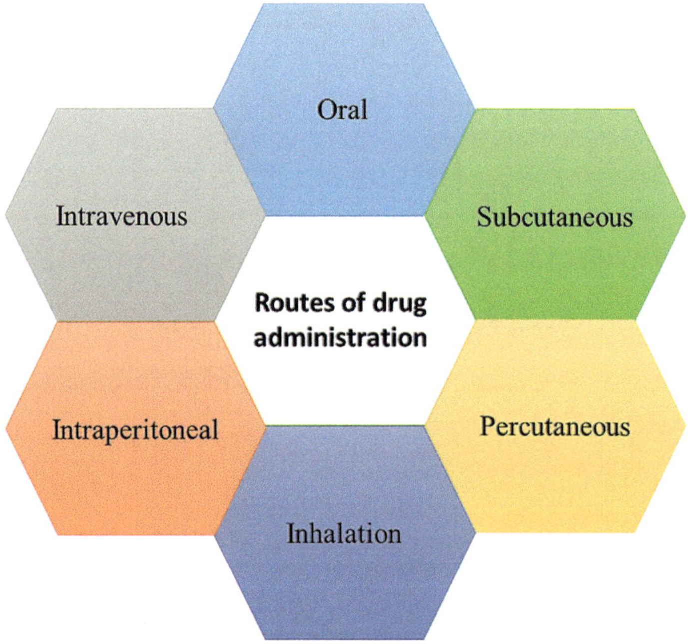

11.1.1 Intravenous

Instantaneous effects are obtained after systemic administration of drugs. The instantaneous effects are beneficial in emergent situations. However, it also involves a significant risk of drug toxicity as plasma levels may reach toxic levels in no time. Of all the available parenteral administration approaches, the intravenous route provides direct access to the systemic circulation with negligible effect on drug absorption. Accordingly, it is prudent that when a drug is administered via an intravenous route, its PK and pharmacodynamics shall be relatively different, as the drug is completely bioavailable. The temporal exposure may rapidly exceed the safety or therapeutic window and precipitate toxic actions. Wherefore, it is absurd to discover the LD_{50} off a compound administered via intravenous route except for Isoniazid. In mice, the oral and parenteral LD_{50} of Isoniazid is 140–160 mg/kg (Walley, 2000). In conclusion, the intravenous route renders easy accessibility to all organs, and any chemical with high potency is more likely to precipitate toxicity rapidly and in a more pronounced manner than any other route of administration.

11.1.2 Intraperitoneal

The intraperitoneal route of drug administration is rarely used in humans, although it is prevalent in the laboratory. However, as is applicable for all routes, drug distribution is quintessential for any drug to exert its effect when administered via the parenteral route. The lethal effects, in such cases, may depend on the parenteral route or sometimes may be independent. As a rule, it is assumed that lethality varies with the route as the rate of drug transfer in different body compartments depends on it. For example, we may assume that the rate of drug transfer from the site of parenteral administration may be so slow as to be superseded by its rate of excretion, rendering the toxicity null and void.

Intraperitoneal injection of chemicals is similar to the enteral route in delivering chemicals via portal circulation to the liver (Miner et al., 1969). This similarity occurs due to the nature of venous circulation that delivers the abdominal blood to the liver through the portal circulation. Therefore, any compound administered intraperitoneally is subjected to metabolism similar to the first-pass effect and may exhibit biliary recirculation. Therefore, any compound toxic to an organ system other than the liver and is subject to significant metabolism by the liver will exhibit greater toxicity if administered via a parenteral route other than the intraperitoneal route. Organic phosphate soman is an example of such compound (Adeyinka et al., 2021; Tambe et al., 2021f).

11.1.3 Oral

The oral route is the most commonly employed in humans for administering drugs or chemicals for therapeutic purposes, including diagnosis. The gastrointestinal (GI) tract is a tube-like structure starting at the mouth and ending at the anus. When administered via the oral route, the chemicals can only affect the mucosal cells lining of the GI tract if they are not absorbed to enter circulation. Acids, alkalis, phenolic substances, and irritants may cause necrosis of the mucosa. Several compounds, including nitroglycerin, alcohol, and several steroids, can be absorbed through the oral mucosa directly into circulation. However, for significant absorption to take place through this route, the compound must be retained in the mouth for a long duration (Abrams, 1985).

Oral toxicity is determined chiefly by the duration of drug therapy and the physiological state of GIT, either fed or fasted. In contrast, extrapolating observation from the animal study for oral toxicity care is to be exercised about how the drug is administered via oral gavage or diet. For instance, dimethylamine (a respiratory stimulant) exhibits a low therapeutic index when given as gavage. At the same time, dixyrazine (a phenothiazine-type drug used as a tranquilizing agent) showed contrasting etiquette (Zhu et al., 2020).

11.1.4 Inhalation route

The inhalation route is felicitous for agents acting on the lungs, and especially it's a boon for targeting the respiratory tract explicitly in children, asthmatic individuals, and geriatric patients (Rajpoot et al., 2021a). Similarly, environmental pollutants can also exert harmful effects on the lungs when subjected to toxic inhalation in polluted air spaces unless air purifiers are utilized to block out the atmospheric contaminants ahead of their infiltration into the respiratory tract (Pauluhn et al., 1996; Parikh et al., 2022). The physical state of the active chemical entity is to be ensured if it is in a gaseous phase and of requisite particle size to prevent it from banishing from the airway to the lungs. Apart from xenobiotics involving medical devices, addictive psychoactive components such as nicotine and cannabis, etc., as well as environmental toxins, can be inhaled either intentionally or unintentionally (Wolfreys et al., 2021; Tiwari et al., 2022).

11.1.5 Subcutaneous

The subcutaneous route, also referred to as a hypodermic administration route, is used to administer small volumes of drugs such as local anesthetics, proteins, peptides, and vaccines (Usach et al., 2019). Several prolonged-release dosage forms (e.g., contraceptives) are also implanted subcutaneously for slow release over long durations. Several factors influence the rate and extended absorption. The physicochemical parameter of the drug, lipophilicity, pH-pKa relation, degree of ionization, formulation parameters such as the type of vehicle, presence of surfactant, viscosity, the particle size of suspension, and dosage parameters such as site and depth of injection, dose, volume administered (should not exceed 2 mL) influence the absorption rate. The drug absorption rate is slower in the subcutaneous region due to its meager vasculature relative to muscle; however, the proportion of drug absorption is equivalent.

11.1.6 Percutaneous

Skin represents a formidable barrier to the entry of environmental chemicals and xenobiotics. The outermost layer comprises aggregation of dead cells called keratinocytes. Descending the keratinocytes, the skin encompasses melanocytes, Langerhans cells, and stem cells, being the lowermost epidermal layer. The hypodermis or the dermis embodies the blood vessels and accessory skin structures like the root of hairs and sebaceous glands. The accessory structures pierce the dermis and have openings on the skin's surface. The multilayered organization of dead keratinocytes complicates the entry of infectious organisms and chemicals (Wester and Maibach, 2012).

The level of skin toxicity depends on the amount of drug applied, in addition to its chemical nature and potency. In some instances, a chemical may elicit an abnormal immune response that may not depend on the quantity of drug applied (i.e., phototoxicity and erythema) (Epstein, 1999; Kim et al., 2015). For conventional drugs, the toxicity depends on the excipients used in the dosage form, such as penetration enhancers (Kovacik et al., 2020). The physicochemical properties of the drug are cardinal in the determination of its skin penetration. In general, liquids penetrate less freely, and solids which are insoluble in water are incapable of penetration to a significant extent. The role of lipid solubility in skin penetration is debatable, e.g., a lipid-soluble insecticide like dichlorodiphenyltrichloroethane (DDT) has very poor skin absorption. However, steroids, vitamin D, vitamin K, and drugs (e.g., nicotine, scopolamine, etc.) are rapidly absorbed. In addition, many other factors that govern drug absorption via the cutaneous route are pH, pKa, molecular weight, and o/w partition coefficient. Physiological factors like skin temperature and blood flow also affect the rate of absorption and the toxicity profile of chemicals. Hence, on a convincing note, a balance of many physicochemical properties and physiological conditions affects the rate and extent of absorption through the skin.

In conclusion, skin toxicity may not be put into a general format. Still, if class toxicity is well-known, then the chemical must be thoroughly screened in multiple animal models to establish its skin toxicity. Nowadays, various in vitro and ex vivo models are proposed, including chip-based technologies, synthetic membranes, and several in silico modeling approaches to screening percutaneous toxicity (Macmillan and Chilton, 2019; Tambe et al., 2021a; Rajpoot et al., 2022a; Polaka et al., 2021b).

The reconstituted human epidermis (RHE) model is used most commonly as the in vitro model for studying skin toxicity (Pham et al., 1990). These RHE models consist of human epidermal keratinocytes. Hence, this model restricts to the toxicologic and pharmacologic evaluation of keratinocytes alone. RHE model systems, when used suitably, can be used for evaluating the biology, pharmacology, and toxicity of candidate drugs. This model can also predict the pharmacological and toxicological effects on the skin in vivo, including clinical toxicity (Hu et al., 2022).

11.2 Relationship between PK and toxicodynamics

Rodent acute toxicity studies play an essential role in drug discovery and regulatory toxicological studies of environmental contaminants. Usually, LD_{50} or the median lethal dose is determined to establish the nature of toxicity. This study involves experimental rodents and is critiqued due to ethical concerns (OECD, 2008; Lagunin et al., 2011). The legislation of Registration, Evaluation, Authorisation, and Restriction of Chemicals (REACH) recommends using quantitative structure-activity relationship (QSAR) for identifying hazardous properties of chemicals (Rybacka et al., 2014). Few QSAR models can predict the acute toxicity of chemicals in rat models (Ballabio et al., 2019; Lunghini et al., 2019). These models make use of the LD_{50} values obtained from databases. QSAR is successfully used in ecotoxicology to accurately predict the toxic effects of numerous chemicals. However, the prediction of LD_{50} value in rats of chemicals with diverse structures is still not achieved due to the lack of suitable models (Sazonovas et al., 2010).

Some of the published QSAR models are strictly developed for single classes of chemicals such as alcohols, phenols, and anilines (Gadaleta et al., 2019). The LD_{50} in rats depends on many variables, and different chemicals have different mechanisms for inducing toxic reactions. This creates difficulty in making accurate predictions using a single QSAR model for diverse chemicals. In addition, QSAR models make accurate predictions for biological systems at a steady state. However, such a steady state is not achieved during acute toxicity studies, making it challenging to predict LD_{50} values in rats a problematic task (Koleva et al., 2011; Chushak et al., 2021).

This nonlinear relationship between the kinetic endpoint ($\log 1/LD_{50}$) and the thermodynamic descriptors of toxicity makes it challenging to model accurate predictions of toxic reactions to environmental toxins in rodents. Any differences in the kinetics of the absorption and metabolism of chemicals due to changes in the route of administration can affect the extent of toxic reactions due to the changes in bioavailability (hence the order of toxicity for the different routes is: intravenous > intraperitoneal > oral). It is difficult for the QSAR models to account for such differences in the predictions for toxic reactions. This warrants the identification and inclusion of additional parameters leading to differences in the rates of absorption and metabolism into the models for better predicts of different routes of administration. A detailed analysis revealed that the incorporation of hydrophobicity and the degree of ionization of chemicals into the model could improve the accuracy in predicting toxicity for different routes of administration. Few attempts are already underway that utilize lethal doses from toxicity studies done in rats exploring oral, IV, and IP routes. In a study by Walum (1998), the correlation in acute toxicities between oral and intravenous administration in mice was examined for 851 aliphatic compounds (Walum, 1998). The result showed that, due to the same mechanisms of the compounds to the same species, toxicities (log $1/LD_{50}$) of mice in the oral route are related to the toxicities in the injection route. However, the first-pass effect was responsible for better safety indices when the drugs were administered orally.

11.3 Organ-specific toxicity

The array of preclinical PK studies carried out in different species during drug discovery provides a valuable database for toxicity predictions as these studies document the metabolic patterns in different models along with the rate of drug clearance, linear or nonlinear. However, there is also a need to perform these studies in association with the toxicity studies to attain better extrapolation or allometry when toxicokinetic data is used instead of PK study (e.g., no-observed-adverse-effect-level (NOAEL) predictions). While performing these studies, many assumptions are made about equilibrium conditions governing the transfer of drugs in different body compartments, and then plasma is sampled for convenience. However, increasing evidence has pointed out opposite directions where concentrations of the drug and its important metabolite (either efficacy or safety point of view) in the target tissue are more critical than in the plasma (Olson et al., 2000).

11.3.1 Skin

All products that employ the cutaneous route of drug delivery have to be evaluated by toxicology testing as per regulatory requirements. Rabbits as laboratory animals serve as the gold standard for these dermal toxicity studies and are widely used to estimate the irritancy of these formulations. The regulatory guidelines have listed guinea pigs as an acceptable species for evaluating dermal toxicity, but they are rarely used. In contrast, guinea pigs are widely used for bioassays involving sensitization studies. The local lymph node assay (LLNA) performed in CBA/Ca, or CBA/J mice, is a modification of the guinea pig assay (Gerberick et al., 2007).

CPC634, a polymeric nanoparticle entrapping docetaxel on intravenous administration, exhibited dose-dependent skin toxicity similar to conventional docetaxel. Histopathological evaluation showed an elevation in the apoptotic cells, mitotic cells with nuclear atypia, micronucleation, and Ki-67 index (Fig. 11.3A–D). In the Napoli trial, severe skin toxicity was observed in a patient administered two cycles of CPC634 at a dose of 80 mg/m^2 without any premedication. Skin biopsy of the patient showed elevated levels in the apoptotic cell population, hyperplasia in the epidermis, hyperkeratosis, hypergranulosis, nuclear hyperchromasia, and erythrocyte extravasation indicative of capillary damage (Fig. 11.3E–F).

11.3.1.1 Irritation

As an outcome of World War II, which involved the development of chemical warfare to a significant extent, a need was observed to provide information for a chemical that was intended for application to the skin. This led to the development of the Draize skin test in

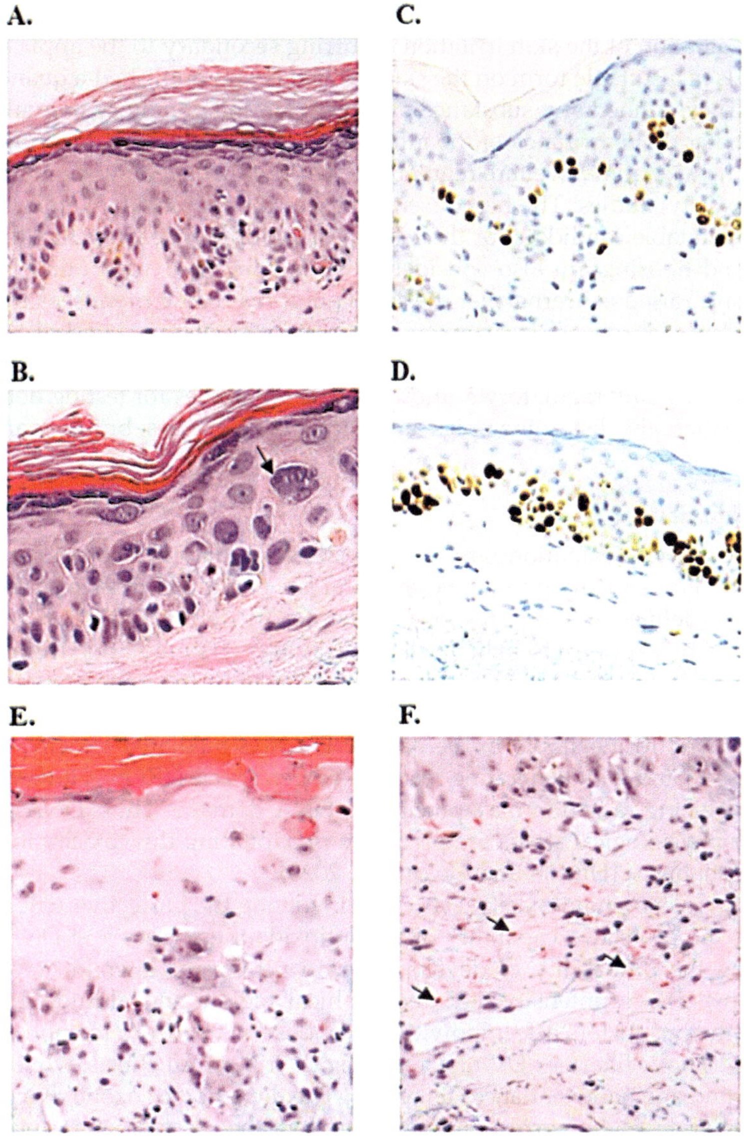

FIGURE 11.3 Histopathological changes in the skin. (**A**) Skin biopsy of a patient posttreatment with CPC634 with epidermis demonstrating hypergranulosis, the influx of lymphocytes, basal vacuolization of keratinocytes, and scattered apoptotic cells along the dermo-epidermal junction (20×magnification). (**B**) This section is a 40× magnification of the same patient showing keratinocyte micronucleation ("grape cells," arrow), also noticing the accompanying apoptosis. Immunohistochemical stain for Ki67 at baseline (**C**) and after CPC634 treatment (**D**) (20× magnification). (**E**) This skin biopsy section of a patient in the Napoli study with skin toxicity shows an epidermis demonstrating vacuolar interface dermatitis with basal vacuolization, the influx of lymphocytes, scattered high apoptosis, and hyper-and parakeratosis (20× magnification). Note the keratinocyte atypia with polymorphic nuclei and prominent nucleoli. (**F**) This section of the same patient shows ectatic capillaries and postcapillary venules of the superficial vascular plexus, a minor lymphohistiocytic perivascular infiltrate, and extensive erythrocyte extravasation (arrow) (20× magnification) (Atrafi et al., 2021). *Adapted from reference Atrafi, F., van Eerden, R.A.G., Koolen, S.L.W., de Bruijn, P., Rijcken, C.J.F., Hanssen, R., et al., 2021. Docetaxel skin exposure and micronucleation contributes to skin toxicity caused by CPC634. Cancers 13 (15), 3741. https://www.ncbi.nlm.nih.gov/pubmed/34359641 under Creative Commons Attribution (CC BY) license. Copyright 2021.*

the mid-20th century. The regulatory agencies were quick to include this in the safety guidelines. For the evaluation of the skin irritation occurring secondary to the application of products or chemicals in a suitable form on the skin, Draize (1944) published a quantitative test of skin irritation. They defined any substance producing an inflammatory dermal reaction as a primary local irritant. The irritancy of the inflammatory reactions was quantified in terms of edema and erythema. Animal welfare regulations worldwide have now mandated cutaneous irritation and toxicity studies. The higher sensitivity of the rabbit skin compared to humans makes it a more suitable candidate for these studies. In addition, ease of handling, availability, breeding, and housing are also considered when compared with other larger species. Some studies have raised concerns over the same point that being more sensitive, the results obtained in such models generally overestimate the toxicity of any chemical, and its clinical relevance is questioned. Taking these into consideration, albino rats are recommended as the preferred species by many regulatory authorities. The guidelines for testing dermal irritation in toxicity evaluation also list guinea pigs as an acceptable species, but they are rarely used (OECD, 2021).

11.3.1.2 Phototoxicity

Dermal phototoxicity evaluations are also crucial as sun bath is a common social practice in many communities, and any phototoxic chemical is a potential threat in such cases. Phototoxicity reaction is defined as a toxic response prompted by dermal or systemic contact with a chemical followed by exposure to light, such as ultraviolet (UV) radiation from sunlight. The longer wavelength (about 10^{-8} to 10^{-6} m) of UV rays restricts their penetration to the superficial layers of the skin and hence has limited biological effects on its own. Abnormalities in melanin production are inevitable in the case of UV-rays-mediated toxicity, which is also thought to be associated with generating reactive oxygen species (ROS). However, prolonged exposures like ionizing radiation may precipitate DNA damage. Thus, DNA repair mechanisms and their physiological status are pivotal in precipitating this toxicity in real-case scenarios (as with sunburn) (Hinton and Goldminz, 2020).

Age has a vital role in phototoxicity, especially involving the protective actions of melanin. Aging weakens the protective capability of the antioxidant enzymes and DNA repair pathways, increasing the probability of developing skin neoplasms later in life. Additionally, clothing, seasons, UV-ray intensity, i.e., geographical region, and altitude are essential in these cases. Numerous factors affect individual response to exposure to sunlight. Moreover, glass, smog, and smoke filter out UV rays reducing their harmful effects, while the reflection of UV rays by sand and snow enhances its effects. The depletion of ozone due to the overuse of chlorofluorocarbons and a corresponding increase in the cases of skin cancer are notable (D'Orazio et al., 2013).

Redness of the skin due to capillary dilation and itching due to histamine release by mast cells is an acute response that usually accompanies UV-light exposure-induced allergic response to certain chemicals. The redness is scored in terms of erythema. These erythematous reactions may involve target (bull's eye-shaped) lesions, macules, nodules, and papules, characterized as a type-IV hypersensitivity reaction. In some cases, a pruritic skin eruption characterized by transient wheels of varying shapes and sizes, with well-defined erythematous margins and pale centers is observed, which is termed urticaria (Dispenza, 2019). The mechanism is the same as discussed above.

Further increase in the severity of the photosensitivity results in the development of bullae, i.e., thin-walled serous fluid-filled blisters on the skin or mucous membranes having a size larger than 1 cm in diameter. The healing of the affected areas involves dehydration, scaling, scarring, fibrosis, and necrosis. Several chemicals include sulfonamides, griseofulvin tetracyclines, thiazide diuretics, coal tar-containing dermal products, salicylic acid, plant derivatives, and components in the formula of cosmetics, soap, or perfumes are examples of agents causing phototoxic reactions (Moore, 2002).

11.3.2 GI tract

The toxicological significance of the gut is enormous as a wide variety of chemicals enter the systemic circulation via this route through diet or beverages and employing a diverse medication. Most of the data available concerning the gut are obtained during the study of the PK of the drug during the discovery process. However, the toxicity is determined by the integrity of the mucosal barrier of the intestine, which is variable in children and geriatric patients, increasing the complexity of the situation. In addition, disease conditions like infections, hypersensitivity reactions, and malnutrition alter gut permeability (Coruzzi, 2010).

GI symptoms are nonspecific, as stressful conditions involving sympathetic activation are known to disturb gut functioning. Similarly, substances may reach systemic circulation via inhalation or cutaneous route causing secondary GI symptoms. It is observed that the majority of the compound for humans tends to have some toxic effects leading to disturbances in the GI tract, such as the development of ulcers. It is evident from the literature that most studies focus on the mechanism of carcinogenic or genotoxic effects of xenobiotics; however, they are also explored for many other aspects (Coruzzi, 2010).

Mucosal biopsies of the GI tract have been commonly performed in humans for many years. These are used to study general morphological features. A more accurate quantification involves the measurement of the depth of the crypt and the height of the villi, calculating the surface areas with light pens, and recording cellular infiltration. Certain cell types, like the mast cell, tend to localize. Monoclonal antibodies are also used to identify a specific subset of the cell population in the GI tract. The introduction of fiber optic endoscopy has facilitated the macroscopic examination, which along with the histological appearances, is an indispensable tool for studying the toxicity patterns of drugs in a real-time scenario. Several compounds like acrylonitrile can promote the development of peptic ulcers as a toxic reaction (Baltrop and Brueton, 1990).

Evaluation of changes in the weights of the organ is another age-old practice in toxicological studies. Such changes are usually occurring in the caecum of the GI tract. One such example is 4-methyl-l-phenylpentan-2-ol, a flavoring agent that increases the caecum's weight in rats. Several physiological processes, such as the change in the microflora and osmotic activity of the contents in the caecum, have been postulated to be the probable mechanism for causing such a change (Abecia et al., 2007; Gultekin et al., 2020). Absorption kinetics is another important parameter useful in toxicological studies, especially toxicokinetics (Rajpoot et al. 2022b, 2022c; Asati et al., 2022). PK studies involving isotope labeling techniques have significantly advanced these studies. In men, after an oral dose of the test substance, analysis of feces, urine, blood, saliva, and expired air can be readily carried out by collecting samples as per the PK profile of the drug.

Further, delayed drug excretion is tracked by extending the study for several days. However, the localized concentration of the compound and its metabolites cannot be identified by whole-body analysis. In animals, the PK of the molecules in different tissues can be evaluated by measuring the time-dependent changes in the radioactivity levels from different tissues and body fluids (Banijamali et al., 2020; Xie et al., 2009).

In addition to the traditional methods described above, there has been a constant search for clinically relevant minimally invasive/noninvasive biomarkers to achieve better prediction and prognosis of GI damage. Nowadays, metabolome-based biomarkers are also being used for this kind of study.

11.3.3 Respiratory tract

Unlike other systems, the respiratory tract is a complex organ system and an incredibly delicate one, both macroscopically and microscopically. Exposure occurs via inhalation, primarily via polluted air, if not during therapy (Parikh et al., 2022). Toxic agents in the form of inhaled particles, gases, or toxins in ingested food can affect the respiratory tract. Factors that affect toxicity are physical and chemical characteristics, dosimetry and sensitivity of the tissue, and host-dependent factors such as health status (Desai et al., 2021), gender (Anup et al., 2021a), and age (Rajpoot et al., 2021a). Any differences in the species and strain (genetic factors) must be considered while interpreting data for risk assessment (Tambe et al., 2021f). Respiratory response to injury induced by toxicants during naturally occurring diseases is nonspecific. Hence, several parameters like the extent and the distribution of lesions, history of the patient, results of ancillary tests as well as histological evaluation have to be evaluated while determining the potential etiologic agents (Casarett, 1971; DeGeorge et al., 1997; Chary et al., 2018; Singh et al., 2021).

11.3.4 Liver

Several liver-derived in vitro model systems, such as slices of liver tissue, perfused liver, primary hepatocytes, immortalized cell lines, isolated microsomes, etc., can be used to evaluate adverse effects of chemicals and drugs. Among these, primary liver cells and immortalized cell lines are used most frequently for testing liver toxicity. These in vitro models' major shortcoming is the loss of viability, loss of liver-specific gene expression and functionality, and poor throughput (Watkins, 2020; Ma et al., 2020).

The field of in vitro hepatotoxicity has some recent development, such as the use of co-cultures of hepatocytes with other cell lines, differentiating stem cells to cells of hepatic lineage, use of 3D organoids and bioartificial liver. To improve the resemblance of cultured liver cells with the physiological conditions novel cell culture systems with incorporated fluid flow, micro-circulation and other organotypic microenvironments have been developed. The use of co-cultures helps in preserving liver-specific morphology and functionality and provides more relevant cell-to-cell communications than can be achieved with pure parenchymal cells. The use of embryonic and adult tissue-derived stem cells from multiple individuals can be an unlimited source of hepatocytes to test individual-specific cytotoxicity. This can significantly improve the reproducibility of liver toxicity testing (Watkins, 2020; Ma et al., 2020; Clemens et al., 2019).

In a study, the researcher evaluated the role of quercitrin in protecting the liver from acetaminophen (APAP)-induced toxicity; balb/c mice were administered quercitrin at a dose of 10 and 50 mg/kg before injection of 300 mg/kg APAP. There was a significant increase in the weight of the liver in the group administered with APAP compared to the control and quercetin alone group in 24 h. Thus, APAP-induced increase in liver weight can be reduced by the peroral preadministration of quercetin (10 and 50 mg/kg) or silymarin (SIL) (50 mg/kg). The toxic effect of high dose of APAP on the liver was also evident from the 14- and a 3-fold increase in serum alanine aminotransferase (ALT) and aspartate aminotransferase (AST) activities on injecting 300 mg/kg of APAP (Fig. 11.4A and B) (Truong et al., 2016).

Pretreatment with quercitrin can be used to protect the liver against elevation in the levels of ALT and AST induced by APAP. This hypothesis was tested in a mouse model using 50 mg/kg of SIL as the positive control (attenuating the ALT and AST activities). Administration of quercetin alone at a dose of 50 mg/kg did not significantly affect the basal activity of ALT and AST, indicating that no liver damage was caused by quercitrin. Histological analysis of the APAP-treated group showed the presence of severe hepatic lesions like inflammation, hydropic degeneration, and hemorrhage can be reduced by pretreatment with quercetin. A similar effect can also be observed in the positive control SIL (Fig. 11.4C) group (Truong et al., 2016).

11.3.5 Immune system

The field of immunotoxicology studies the potential adverse effects on the immune system bought by xenobiotics. This field has undergone consistent evolution due to intensive research focusing on the national and international communities over the last two decades. To support the toxicological testing to align with the requirements of the approval process the regulatory authorities of the US, European, and Japan circulated the guidelines for testing immunotoxicity (Hastings, 2018).

Immunotoxicity impairs the ability of the host to fight against infectious diseases or neoplastic growth (immunosuppression) or causes damage to the host tissue (autoimmunity, hypersensitivity, or chronic inflammation). This definition incorporates the concept that the immune system is a complex balance that includes interactions with other systems (e.g., nervous and endocrine) that may utilize or be affected by the same biological mediators (e.g., neuropeptide and steroid hormones) (Peyton Myers, 2018).

All the data available from the preclinical studies, clinical trials, and the patient response has to be considered in deciding the immunotoxic potential of a material or device. Because the available data will often be less than conclusive, good judgment will play an essential part in immunotoxic risk assessment (Anderson and Shane, 2018).

11.3.6 Kidney

The excretory system is vital in toxicology due to some fundamental reasons, for instance, the role of the kidney in receiving 20%–25% of the resting cardiac output, thereby resulting in increased drug exposure. The tubules of the kidneys concentrate the filtrate, and hence, higher concentrations of drugs cause localized toxic effects. The presence of transporters can further elevate the intracellular concentrations of drugs by accumulation, and the higher

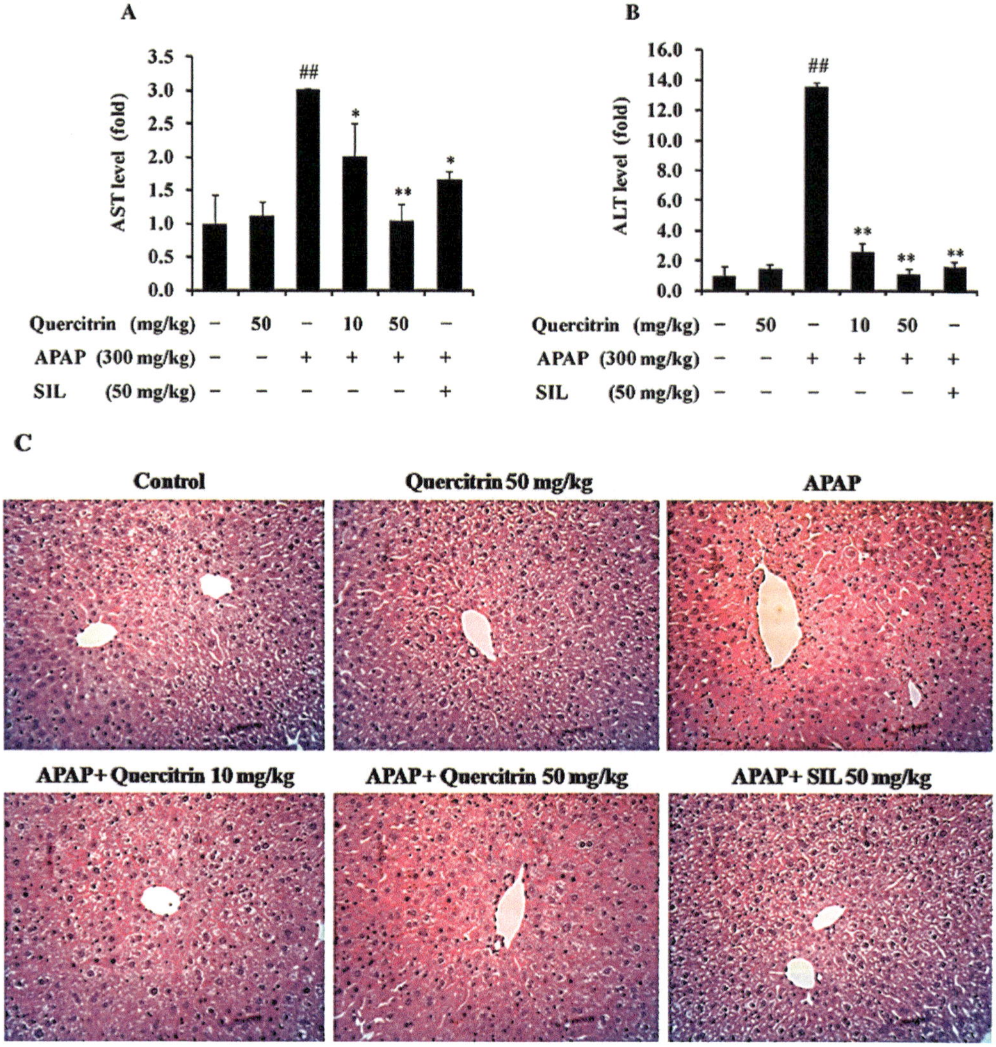

FIGURE 11.4 Protective effects of quercitrin on APAP intoxicated mice. Mice were orally administered quercitrin of 10 or 50 mg/kg once a day for 7 days. The control group received the same volume of saline. After the seventh gavage of quercitrin or saline, animals received a single injection of APAP (300 mg/kg). All mice were sacrificed at 24 h after APAP injection to obtain blood and liver. Serum ALT (**A**) and AST (**B**) levels; and H&E staining (**C**) All data represent the means ± SD of five mice in each group. Significant differences were (##) $P < .01$ as compared with the control; (**) $P < .01$ or (*) $P < .05$ as compared with the APAP group. *Adapted from reference Truong, V.L., Ko, S.Y., Jun, M., Jeong, W.S., 2016. Quercitrin from Toona sinensis (Juss.) M. Roem. Attenuates acetaminophen-induced acute liver toxicity in HepG2 cells and mice through induction of antioxidant machinery and inhibition of inflammation. Nutrients 8 (7), 431. https://www.ncbi.nlm.nih.gov/pubmed/27428996 under Creative Commons Attribution (CC BY) license. Copyright 2016.*

energy requirements of the tubules make them susceptible to nephrotoxic injury. Drug-induced kidney injury is commonly encountered during drug development (Barnett and Cummings, 2018; Xu et al., 2016).

A standard animal model for kidney injury can be developed by thioacetamide (TAA) intoxication. TAA is metabolized by a phase I oxidation reaction, which causes damage that eventually leads to kidney failure. The remarkable antioxidant function of wheat germ oil helps antagonize the free radicals produced during the metabolism of TAA and can have protective effects on kidney function.

Histopathological sections of the kidneys are depicted in Fig. 11.5. Groups I, IV, and V experimental mice showed normal cuboidal cells with a perfect nucleus and eosinophilic cytoplasm. The histology of kidneys treated with TAA (Group II) and TAA followed by olmutinib (Group III) showed an increase in hematopoiesis. In addition, there was a fusion of individual cell margins detected with fuzzy membranes of cells. Furthermore, vascular degeneration and pyknotic nuclei were observed in the TAA and olmutinib groups. WGO treatments reversed all degenerative changes in kidney tubules, with normal cuboidal cells having prominent nuclei (Alamery et al., 2022).

11.3.7 Central nervous system (CNS)

"Neurotoxicology is the study of the adverse effects of chemical, biological, and certain physical agents on the nervous system and/or behavior during development and in

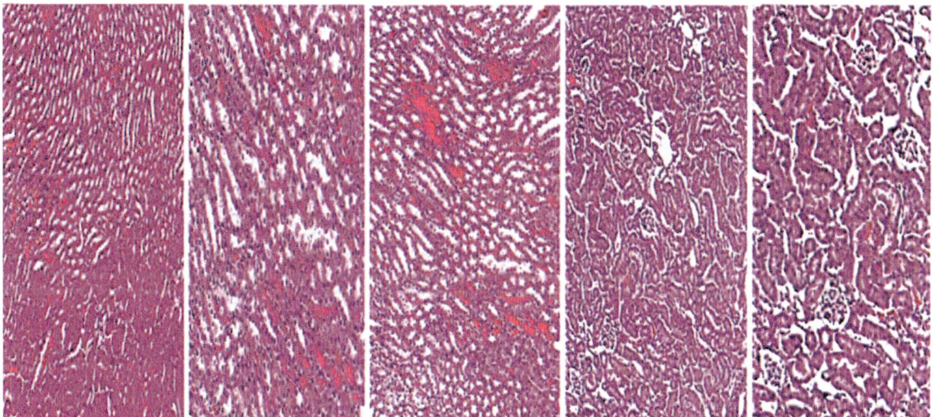

FIGURE 11.5 Images of H&E staining of kidneys of all experimental groups of mice (10×). Group I (control kidney), Group II (TAA with further TAA treatment), Group III (TAA with olmutinib treatment), Group IV (TAA treated with WGO), and Group V (TAA treated with olmutinib + WGO). Groups I, IV, and V show normal histology, while Groups II and III show pyknosis of the nucleus in renal tubular cells with cell membranes and lesion shrinkage. *Adapted from reference Alamery, S., Zargar, S., Yaseen, F., Wani, T.A., Siyal, A. 2022. Evaluation of the effect of wheat germ oil and olmutinib on the thioacetamide-induced liver and kidney toxicity in mice. Life 12 (6) 900. https://www.ncbi.nlm.nih.gov/pubmed/35743930 under Creative Commons Attribution (CC BY) license. Copyright 2022.*

maturity." Examples of common substances with neurotoxic potential include pesticides, ethanol, and heavy metals like lead and mercury.

The data from neurotoxicity analysis is an essential element in toxicity analysis during regulatory filings. It encompasses a battery of tests targeting the CNS. It is sometimes considered a component of organ toxicity studies since CNS is one of the target organs. Exposure to neurotoxins in utero can adversely affect the CNS development of the fetus and is referred to as developmental neurotoxicity (DNT) (Grandjean and Landrigan, 2014; Danish and Santomasso, 2021).

11.3.8 Endocrine system

The complex nature of the endocrine system makes it challenging to tailor standardized testing protocols that can effectively identify chemicals with potential toxicity. The US Environmental Protection Agency (EPA) developed a two-tiered testing system for its Endocrine Disruptor Screening Program (EDSP). The 11 tests in tier 1 and three tests in tier 2 can identify chemicals acting as agonists or antagonists on receptors for thyroid hormone, estrogen, progesterone, and those interfering with steroidogenesis. However, several issues have been identified in this approach of identifying endocrine-disrupting chemicals (EDCs), thereby exposing the public to known EDCs (Gore et al., 2015).

11.4 Mechanism of toxicity

A thorough knowledge of the toxicity mechanisms can help develop a more rational basis for interpreting the toxicity data. The cellular mechanisms contributing to the manifestation of toxicities are overviewed by relating a series of events that begins with exposure, involve many interactions between the invading toxicant and the organism, and culminate in a toxic effect. As a result of the vast number of potential toxicants and the multitude of biological structures and processes that can be impaired, many possible pathways may lead to toxicity. Commonly, a toxicant is delivered to its target, and reacts with it, and the resultant cellular dysfunction manifests itself in toxicity. Sometimes a xenobiotic does not react with a specific target molecule, but adversely influences the biological environment, causing molecular, organellar, cellular, or organ dysfunction leading to harmful effects. Biotransformation to harmful products is called toxication or metabolic activation. Biotransformation reactions that eliminate the ultimate toxicant or prevent its formation are called detoxications. Apoptosis, or programmed cell death, is a tightly controlled, organized process whereby individual cells break into tiny fragments that are phagocytosed by adjacent cells or macrophages without producing an inflammatory response (Zhang, 2018).

Sustained elevation of intracellular Ca^{2+} is harmful because it can result in (1) depletion of energy reserves by inhibiting the ATPase used in oxidative phosphorylation, (2) dysfunction of microfilaments, (3) activation of hydrolytic enzymes, and (4) generation of ROS and reactive nitrogen species (RNS). Cell injury progresses toward cell necrosis (death) if molecular repair mechanisms are inefficient or the molecular damage is not readily reversible. Chemical carcinogenesis involves the impaired function of various repair mechanisms, including (1) failure of DNA repair, (2) failure of apoptosis (programmed cell death), and (3) failure to terminate cell proliferation (Kennedy and Salama, 2020).

11.5 Conclusion

In conclusion, toxicological investigations have come of age. Now, every chemical being put to use in a human being is thoroughly investigated for all its potential effects on the human system in validated models employing different animal species. Finding a surrogate chemical entity with a noticeably reduced risk for organ-specific toxicity may be made possible with cognizance of the toxicokinetic profile of that toxin. A possible strategy needs to be developed to ratify identical toxicity that alternative medicine does not have, by focusing the studies on determining the tissue load of the medication and its byproducts.

11.6 List of abbreviations

ALT alanine aminotransferase
APAP acetaminophen
AS aspartate aminotransferase
CNS central nervous system
CSF cerebrospinal fluid
DDT dichlorodiphenyltrichloroethane
DNT developmental neurotoxicity
EDCs endocrine-disrupting chemicals
EDSP endocrine disruptor screening program
EPA Environmental Protection Agency
GI gastrointestinal
IM intramuscular
IP intraperitoneal
IV intravenous
LD50 median lethal dose
LLNA local lymph node assay
NOAEL no-observed-adverse-effect-level
OECD organization for economic co-operation and development
PK pharmacokinetics
QSAR quantitative structure-activity relationship
REACH registration, evaluation, authorisation, and restriction of chemicals
RHE reconstituted human epidermis
ROS reactive oxygen species
SIL silymarin
TAA thioacetamide
UV ultraviolet
WGO wheat germ oil

References

Abbott, A., 1993. Paracelsus. Nature 366 (6451), 98. https://www.ncbi.nlm.nih.gov/pubmed/8232565.

Abecia, L., Fondevila, M., Balcells, J., Lobley, G.E., McEwan, N.R., 2007. The effect of medicated diets and level of feeding on caecal microbiota of lactating rabbit does. J. Appl. Microbiol. 103 (4), 787–793. https://www.ncbi.nlm.nih.gov/pubmed/17897180.

Abrams, J., 1985. Pharmacology of nitroglycerin and long-acting nitrates. Am. J. Cardiol. 56 (2), 12A–18A. https://www.ncbi.nlm.nih.gov/pubmed/3925750.

Achanta, N.S.K., Rajpoot, K., Tekade, R.K., 2021. Drug metabolic kinetics. In: Tekade, R.K. (Ed.), Biopharmaceutics and Pharmacokinetics Considerations. Elsevier, Academic Press, pp. 335–353.

Adeyinka, A., Mandal, Y., Mohammad Ashraf, H., Pierre, L., Kondamudi, N., 2021. A rare cause of post-traumatic right lower extremity swelling in an adolescent male. Cureus 13 (9), e17726. https://www.ncbi.nlm.nih.gov/pubmed/34659940.

Alamery, S., Zargar, S., Yaseen, F., Wani, T.A., Siyal, A., 2022. Evaluation of the effect of wheat germ oil and olmutinib on the thioacetamide-induced liver and kidney toxicity in mice. Life 12 (6), 900. https://www.ncbi.nlm.nih.gov/pubmed/35743930.

Anderson, S.E., Shane, H.L., 2018. Investigative immunotoxicology. In: Methods in Molecular Biology. Springer, New York. https://doi.org/10.1007/978-1-4939-8549-4_3.

Anup, N., Desai, N., Rajpoot, K., Tekade, R.K., 2021a. Kinetics of maternal–fetal drug transfer. In: Tekade, R.K. (Ed.), Biopharmaceutics and Pharmacokinetics Considerations, pp. 145–162. https://doi.org/10.1016/B978-0-12-814425-1.00007-3.

Anup, N., Gadeval, A., Rajpoot, K., Tekade, R.K., 2021b. Software used in ADME computation. In: Tekade, R.K. (Ed.), Biopharmaceutics and Pharmacokinetics Considerations. Elsevier, Academic Press, pp. 699–708.

Anup, N., Rajpoot, K., Tekade, R.K., 2021c. Overview of biopharmaceutics and pharmacokinetics. In: Tekade, R.K. (Ed.), Biopharmaceutics and Pharmacokinetics Considerations, vol. 1. Elsevier, Academic Press, pp. 1–16.

Asati, S., Pandey, V., Gour, V., Tiwari, R., Soni, V., Rajpoot, K., Tekade, M., Sharma, M.C., Tekade, R.K., 2022. Toxicity and toxicokinetic considerations in product development and drug research. In: Pharmacokinetics and Toxicokinetic Considerations, vol. 2. Elsevier. https://doi.org/10.1016/b978-0-323-98367-9.00001-9.

Atrafi, F., van Eerden, R.A.G., Koolen, S.L.W., de Bruijn, P., Rijcken, C.J.F., Hanssen, R., Eskens, F., Lolkema, M.P., Oomen-de Hoop, E., Damman, J., Mathijssen, R.H.J., 2021. Docetaxel skin exposure and micronucleation contributes to skin toxicity caused by CPC634. Cancers 13 (15), 3741. https://www.ncbi.nlm.nih.gov/pubmed/34359641.

Ballabio, D., Grisoni, F., Consonni, V., Todeschini, R., 2019. Integrated QSAR models to predict acute oral systemic toxicity. Mol. Inform. 38 (8–9), e1800124. https://www.ncbi.nlm.nih.gov/pubmed/30549437.

Baltrop, D., Brueton, M.J., 1990. The gastrointestinal tract and short term toxicity tests. In: Bourdeoui, P. (Ed.), Short Term Toxicity Tests for Non-genotoxic Effects. John Wiley and Sons, p. 99.

Banijamali, A.R., Carvalho, A.E., Wakefield, J.D., Germano, P., Barden, T.C., Tobin, J.V., Zimmer, D.P., Masferrer, J.L., Profy, A.T., Currie, M.G., Todd Milne, G., 2020. Pharmacokinetics, mass balance, tissue distribution, metabolism, and excretion of praliciguat, a clinical-stage soluble guanylate cyclase stimulator in rats. Pharmacol. Res. Perspect. 8 (2), e00579.

Barnett, L.M.A., Cummings, B.S., 2018. Nephrotoxicity and renal pathophysiology: a contemporary perspective. Toxicol. Sci. 164 (2), 379–390. https://www.ncbi.nlm.nih.gov/pubmed/29939355.

Boroujerdi, M., 2015. The influence of routes of administration on ADME. In: Pharmacokinetics and Toxicokinetics. CRC Press. https://doi.org/10.1201/b18133-2.

Casarett, L.J., 1971. Toxicology: the respiratory tract. Annu. Rev. Pharmacol. 11 (1), 425–446. https://www.ncbi.nlm.nih.gov/pubmed/4948843.

Chary, A., Hennen, J., Klein, S.G., Serchi, T., Gutleb, A.C., Blomeke, B., 2018. Respiratory sensitization: toxicological point of view on the available assays. Arch. Toxicol. 92 (2), 803–822. https://www.ncbi.nlm.nih.gov/pubmed/29038838.

Choudhary, D., Goykar, H., Rajpoot, K., Tekade, R.K., 2021. Chronopharmacokinetics. In: Tekade, R.K. (Ed.), Biopharmaceutics and Pharmacokinetics Considerations. Elsevier, Academic Press, pp. 163–194.

Chushak, Y., Gearhart, J.M., Ott, D., 2021. In silico assessment of acute oral toxicity for mixtures. Chem. Res. Toxicol. 34 (2), 345–354. https://www.ncbi.nlm.nih.gov/pubmed/33206501.

Clemens, M.M., McGill, M.R., Apte, U., 2019. Mechanisms and biomarkers of liver regeneration after drug-induced liver injury. Adv. Pharmacol. 85, 241–262. https://www.ncbi.nlm.nih.gov/pubmed/31307589.

Coruzzi, G., 2010. Overview of gastrointestinal toxicology. Curr. Protoc. Toxicol. 43 (1), 21. https://www.ncbi.nlm.nih.gov/pubmed/20967743.

D'Orazio, J., Jarrett, S., Amaro-Ortiz, A., Scott, T., 2013. UV radiation and the skin. Int. J. Mol. Sci. 14 (6), 12222–12248. https://www.ncbi.nlm.nih.gov/pubmed/23749111.

Danish, H., Santomasso, B.D., 2021. Neurotoxicity biology and management. Cancer J. 27 (2), 126–133. https://www.ncbi.nlm.nih.gov/pubmed/33750072.

DeGeorge, J.J., Ahn, C.H., Andrews, P.A., Brower, M.E., Choi, Y.S., Chun, M.Y., Du, T., Lee-Ham, D.Y., McGuinn, W.D., Pei, L., Sancilio, L.F., Schmidt, W., Sheevers, H.V., Sun, C.J., Tripathi, S., Vogel, W.M., Whitehurst, V., Williams, S., Taylor, A.S., 1997. Considerations for toxicology studies of respiratory drug products. Regul. Toxicol. Pharmacol. 25 (2), 189–193. https://www.ncbi.nlm.nih.gov/pubmed/9185894.

Desai, N., Koppisetti, H., Rajpoot, K., Tekade, M., Sharma, M.C., Tekade, R.K., 2021. Influence of fever on pharmacokinetics of drugs. In: Tekade, R.K. (Ed.), Biopharmaceutics and Pharmacokinetics Considerations, first ed. Elsevier, pp. 451–463. https://doi.org/10.1016/B978-0-12-814425-1.00011-5.

Dispenza, M.C., 2019. Classification of hypersensitivity reactions. Allergy Asthma Proc. 40 (6), 470–473. https://www.ncbi.nlm.nih.gov/pubmed/31690397.

Draize, J.H., 1944. Methods for the study of irritation and toxicity of substances applied topically to the skin and mucous membranes. J. Pharmacol. Exp. Therapeut. 82, 377–390.

Epstein, J.H., 1999. Phototoxicity and photoallergy. Semin. Cutan. Med. Surg. 18 (4), 274–284. https://www.ncbi.nlm.nih.gov/pubmed/10604793.

Gadaleta, D., Vukovic, K., Toma, C., Lavado, G.J., Karmaus, A.L., Mansouri, K., Kleinstreuer, N.C., Benfenati, E., Roncaglioni, A., 2019. SAR and QSAR modeling of a large collection of LD50 rat acute oral toxicity data. J. Cheminf. 11 (1), 58. https://www.ncbi.nlm.nih.gov/pubmed/33430989.

Gerberick, G.F., Ryan, C.A., Dearman, R.J., Kimber, I., 2007. Local lymph node assay (LLNA) for detection of sensitization capacity of chemicals. Methods 41 (1), 54–60. https://www.ncbi.nlm.nih.gov/pubmed/16938465.

Gore, A.C., Chappell, V.A., Fenton, S.E., Flaws, J.A., Nadal, A., Prins, G.S., Toppari, J., Zoeller, R.T., 2015. EDC-2: the endocrine society's second scientific statement on endocrine-disrupting chemicals. Endocr. Rev. 36 (6), E1–E150. https://www.ncbi.nlm.nih.gov/pubmed/26544531.

Grandjean, P., Landrigan, P.J., 2014. Neurobehavioural effects of developmental toxicity. Lancet Neurol. 13 (3), 330–338. https://www.ncbi.nlm.nih.gov/pubmed/24556010.

Gultekin, F., Oner, M.E., Savas, H.B., Dogan, B., 2020. Food additives and microbiota. North. Clin. Istanb. 7 (2), 192–200. https://www.ncbi.nlm.nih.gov/pubmed/32259044.

Gupta, R., Polaka, S., Rajpoot, K., Tekade, M., Sharma, M.C., Tekade, R.K., 2022a. Importance of toxicity testing in drug discovery and research. In: Pharmacokinetics and Toxicokinetic Considerations, vol. 2. Elsevier. https://doi.org/10.1016/b978-0-323-98367-9.00016-0.

Gupta, R., Rajpoot, K., Tekade, M., Sharma, M.C., Safavi, M., Tekade, R.K., 2022b. Factors influencing drug toxicity. In: Pharmacokinetics and Toxicokinetic Considerations, vol. 2. Elsevier. https://doi.org/10.1016/b978-0-323-98367-9.00014-7.

Gupta, R., Rajpoot, K., Tekade, M., Sharma, M.C., Tekade, R.K., 2022c. Methods and models for in vitro toxicity. In: Pharmacokinetics and Toxicokinetic Considerations, vol. 2. Elsevier. https://doi.org/10.1016/b978-0-323-98367-9.00006-8.

Hastings, K.L., 2018. Immunotoxicology: a brief history. In: Methods in Molecular Biology. Springer, New York. https://doi.org/10.1007/978-1-4939-8549-4_1.

Hinton, A.N., Goldminz, A.M., 2020. Feeling the burn: phototoxicity and photoallergy. Dermatol. Clin. 38 (1), 165–175. https://www.ncbi.nlm.nih.gov/pubmed/31753189.

Hu, F., Santagostino, S.F., Danilenko, D.M., Tseng, M., Brumm, J., Zehnder, P., Wu, K.C., 2022. Assessment of skin toxicity in an in vitro reconstituted human epidermis model using deep learning. Am. J. Pathol. 192 (4), 687–700. https://www.ncbi.nlm.nih.gov/pubmed/35063406.

Kennedy, L.B., Salama, A.K.S., 2020. A review of cancer immunotherapy toxicity. CA A Cancer J. Clin. 70 (2), 86–104. https://www.ncbi.nlm.nih.gov/pubmed/31944278.

Kim, K., Park, H., Lim, K.M., 2015. Phototoxicity: its mechanism and animal alternative test methods. Toxicol. Res. 31 (2), 97–104. https://www.ncbi.nlm.nih.gov/pubmed/26191378.

Koleva, Y.K., Cronin, M.T., Madden, J.C., Schwobel, J.A., 2011. Modelling acute oral mammalian toxicity. 1. Definition of a quantifiable baseline effect. Toxicol. Vitro 25 (7), 1281–1293. https://www.ncbi.nlm.nih.gov/pubmed/21557997.

Kovacik, A., Kopecna, M., Vavrova, K., 2020. Permeation enhancers in transdermal drug delivery: benefits and limitations. Expert Opin. Drug Deliv. 17 (2), 145–155. https://www.ncbi.nlm.nih.gov/pubmed/31910342.

Kumawat, A., Raval, N., Reddy, G., Rajpoot, K., Tekade, R.K., 2020. Gene delivery to tackle diabetic nephropathy. In: Tekade, R.K. (Ed.), The Future of Pharmaceutical Product Development and Research, vol. 1. Academic Press, pp. 515–537. http://www.sciencedirect.com/science/article/pii/B9780128144558000153.

Lagunin, A., Zakharov, A., Filimonov, D., Poroikov, V., 2011. QSAR modelling of rat acute toxicity on the basis of PASS prediction. Mol. Inform. 30 (2–3), 241–250. https://doi.org/10.1002/minf.201000151.

Lunghini, F., Marcou, G., Azam, P., Horvath, D., Patoux, R., Van Miert, E., Varnek, A., 2019. Consensus models to predict oral rat acute toxicity and validation on a dataset coming from the industrial context. SAR QSAR Environ. Res. 30 (12), 879–897. https://www.ncbi.nlm.nih.gov/pubmed/31607169.

Ma, X., McKeen, T., Zhang, J., Ding, W.X., 2020. Role and mechanisms of mitophagy in liver diseases. Cells 9 (4), 837. https://www.ncbi.nlm.nih.gov/pubmed/32244304.

Macmillan, D.S., Chilton, M.L., 2019. A defined approach for predicting skin sensitisation hazard and potency based on the guided integration of in silico, in chemico and in vitro data using exclusion criteria. Regul. Toxicol. Pharmacol. 101, 35–47. https://www.ncbi.nlm.nih.gov/pubmed/30439387.

Matzneller, P., Krasniqi, S., Kinzig, M., Sorgel, F., Huttner, S., Lackner, E., Muller, M., Zeitlinger, M., 2013. Blood, tissue, and intracellular concentrations of azithromycin during and after end of therapy. Antimicrob. Agents Chemother. 57 (4), 1736–1742. https://www.ncbi.nlm.nih.gov/pubmed/23357769.

Miner, N.A., Koehler, J., Greenaway, L., 1969. Intraperitoneal injection of mice. Appl. Microbiol. 17 (2), 250–251. https://www.ncbi.nlm.nih.gov/pubmed/5775909.

Moore, D.E., 2002. Drug-induced cutaneous photosensitivity: incidence, mechanism, prevention and management. Drug Saf. 25 (5), 345–372. https://www.ncbi.nlm.nih.gov/pubmed/12020173.

Ning, Z.H., Long, S., Zhou, Y.Y., Peng, Z.Y., Sun, Y.N., Chen, S.W., Su, L.M., Zhao, Y.H., 2015. Effect of exposure routes on the relationships of lethal toxicity to rats from oral, intravenous, intraperitoneal and intramuscular routes. Regul. Toxicol. Pharmacol. 73 (2), 613–619. https://www.ncbi.nlm.nih.gov/pubmed/26361856.

OECD, 2008. OECD. In: Kirch, W. (Ed.), Encyclopedia of Public Health. Springer Netherlands, Dordrecht, pp. 1034–1035. https://doi.org/10.1007/978-1-4020-5614-7_2421.

OECD, 2010. Test No. 417: Toxicokinetics. OECD Guidelines for the Testing of Chemicals, Section 4. OECD Publishing Paris. https://doi.org/10.1787/9789264070882-en.

OECD, 2021. Test No. 405: Acute Eye Irritation/Corrosion. OECD Guidelines for the Testing of Chemicals, Section 4. https://www.oecd-ilibrary.org/content/publication/9789264185333-en.

Olson, H., Betton, G., Robinson, D., Thomas, K., Monro, A., Kolaja, G., Lilly, P., Sanders, J., Sipes, G., Bracken, W., Dorato, M., Van Deun, K., Smith, P., Berger, B., Heller, A., 2000. Concordance of the toxicity of pharmaceuticals in humans and in animals. Regul. Toxicol. Pharmacol. 32 (1), 56–67. https://www.ncbi.nlm.nih.gov/pubmed/11029269.

Padiyar, A., Agrawal, O.P., Rajpoot, K., Tekade, R.K., 2020. Hydrotropy, mixed hydrotropy, and mixed solvency as trending concept for solubilization of lipophilic drugs. In: Tekade, R.K. (Ed.), The Future of Pharmaceutical Product Development and Research. Academic Press, pp. 145–178. http://www.sciencedirect.com/science/article/pii/B9780128144558000050.

Parikh, K.J., Christian, J.R., Rajpoot, K., Tekade, R.K., 2022. Environmental and safety aspects of bionanotechnology. In: Pharmacokinetics and Toxicokinetic Considerations, vol. 2. Elsevier. https://doi.org/10.1016/b978-0-323-98367-9.00022-6.

Pauluhn, J., Bury, D., Fost, U., Gamer, A., Hoernicke, E., Hofmann, T., Kunde, M., Neustadt, T., Schlede, E., Schnierle, H., Wettig, K., Westphal, D., 1996. Acute inhalation toxicity testing: considerations of technical and regulatory aspects. Arch. Toxicol. 71 (1–2), 1–10. https://www.ncbi.nlm.nih.gov/pubmed/9010579.

Peloquin, C.A., Berning, S.E., Nitta, A.T., Simone, P.M., Goble, M., Huitt, G.A., Iseman, M.D., Cook, J.L., Curran-Everett, D., 2004. Aminoglycoside toxicity: daily versus thrice-weekly dosing for treatment of mycobacterial diseases. Clin. Infect. Dis. 38 (11), 1538–1544. https://www.ncbi.nlm.nih.gov/pubmed/15156439.

Peyton Myers, L., 2018. Clinical immunotoxicology. In: Methods in Molecular Biology. Springer, New York. https://doi.org/10.1007/978-1-4939-8549-4_2.

Pham, M.A., Magdalou, J., Siest, G., Lenoir, M.C., Bernard, B.A., Jamoulle, J.C., Shroot, B., 1990. Reconstituted epidermis: a novel model for the study of drug metabolism in human epidermis. J. Invest. Dermatol. 94 (6), 749–752. https://www.ncbi.nlm.nih.gov/pubmed/2113070.

Polaka, S., Desai, N., Kshirsagar, B., Rajpoot, K., Tekade, R.K., 2021a. Revamping the pharmacokinetics of poorly soluble drugs using different formulations. In: Tekade, R.K. (Ed.), Biopharmaceutics and Pharmacokinetics Considerations, first ed. Elsevier, pp. 387–413. https://doi.org/10.1016/B978-0-12-814425-1.00005-X.

Polaka, S., Makwana, V., Vasdev, N., Sheth, A., Rajpoot, K., Sengupta, P., Tekade, R.K., 2022a. Engineering immunity via skin-directed drug delivery devices. J. Contr. Release 345, 385–404. https://www.ncbi.nlm.nih.gov/pubmed/35283256.

Polaka, S., Rajpoot, K., Tekade, M., Sharma, M.C., Tekade, R.K., 2022b. Food—drug interactions and their implications on oral drug bioavailability. In: Pharmacokinetics and Toxicokinetic Considerations, vol. 2. Elsevier. https://doi.org/10.1016/b978-0-323-98367-9.00002-0.

Polaka, S., Swetha, K.L., Dittakavi, S., Rajpoot, K., Tekade, R.K., 2021b. Bioanalytical method development and validation for establishing bioavailability and bioequivalence. In: Tekade, R.K. (Ed.), Biopharmaceutics and Pharmacokinetics Considerations. Elsevier, pp. 487—516. https://doi.org/10.1016/B978-0-12-814425-1.00001-2.

Rajpoot, K., Desai, N., Koppisetti, H., Tekade, M., Sharma, M.C., Behera, S.K., Tekade, R.K., 2022a. In silico methods for the prediction of drug toxicity. In: Pharmacokinetics and Toxicokinetic Considerations, vol. 2. Elsevier. https://doi.org/10.1016/b978-0-323-98367-9.00012-3.

Rajpoot, K., Katare, P., Tekade, M., Sharma, M.C., Polaka, S., Sengupta, P., Tekade, R.K., 2022b. Toxicokinetic and toxicodynamic considerations in drug research. In: Pharmacokinetics and Toxicokinetic Considerations, vol. 2. Elsevier. https://doi.org/10.1016/b978-0-323-98367-9.00026-3.

Rajpoot, K., Tekade, M., Sharma, M.C., Arafat, B., Tekade, R.K., 2022c. Principles and concepts in toxicokinetic. In: Pharmacokinetics and Toxicokinetic Considerations, vol. 2. Elsevier. https://doi.org/10.1016/b978-0-323-98367-9.00023-8.

Rajpoot, K., Tekade, M., Sharma, M.C., Sreeharsha, N., Sharma, A., Tekade, R.K., 2020b. Recombinant blood products and therapeutic enzymes: an update. In: Tekade, R.K. (Ed.), The Future of Pharmaceutical Product Development and Research. Academic Press, pp. 447—482. http://www.sciencedirect.com/science/article/pii/B978012814455800013X.

Rajpoot, K., Tekade, M., Sreeharsha, N., Sharma, M.C., Tekade, R.K., 2020c. Recent advancements in solubilization of hydrophobic drugs. In: Tekade, R.K. (Ed.), The Future of Pharmaceutical Product Development and Research. Academic Press, pp. 109—144. http://www.sciencedirect.com/science/article/pii/B9780128144558000049.

Rajpoot, K., Tekade, R.K., Chatterjee, B., Sharma, M.C., Tekade, M., 2021a. Biopharmaceutical considerations in the pediatric and geriatric formulation development. In: Tekade, R.K. (Ed.), Biopharmaceutics and Pharmacokinetics Considerations, vol. 1. Elsevier, Academic Press, pp. 109—144.

Rajpoot, K., Tekade, R.K., Sharma, M.C., Safavi, M., Tekade, M., 2021b. Pharmacokinetics modeling in drug delivery. In: Tekade, R.K. (Ed.), Biopharmaceutics and Pharmacokinetics Considerations. Elsevier, Academic Press, pp. 279—334.

Rajpoot, K., Tekade, R.K., Sharma, M.C., Tekade, M., 2021c. Pharmacokinetics and biopharmaceutics: "a leader or attendant". In: Tekade, R.K. (Ed.), Biopharmaceutics and Pharmacokinetics Considerations. Elsevier, Academic Press, pp. 17—27.

Rybacka, A., Ruden, C., Andersson, P.L., 2014. On the use of in silico tools for prioritising toxicity testing of the low-volume industrial chemicals in REACH. Basic Clin. Pharmacol. Toxicol. 115 (1), 77—87. https://www.ncbi.nlm.nih.gov/pubmed/24428755.

Sazonovas, A., Japertas, P., Didziapetris, R., 2010. Estimation of reliability of predictions and model applicability domain evaluation in the analysis of acute toxicity (LD50). SAR QSAR Environ. Res. 21 (1), 127—148. https://www.ncbi.nlm.nih.gov/pubmed/20373217.

Singh, A.V., Romeo, A., Scott, K., Wagener, S., Leibrock, L., Laux, P., Luch, A., Kerkar, P., Balakrishnan, S., Dakua, S.P., Park, B.W., 2021. Emerging technologies for in vitro inhalation toxicology (adv. Healthcare mater. 18/2021). Adv. Healthc. Mater. 10 (18), 2170082. https://doi.org/10.1002/adhm.202170082.

Tambe, V., Desai, N., Rajpoot, K., Tekade, R.K., 2021a. "Organ-on-a-chip"-based physiologically relevant pharmacokinetic models. In: Tekade, R.K. (Ed.), Biopharmaceutics and Pharmacokinetics Considerations, first ed. Elsevier, pp. 643—673. https://doi.org/10.1016/B978-0-12-814425-1.00024-3.

Tambe, V., Ditani, A., Rajpoot, K., Tekade, R.K., 2021b. Pharmacokinetics aspects of structural modifications in drug design and therapy. In: Tekade, R.K. (Ed.), Biopharmaceutics and Pharmacokinetics Considerations, vol. 1. Elsevier, Academic Press, pp. 83—108.

Tambe, V., Kathar, U., Raval, N., Rajpoot, K., Shilpi, S., Khatri, K., Tekade, R.K., 2021c. Positron emission tomography as a non-invasive tool in pharmacokinetic studies. In: Tekade, R.K. (Ed.), Biopharmaceutics and Pharmacokinetics Considerations. Elsevier, Academic Press, pp. 617—641.

Tambe, V., Pande, S., Gadeval, A., Rajpoot, K., Raval, N., Tekade, R.K., 2021d. Microdialysis: an emerging technique for pharmacokinetic—pharmacodynamic profiling. In: Tekade, R.K. (Ed.), Biopharmaceutics and Pharmacokinetics Considerations, first ed. Elsevier, pp. 601—616. https://doi.org/10.1016/B978-0-12-814425-1.00018-8.

Tambe, V., Shukla, H., Rajpoot, K., Pandey, M.M., Tekade, R.K., 2021e. Pharmacokinetics aspects of biotechnological products. In: Tekade, R.K. (Ed.), Biopharmaceutics and Pharmacokinetics Considerations. Elsevier, Academic Press, pp. 539–565.

Tambe, V., Sirsat, B., Rajpoot, K., Gadeval, A., Tekade, R.K., 2021f. Pharmacogenomics and drug metabolism. In: Tekade, R.K. (Ed.), Biopharmaceutics and Pharmacokinetics Considerations, vol. 1. Elsevier, Academic Press, pp. 355–385.

Tekade, M., Koppisetti, H., Sharma, M.C., Rajpoot, K., Sengupta, P., Kumar, M., Tekade, R.K., 2022. Understanding the concept of signal toxicity and its implications on human health. In: Pharmacokinetics and Toxicokinetic Considerations, vol. 2. Elsevier. https://doi.org/10.1016/b978-0-323-98367-9.00020-2.

Tiwari, A., Joshi, M., Salvi, N., Gupta, D., Gandhi, S., Rajpoot, K., Tekade, R.K., 2022. Toxicity of pharmaceutical azo dyes. In: Pharmacokinetics and Toxicokinetic Considerations, vol. 2. Elsevier. https://doi.org/10.1016/b978-0-323-98367-9.00004-4.

Truong, V.L., Ko, S.Y., Jun, M., Jeong, W.S., 2016. Quercitrin from Toona sinensis (Juss.) M. Roem. Attenuates acetaminophen-induced acute liver toxicity in HepG2 cells and mice through induction of antioxidant machinery and inhibition of inflammation. Nutrients 8 (7), 431. https://www.ncbi.nlm.nih.gov/pubmed/27428996.

Usach, I., Martinez, R., Festini, T., Peris, J.E., 2019. Subcutaneous injection of drugs: literature review of factors influencing pain sensation at the injection site. Adv. Ther. 36 (11), 2986–2996. https://www.ncbi.nlm.nih.gov/pubmed/31587143.

Vasdev, N., Rajpoot, K., Tekade, R.K., 2021. Molecular mechanisms of circadian rhythm and its influence on the pharmacokinetics of drugs. In: Tekade, R.K. (Ed.), Biopharmaceutics and Pharmacokinetics Considerations. Elsevier, Academic Press, pp. 415–449.

Walley, T.J., 2000. Davies textbook of adverse drug reactions. Postgrad. Med. 76 (901), 741E. https://www.ncbi.nlm.nih.gov/pubmed/11060180.

Walum, E., 1998. Acute oral toxicity. Environ. Health Perspect. 106 (Suppl. 2), 497–503.

Watkins, P.B., 2020. Quantitative systems toxicology approaches to understand and predict drug-induced liver injury. Clin. Liver Dis. 24 (1), 49–60. https://www.ncbi.nlm.nih.gov/pubmed/31753250.

Wester, R.C., Maibach, H.I., 2012. Erratum to percutaneous absorption of drugs. Clin. Pharmacokinet. 24 (1), 70. https://doi.org/10.1007/bf03259380.

Wolfreys, A., Kilgour, J., Allen, A.D., Dudal, S., Freke, M., Jones, D., Karantabias, G., Krantz, C., Moore, S., Mukaratirwa, S., Price, M., Tepper, J., Cauvin, A., Manetz, S., Robinson, I., 2021. Review of the technical, toxicological, and PKPD considerations for conducting inhalation toxicity studies on biologic pharmaceuticals-the outcome of a cross-industry working group survey. Toxicol. Pathol. 49 (2), 261–285. https://www.ncbi.nlm.nih.gov/pubmed/33535023.

Xie, L.H., Li, Q., Zhang, J., Weina, P.J., 2009. Pharmacokinetics, tissue distribution and mass balance of radiolabeled dihydroartemisinin in male rats. Malar. J. 8, 112.

Xu, X.L., Yang, L.J., Jiang, J.G., 2016. Renal toxic ingredients and their toxicology from traditional Chinese medicine. Expert Opin. Drug Metabol. Toxicol. 12 (2), 149–159. https://www.ncbi.nlm.nih.gov/pubmed/26670420.

Zhang, Y., 2018. Cell toxicity mechanism and biomarker. Clin. Transl. Med. 7 (1), 34. https://www.ncbi.nlm.nih.gov/pubmed/30374795.

Zhu, Q., Yang, Y., Lao, Z., Zhong, Y., Zhang, K., Zhao, S., 2020. Acute and chronic toxicity of deltamethrin, permethrin, and dihaloacetylated heterocyclic pyrethroids in mice. Pest Manag. Sci. 76 (12), 4210–4221. https://www.ncbi.nlm.nih.gov/pubmed/32596996.

Further reading

Mathaes, R., Koulov, A., Joerg, S., Mahler, H.C., 2016. Subcutaneous injection volume of biopharmaceuticals-pushing the boundaries. J. Pharm. Sci. 105 (8), 2255–2259. https://www.ncbi.nlm.nih.gov/pubmed/27378678.

Rajpoot, K., Tekade, M., Pandey, V., Nagaraja, S., Youngren-Ortiz, S.R., Tekade, R.K., 2020a. Self-microemulsifying drug-delivery system: ongoing challenges and future ahead. In: Tekade, R.K. (Ed.), Drug Delivery Systems. Academic Press, pp. 393–454. http://www.sciencedirect.com/science/article/pii/B9780128144879000090.

Rajpoot, K., Tekade, R.K., 2019. Microemulsion as drug and gene delivery vehicle: an inside story. In: Tekade, R.K. (Ed.), Drug Delivery Systems. Academic Press, pp. 455–520. http://www.sciencedirect.com/science/article/pii/B9780128144879000107.

CHAPTER

12

Drug-induced nephrotoxicity and its biomarkers

Suryanarayana Polaka[1], *Lakshmi Vineela Nalla*[1,2], *Rana Dhwani Kalpeshkumar*[1], *Paritala Sree Teja*[1], *Anand More*[1], *Muktika Tekade*[3], *Dinesh Kumar Chellappan*[4] and *Rakesh Kumar Tekade*[1]

[1]National Institute of Pharmaceutical Education and Research (NIPER)- Ahmedabad, An Institute of National Importance, Government of India, Department of Pharmaceuticals, Ministry of Chemicals and Fertilizers, Palaj, Gandhinagar, Gujarat, India; [2]Department of Pharmacy, Koneru Lakshmaiah Education Foundation, Vaddeswaram, Andhra Pradesh, India; [3]School of Pharmacy, Devi Ahilya Vishwavidyalaya, Indore, Madhya Pradesh, India; [4]Department of Life Sciences, School of Pharmacy, International Medical University, Kuala Lumpur, Malaysia

12.1 Introduction

The kidney is one of the most vital organs in the human body. It is where the homeostasis of the body is maintained by regulating electrolytes, water, and excretion of waste products produced during metabolism. It also maintains the acid-base balance. The kidney produces essential hormones like renin and erythropoietin to control the renin-angiotensin-aldosterone hormonal system (Jose et al., 2017). Since the kidney is involved in the excretion of many xenobiotics, it is considered the most susceptible organ to chemical toxicity. It is known to be affected by the medications delivered to treat various diseases (Altınkaynak et al., 2018). It has been reported that around 19% of the subjects who were admitted to the intensive care unit (ICU) were suffering from complications of acute renal failure (ARF) related to drugs (Hoste et al., 2015).

Recently, it has been believed that drug-induced nephrotoxicity is the primary reason for renal damage (Jose et al., 2017). Sometimes co-administered herbs, drugs, food and excipients

Essentials of Pharmatoxicology in Drug Research, Volume 1
https://doi.org/10.1016/B978-0-443-15840-7.00011-7

affect the pharmacokinetics and pharmacodynamics of the other drugs, which subsequently leads to some adverse effects in the human body (Niguram et al., 2020; Polaka et al., 2021a,b,c,d; Polaka et al., 2022a,b,c,d,e,f). Therefore, there is an urgent need to understand drug-induced nephrotoxicity along with the mechanisms and biomarkers involved. These strategies can help mitigate drug-induced nephrotoxicity at the early stage of drug development. When we look into the physical characteristics, with a granular surface, the nephrotoxic kidney is small and has restricted functions. Histologically, the nephrotoxic kidney exhibits larger glomerular space (Fig. 12.1).

The kidney's primary function is to concentrate and eliminate drugs and metabolite toxins. Hence, kidney is considered the most vulnerable target for drug-induced toxicity upon chronic drug exposure. In hospital settings, it was reported that the drug toxicants majorly

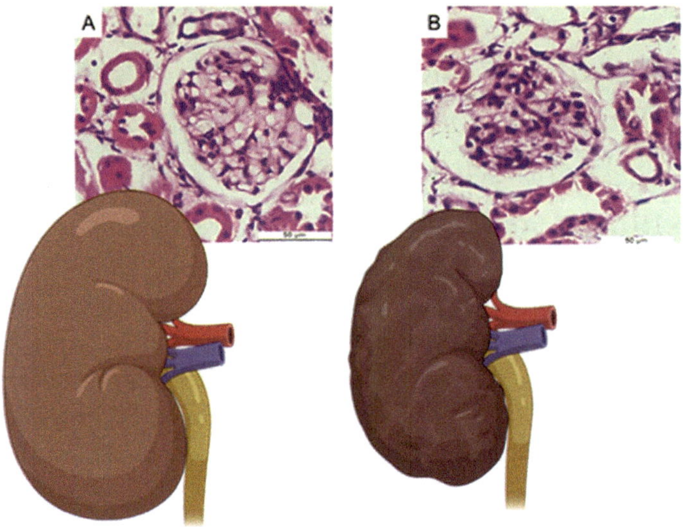

FIGURE 12.1 Differences between the (A) healthy and (B) nephropathic kidneys. Therapeutic interventions are needed to treat most ailments; adverse reactions from the given medications often lead to severe complications. Drug-induced nephrotoxicity is a substantial complication observed in medical practice, and the incidence of drug-related acute kidney injury (AKI) accounts for over 60% (Ghane Shahrbaf and Assadi, 2015). In older adults, drug-induced nephrotoxicity was reported as high as 66% (Kohli et al., 2000; Naughton, 2008). Drug-associated nephrotoxicity is usually prevalent among several patients and specific clinical settings, where community-acquired and hospitalization are significant grounds. Most of the water soluble drugs (molecular weight less than 500 Da) pass through the kidney freely, increasing the risk on the kidney and making it vulnerable for developing drug toxicity; the significant factor that needs to be considered include the total amount of blood that reaches the kidney is 25% of cardiac output that corresponds to 50 times the exposure of the drug to the kidney (Sharfuddin and Molitoris, 2011). Kidney has the largest endothelial surface per gram of tissue compared to any other organ (Verma and Molitoris, 2015). The urine is concentrated at the distal convoluted tubule, which increases the major risk of precipitation of crystals (Pazhayattil and Shirali, 2014). *Adapted with permission from reference Raval, N., et al., 2021. Engineered nanoplex mediated targeted miRNA delivery to rescue dying podocytes in diabetic nephropathy. Int. J. Pharm. 605, 120842.*

contributed to acute kidney injury (8%–60%) (2012). Many drugs suffer from side effects of nephrotoxicity. Such side effects of drugs restrict drug use and result in severe adverse reactions. Understanding the molecular mechanism behind drug-induced nephrotoxicity can help avert this toxicity and enhance the patient's tolerability to higher drug doses for prolonged periods (Shayan and Elyasi, 2020). A vast number of therapeutics available in the market, either prescribed or over-the-counter (OTC), have the potential to induce nephrotoxicity, thus reducing their clinical use (Tiong et al., 2014).

Drug-induced nephrotoxicity is counted as one of the significant challenges in hospital settings. Due to the lack of standard nephrotoxic prediction tools and preclinical models, it is challenging to develop less nephrotoxic drugs at the early stages of drug development (Fisel et al., 2014). As a result, drug-induced nephrotoxicity will be distinguished at the later stages of drug development and is associated with substantial economic expenditures (Redfern and Valentin, 2011). Hence, it is imperative to identify nephrotoxicity at the initial stages of drug development to enhance the health outcomes of patients. This chapter reviews different aspects of drug-induced nephrotoxicity, the mechanism of drug-induced nephrotoxicity, few case studies, biomarkers for early detection of nephrotoxicity, and several novel methods to identify biomarkers.

12.2 Mechanisms of drug-induced nephrotoxicity

Nephrotoxicity insinuates precipitous deterioration of kidney functions, a common complication observed due to the toxic effects of several medications and chemicals (Nolin and Himmelfarb, 2010; Al-Naimi et al., 2019). Drug-induced nephrotoxicity is close to 20% of all nephrotoxicity-related incidences, and this percentage is slightly higher in the elderly owing to underlying conditions and poly-medications (Al-Naimi et al., 2019). The drugs causing nephrotoxicity act by one or more of the following mechanisms.

12.2.1 Tubular epithelial cell damage

Continuous exposure to drugs such as antibiotics to proximal convoluted tubule (PCT) causes tubular epithelial cell damage. Reabsorption and concentration of drugs take place in PCT through the glomerulus. Accumulation of aminoglycosides, amphotericin B, gentamicin, and vancomycin in tubular epithelial cells lead to cytotoxicity causing damage to basal membranes. Reabsorption of these drugs is dose-dependent across the tubular cell membranes (Downes et al., 2020). The concentration of drugs in the tubular cell membrane and organelles, such as the endoplasmic reticulum, golgi complex, and lysosomes, leads to endocytosis and tubular cell damage, thereby inhibiting the phospholipase activity. Acute tissue necrosis results when threshold levels cause mitochondrial destruction, leading to cellular oxidative stress, generating oxygen-free radicals, and ultimately tissue damage.

Tubular cell injury also leads to renal insufficiency by obstructing the renal tubules through spillage of cellular components and impaired renal absorption by a complex known as a tubuloglomerular feedback loop (Fig. 12.2) (Lopez-Novoa et al., 2011). It causes the excess distribution of water as well as electrolytes to the distal nephron by increasing the

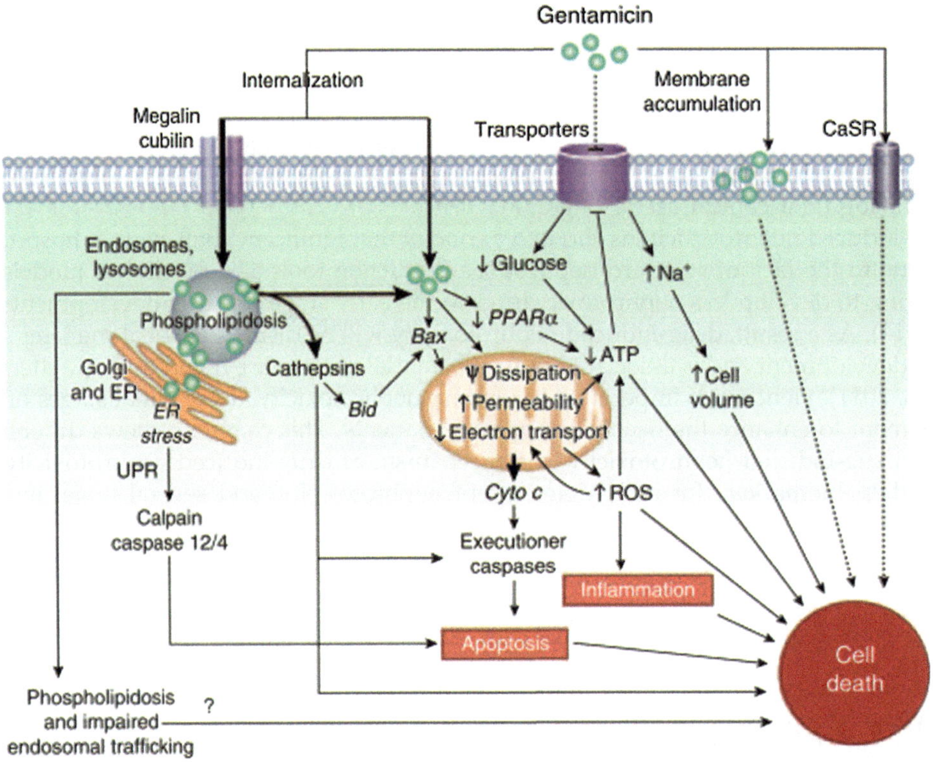

FIGURE 12.2 Gentamicin-induced cell death and inflammation in tubular epithelial cells of the kidney. *Adapted from Lopez-Novoa, J. M., et al., 2011. New insights into the mechanism of aminoglycoside nephrotoxicity: an integrative point of view. Kidney Int. 79 (1), 33–45.*

hydrostatic pressure. This phenomenon triggers the vascular feedback mechanism, reducing the glomerular filtration rate, renal flow, and electrolyte losses. In some conditions, vacuolization and swelling might be observed in PCT with osmotic nephrosis (Perazella, 2005).

12.2.2 Inflammation

One of the pathways of drug-induced nephrotoxicity is the induction of inflammatory response by the host, targeting the glomerulus, proximal tubules, and surrounding interstitium (Naughton, 2008; Perazella, 2018). Aminoglycosides, especially gentamicin-induced inflammation, include impaired mitochondrial ATP production, releasing excessive ROS-inducing inflammation (Fig. 12.2) (Lopez-Novoa et al., 2011). These inflammatory changes result in renal scarring and fibrosis of the kidney tissues, ultimately leading to toxicity induction, including glomerulonephritis, acute interstitial nephritis, and chronic interstitial nephritis (Kim and Moon, 2012). Glomerulonephritis is known to have an association with proteinuria in the nephrotic range (Perazella, 2005). Acute interstitial nephritis results from an allergic response to medications binding to renal antigens or medications acting as antigens. These antigens are known to deposit in the interstitium, causing the induction of an immune reaction (Rossert, 2001). Acute interstitial nephritis might be associated with around 15% of subjects hospitalized for acute renal failure (Kodner and Kudrimoti, 2003). Chronic interstitial nephritis is an implication observed by long-term usage of certain drugs like NSAIDs and analgesic agents. The eventual complications observed are recurrent papillary necrosis and chronic renal failure (Paller, 1990).

12.2.3 Intraglomerular hemodynamic changes

The glomerulus is a network of tiny blood capillaries situated at the initial part of the nephron, which consists of two blood vessels: the afferent arteriole and the efferent arteriole. The primary function of the glomerulus is to maintain the glomerular filtration rate (GFR). The standard GFR is 120 mL/min in a healthy individual (Kim and Moon, 2012). This process is regulated by vasodilation of the afferent and vasoconstriction of the efferent arterioles. Angiotensin II regulates hemodynamics in the nephron. ACE inhibitors are known to prevent the transformation of angiotensin I to angiotensin II, which results in decreased blood flow and blood pressure. This results in vasoconstriction of afferent arteriole and vasodilation of efferent arteriole, thereby altering the hemodynamics of the kidney resulting in reduced blood flow and renal volume insufficiency (Nolin and Himmelfarb, 2010; Chen and Busse, 2017) (Fig. 12.3A). There are circulating prostaglandins that regulate the process of vasodilation of afferent arteriole across the glomerulus. Usage of NSAIDS like COX-1 inhibitor

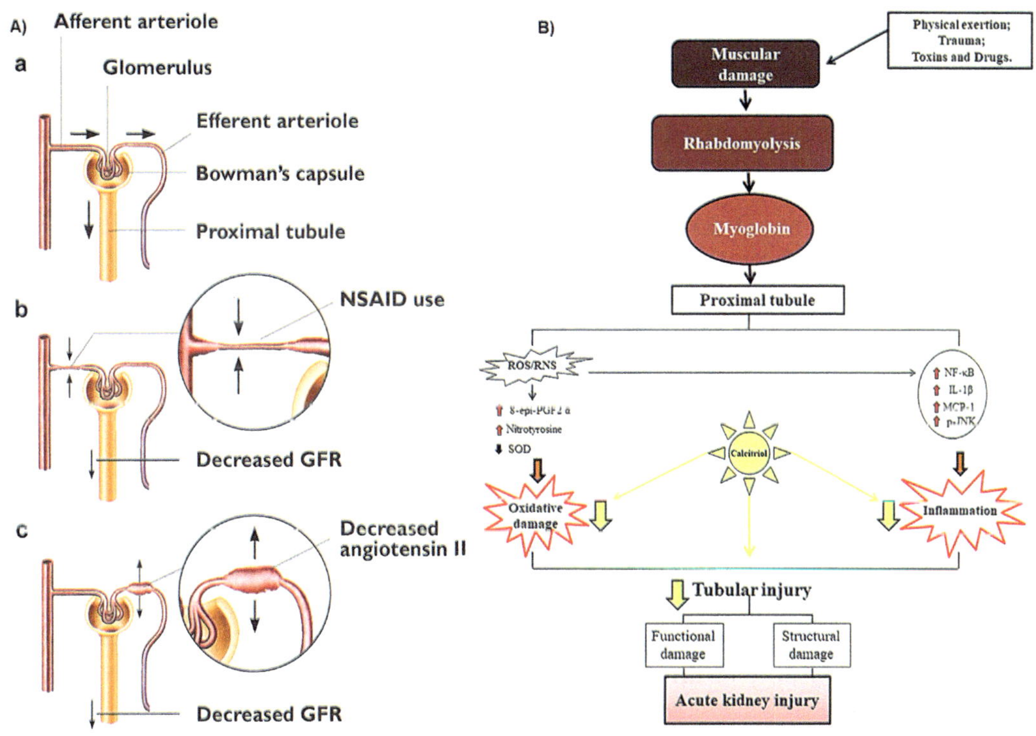

FIGURE 12.3 (A) (a) in normal human physiology, (b) vasoconstriction induced with NSAID use, (c) vasodilation with angiotensin II deficiency; (B) drug-induced rhabdomyolysis causing AKI. *(A) Adapted from Chen, H., Busse, L.W., 2017. Novel therapies for acute kidney injury. Kidney Inter. Rep. 2 (5), 785–799. (B) Adapted from Reis, N.G., et al., 2019. Protective effect of calcitriol on rhabdomyolysis-induced acute kidney injury in rats. Sci. Rep. 9 (1), 1–10 under common creative license.*

(aspirin) COX-2 inhibitors (ibuprofen, diclofenac, naproxen) inhibits the prostaglandin synthesis causing vasoconstriction of afferent arteriole due to decreased production of PGE2, leading to decreased renal blood volume, renal output, and renal ischemia (Chen and Busse, 2017; Wu and Huang, 2018) (Fig. 12.3A). Decreased blood flow causes auto secretion of renin, resulting in increased blood flow and GFR. Continuous use of ACEs and ARBs results in decreased blood flow, blood pressure, and excess diuresis causing hypotension and electrolyte imbalances leading to nephrotoxicity, AKI, and renal failure. Proper monitoring of renal outcomes must be maintained for patients undergoing such treatment.

12.2.4 Rhabdomyolysis

Rhabdomyolysis, a clinical and biochemical syndrome, is the breakdown of skeletal muscle leading to the release of large quantities of intracellular myocyte components into the plasma. Lysis of myocytes leads to leakage of muscle contents such as myoglobin and creatinine kinase into the extracellular fluids and circulation. The released myoglobin results in the induction of tubular obstruction, alterations in glomerular filtration rates, and renal injury secondary to direct toxic effects on myocytes, ultimately resulting in acute tubular necrosis or renal failure (Sauret et al., 2002; Coco and Klasner, 2004; Naughton, 2008; Kim and Moon, 2012). More than 150 medications and toxins are reported to cause skeletal muscle injury (Coco and Klasner, 2004). These medications cause rhabdomyolysis by inhibiting calcium metabolism employing the sarcoplasmic reticulum, cell membrane disruption due to impaired production of adenosine triphosphate, and changes in carbohydrate metabolism. Drug-induced coma also leads to more oxygen demands due to prolonged muscle immobilization. A study conducted in AKI rats treated with calcitriol showed a protective effect by decreasing the ROS and inflammatory markers in rhabdomyolysis-induced AKI (Reis et al., 2019) (Fig. 12.3B).

Further, prolonged muscle immobilization causes more oxygen demands; the implications are due to drug-induced coma (Prendergast and George, 1993; Coco and Klasner, 2004). Some of the common medications causing rhabdomyolysis are listed in Table 12.1. Consumption of alcohol is the most common cause among others and contributes to around 81% of cases of rhabdomyolysis, and 50% of patients consequently develop ARF (Naughton, 2008).

12.2.5 Crystal growth in nephron

Crystal nephropathy refers to the precipitation of crystals from various therapeutic agents and their derivatives within the distal tubular lumens owing to their comparative insolubility in human urine. Accumulating insoluble crystals lead to tubular obstruction and acute renal injury eliciting interstitial reactions. Certain medications may also cause endogenous substances to precipitate, inducing renal injury (Perazella, 2005; Naughton, 2008; Yarlagadda and Perazella, 2008; Kim and Moon, 2012). The concentration of drugs in the urine as well as the pH of urine (acidity of urine) governs the formation of insoluble crystals (Perazella, 1999; Naughton, 2008; Kim and Moon, 2012). Studies with kidney biopsy findings from patients who intervened with different medications like sulfadiazine, methotrexate, indinavir, and triamterene displayed different shaped crystals in the urine (Fig. 12.4) (Perazella and

TABLE 12.1 Drugs implicating nephrotoxicity.

Types of nephrotoxicity	Medications causing renal conditions	References
Glomerulonephritis	Lithium, NSAIDs, propyl thiouracil, gold therapy, hydralazine, interferon-alfa, pamidronate, cyclooxygenase-2 inhibitors, ampicillin, penicillin	Naughton (2008), Nolin and Himmelfarb (2010), Frazier and Obert (2018)
Acute interstitial nephritis	Allopurinol, rifampicin, sulfonamide, lansoprazole, phenytoin, quinolones, loop diuretics (furosemide, bumetanide, torsemide), thiazide diuretics, proton pump inhibitors (lansoprazole, omeprazole, pantoprazole), H_2 blockers (cimetidine, ranitidine), beta-lactams (penicillin, cephalosporins), abacavir, acyclovir, atazanavir, indinavir, NSAIDs, a selective COX-2 inhibitor, 5-aminosalicylates	Rossert (2001), Perazella (2005), Naughton (2008)
Chronic interstitial nephritis	Acetaminophen, aspirin, NSAIDs (>1 g/day) for 2 years, calcineurin, lithium, cyclosporine, tacrolimus, Chinese herbal medicine, aristolochic acid, chemotherapeutics (carmustine)	Olyaei et al. (1999), Fored et al. (2001), Naughton (2008), Nolin and Himmelfarb (2010), Rodríguez-Iturbe and García (2010), Al-Naimi et al. (2019)
Rhabdomyolysis	Haloperidol, propofol, leflunomide, fluoxetine, amitriptyline, statins, lithium, trabectedin, daptomycin, benzodiazepines, ethanol, methanol, isoniazid, hydrocortisone, caffeine, prednisone, strychnine, loxapine, baclofen, serotonin antagonists, ketamine **Drug of abuse:** narcotics, cocaine, heroin, ketamine, methamphetamine, methadone, marijuana **Antihistamine:** diphenhydramine	Coco and Klasner (2004), Naughton (2008), Hohenegger (2012), Torres et al. (2015), Matsubara et al. (2018)
Crystal nephropathy	Methotrexate, diuretic-triamterene, indinavir, quinolones, ganciclovir, acyclovir, foscarnet, sulphonamides (sulfadiazine, sulfamethoxazole), nitrofurantoin, aminopenicillins (amoxicillin, ampicillin), quinolones (ciprofloxacin, norfloxacin), orlistat, oral sodium phosphate solution	Perazella (2005), Naughton (2008), Yarlagadda and Perazella (2008)
Obstructive nephropathy	Acyclovir, sulphonamides-sulfadiazine, methotrexate, triamterene, indinavir, nelfinavir, forcarnet, ciprofloxacin, amoxicillin, nitrofurantoin thrombolytic agents, norephedrine, pseudoephedrine and ephedrine	Daudon and Jungers (2004), Taber and Pasko (2008), Nolin and Himmelfarb (2010)
Osmotic nephropathy	Dextran, mannitol, radiographic contrast media, propylene glycol, and sucrose	Perazella (2005)
Thrombotic macroangiopathy	Ticlopidine, cyclosporine, clopidogrel, quinine, mitomycin C	Pisoni et al. (2001)

Herlitz, 2021). Various antibiotics, antivirals, and other medications causing crystal nephropathy are mentioned in Table 12.1.

12.2.6 Obstructive nephropathy

Obstructive nephropathy is the presence of functional and structural changes that cause mechanical obstruction of urine following glomerular filtration, impeding normal urine flow (Klahr, 2000; Taber and Pasko, 2008). In the events of obstructive nephropathy, increased pressure in the bowman's space impedes the intratubular filtration pressure, thereby decreasing the intraglomerular blood flow (Fig. 12.5A) (Chávez-Iñiguez et al., 2020). Medications and/or their metabolites precipitating in the intratubular region and lower urinary tract cause obstructive nephropathy, leading to AKI. Intratubular precipitation is the leading cause of drug-induced rhabdomyolysis, among other factors. Abnormal crystal precipitation in the renal collecting system, called nephrolithiasis, is also a common type of obstructive nephropathy (Nolin and Himmelfarb, 2010). Various medications (Table 12.1) are known to cause obstructive nephropathy leading to urinary tract dilatation, an impedance of urine flow, pressure difference within the tubular system of the kidney, and impaired kidney functions (Liji Thomas, 2019).

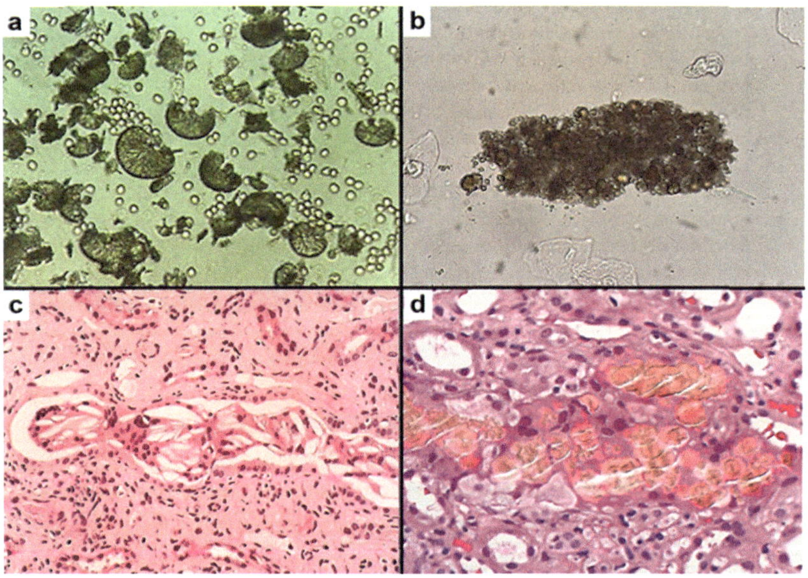

FIGURE 12.4 (A) fan-shaped sulfadiazine crystals in the urine, (B) brown-colored methotrexate crystals are observed within a urinary cast, (C) indinavir crystals within the tubular lumens of the kidney, and (D) triamterene crystals are noted within the tubular lumens of the kidney. *Adapted from Perazella, M.A., Herlitz, L.C., 2021. The crystalline nephropathies. Kidney Inter. Rep. 6 (12), 2942–2957.*

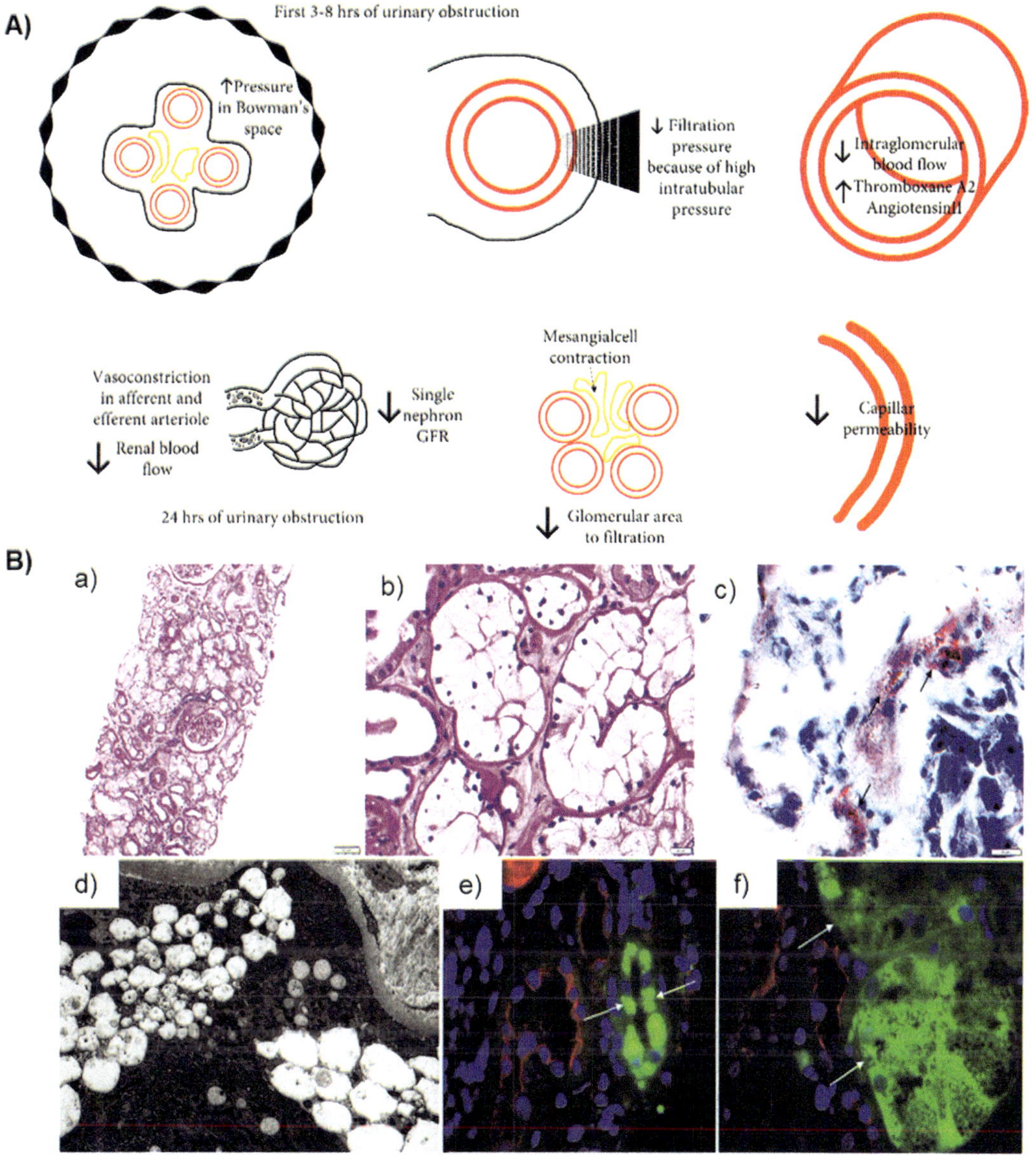

FIGURE 12.5 (A) Glomerular changes during obstructive nephropathy. (B) Proximal tubules with osmotic tubulopathy at a: Low (10×) and b: High (40×) magnifications using periodic acid–Schiff stain; c: Lipid deposits in proximal tubule using Oil Red O staining, d: Ultrastructural studies show clear vacuoles within the proximal tubules and immunofluorescence of e: aldose reductase, and f: fructokinase. *(A) Adapted from Chávez-Iñiguez, J. S., et al., 2020. Acute kidney injury caused by obstructive nephropathy. Inter. J. Nephrol. 2020. (B) Adapted from Phadke, G., et al., 2020. Osmotic nephrosis and acute kidney injury associated with SGLT2 inhibitor use: a case report. Am. J. Kidney Dis. 76 (1), 144–147 under common creative license.*

12.2.7 Osmotic nephropathy

Drugs like dextran, mannitol, radiographic contrast media, or solvents like propylene glycol and sucrose (as a career combined with IV immunoglobulin) cause osmotic nephropathy. They are closely related to vacuolization, swelling, and necrosis of PCT epithelial cells with decreased kidney function (Perazella, 2005). Due to the hypertonic and osmotic effects of these agents, a decline in renal function may occur. Intravenous immunoglobulin solution of sucrose (hyper molar) is associated with osmotic nephrosis, and acute kidney injury is typically reversed following cessation of therapy (Orbach et al., 2004). They are absorbed by the proximal tubule and not metabolized because of their characteristic structure. Cell edema occurs due to the inhibition of lysosome function vacuolization of cells, resulting in a block of tubules (Dickenmann et al., 2008). Hydroxyethyl starch is also associated with osmotic nephropathy. Mannitol causes oligoanuric kidneys in rare cases (Choudhury and Ahmed, 2006). Further, a case report of a patient treated with an SGLT2 inhibitor (Canagliflozin) displayed osmotic nephrosis and AKI. Clear vacuoles were observed in the PCT (Fig. 12.5B) (Phadke et al., 2020).

12.2.8 Thrombotic macroangiopathy

Drugs like ticlopidine, cyclosporine, clopidogrel, quinine, and mitomycin C cause vascular endothelial toxicity by inducing immune reaction that leads to platelet clump formation, i.e., thrombotic thrombocytopenic purpura that occurs in microcirculation. The drug induces an immune response or is directly toxic to vascular endothelial cells (Pisoni et al., 2001).

12.3 Case studies of drug-induced nephrotoxicity

Liu et al. conducted a multicenter cross-sectional survey on drug-induced hospital-acquired acute kidney injuries in China. They screened 280,255 admitted subjects, suggesting 1960 cases of hospital-acquired AKI. Of these, 735 cases were demarcated as drug-induced acute kidney injury (D-AKI) (37.50%, 735/1960) with an in-hospital death rate of 13.88% and 54.34%, and the fighters were unable to achieve complete renal recovery. A total of 1642 drugs were associated with AKI in these subjects, most of them being anti-infective, diuretics, and proton pump inhibitors (66.63% cumulatively) (Liu et al., 2021).

Similarly, Nash et al. performed a hospital-acquired renal insufficiency (HARI) survey wherein the study involved follow-ups from 4622 patients admitted to the hospital. Data suggested the development of acute deterioration in 7.2% of patients. Observations showed a lesser occurrence of hospital-acquired renal failure in women and blacks. Among the causes of HARI, 16% (61 episodes) of incidences were attributed to drug-induced renal complications. The medications were associated with nephrotoxicity, intestinal nephritis, and elevated serum creatinine levels. Aminoglycosides are attributed to 29.5% (18 episodes) of drug-induced events. NSAIDs (Nonsteroidal anti-inflammatory drugs) accounted for 21% (13 episodes), followed by piperacillin/tazobactam accounting for 11.4% (7 episodes). Amphotericin B and trimethoprim/sulfa implicated incidences were at 9.83% each (6 episodes each), whereas cyclosporine was involved in three episodes (4.91%). Angiotensin-converting enzyme inhibitors and multiple nephrotoxins were responsible for two episodes each, resulting in 6.54% of the incidences. Ciprofloxacin, cis-platinum, acyclovir, and ceftazidime were involved in 1.64% of total episodes. Apart from the medications, radioactive contrast media reported 11% (43 episodes), mainly computed tomographic (CT) scans and angioplasties. Of all, 22.6% of patients showed partial recovery, while a total death rate of 19.4% was observed (Nash et al., 2002).

A hospital-based prospective study on treatment-related ARF in the elderly (>60 years) over 12 months was undertaken by Kohli et al. Of the 4176 elderly patients, 59 had ARF in the hospital setting. Among them, ARF in 39 patients resulted from using nephrotoxic drugs (66%) (Kohli et al., 2000).

Likewise, Kaufman et al. conducted a prospective study of hospitalized patients with raised serum creatinine levels to study the implication of community-acquired ARF. In this 17-month study period, 100 patients with serum creatinine levels of more than 177 μmol/L (2 mg/dL) were screened. Of the admitted patients, 70% had prerenal azotemia, 17% had obstruction, 11% had intrinsic ARF, and 2% were ungrouped. In prerenal azotemia cases, drugs were the primary cause in almost 14 cases. Among these, angiotensin-converting enzyme inhibitors were the contributing cause in six patients, while ACE inhibitors were the cause in four patients with acute renal failure. Observations revealed a decrease in serum creatinine levels after discontinuation of ACE inhibitors in all six patients, usually within 2–4 days. It was observed that two patients taking demeclocycline developed prerenal azotemia, and one patient undergoing sulindac therapy reported developing ARF. It was also observed that cisplatin contributed to renal failure in two patients, rifampicin in one patient, and glyburide in one patient. The mortality rate in patients admitted with ARF was 15%, compared to a death rate of 3.9% among all hospital admissions. Overall, it was concluded that drugs were critical precipitating factors in 19% of the subjects, captopril being the most widespread offending cause. The findings concluded that diuretics and antihypertensives also led to ARF apart from ACE inhibitors. This prospective study implicated that a diversity of medications was accountable for the community-acquired ARF, either as direct nephrotoxins or resulting in reduced renal perfusion. In hospital-acquired renal insufficiency, drugs were the cause for 20% of the incidents, with contrast media and aminoglycosides as the primary causative agents (Kaufman et al., 1991).

Incidents of drug-induced renal failures (DIRF) are difficult to ascertain. Data suggest that DIRF contributes to 18%–27% of ARF in hospitalized patients, while around 20% of hospital admissions for ARF are caused by drugs, mainly NSAIDs. NSAIDs and ACE inhibitors implicate renal hypoperfusion, whereas drugs such as antibiotics, antivirals, and immunosuppressants are connected with the development of interstitial nephritis (Hannah, 2007).

12.4 Biomarkers for nephrotoxicity

The nephron is the fundamental kidney unit, and it mainly performs the excretion of waste materials and toxic metabolites from the body. Molecular movement across the nephron is highly restricted under normal conditions. But under some pathological conditions such as nephrotoxicity or any other renal injuries, the molecules freely move across the nephron leading to alterations in the excretory process and promoting the elimination of essential ions, water, and other proteins from the body. This damage to renal function may be caused due to many factors, and one among them is drug-induced nephrotoxicity. So, it is vital to identify renal damage at very early stages.

Biomarkers are the biological components that alter in response to physiological damage or organ dysfunction. Proteins that are excreted through urine are considered a potential marker for drug-induced nephrotoxicity (Al-Naimi et al., 2019). Serum creatinine and urinary output are considered traditional biomarkers, but they are accompanied by limitations such as low sensitivity and specificity (Edelstein, 2017). This led to the development of novel biomarkers that help diagnose kidney injury at an early stage.

12.4.1 Protein-based biomarkers

Many biological and molecular changes have been reported in kidney injury, and the use of biomarkers has been suggested. These biomarkers detect kidney injury at an early stage before the creatinine levels rise in serum. These biomarkers aid in tracing the toxicity of a drug or any other substance, assessing potential effects, and helping in the recovery of the kidney after renal injury. The potentiality of a biomarker to detect the AKI priorly is usually represented graphically by using the receiver operating characteristic curve (ROC). The area under the curve (AUC) of the ROC curve determines the predictive ability of a biomarker. The ROC helps determine the sensitivity and specificity of biomarkers (Ghatanatti et al., 2014).

As the concentration of biomarkers depends on the urinary samples of patients, it becomes challenging to measure the concentration of the biomarker in anuric patients. Contrary to this, serum biomarkers can overcome the disadvantages of urinary biomarkers, but there might be nonrenal sources that generate false results (Devarajan and Murray, 2014). A single biomarker cannot produce overall results related to kidney injury because of the diversity of nephrons. So, several biomarkers have been identified for a specific nephron region. Tubular damage is detected by increased urinary excretion of proximal tubule proteins, whereas decreased reabsorption of filtered proteins indicates the dysfunction of the proximal tubule (Redahan and Murray, 2017). Protein biomarkers are enlisted in Fig. 12.6.

12.4.1.1 Albumin

The progression of renal disease occurs due to microalbuminuria, a pathological condition categorized by the excretion of albumin in the range of 30–300 mg in 24 h (Basi et al., 2008). Because albumin has a negative charge, it cannot be filtered via the glomerulus. As a result, microalbuminuria is a good diagnostic feature for proximal tubule injury. It is also one of the FDA/EMA-qualified biomarkers for AKI. Albuminuria is also a diagnostic agent in drug-induced renal tubular injury (Tugay et al., 2006). Conditions such as hematuria, urinary tract infections (UTI), and dehydration also lead to the development of microalbuminuria, limiting its usage due to its nonspecific nature.

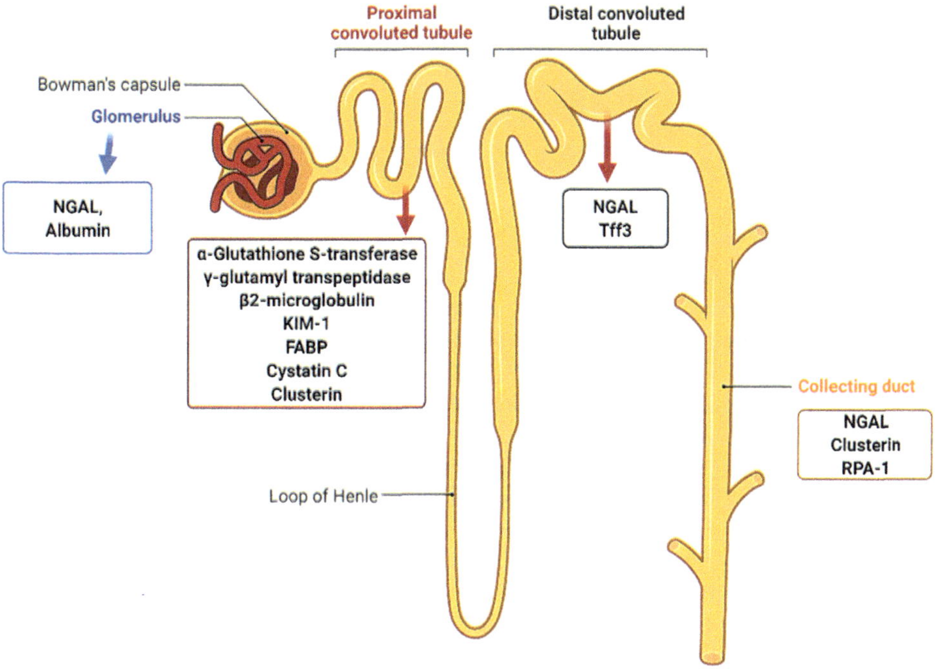

FIGURE 12.6 List of protein biomarkers form different parts of the nephron.

12.4.1.2 *β2-microglobulin*

The glomerulus filters most of the β2-microglobulin, which gets reabsorbed and broken down by proximal tubular cells. Pathological conditions, including renal tubule injury, lupus nephritis, pyelonephritis, kidney transplantation, and medications like tenofovir, can increase β2-microglobulin excretion, making it valuable as a diagnostic agent. β2-microglobulin is often unstable at ambient temperature and in acidic environments; thus, it has limited usage (Kang et al., 2015).

12.4.1.3 *Clusterin*

In response to stress, the expression levels of two isoforms of Clusterin 2 [nuclear form (nCLU) and secretory form] are increased. Pathological conditions like subtotal nephrectomy, ischemia/reperfusion injury, unilateral ureteral obstruction drug-induced kidney injury promote the expression of clusterin (Davis et al., 2004). This is also among the FDA/EMA-qualified biomarkers, as the levels of urinary CLU correlate with the severity of proximal tubular injury in rats. Although clusterin has activity as a biomarker, there is still ambiguity in considering it as an efficient biomarker because of the inconsistency in data obtained from clinical and preclinical studies (Dieterle et al., 2010).

12.4.1.4 *Cystatin-C*

Cystatin-C (Cys-C) is filtered via glomerulus followed by reabsorption, thereby preventing its secretion into tubules. Elevated levels of urinary Cys-C were observed in subjects with tubular dysfunction. Urinary Cys-C and β2 microglobulin were detected due to the impairment of tubular reabsorption resulting from glomerular damage (Togashi et al., 2013). Two recent meta-analysis studies included urinary Cys-C as a biomarker for AKI following cardiac surgery (>5000 patients from 28 studies) and also for CKD (>3000 patients from 19 studies), which has proven an overall good performance in medical situations (Wei et al., 2015).

12.4.1.5 Fatty acid-binding proteins

Fatty acid-binding proteins (FAPBs) mainly facilitate the transportation of free fatty acids from the plasma membrane to intracellular organelles such as mitochondria or peroxisomes. There are two isoforms of FAPB: heart-type FABP in the distal tubule and liver-type FABP in the proximal tubule (Oyama et al., 2005). H-FABP acts as a prognostic biomarker in aminoglycoside-induced nephrotoxicity in rats. Elevated H-FAPB and L-FAPB were observed in patients undergoing surgery for abdominal aortic aneurysms, revealing their role in predicting tubular injury. L-FAPB also helps predict the requirement for renal transplantation in patients suffering from AKI. L-FABP was considered one of the five tubular biomarkers for AKI and diabetic nephropathy reported in a Japan-based toxicity study conducted in mice. L-FAPB levels were elevated in patients with interstitial ischemia and might be influenced by the upregulation of L-FABP levels in serum in liver disease (Kokot et al., 2014).

12.4.1.6 Glutathione S-transferases (GST)

GST are cytosolic enzymes that have α GST and π GST isomers expressed in the tubular region of the nephron. Proteinuria-related damage to the brush border lining of the kidney is caused by increased excretion of these isomeric forms. These GST isomers are thought to be a predictor of polyene-induced kidney damage. They are also concerned with the progression of various stages of AKI in subjects after cardiac surgery. Although they are precise and sensitive biomarkers, their urinary instability is a drawback (Koyner et al., 2010).

12.4.1.7 Kidney injury molecule 1 (KIM-1)

Elevated levels of KIM-1 mRNA in the proximal tubule were observed in association with kidney damage. KIM-1 expression promotes the transformation of PCT cells into macrophages that promote the phagocytosis of damaged cells, providing nephroprotective activity after renal injury. Urinary KIM-1 was a predictive biomarker in several animal models of drug-induced nephrotoxicity in early kidney injury. KIM helps in the early diagnosis of kidney damage in humans. KIM-1 tends to be a prominent biomarker to predict proximal tubular injury, and it is often associated with a decrease in renal function. KIM-1 expression endorses kidney fibrosis that leads to chronic kidney damage. KIM-1 acts as a predictive and most sensitive biomarker in preclinical studies, unlike a clinical AKI biomarker (Ichimura et al., 2008).

12.4.1.8 Neutrophil gelatinase-associated lipocalin (NGAL)

NGAL is a monomeric molecule that is secreted by tubular cells of the kidney. Studies performed in animal models revealed that the expression of NGAL is upregulated in conditions of ischemia or drug-induced AKI. NGAL also acts as a biomarker for AKI in patients undergoing cardiac corrective surgery. It also helps predict graft rejection in patients undergoing kidney transplantation (Cai et al., 2010).

12.4.1.9 Renal papillary antigen (RPA-1)

Renal papillary antigen (RPA-1) is selective for CD of the nephron and predicts any damage within it. Initially, monoclonal antibodies were elevated compared to proteins released in rats treated with nephrotoxic agents, and corresponding antibodies were generated. Being a glycoprotein, RPA-1 was proved to be a predictive biomarker for renal papillary necrosis and collecting duct injury. Preclinical studies done in rats treated with drugs inducing kidney toxicity proved the role of RPA-1 as a predictive urinary biomarker. It also helps to trace the advancement of CKD in hypertensive and obese rat models. But the role of RPA-1 is limited only to animal models. Their role in humans is still under investigation (Price et al., 2010; Sasaki et al., 2011).

12.4.1.10 Trefoil factor 3

Trefoil factor 3 is mainly associated with respiratory, intestinal, and urogenital tract epithelial cells, which help maintain, protect, and repair. It lines the basal and intermediate layers of different parts of a nephron. Dose-dependent decrease of urinary TFF4-3 was correlated with AKI in preclinical studies using three nephrotoxic agents. Higher levels of TFF-3 in urine and serum were associated with chronic inflammatory diseases such as CKD, but TFF-3 can moderately predict delayed graft rejection compared to TIMP-2. Further clinical studies have to be conducted to explore the activity of TFF-3 as a biomarker of kidney injury (Rinnert et al., 2010; Yu et al., 2010). All the biomarkers related to the drug-induced kidney injury is enlisted in Table 12.2.

12.4.2 MicroRNA-based biomarkers for glomerular injury

Recent literature sheds light on a particular group of nucleic acids that has been gaining significant attention in glomerular injury as biomarkers-microRNAs. MicroRNAs (miRNAs) are short, noncoding, 18–24 nucleotide length RNA segments that regulate the post-transcriptional process of several proteins involved in diverse physiological and pathological conditions. They bind to the 3′ UTR region of target mRNA and regulate the gene expression (O'Brien et al., 2018; Gajula et al., 2020). Maximum miRNAs are transcribed from DNA. The transcripts undergo a series of processing steps such as endonucleolytic cleavage, nuclear export, and a strand selection procedure. Then they are converted to pri-miRNA and pre-miRNA that is eventually cleaved, forming matured miRNA (Zeng, 2006; Nalewajska et al., 2019). Studies estimate that 50% of the mammalian protein-coding genes are regulated by the miRNAs (Krol et al., 2010). Generally, the miRNAs are packed into exosomes and microvesicles in cells, rendering their degradation from extracellular RNA-degrading enzymes (Hoy and Buck, 2012). These extracellular microRNAs secreted in the extracellular fluids, namely blood serum and urine, are known to be potential biomarkers for various diseases, the renal disorder being one among them.

According to the FDA's description, extracellular miRNAs fit all the criteria as a biomarker as they have remarkable stability and easy accessibility in body fluids, which can be analyzed

TABLE 12.2 Biomarkers for drug-induced kidney injury.

Protein name	Presumed marker for	Supportive experimental results	Clinical trial data	Detection system	Clinical utility	References
α-glutathione-S-transferase	Proximal convoluted tubule	Elevated levels of α-GST were observed in rats administered with valproic acid.	Studies performed in rats administered with 20 mg/kg of valproic acid showed a slight increase in α-GST, whereas a gradual rise in α-GST was observed in rats administered with 5omg/kg and 100 mg/kg dose of valproic acid, respectively.	ELISA	Nephrotoxic, kidney transplantation, ischemia, sepsis	Lee et al. (2009)
ϒ-glutamyl transpeptidase	Proximal convoluted tubule	Elevated levels of urinary ϒ-glutamyl transpeptidase were observed in dogs with AKI.	Studies performed on dogs with AKI exhibited high levels of urinary ϒ-glutamyl transpeptidase.	Colorimetry	AKI, sepsis	Nivy et al. (2017)
NGAL	Glomerulus, PCT, DCT, CD	Elevated levels of urinary NGAL were detected in patients induced with cisplatin.	Studies on patients revealed that urinary NGAsL levels were observed higher within 2 h of cisplatin induction.	ELISA, Luminex-based assay.	Nephrotoxicity ischemia, sepsis	Karademir et al. (2016)
β2-microglobulin	Proximal convoluted tubule damage	Elevated in conditions of unilateral nephrectomy in diabetic rats.	There will be upregulation of β2-microglobulin levels in patients suffering from drug-induced kidney injury or renal replacement therapy associated with tubulointerstitial rejection.	ELISA, nephelometer	Nephrotoxicity ischemia sepsis renal transplantation	Fels et al. (2019), Atef et al. (2021)
		Increased exposure to Cd^{+2} leading to megalin-cubilin dependent renal toxicity.	Elevated in patients who are exposed to Cd^{+2} present in food and tobacco.			
KIM-1		Upregulation of KIM-1 was observed	Patients with kidney transplantation and		Nephrotoxicity ischemia, sepsis	Luo et al. (2016)

TABLE 12.2 Biomarkers for drug-induced kidney injury.—cont'd

Protein name	Presumed marker for	Supportive experimental results	Clinical trial data	Detection system	Clinical utility	References
	Proximal tubule damage	due to the induction of gentamicin, sevoflurane, cisplatin, and bacitracin by increasing the mRNA expression and exposure to metals such as mercury, chromium, and cadmium.	acute kidney injury exhibit high levels of KIM-1.	ELISA, Luminex-based assays.	renal transplantation	
		p-ERK associated upregulation of KIM-1 levels was observed in gentamicin and lead acetate-induced rats.	Studies performed on rats administered with lead acetate and gentamycin revealed a correlation between p-ERK levels and KIM-1 levels that helps in the early detection of renal damage.			Ruiz-Ramirez et al. (2021)
		Elevated levels are observed in rats after treatment with vancomycin.	Studies performed on rats administered with vancomycin showed upregulation of KIM-1 and clusterin on 1st day. Later on, upregulation of KIM-1 and clusterin helps in predicting the histopathological changes within 3−6 days.			Pais et al. (2019)
Fatty acid-binding protein (FABP)	Proximal convoluted tubule	Upregulation of urinary FABP was observed in puromycin and N-Phenylanthranylic acid dosed Wistar rats.	Wister rats showed increased urinary FABP within 1−3 days after treatment with NPAA and 14−28 days after treatment with puromycin.	ELISA	Nephrotoxicity, renal transplantation	Obajdin et al. (2018)

(*Continued*)

TABLE 12.2 Biomarkers for drug-induced kidney injury.—cont'd

Protein name	Presumed marker for	Supportive experimental results	Clinical trial data	Detection system	Clinical utility	References
Cystatin C	Proximal tubule damage	Upregulation of Cys-C levels was observed due to subtotal or unilateral nephrectomy and chromium nephropathy in diabetic rats.	Patients with acute kidney injury or tubular damage would exhibit high levels of Cys-C.	ELISA		Uchida and Gotoh (2002), Larki et al. (2018)
		Elevated levels in response to colistin.	There was an increase in the concentration of Cys C after 5 days of treatment with colistin.			
Albumin	Glomerulus	Elevated levels were observed in cancer patients treated with cisplatin.	The cumulative effect of cisplatin was detected by evaluating markers at different cycles from I to IV in samples 0 to 4. Albumin and albumin to creatinine levels were increased statistically and are significant in cycles II, III, and IV.	ELISA	Nephrotoxicity, septic acute kidney injury, ischemia.	Florova et al. (2020)
Tff 3	Distal convoluted tubule, collecting duct.	TFF3 levels were up-regulated in patients receiving cisplatin therapy.	Studies performed on cancer patients receiving cisplatin revealed an increase in TFF3 after 3 days, and this level was consistent in subsequent phases of cisplatin chemotherapy.	ELISA and Luminex	N/A	George et al. (2020)
Clusterin	Proximal tubule and collecting duct damage	Urinary clusterin levels were upregulated due to proximal tubular injury induced by administering drugs	Studies performed on animals indicate that urinary clusterin has the highest diagnostic power indicated by AUC	ELISA	N/A	Dieterle et al. (2010)

TABLE 12.2 Biomarkers for drug-induced kidney injury.—cont'd

Protein name	Presumed marker for	Supportive experimental results	Clinical trial data	Detection system	Clinical utility	References
		such as gentamycin, vancomycin, and lithium.	for inclusion analysis value of 0.88 and thus helps detect proximal tubular damage.			
RPA-1	Collecting duct damage	Increased RPA-1 levels were observed in the urine and tissue of rats treated with BEA, propylene imine, and indomethacin.	Increased levels of RPA-1 were observed in preclinical studies of rats, indicating the role of RPA-1 as a predictive biomarker for CD damage.	ELISA	N/A	Price et al. (2010)

and quantified with sensitive methods like RT-qPCR. In addition, these are conserved across species and even associated with pathological states (Califf, 2018). These exclusive features portray miRNAs as excellent noninvasive diagnostic and prognostic biomarkers. The levels of miRNAs can be distinguished in all the biological fluids together with the chief body fluids like blood and urine (Tölle et al., 2018). Further, these are organ-specific and show high conservation across species. Serum creatinine, proteinuria, estimated glomerular filtration rate (eGFR), and albuminuria are the standard biomarkers for kidney injury but lack specificity and sensitivity (Cavanaugh and Okusa, 2020). miRNA-based novel biomarkers might shift the treatment paradigm by providing initial warning signs as well as crucial information on the progression of the disease (Trionfini and Benigni, 2017).

Several miRNAs, such as miR-216, miR-192, miR-27b, miR-194, miR-215, and miR-204, have been recognized as renal-specific molecules. Wu et al. discovered a plasma miRNA signature involving four upregulated miRNAs in Immunoglobulin A nephropathy (IgAN). Initially, the study involved the identification of 48 miRNAs using quantitative reverse transcription-polymerase chain reaction (qRT-PCR) and ultimately discovering four upregulated miRNAs in subjects with IgAN responsible for renal lesions. They found a significant correlation between miR-425-3p, miR-148a-3p, miR-20a-5p, miR-150-5p, and eGFR, revealing their possible roles in the pathophysiology and development of IgAN (Wu et al., 2018). Chorley et al. conducted a cross-sectional study to identify and characterize urinary miRNA patterns in drug-induced kidney injury (DIKI). Segment selective nephron toxicants are known to instigate damage to individual sections of the nephron: the glomerulus (puromycin), proximal tubule (potassium dichromate, cisplatin, and gentamicin), thick ascending limb (TAL) of the loop of Henle (2 proprietary compounds X and Y) and collecting duct (CT) (N-phenylanthranilic acid-NPAA and the proprietary compound Z). These chemical substances were administered to rats, and the meta-analysis revealed the presence of potential miRNA biomarkers. Following this exposure to nephron toxicants, elevated levels of various miRNAs were observed in rat urine with minimal variations in serum creatinine as well as blood urea nitrogen (BUN) levels. The findings revealed the role of miR-23a-3p (glomerulus), miR-192-5p (proximal tubule), miRs-221-3p, miRs-22-3p, and miRs-210-3p (TAL), miR-210-3p (CD) as specific biomarkers useful for discrimination of drug-induced kidney lesions (Chorley et al., 2021).

Circulating miRNA biomarkers for organ injury has been gaining attention recently. Similar to the study mentioned above, Kagawa et al. investigated biomarkers for drug-induced glomerular injury (puromycin 120 mg/kg, doxorubicin 7.5 mg/kg) in Sprague–Dawley rats. Time-related variations of plasma miRNA expression profiles were performed using miRNA sequencing in drug-induced acute kidney injury models. Results were suggestive for the downregulation of miR-143-3p and miR-122-5p in glomerular injury models. Another glomerular injury biomarker candidate, miR-3473, was also acknowledged to be explicitly upregulated (Kagawa et al., 2019). More studies involving miRNAs as biomarkers in kidney injury are listed in Table 12.3.

TABLE 12.3 miRNAs as biomarkers in kidney injury.

MiRNAs	Study model	Sample collection	References
MicroRNA-10a, MicroRNA-30d	Ischemia-reperfusion and streptozotocin (STZ)-induced renal injury	Urine	Wang et al. (2012)
MicroRNA-34c-3p	Doxorubicin-induced glomerular injury	Urine	Church et al. (2014)
Let-7g-5p and miR-191-5p	Patients with CKD and hypertension	Plasma	Berillo et al. (2020)
miR-452	AKI in sepsis patients	Serum and urine	Song et al. (2020)
MicroRNA-30c-5p and MicroRNA-192-5p	Ischemia-reperfusion-induced kidney injury	Urine	Zou et al. (2017)
MiR-223-3p and miR-93-5p	CKD patients	Serum	Ulbing et al. (2017)
microRNAs miR-15b and miR-30a	Gentamicin-induced acute kidney injury	Urine	Sun et al. (2021)
miRNA-188, miRNA-30a, and miRNA-30e	Contrast-induced acute kidney injury	Plasma	Gurm (2020)
MicroRNA-423-5p	AKI in patients with acute decompensated heart failure	Serum and urine	Zhang et al. (2021)
miR-21	Hypertensive kidney injury and fibrosis	Urine	Chen et al. (2017)
miR-652-3p	Patients with acute decompensated heart failure and acute kidney injury	Serum and urine	Liu et al. (2020)
miRNA-122	Kidney injury and sepsis in CD-1 mouse model	Serum	Leelahavanichkul et al. (2015)

12.4.2.1 Challenges of miRNAs as biomarkers

Even though miRNAs can be considered promising biomarkers for prognostic and diagnostic approaches in kidney injury, their quantification and validation are limited by the following challenges. Firstly, there is a lack of standardization in miRNA isolation and quantification methods (El-Khoury et al., 2016). Secondly, serum creatinine (SCr) is considered the gold standard for kidney injury in clinical studies. The usage of other biomarkers for kidney injury is well-defined, primarily based on increased SCr levels (Pavkovic et al., 2015). Further, establishing reference ranges for miRNAs is essential, but their levels were age and sex-dependent in preclinical and clinical settings (Kwekel et al., 2015). Therefore, accelerating the standardization and quantification techniques may progress miRNA interpretation as biomarkers from preclinical and clinical studies.

12.5 Methods to evaluate biomarkers

Biomarkers are biomolecules that can be used to help in early disease diagnosis. As a result, for accurate diagnosis, sensitive detection technologies are required. These markers should also be plentiful enough to identify damaged organ locations in connection to injury phenotypes without compromising specificity or stability. The use of detection tools will help to better understand the cause of nephrotoxicity and enhance the screening and disease prognosis. The approaches that are often utilized to detect possible biomarkers implicated in nephrotoxicity are discussed in the next section.

12.5.1 ELISA

Enzyme-linked immunoassays (ELISA) are mainly used to detect single analytes. ELISAs are available for biomarkers such as Kim-1 and Clusterin. BioPorto had developed some specialized ELISAs and test kits that made the detection of NGAL possible in humans, rats, monkeys, mice, dogs, and donkeys.

12.5.2 Dipstick assay

Dipstick assay is a rapid detection method for Kim-1, the most predictive biomarker in AKI. The dipstick assay is now available under the name RENA-Strips, established on gold-sol conjugates and lateral flow assays (Dieterle et al., 2010).

12.5.3 Multiplex assays

Multiplex assays, based on bead-based technology, provide a platform for simultaneously analyzing many biomarkers from a single sample. In terms of cost and time, it appears to be a cost-effective tool for investigators. It compares with ELISA in terms of sensitivity and repeatability. Although ELISA has made detecting biomarkers easier, they are limited to only a single analyte. To overcome this limitation, multiplex analyzing assays have been developed, which helps to detect multiple analytes.

12.5.3.1 *Luminex xMAP*

The Luminex xMAP is based mainly on the flow cytometry of antibodies specific to an analyte and coated on a microsphere bead. Further secondary antibody addition is done, which helps form bead-analyte-fluorophore conjugate identified through Luminex compact analyzer. This technology has allowed the development of multiple unique assays using a single analyte. A service provider termed rule-based medicine (RBM) was developed to discover and accept the existing biomarkers.

12.5.3.2 *Mesoscale Discovery*

Mesoscale Discovery (MSD) is another type of multiplex system that helps detect novel biomarkers using a solid phase instead of a liquid array of Luminex xMAP. A solid carbon surface having a multiwell plate is available on which the antibodies against specific analytes may be coated. The light emitting from the surface of microplates will be recognized by the detectors. This light-sensing technology plays a significant role in high-throughput screening. High-throughput screening uses this technique as it takes little time to generate the result (Alexopoulos et al., 2009).

12.5.3.3 *FirePlex particle technology*

FirePlex porous bio-inert hydrogels are a crucial component of FirePlex particle technology. These particles have the following features: (1) 100 times more binding sites per particle than previous bead-based technologies, (2) picomolar sensitivity and excellent specificity, and (3) the ability to identify 65 miRNAs from a single well without the need for RNA purification. Flow cytometry may be used to produce results, which can then be analyzed (Tackett and Diwan, 2017).

12.6 Conclusions

Drug-induced nephrotoxicity is very closely linked with AKI and chronic kidney injury. Though it is impossible to describe all the drugs in use and their nephrotoxicity potential, various important classes of drugs that induce nephrotoxicity have been discussed in this chapter. In addition, the mechanism of drug-induced nephrotoxicity has also been discussed with the help of some specific drugs that are widely used in clinics.

Traditional biomarkers used in the clinic, such as blood urea and serum creatinine, do not have sufficient sensitivity. They do not provide important information about drug-induced nephrotoxicity after significant loss of kidney function. Significant efforts has been made to find novel biomarkers through which diagnosis of drug-induced nephrotoxicity can be made at an early stage of drug development. Novel methods to determine the proteins and miRNA-based novel biomarkers are on their way to provide in-depth information about drug-induced nephrotoxicity at an early stage of drug development, thereby reducing the cost burden during the safety assessment of new drug molecules. Moreover, novel methods to determine the protein and miRNA biomarkers have also been deliberated. Future research must focus on developing highly selective and sensitive methods for determining both conventional and novel biomarkers with less cost and time. However, further research on highly effective biomimetic in vivo and in vitro model development needs more attention to make them cheaper future alternative techniques for biomarker analysis.

12.6 List of abbreviations

3′ UTR Three prime untranslated regions
ACE Angiotensin-converting enzyme
AKI Acute kidney injury
ARB's Angiotensin receptor blockers
ARF Acute renal failure
AUC Area under the curve
BEA Beauvericin
BUN Blood urea nitrogen
CD Collecting duct
CKD Chronic kidney disease
COX-1 Cyclooxygenase 1
COX-2 Cyclooxygenase 2
CT Computed tomographic
Cys-C Cystatin-C
D-AKI Drug-induced acute kidney injury
DCT Distal convoluted tubule
DIRF Drug-induced renal failures
DNA Deoxyribonucleic acid
ELISA Enzyme-linked immunosorbent assay
EMA European Medicines Agency
FAPB Fatty acid-binding proteins
FDA Food and Drug Administration
GFR Glomerular filtration rate
GST Glutathione S-transferases
HARI Hospital-acquired renal insufficiency
ICU Intensive care unit
IgAN Immunoglobulin A nephropathy
KIM-1 Kidney Injury Molecule 1
miRNA micro-RNA
mRNA Messenger RNA
NGAL Neutrophil gelatinase-associated lipocalin
NPAA N-phenylanthranilic acid
NSAIDS Nonsteroidal anti-inflammatory drugs
OTC Over the counter
p-ERK Phosphorylated extracellular-signal-regulated kinase
PCT Proximal convoluted tubule
PGE2 Prostaglandin E2
RNA Ribonucleic Acid
ROC Receiver operating characteristic curve
RPA-1 Renal Papillary Injury 1
RT-qPCR Reverse transcription-quantitative polymerase chain reaction
SCr Serum creatinine
STZ Streptozotocin
TAL Thick ascending limb
TFF3 Trefoil factor 3
UTI Urinary tract infection

References

Al-Naimi, M.S., et al., 2019. Nephrotoxicity: role and significance of renal biomarkers in the early detection of acute renal injury. J. Adv. Pharm. Technol. Res. (JAPTR) 10 (3), 95.

Alexopoulos, L.G., et al., 2009. High throughput protein-based technologies and computational models for drug development, efficacy and toxicity. In: Drug Efficacy, Safety, Biologics Discovery: Emerging Technologies Tools. Wiley, pp. 29–52.

Altınkaynak, Y., et al., 2018. Protective effects of L-theanine against doxorubicin-induced nephrotoxicity in rats. Biomed. Pharmacother. 108, 1524–1534.

Atef, M., et al., 2021. Is urinary beta2-microglobulin a reliable marker for assessment of renal tubular dysfunction in chronic hepatitis B patients receiving tenofovir therapy. Eur. J. Gastroenterol. Hepatol. 33 (1S), e992–e998.

Basi, S., et al., 2008. Microalbuminuria in type 2 diabetes and hypertension: a marker, treatment target, or innocent bystander? Diabetes Care 31 (Suppl. 2), S194–S201.

Berillo, O., et al., 2020. Circulating let-7g-5p and miR-191-5p are independent predictors of chronic kidney disease in hypertensive patients. Am. J. Hypertens. 33 (6), 505–513.

Cai, L., et al., 2010. The origin of multiple molecular forms in urine of HNL/NGAL. Clin. J. Am. Soc. Nephrol. 5 (12), 2229–2235.

Califf, R.M., 2018. Biomarker definitions and their applications. Exp. Biol. Med. 243 (3), 213–221.

Cavanaugh, C., Okusa, M.D., 2020. The evolving role of novel biomarkers in glomerular disease: a review. Am. J. Kidney Dis. 77 (1), 122–131.

Chávez-Iñiguez, J.S., et al., 2020. Acute kidney injury caused by obstructive nephropathy. Inter. J. Nephrol. 2020.

Chen, H., Busse, L.W., 2017. Novel therapies for acute kidney injury. Kidney Inter. Rep. 2 (5), 785–799.

Chen, C., et al., 2017. Urinary miR-21 as a potential biomarker of hypertensive kidney injury and fibrosis. Sci. Rep. 7 (1), 1–9.

Chorley, B.N., et al., 2021. Urinary miRNA biomarkers of drug-induced kidney injury and their site specificity within the nephron. Toxicol. Sci. 180 (1), 1–16.

Choudhury, D., Ahmed, Z., 2006. Drug-associated renal dysfunction and injury. Nat. Clin. Pract. Nephrol. 2 (2), 80–91.

Church, R.J., et al., 2014. MicroRNA-34c-3p is an early predictive biomarker for doxorubicin-induced glomerular injury progression in male Sprague-Dawley rats. Toxicol. Res. 3 (5), 384–394.

Coco, T.J., Klasner, A.E., 2004. Drug-induced rhabdomyolysis. Curr. Opin. Pediatr. 16 (2), 206–210.

Daudon, M., Jungers, P., 2004. Drug-induced renal calculi. Drugs 64 (3), 245–275.

Davis II, J.W., et al., 2004. Quantitative gene expression analysis in a nonhuman primate model of antibiotic-induced nephrotoxicity. Toxicol. Appl. Pharmacol. 200 (1), 16–26.

Devarajan, P., Murray, P., 2014. Biomarkers in acute kidney injury: are we ready for prime time? Nephron Clin. Pract. 127 (1–4), 176–179.

Dickenmann, M., et al., 2008. Osmotic nephrosis: acute kidney injury with accumulation of proximal tubular lysosomes due to administration of exogenous solutes. Am. J. Kidney Dis. 51 (3), 491–503.

Dieterle, F., et al., 2010. Urinary clusterin, cystatin C, β2-microglobulin and total protein as markers to detect drug-induced kidney injury. Nat. Biotechnol. 28 (5), 463–469.

Downes, K.J., et al., 2020. Mechanisms of antimicrobial-induced nephrotoxicity in children. J. Antimicrob. Chemother. 75 (1), 1–13.

Edelstein, C.L., 2017. Biomarkers in acute kidney injury. In: Biomarkers of Kidney Disease, pp. 241–315.

El-Khoury, V., et al., 2016. Assessing cellular and circulating miRNA recovery: the impact of the RNA isolation method and the quantity of input material. Sci. Rep. 6 (1), 1–14.

Fels, J., et al., 2019. Cadmium complexed with β2-microglubulin, albumin and lipocalin-2 rather than metallothionein cause megalin: cubilin dependent toxicity of the renal proximal tubule. Int. J. Mol. Sci. 20 (10), 2379.

Fisel, P., et al., 2014. Solute carrier transporter and drug-related nephrotoxicity: the impact of proximal tubule cell models for preclinical research. Expet Opin. Drug Metabol. Toxicol. 10 (3), 395–408.

Florova, B., et al., 2020. NGAL, albumin and cystatin C during cisplatin therapy. Physiol. Res. 69 (2), 307–317.

Fored, C.M., et al., 2001. Acetaminophen, aspirin, and chronic renal failure. N. Engl. J. Med. 345 (25), 1801–1808.

Frazier, K.S., Obert, L.A., 2018. Drug-induced glomerulonephritis: the spectre of biotherapeutic and antisense oligonucleotide immune activation in the kidney. Toxicol. Pathol. 46 (8), 904–917.

Gajula, S.N.R., et al., 2020. Analytical and Omics Approaches in the Identification of Oxidative Stress-Induced Cancer Biomarkers, pp. 1–24.

George, B., et al., 2020. Time-dependent changes in kidney injury biomarkers in patients receiving multiple cycles of cisplatin chemotherapy. Toxicol. Rep. 7, 571–576.

Ghane Shahrbaf, F., Assadi, F., 2015. Drug-induced renal disorders. J. Ren. Inj. Prev. 4 (3), 57–60.

Ghatanatti, R., et al., 2014. Role of renal biomarkers as predictors of acute kidney injury in cardiac surgery. Asian Cardiovasc. Thorac. Ann. 22 (2), 234–241.

Gurm, H.S., 2020. Renal Disease and Coronary, Peripheral and Structural Interventions, an Issue of Interventional Cardiology Clinics. E-Book. Elsevier Health Sciences.

Hannah, R., Howell, M.L.B., Langworthy, L., 2007. Drug-induced acute renal failure. U.S. Pharm. 32 (3), 45–50.

Hohenegger, M., 2012. Drug induced rhabdomyolysis. Curr. Opin. Pharmacol. 12 (3), 335–339.

Hoste, E.A., et al., 2015. Epidemiology of acute kidney injury in critically ill patients: the multinational AKI-EPI study. Intensive Care Med. 41 (8), 1411–1423.

Hoy, A.M., Buck, A.H., 2012. Extracellular small RNAs: what, where, why? Biochem. Soc. Trans. 40 (4), 886–890.

Ichimura, T., et al., 2008. Kidney injury molecule–1 is a phosphatidylserine receptor that confers a phagocytic phenotype on epithelial cells. J. Clin. Invest. 118 (5), 1657–1668.

Jose, S.P., et al., 2017. Nephro-protective effect of a novel formulation of unopened coconut inflorescence sap powder on gentamicin induced renal damage by modulating oxidative stress and inflammatory markers. Biomed. Pharmacother. 85, 128–135.

Kagawa, T., et al., 2019. A scrutiny of circulating microRNA biomarkers for drug-induced tubular and glomerular injury in rats. Toxicology 415, 26–36.

Kang, J., et al., 2015. Urine alpha1-microglobulin is a better marker for early tubular dysfunction than beta2-microglobulin among tenofovir-exposed human immunodeficiency virus-infected men who have sex with men. Braz. J. Infect. Dis. 19, 410–416.

Karademir, L.D., et al., 2016. The efficacy of theophylline in preventing cisplatin-related nephrotoxicity in patients with cancer. Ren. Fail. 38 (5), 806–814.

Kaufman, J., et al., 1991. Community-acquired acute renal failure. Am. J. Kidney Dis. 17 (2), 191–198.

Kim, S.Y., Moon, A., 2012. Drug-induced nephrotoxicity and its biomarkers. Biomol. & Ther. 20 (3), 268.

Klahr, S., 2000. Obstructive nephropathy. Intern. Med. 39 (5), 355–361.

Kodner, C., Kudrimoti, A., 2003. Diagnosis and management of acute interstitial nephritis. Am. Fam. Phys. 67 (12), 2527–2534.

Kohli, H.S., et al., 2000. Treatment-related acute renal failure in the elderly: a hospital-based prospective study. Nephrol. Dial. Transplan. 15 (2), 212–217.

Kokot, M., et al., 2014. Assessment of subclinical acute kidney injury after abdominal aortic aneurysm surgery using novel markers: L-FABP and H-FABP. Nefrologia 34 (5), 628–636.

Koyner, J.L., et al., 2010. Urinary biomarkers in the clinical prognosis and early detection of acute kidney injury. Clin. J. Am. Soc. Nephrol. 5 (12), 2154–2165.

Krol, J., et al., 2010. The widespread regulation of microRNA biogenesis, function and decay. Nat. Rev. Genet. 11 (9), 597–610.

Kwekel, J.C., et al., 2015. Age and sex differences in kidney microRNA expression during the life span of F344 rats. Biol. Sex Differ. 6 (1), 1–16.

Larki, R.A., et al., 2018. Serum cystatin C for evaluation of acute kidney injury in adults treated with colistin. J. Res. Pharm. Pract. 7 (4), 178.

Lee, M.S., et al., 2009. The relationship between glucuronide conjugate levels and hepatotoxicity after oral administration of valproic acid. Arch Pharm. Res. (Seoul) 32 (7), 1029–1035.

Leelahavanichkul, A., et al., 2015. Serum miRNA-122 in acute liver injury induced by kidney injury and sepsis in CD-1 mouse models. Hepatol. Res. 45 (13), 1341–1352.

Dr Liji Thomas, M., February 27, 2019. Obstructive Nephropathy - Uropathy. Available from: https://www.news-medical.net/health/Obstructive-Nephropathy-Uropathy.aspx.

Liu, J., et al., 2020. Diagnostic and prognostic significance of aberrant miR-652-3p levels in patients with acute decompensated heart failure and acute kidney injury. J. Int. Med. Res. 48 (11), 0300060520967829.

Liu, C., et al., 2021. Drug-induced hospital-acquired acute kidney injury in China: a multicenter cross-sectional survey. Kidney Dis. 7 (2), 110–122.

Lopez-Novoa, J.M., et al., 2011. New insights into the mechanism of aminoglycoside nephrotoxicity: an integrative point of view. Kidney Int. 79 (1), 33–45.

Luo, Q.-H., et al., 2016. Evaluation of KIM-1 and NGAL as early indicators for assessment of gentamycin-induced nephrotoxicity in vivo and in vitro. Kidney Blood Pres. Res. 41 (6), 911–918.

Matsubara, A., et al., 2018. Establishment of a drug-induced rhabdomyolysis mouse model by co-administration of ciprofloxacin and atorvastatin. Toxicol. Lett. 291, 184–193.

Nalewajska, M., et al., 2019. The role of microRNAs in selected forms of glomerulonephritis. Int. J. Mol. Sci. 20 (20), 5050.

Nash, K., et al., 2002. Hospital-acquired renal insufficiency. Am. J. Kidney Dis. 39 (5), 930–936.

Naughton, C.A., 2008. Drug-induced nephrotoxicity. Am. Fam. Phys. 78 (6), 743–750.

Niguram, P., et al., 2020. Update on compatibility assessment of empagliflozin with the selected pharmaceutical excipients employed in solid dosage forms by thermal, spectroscopic and chromatographic techniques. Drug Dev. Ind. Pharm. 46 (2), 209–218.

Nivy, R., et al., 2017. Utility of urinary alkaline phosphatase and γ-glutamyl transpeptidase in diagnosing acute kidney injury in dogs. Vet. J. 220, 43–47.

Nolin, T.D., Himmelfarb, J., 2010. Mechanisms of drug-induced nephrotoxicity. Adv. Drug React. 111–130.

O'Brien, J., et al., 2018. Overview of microRNA biogenesis, mechanisms of actions, and circulation. Front. Endocrinol. 9, 402.

Obajdin, J., et al., 2018. Fatty-acid binding protein 4 (FABP4) as a potential preclinical biomarker of drug-induced kidney injury. Toxicol. Sci. 166 (2), 441–450.

Olyaei, A.J., et al., 1999. Immunosuppressant-induced nephropathy. Drug Saf. 21 (6), 471–488.

Orbach, H., et al., 2004. Intravenous immunoglobulin and the kidney—a two-edged sword. In: Seminars in Arthritis and Rheumatism. Elsevier.

Oyama, Y., et al., 2005. Evidence for megalin-mediated proximal tubular uptake of L-FABP, a carrier of potentially nephrotoxic molecules. Lab. Invest. 85 (4), 522–531.

Pais, G.M., et al., 2019. Comparative performance of urinary biomarkers for vancomycin-induced kidney injury according to timeline of injury. Antimicrob. Agents Chemother. 63 (7) e00079–19.

Paller, M.S., 1990. Drug-induced nephropathies. Med. Clin. 74 (4), 909–917.

Pavkovic, M., et al., 2015. Glomerulonephritis-induced changes in urinary and kidney microRNA profiles in rats. Toxicol. Sci. 145 (2), 348–359.

Pazhayattil, G.S., Shirali, A.C., 2014. Drug-induced impairment of renal function. Int. J. Nephrol. Renovascular Dis. 7, 457.

Perazella, M.A., 1999. Crystal-induced acute renal failure. Am. J. Med. 106 (4), 459–465.

Perazella, M.A., 2005. Drug-induced nephropathy: an update. Expet Opin. Drug Saf. 4 (4), 689–706.

Perazella, M.A., 2018. Pharmacology behind common drug nephrotoxicities. Clin. J. Am. Soc. Nephrol. 13 (12), 1897–1908.

Perazella, M.A., Herlitz, L.C., 2021. The crystalline nephropathies. Kidney Inter. Rep. 6 (12), 2942–2957.

Phadke, G., et al., 2020. Osmotic nephrosis and acute kidney injury associated with SGLT2 inhibitor use: a case report. Am. J. Kidney Dis. 76 (1), 144–147.

Pisoni, R., et al., 2001. Drug-induced thrombotic microangiopathy. Drug Saf. 24 (7), 491–501.

Polaka, S., et al., 2021. Revamping the pharmacokinetics of poorly soluble drugs using different formulations. In: Tekade, R.K. (Ed.), Biopharmaceutics and Pharmacokinetics Considerations. Elsevier, pp. 387–413.

Polaka, S., et al., 2021. Factors affecting the pharmacokinetics of the liposomal drugs. In: Biopharmaceutics and Pharmacokinetics Considerations. Elsevier, pp. 567–599.

Polaka, S., et al., 2021. Bioanalytical method development and validation for establishing bioavailability and bioequivalence. In: Biopharmaceutics and Pharmacokinetics Considerations. Elsevier, pp. 487–516.

Polaka, S., et al., 2021. Factors affecting the stability of drugs and their metabolites in biological matrices. In: Biopharmaceutics and Pharmacokinetics Considerations. Elsevier, pp. 517–537.

Polaka, S., et al., 2022. Clinical importance of herb–drug interaction. In: Pharmacokinetics and Toxicokinetic Considerations. Elsevier, pp. 323–356.

Polaka, S., et al., 2022. Pharmaceutical excipients: special focus on adverse interactions. In: Pharmacokinetics and Toxicokinetic Considerations. Elsevier, pp. 513–542.

Polaka, S., et al., 2022. Drug−drug interactions and their implications on the pharmacokinetics of the drugs. In: Pharmacokinetics and Toxicokinetic Considerations. Elsevier, pp. 291−322.

Polaka, S., et al., 2022. Emerging role of novel excipients in drug product development and their safety concerns. In: Pharmacokinetics and Toxicokinetic Considerations. Elsevier, pp. 543−567.

Polaka, S., et al., 2022. Food−drug interactions and their implications on oral drug bioavailability. In: Pharmacokinetics and Toxicokinetic Considerations. Elsevier, pp. 263−289.

Polaka, S., et al., 2022. Impact of ageing on the pharmacokinetics and pharmacodynamics of the drugs. In: Pharmacokinetics and Toxicokinetic Considerations. Elsevier, pp. 241−261.

Prendergast, B., George, C., 1993. Drug-induced rhabdomyolysis–mechanisms and management. Postgrad. Med. 69 (811), 333.

Price, S.A., et al., 2010. Characterization of renal papillary antigen 1 (RPA-1), a biomarker of renal papillary necrosis. Toxicol. Pathol. 38 (3), 346−358.

Raval, N., et al., 2021. Engineered nanoplex mediated targeted miRNA delivery to rescue dying podocytes in diabetic nephropathy. Int. J. Pharm. 605, 120842.

Redahan, L., Murray, P.T., 2017. Biomarkers of drug-induced kidney injury. Curr. Opin. Crit. Care 23 (6), 463−469.

Redfern, W.S., Valentin, J.-P., 2011. Trends in safety pharmacology: posters presented at the annual meetings of the Safety Pharmacology Society 2001−2010. J. Pharmacol. Toxicol. Methods 64 (1), 102−110.

Reis, N.G., et al., 2019. Protective effect of calcitriol on rhabdomyolysis-induced acute kidney injury in rats. Sci. Rep. 9 (1), 1−10.

Rinnert, M., et al., 2010. Synthesis and localization of trefoil factor family (TFF) peptides in the human urinary tract and TFF2 excretion into the urine. Cell Tissue Res. 339 (3), 639−647.

Rodríguez-Iturbe, B., García, G.G., 2010. The role of tubulointerstitial inflammation in the progression of chronic renal failure. Nephron Clin. Pract. 116 (2), c81−c88.

Rossert, J., 2001. Drug-induced acute interstitial nephritis. Kidney Int. 60 (2), 804−817.

Ruiz-Ramirez, C., et al., 2021. Correlation between urinary KIM-1 and kidney protein expression of p-ERK following damage in rats exposed to gentamicin or lead acetate. J. Biochem. Mol. Toxicol. e22875.

Sasaki, D., et al., 2011. Comparison of the course of biomarker changes and kidney injury in a rat model of drug-induced acute kidney injury. Biomarkers 16 (7), 553−566.

Sauret, J.M., et al., 2002. Rhabdomyolysis. Am. Fam. Physician 65 (5), 907.

Sharfuddin, A.A., Molitoris, B.A., 2011. Pathophysiology of ischemic acute kidney injury. Nat. Rev. Nephrol. 7 (4), 189−200.

Shayan, M., Elyasi, S., 2020. Cilastatin as a protective agent against drug-induced nephrotoxicity: a literature review. Expet Opin. Drug Saf. 19 (8), 999−1010.

Song, X., et al., 2020. Antibacterial effects and mechanism of Mandarin (Citrus reticulata L.) essential oil against *Staphylococcus aureus*, 25 (21), 4956.

Sun, B., et al., 2021. Urinary microRNAs miR-15b and miR-30a as novel noninvasive biomarkers for gentamicin-induced acute kidney injury. Toxicol. Lett. 338, 105−113.

Taber, S.S., Pasko, D.A., 2008. The epidemiology of drug-induced disorders: the kidney. Expet Opin. Drug Saf. 7 (6), 679−690.

Tackett, M.R., Diwan, I., 2017. Using Fireplex™ Particle Technology for Multiplex MicroRNA Profiling without RNA Purification. Functional Genomics. Springer, pp. 209−219.

Tiong, H.Y., et al., 2014. Drug-induced nephrotoxicity: clinical impact and preclinical in vitro models. Mol. Pharm. 11 (7), 1933−1948.

Togashi, Y., et al., 2013. Urinary cystatin C as a renal biomarker and its immunohistochemical localization in anti-GBM glomerulonephritis rats. Exp. Toxicol. Pathol. 65 (7−8), 1137−1143.

Tölle, A., et al., 2018. Circulating miRNAs in blood and urine as diagnostic and prognostic biomarkers for bladder cancer: an update in 2017. Biomarkers Med. 12 (6), 667−676.

Torres, P.A., et al., 2015. Rhabdomyolysis: pathogenesis, diagnosis, and treatment. Ochsner J. 15 (1), 58−69.

Trionfini, P., Benigni, A., 2017. MicroRNAs as master regulators of glomerular function in health and disease. J. Am. Soc. Nephrol. 28 (6), 1686−1696.

Tugay, S., et al., 2006. Acute effects of gentamicin on glomerular and tubular functions in preterm neonates. Pediatr. Nephrol. 21 (10), 1389−1392.

Uchida, K., Gotoh, A., 2002. Measurement of cystatin-C and creatinine in urine. Clin. Chim. Acta 323 (1−2), 121−128.

Ulbing, M., et al., 2017. MicroRNAs 223-3p and 93-5p in patients with chronic kidney disease before and after renal transplantation. Bone 95, 115–123.

Verma, S.K., Molitoris, B.A., 2015. Renal endothelial injury and microvascular dysfunction in acute kidney injury. Semin. Nephrol. 35 (1), 96–107.

Wang, N., et al., 2012. Urinary microRNA-10a and microRNA-30d serve as novel, sensitive and specific biomarkers for kidney injury. PLoS One 7 (12), e51140.

Wei, L., et al., 2015. Diagnostic accuracy of serum cystatin C in chronic kidney disease: a meta-analysis. Clin. Nephrol. 84 (2), 86–94.

Wu, H., Huang, J., 2018. Drug-induced nephrotoxicity: pathogenic mechanisms, biomarkers and prevention strategies. Curr. Drug Metabol. 19 (7), 559–567.

Wu, J., et al., 2018. Plasma microRNA signature of patients with IgA nephropathy. Gene 649, 80–86.

Yarlagadda, S.G., Perazella, M.A., 2008. Drug-induced crystal nephropathy: an update. Expet Opin. Drug Saf. 7 (2), 147–158.

Yu, Y., et al., 2010. Urinary biomarkers trefoil factor 3 and albumin enable early detection of kidney tubular injury. Nat. Biotechnol. 28 (5), 470–477.

Zeng, Y., 2006. Principles of micro-RNA production and maturation. Oncogene 25 (46), 6156–6162.

Zhang, H., et al., 2021. MicroRNA-423-5p as a biomarker for early diagnosis and outcome prediction of acute kidney injury in patients with acute decompensated heart failure. Int. J. Urol. 28 (1), 25–32.

Zou, Y.-F., et al., 2017. Urinary microRNA-30c-5p and MicroRNA-192-5p as potential biomarkers of ischemia–reperfusion-induced kidney injury. Exp. Biol. Med. 242 (6), 657–667.

CHAPTER

13

Mechanism of drug-induced neurotoxicity and its management

Rachna Gupta[1], *Muktika Tekade*[2], *Nupur Vasdev*[1], *Tanisha Gupta*[1], *Bhakti Pawar*[1], *Kuldeep Kumar Bansal*[3] and *Rakesh Kumar Tekade*[1]

[1]National Institute of Pharmaceutical Education and Research (NIPER)- Ahmedabad, An Institute of National Importance, Government of India, Department of Pharmaceuticals, Ministry of Chemicals and Fertilizers, Palaj, Gandhinagar, Gujarat, India; [2]School of Pharmacy, Devi Ahilya Vishwavidyalaya, Indore, Madhya Pradesh, India; [3]Pharmaceutical Sciences Laboratory, Faculty of Science and Engineering, Åbo Akademi University, Turku, Finland

13.1 Introduction

Neurotoxicity is defined as the adverse effects of drugs or chemicals that cause damage to the structure and function of the central and peripheral nervous systems of humans and animals. Maximum biological, chemical, and physical agents exhibit neurotoxic effects directly on neural cells, while others interact with metabolic activities of the nervous system. They also malfunction the adult nervous system, wherein Alzheimer's and Parkinson's diseases result from neurotoxic effects. These neurotoxic effects can also be accompanied by neurocognitive disorders depending on the particular areas or extreme neurotoxic damage. The drugs with neurotoxic potential are known as neurotoxins, whose toxic efficacy depends on the extent of exposure. There is a substantial delay between the exposure and the occurrence of neurotoxic effects.

Natural biological agents or drugs with high target specificity and neurotoxic potency are found in microbes, insects, and other organisms, for example, vitamin A, diphtheria toxin, apamin, palytoxin, and scorpion toxin (Pereira et al., 2017). Heavy metals and synthetic chemicals having neurotoxic potential are lead, mercury, arsenic, pesticides, acrylamide (pyrolysis products), pyridinethione (antidandruff shampoos), ethanol, amphetamines, cocaine,

https://doi.org/10.1016/B978-0-443-15840-7.00006-3

and opiates (Ijomone et al., 2020). Besides this, cardiovascular and chemotherapeutic agents are also neurotoxins. The numerous other drugs or chemicals with their varied neurotoxic effects are discussed in Table 13.1.

The nervous system exhibits a wide range of functional reactions to drug or chemical stress that leads to an excess of neurological and psychiatric occurrences, wherein many are treated as diseases induced by nontoxic agents. Neurotoxic effects caused by chemicals vary depending on their molecular structural activity (Schwarcz et al., 1978). For instance, a high dose of ethanol influences functional variations in the organism that appear for a short or long duration (Grobin et al., 1998). In contrast, the toxic effects of methanol are liable to the activity of its metabolite, formate (Moral et al., 2015). Anticholinesterase agents cause parasympathomimetic effects, which can be reverted to normal by replacing or reactivating acetylcholinesterase. Most neurotoxins initiate brain damage by triggering numerous neurotransmitter (NT) systems (Cadet et al., 2014). The neurotoxin changes NT release, concentration, and retention time and acts as an agonist or antagonist at a postsynaptic receptor. These

TABLE 13.1 Examples of the drugs having neurotoxic potential.

Neurotoxin	Neurotoxic effect type	References
Carbon tetrachloride	Acute encephalopathy, visual damage	Wang et al. (2017)
Methylmercury	Tunnel vision, peripheral neuropathy, teratogenesis, chronic encephalopathy	Ceccatelli et al. (2013)
Pesticides	Acetylcholinesterase inhibition, peripheral neuropathy, motor nerve dysfunction	Costa et al. (2008)
Phenytoin	Cerebellar syndrome, peripheral neuropathy, cognitive disorders, fetal phenytoin syndrome, extrapyramidal problem	Keppel Hesselink and Kopsky (2017)
Amiodarone	Sensory and motor chronic	Kang et al. (2007)
Platinum compounds	Acute and chronic sensory neuropathy	Hartmann and Lipp (2003)
Arsenic trioxides	Chronic motor and sensory polyneuropathy	Helso et al. (2020)
Ethambutol	Optic neuropathy	Mukherjee et al. (2022)
Isoniazid	Sensory peripheral nervous system	Zaoui et al. (2012)
Metronidazole	Optic and automatic neuropathy	Sarna et al. (2009)
Interferons	Demyelinating polyneuropathy, axonal and vasculitic neuropathy	Meriggioli and Rowin (2000)
Leflunomide	Distal axonal and sensorimotor polyneuropathy	Bonnel and Graham (2004)
Triazole	Axonal and sensory neuropathy	Kanafani (2011)
Levodopa	Sensory peripheral neuropathy	Romagnolo et al. (2019)

variations result in neurotoxicity, where the drug or agents interact with acetylcholinesterase and dismiss the NT activity at the neuromuscular junction.

Another target for drugs having neurotoxic potential is acetylcholine, glutamate, and glycine receptors. The neurotoxins can be antagonists or agonists for these receptors. D-Tubocurarine is an antagonist, while anatoxin-α is an agonist for the nicotinic acetylcholine receptor. The chemicals linked with glutamate receptors are responsible for central nervous system (CNS) degeneration and neuronal excitotoxicity, such as domoic acid derived from dinoflagellate. Strychnine and hydrastine are antagonists against glycine receptors that take part in inhibitory NT in the brainstem and spinal cord, causing hyperreflexia and tetanic muscle contraction. Therefore, such drug-induced impairments can result in severe changes in neurocognitive activities, including attention, memory, decision-making, movements, and others (Table 13.1).

Apart from these drugs or chemicals, chemotherapy agents, including platinum compounds (e.g., Cisplatin), taxanes (e.g., Paclitaxel), and vinca alkaloids (e.g., Vincristine, Vinblastine), are well known for inducing damage to the peripheral as well as the central nervous system in cancer patients (Banach et al., 2017). These chemotherapy agents hamper the sensory and motor nerves that directly contribute to movement activity, and this impairment reduces the life value of cancer survivors after treatment (Quasthoff and Hartung, 2002). In general, the incidence of symptoms takes a week or month, depending on the neurotoxin concentration in the bloodstream. In addition, various risk factors are also involved that affect the neurotic effects of drugs, including age, gender, temperature, nutrition status, and others. This chapter aims to provide information on drug-induced neurotoxicity to find the areas of research required to improve the evaluation and treatments for neurodegenerative disorders and movement dysfunction.

13.2 Mechanisms involved in drug-induced neurotoxicity

The drug induces neurotoxicity through numerous cellular and molecular mechanisms and routes. The effective mechanisms in neurotoxicity induced by chemicals or drugs are oxidative stress, apoptosis, covalent modification, inflammatory responses, channelopathies, and other biochemical pathways. Moreover, neurotoxic effects have also arisen through NT dysfunction and loss of signaling pathways. The mechanisms mentioned above are explained briefly next.

13.2.1 Oxidative stress

The neurotoxicity of drugs is triggered by the immense generation of reactive oxygen species (ROS) such as superoxide radicals (O_2^-), hydrogen peroxide (H_2O_2), hydroxyl radicals (•OH), and singlet oxygen (O_2). This ROS accumulation results in oxidative stress responsible for changes in protein, lipids, and nucleic acids (Gupta et al., 2022a). Many reports are available that exhibit the involvement of oxidative stress in causing neural damage. For instance, methamphetamine (METH) and methylenedioxymethamphetamine (MDMA) cause neurodegenerative damage owing to the increased production of ROS in monoaminergic brain areas (Cadet and Brannock, 1998). This ROS oxidizes the enhanced dopamine to

6-hydroxydopamine resulting in Parkinson's disease via degenerating neural cells. METH not only dysregulates dopamine but also causes mitochondrial dysfunction as well as DNA damage. This neurotoxin affects the dopaminergic terminals (dopamine transporter and tyrosine hydroxylase marker) in the striatum, but the activation of dopamine receptors reduces its neurotoxicity.

Amiodarone, an anti-arrhythmic agent, encourages sensory and motor deficits via increasing oxidative stress within the Schwann cells, exhibiting dose and time-dependent effects (Niimi et al., 2016). Another study exhibits the neurotoxic effect of cocaine based on oxidative stress, which is responsible for enhancing H_2O_2 and reducing catalase activity in rat's prefrontal cortex and striatum area (Dietrich et al., 2005). Moreover, through oxidative stress, heroin induces deoxyribonucleic acid (DNA) damage, protein oxidation, and lipid peroxidation due to high oxygen utilization and metabolic action of neurons. In contrast, morphine decreases the concentration of fatty acid in the spinal cord and brain via triggering oxidative stress, which in turn results in their abnormal development (Özmen et al., 2007).

13.2.2 Apoptosis progressions

Like oxidative stress, apoptotic progression is another effective mechanism in neurotoxicity induced by some drug abuse. In the apoptosis process, cells undergo morphological and biochemical changes, including cell shrinkage, chromatin condensation, and nuclear and DNA fragmentation. The pathways involved in apoptosis are responsible for activating death receptors, caspase-related or unrelated events, and increasing mitochondrial membrane permeability (Jayanthi et al., 2005). For instance, several reports exhibit a neuronal loss in dorsal root ganglion (DRG) and DNA damage by platinum compounds inducing apoptosis in in vivo and in vitro models (Alaedini et al., 2008).

Cisplatin, a platinum-based agent, allows the reentry of neurons from the G0 phase to the cell cycle and causes neuronal cell death. Membrane transporters, copper transporter-1 (CTR1), and organic cation transporter-2 (OCT2) permit the cellular uptake of cisplatin or oxaliplatin. Moreover, cisplatin also increased calcium levels in rat DRG neurons that induced apoptosis and caspase-3 activation, as shown in Fig. 13.1 (Tomaszewski and Büsselberg, 2007). Like cisplatin, bortezomib generates apoptotic neuronal cell death through calcium release activity and Transcription Factor three stimulation in DRG neurons (Yin et al., 2019).

Another study demonstrates the neurotoxic effect of amphetamine and its derivatives that induces apoptosis in various parts of the brain areas (Cadet et al., 2007). These drugs influence death events because of p53 activation, caspase activation, cytochrome *c* release, mitochondrial DNA damage, and enhanced Bax/Bcl2 fractions (Warren et al., 2007). In addition, other significant studies have suggested the apoptotic death of neuronal cells by heroin and paraquat herbicide which is mediated through the Fas pathway in the cortex and hippocampus region of the brain (Tramullas et al., 2008). Ethanol exposure brings about neuronal damage via apoptosis, leading to various functional deficits in the neonatal rodent brain. Due to its N-methyl-D-aspartate (NMDA) antagonist and γ-Aminobutyric acid imitator activities, neuronal cell death increased compared to a substance containing any of these activities (Paus et al., 2008).

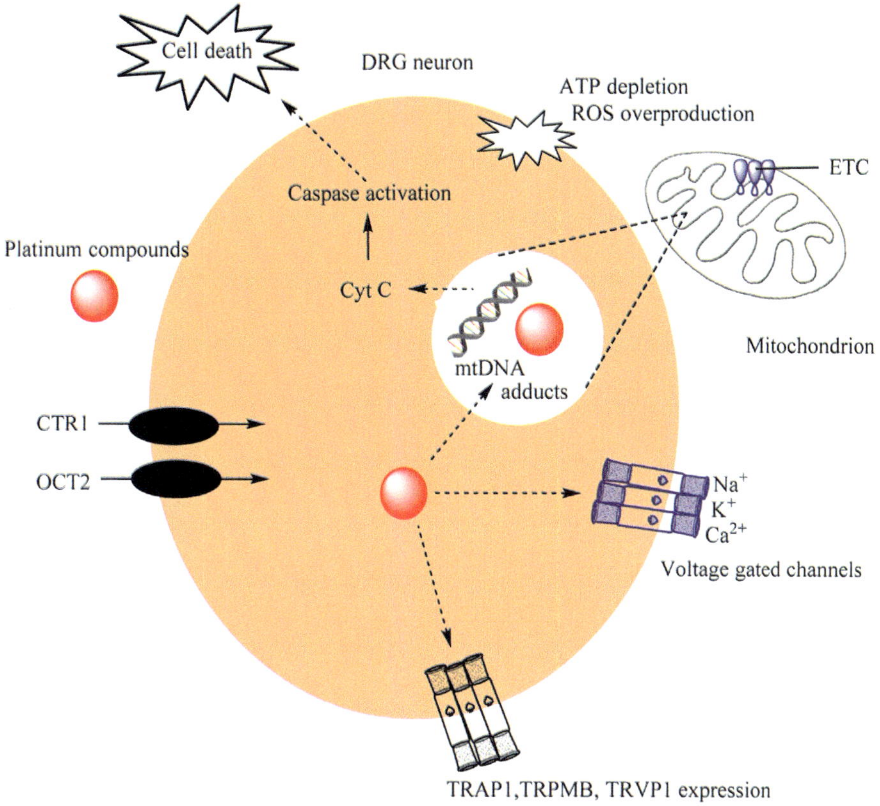

FIGURE 13.1 Proposed mechanism of platinum-induced neurotoxicity where dorsal region ganglion neuron is a chief target for platinum drugs causing mitochondrial DNA damage and voltage-gated channels dysfunction that ultimately result in apoptotic neuronal cell death.

13.2.3 Covalent modification

The drugs or chemicals can bind with DNA molecules and cause changes in the DNA structure or function, leading to a loss of neurons or functional deficit in brain regions. Such activity produces covalent modification. One of the best examples is drugs consisting of platinum, such as cisplatin and oxaliplatin, attached to DRG DNA with higher affinity than neuron-like dividing cell lines. They interact with DNA replication and cause sensory neuropathy (McDonald et al., 2005). Contrary to oxaliplatin, cisplatin produces three times higher DNA adducts, and thereby, oxaliplatin is considered less effective for neuronal cell death. This covalent modification also prompts apoptosis by activating p53 and other pro-apoptotic transcriptional factors that occur through blocking DNA replication (Roos and Kaina, 2006). These agents damage nuclear DNA and affect mitochondrial DNA directly, resulting in mitochondrial dysfunction in neurons. Improper mitochondrial transport leads to adenosine triphosphate (ATP) depletion and calcium accumulation in neurons (Fig. 13.1) (Podratz et al., 2011). Besides this, high expression of transient receptor potential channels like transient receptor potential ankyrin-1 (TRPA1), transient receptor potential melastatin

8 (TRPM8), and transient receptor potential vanilloid 1 (TRPV1) also exhibits a significant role in platinum-induced neurotoxicity.

13.2.4 Organelle deterioration

Amongst organelles, mitochondria and endoplasmic reticulum (ER) are the most affected organelle in neurotoxicity caused by drug abuse. Chemotherapeutic agents such as taxanes, epothilones, bortezomib, and thalidomide induce microtubule depolarization (Fig. 13.2). Due to this, calcium channels in ER are open, affecting the mitochondrial membrane permeability and producing ROS and cytochrome C. Such species release causes neuronal cell death with intracellular inflammation in the nerve (Jones et al., 2020). Organelle damage also affects the

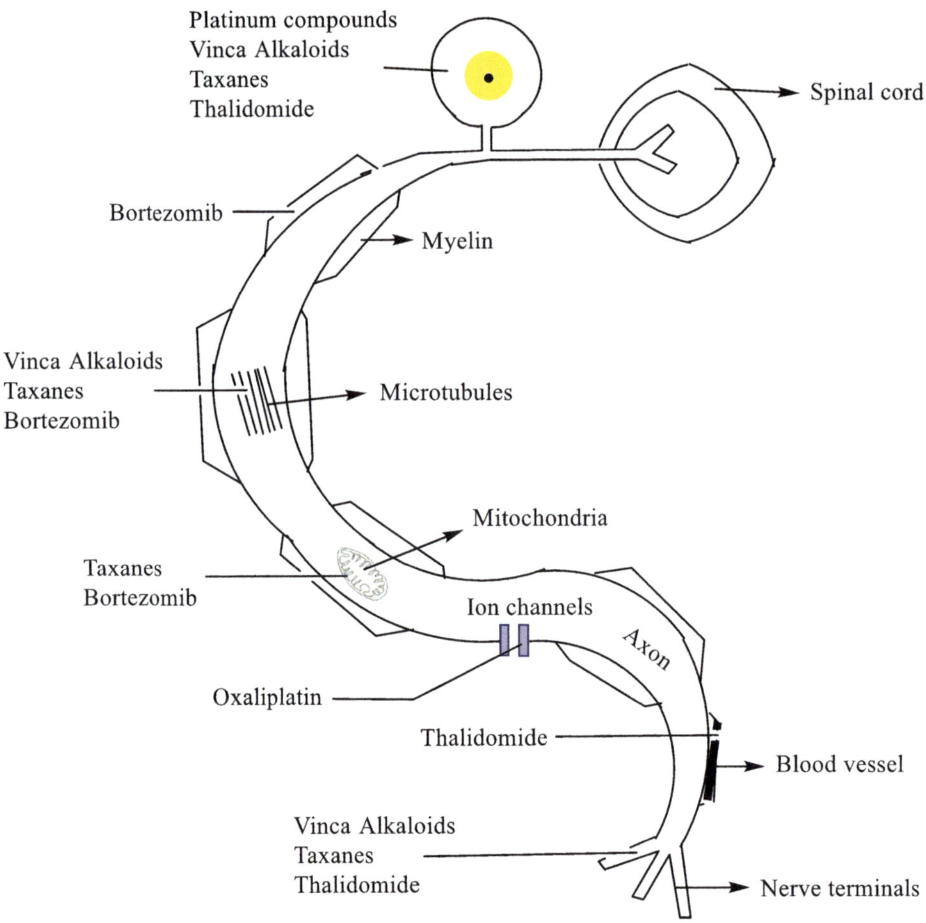

FIGURE 13.2 Site of chemotherapy causing neurotoxic effects in the nerve cell where chemotherapeutic agents (taxanes, epothilones, bortezomib, thalidomide, and oxaliplatin) induce microtubule depolarization, mitochondrial and ion channel dysfunction.

transport of materials along axons resulting in axonal degeneration and microtubule dysfunction (Meregalli et al., 2014) (Fig. 13.2).

13.2.5 Excitotoxic activation

Drug-induced neuronal cell death is also mediated through the excitotoxic effects of amino acids and other components. Owing to the excess Ca^{2+} influx, the NMDA receptors undergo overactivation by releasing glutamate that exhibits excitotoxicity (McCann and Ricaurte, 2004). However, the introduction of glutamate receptor antagonists like MK-801 is responsible for reducing methamphetamine-related neuronal damage in various brain regions (Chipana et al., 2008; Sekine et al., 2008). Like methamphetamine, amphetamine, cocaine, crack, and other chemotherapeutic drugs also enhance glutamate activity in the cortex, ventral tegmental area, striatum, and accumbens region of the brain (Williams and Steketee, 2004). Therefore, this results in alterations of synaptic plasticity, glutamate homeostasis, and postsynaptic glutamatergic signaling with increased intracellular Ca^{2+} levels.

Moreover, Ca^{2+} incrementally destroys proteins, phospholipids, and nucleic acids by activating Ca^{2+}-dependent enzymes. Paraquat substance also generates excitotoxicity by increasing nitric oxide concentration with the influence of glutamate activity on the NMDA receptors. This release of nitric oxide leads to the long-lasting overflow of dopamine and ultimately causes neurodegeneration (Shimizu et al., 2003). Apart from this, thiamine or vitamin B1 shortage is also one of the reasons for hyperexcitability and glutamate excitotoxicity, which results in convulsions and neuronal dysfunction (Inaba et al., 2016).

13.2.6 Channelopathies

Voltage-gated ion channels are essential in the normal functioning of axons, neurons, muscles, and glial cells. These ion channels target neurotoxins, causing neuronal damage, and the dysfunction of these channels is termed channelopathies. Tetrodotoxin is an agent that interferes with voltage Na^{+} channels and inhibits ion influx present in fish, octopus, and salamanders. Like tetrodotoxin, oxaliplatin also remarkably influences Na^{+} channels by weakening their inactivation and decreasing the Na^{+} peak current (Figs. 13.1 and 13.3). Such activity increases the relative refractory period of sensory neurons (Wu et al., 2009; Park et al., 2011). It also exhibits an indirect effect on voltage Na^{+} channels by interacting with extracellular Ca^{2+} through its metabolite oxalate, bringing about hyperexcitation of sensory neurons and causing impulsive ectopic ejections (Adelsberger et al., 2000).

Besides Na^{+} channels, K^{+} channels are also affected by oxaliplatin which slows down neuronal actions via failure of gap junction channels and hemichannels in myelinated fibers (Tong et al., 2015). However, the long-lasting opening of these channels causes a massive accumulation of K^{+} in the periaxonal cavity, and its osmotic distension results in K^{+} channel dysfunction. Other K^{+} channel blockers are thallium, bromine, and venom of snakes, bees, and scorpions that significantly cause neuron dysfunction. Unlike oxaliplatin, cisplatin primarily affects Ca^{2+} channels via increasing intracellular Ca^{2+} influx that activates caspase three and ultimately results in apoptosis.

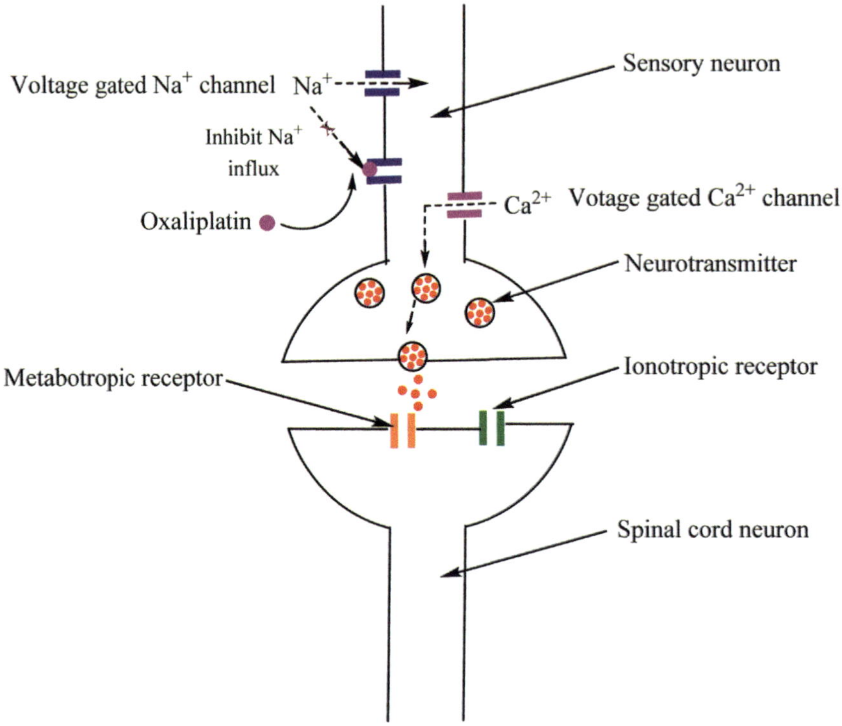

FIGURE 13.3 Voltage-gated Na$^+$ channel dysfunction on exposure of oxaliplatin inducing sensory neuron hyper excitation.

13.2.7 Microglial activation

Microglial cell activation is another biochemical pathway triggered by drug abuse inducing neurotoxicity. For instance, exposure to oxaliplatin, methamphetamine, and other agents causes microglial activation responsible for releasing pro-inflammatory chemicals in the spinal cord or dorsal striatum (Thomas et al., 2004). These microglial cells exhibit both neurotoxic and neuroprotective functions. However, the overactivation of microglial cells leads to inflammation and facilitates neuronal damage. To reduce the neurotoxic microglial activation, inhibitors such as minocycline can hinder microglial activation but not for oxaliplatin-dependent neuropathy (Thomas et al., 2004).

13.3 Factors affecting drug-related neurotoxicity

The chemicals or substances can be considered drugs or poison based on several factors, including dosage, exposure duration, age, gender, nutritional condition, temperature, metabolites, and others (Fig. 13.4). Metabolism is a critical factor that converts the drug into active metabolites having neurotoxic potential. These factors are responsible for causing changes in

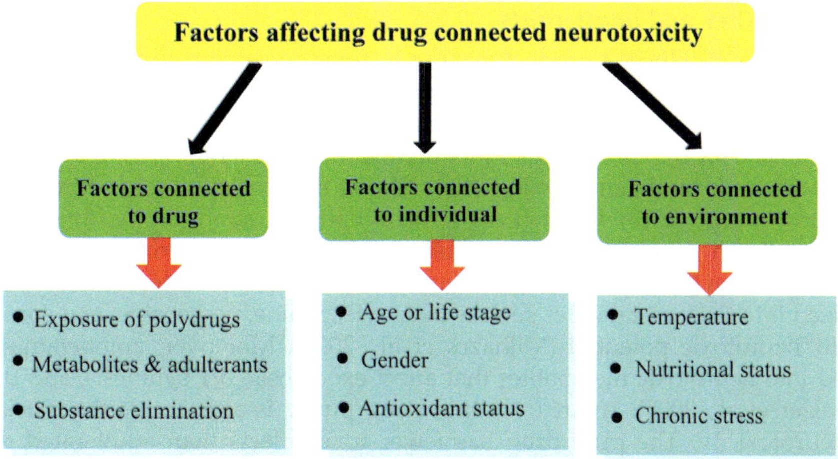

FIGURE 13.4 Schematic diagram depicts the various factors affecting drug-induced neurotoxicity.

several NT systems that result in neuronal damage induced by drug abuse. The factors mentioned above are briefly discussed next.

13.3.1 Factors connected to drug

The factors associated with a drug are dependent on its structural and chemical activities, including exposure to multiple drugs, purity, drug metabolism, and elimination. These factors significantly impact the neurotoxic potency of drugs, which are described in the following sections.

13.3.1.1 Exposure to polydrugs

By using multiple drugs, patients suffer from serious health issues caused due to the adverse effect of drugs (Connor et al., 2014). Polydrug users have a higher risk of neurotoxic effects compared to single-drug users. On polydrug exposure, one drug affects the biochemical property of another drug and increases its neurotoxic potential. For instance, the combined use of opioids and benzodiazepines enhances the risk of neurotoxicity (Jones et al., 2012). To prevent patients from the harmful effects of overuse of opioids, benzodiazepines are used as effective therapeutic agents for treating anxiety syndromes (i.e., confusion, drowsiness, hallucination) and many neurological disorders (i.e., seizures, delirium). However, their combination proved to be an abusive drug as both exhibit modulatory influences upon each other.

Diazepam is a type of benzodiazepine that changes the pharmacokinetics of opioids. It acts as a noncompetitive and competitive inhibitor for methadone metabolism and hepatic N-demethylation of methadone, respectively (Shah et al., 1979). So, for this reason, methadone dosage increases in CNS and ultimately boosts its neurotoxic potential. Another example is Mephedrone which enhances the neurotoxic potential of other drugs, such as methamphetamine and amphetamine, without exhibiting neuronal death by itself.

13.3.1.2 *Metabolites and adulterants*

Drug metabolism produces a product that can be toxic depending on the bioactivation process. In the bioactivation methods, the drug is metabolized into metabolites in the presence of enzyme activities. These toxic and active metabolites cause neurotoxicity by crossing the blood-brain barrier (BBB). For example, β-N-methylamino-L-alanine (L-BMAA) is converted to toxic formaldehyde by the metabolic action of brain tissue, resulting in neurodegenerative diseases (Delcourt et al., 2018). Like L-BMAA, methyl phenyl tetrahydropyridine (MPTP) also produces neurotoxin products via metabolizing into mitochondrial toxin N-methyl-4-phenylpyridinium ion (MPP^+) that targets neuromelanin and causes neuronal death. Cocaine is metabolized into toxic metabolites such as benzoylecgonine, norcocaine, and cocaethylene, having their neurotoxic potential (Milhazes et al., 2006). Moreover, amphetamine is also metabolized into neurotoxic metabolites that affect exocytosis, NT synthesis, and uptake inhibition (Sulzer et al., 2005). Apart from this, drug purity is also one of the crucial factors affecting neurotoxicity. The pure drug has fewer toxic effects than adulterated drug. For example, organophosphates in any drug or substance enhance neurotoxicity by inhibiting neurotoxic esterase (Misra and Kalita, 2009). Another study revealed that b-cyanoalanine and c-glutamyl b-cyanoalanine are used as lentil adulterants and are involved in neuropathy (Ghasemi, 2017). Similarly, impure heroin generates higher toxicity in PC12 cells via increasing caspase activation than pure ones (Cunha-Oliveira et al., 2007).

13.3.1.3 *Substance elimination*

Substance or drug removal from addicts for a long time can enhance the brain's sensitivity to excitotoxic destruction. Ethanol elimination enhanced the NMDA-related neuronal apoptosis by modifying the fraction among GluN2A and GluN2B NMDA receptor subunits (Rubio et al., 2011). Similarly, methamphetamine withdrawal reduces the Mg^{2+} blockade of NMDA receptors and enhances this receptor-mediated excitatory postsynaptic activities in the neostriatum (Moriguchi et al., 2002).

13.3.2 Factors connected to individual

Drug toxic responses vary depending on different groups of organisms, their age or life stage, sex, and antioxidant status. These factors are related to individuals that have adverse effects on the neurotoxicity of chemicals and are briefly discussed next.

13.3.2.1 *Age or life stage*

The age or life stage of organisms plays a significant role in determining their response to neurotoxins. Age in humans is connected with enhanced vulnerability to chemical drugs massively due to the weakening of biotransformation, excretion, and renal clearance (Gupta et al., 2022b). The infant life stage is more susceptible than the late stage. However, it is not necessary always that young people will be more prone to neurotoxicity than older ones. In a few cases, old-aged individuals have a higher risk of neurotoxicity than young aged. For instance, in one study, old-aged rats exhibited higher methamphetamine neurotoxic effects than young ones (Krasnova and Cadet, 2009). In addition, at low drug dosages, old rats deal with more toxicity than young ones having negligible toxicity at high doses of the drug (Miller et al., 2000). Neuronal function varies as per the age of individuals (Lotti, 2002).

As with growing age, neuronal DNA damage, loss of nerve cells, and axonal pathology increase. Dopamine showed age-related neurotoxicity wherein middle-aged rats experienced motor neuron deficits more than young-aged rats (Cantuti-Castelvetri et al., 2003).

13.3.2.2 Gender/sex

Both males and females are metabolically and hormonally dissimilar, so they respond differently to chemical substances or drugs. Besides metabolic differences, females' low body weight, slow renal clearance, and hormonal imbalance affect kidney activity and gastrointestinal movement, making them different in pharmacokinetics from males. Depending on the species, their metabolic rate as well as neurotoxic response against drugs also differs. For example, male rodents are more susceptible to organophosphate pesticides than females. In contrast, in humans, females have a higher risk of pesticide-mediated neurotoxic potential than males (Astiz et al., 2014). In both rats and mice, females are more prone to ethanol than males (Sharrett-Field et al., 2013; Sherrill et al., 2011). Like ethanol, cocaine also induces higher neurotoxicity in females than males (Becker et al., 2017).

13.3.2.3 Antioxidant status

An antioxidant is a biochemical agent that prevents the cells from the neurotoxic potential of toxicants via scavenging the free radicals causing oxidative damage to neurons. Antioxidant enzymes such as superoxide dismutase, catalase, glutathione peroxidase, and superoxide reductase play a critical function in avoiding neurotoxicity. However, deactivating these enzymes may result in drastic neuron function changes leading to neurodegenerative diseases. For instance, in one report, researchers revealed that mice with glutathione peroxidase deficiency are more prone to neurotoxicity due to excess free radicals produced from neurotoxin activity (Zhang et al., 2000). Another study demonstrated that the high expression of CuZn-superoxide dismutase in mice could exhibit a positive response against the toxic effects of methamphetamine and MDMA (Cadet et al., 1994). Similarly, decreased activity of glutathione results in oxidative stress-inducing neuronal death in the presence of methylmercury (Farina and Aschner, 2019).

13.3.3 Factors connected to the environment

Environmental factors such as temperature, nutrition status, and chronic stress affect the drug's neurotoxic effects. These factors depend on the species type, metabolic drug nature, the quantity of nutritional components, response, and developments. These are briefly discussed in the following sections.

13.3.3.1 Temperature

Temperature is the significant determinant of the response that occurs in the nervous system against drug exposure. Metabolic activity, absorption, excretion, and detoxification vary with changing temperatures affecting the drug's neurotoxicity. In addition, it also influences the toxicity of drug abuse *by* relying on the species type, drug nature, response, and developments. High body temperature enhances methamphetamine-related dopamine neurotoxicity, while low temperature reduces the neurotoxic effects of methamphetamine (Thomas et al., 2004). Likewise, environmental temperature variations exhibit an excellent effect on neurotoxicity induced by methamphetamine, which is equal to a high drug dosage (Miller and O'Callaghan, 2003). However, in contrast to hyperthermia, hypothermia protects against neuronal deficits caused by drug abuse (Johnson et al., 2000). In one of the findings, hypothermia protected asphyxiated newborns from iron-induced neurotoxicity (Caputa et al., 2001).

13.3.3.2 *Nutritional status*

Nutritional status is another important deciding factor for drug neurotoxicity. Individuals who lack nutrition are more susceptible to the drug-causing neuronal death than healthy people. Vitamin E deficiency promotes neurotoxic effects induced by MDMA that generate free radical molecules involved in oxidative stress (Johnson et al., 2002). The mice with sufficient vitamin E have a high potency to fight against free radicals compared to the vitamin E-lacking group. Alcoholic individuals who suffer from thiamine deficiency impart mitochondrial impairment, oxidative stress, and glutamate excitotoxicity in various brain regions (Kopelman et al., 2009). This is due to the interaction of the alcohol with the nutrient's absorption activity. Moreover, excessive intake of nutritional components is also responsible for producing several severe neurotoxic effects. For example, high contents of vitamin A in the diet lead to neurological deficits, but the precise mechanism involved in neurotoxicity is not yet known (Snodgrass, 1992). Therefore, a balanced nutrition diet is necessary to reduce the neurotoxic effects caused by drug abuse.

13.3.3.3 *Chronic stress*

Chronic stress exposure significantly changes the volume of the hippocampus, frontal cortex, and amygdala, resulting in adverse effects on the brain. It also enhances motor deficits *by* reducing the NT, dopamine, serotonin, and other agents released in motor neurons. Besides this, chronic stress also plays a crucial role in affecting the neurotoxic potential of the drug. For instance, in one finding, chronic stress enhances the MDMA-induced dopamine and serotonin release in the ventral tegmental region of the brain and causes long-term impairment in 5-HT ends (Amato et al., 2007). Another study revealed the promoting activity of chronic stress toward methamphetamine toxicity causing long-term excitotoxic injury through increasing the glutamate release in the striatum (Tata and Yamamoto, 2008). Similarly, other findings also demonstrated the increased susceptibility of the neuron to methamphetamine under the influence of chronic stress (Matuszewich and Yamamoto, 2004). In addition, stress encourages hyperthermia responses in stressed rats compared to nonstressed models.

13.4 Drug-induced neurological disorders

Most of the powerful drugs that are used for treating cancer, cardiovascular and respiratory diseases have side effects which bring about severe alterations in human behavior. Drug practices cannot predict every incidental interaction or defect, so pharmaceutical research must be continued for drug improvement. Doctors must improve their skills in applied therapeutics to assist pharmacists, colleagues, and medical representatives concerning the drug's adverse effects. The following discussion on drug-induced neurological disorders is needed for understanding and identifying the symptoms that deal with drugs causing neuronal damage.

13.4.1 Drug-induced schizophrenia/psychosis

Both schizophrenia and psychosis are chronic mental illnesses that occur due to drug abuse and have similar psychotic symptoms, such as hallucinations, delusions, difficulty in decision-making, agitation, decreased feelings of pleasure, and incapability to separate thoughts, observations, and reality (Ham et al., 2017). Nearly 1.1% of people worldwide are affected by such disorders. However, drug-induced psychosis is not schizophrenia, as schizophrenia is only a misnomer. Patients with schizophrenia take more than 6 months to recover, while psychosis is temporary. These syndromes are not a disease but acute problems that can be reduced by avoiding drug usage such as cocaine, hallucinogens, alcohol, amphetamine, cannabis, marijuana, and opioids. The prolonged use or overdoses of these drugs may cause severe alterations in the neurotransmitter levels of the brain.

13.4.2 Drug-induced bipolar disorder

Bipolar or mood disorders arise from exposure to a substance or prescribed medication that causes manic, hypomanic, and depressive symptoms. These symptoms involve changes in cerebral structures and neurotransmitter function (Kosten et al., 1998). Drugs contributing to bipolar or manic include cocaine, alcohol, opioids, interferon (IFN), corticosteroids, digoxin, and antiepileptic substances. Depression or mood disorders lead to an increased risk of suicide attempts owing to such drug abuse. Terminating severe intoxication and acute withdrawal from these substances can resolve bipolar disorders in 1 month. Stimulant use (cocaine, amphetamines, and others) can imitate bipolar disorders by generating euphoria, increased energy, anorexia, grandiosity, and paranoia. In contrast, stimulant withdrawal can result in anhedonia, apathy, depressed mood, and suicidal ideation (Quello et al., 2005).

13.4.3 Drug-induced parkinsonism

Drug-causing PD symptoms are referred to as drug-induced parkinsonism (DIP). DIP and PD have similar clinical features, so patients with DIP are misdiagnosed by antipsychotics, gastrointestinal prokinetics, and antiepileptic drugs for a long time. These drugs affect dopamine receptors that reduce dopamine concentrations in the nerve cells and cause movement disorders (Shin and Chung, 2012). Other parkinsonism symptoms include resting tremors, muscle stiffness, dementia, hallucinations, impaired speech, and posture. Drugs involved in DIP are fluphenazine, perphenazine, pimozide, chlorpromazine, metoclopramide, levosulpiride, diltiazem, and others. After cessation of these drugs, patients with DIP may be recovered, but it can quicken PD in people suffering from DIP.

13.4.4 Drug-induced tremor

This tremor is a rhythmic, involuntary action like shaking, twitching, or quivering that is uncontrollable. It generally occurs in the hands, fingers, arms, legs, and face for 6–10 s. The tremor caused by DIP is in resting condition and controllable, which makes it different from drug-induced tremors. The drugs connected with tremors are amiodarone, lithium, serotonin, amitriptyline, β-adrenoceptor agonists, dopamine receptor antagonists, ethanol, cocaine, and others (Morgan and Sethi, 2005). Besides these drugs, anticonvulsants are one of the most common drugs causing tremors as well as bipolar disorders. Tremor affects both the left and right sides of the arms compared to PD, causing one side only, and also, there is no brain degeneration in drug-induced tremors (Morgan and Sethi, 2005).

13.4.5 Drug-induced dyskinesia

Like DIP, dyskinesia is also an involuntary movement disorder that occurs on exposure to drugs used in treating PD for a long duration, such as antipsychotic drugs and levodopa. Motion disorders of the mouth, face, jaw, limbs, and trunk are the common symptoms of dyskinesia. It is classified into dystonic, ballistic, choreic, and myoclonic based on the administration time interval of dopaminergic medication (Nutt, 2001). Tardive dyskinesia is another essential type that results from dopamine-blocking agent usage and exhibits permanent adverse effects (Cloud et al., 2014). It affects mainly the mouth, face, and tongue and has less influence on the legs and trunk. Most women suffer from such disorder, yet no treatment successfully reduces tardive dyskinesia.

13.4.6 Drug-induced dystonia

Dystonia too occurs on exposure to dopamine-blocking agents that reduce dopamine levels in the brain resulting in muscle spasms and abnormal postures within hours or days of starting such drugs. In this neurological disorder, the tongue protrudes with a tilted head, the eyes are turned upwards, and the mouth is forcibly opened. Treatment with anticholinergics or antihistamines (i.e., diphenhydramine) and the ceasing of dopamine-blocking drugs can decrease the adverse effects of dystonia within 12–48 h (van Harten et al., 1999).

13.4.7 Drug-induced seizure

Drugs associated with seizures are antidepressants, antipsychotics, antiepileptic drugs (overdose or discontinuation), antibiotics, immunosuppressants and immunomodulators, antitumor agents, analgesics, central nervous system stimulators, anesthetics, and others. Typically, seizure arises due to scarce inhibitory impacts (i.e., gamma-aminobutyric acid, GABA) and sufficient excitatory stimulation (i.e., glutamate). Maximum drug-induced seizures are self-restricted and vary depending on geographic area. For instance, in Australia and Iran, a high dose of tramadol is a reason for seizures, while in the United States, bupropion was the cause of this disorder (Shadnia et al., 2012; Ryan and Isbister, 2015). An individual can be prevented from such disorders by using an optimal dose of these drugs and evading the simultaneous administration of various drugs that stimulate the CNS.

13.5 Preventive approaches against drug neurotoxicity

Different approaches were used to reduce neurotoxic effects induced by drug abuse, including scavenging, antiapoptotic, anti-inflammatory, receptor antagonist, drug rotation, and thermoregulation. Such approaches have proved beneficial in understanding the reason or the mechanism behind the neurotoxicity of chemicals. With the help of these strategies, researchers can tailor appropriate treatment for neurologic diseases occurring from drug exposure. The following preventive approaches are discussed next.

13.5.1 Free radicals scavenging approach

Free radicals cause oxidative stress that damages neuronal cells and thus, to protect the cells from such effects, these free radical species are needed to be reduced via antioxidant molecules. Antioxidants including N-acetyl-L-cysteine, ascorbic acid, vitamin C, selenium, and melatonin are capable of scavenging free radicals and prevent against psychostimulant related neurotoxic effects (Sharma et al., 2007). Pretreatment of an animal model with compound H-290/51, a new potent antioxidant has reduced the BBB disturbance induced by neurotoxic drugs. Not only synthetic antioxidants but natural antioxidants also showed a remarkable neuroprotective result. Thymoquinone or geraniol, a natural antioxidant, has protected cisplatin-related neurotoxic effects in rats by minimizing memory and learning deficits (Kandeil et al., 2020).

Likewise, lycopene is one of the carotenoids isolated from red plants that exhibited excellent neuroprotection in Wistar rats where neuropathy was induced by acrylamide (Aboubakr et al., 2021). Moreover, a combination of iron oxide nanoparticles (NPs) with quercetin also prevented the neurotoxic influence of aluminum chloride on rat brain tissue. Quercetin nanoparticles improved its bioavailability, and the controlled balance of antioxidant enzymes in the hippocampus of rats results in protective effect in animal suffering from Alzheimer's disease (Esmaeili et al., 2020). Besides this, many other antioxidant agents are also involved in reducing the neurotoxic effects induced by platinum drugs (Stankovic et al., 2020).

13.5.2 Antiapoptotic approach

Deactivation of apoptotic pathways is one of the crucial tactics to fight against drug-induced neurotoxic effects. Researchers have made remarkable efforts to develop an effective antiapoptotic method. For instance, recently, the involvement of curcumin has been one of the effective approaches to inhibiting apoptosis pathways that promote acrylamide-induced neurotic effects in rats (Guo et al., 2020). Curcumin-treated acrylamide rats had shown less neurotic effects than the non-curcumin treated group. The reason behind this is linked with the upregulation of telomerase reverse transcriptase associated with antiapoptotic activity by curcumin. In another study, researchers revealed the antiapoptotic activity of L-carnitine against caffeine-related neuronal cell death in the SH-SY5Y neuroblastoma cell line (Bavari et al., 2016). Their results indicated that L-carnitine had protected the neural cells via inhibiting oxidative stress-related cell apoptosis and mitochondria disturbance. Melatonin and dopamine type 1 receptors had also successfully aided Caspase and Fas facilitated cell apoptosis induced by methamphetamine (Wisessmith et al., 2009).

Similarly, the introduction of Calpastatin also reverses the cytotoxicity induced by methamphetamine via reducing the phosphorylation of transcription factor, c-Jun, and Bax/Bcl-2 ratio levels in neuroblastoma cell lines (Chetsawang et al., 2012).

13.5.3 Anti-inflammatory approach

Like the antioxidant approach, anti-inflammatory strategies have also been proven effective in preventing drug-induced neurotoxic effects. Many anti-inflammatory drugs have been applied as therapeutic agents to reduce the negative effect of inflammation on brain tissues caused by drug abuse. This approach can be successfully developed for neuroprotection by modifying the interaction among the proinflammatory cytokines and their targets, altering peripheral inflammation and CNS interface, and changing inflammasome expression in CNS regions. Cyclooxygenase inhibitors such as nimesulide and indomethacin have made it possible to inhibit the contact between the peripheral inflammatory cells and CNS, preventing neurodegeneration disorders.

Ketoprofen and indomethacin as anti-inflammatory drugs have protected the neural cells from neurotoxicity induced by methamphetamine. For neuroprotection, inhibition of proinflammatory cytokine synthesis using specific IL-1 receptor antagonists and sitagliptin significantly increased anti-inflammatory cytokine formation in the mouse model (Veltkamp and Gill, 2016). Apart from this, numerous polyphenol constituents of plants have anti-inflammatory potency that makes them suitable therapeutic agents for treating neurodegenerative diseases (Luo et al., 2020). These phytochemicals, such as terpenoids, flavonoids, steroids, and alkaloids, inhibit the amyloid β peptide-associated nuclear factor-kappa B signaling pathway that regulates the gene or protein expression involved in neurotoxicity (Park et al., 2016). In addition, they can cross BBB to protect cells from neurotic effects (Kam et al., 2012).

13.5.4 Receptor antagonist

A receptor antagonist is a drug or receptor ligand that deactivates the receptor's response by binding to it. Such antagonism activity of the drug can protect the neuronal cells from chemical-driven toxicity. The cells can be prevented from NMDA receptor-driven neurotoxicity using its antagonist. For example, MK801, an NMDA receptor antagonist, significantly reduced the neurotoxic effects in the canine model, and its activity is further improved via conjugating with dendrimer NPs (Giuliano et al., 2021). Ketamine and Memantine are other NMDA receptor antagonists that protect animals or humans from opioid-induced neurotoxicity and Alzheimer's disease, respectively (Bruera and Kim, 2003). Apart from NMDA receptor antagonists, adenosine A_{2A} receptor and metabotropic glutamate receptor 5 antagonism have also proved to be effective approaches to neuroprotection (Gołembiowska et al., 2003). Additionally, muscarinic receptor antagonists such as pirenzepine, VU0255035, or muscarinic toxin 7 had reversed peripheral neuropathy triggered by dichloroacetate and paclitaxel (Calcutt et al., 2017).

13.5.5 Drug rotation

Drug rotation is a method to replace one drug with another with similar characteristics to the former. This process has made it possible to reduce the neurotoxic effects induced by neurotoxicants. For instance, rotating one opioid with another alternative opioid prevented neurotoxicity induced by opioids (Knotkova et al., 2009). Patients with neurotoxic effects induced by morphine were protected by shifting morphine to methadone. Both drugs are opioids, and their rotation to each other, has reduced the morphine-related adverse effects. In the drug rotation approach, an appropriate dose of other drugs must be chosen that does not cause toxicity and can decrease adverse effects (Knotkova et al., 2009). Different kinds of opioids with suitable doses can be exchanged in opioid rotation for neuroprotection. Interestingly, opioid rotation inhibits drug-induced neurotoxicity and reduces metabolites-related adverse effects (Corli et al., 2019). However, further research is still needed to find out newer effective opioids using this approach in preventing drug-induced neurotoxicity.

Like opioids, tacrolimus, an immunosuppressant, also causes neurological damage in a patient having a renal transplant. Nearly 25% of patients undergo tremors, confusion, headache, reduced spontaneity and speech, lethargy, convulsions, and others on exposure to tacrolimus. To minimize its neurotoxic effects, tacrolimus is exchanged with a different immunosuppressant, such as cyclosporine, prednisone, and mycophenolic acid, having negligible neurotoxic effects. Such a drug rotation technique has remarkably prevented neurological damage (Group, 1994).

13.5.6 Thermoregulatory approach

An elevated body temperature exerts adverse effects on the brain tissue, while a lower temperature helps to protect the neuronal cells from toxicity induced by drugs. Therefore, the regulation of temperature is a crucial approach to neuroprotection. Hypothermia strategy or cooling of targeted tissue to 32–34°C has improved the reduction of adverse effects in hyperthermia patients (Pietrini et al., 2012). Hypothermia therapy induction enhances the prevention of drug-related neurological diseases through attenuating metabolism, free radical's production, excitotoxicity, apoptosis, and inflammation. Mainly, eight kinds of hypothermia-inducing drugs are employed to treat brain damage, including cannabinoids, opioid receptor activators, transient receptor potential vanilloid, neurotensins, thyroxine derivatives, dopamine receptor activators, hypothermia-inducing gasses, adenosine, and adenine nucleotides (Zhang et al., 2013). L-Lobeline is one of the nicotinic receptor ligands that acts as neuroprotectants in hyperthermia rats induced by methamphetamine. This drug reduces toxicity related to methamphetamine via decreasing body temperature that declines the vesicular monoamine transporter 2, dopamine and serotonin concentration in rat striatum (Eyerman and Yamamoto, 2005). In addition, MK-801, diazepam, and phenobarbital are other well-known drugs that induce hypothermia for neuroprotection (Zhou et al., 2021).

13.6 Nanoparticles-induced neurotoxicity

The emergence of NPs in the biomedical, industrial, agricultural, and pharmaceutical fields has created great attention among researchers owing to their nanosized with large surface area to volume ratio properties (Gupta et al., 2019a, 2019b). Their different shapes, sizes, and structures make them unusual in physical, chemical, and biological activities (Gupta and Singh, 2021; Gadekar et al., 2021; Gorain et al., 2016; Muniswamy et al., 2019; Prajapati et al., 2009). They are classified into organic, inorganic, and carbon-dependent NPs. Polymeric NPs are organic, biodegradable, and nontoxic, while silver, gold, zinc, copper,

TABLE 13.2 Few of the nanoparticles and their neurotoxic effects.

Nanoparticles (NPs)	Neurotoxicity	References
Silver	Mitochondrial damage, ROS production, and elevated Ca^{2+} levels	Xu et al. (2015)
Titanium oxide	Genotoxicity, inflammation, DNA and organelles damage, oxidative stress	Jia et al. (2017)
Gold	Enhance the number of astrocytes, seizure function, and cognition defects	Teleanu et al. (2019)
Iron oxide	Synaptic transmission and nerve conduction disturbance, variation in immune cell infiltration	Valdiglesias et al. (2015)
Silica	Negative effects on dopaminergic neurons, microglial and cognitive dysfunction, synaptic injury	Zhou et al. (2016)
Polymeric	Elevated oxidative stress, inflammation, and neuronal apoptosis	Yuan et al. (2015)
Carbon nanotubes	Changes in mitochondrial membrane potential, cell proliferation inhibition, astrogliosis, and lipid peroxidation	Win-Shwe and Fujimaki (2011)

iron, zinc oxide, titanium oxide, and others are inorganic NPs. Graphene, fullerene, and carbon nanotubes are carbon-based NPs. These NPs are highly applied in diagnosing and treating diseases as drug delivery systems, biosensors, bioimaging, hyperthermia, and photoablation (Malik et al., 2021). This is because of their enhanced stability, functionalization, absorption efficacy, quantum confinement, and magnetic and optical assets. Besides this, they may cause toxicity to individuals, especially damage to the brain tissue, because of their high reactivity and ability to pass through BBB (Oberdörster et al., 2009).

NPs induced neurotoxicity by gathering in particular brain areas, wherein they come in contact with neurons, astrocytes, and microglia after crossing the BBB (Win-Shwe and Fujimaki, 2011). Like other therapeutic drugs, NPs also cause neurotoxic effects via cell apoptosis, oxidative stress, inflammation, and excitotoxicity (Win-Shwe and Fujimaki, 2011; Youngren et al., 2013; Tekade and Chougule, 2013). Silver, gold, silica, graphene, fullerene, titanium oxide, iron oxide, and polymeric NPs have been widely studied for neurotoxicity, which is discussed in Table 13.2.

13.7 Conclusion

Neurotoxic effects of drugs used in diagnosing and treating diseases are self-limiting and progressive depending on the drug exposure extent. Besides their beneficial role, these drugs exert adverse effects on brain tissue that are manifested through several mechanisms, such as cell apoptosis, oxidative stress, mitochondrial dysfunction, inflammation, excitotoxicity, and other biological pathways. A drug's neurotoxic potential varies because of many factors associated with the drug's nature, environment, age, sex, and nutritional status. Maximum drugs used for treating PD, liver, kidney, and cancer diseases have CNS-related severe side effects that hamper the movements of body parts and cause mental illness. Such drugs induce numerous neurological disorders like DIP, dyskinesia, dystonia, seizure, bipolar, psychosis, and others.

Various preventive methods are developed to protect against neurological diseases caused by drug abuse. Alongside this, knowledge must be provided among the patients, caretakers, and health care providers about the identification and response to symptoms of drug-induced neurotoxicity. Doctors must improve their skills in applied therapeutics to assist pharmacists, colleagues, and medical representatives concerning the drug's adverse effects. But still, further investigations are required to explore new approaches to protect and treat these neurotoxic effects induced by drugs. Like other therapeutic drugs, NPs also have positive and negative effects on the nervous system's health. Depending on their unique characteristics and small size, they can easily cross BBB and affect brain areas. Therefore, the advancement of toxicological research is vital for improving brain retrieval.

13.8 List of abbreviations

ATP Adenosine triphosphate
BBB Blood-brain barrier
CNS Central nervous system
CTR1 Copper transporter-1
DIP Drug-induced Parkinsonism
DNA Deoxyribonucleic acid
DRG Dorsal root ganglion
ER Endoplasmic reticulum
GABA Gamma aminobutyric acid
H_2O_2 Hydrogen peroxide
L-BMAA β-N-methylamino-L-alanine
MDMA Methylenedioxymethamphetamine
METH Methamphetamine
MPP^+ N-methyl-4-phenylpyridinium ion
MPTP Methylphenyltetrahydropyridine
NMDA N-methyl-D-aspartate
NPs Nanoparticles
NT Neurotransmitter
O_2 Oxygen
O_2^- Superoxide
OCT2 Organic cation transporter-2
PD Parkinson disease
ROS Reactive oxygen species
TRPA1 Transient receptor potential ankyrin-1
TRPM8 Transient receptor potential melastatin-8
TRPV1 Transient receptor potential vanilloid-1
• OH Hydroxyl

References

Aboubakr, M., Elshafae, S.M., Abdelhiee, E.Y., Fadl, S.E., Soliman, A., Abdelkader, A., Abdel-Daim, M.M., Bayoumi, K.A., Baty, R.S., Elgendy, E., 2021. Antioxidant and anti-inflammatory potential of thymoquinone and lycopene mitigate the chlorpyrifos-induced toxic neuropathy. Pharmaceuticals 14, 940.

Adelsberger, H., Quasthoff, S., Grosskreutz, J., Lepier, A., Eckel, F., Lersch, C., 2000. The chemotherapeutic oxaliplatin alters voltage-gated Na+ channel kinetics on rat sensory neurons. Eur. J. Pharmacol. 406, 25–32.

Alaedini, A., Xiang, Z., Kim, H., Sung, Y.-J., Latov, N., 2008. Up-regulation of apoptosis and regeneration genes in the dorsal root ganglia during cisplatin treatment. Exp. Neurol. 210, 368–374.

Amato, J.L., Bankson, M.G., Yamamoto, B.K., 2007. Prior exposure to chronic stress and MDMA potentiates mesoaccumbens dopamine release mediated by the 5-HT1B receptor. Neuropsychopharmacology 32, 946–954.

Astiz, M., Acaz-Fonseca, E., Garcia-Segura, L.M., 2014. Sex differences and effects of estrogenic compounds on the expression of inflammatory molecules by astrocytes exposed to the insecticide dimethoate. Neurotox. Res. 25, 271–285.

Banach, M., Juranek, J.K., Zygulska, A.L., 2017. Chemotherapy-induced neuropathies—a growing problem for patients and health care providers. Brain Behav. 7, e00558.

Bavari, M., Tabandeh, M.R., Najafzadeh Varzi, H., Bahramzadeh, S., 2016. Neuroprotective, antiapoptotic and antioxidant effects of l-carnitine against caffeine-induced neurotoxicity in SH-SY5Y neuroblastoma cell line. Drug Chem. Toxicol. 39, 157–166.

Becker, J.B., Mcclellan, M.L., Reed, B.G., 2017. Sex differences, gender and addiction. J. Neurosci. Res. 95, 136–147.

Bonnel, R.A., Graham, D.J., 2004. Peripheral neuropathy in patients treated with leflunomide. Clin. Pharmacol. Therapeut. 75, 580–585.

Bruera, E., Kim, H.N., 2003. Cancer pain. JAMA 290, 2476–2479.

Cadet, J.L., Bisagno, V., Milroy, C.M., 2014. Neuropathology of substance use disorders. Acta Neuropathol. 127, 91–107.

Cadet, J.L., Brannock, C., 1998. Invited review free radicals and the pathobiology of brain dopamine systems. Neurochem. Int. 32, 117–131.

Cadet, J.L., Krasnova, I.N., Jayanthi, S., Lyles, J., 2007. Neurotoxicity of substituted amphetamines: molecular and cellular mechanisms. Neurotox. Res. 11, 183–202.

Cadet, J.L., Sheng, P., All, S., Rothman, R., Carlson, E., Epstein, C., 1994. Rapid communication: attenuation of methamphetamine-induced neurotoxicity in copper/zinc superoxide dismutase transgenic mice. J. Neurochem. 62, 380–383.

Calcutt, N.A., Smith, D.R., Frizzi, K., Sabbir, M.G., Chowdhury, S.K.R., Mixcoatl-Zecuatl, T., Saleh, A., Muttalib, N., van der Ploeg, R., Ochoa, J., 2017. Selective antagonism of muscarinic receptors is neuroprotective in peripheral neuropathy. J. Clin. Invest. 127, 608–622.

Cantuti-Castelvetri, I., Shukitt-Hale, B., Joseph, J.A., 2003. Dopamine neurotoxicity: age-dependent behavioral and histological effects. Neurobiol. Aging 24, 697–706.

Caputa, M., Rogalska, J., Nowakowska, A., 2001. Effect of temperature on postanoxic, potentially neurotoxic changes of plasma pH and free iron level in newborn rats. Brain Res. Bull. 55, 281–286.

Ceccatelli, S., Bose, R., Edoff, K., Onishchenko, N., Spulber, S., 2013. Long-lasting neurotoxic effects of exposure to methylmercury during development. J. Intern. Med. 273, 490–497.

Chetsawang, J., Suwanjang, W., Pirompul, N., Govitrapong, P., Chetsawang, B., 2012. Calpastatin reduces methamphetamine-induced induction in c-Jun phosphorylation, Bax and cell death in neuroblastoma SH-SY5Y cells. Neurosci. Lett. 506, 7–11.

Chipana, C., Torres, I., Camarasa, J., Pubill, D., Escubedo, E., 2008. Memantine protects against amphetamine derivatives-induced neurotoxic damage in rodents. Neuropharmacology 54, 1254–1263.

Cloud, L.J., Zutshi, D., Factor, S.A., 2014. Tardive dyskinesia: therapeutic options for an increasingly common disorder. Neurotherapeutics 11, 166–176.

Connor, J.P., Gullo, M.J., White, A., Kelly, A.B., 2014. Polysubstance use: diagnostic challenges, patterns of use and health. Curr. Opin. Psychiatr. 27, 269–275.

Corli, O., Roberto, A., Corsi, N., Galli, F., Pizzuto, M., 2019. Opioid switching and variability in response in pain cancer patients. Support. Care Cancer 27, 2321–2327.

Costa, L.G., Giordano, G., Guizzetti, M., Vitalone, A., 2008. Neurotoxicity of pesticides: a brief review. Front. Biosci.-Landmark 13, 1240–1249.

Cunha-Oliveira, T., Rego, A.C., Garrido, J., Borges, F., Macedo, T., Oliveira, C.R., 2007. Street heroin induces mitochondrial dysfunction and apoptosis in rat cortical neurons. J. Neurochem. 101, 543–554.

Delcourt, N., Claudepierre, T., Maignien, T., Arnich, N., Mattei, C., 2018. Cellular and molecular aspects of the β-N-Methylamino-l-alanine (BMAA) mode of action within the neurodegenerative pathway: facts and controversy. Toxins 10, 6.

Dietrich, J.-B., Mangeol, A., Revel, M.-O., Burgun, C., Aunis, D., Zwiller, J., 2005. Acute or repeated cocaine administration generates reactive oxygen species and induces antioxidant enzyme activity in dopaminergic rat brain structures. Neuropharmacology 48, 965–974.

Esmaeili, A., Rahgozar, S., Noorbakhshnia, M., 2020. Quercetin-conjugated superparamagnetic iron oxide nanoparticles protect AlCl 3-induced neurotoxicity in a rat model of alzheimer's disease via antioxidant genes, APP gene, and miRNA-101. Front. Neurosci. 14, 598617.

Eyerman, D.J., Yamamoto, B.K., 2005. Lobeline attenuates methamphetamine-induced changes in vesicular monoamine transporter 2 immunoreactivity and monoamine depletions in the striatum. J. Pharmacol. Exp. Therapeut. 312, 160–169.

Farina, M., Aschner, M., 2019. Glutathione antioxidant system and methylmercury-induced neurotoxicity: an intriguing interplay. Biochim. Biophys. Acta Gen. Subj. 1863, 129285.

Gadekar, V., Borade, Y., Kannaujia, S., Rajpoot, K., Anup, N., Tambe, V., Kalia, K., Tekade, R.K., 2021. Nanomedicines accessible in the market for clinical interventions. J. Contr. Release 330, 372–397.

Ghasemi, N., 2017. Synthesis of 13C labeled β-cyano-L-alanine. Org. Commun. 10, 6.

Giuliano, K., Etchill, E., Zhou, X., Lui, C., SUAREZ-Pierre, A., Sharma, R., Wilson, M.A., Blue, M.E., Troncoso, J.C., Kannan, S., 2021. NMDA receptor antagonism for neuroprotection in a canine model of hypothermic circulatory arrest. J. Surg. Res. 260, 177–189.

Gołembiowska, K., Konieczny, J., Wolfarth, S., Ossowska, K., 2003. Neuroprotective action of MPEP, a selective mGluR5 antagonist, in methamphetamine-induced dopaminergic neurotoxicity is associated with a decrease in dopamine outflow and inhibition of hyperthermia in rats. Neuropharmacology 45, 484–492.

Gorain, B., Choudhury, H., Tekade, R.K., Karan, S., Jaisankar, P., Pal, T.K., 2016. Comparative biodistribution and safety profiling of olmesartan medoxomil oil-in-water oral nanoemulsion. Regul. Toxicol. Pharmacol. 82, 20–31.

Grobin, A.C., Matthews, D.B., Devaud, L.L., Morrow, A.L., 1998. The role of GABA(A) receptors in the acute and chronic effects of ethanol. Psychopharmacology (Berl) 139, 2–19.

Group, U.M.F.L.S., 1994. A comparison of tacrolimus (FK 506) and cyclosporine for immunosuppression in liver transplantation. N. Engl. J. Med. 331, 1110–1115.

Guo, J., Cao, X., Hu, X., Li, S., Wang, J., 2020. The anti-apoptotic, antioxidant and anti-inflammatory effects of curcumin on acrylamide-induced neurotoxicity in rats. BMC Pharmacol. Toxicol. 21, 1–10.

Gupta, R., Das, N., Singh, M., 2019a. Fabrication and surface characterisation of c-ZnO loaded TTDMM dendrimer nanocomposites for biological applications. Appl. Surf. Sci. 484, 781–796.

Gupta, R., Malik, P., Das, N., Singh, M., 2019b. Antioxidant and physicochemical study of Psidium guajava prepared zinc oxide nanoparticles. J. Mol. Liq. 275, 749–767.

Gupta, R., Polaka, S., Rajpoot, K., Tekade, M., Sharma, M.C., Tekade, R.K., 2022a. Importance of toxicity testing in drug discovery and research. Pharmacokinetics and Toxicokinetic Considerations. Elsevier, pp. 117–144.

Gupta, R., Rajpoot, K., Tekade, M., Sharma, M.C., Safavi, M., Tekade, R.K., 2022b. Factors Influencing Drug Toxicity. Pharmacokinetics and Toxicokinetic Considerations. Elsevier, pp. 27–50.

Gupta, R., Singh, M., 2021. Physicochemical properties of sustainable caped ZnO-Dendrimer nanocomposite with aqueous DMSO interfaces from 298.15–313.15 K. J. Mol. Liq. 322, 114936.

Ham, S., Kim, T.K., Chung, S., Im, H.I., 2017. Drug abuse and psychosis: new insights into drug-induced psychosis. Exp. Neurobiol. 26, 11–24.

Hartmann, J.T., Lipp, H.-P., 2003. Toxicity of platinum compounds. Expert Opin. Pharmacother. 4, 889–901.

Helso, S.N., Roug, A.S., Mork, M., Maksten, E.F., Severinsen, M.T., 2020. Severe peripheral neuropathy from treatment with arsenic trioxide in a patient suffering from acute promyelocytic leukemia. J. Hematol. 9, 89.

Ijomone, O.M., Ifenatuoha, C.W., Aluko, O.M., Ijomone, O.K., Aschner, M., 2020. The aging brain: impact of heavy metal neurotoxicity. Crit. Rev. Toxicol. 50, 801–814.

Inaba, H., Kishimoto, T., Oishi, S., Nagata, K., Hasegawa, S., Watanabe, T., Kida, S., 2016. Vitamin B1-deficient mice show impairment of hippocampus-dependent memory formation and loss of hippocampal neurons and dendritic spines: potential microendophenotypes of Wernicke–Korsakoff syndrome. Biosci. Biotechnol. Biochem. 80, 2425–2436.

Jayanthi, S., Deng, X., Ladenheim, B., Mccoy, M.T., Cluster, A., Cai, N.-S., Cadet, J.L., 2005. Calcineurin/NFAT-induced up-regulation of the Fas ligand/Fas death pathway is involved in methamphetamine-induced neuronal apoptosis. Proc. Natl. Acad. Sci. USA 102, 868–873.

Jia, X., Wang, S., Zhou, L., Sun, L., 2017. The potential liver, brain, and embryo toxicity of titanium dioxide nanoparticles on mice. Nanoscale Res. Lett. 12, 1–14.

Johnson, E.A., Sharp, D.S., Miller, D.B., 2000. Restraint as a stressor in mice:: against the dopaminergic neurotoxicity of d-mdma, low body weight mitigates restraint-induced hypothermia and consequent neuroprotection. Brain Res. 875, 107–118.

Johnson, E.A., Shvedova, A.A., Kisin, E., O'callaghan, J.P., Kommineni, C., Miller, D.B., 2002. d-MDMA during vitamin E deficiency: effects on dopaminergic neurotoxicity and hepatotoxicity. Brain Res. 933, 150–163.

Jones, J.D., Mogali, S., Comer, S.D., 2012. Polydrug abuse: a review of opioid and benzodiazepine combination use. Drug Alcohol Depend. 125, 8–18.

Jones, M.R., Urits, I., Wolf, J., Corrigan, D., Colburn, L., Peterson, E., Williamson, A., Viswanath, O., 2020. Drug-induced peripheral neuropathy: a narrative review. Curr. Clin. Pharmacol. 15, 38–48.

Kam, A., M Li, K., Razmovski-Naumovski, V., Nammi, S., Chan, K., Li, Y., Q Li, G., 2012. The protective effects of natural products on blood-brain barrier breakdown. Curr. Med. Chem. 19, 1830–1845.

Kanafani, Z.A., 2011. Peripheral neuropathy in patients on long-term triazole antifungal therapy. J. Invasive Fungal Infect. 5, 127.

Kandeil, M.A., Gomaa, S.B., Mahmoud, M.O., 2020. The effect of some natural antioxidants against cisplatin-induced neurotoxicity in rats: behavioral testing. Heliyon 6, e04708.

Kang, H.M., Kang, Y.S., Kim, S.H., Seong, J.K., Kang, D.Y., Lee, H.Y., Lee, B.S., 2007. Amiodarone-induced hepatitis and polyneuropathy. Korean J. Intern. Med. 22, 225.

Keppel Hesselink, J.M., Kopsky, D.J., 2017. Phenytoin: neuroprotection or neurotoxicity? Neurol. Sci. 38, 1137–1141.

Knotkova, H., Fine, P.G., Portenoy, R.K., 2009. Opioid rotation: the science and the limitations of the equianalgesic dose table. J. Pain Symptom Manag. 38, 426–439.

Kopelman, M.D., Thomson, A.D., Guerrini, I., Marshall, E.J., 2009. The Korsakoff syndrome: clinical aspects, psychology and treatment. Alcohol Alcohol. 44, 148–154.

Kosten, T.R., Markou, A., Koob, G.F., 1998. Depression and stimulant dependence: neurobiology and pharmacotherapy. J. Nerv. Ment. Dis. 186, 737–745.

Krasnova, I.N., Cadet, J.L., 2009. Methamphetamine toxicity and messengers of death. Brain Res. Rev. 60, 379–407.

Lotti, M., 2002. Age-related sensitivity of the nervous system to neurotoxic insults. Toxicol. Lett. 127, 183–187.

Luo, Z., Yu, G., Chen, X., Liu, Y., Zhou, Y., Wang, G., Shi, Y., 2020. Integrated phytochemical analysis based on UHPLC-LTQ–Orbitrap and network pharmacology approaches to explore the potential mechanism of Lycium ruthenicum Murr. for ameliorating Alzheimer's disease. Food Funct. 11, 1362–1372.

Malik, P., Gupta, R., Malik, V., Ameta, R.K., 2021. Emerging nanomaterials for improved biosensing. Meas. Sensors 16, 100050.

Matuszewich, L., Yamamoto, B., 2004. Chronic stress augments the long-term and acute effects of methamphetamine. Neuroscience 124, 637–646.

Mccann, U.D., Ricaurte, G.A., 2004. Amphetamine neurotoxicity: accomplishments and remaining challenges. Neurosci. Biobehav. Rev. 27, 821–826.

Mcdonald, E.S., Randon, K.R., Knight, A., Windebank, A.J., 2005. Cisplatin preferentially binds to DNA in dorsal root ganglion neurons in vitro and in vivo: a potential mechanism for neurotoxicity. Neurobiol. Dis. 18, 305–313.

Meregalli, C., Chiorazzi, A., Carozzi, V.A., Canta, A., Sala, B., Colombo, M., Oggioni, N., Ceresa, C., Foudah, D., LA Russa, F., 2014. Evaluation of tubulin polymerization and chronic inhibition of proteasome as citotoxicity mechanisms in bortezomib-induced peripheral neuropathy. Cell Cycle 13, 612–621.

Meriggioli, M.N., Rowin, J., 2000. Chronic inflammatory demyelinating polyneuropathy after treatment with interferon-α. Muscle Nerve Off. J. Am. Associat. Electrodiagn. Med. 23, 433–435.

Milhazes, N., Cunha-Oliveira, T., Martins, P., Garrido, J., Oliveira, C., Rego, C., Borges, F., 2006. Synthesis and cytotoxic profile of 3, 4-methylenedioxymethamphetamine ("Ecstasy") and its metabolites on undifferentiated PC12 cells: a putative Structure– toxicity relationship. Chem. Res. Toxicol. 19, 1294–1304.

Miller, D.B., O'callaghan, J.P., Ali, S.F., 2000. Age as a susceptibility factor in the striatal dopaminergic neurotoxicity observed in the mouse following substituted amphetamine exposure. Ann. N. Y. Acad. Sci. 914, 194–207.

Miller, D.B., O'callaghan, J.P., 2003. Elevated environmental temperature and methamphetamine neurotoxicity. Environ. Res. 92, 48–53.

Misra, U.K., Kalita, J., 2009. Toxic neuropathies. Neurol. India 57, 697.

Moral, A.R., Çankayalı, İ., Sergin, D., BoyaCılar, Ö., 2015. Neuromuscular functions on experimental acute methanol intoxication. Turk. J. Anaesthesiol. Reanim. 43, 337–343.

Morgan, J.C., Sethi, K.D., 2005. Drug-induced tremors. Lancet Neurol. 4, 866–876.

Moriguchi, S., Watanabe, S., Kita, H., Nakanishi, H., 2002. Enhancement of N-methyl-D-aspartate receptor-mediated excitatory postsynaptic potentials in the neostriatum after methamphetamine sensitization. Exp. Brain Res. 144, 238–246.

Mukherjee, S., Era, N., Chatterjee, M., Mukherjee, M., 2022. Ethambutol-induced optic neuritis in a case of pulmonary tuberculosis. TNOA J. Ophthalmic Sci. Res. 60, 83.

Muniswamy, V.J., Raval, N., Gondaliya, P., Tambe, V., Kalia, K., Tekade, R.K., 2019. 'Dendrimer-Cationized-Albumin' encrusted polymeric nanoparticle improves BBB penetration and anticancer activity of doxorubicin. Int. J. Pharm. 555, 77–99.

Niimi, N., Yako, H., Tsukamoto, M., Takaku, S., Yamauchi, J., Kawakami, E., Yanagisawa, H., Watabe, K., Utsunomiya, K., Sango, K., 2016. Involvement of oxidative stress and impaired lysosomal degradation in amiodarone-induced schwannopathy. Eur. J. Neurosci. 44, 1723–1733.

Nutt, J.G., 2001. Motor fluctuations and dyskinesia in Parkinson's disease. Park. Relat. Disord. 8, 101–108.

Oberdörster, G., Elder, A., Rinderknecht, A., 2009. Nanoparticles and the brain: cause for concern? J. Nanosci. Nanotechnol. 9, 4996–5007.

Özmen, İ., NAZıroğlu, M., Alici, H.A., Sahin, F., Cengiz, M., Eren, I., 2007. Spinal morphine administration reduces the fatty acid contents in spinal cord and brain by increasing oxidative stress. Neurochem. Res. 32, 19–25.

Park, S.B., Lin, C.S., Krishnan, A.V., Goldstein, D., Friedlander, M.L., Kiernan, M.C., 2011. Dose effects of oxaliplatin on persistent and transient Na+ conductances and the development of neurotoxicity. PLoS One 6, e18469.

Park, S.K., Ha, J.S., Kim, J.M., Kang, J.Y., Lee, D.S., Guo, T.J., Lee, U., Kim, D.-O., Heo, H.J., 2016. Antiamnesic effect of broccoli (*Brassica oleracea* var. italica) leaves on amyloid beta (Aβ) 1–42-induced learning and memory impairment. J. Agric. Food Chem. 64, 3353–3361.

Paus, T., Keshavan, M., Giedd, J.N., 2008. Why do many psychiatric disorders emerge during adolescence? Nat. Rev. Neurosci. 9, 947–957.

Pereira, M.M.A., Mahú, I., Seixas, E., Martinéz-Sánchez, N., Kubasova, N., Pirzgalska, R.M., Cohen, P., Dietrich, M.O., López, M., Bernardes, G.J.L., Domingos, A.I., 2017. A brain-sparing diphtheria toxin for chemical genetic ablation of peripheral cell lineages. Nat. Commun. 8, 14967.

Pietrini, D., Piastra, M., Luca, E., Mancino, A., Conti, G., Cavaliere, F., DE Luca, D., 2012. Neuroprotection and hypothermia in infants and children. Curr. Drug Targets 13, 925–935.

Podratz, J.L., Knight, A.M., Ta, L.E., Staff, N.P., Gass, J.M., Genelin, K., Schlattau, A., Lathroum, L., Windebank, A.J., 2011. Cisplatin induced mitochondrial DNA damage in dorsal root ganglion neurons. Neurobiol. Dis. 41, 661–668.

Prajapati, R.N., Tekade, R.K., Gupta, U., Gajbhiye, V., Jain, N.K., 2009. Dendimer-mediated solubilization, formulation development and in vitro-in vivo assessment of piroxicam. Mol. Pharm. 6, 940–950.

Quasthoff, S., Hartung, H.P., 2002. Chemotherapy-induced peripheral neuropathy. J. Neurol. 249, 9–17.

Quello, S.B., Brady, K.T., Sonne, S.C., 2005. Mood disorders and substance use disorder: a complex comorbidity. Sci. Practice Perspect. 3, 13.

Romagnolo, A., Merola, A., Artusi, C.A., Rizzone, M.G., Zibetti, M., Lopiano, L., 2019. Levodopa-induced neuropathy: a systematic review. Mov. Disord. Clin. Pract. 6, 96–103.

Roos, W.P., Kaina, B., 2006. DNA damage-induced cell death by apoptosis. Trends Mol. Med. 12, 440–450.

Rubio, M., Villain, H., Docagne, F., Roussel, B.D., Ramos, J.A., Vivien, D., Fernandez-Ruiz, J., Ali, C., 2011. Pharmacological activation/inhibition of the cannabinoid system affects alcohol withdrawal-induced neuronal hypersensitivity to excitotoxic insults. PLoS One 6, e23690.

Ryan, N.M., Isbister, G.K., 2015. Tramadol overdose causes seizures and respiratory depression but serotonin toxicity appears unlikely. Clin. Toxicol. 53, 545–550.

Sarna, J.R., Brownell, A.K.W., Furtado, S., 2009. Reversible cerebellar syndrome caused by metronidazole. CMAJ (Can. Med. Assoc. J.) 181, 611–613.

Schwarcz, R., Scholz, D., Coyle, J., 1978. Structure-activity relations for the neurotoxicity of kainic acid derivatives and glutamate analogues. Neuropharmacology 17, 145–151.

Sekine, Y., Ouchi, Y., Sugihara, G., Takei, N., Yoshikawa, E., Nakamura, K., Iwata, Y., Tsuchiya, K.J., Suda, S., Suzuki, K., 2008. Methamphetamine causes microglial activation in the brains of human abusers. J. Neurosci. 28, 5756–5761.

Shadnia, S., Brent, J., Mousavi-Fatemi, K., Hafezi, P., Soltaninejad, K., 2012. Recurrent seizures in tramadol intoxication: implications for therapy based on 100 patients. Basic Clin. Pharmacol. Toxicol. 111, 133–136.

Shah, N., Patel, V., Donald, A., 1979. Effect of diazepam, desmethylimipramine, and SKF 525-A on the disposition of levo-methadone in mice after single or double injection. Drug Metabol. Dispos. 7, 241–242.

Sharma, H.S., Sjoquist, P.-O., Ali, S.F., 2007. Drugs of abuse-induced hyperthermia, blood-brain barrier dysfunction and neurotoxicity: neuroprotective effects of a new antioxidant compound H-290/51. Curr. Pharmaceut. Des. 13, 1903–1923.

Sharrett-Field, L., Butler, T.R., Reynolds, A.R., Berry, J.N., Prendergast, M.A., 2013. Sex differences in neuroadaptation to alcohol and withdrawal neurotoxicity. Pflueg. Arch. Eur. J. Physiol. 465, 643–654.

Sherrill, L.K., Berthold, C., Koss, W.A., Juraska, J.M., Gulley, J.M., 2011. Sex differences in the effects of ethanol pre-exposure during adolescence on ethanol-induced conditioned taste aversion in adult rats. Behav. Brain Res. 225, 104–109.

Shimizu, K., Matsubara, K., Ohtaki, K., Fujimaru, S., Saito, O., Shiono, H., 2003. Paraquat induces long-lasting dopamine overflow through the excitotoxic pathway in the striatum of freely moving rats. Brain Res. 976, 243–252.

Shin, H.W., Chung, S.J., 2012. Drug-induced parkinsonism. J. Clin. Neurol. 8, 15–21.

Snodgrass, S.R., 1992. Vitamin neurotoxicity. Mol. Neurobiol. 6, 41–73.

Stankovic, J.S.K., Selakovic, D., Mihailovic, V., Rosic, G., 2020. Antioxidant supplementation in the treatment of neurotoxicity induced by platinum-based chemotherapeutics—a review. Int. J. Mol. Sci. 21, 7753.

Sulzer, D., Sonders, M.S., Poulsen, N.W., Galli, A., 2005. Mechanisms of neurotransmitter release by amphetamines: a review. Prog. Neurobiol. 75, 406–433.

Tata, D.A., Yamamoto, B.K., 2008. Chronic stress enhances methamphetamine-induced extracellular glutamate and excitotoxicity in the rat striatum. Synapse 62, 325–336.

Tekade, R.K., Chougule, M.B., 2013. Formulation development and evaluation of hybrid nanocarrier for cancer therapy: taguchi orthogonal array based design. BioMed Res. Int. 2013, 712678.

Teleanu, D.M., Chircov, C., Grumezescu, A.M., Teleanu, R.I., 2019. Neurotoxicity of nanomaterials: an up-to-date overview. Nanomaterials 9, 96.

Thomas, D.M., Walker, P.D., Benjamins, J.A., Geddes, T.J., Kuhn, D.M., 2004. Methamphetamine neurotoxicity in dopamine nerve endings of the striatum is associated with microglial activation. J. Pharmacol. Exp. Therapeut. 311, 1–7.

Tomaszewski, A., Büsselberg, D., 2007. Cisplatin modulates voltage gated channel currents of dorsal root ganglion neurons of rats. Neurotoxicology 28, 49–58.

Tong, X., Han, X., Yu, B., Yu, M., Jiang, G., Ji, J., Dong, S., 2015. Role of gap junction intercellular communication in testicular leydig cell apoptosis induced by oxaliplatin via the mitochondrial pathway. Oncol. Rep. 33, 207–214.

Tramullas, M., Martínez-Cué, C., Hurlé, M.A., 2008. Chronic administration of heroin to mice produces up-regulation of brain apoptosis-related proteins and impairs spatial learning and memory. Neuropharmacology 54, 640–652.

Valdiglesias, V., Kiliç, G., Costa, C., Fernández-Bertólez, N., Pásaro, E., Teixeira, J.P., Laffon, B., 2015. Effects of iron oxide nanoparticles: cytotoxicity, genotoxicity, developmental toxicity, and neurotoxicity. Environ. Mol. Mutagen. 56, 125–148.

van Harten, P.N., Hoek, H.W., Kahn, R.S., 1999. Acute dystonia induced by drug treatment. Br. Med. J. 319, 623–626.

Veltkamp, R., Gill, D., 2016. Clinical trials of immunomodulation in ischemic stroke. Neurotherapeutics 13, 791–800.

Wang, W.-W., Zhang, Y., Huang, X.-B., You, N., Zheng, L., Li, J., 2017. Fecal microbiota transplantation prevents hepatic encephalopathy in rats with carbon tetrachloride-induced acute hepatic dysfunction. World J. Gastroenterol. 23, 6983.

Warren, M.W., Larner, S.F., Kobeissy, F.H., Brezing, C.A., Jeung, J.A., Hayes, R.L., Gold, M.S., Wang, K.K., 2007. Calpain and caspase proteolytic markers co-localize with rat cortical neurons after exposure to methamphetamine and MDMA. Acta Neuropathol. 114, 277–286.

Williams, J.M., Steketee, J.D., 2004. Cocaine increases medial prefrontal cortical glutamate overflow in cocaine-sensitized rats: a time course study. Eur. J. Neurosci. 20, 1639–1646.

Win-Shwe, T.-T., Fujimaki, H., 2011. Nanoparticles and neurotoxicity. Int. J. Mol. Sci. 12, 6267–6280.

Wisessmith, W., Phansuwan-Pujito, P., Govitrapong, P., Chetsawang, B., 2009. Melatonin reduces induction of Bax, caspase and cell death in methamphetamine-treated human neuroblastoma SH-SY5Y cultured cells. J. Pineal Res. 46, 433–440.

Wu, S.-N., Chen, B.-S., Wu, Y.-H., Peng, H., Chen, L.-T., 2009. The mechanism of the actions of oxaliplatin on ion currents and action potentials in differentiated NG108-15 neuronal cells. Neurotoxicology 30, 677–685.

Xu, L., Shao, A., Zhao, Y., Wang, Z., Zhang, C., Sun, Y., Deng, J., Chou, L.L., 2015. Neurotoxicity of silver nanoparticles in rat brain after intragastric exposure. J. Nanosci. Nanotechnol. 15, 4215–4223.

Yin, Y., Qi, X., Qiao, Y., Liu, H., Yan, Z., Li, H., Liu, Z., 2019. The association of neuronal stress with activating transcription factor 3 in dorsal root ganglion of in vivo and in vitro models of bortezomib-induced neuropathy. Curr. Cancer Drug Targets 19, 50–64.

Youngren, S.R., Tekade, R.K., Gustilo, B., Hoffmann, P.R., Chougule, M.B., 2013. STAT6 siRNA matrix-loaded gelatin nanocarriers: formulation, characterization, and ex vivo proof of concept using adenocarcinoma cells. BioMed Res. Int. 2013, 858946.

Yuan, Z.-Y., Hu, Y.-L., Gao, J.-Q., 2015. Brain localization and neurotoxicity evaluation of polysorbate 80-modified chitosan nanoparticles in rats. PLoS One 10, e0134722.

Zaoui, A., Abdelghani, A., BEN Salem, H., Quanta, W., Hayoum, A., Khachnaoui, N., Rejeb, N., Benzartr, M., 2012. Early-onset severe isoniazid-induced motor-dominant neuropathy: a case report. East. Mediterr. Health J. 18 (3), 298–299.

Zhang, J., Graham, D.G., Montine, T.J., Ho, Y.-S., 2000. Enhanced N-methyl-4-phenyl-1, 2, 3, 6-tetrahydropyridine toxicity in mice deficient in CuZn-superoxide dismutase or glutathione peroxidase. J. Neuropathol. Exp. Neurol. 59, 53–61.

Zhang, M., Wang, H., Zhao, J., Chen, C., Leak, R.K., Xu, Y., Vosler, P., Chen, J., Gao, Y., Zhang, F., 2013. Drug-induced hypothermia in stroke models: does it always protect? CNS Neurol. Disord. Drug Targets 12, 371–380.

Zhou, K.Q., Mcdouall, A., Drury, P.P., Lear, C.A., Cho, K.H., Bennet, L., Gunn, A.J., Davidson, J.O., 2021. Treating seizures after hypoxic-ischemic encephalopathy—current controversies and future directions. Int. J. Mol. Sci. 22, 7121.

Zhou, M., Xie, L., Fang, C.-J., Yang, H., Wang, Y.-J., Zhen, X.-Y., Yan, C.-H., Wang, Y., Zhao, M., Peng, S., 2016. Implications for blood-brain-barrier permeability, in vitro oxidative stress and neurotoxicity potential induced by mesoporous silica nanoparticles: effects of surface modification. RSC Adv. 6, 2800–2809.

CHAPTER

14

Thermal processing and food-related toxicants

Bhakti Pawar[1], *Sneha A. Dhamne*[2], *Prashant L. Pingale*[2], *Anjani Sheth*[1], *Muktika Tekade*[3], *Randa SH. Mansour*[4] and *Rakesh Kumar Tekade*[1]

[1]National Institute of Pharmaceutical Education and Research (NIPER)- Ahmedabad, An Institute of National Importance, Government of India, Department of Pharmaceuticals, Ministry of Chemicals and Fertilizers, Palaj, Gandhinagar, Gujarat, India; [2]Department of Pharmaceutics, GES's Sir Dr. M. S. Gosavi College of Pharmaceutical Education and Research, Nashik, Maharashtra, India; [3]School of Pharmacy, Devi Ahilya Vishwavidyalaya, Indore, Madhya Pradesh, India; [4]Faculty of Pharmacy, Philadelphia University, Amman, Jordan

14.1 Introduction

In day-to-day life, home cooking techniques have produced a wide range of distinct ways to use heat treatment to produce particular food qualities. Thermal processing of food is practiced for improving the organoleptic properties, imparting antimicrobial effect to preserve the food, in addition to improving food quality and consumer compliance. Such processing changes the physical and chemical structure of nutrients present in the food. It induces the generation of new chemical molecules, which can be beneficial as antioxidating agents and immunomodulators.

On the other hand, there has been evidence of the formation of certain chemical intermediates which result in a threat to human health as they can be mutagenic and carcinogenic byproducts, for example, heterocyclic aromatic amines, chloropropanols, polycyclic hydrocarbons, and 5-hydroxyfurfural that have been reported to be carcinogenic (Mogol and Gökmen, 2016; Jägerstad and Skog, 2005). These byproducts interact with the DNA and form the DNA adducts. These DNA adducts are responsible for showing DNA mutations that further lead to cancer (Jägerstad and Skog, 2005).

Essentials of Pharmatoxicology in Drug Research, Volume 1
https://doi.org/10.1016/B978-0-443-15840-7.00022-1

The International Agency for Research on Cancer (IARC) consistently evaluated the genotoxicity and carcinogenicity of these toxicants generated in the thermal processing of food. It focused primarily on high-dose, long-term animal studies as well as in vitro and in vivo genotoxicity tests has determined the number of these toxicants possibly (2A) or presumably (2B) carcinogenic to humans (Verma and Yadav, 2020).

Frying, dry heat, and moist heat preparation methods are usually involved in thermal food processing. Frying involves simultaneous heat and mass transfer mechanisms to impart specific sensory characteristics to the food. The special case with the frying of food is in the presence of oxygen and moisture. The oil undergoes harmful reactions, precisely due to the presence of water causing hydrolysis of oil. The presence of oxygen and high temperature causes oxidation and thermal alterations in the food (Dasa and Abera, 2019).

Similarly, dry and moist heat food preparation methods are widely used to preserve food items. The dry heat method, in which the food is exposed to a high temperature ranging from 150 to 250°C, includes baking, roasting, and grilling. Moist heat method includes steaming, boiling, and blanching, where food is exposed to a temperature ranging from 65 to 100°C (Ramesh, 2003). Additionally, modern methods like microwave irradiations generate toxic compounds such as polycyclic aromatic amines, acrylamide, heterocyclic aromatic amines, chloropropanols, etc. (Koszucka and Nowak, 2019).

Various food-related changes caused by thermal processing technologies are highlighted in this chapter. The formation of different toxicants during thermal heating, the hazards associated with them, and techniques to analyze them are comprehensively discussed. In addition, possible ways to minimize the formation of these toxicants are mentioned.

14.2 Thermal processing technologies

14.2.1 Enzyme inactivation

Enzyme inactivation is one of the significant factors to be considered during food storage. Widely used thermal processing technology for enzyme inactivation involves various events such as breaking into subunits, aggregation, or structural changes and usually results in the deterioration of nutritional components.

Enzyme inactivation can be understood from its fundamental aspects, including kinetics, mathematical modeling, and the effect of enzyme activity on the quality of food stuff. The kinetics involved with enzyme inactivation can be defined by measuring enzyme activity based on enzyme reaction under particular conditions, whereas mathematical modeling in thermally treated food studies the residual activity of enzymes related to quality based on time versus temperature profile and enzyme inactivation kinetics. The time versus temperature profile data is examined with activation energy to determine the inactivation process at a reference temperature. This will lead to the determination of the amount of residual enzyme activity related to the process that is being modeled (Adams, 1991).

Heat-treated enzyme inactivation is favored mainly in dairy industries, where enzyme activation causes deleterious and harmful effects. Deeth and coworkers has reviewed the thermal stability of many enzymes in milk and dairy products. Hexose isomerase and lipoprotein lipase were found to be inactivated or almost inactivated at temperatures ranging from about 55 to 90°C. In contrast, plasmin and cathepsin D required high-temperature exposure above 90°C to get inactivated (Deeth, 2021).

14.2.2 Microbial destruction

Microbial contamination leads to substantial economic loss as well as food-borne diseases. Thermal processing is lethal for microorganisms and thus employed for food preservation. Conventional thermal methods to reduce the microbial load in food are based on heat convection. Heat exposure is based on the type of food as a solid long time of heat exposure is required to ensure sterilization and extend shelf life. For viscous liquid food, long-term heat exposure can lead to overprocessing and loss of quality. To overcome this issue, alternative processing technologies have been proposed, one of which is Ohmic heating. In Ohmic heating, heat is directly produced within the food when an electric current passes through it, and the energy generated causes an increase in temperature (Tian et al., 2018).

For food preservation, two temperature categories are generally used: pasteurization and sterilization. In pasteurization, food is treated with mild heat, usually below 100°C. The required heat intensity is determined by the D value, which represents the time to reduce 90% of the initial microbial count. Alkaline phosphatase, an enzyme present in raw milk, has a D value similar to that of heat-resistant pathogens; therefore, it can be used as an indicator to evaluate the effectiveness of pasteurization (Chiozzi et al., 2022).

Nowadays, sterilization is another food preservation technique used. It can be thermal or nonthermal. The former being most commonly employed. Different sterilization temperatures are used per the requirement within the range 135–302°F, as shown in Table 14.1. However, thermal sterilization causes loss of nutrients and spoilage of food qualities, and also, sometimes, it is ineffective against certain bacteria (Sevenich et al., 2013).

14.2.3 Chemical changes in protein

Chemical changes in proteins due to thermal processing are one of the major factors for the loss of nutritional value in overcooked food. Such chemical changes include precipitation, aggregation, or gelation. One of the most critical processes that occur during the preparation and preservation of food is browning. Depending upon the type of food, both enzymatic

TABLE 14.1 Temperature and heat exposure time for sterilization.

Temperature (°F)	Time
135	45 min
145	30 min (low-temperature long-time method)
162	15 s (high-temperature short-time method)
280–302	1–2 s (ultra-high temperature (UHT))

and nonenzymatic browning can have a favorable or detrimental effect on food quality (Tessier, 2021). Enzymatic browning involves the conversion of phenolic compounds into quinones with the help of phenolic oxidase. Different seafood, fish, and vegetables are prone to this reaction.

On the other hand, nonenzymatic browning is known as the Maillard reaction. It occurs between the amino group from amino acids, proteins, or peptides and the carbonyl group from reducing sugars, giving an undesired aroma (Liu et al., 2022). Food browning can also be seen in the case of caramelization which is the product of the degradation of carbohydrates (Nath et al., 2022). The thermal processing of protein-containing food causes disturbance in the stability of the product, thereby losing nutritional value.

14.2.3.1 Precipitation, aggregation, and gelation

Thermal processing may alter the functional properties of food due to changes in protein structure and altered spatial organization, which may result in precipitation, aggregation, gelation, and degradation of proteins (López-Pedrouso et al., 2019).

At higher temperatures, proteins have the property to form aggregation, which is considered a reversible cellular response. Protein aggregation is observed during food processing, including mixing, refining, and storage. Aggregation depends on factors such as protein structure or processing and storage conditions. Temperature change is considered to be the extrinsic factor. An increase in temperature may lead to an increase in hydrophobic interaction and a decrease in activation energy, resulting in a more molecular collision and accelerated formation of aggregates (Wang et al., 2010). The thermal stability of the Pea Protein Isolate was examined under different conditions by Bogahawaththa et al. (2019). Insoluble protein aggregates were observed to form by noncovalent interactions when exposed to 140°C for 4 s and when subjected to 121°C for 2.8 min, whereas soluble aggregates were formed due to covalent interactions. Heat-induced aggregation of hen egg white protein (EWP) in the presence of different inorganic salts was studied by Iwashita et al. (2015). NaSCN was observed to form protein aggregates with an increase in temperature. Also, the temperature for aggregation reduced as the concentration of EWP increased, whereas Na_2SO_4 did not alter the aggregation temperature.

The aggregation process resulting from protein-protein interaction in which one of the protein structures gets altered can be responsible for irreversible gelation. Most of the proteins that result in gelation are present in whey proteins, plant globulins, and egg white proteins, which commonly consist of globular proteins. Irreversible aggregation occurs for globular proteins denatured in aqueous media, exposing the amino acids located in the interior part of the protein. These amino acids then become available to form a bond with other proteins (Nicolai, 2019).

14.2.3.2 Maillard reaction

Maillard reaction (MR) was first discovered by Louis C. Maillard in 1912. It is commonly known as a nonenzymatic browning reaction resulting from the interaction between carbonyl compounds, which may include reducing sugars with compounds having a free amino

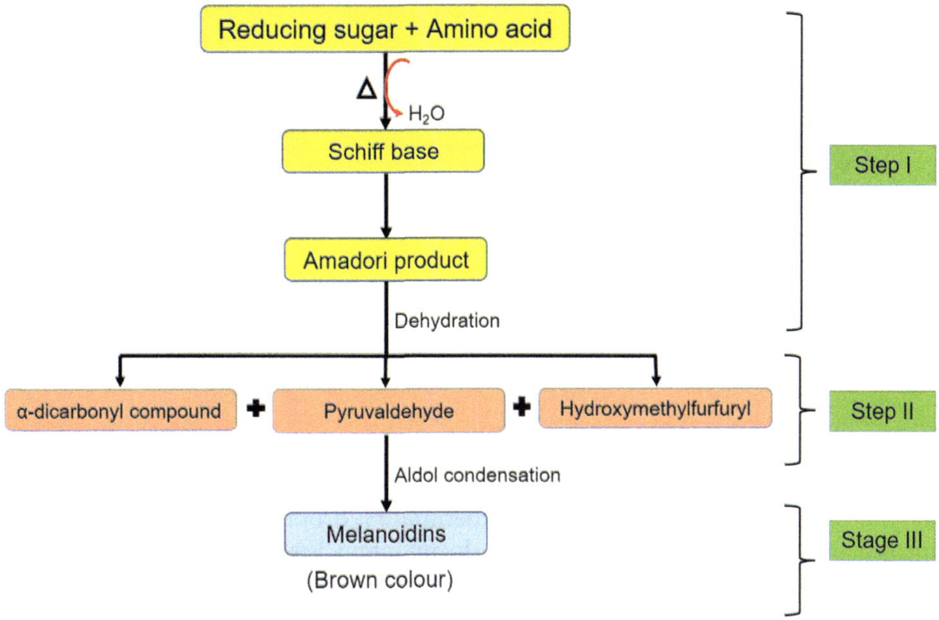

FIGURE 14.1 Simplified diagram of milliard reaction.

group. Maillard reaction is not only responsible for nutritional damage but also the development of aroma and color in the thermal processing of food (Tamanna and Mahmood, 2015).

MR comprises three stages: (i) initial, (ii) intermediate, and (iii) final. The early phase of the reaction leads to the formation of early glycation Amadori adduct. In the intermediate stage, the further reaction of the Amadori adduct leads to the formation of hydroxy methyl furfural, pyruvaldehyde, and α-dicarbonyl compounds. These compounds are called Milliard Reaction Products (MRPS) and are yellow or colorless with strong UV absorption. In the final stage, melanoidins are produced, having brown color, and are responsible for the aroma and flavor (ALjahdali and Carbonero, 2019) (Fig. 14.1).

Various experiments have been studied by scientists to reduce and inhibit the Maillard reaction. Zhang et al. (2018) have studied the inhibition of MR by replacement of the monosaccharide. Galactose is very reactive during MR; therefore, monosaccharides are replaced by β-galactosidase, which inhibits the release of galactose and converts lactose to galacto-oligosaccharides. Galacto-oligosaccharides were observed to react less in MR (Liu et al., 2018). The formation of red color was observed in spray-dried powder of whey protein isolate and ascorbic acid due to the occurrence of MR. Storage conditions were found to have a major impact on MR. At 20°C, the reaction rate was observed to occur fast in the spray-dried powders (Zhong et al., 2019). Researchers have summarized the targeting of various reactive intermediates and products to reduce MR. One such target is the modification of reducing sugars by the fermentation process, leading to their conversion to nonreducing sugar. This results in the prevention of browning (Lund and Ray, 2017).

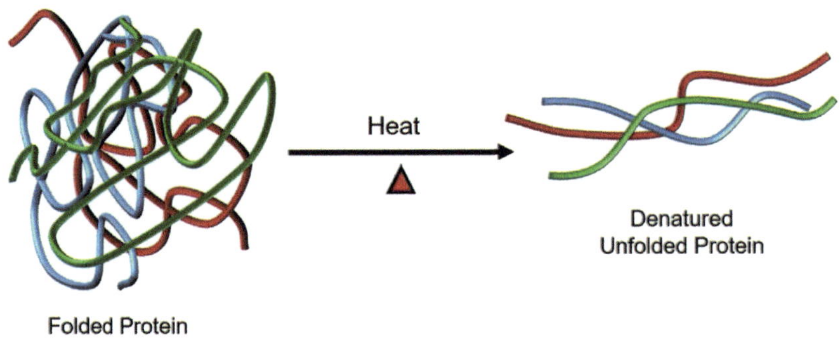

FIGURE 14.2 Illustration of protein denaturation due to heat.

14.2.3.3 *Protein denaturation by heat*

Heat causes protein denaturation (Fig. 14.2) due to the unfolding of quaternary, tertiary, or secondary structures as a response to hyperthermia. Hydrophobic interactions are responsible for the stability of protein as it allows to maintain less surface area of protein and decrease undesired interactions with the polar environment. Denaturation may cause breakage of hydrogen-disulfide bonding and hydrophobic interactions, damaging protein structure.

Denaturation temperatures of the different proteins studied by the researchers in the animal-derived milk products, such as bovine serum albumin, α-lactalbumin, β-lactoglobulin, are mentioned in Table 14.2.

Different proteins have different noncovalent bonds; therefore, they react differently to thermal exposure, and each protein reacts differently to the same type of food components in the food system. Possible alterations of amino acids found in cooked meat involve conversion to protein carbonylation and changes in the structures of aromatic residues. Meat protein components such as myofibrillar, sarcoplasmic, and stromal have a heat capacity ranging from 20 to 90°C (Yu et al., 2017). Sergius-Sergius-Ronot et al. conducted studies comparing protein denaturation in human milk protein concentrate occurring through high temperature and high pressure. It was concluded that thermal treatment induced more protein denaturation comparatively and the aggregates obtained mainly consisted of lactoferrin and α-lactalbumin (Sergius-Ronot et al., 2022).

TABLE 14.2 Denaturation temperatures of some proteins found in animal-derived milk products.

Protein	Denaturation temperature (°C)	Investigators
Bovine serum albumin	64	Ameseder et al. (2018)
α-lactalbumin	62	Lam and Nickerson (2015)
β-lactoglobulin	80	Roefs and De Kruif (1994)

14.3 Toxicant formation in food

The generation of some of the chemical substances in cooking has long been suspected of posing a health danger to humans. Advancements in technology and the use of different commercial and home cooking practices have resulted in various diverse methods for using heat decomposition to obtain particular food attributes, including pleasant odors, pigments, and flavors of active substances, improved nutritional quality, increased shelf life, the release of bioactive components, and increased digestibility and bioavailability of nutrients. The latter effect results from altering the physiochemical content of crucial nutrients, such as carbohydrates and proteins. Unfortunately, heat treatment possibly produces carcinogenicity and mutagenicity in products as it stimulates oxidation reactions in proteins and lipids by boosting free radical formation while diminishing the protection of dietary antioxidants.

Heterocyclic aromatic amines, N-nitroso compounds, acrylamide, polycyclic aromatic hydrocarbons, 5-Hydroxymethyl furfural, acrolein, chloropropanols, chloroesters, and dietary furan are some of the toxicants produced in food products as a result of thermal processing. The formation of these chemical compounds is responsible for the aroma produced and the color developed after thermal processing. To reduce these toxicants, it is necessary to have a brief understanding of the mechanism of the generation of these toxicants in processed food. Heat-induced dietary toxins that arise through the normal thermal activity of foods are given next (Koszucka and Nowak, 2019).

14.3.1 Heterocyclic aromatic amines (HAA)

The formation of hazardous chemicals such as HAAs is an unintended adverse outcome of thermal food processing (Zamora and Hidalgo, 2020). HAAs are toxic chemicals that occur when protein-rich foods, like meat and fish, are cooked for a long time. Several studies have found that the high temperature of various cooking operations, such as roasting, grilling, barbecuing, frying, and smoking, adds to the development of HAAs when meat-based items are cooked (Barzegar et al., 2019).

HAAs are categorized into two groups according to their formation: (i) thermic and (ii) pyrolytic. Thermic HAAs are produced in the temperature range of 100 to 300°C. They are further differentiated into two subgroups based on their structure, imidazoquinolones, and imidazoquinoxalines. Pyrolytic HAAs are formed at temperatures above 300°C (Barzegar et al., 2019). Various factors, such as the cooking process, pH, lipid content, free amino acids, etc., affect the formation of HAAs. They are absorbed in the small intestine, after which it is transported to the liver and then to other organs, where they are metabolized. The metabolic activation begins with N-oxidation by cytochrome enzymes, followed by acetylation producing N-acetoxyamine as the final product. It has been proven to cause DNA damage and mutations (Barzegar et al., 2019). International Agency for Research on Cancer (IARC) has classified HAAs as possible human carcinogens (Group 2B) and probable human carcinogens (Group 2A) (Table 14.3).

14.3.1.1 HAA formation in proteinaceous food

In proteinaceous foods, about 25 HAAs have been discovered. They are divided into two groups: carbolines (pyrolytic HAAs) and aminoimidazoazaarenes.

14.3.1.1.1 Pyrolytic HAAs formation

Pyrolytic HAAs are generated at high temperatures (more than 250°C) and are classified into one of five classes based on their structures: pyridoindoles (harman, nor Harman, AαC, MeAαC, Trp-P-1, Trp-P-2), pyridoimidazoles (Glu-P-1, Glu-P-2), phenylpyridines (Phe-P-1), tetraazofluoranthenes (Orn-P-1), or benzimidazoles (Cre-P-1). They are made up of precursors of amino acids such as tryptophan, phenylalanine, glutamic acid, or ornithine, as well as casein and soybean globulin from pyrolysis. Deaminated and decarboxylated complexes, along with reactive radicals, are produced at high temperatures. The pyrolytic HAAs are formed when these various chemicals react together (Wang et al., 2021b).

14.3.1.1.2 Amino imidazoazaarenes formation

At normal cooking temperatures (150–200°C), the aminoimidazoazaarenes are produced through the Maillard reaction. The Skeleton of HAA is produced by Strecker breakdown molecules through the Maillard reaction between amino acid and hexose, and it can be made from various precursors. Depending on the core structure of the intermediates generated during this phase, specific HAAs will result pyrazines, quinoxalines, and pyrido imidazoles. During the process, creatinine is used to synthesize the imidazole moiety (Meurillon and Engel, 2016).

14.3.2 N-nitroso compounds (N–NA)

N-nitroso (N–NA) compounds are one of the major toxic chemical substances that are proved to be carcinogenic. These compounds may even lead to various diseases, including

TABLE 14.3 Structures of various HAAs, their carcinogen activity, and classification according to IARC.

Structure	Chemical name	Carcinogen activity
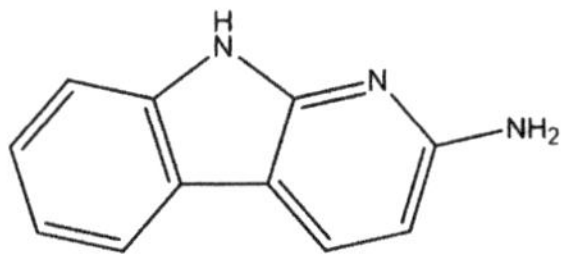	2-Amino-9H-pyrido[2,3-b] indole	Group 2B
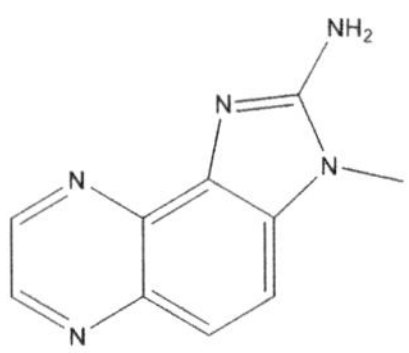	2-Amino-3-methylimidazo[4,5-*f*] quinoxaline	Group 2A
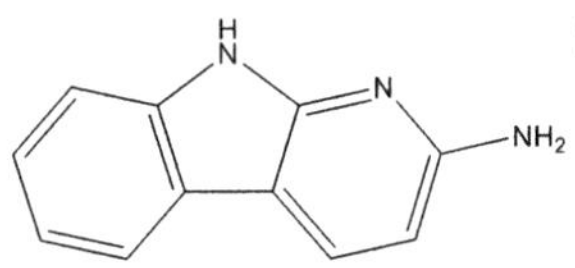	2-Amino-9H-pyrido[2,3-b] indole	Group 2B

TABLE 14.3 Structures of various HAAs, their carcinogen activity, and classification according to IARC.—cont'd

Structure	Chemical name	Carcinogen activity
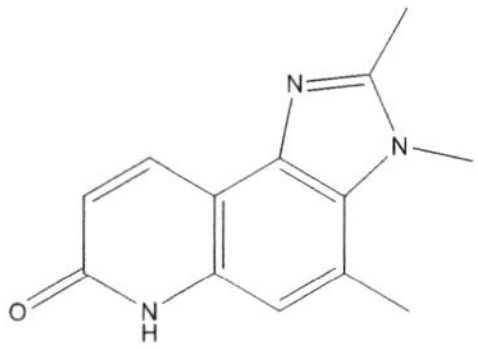	2-Amino-3,4-dimethylimidazo[4,5-f] quinolone	Group 2B
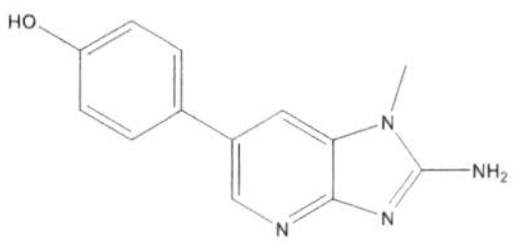	2-Amino-1-methyl-6-(4'hydroxyphenyl)-imidazo[4,5-b] pyridine	Group 2B
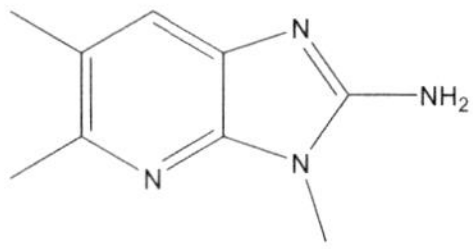	2-Amino-3,5,6-trimethylimidazo[4,5-b] pyridine	Group 2B
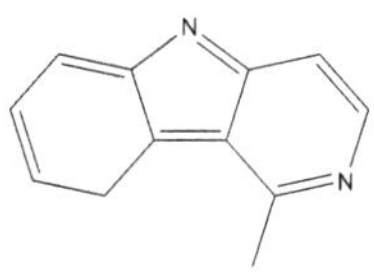	1-Methyl-9H-pyrido[4,3-b] indole	Group 2B

colorectal, gastric, hepatocellular, and esophageal cancer (Zheng et al., 2021; Lee et al., 2006). According to animal research, N−NA compounds have been shown to cause cancer in various organs, including the pancreas. N−NA compounds are divided into two sets: N-nitrosamides and N-nitrosamines. N-nitrosodimethyl amine (NDMA) and N-nitrosodiethyl amine (NDEA), two of hundreds studied, are the most common chemicals in foods (Zheng et al., 2019) and are carcinogenic to the liver (Zheng et al., 2019), and were classed as possible human carcinogens (Zheng et al., 2019). In a study by Nowak et al. (2014), considerable evidence has been collected regarding the generation of the carcinogenic process by a particular group of carcinogens, such as methyl benzyl nitrosamine, which is linked to the metabolic conversion of these carcinogens to mutagenic metabolites and its binding to DNA. In a study carried out by García et al. (2008), it was observed that in the HL-60 human leukemia cell line, N-nitrosopiperadine and N-nitrosodibutyl amine caused apoptotic cell death, which was characterized by several parameters.

Thermal processing of food is considered the primary source of these compounds. The heating of food products such as cured meat, sea fish, and even drinking water above 130°C leads to their formation. The formation of nitrosamine has been authenticated by the formation of nitrosating reagents by nitrites or nitrogen oxide with the compounds naturally containing nitrogen while undergoing a nitrosation reaction (Yurchenko and Mölder, 2005).

For example, nitrites react with secondary amines to create (N—NA) in meat. Due to this, nitrites and nitrates are being used precisely in a controlled way in meat-based thermal food processing industries. The European Commission has set a limit of 150 ppm for nitrite in meat products (van Breda et al., 2021). (N—NA) are being classified by International Agency for Research on Cancer (IARC) based on various studies in which NDBA, NPYR, NMOR, and NPIP are classified in Group 2B (possibly carcinogenic to human beings) while NDMA and NDEA are classified in to Group 2A (probably carcinogenic to human beings) (Table 14.4).

The consumption of compounds containing nitrosamine as a chemical plays a significant role in enhancing nitrosamine-based cancer. Dietary intake of nitrite and amines react together and result in the formation of various nitrosamines in the GIT. Consumption of tobacco that contains nicotine as a major compound leads to breast cancer by causing DNA mutations (Gankhuyag et al., 2017).

TABLE 14.4 Various nitrosamines classified according to IARC.

Structure	Chemical name	IARC classification
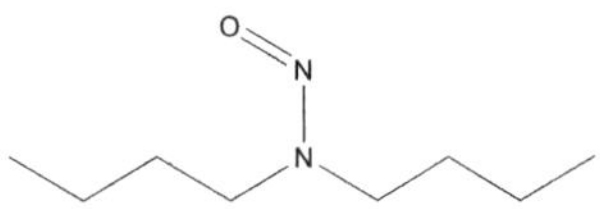	NDBA, N-nitrosodibutyl amine	Group 2B
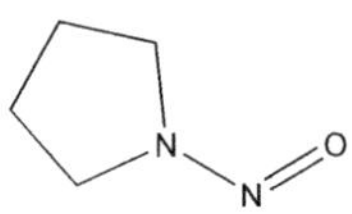	NPYR, N-nitroso pyrrolidine	Group 2B
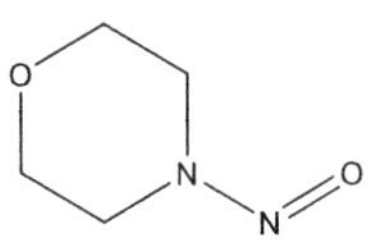	NMOR, N-nitrosomorpholine	Group 2B
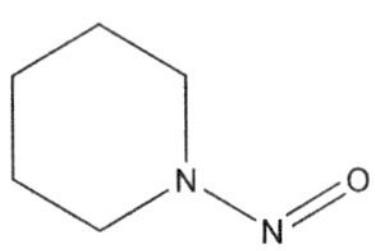	NPIP, N-nitrosopiperidine	Group 2B
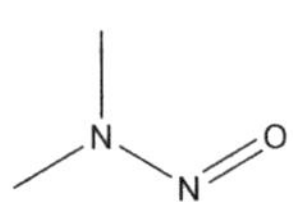	NDMA, N-nitrosodimethylamine	Group 2A
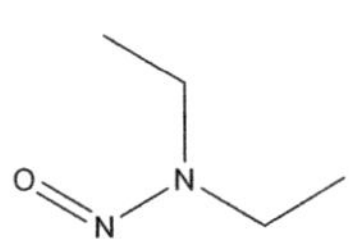	NDEA, N-nitrosodiethylamine	Group 2A

14.3.3 Acrylamide (AA)

Acrylamide is a low molecular weight (71.08 kDa) compound with a functional group of unsaturated amides. It is a commonly used monomer to synthesize polyacrylamides which are generally used in electrophoresis and as a constituent in products like paper, textiles, cosmetics, etc. Despite having many applications, acrylamide concentrations above minimum safety levels are found to be causing hepatotoxicity, neurotoxicity, and also it has potential genotoxic nature. It has been found that acrylamide occurs as an intermediate product of the Maillard reaction in heat-processed food products; this process is known as browning (Zamani et al., 2017).

The formation of AA in food has two main pathways that are widely studied: the N-glycoside (Strecker pathway) and the Acrolein pathway.

According to the Strecker pathway, heat treatment of food rich in proteins and carbohydrates containing asparagine at a temperature >120°C leads to synthesizing Schiff base. The base can be decarboxylated to azomethine ylide or converted into Amadori compounds. AA may be manufactured after azomethine ylide, by b-elimination of a decarboxylated Amadori molecule, and by hydrolysis of the ylide trailed by 3-amino propionamide's (3-APA) deamination. On the other hand, according to the Acrolein pathway, the decomposition of lipids and dehydration of glycerol produces acrolein and acrylic acids, which are combined with ammonia obtained after the breakdown of asparagine and different amino acids to produce acrylamide. Acrylamide formation is affected by different parameters, together with the amount of precursor, temperature, time, heat treatment, and pH (Khorshidian et al., 2020).

AA is quickly circulated and absorbed all over the body following oral consumption. It is usually excreted in the urine within 24 h. AA undergoes enzymatic modifications. It is oxidized to glycinamide (2,3-epoxy propionamide; GA) at cytochrome P450 2E1 (CYP2E1), which is considered an activation pathway. Both AA and GA have the potential to attach proteins, hemoglobin, DNA, and blood plasma albumins (Duda-Chodak et al., 2016).

Due to its genotoxic effect, AA can induce neurotoxicity by disrupting microtubules in the central and peripheral nervous systems (El-Assouli, 2009). AA is also observed to cause gene mutation and DNA damage over an extended duration of exposure. It has also been found to form covalent adducts with protaminase in the germ cells of mice. Therefore, acrylamide has been classified under Group 2A (probable human carcinogen) by The International Agency for Research on Cancer (IARC). "Acrylamide Toolbox" is a compilation of scientific publications which includes information about the guidelines intended to reduce the formation of acrylamide specifically for industrial food application (Confederation of the Food and Drink Industry of the EU, 2011).

14.3.4 Polycyclic aromatic hydrocarbons (PAHs)

Polycyclic aromatic hydrocarbon (PAH) is a chemical compound containing multiple fused aromatic rings having only carbon and hydrogen. A few such compounds include naphthalene (having two aromatic rings), phenanthrene, and anthracene (three-ring compounds). PAHs with up to six aromatic rings are considered "small PAHs," and fusion of more than six aromatic rings is considered "large PAHs." Most PAHs tend to dissolve in water weakly and can be readily photo-oxidized. PAHs are produced when the combustion of some organic substances, gas, tobacco, and oil is incomplete, and food constituents are processed above 120°C. Its mechanism involves the condensation of certain organic compounds by pyro synthesis. According to European Food Safety Authority (EFSA), they are considered ubiquitous pollutants and food contaminants. Various PAHs tend to be produced by themselves and are already observed in plants.

The solubility of PAHs reduces as their molecular weight increases and their toxicity rises. US Environmental Protection Agency has recognized 16 PAHs as contaminants, counting (NAP) Naphthalene, (ACE) Acenaphthene, (ACY) Acenaphthylene, (FLO) Fluorene, (PHE) Phenanthrene, (ANT) Anthracene, (FLA) Fluoranthene, (PYR) Pyrene, (BaA) Benza(α)anthracene, (CHR) Chrysene, (BbF) Benzo(b)fluoranthene, (BkF) Benzo (k) fluoranthene, (BaP) Benzo(α)pyrene, (IcdP) Indeno(1,2,3-cd) pyrene, (DahA) Ibenz (α, h) anthracene, and (BghiP) Benzo(g,h,i)perylene (Zhang and Chen, 2017). PAH exposure has been associated with oxidative stress, diabetes, inflammation, infertility, cardiovascular disease, poor fetal development, reproductive disorders (Bolden et al., 2017), irritation of the skin and eye, nausea and vomiting, and inflammation are temporary health impacts, while stable health condition contains different malignancies, protein and DNA damage, and gene mutation. Although unmetabolized PAHs are poisonous, their reactive metabolites can bind to cellular DNA and proteins, which is a big issue that results in mutations, developmental abnormalities, tumors, and cancer (Gao et al., 2018).

The binding of epoxides and dihydrodiols to DNA is one of the significant concerns related to PAHs as it results in biochemical disruptions and mutations resulting in cancer (Ledesma et al., 2015).In studies conducted by (Daniel et al., 2011), through histological studies, it can be observed that consuming heat-processed meat increased the risk of renal cell carcinoma. Alterations in reproduction and cellular functions have been caused due to benzo[a]pyrene (Essumang et al., 2013). In an investigation carried out by (Alomirah et al., 2011), the presence of high proportions of PAHs, including the highest level of phenanthrene, was found in smoked food, which is the primary cause of genotoxicity. High levels of PAHs were found in whole grilled chicken, grilled vegetables, and shish tauk, which are the primary dietary intake leading to increased PAH levels in children and adolescents. It was also reported that exposure to PAHs increases cancer risk by 3.1×10^{-5} times worldwide (Shen et al., 2014).

14.3.5 5-Hydroxymethyl furfural (HMF)

5-Hydroxymethyl furfural ($C_6H_6O_3$) is an organic compound with a low melting point (30–34°C) and a common intermediate product of over-heated food products. HMF is produced due to the dehydration of hexose sugars in an acidic environment, and this process is termed caramelization. The most common way of HMF production is by directly heating foodstuff above 150°C, and also it can result from the Maillard reaction, which contributes to desired color and aroma. 3-deoxyosone is the primary, intermediate product formed by 1,2 enolization of glucose and fructose, which on further dehydration and cyclization forms 5-hydroxymethyl furfural.

5-HMF can also be formed when sugars are subjected to acidic environments during heat processing. The fructofuranosyl cation is formed by acid-catalyzed fructose breakdown, and then mainly in dry conditions, a positively charged ion can be transformed to 5-HMF.

Additionally, by 1, 2-enolization, and dehydration, reducing sugars can generate 3-DG, which can then be dehydrated and cyclized to yield 5-HMF (Lee et al., 2019).

HMF is commonly found in bakery products, malt, vinegar, and coffee in about 2–1900 mg/kg range and in milk products such as milk powder, infant formulas, and milk-based baby food ranging up to 3 mg/kg. A high level of 5-HMF has also been found in fruit juices, bread toast, breakfast cereals, honey, and red wine (Capuano and Fogliano, 2011).

In a study performed on the Caco2 cell line by Delgado-Andrade et al. (2008), it was found that the absorption and transport of HMF depend on its concentration. As the concentration increases, its absorption and transport also increase, but a few factors may alter its absorption, like the presence of fibers in the diet alters HMF uptake. Furthermore, it has been reported that bacterial strains present in small intestines convert HMF to furfuryl alcohol.

The metabolism pathway of HMF comprises the formation of 5-hydroxymethyl 2-furanoic acid (HMFA) and its composite with glycine resulting in N-(5-hydroxymethyl-2-furoyl glycine) (HMFG). HMF in elevated concentration causes severe toxicities such as eye irritation, respiratory tract damage, and skin disorders. There has been evidence that the conversion of HMF to 5-Sulfoxymethylfurfural (5-SMF) is mutagenic as well as genotoxic. Studies comprising ^{14}C labeled HMF administered in rodents observed it absorbed and rapidly excreted in urine or metabolized (Lee et al., 2019). Sufficient evidence is still not obtained about HMF being carcinogenic; therefore, HMF is still not categorized into group 2A or 2B by IARC.

14.3.6 Acrolein

Acrolein is a thiol-reactive electrophile (Gupta et al., 2021). In its pure form, acrolein (2-propenal, $CH_2 = CHCHO$) is a colorless, volatile liquid (B.P. 53°C), with a foul smell described initially by Berzelius in 1839 after a thorough breakdown of glycerine (Gupta et al., 2020). It has $LD_{50} = 175$ ppm (mouse, 10 min) and 375 ppm (rat, 10 min). Acrolein is formed by thermal processing at above 150°C of protein and carbohydrate-containing food products such as fish and cheese, and also its presence is found in fruits like grapes and berries. Moreover, it is also observed in spirits and wines (Moghe et al., 2015).

Acrolein toxicity is linked mainly with CNS and CVS disorders, namely Alzheimer's disease, spinal cord injury (SCI), atherosclerosis, and lung-associated disorders, mainly COPD, which also irritates the skin and eyes (Arntz et al., 2007). Exposure of acrolein to the eye in a battle zone induces instant eye closure, discomfort, and lacrimation, rendering the enemy incapacitated on the battlefield. Depending on the dose and duration, acrolein exposure can cause corneal erosions, anterior chamber inflammation, and corneal neovascularization. It can also lead to a limbal stem cell deficit in the long term. Acrolein exposure to the cornea can cause rapid incapacitation, which can be avoided by short-term therapy with local anesthetics and anti-inflammatory medicines. Because of the unknown chemical pathways that induce acrolein toxicity in the cornea, there is currently no definite remedy for acrolein toxicity (Gupta et al., 2021).

The World Health Organization has set permissible limits for oral intake of acrolein of 7.5 μg each day per kg body weight (Abraham et al., 2011). The metabolism pathway through which acrolein is metabolized is initiated through forming conjugate with glutathione, cysteine, and thioredoxin, which may lead to the formation of the adduct of thiol groups and −NH groups of proteins and nucleic acids and result in DNA damage (Cai et al., 2009; Ou et al., 2020). Other mechanisms include the production of ROS and initiation of mitochondrial and endoplasmic reticulum stress.

In studies conducted by Conklin et al. (2017), mice were exposed to an equivalent amount of acrolein found in tobacco. It was observed that there are threefold rise in urine metabolites and an increase in enzymes present at a pulmonary level for the metabolism of acrolein. Moreover, it was examined by Stevens and Maier (2008) that acrolein can alter many signaling pathways that require NF-κB, conversion of macrophages to foam cells, and transcription factors.

Further investigations are going on to confirm if acrolein has mutagenic properties; henceforth, IARC has categorized it under group 3.

14.3.7 Chloropropanols and chloro esters

Chloropropanols are toxicants generated during heat processing of foodstuff above 150°C. Eight isomers of chloropropanols, of which 1,3-DCP and 3-MCPD are more carcinogenic and genotoxic. Earlier in the 1980s, they were discovered in hydrolyzed vegetable proteins (HVPs). Still, on further investigations, they were also found in heated and smoked food and food ingredients, which were grains derived, such as bread, toast, doughnuts, and French fries. The reaction between chloride ions of hydrochloric acid and lipid constituents of hydrolyzed vegetable proteins results in chloro propanol and its isomers (Arisseto et al., 2013).

Refining procedures seem to be responsible for the synthesis of 3-MCPD and esters in consumable oils. The number of 3-MCPD esters is increased when heat is supplied during the deodorization stage. In acid HVP-based and other heat-treated meals, one reaction occurs between the lipid compounds and chloride ions, resulting in 3-MCPD esters. 3-MCPD is produced by smoking and also by enzymatic hydrolysis. The occurrence of 3-MCPD in foods is a public health hazard having Kidney dysfunction, benign cysts, nephritis, and tubular hyperplasia. The daily intake for 3-MCPD is 2 μg/kg bw/day, although (EFSA) European Food Safety Authority has fixed a consumption threshold of 0.82 μg/kg bw/day. For HVP with soy sauce, European Commission (EC) set a limit dose of 3-MCPD of 0.02 mg/kg (20 μg/kg) (on a 40% dry matter basis) (Ahmad et al., 2020). To minimize the development of 3-MCPD, 2-MCPD, and MCPD in biscuits, a current study advises reducing the heat burden or restricting chloride content. When salt was removed from the formula in biscuits, the 2 MCPD and 3 MCPD were reduced by 57.5% and 85.4% sequentially (Mogol and Gökmen, 2016).

In a research experiment to study the effect of free 3-MCPD using an HK-2 cell line, significant cytotoxicity was observed at the highest tested treatment concentration (Mossoba et al., 2020). Cellular metabolic activity was found to be decreased in cytotoxicity studies performed using Alamar blue assay on HUVEC/Ter2 cell lines (Moser et al., 2021). IARC has classified chloropropanols under group 2B. The permissible range that can be tolerable for daily oral intake is determined to be 2 μg/kg decided by The Scientific Committee on Food, 2011. This limit was further approved by the WHO Committee of Food Additives.

Data on 1,3-DCP being mutagenic and carcinogenic is gathered by the Joint FAO/WHO Expert Committee on Food and Additives. Hepatotoxicity and carcinogenicity of 1,3-DCP were concluded through various animal studies, and its genotoxicity was confirmed by in vitro studies. In a study, the adverse effect of 1,3-DCP was examined by exposing it to pregnant Sprague Dawley rats (Lee et al., 2009). At the highest dose (90 mg/mg/kg), a decrease in fetal body weight and initiation of toxic effects was observed, and also, at 30 mg/kg dose, no maternal toxicity was reported. More in vivo investigation is suggested to investigate the carcinogenicity and set the limits for daily intake of 1,3-DCP.

14.3.8 Dietary furan

Furan (C_4H_4O) is a highly volatile (31°C) organic compound consisting of five-membered heterocyclic rings. It is found in various food products, including coffee, soups, fruit juices, and baby food. The presence of furan in heat-processed food was first found in the 1960s. Its toxic concentrations are found in ground roasted coffee (up to 1912 μg/kg), food stuffs obtained from cereals and vegetables, and beverages. Furan, 2-methyl furan, 3-methyl furan, 2,5-dimethylfuran, and 2,3-dimethylfuran, together known as furan derivatives, have been found in coffee. Furan derivatives are produced by thermal breakdown during roasting (Rahn and Yeretzian, 2019). Among various pathways, the formation of furan through thermal degradation of carbohydrates, amino acids (observed in the Maillard reaction), and oxidation of ascorbic acid and PUFA (Poly Unsaturated Fatty Acids) due to exposure to elevated temperature (Conklin et al., 2017).

Due to Maillard's reactions, fried food palatability is linked to specific sensory features such as brown color, crunchy texture, and other desired flavors and tastes. Because of the mass transfer between the frying vehicle and the fat of the food, the frying process causes significant changes in the food, such as water loss, melanoidin development, increased fat content, and changes in the fatty acid profile. The Maillard process also creates volatile chemicals that give roasted and fried meals with a distinct scent and flavor. Furan and furanic chemicals, for example, can considerably impact the sensory qualities of heat-treated meals. On the other hand, furan is a very volatile chemical that IARC has categorized as a probable carcinogen to people (group 2B). Furan exposure through diet is a public health hazard (Juániz et al., 2016).

Furans are synthesized in various ways with the help of precursors, including ascorbic acid, amino acids, sugars, unsaturated fatty acids, and carotenoids. For example, the unsaturated fatty acid oxidation and the Strecker reaction are two chemical changes that might result from traditional food heat processing. Maillard reaction, amino acid heat dissociation such as cysteine and serine, and polyunsaturated fatty acid oxidation are some of the mechanisms that cause furan formation (PUFA). The carbohydrate breakdown process begins with the formation of aldotetrose derivatives, which are then cyclized into Furan. In the Maillard reaction, reducing sugars, particularly hexoses containing amino acids, are involved in synthesizing intermediate molecules, such as 1-deoxy- and 3-deoxyosones. Through alpha-dicarbonyl cleavage, 1-deoxyosone yields aldotetrose. However, in a lack of amino acids, aldotetrose is formed in minor quantities by retroaldol degradation. Next, a dehydration reaction produces 2-deoxy-3-keto-aldotetrose. Finally, alpha-dicarbonyl cleavage converts 3-deoxyosone to 2-deoxyaldotetrose, which is then oxidized and decarboxylated. As a result, all aldotetrose compounds can be easily converted to Furan. By interacting with amino acids or dehydrating the C-3 hydroxyl group of pentoses, such as hexoses, 3-deoxyosone derivatives can be produced. The intermediate is transformed to 2-deoxyaldotetrose when alpha-dicarbonyl, a predecessor of furan, is broken down (Javed et al., 2021).

Carcinogenicity of furans was examined on F344 rats by Ding et al. (2012). Rats exposed to higher doses (12 and 16 mg/kg) died after 3 hours with more DNA damage in the liver (Jestoi et al., 2009). The estimated concentration of Furan in baby food samples purchased from finished markets showed that samples derived from fruit had the lowest concentration of Furan as compared to other products. According to The European Food Safety Authority (2008), the active metabolite of Furan that is cis-2-butene-1,4-dial is the reason for causing genotoxicity. But no sufficient data is available to conclude it, further demanding more research in this field. IARC has classified Furan under group 2B (Seok et al., 2015).

14.4 Hazards associated with toxicants of thermal processing

Cooking methods and dietary routines greatly influence the risk of adverse effects resulting in carcinogenesis, mutation, genotoxicity, and various other disorders associated with the liver, cardiovascular system, and central nervous system. Table 14.5 lists some possible mutagens in thermally processed food. Even the ways of heat processing, like roasting, microwave heating, frying, grilling, boiling, pasteurization, etc., affect the level of toxicity. Constituents in the foodstuff act as a substrate and carry out chemical reactions when exposed to favorable conditions. Such reactions result in desired aroma, color, and hazardous chemical substances that may cause severe health-related problems (Koszucka and Nowak, 2019).

Fried foods, including potato chips, French fries, extended snacks, roasted almonds, extruded noodles, doughnuts, and fried fish and fowl, have become extremely popular worldwide. During food frying, heat produces food toxicants such as acrylamide, hydroxymethylfurfural (HMF), heterocyclic amine (2-2-amino-1-methyl-6-phenylimidazo-pyridine), nitrosamines, and polyaromatic hydrocarbons such as benzoapyrene and chloropropanols (for example, 3-monochloropropane-1-diol, 3-MCPD) (Nabil et al., 2021; Stadler, 2012). Different types of DNA damage, such as nucleotide changes and extensive chromosomal abnormalities, are caused by such chemicals.

Some Maillard reaction products (MRPs) are harmful, like heterocyclic amines (HCAs), acrylamide (AA), and end products of advanced glycation (AGEs). In contrast, others stimulate the manufacturing of flavor elements like pyrazine, furan, and pyridine. Although these hazardous MRPs occur at extremely low concentrations (ppb), several of them have been shown to be carcinogenic in animal experiments and have significant mutagenicity in bacterial assays. Furthermore, epidemiological studies show a link between dangerous MRPs use and the development of various cancers (Ahmad et al., 2019).

Some HCAs have been shown to cause tumors in 'various organs of mice, and epidemiological research supports a link between dietary HCA intake and the risk of specific cancers. Long-term exposure to acrylamide has been demonstrated to harm the peripheral and central neurological systems, generating gene mutations and chromosomal abnormalities and

TABLE 14.5 Mutagens and their toxicity.

Mutagens	Source	Toxic effects	Toxic concentration
Acrylamide	Cake, bread, French fries, chips, coffee, canned black olives	• Classified as group 2A • mothers and infants are most prone to the toxicity • Alteration in hepatic functioning • Result in mutations that lead to chromosome segregation during cell mitosis • Intracellular ROS genesis • DNA damage	16 mg/kg/d
Acrolein	Fish products, cheese, grapes, berries	• Classified as group 3 • Induction of apoptosis • cardiac dysfunction • Alzheimer's, atherosclerosis, and lungs associated disorders • Skin irritation	>7.5 μg/kg body weight/ day
Nitrosamines	Cured meat, sea fish	• Classified as a potent carcinogen • Liver damage • hepatic fibrosis • Interference in glucose metabolism • ROS production	26 ng/day
Chloropropanols and chloroesters	Bread, toast, doughnuts, French fries	• Classified as group 2B • Reduction in cell growth and body weight • Increase in apoptosis and weight of kidney • Anemia	>2.1 mg/kg body weight
5-HMF	Bakery products, malt, vinegar, coffee, milk powder, infant formulas	• Classified as a potential carcinogen • Conversion to sulphoxymethyl furfural (SMF) induces a genotoxic effect • Evidence of colon cancer • Skin disorders • Eye irritation	80–100 mg/kg body weight
PAHs	Tobacco, whole grilled chicken, grilled vegetables, shish tauk	• Classified as Group 2A • DNA damage	>3.5 μg/kg body weight
HAAs	Cooked meat, beef, pork, sea fish	• Classified as Group 2B • Various histological tumors were observed in different organs after being administered orally • Increase in levels of DNA adducts observed	0.1–64.6 mg/ kg/day in rodents
Dietary furan	Coffee, soups, fruit juice, baby food	• Classified as group 2B • Evidences of hepatotoxicity and hepatocarcinogenesis • Reduction in serum testosterone level	>2 mg/kg/ body weight in rodents

demonstrating its mutagenic potential (Bin-Jumah et al., 2021). AGEs may accumulate in the human body and are associated with the progression of different diseases, including diabetes, neurodegenerative disease, and cardiovascular disease (Dariya and Nagaraju, 2020).

Humans at the top of the food chain may be exposed to health concerns due to eating seafood contaminated with MPs and hazardous chemicals (Wang et al., 2018). HAAs are one of the primary causes of breast, colon, pancreatic, and other cancers, according to the findings of several epidemiological studies. HAAs may raise the threat of long-lasting diseases like cardiovascular diseases and obesity, as well as cancer, by initiating oxidative stress mechanisms at the metabolic level (Cao et al., 2020).

Alzheimer's disease, thyroid eruptions, ovarian problems, breast cancer, nerve damage, testicular carcinoma, obesity, and schizophrenia come from endocrine disrupting chemicals (EDCs) that are emitted by the packaging industry, insecticides, and food additives have resulted in significant risks for human (Maqbool et al., 2016). Consumption of fried meals was linked to a higher prevalence of hypertension in a cross-sectional study (Dasa and Abera, 2019).

Different processing parameters interfere in the synthesis of the Maillard reaction, thus affect the formation of MRPs. For example, the precursor type and content affect the formation of MRPs. HCA precursors such as creatinine, reducing sugars, and amino acids may substantially impact HCA synthesis. The amount of added sugar could have very different effects. For example, adding 19% sugar inhibited HCA development, whereas adding 9% and 14% increased HCA formation by 85% and 15%, respectively.

The temperature and duration of heating are also two of the essential factors that influence the production of MRPs. HCA production is often aided by elevated temperature and excessive cooking times. For example, when meat essence was heated at 200°C for 30 min, the concentration of HCAs started growing, whereas at 100°C and 150°C, very few HCAs formed (Olalekan Adeyeye and Ashaolu, 2021). Minor water content (4%) was more favorable for acrylamide production than high water content (16%) in a fat-rich model system. Also, changes in pH have an impact on the production of AA. The cooking method, such as frying, roasting, heating, etc., plays an essential role in forming these harmful toxicants. A comparison of several cooking methods for chicken chops and fish fillets, comprising microwave, barbecuing, oven baking, and hot plate, revealed that grilling produced the greatest HCA concentration (8.13 ng/g) in chunks of a hen. Panfrying yielded a maximum HCA concentration (5.89 ng/g) in the fish testers, which was unnoticeable in those heated with a hot plate or a microwave. To reduce the creation of HCAs, it is typically suggested to practice microwave cooking, boiling, and steaming meat and fish instead of barbecuing or frying. Exogenous additives such as polyphenols, vitamins, and organosulfur compounds that come under natural products have been shown in several studies to inhibit the development of HCAs because of their antioxidant property and thus interfere with the Maillard process (Zhang et al., 2021; Barzegar et al., 2019).

14.5 Analysis of thermally processed toxicants

Identifying and determining the concentration of the genotoxic and carcinogenic substances produced during the heat processing of food substances is essential for safety purposes. Hyphenated techniques of liquid chromatography along with mass spectrometry

(LC-MS) and gas chromatography hyphenated with mass spectrometry (GC-MS) are the standard methods to quantify and analyze toxicants that are formed during the thermal processing of food. Though these systems are costly and slow to operate, they provide accurate information of the best quality because of their extraordinary sensitivity and selectivity.

Factors that affect the analysis include the nature of the analyte to be examined, the procedure of sample preparation, and the concentration of the sample. Determination of toxicants consists of three phases: (i) sampling, (ii) sampling procedure, and (iii) analyzing (Beekman et al., 2019). In the next section, we have briefly discussed the different techniques that have been used to quantify food toxicants.

14.5.1 MS, LC-MS, and GC-MS

The principal method for detecting toxicants such as AA in foods is mass spectrometry (MS), which could be coupled with high-performance liquid chromatography (LC) or gas chromatography (GC). These methods are of utmost dependable analysis and detection since they have high accuracy and sensitivity, as well as strong stability and repeatability (Pan et al., 2020).

14.5.2 Capillary electrophoresis (CE)

CE is a helpful technology for analyzing trace components in foods because of its fast analytical speed, high separation efficiency, and the fact that it only requires a minimal amount of material (Pan et al., 2020).

14.5.3 Immunoassay method

This is a brand-new, high-throughput analytical technique based on a specific antigen (Ag) and antibody combination (Ab). After nearly 2 decades of research, the immunoassay has evolved into enzyme-linked immunoassays (ELISA) (Cui et al., 2019), fluorescent immunoassays (Chen et al., 2019), and other types of immunoassays widely employed in food analysis particularly in the field of quick detection (Pan et al., 2020).

14.5.4 Sensor analysis technique

To fulfill the goal of analysis and detection, sensors can monitor the critical response between the tested chemical and the identification element in real time and transform the resulting binding signal into a signal that can be analyzed quantitatively, such as electricity, light, or mass. Two types of sensing analysis have been established, electrochemical and fluorescence sensing analysis methods (Pan et al., 2020).

14.5.5 Thermal lens spectrometry (TLS) approaches for fast screening

This spectroscopic technique is widely regarded as a susceptible method for liquid estimation. TLS can measure less than 10 optical absorbances because of its intrinsic sensitivity. It also probes tiny (sub-picolitre) quantities on millisecond time measure. It gives a comparatively rapid signal response for liquid estimation and allows for online detection in flowing samples. TLS is mainly used in separation methods as a detection technique that gives the desired selectivity, such as capillary electrophoresis (CE), ion chromatography (IC), and high-performance liquid chromatography (HPLC). Using bioanalytical assays or specified colorimetric reactions, we can add high specificity to TLS measurements (Proskurnin et al., 2016). When TLM or TLS are used in conjunction with bioanalytical techniques, the sensitivity and selectivity of analyte determination improve significantly (Franko et al., 2016).

14.5.5.1 *TLS detection: flow-injection manifolds (FIA)*

When FIA manifolds are used in conjunction with TLS, multiple chemical processes are essential for the ultimate recognition of an analyte, and they can be performed online. Chemical transformations of the analyte, such as reduction/oxidation reactions and/or other derivatization methods (coloring reactions), and connectivity to specific antibodies or enzymes, are all possible (Boškin et al., 2009; Franko et al., 2016).

14.5.5.2 *Microfluidic systems: thermal lens microscopy*

Thermal lens microscopy (TLM) has one probe beam and distinct coaxial geometry for excitation. A solitary objective chromatic microscopic lens is focused on this arrangement. Chromatic aberration of microscopic objective lenses causes few millimeter movements in the probe beam foci and excitation, which is required to evaluate the thermal lens' effect on the probe beam. It allows for analyte recognition, which is impossible with a transverse mode (Franko et al., 2016).

14.5.5.3 *TLS and TLM future outlooks*

This will use a few of the previously established TLM detection principles in conjunction with biological cells on microchips and chemistry to determine new developing contaminants such as pharmaceuticals, allergies, and toxicogenic chemicals in drinking water and meals (Franko et al., 2016).

14.6 Techniques to minimize the toxicants

For a long time, scientists worldwide, along with agencies, namely Food and Agriculture Organization and World Health, have been working on strategies to reduce the toxicants in thermally processed foodstuffs. To minimize the toxic concentration of AA, various methods, such as soaking, fermentation, and the use of antioxidants, have been reported (Rifai and Saleh, 2020). Various cooking processes were studied to screen the method which produces the least amount of heterocyclic aromatic amines. Combined microwave heating with the infrared grilling of beef showed maximum reduction in the content of heterocyclic aromatic amine compared to only microwave heating and without the change in visual appearance. The reduction in HAAs was observed due to moisture content and oxidation of the lipidic contents (Wang et al., 2021a).

The techniques for reducing toxicants can be established based on understanding the mechanism of toxicant formation. The food industries have developed and are practicing various nonthermal food processing methods. Cold plasma technology is one of the widely used nonthermal food processing technology. Various ongoing studies have proved that it is a superior technology for surface decontamination without altering the food constituents (Mandal et al., 2018). Another approach is the use of high hydrostatic pressure. This technique prevents the activation of pathogenic microorganisms and the spoilage of food. It is also approved by the US FDA and US Department of Agriculture as the alternate approach for pasteurization (Wang et al., 2016).

The cooking style also has a role, as greater temperature procedures (barbecuing/grilling, pan frying, and cooking in the oven) have been shown to produce the largest HAA concentrations. On the other hand, preliminary treatment with microwave results in little HAA production. The coating of microwave oven-based utensils may further limit the production of HAA by acting as an insulator between the thermal source and meat, preventing direct exposure (Meurillon et al., 2018). To minimize the effect of HAAs, two approaches could be taken: (i). minimize HAA production during the cooking process before consumption, and (ii) lower its bioavailability or metabolization in the body after consumption (Engel et al., 2015). It is hypothesized that HAAs are only mutagenic or carcinogenic after they have undergone metabolic activation, which includes phase I N-hydroxylation by several cytochrome P450 isoenzymes mostly (CYP1A2) and phase II esterification of the exocyclic amino group; thus the enzymatic inactivation can help lower the bioavailability of HAAs (Woziwodzka et al., 2013).

14.7 Conclusion

This chapter discusses the current scenario of food toxicants generated while performing different cooking methods. A variety of thermal processing technologies used in cooking are discussed in the above sections. It was also found that overcooking food loses its nutritional content. Also, various chemical changes were seen, such as denaturation of the protein content and formation of the Maillard reaction product during food processing. Researchers have studied the effect of temperature on the protein; the results were aggregation, gelation, and denaturation. Majorly studied food toxicants such as heterocyclic aromatic amines (HAA), acrylamide (AA), N-nitroso compounds, etc., are comprehensively studied in the above discussion. The side effects caused by these chemicals on different organs have been explored. The finding of toxicants is equally vital to the analysis of toxicants, so we have given a brief description of the utmost critical analytical techniques, such as thermal lens spectrometry (TLS), microfluidic systems, etc. There are various techniques by which we can at least try to minimize the formation of such harmful toxicants. Because every cooking style has pros and cons, it's time to find better minimization techniques to avoid food toxicants. It needs time to develop advanced techniques to help minimize food toxicants generation.

14.8 Abbreviations used

5-SMF 5-Sulfoxymethylfurfural
AA acrylamide
Advanced AGEs Advanced glycated end products

CE Capillary Electrophoresis
EC European Commission
EDCs endocrine disrupting chemicals
EWP egg white protein
FIA Flow-injection Manifolds
GC gas chromatography
GC-MS gas chromatography-mass spectrometry
HAA heterocyclic aromatic amines
HCAs Heterocyclic amines
HMF hydroxymethylfurfural
HMFA 5-hydroxymethyl 2-furanoic acid
HVPs hydrolyzed vegetable proteins
IARC International Agency for Research on Cancer
LC-MS liquid chromatography along with mass spectrometry
MR Maillard reaction
MRPs Maillard reaction products
NDEA N-nitrosodiethyl amine
NDMA N-nitrosodimethyl amine
PUFA polyunsaturated fatty acid
TLM Thermal lens Microscopy
TLS Thermal lens Spectrometry

References

Abraham, K., Andres, S., Palavinskas, R., Berg, K., Appel, K.E., Lampen, A., 2011. Toxicology and risk assessment of acrolein in food. Mol. Nutr. Food Res. 55, 1277–1290.

Adams, J., 1991. Enzyme inactivation during heat processing of food-stuffs. Int. J. Food Sci. Technol. 26, 1–20.

Ahmad, N., Shabbir, M.A., Butt, M.S., Shahid, M., Robert, T.H., 2020. Quantification of 3-monochloropropane-diol fatty acid esters by liquid chromatography-mass spectrometry method with their subsequent reduction in processed foods. Pakistan J. Agric. Sci. 57.

Ahmad, S., Masood, F., Khatoon, K., Malik, A., 2019. Risk Management of Chemical Hazards Arising during Food Manufacturing. *Health and Safety Aspects of Food Processing Technologies*. Springer.

Aljahdali, N., Carbonero, F., 2019. Impact of Maillard reaction products on nutrition and health: current knowledge and need to understand their fate in the human digestive system. Crit. Rev. Food Sci. Nutr. 59, 474–487.

Alomirah, H., Al-Zenki, S., Al-Hooti, S., Zaghloul, S., Sawaya, W., Ahmed, N., Kannan, K., 2011. Concentrations and dietary exposure to polycyclic aromatic hydrocarbons (PAHs) from grilled and smoked foods. Food Control 22, 2028–2035.

Ameseder, F., Radulescu, A., Holderer, O., Falus, P., Richter, D., Stadler, A.M., 2018. Relevance of internal friction and structural constraints for the dynamics of denatured bovine serum albumin. J. Phys. Chem. Lett. 9, 2469–2473.

Arisseto, A.P., Vicente, E., Furlani, R.P.Z., Toledo, M.C.D.F., 2013. Estimate of dietary intake of chloropropanols (3-MCPD and 1, 3-DCP) and health risk assessment. Food Sci. Technol. 33, 125–133.

Arntz, D., Achin, F., Höpp, M., Jacobi, S., Sauer, J., Ohara, T., Sato, T., Shimizu, N., Schwind, H., 2007. Acrolein and methacrolein. Ullmann's Encyclopedia of Industrial Chemistry, pp. 329–346.

Barzegar, F., Kamankesh, M., Mohammadi, A., 2019. Heterocyclic aromatic amines in cooked food: a review on formation, health risk-toxicology and their analytical techniques. Food Chem. 280, 240–254.

Beekman, J.K., Granvogl, M., Macmahon, S., 2019. Analysis and occurrence of MCPD and glycidyl esters in infant formulas and other complex food matrices. In: Food-Borne Toxicants: Formation, Analysis, and Toxicology. ACS Publications.

Bin-Jumah, M., Abdel-Fattah, A.-F.M., Saied, E.M., El-Seedi, H.R., Abdel-Daim, M.M., 2021. Acrylamide-induced peripheral neuropathy: manifestations, mechanisms, and potential treatment modalities. Environ. Sci. Pollut. Control Ser. 28, 13031–13046.

Bogahawaththa, D., Chau, N.H.B., Trivedi, J., Dissanayake, M., Vasiljevic, T., 2019. Impact of selected process parameters on solubility and heat stability of pea protein isolate. Lebensm. Wiss. & Technol. 102, 246–253.

Bolden, A.L., Rochester, J.R., Schultz, K., Kwiatkowski, C.F., 2017. Polycyclic aromatic hydrocarbons and female reproductive health: a scoping review. Reprod. Toxicol. 73, 61–74.

Boškin, A., Tran, C.D., Franko, M., 2009. Oxidation of organophosphorus pesticides with chloroperoxidase enzyme in the presence of an ionic liquid as co-solvent. Environ. Chem. Lett. 7, 267–270.

Cai, J., Bhatnagar, A., Pierce Jr., W.M., 2009. Protein modification by acrolein: formation and stability of cysteine adducts. Chem. Res. Toxicol. 22, 708–716.

Cao, H., Chen, B.H., Inbaraj, B.S., Chen, L., Alvarez-Rivera, G., Cifuentes, A., Zhang, N., Yang, D.J., Simal-Gandara, J., Wang, M., 2020. Preventive potential and mechanism of dietary polyphenols on the formation of heterocyclic aromatic amines. Food Front. 1, 134–151.

Capuano, E., Fogliano, V., 2011. Acrylamide and 5-hydroxymethylfurfural (HMF): a review on metabolism, toxicity, occurrence in food and mitigation strategies. *LWT-Food Sci. Technol.* 44, 793–810.

Chen, E., Xu, Y., Ma, B., Cui, H., Sun, C., Zhang, M., 2019. Carboxyl-functionalized, Europium nanoparticle-based fluorescent immunochromatographic assay for sensitive detection of citrinin in monascus fermented food. Toxins 11, 605.

Chiozzi, V., Agriopoulou, S., Varzakas, T., 2022. Advances, applications, and comparison of thermal (pasteurization, sterilization, and aseptic packaging) against non-thermal (ultrasounds, UV radiation, ozonation, high hydrostatic pressure) technologies in food processing. Appl. Sci. 12, 2202.

Conklin, D.J., Malovichko, M.V., Zeller, I., Das, T.P., Krivokhizhina, T.V., Lynch, B.H., Lorkiewicz, P., Agarwal, A., Wickramasinghe, N., Haberzettl, P., Sithu, S.D., Shah, J., O'toole, T.E., Rai, S.N., Bhatnagar, A., Srivastava, S., 2017. Biomarkers of chronic acrolein inhalation exposure in mice: implications for tobacco product-induced toxicity. Toxicol. Sci. 158, 263–274.

Cui, Y., Zhao, J., Zhou, J., Tan, G., Zhao, Q., Zhang, Y., Wang, B., Jiao, B., 2019. Development of a sensitive monoclonal antibody-based indirect competitive enzyme-linked immunosorbent assay for analysing nobiletin in citrus and herb samples. Food Chem. 293, 144–150.

Daniel, C., Schwartz, K., Colt, J., Dong, L., Ruterbusch, J., Purdue, M., Cross, A., Rothman, N., Davis, F., Wacholder, S., 2011. Meat-cooking mutagens and risk of renal cell carcinoma. Br. J. Cancer 105, 1096–1104.

Dariya, B., Nagaraju, G.P., 2020. Advanced glycation end products in diabetes, cancer and phytochemical therapy. Drug Discov. Today 25, 1614–1623.

Dasa, F., Abera, T., 2019. Why fried food is Unhealthy: heat induced food toxicants and associated health risks. J. Agric. Sci. Food Technol. 5, 32–41.

Deeth, H.C., 2021. Heat-induced inactivation of enzymes in milk and dairy products. A review. Int. Dairy J. 105104.

Delgado-Andrade, C., Seiquer, I., Navarro, M.P., Morales, F.J., 2008. Estimation of hydroxymethylfurfural availability in breakfast cereals. Studies in Caco-2 cells. Food Chem. Toxicol. 46, 1600–1607.

Ding, W., Petibone, D.M., Latendresse, J.R., Pearce, M.G., Muskhelishvili, L., White, G.A., Chang, C.-W., Mittelstaedt, R.A., Shaddock, J.G., Mcdaniel, L.P., 2012. In vivo genotoxicity of Furan in F344 rats at cancer bioassay doses. Toxicol. Appl. Pharmacol. 261, 164–171.

Duda-Chodak, A., Tarko, T., Sroka, P., Satora, P., 2016. A review of the interactions between acrylamide, microorganisms and food components. Food Funct. 7, 1282–1295.

El-Assouli, S.M., 2009. Acrylamide in selected foods and genotoxicity of their extracts. Egypt. Public Health Assoc. 84, 371–392.

Engel, E., Ratel, J., Bouhlel, J., Planche, C., Meurillon, M., 2015. Novel approaches to improving the chemical safety of the meat chain towards toxicants. Meat Sci. 109, 75–85.

Essumang, D., Dodoo, D., Adjei, J., 2013. Effect of smoke generation sources and smoke curing duration on the levels of polycyclic aromatic hydrocarbon (PAH) in different suites of fish. Food Chem. Toxicol. 58, 86–94.

Franko, M., Liu, M., Boškin, A., Delneri, A., Proskurnin, M.A., 2016. Fast screening techniques for neurotoxigenic substances and other toxicants and pollutants based on thermal lensing and microfluidic chips. Anal. Sci. 32, 23–30.

Gankhuyag, N., Lee, K.-H., Cho, J.-Y., 2017. The role of nitrosamine (NNK) in breast cancer carcinogenesis. J. Mammary Gland Biol. Neoplasia 22, 159–170.

Gao, P., Da Silva, E., Hou, L., Denslow, N.D., Xiang, P., Ma, L.Q., 2018. Human exposure to polycyclic aromatic hydrocarbons: metabolomics perspective. Environ. Int. 119, 466–477.

García, A., Morales, P., Arranz, N., Delgado, E., Rafter, J., Haza, A.I., 2008. Induction of apoptosis and reactive oxygen species production by N-nitrosopiperidine and N-nitrosodibutylamine in human leukemia cells. J. Appl. Toxicol.: Int. J. 28, 455–465.

Gupta, S., Fink, M.K., Martin, L.M., Sinha, P.R., Rodier, J.T., Sinha, N.R., Hesemann, N.P., Chaurasia, S.S., Mohan, R.R., 2020. A rabbit model for evaluating ocular damage from acrolein toxicity in vivo. Ann. N. Y. Acad. Sci. 1480, 233–245.

Gupta, S., Kamil, S., Sinha, P.R., Rodier, J.T., Chaurasia, S.S., Mohan, R.R., 2021. Glutathione is a potential therapeutic target for acrolein toxicity in the cornea. Toxicol. Lett. 340, 33–42.

Iwashita, K., Inoue, N., Handa, A., Shiraki, K., 2015. Thermal aggregation of hen egg white proteins in the presence of salts. Protein J. 34, 212–219.

Jägerstad, M., Skog, K., 2005. Genotoxicity of heat-processed foods. Mutat. Res. 574, 156–172.

Javed, F., Shahbaz, H.M., Nawaz, A., Olaimat, A.N., Stratakos, A.C., Wahyono, A., Munir, S., Mueen-Ud-Din, G., Ali, Z., Park, J., 2021. Formation of Furan in baby food products: identification and technical challenges. Compr. Rev. Food Sci. Food Saf. 20, 2699–2715.

Jestoi, M., Järvinen, T., Järvenpää, E., Tapanainen, H., Virtanen, S., Peltonen, K., 2009. Furan in the baby-food samples purchased from the Finnish markets—Determination with SPME—GC—MS. Food Chem. 117, 522–528.

Juániz, I., Zocco, C., Mouro, V., Cid, C., De Peña, M.P., 2016. Effect of frying process on furan content in foods and assessment of furan exposure of Spanish population. LWT Food Sci. Technol. 68, 549–555.

Khorshidian, N., Yousefi, M., Shadnoush, M., Siadat, S.D., Mohammadi, M., Mortazavian, A.M., 2020. Using probiotics for mitigation of acrylamide in food products: a mini review. Curr. Opin. Food Sci. 32, 67–75.

Koszucka, A., Nowak, A., 2019. Thermal processing food-related toxicants: a review. Crit. Rev. Food Sci. Nutr. 59, 3579–3596.

Lam, R.S., Nickerson, M.T., 2015. The effect of pH and temperature pre-treatments on the structure, surface characteristics and emulsifying properties of alpha-lactalbumin. Food Chem. 173, 163–170.

Ledesma, E., Rendueles, M., Díaz, M., 2015. Spanish smoked meat products: benzo (a) pyrene (BaP) contamination and moisture. J. Food Compos. Anal. 37, 87–94.

Lee, C.-H., Chen, K.-T., Lin, J.-A., Chen, Y.-T., Chen, Y.-A., Wu, J.-T., Hsieh, C.-W., 2019. Recent advances in processing technology to reduce 5-hydroxymethylfurfural in foods. Trends Food Sci. Technol. 93, 271–280.

Lee, J., Shin, I., Ahn, T., Kim, K., Moon, C., Kim, S., Shin, D., Park, S., Kim, Y., Kim, J., 2009. Developmental toxic potential of 1, 3-dichloro-2-propanol in Sprague—Dawley rats. Regul. Toxicol. Pharmacol. 53, 63–69.

Lee, S.Y., Munerol, B., Pollard, S., Youdim, K.A., Pannala, A.S., Kuhnle, G.G., Debnam, E.S., Rice-Evans, C., Spencer, J.P., 2006. The reaction of flavanols with nitrous acid protects against N-nitrosamine formation and leads to the formation of nitroso derivatives which inhibit cancer cell growth. Free Radic. Biol. Med. 40, 323–334.

Liu, J., Du, P., Mao, H., Zhang, L., Ju, H., Lei, J., 2018. Dual-triggered oxygen self-supply black phosphorus nanosystem for enhanced photodynamic therapy. Biomaterials 172, 83–91.

Liu, X., Chen, D., Yang, Z., Chen, F., Hu, X., Xiao, Z., Ji, J., Ma, L., 2022. Non-enzymatic browning induced by chlorogenic acid quinone mediated catechin oxidation. Food Res. Int. 111297.

López-Pedrouso, M., Lorenzo, J.M., Zapata, C., Franco, D., 2019. Proteins and Amino Acids. *Innovative Thermal and Non-thermal Processing, Bioaccessibility and Bioavailability of Nutrients and Bioactive Compounds*. Elsevier.

Lund, M.N., Ray, C.A., 2017. Control of Maillard reactions in foods: strategies and chemical mechanisms. J. Agric. Food Chem. 65, 4537–4552.

Mandal, R., Singh, A., Singh, A.P., 2018. Recent developments in cold plasma decontamination technology in the food industry. Trends Food Sci. Technol. 80, 93–103.

Maqbool, F., Mostafalou, S., Bahadar, H., Abdollahi, M., 2016. Review of endocrine disorders associated with environmental toxicants and possible involved mechanisms. Life Sci. 145, 265–273.

Meurillon, M., Engel, E., 2016. Mitigation strategies to reduce the impact of heterocyclic aromatic amines in proteinaceous foods. Trends Food Sci. Technol. 50, 70–84.

Meurillon, M., Ratel, J., Engel, E., 2018. How to secure the meat chain against toxicants? Innovat. Food Sci. Emerg. Technol. 46, 74–82.

Moghe, A., Ghare, S., Lamoreau, B., Mohammad, M., Barve, S., Mcclain, C., JOSHI-Barve, S., 2015. Molecular mechanisms of acrolein toxicity: relevance to human disease. Toxicol. Sci. 143, 242–255.

Mogol, B.A., Gökmen, V., 2016. Thermal process contaminants: acrylamide, chloropropanols and furan. Curr. Opin. Food Sci. 7, 86–92.

Moser, D., Leitner, P., Filipek, P.A., Hussain, S., Rainer, M., Jakschitz, T., Rode, B.M., Bonn, G.K., 2021. Quantification and cytotoxicity of degradation products (chloropropanols) in sucralose containing e-liquids with propylene glycol and glycerol as base. Toxicol. Appl. Pharmacol. 430, 115727.

Mossoba, M.E., Mapa, S.T.M., Magali, A., Yang, Z., et al., 2020. In vitro toxicological assessment of free 3-MCPD and select 3-MCPD esters on human proximal tubule HK-2 cells. Cell Biol. Toxicol. 36 (3), 209–221.

Nabil, S.K., Mustari, N., Khan, M.S., 2021. Sources and health impacts of chemical contaminants in foods. In: Techniques to Measure Food Safety and Quality. Springer.

Nath, P., Pandey, N., Samota, M., Sharma, K., Kale, S., Kannaujia, P., Sethi, S., Chauhan, O., 2022. Browning reactions in foods. In: Advances in Food Chemistry. Springer.

Nicolai, T., 2019. Gelation of food protein-protein mixtures. Adv. Colloid Interface Sci. 270, 147–164.

Nowak, A., Kuberski, S., Libudzisz, Z., 2014. Probiotic lactic acid bacteria detoxify N-nitrosodimethylamine. Food Addit. Contam. 31, 1678–1687.

Olalekan Adeyeye, S.A., Ashaolu, T.J., 2021. Heterocyclic amine formation and mitigation in processed meat and meat products: a mini-review. J. Food Protect. 84, 1868–1877.

Ou, J., Zheng, J., Huang, J., Ho, C.-T., Ou, S., 2020. Interaction of acrylamide, acrolein, and 5-hydroxymethylfurfural with amino acids and DNA. J. Agric. Food Chem. 68, 5039–5048.

Pan, M., Liu, K., Yang, J., Hong, L., Xie, X., Wang, S., 2020. Review of research into the determination of acrylamide in foods. Foods 9, 524.

Proskurnin, M., Bendrysheva, S., Smirnova, A., 2016. Thermal lens spectrometry in electromigration methods of analysis. J. Anal. Chem. 71, 431–458.

Rahn, A., Yeretzian, C., 2019. Impact of consumer behavior on Furan and furan-derivative exposure during coffee consumption. A comparison between brewing methods and drinking preferences. Food Chem. 272, 514–522.

Ramesh, M.N., 2003. Sterilization of foods. In: Caballero, B. (Ed.), Encyclopedia of Food Sciences and Nutrition, second ed. Academic Press, Oxford.

Rifai, L., Saleh, F.A., 2020. A review on acrylamide in food: occurrence, toxicity, and mitigation strategies. Int. J. Toxicol. 39, 93–102.

Roefs, S.P., De Kruif, K.G., 1994. A model for the denaturation and aggregation of β-lactoglobulin. Eur. J. Biochem. 226, 883–889.

Seok, Y.-J., Her, J.-Y., Kim, Y.-G., Kim, M.Y., Jeong, S.Y., Kim, M.K., Lee, J.-Y., Kim, C.-I., Yoon, H.-J., Lee, K.-G., 2015. Furan in thermally processed foods-a review. Toxicol. Res. 31, 241–253.

Sergius-Ronot, M., Pitino, M.A., Suwal, S., Shama, S., Unger, S., O'connor, D.L., Pouliot, Y., Doyen, A., 2022. Impact of holder, high temperature short time and high hydrostatic pressure pasteurization methods on protein structure and aggregation in a human milk protein concentrate. Food Chem. 374, 131808.

Sevenich, R., Bark, F., Crews, C., Anderson, W., Pye, C., Riddellova, K., Hradecky, J., Moravcova, E., Reineke, K., Knorr, D., 2013. Effect of high pressure thermal sterilization on the formation of food processing contaminants. Innovat. Food Sci. Emerg. Technol. 20, 42–50.

Shen, H., Tao, S., Liu, J., Huang, Y., Chen, H., Li, W., Zhang, Y., Chen, Y., Su, S., Lin, N., 2014. Global lung cancer risk from PAH exposure highly depends on emission sources and individual susceptibility. Sci. Rep. 4, 1–8.

Stadler, R., 2012. Heat-generated toxicants in foods: acrylamide, MCPD esters and Furan. In: Chemical Contaminants and Residues in Food. Elsevier.

Stevens, J.F., Maier, C.S., 2008. Acrolein: sources, metabolism, and biomolecular interactions relevant to human health and disease. Mol. Nutr. Food Res. 52, 7–25.

Tamanna, N., Mahmood, N., 2015. Food processing and maillard reaction products: effect on human health and nutrition. Int. J. Food Sci. Technol. 2015.

Tessier, F.J., 2021. Browning: the glycation and maillard reactions—major non-enzymatic browning reactions in food. In: Handbook of Molecular Gastronomy. CRC Press.

Tian, X., Yu, Q., Wu, W., Dai, R., 2018. Inactivation of microorganisms in foods by ohmic heating: a review. J. Food Protect. 81, 1093–1107.

Van Breda, S.G., Mathijs, K., Pieters, H.J., Sági-Kiss, V., Kuhnle, G.G., Georgiadis, P., Saccani, G., Parolari, G., Virgili, R., Sinha, R., 2021. Replacement of nitrite in meat products by natural bioactive compounds results in reduced exposure to N-Nitroso compounds: the phytome project. Mol. Nutr. Food Res. 65, 2001214.

Verma, V., Yadav, N., 2020. Genotoxicity of heat induced contaminants in food. Plant Archives 20, 36–41.

Wang, C.-Y., Huang, H.-W., Hsu, C.-P., Yang, B.B., 2016. Recent advances in food processing using high hydrostatic pressure technology. Crit. Rev. Food Sci. Nutr. Res. 56, 527–540.

Wang, F., Wong, C.S., Chen, D., Lu, X., Wang, F., Zeng, E.Y., 2018. Interaction of toxic chemicals with microplastics: a critical review. Water Res. 139, 208–219.

Wang, W., Dong, L., Zhang, Y., Yu, H., Wang, S., 2021a. Reduction of the heterocyclic amines in grilled beef patties through the combination of thermal food processing techniques without destroying the grilling quality characteristics. Foods 10, 1490.

Wang, W., Nema, S., Teagarden, D., 2010. Protein aggregation—pathways and influencing factors. Int. J. Pharm. 390, 89—99.

Wang, Y., Liu, Y., Huang, X., Xiao, Z., Yang, Y., Yu, Q., Chen, S., He, L., Liu, A., Liu, S., 2021b. A review on mechanistic overview on the formation of toxic substances during the traditional fermented food processing. Food Rev. Int. 1—18.

Woziwodzka, A., Gołuński, G., Piosik, J., 2013. Heterocyclic Aromatic Amines Heterocomplexation with Biologically Active Aromatic Compounds and its Possible Role in Chemoprevention. International Scholarly Research Notices.

Yu, T.Y., Morton, J.D., Clerens, S., Dyer, J.M., 2017. Cooking-induced protein modifications in meat. Compr. Rev. Food Sci. Food Saf. 16, 141—159.

Yurchenko, S., Mölder, U., 2005. N-nitrosodimethylamine analysis in Estonian beer using positive-ion chemical ionization with gas chromatography mass spectrometry. Food Chem. 89, 455—463.

Zamani, E., Shokrzadeh, M., Fallah, M., Shaki, F., 2017. A review of acrylamide toxicity and its mechanism. Pharm. Biomed. Res. 3, 1—7.

Zamora, R., Hidalgo, F.J., 2020. Formation of heterocyclic aromatic amines with the structure of aminoimidazoazarenes in food products. Food Chem. 313, 126128.

Zhang, N., Zhou, Q., Fan, D., Xiao, J., Zhao, Y., Cheng, K.-W., Wang, M., 2021. Novel roles of hydrocolloids in foods: inhibition of toxic maillard reaction products formation and attenuation of their harmful effects. Trends Food Sci. Technol. 111, 706—715.

Zhang, P., Chen, Y., 2017. Polycyclic aromatic hydrocarbons contamination in surface soil of China: a review. Sci. Total Environ. 605, 1011—1020.

Zheng, J., Daniel, C.R., Hatia, R.I., Stuff, J., Abdelhakeem, A.A., Rashid, A., Chun, Y.S., Jalal, P.K., Kaseb, A.O., Li, D., 2021. Dietary N-nitroso compounds and risk of hepatocellular carcinoma: a USA-based study. Hepatology 74 (6), 3161—3173.

Zheng, J., Stuff, J., Tang, H., Hassan, M.M., Daniel, C.R., Li, D., 2019. Dietary N-nitroso compounds and risk of pancreatic cancer: results from a large case—control study. Carcinogenesis 40, 254—262.

Zhong, C., Tan, S., Langrish, T., 2019. Redness generation via Maillard reactions of whey protein isolate (WPI) and ascorbic acid (vitamin C) in spray-dried powders. J. Food Eng. 244, 11—20.

CHAPTER

15

Medication errors and approaches for its prevention

Ankit Mishra[1], *Nimeet Desai*[2], *Muktika Tekade*[3], *Kuldeep Rajpoot*[2], *Anuradha Gadeval*[2], *Manish Sharma*[4] *and Rakesh Kumar Tekade*[2]

[1]VNS Group of Institutions, Bhopal, Madhya Pradesh, India; [2]National Institute of Pharmaceutical Education and Research (NIPER)- Ahmedabad, An Institute of National Importance, Government of India, Department of Pharmaceuticals, Ministry of Chemicals and Fertilizers, Palaj, Gandhinagar, Gujarat, India; [3]School of Pharmacy, Devi Ahilya Vishwavidyalaya, Indore, Madhya Pradesh, India; [4]Dept of Pharmacy Practice, University of Nebraska Medical Center, Omaha, NE, United States

15.1 Introduction

Medication errors (MEs) are extensively scrutinized in the healthcare profession and is the most critical subject. Since the 1960s, several studies have been conducted internationally, providing ample evidence on medical and ME on all medical premises approximately daily. For instance, 40,000 MEs were noticed in 173 hospital trusts in England and Wales in the 12 months. This data was recorded by the National Patient Safety Agency, where it showed approximately 15% slight harm while 5% moderate or severe harm (BBC News, 2006). On the other hand, other investigations carried out in the US revealed that nearly 1.7% of prescriptions dispensed by community pharmacies reported MEs (Flynn et al., 2003; Aronson, 2009).

The outcomes of these studies suggest that ME has more lethality than existing, not curable diseases like cancer or acquired immunodeficiency syndrome. The report mentioned above suggests that even without intentions, 20% of the patients were harmed due to ME (Aronson, 2009). The prevention of these errors is required to improve patient care, enhance efficacy, and save lives.

These MEs can be prevented by talking to the patient, confirming their knowledge of the dosage/drug allergies, and examining any other drugs they may be taking

Essentials of Pharmatoxicology in Drug Research, Volume 1
https://doi.org/10.1016/B978-0-443-15840-7.00003-8

(Isaacs et al., 2021). Additionally, the pharmacist's duties frequently involve monitoring patients' prescription regimens and alerting the medical staff when an error has occurred. The majority of prescription inconsistencies are discovered upon discharge, underlining the necessity of a pharmacist helping with discharge (Gillani et al., 2021). Furthermore, some common MEs can be corrected by delivering the correct dosage, identifying contraindications to drug therapy and any drug allergic reactions, monitoring drugs with narrow therapeutic indexes, recognizing drug interactions, and improving knowledge deficits (Tariq et al., 2022).

ME can be prevented using a technologically advanced system that can detect it accurately. For example, applying checklists, fail-safe measures, and computerized alerts can help avoid some technical MEs, including adding the incorrect amount of potassium chloride to an infusion container. Another example is knowing that the patient is allergic to penicillin but failing to remember. These are difficult to prevent, but automated prescription systems and cross-checking can identify them (Aronson, 2009). However, these systems must be inexpensive and ready to be adaptable by most hospitals and staff working there.

15.1.1 MEs

ME is any preventable event that may cause or lead to inappropriate medication use or patient harm while the medication is controlled by the health care professional, patient, or consumer (Cousins and Heath, 2008). In nontechnical language, it can be called failure in the treatment, which may or can cause maltreatment to the patient. Here the treatment term is commonly used to treat the symptoms or the causes of symptoms, prevention, and diagnosis of the disease or pathophysiological changes. The term also contains prescribing, some-time transcribing, dispensing, compounding, administering, and monitoring. Lack of benefit to the patient is also included in maltreatment (Ferner and Aronson, 2006).

A study performed on ME reported that about 5%–14% of dispensed drug doses lead to one or even more MEs. ME combined with avoidable adverse drug events (ADEs) can affect the patient's health-related decisions, may lead to improved resident time in the hospital, unfavorable situations like partial or complete damage to the patient's body organs, and even death (Bates et al., 1995; Crespin et al., 2010). MEs, which may lead to the patient's injury, are considered potential ADE.

Preventable events are any event that might result in improper drug usage or patient injury when the medicine is under the medical practitioner, patient, or user's control. Such occurrences may be associated with medical practices, healthcare items, methods, and systems, such as prescription writing, order communication, product labeling, packaging, as well as nomenclature, compounding, dispensing, distribution, administration, instruction, surveillance, and usage (Zirpe et al., 2020; Ibrahim et al., 2020; Aseeri et al., 2020). On the other hand, nonpreventable events are adverse drug reactions, which are expected to show adverse effects that are a natural consequence of the drug's pharmacologic activity and are not always avoidable (Neal et al., 2021; Kefale et al., 2020). For example, an overdose of gentamicin sulfate administered to a person without any sequential disease or injury can be considered a potential ADE-based ME, which can be prevented by correcting the dose. At the same time, after administration of cefazolin sodium, the development of rashes in patients owing to cephalosporin allergy is an example of nonpreventable ADRs (Kaushal et al., 2001). However, some ADRs can be prevented by understanding drug-drug or food-drug interactions (Polaka et al., 2022a,b). Aromatic polyanhydride and polyesters based on lactic acid and caprolactone showed interaction with the amine derivatives at pH 7.4; however, it can be prevented by using appropriate salt derivatives of the amines (Domb et al., 1994). Fig. 15.1 shows the relationship between adverse events, ADRs, and MEs.

15.2 History and scope

Many research teams have meticulously recorded, studied, analyzed, and published the magnitude and scope of MEs (Ganeshpurkar et al., 2018). For instance, in 2000, a critical study was published as "To Err is Human: Building a Safe Health System," conducted at the Institute of Medicine (now known as the National Academy of Medicine) in Washington DC. This study highlighted the existence, clinical significance, and economic burdens of ADEs due to ME hospitals (Donaldson et al., 2000).

Back in 1975, Institute for Safe Medication Practices (ISMP), Pennsylvania, developed a voluntary ME reporting system. This development was under the MEs Reporting Program of the ISMP. This system was the first of its kind, well-organized ME reporting system. ISMP is a global leader in providing information, data, and prevention of ADEs. After 1991, the MEs reporting program was transferred to the United States Pharmacopeia (USP) for further execution. The Food and Drug Administration (FDA) initiated a Medical Device Reporting program in 1984 for reporting device-related adverse events by the manufacturer to the FDA (Vaida, 2015a; Cohen, 2002).

After the amendment of the Safe Medical Device Act in 1990, all hospitals, nursing homes, and other such user facilities must report device-related severe injuries and death to the FDA as well as to the manufacturer. Under the Secretariat of USP and the various member organizations involved in health care, the National Coordinating Council for ME reporting and prevention (NCCMERP) was established in 1995. The Council has clear strategies for

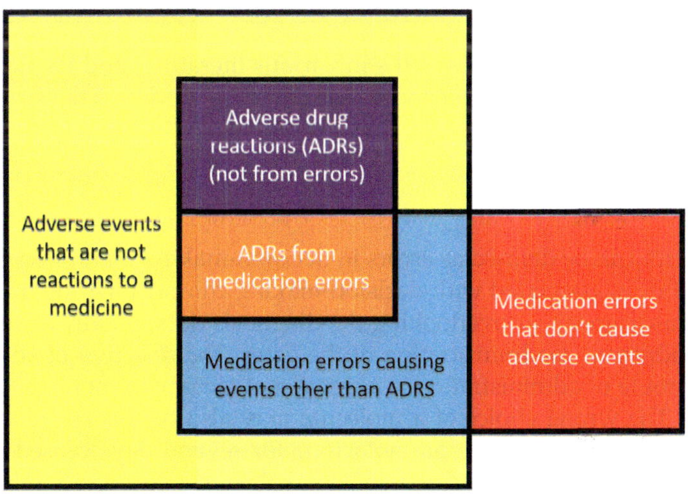

FIGURE 15.1 A venn diagram showing the relation between adverse events, adverse drug reactions, and MEs.

reporting, understanding, and preventing ME. The Council also established a record of reporting models. This establishment of the record is a noteworthy contribution, as it utilizes a computer-based tracking system to avoid ME in the entire healthcare system (Cousins and Heath, 2008).

In 1996, a US-based nonprofit organization, the Joint Commission on the Accreditation of Healthcare Organizations, initiated a sentinel event reporting system for hospitals. This organization accredits nearly 22,000 US healthcare organizations today. The National Academy for State Health Policy surveyed 50 states of the US in February 2000. The study found many ME reporting systems are categorized as mandatory by the state governments. These systems were also designed to track ADEs (Billstein-Leber et al., 2018; Cohen et al., 2018).

15.3 Consequences of MEs

On both the personal and corporate levels, ME has substantial consequences. However, personal-level consequences can be exemplified by more suffering, increased stay in the hospital, financial losses, a level of family and social disruption, loss of income sources, disabilities, or death. Not only the person but also the family suffer from the emotional and financial load. One must also remember the direct influence of ME on the healthcare professional. After the ME, healthcare professionals, especially nurses, reported a feeling of guilt and fear. Fear of disciplinary action and litigations after the incidence is another major problem faced by healthcare professionals. They also report the loss of self and clinical confidence and difficulties in recovering to a normal state due to the feeling of guilt and fear due to disciplinary action. Additional resource consumption and bed occupancy are also associated with financial burdens at the corporate level (Crossman, 2009).

15.4 Common types of MEs

Various researchers have classified MEs in various literature, and the number of ME classes is continuously increasing as per the individual case studies. The list of some common types of MEs is given in Fig. 15.2.

15.4.1 Prescribing errors

Prescribing error can be defined as errors in decision-making and/or writing prescriptions by a physician. Errors associated with decision-making comprise wrong drug choices for the patient due to misdiagnosis or overlooking the diagnosis data, mainly about the functioning of the liver or kidney or coadministration of the drug. The selection of an incorrect dose or nonappropriate route of administration is a significant factor commonly associated with prescription errors. The wrong choice of a molecule may also be associated with allergies and ADEs; for instance, a total dose of spironolactone for several days caused potassium depletion due to Liddle's syndrome and led to hypokalaemia. To correct this, when she took

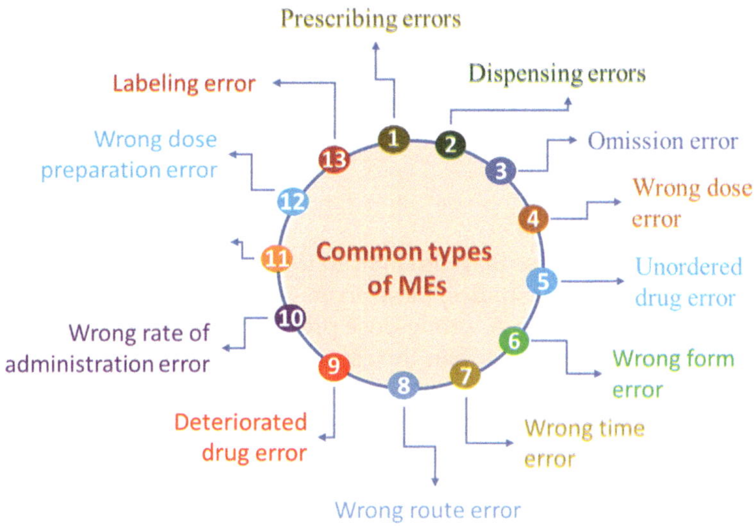

FIGURE 15.2 A list of some common types of MEs.

amiloride instead of spironolactone, her blood potassium level quickly increased to the normal range (Aronson, 2009). Errors associated with writing a prescription include unclear abbreviations, unreadability, inadequate information (e.g., prescribing date, route of administration, dose and dosing frequency), etc. (Dean et al., 2000).

15.4.2 Dispensing errors

Dispensing errors can be defined as errors in the wrong interpretation of prescriptions and/or inaccurate calculations in dispensing. These errors are referred to as pharmacy-linked MEs. However, dispensing errors due to inaccurate calculations are almost eliminated nowadays due to the reduced, almost ancient practice of dispensing prescriptions. Dispensing errors comprise the errors of commission and omission. For instance, errors of commission are due to dispensing the incorrect drug or the incorrect dose.

On the other hand, errors of omission are due to failure to counsel the patient about the safe use of the drug. Dispensing of the incorrect dosage form is also a common dispensing error. Investigators identified four prominent causes for dispensing errors: poor unreadable handwriting, look-alike or sound-alike drugs, ineffective controls, and poor alertness owing to interruptions. Further, dispensing errors are likely to be seen if ineligible prescriptions or verbal medication orders are given. These dispensing errors are commonly seen at the end of pharmacists if the drugs are look-alike or sound-alike (Roy et al., 2006). A study performed in the USA suggested that the workload of the pharmacist, as well as the automated telephone systems for prescription orders, were strongly responsible for dispensing medication errors and causing possible drug-drug interactions (Malone et al., 2007).

15.4.3 Omission error

This error may be seen when a hospital doctor forgets to order a crucial medicine that the patient is taking at home, when a nurse misses delivering a medication as directed, or when a chemist forgets to dispense a prescribed medication.

15.4.4 Wrong dose error

If a pharmacist provides a dose that differs from the ordered one is called an inappropriate dose error. In the various global studies, these errors were >17% for nonparenteral and more than 10% for parenteral products. A wrong dose prescribing error was reported in pediatrics as a dose that is 25% greater or less than the recommended dose (Ghaleb et al., 2005). Elsewhere, authors have suggested upper and lower limits for dose beyond which doses can be deemed inappropriate, such as infusion rates higher than 15% of the intentional rate, gentamicin as well as vancomycin doses less than or equal to 10% and 20% of the doses advised by guidelines, and doses of oral liquid medications less than or equal to 17% of the dose prescribed (Westbrook et al., 2011; Hamad et al., 2015; Allan and Barker, 1990).

15.4.5 Unordered drug error

If a drug is administered to a patient that is not prescribed for him is called an unordered drug error.

15.4.6 Wrong dosage form error

If a patient is given a different dosage form, then this error is called the wrong dosage form error.

15.4.7 Wrong time error

If the patient is administered the same drug and dose as prescribed but with a time deviation of more than 30 min is considered a wrong time error.

15.4.8 Wrong route error

If the patient is administered the same drug in the correct dose size but by a route other than ordered is called a wrong route error.

15.4.9 Deteriorated or expired drug error

It is called a deteriorated drug error if a patient is administered an expired or physically deteriorated drug dosage form. Usually, this type of error occurs owing to improper storage of formulations like wrong environmental conditions (i.e., temperature, humidity, etc.) and improper handling, which lead to deterioration or expiration of products.

15.4.10 Wrong rate of administration error

This error occurs when intravenous fluids or infusions are administered to a patient other than the prescribed rate.

15.4.11 Wrong administration technique error

Suppose the appropriate technique is not followed for administering the drug, for example, failing to wipe an injection site with alcohol before administering an injection. In that case, this error is termed the wrong administration technique error.

15.4.12 Wrong dose preparation error

Suppose a patient is administered the wrong dose at the time of drug administration. For example, administering an oral suspension without shaking the container is termed the wrong dose preparation error. In addition, the improper proportional mixing of solutions and powder as prescribed for pediatric patients will result in wrong dose preparation errors.

15.4.13 Labeling error

This type of error can be defined as if the formulation is labeled with incomplete or wrong labeling information. For instance, some ingredients are not printed, or the quantity of ingredients is missing, or the printed label is not correctly readable due to faint color. In addition, label missing any essential information regarding storage or usage instructions will also lead to labeling errors. Exchange of the labels is also possible. ME is possible due to failure to follow label instructions, for instance:

- **i.** Failure to "shake well."
- **ii.** Medications are taken with food or antacids.
- **iii.** Tablets to be used in the oral cavity should not be swallowed.
- **iv.** Use of inappropriate solvents, etc.

15.5 Causes of ME

Although possibilities of ME are at every step, from prescribing to use, it may be lethal for the patient. One must know the various causes behind it is to provide the patient the errorless therapy (Fig. 15.3). Some of the critical areas of potential causes of ME were identified by ISMP (ISMP, 2021).

15.5.1 Failed communication

It possibly causes ME due to unreadable handwriting or oral communications (majorly via telephonic), similar drug names (e.g., digoxin or digitoxin, epinephrine or nor

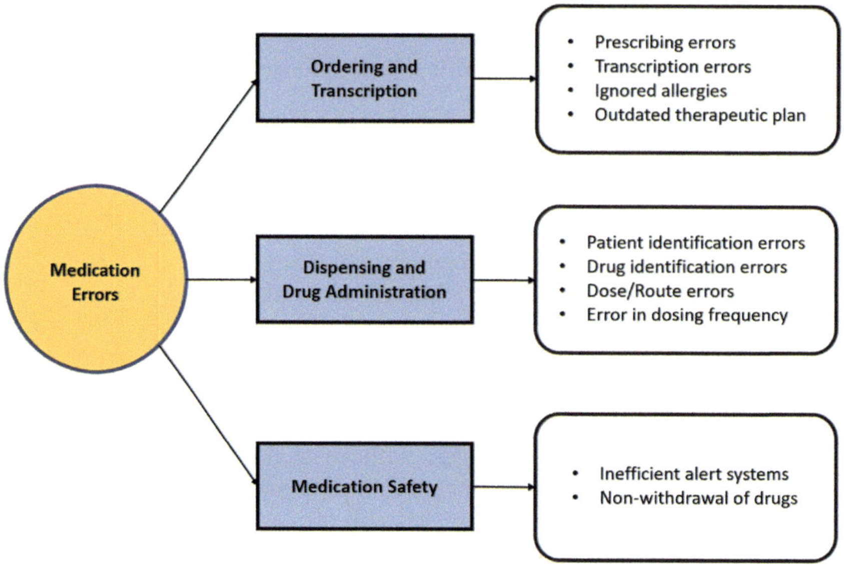

FIGURE 15.3 MEs commonly observed in any clinical setting along with their types.

epinephrine etc.), misplaced or missing zero or decimal points, and confusion between old and new measurements.

15.5.2 Incomplete patient information

If unknown or ignored, the medical information of the patient can cause ME, for example, coadministration of other drugs or ongoing drug therapies, allergic conditions, previous disease and therapies, pathological conditions, etc. Some fundamental causes of MEs are poor drug distribution practices, environmental conditions (e.g., extreme heat, moisture, and cold), workplace environment (e.g., job stress), technology design (e.g., poor or complex design), whether the drug access is provided to the nonpharma person, miscalculation of the dose, limited or incomplete information to the prescriber, and if the patient is lacking in understanding the therapy.

15.5.3 Possible factors for MEs by a pharmacist

There are various pharmacist-related factors that may lead to MEs (Fig. 15.4).

15.6 ME rate

The percentage error in treatment is expressed in terms of the ME rate. It is the ratio of total observed errors to the opportunities of error. Opportunities for errors include errors observed

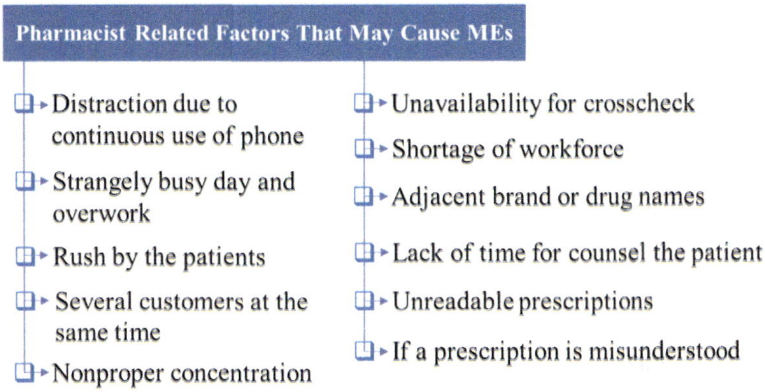

FIGURE 15.4 Various pharmacist-related factors that may cause MEs.

in the dose administered and in doses ordered but not administered. The ME rate can be determined by using the equation given below:

$$\text{ME rate} = \frac{\text{Number of Errors Observed}}{\text{Opportunities for Errors}} \times 100$$

15.7 Prevention of MEs

The top priority of a health professional is to prevent MEs. Prevention of ME is possible by the collective efforts of individuals and the use of technologies. In 1992, McGovern suggested 10 golden rules for safe drug administration (Fig. 15.5) (McGovern, 1992). The ISMP and

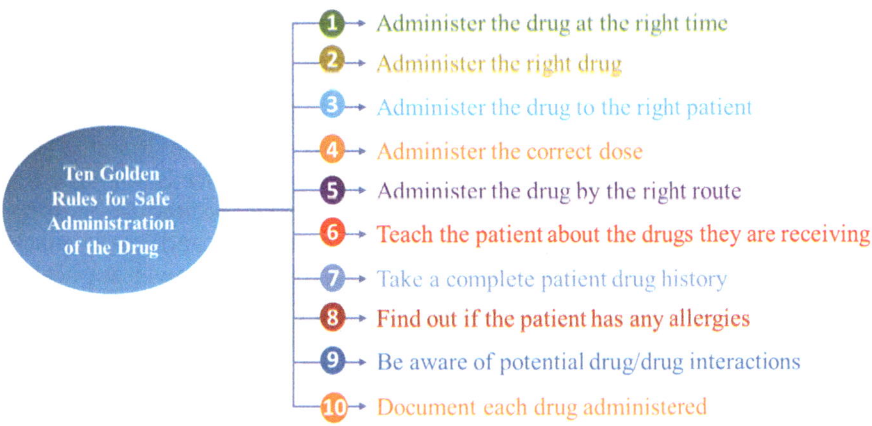

FIGURE 15.5 Ten golden rules for safe administration of the drug.

NCCMERP highlight the unreadable and unclear prescriptions that may result in injuries, short time, long time, partial or complete disabilities, or death of the patient (Vaida, 2015b).

15.7.1 Recommendations to enhance the accuracy of dispensing medications

The NCCMERP council issued recommendations for pharmacy staff involved in dispensing or dispatching the medications. These recommendations also apply to nursing staff that uses automated dispensing technologies and the nurses or healthcare managers that use pharmacy stock after hours. The points recommended by the NCCMERP council are given below:

i. To properly review the prescription or dispensing order by the pharmacist before dispensing.

ii. Unreadable, incomplete, or any other concern must be made clear by any established communication method between the prescriber and the pharmacist.

iii. To ensure the patient's recent profile, ensure sufficient information about him in the profile, which helps in deciding the prescription's appropriateness.

iv. To ensure the selection of appropriately designed areas for dispensing to prevent errors. An appropriate ideal area must contain sufficient light, air conditioning, and minimum noise level. These ergonomic features help in reducing fatigue conditions. In the ideal dispensing area, distraction can be minimized by avoiding the telephone, other personal interactions, and unrelated tasks. Sufficient staff and resources must also be provided in dispensing area for proper workload distribution.

v. To ensure the product inventory and its arrangements, which helps to differentiate medications from one another. The use of visual discriminations like markings and signs is recommended to identify the proper medicament. The importance of visual signs is highly impacted if confusion exists between strengths, a name that appears or sounds similar, or labels that look alike.

vi. To ensure the series of checks assigned to evaluate the dispensing process's accuracy before providing the medication to the patient. A compulsory check by the second individual is always recommended. With the increasing use of technologies, barcoding systems and computers are also included in record maintenance.

vii. Ensure the proper medicament by reading the labels of the containers thrice, initially while selecting, followed by at the time of dispensing, and finally while returning the container to the shelf.

viii. To ensure the replenishment of medication stock by either an automated dispensing machine or manually by pharmacy staff. Manual maintenance is suggested as a triple-check to confirm the accuracy of the product. This triple check must be done while selecting, after just before the product leaves the pharmacy, and finally placing the product in an automated dispensing machine or cabinet, wherever applicable.

ix. To ensure the proper counsel to the patient during product handover. Counseling is an excellent opportunity to recognize the patient's understanding of the proper use of medication. Counseling also provides an opportunity for the pharmacist to cross-check the dispensed medicines. Important points to be covered during counseling are described in Fig. 15.6.

x. To ensure the collection and analysis of data for potential and/or actual errors, which helps to improve the quality. An essential responsibility of the pharmacies includes providing feedback to the prescribers about errors and reporting the same to the national reporting programs and databases.

xi. To ensure the proper training of initial and ongoing staff. This training must comply with accepted standards of practice for dispensing procedures and include efforts to reduce ME.

xii. To ensure the establishment of policies and their implementation for dispensing medications. Policies must ensure that all the individuals involved, i.e., pharmacists, support, and relieving staff, must be informed of the dispensing procedure's expectations.

15.7.2 Recommendations to reduce MEs associated with verbal medication orders

Verbal medication orders are orders communicated orally between the receiver and sender directly, face-to-face, telephonically, or by any other auditory device. Although these types of orders are never encouraged as the medicines are lifesaving chemicals, considering the patient's situation and the nature of the therapy, verbal medication orders may sometimes be excepted. To reduce the ME, the following recommendations are advised:

i. The practice of verbal medication orders must be limited to urgent situations and avoided if immediate writing or electronic communication is available.

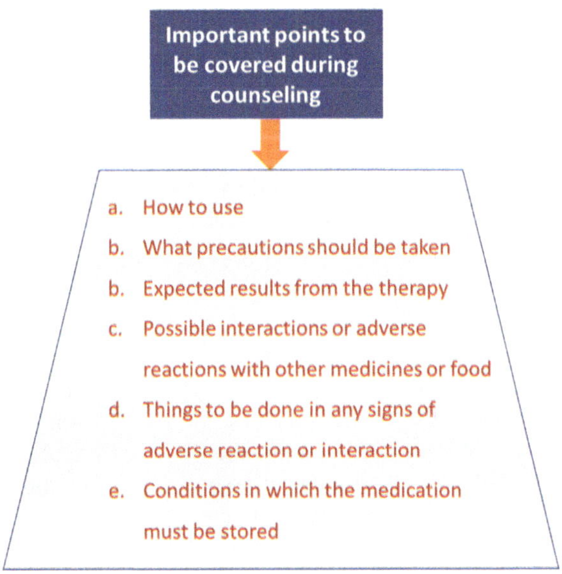

FIGURE 15.6 Important points to be covered during counseling of patients.

ii. Healthcare organizations must establish firm policies and procedures *by* considering some critical points, as described in Fig. 15.7.

iii. A culture in which pharmacists or other staff can question the prescriber when there is a query and/or disagreement should be vigorously promoted by the organizations, especially with verbal orders. Resolving the query related to verbal or any other medication order is a necessary step in the path of human health.

iv. As chemotherapeutic agents have a narrow margin of safety and are not used in emergencies, verbal communication should never be accepted in the case of medicines used for cancer therapy. The essentials to be included in a verbal order are listed in Fig. 15.8.

v. The content clarity in the communicated verbal orders should always be present.

a. The name of the drug should be confirmed by all the following means:
- Clear pronunciation and spelling
- Both brand and generic names can be asked
- Therapeutical use of the drug

b. Confusion in the spoken numbers must be avoided with clear discussions, like a dose such as 60 mg should be dictated as "60 milligrams or six 0 milligrams" to be differentiated from "16 milligrams or one 6 milligrams."

c. Additional spelling assistance is recommended to avoid confusion in drug name modifiers like prefixes and suffixes—an example of such can be "Pantop-D," D for Delhi.

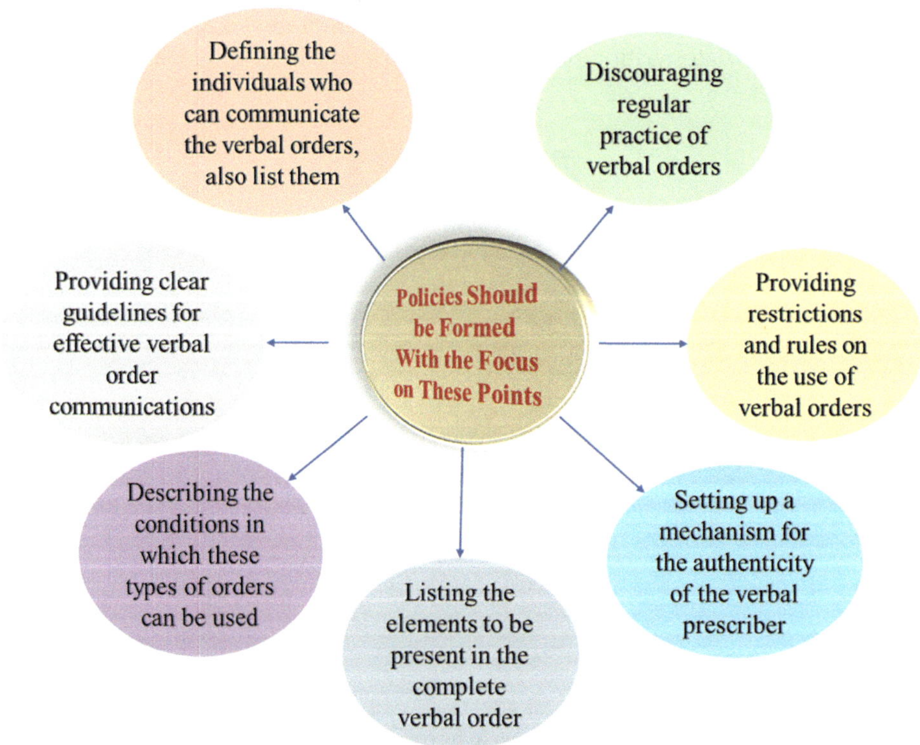

FIGURE 15.7 Policies should be formed with a focus on these points.

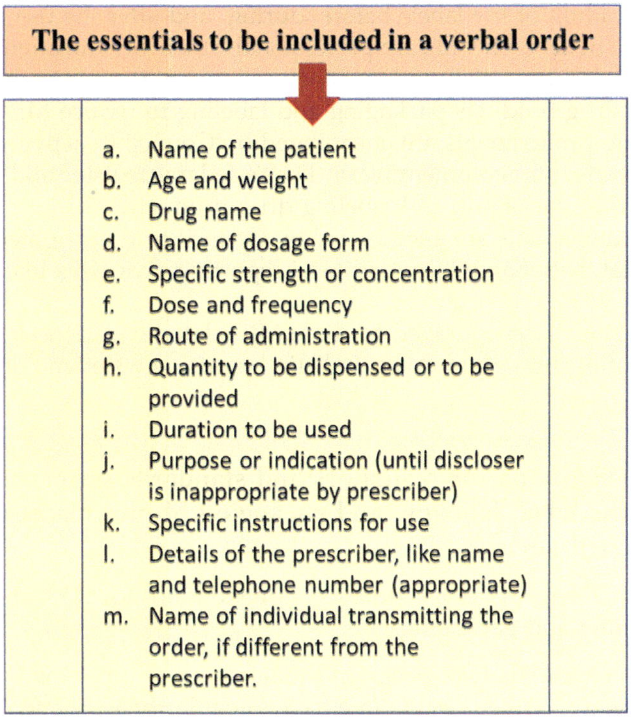

FIGURE 15.8 The list showing essentials to be included in a verbal order.

- **d.** With verbal medication orders, abbreviations should be avoided, especially in instructions for use. For example, the recommendation is to use "Take/give one tablet three times daily" in staid of "1 tab tid."
- **e.** If possible, the receiver of the verbal medication order should note down the complete order to enter the details in the computer and read it back for confirmation from the receiver.

vi. Verbal medication orders are recommended to be converted into written orders soon and signed by the receiver of the order.

vii. Documentation of countersigned verbal orders in the patient's medical record should be done as soon as possible.

15.7.3 Recommendations for healthcare professionals to reduce MEs associated with the label, labeling, and packaging of pharmaceutical (drug) products and related devices

Regulatory authorities such as the FDA, USP, and experts have provided recommendations for prescribers, including physicians, pharmacists, nurses, and other health professionals handling prescriptions and medicines.

i. Three times reading of the labels before, during, and after the use is recommended.
ii. Collaborations between healthcare professionals, their organizations, pharmaceutical industries, regulating bodies, and standard-setters are recommended to simplify the design of the drug products packaging and labeling to reduce ME.
iii. The health care professionals are encouraged by Council to active participation in proposing, reviewing, and commenting on FDA's federal register and US pharmacopeial forums related to packaging and labeling drug products.
iv. Healthcare professionals are encouraged by Council to report potential and actual ME to international, national, internal, or local reporting programs like MedWatch or USP-ISMP.
v. Council members are encouraged to share ME-related experiences, case studies, or other such stories through journals, bulletin boards, newsletters, or the internet.

15.7.4 Recommendations for regulators and standards setters to prevent MEs associated with the label, labeling, and packaging of pharmaceutical (drug) products and related devices

NCCMERP council has suggested some recommendations for FDA and USP to reduce the ME related to labeling and packaging.

i. The error prevention analysis program's maintenance by FDA is fortified by the NCCMERP council, which results in effective regularity assessment of the packaging and labeling of drug products to reduce the ME associated with product design.
ii. The size of the company logo is an excellent strategy for brand marketing, but its size on the printed label should not be larger than the typed size of the drug name; it helps to reduce the ME. The Council recommends that the FDA takes care of the same at the end of pharmaceutical manufacturers.
iii. Innovative labeling, which helps distinguish between drug products, must be encouraged by standard setters and regulators recommended by Council.
iv. The Council recommends that FDA encourage printing of both brand and generic drug names and dose/strength on both sides of containers and overwraps. In large-volume parenteral, the name and strength should be readable in upright and inverted positions.
v. Council recommends advisability and examination feasibility of tactile signs (any sign that can be read by touch) in the packaging container of the drug product by the FDA and USP. Cues can be included in the label if not designed in the containers.
vi. The formation of an advisory panel jointly or individually by the FDA or/and USP is recommended by Council, especially for simplifying labeling for injections.
vii. Consideration by the FDA and USP for expanding the simplification concept in the packaging and labeling of drug products is encouraged by the Council.
viii. Alerting the healthcare professionals about proposed regulations and standards by FDA and USP is encouraged by Council.

ix. The Council encourages collaboration among standards-setters, regulators, manufacturers, healthcare organizations, and professionals to enable the design of packaging and labeling of drug products to help minimize ME.

15.7.5 Roles of pharmacists to prevent MEs according to American society of Health-System Pharmacist guidelines

The pharmacist is the direct link between the prescriber and patients, and he plays a vital role in dispensing and patient compliance with drug safety and rational use. The pharmacist is best positioned to inform other health professionals about ME and how to prevent it. Participation of the pharmacist in various policies for patient care development is required to raise the points of one of the most critical patient prescriber links. Every healthcare organization must establish a minimum acceptable level of participation by the pharmacist in preventing errors in the care of patients (Kohler et al., 2002; Billstein-Leber et al., 2018). This participation must be but is not limited to, proactively reviewing medication orders, screening laboratory results, conveying information related to drugs, patient counseling, and reviewing drug storage conditions. Participation of pharmacists should be recommended in the following areas:

i. Educate the other healthcare professionals (e.g., nurses, pharmacists, etc.) about ME.
ii. Verification of medication dosages, schedules, and routes of administration, independently.
iii. Contribute to multidisciplinary efforts to create drug-specific application constraints, especially in deciding maximum dose and dosage regimens for medications.
iv. Contribute to multidisciplinary efforts to regulate the prescribing terminology (e.g., OD, BD, etc.).
v. Contribute to multidisciplinary efforts to educate patients and their families.
vi. Contribute to improving communication between patients and health care providers.

15.8 Use of computers and information technology in error prevention

Computer use in our day-to-day life and healthcare organizations is gaining pace with increasing advances in computer-based technologies. A few advantages of computerized prescribing systems are legible and complete, a precise selection of standard dosages, and a prescriber's identification. Error-prone manual paper transcriptions can be eliminated due to the use of these computerized prescribing systems. These systems also offer control on effective drug administration through regular entries by the health care staff, usually done after every dose given to every patient. Drug-drug interactions and warnings associated with them can be highlighted by incorporating artificial intelligence (AI) through these systems. Fig. 15.9 shows various applications of computer-based technologies in the prevention of ME.

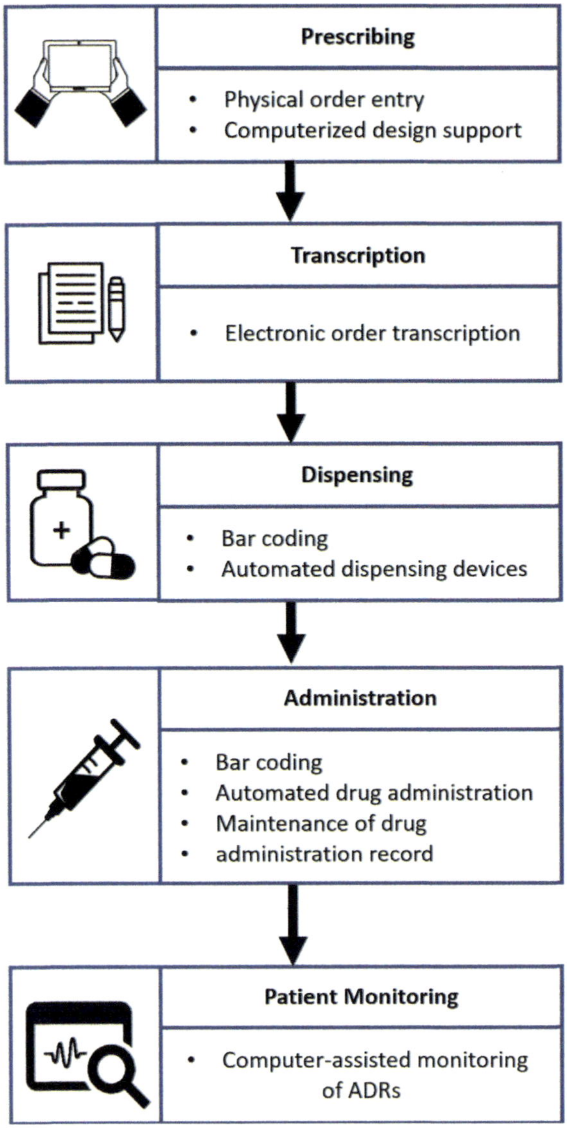

FIGURE 15.9 Role of computers and information technology (by stage) in ME prevention. *ADRs*, adverse drug reactions.

15.8.1 For in-patient setting

ME can be reduced with the help of the powerful tool of information technology. Examples of interventions include:

i. Computerized physician order entry (CPOE) and decision support.
ii. Computerized medication administration records.

iii. Automated pharmacy systems.
iv. Barcoding.
v. "Smart" intravenous devices and computerized discharge prescriptions and instructions.

15.8.1.1 CPOE and decision support

Improved drug safety can be mediated by the powerful practice of computerization of medical orders. Handwritten orders may be incorrect or incomplete in dose, route, or dosage regimen. These handwritten orders may also contain illegible orders or nonstandard terminology (Koppel et al., 2008). Such MEs can be logically intervened by computerized medication order as it is in a standard format. Today's latest technologies combined with AI, like clinical decision support, incorporate significant value to CPOE by giving opinions to the doctor. At the same time, preparation of medical orders.AI can help analyze the ordered drug with characteristics of patients such as weight, co-administered drugs, reported or potential allergies, and laboratory test values. AI also helps to reduce prescribing errors by suggesting appropriate doses, routes, and dosage regimens to prescribers.

A well-known case of ME leading to an infant's death due to an incorrect administration route as prescribing error occurred in Denver in 1996, as benzathine penicillin was administered IV instead of IM. The incidence could have been prevented if the computerized forcing function had been used during the ordering medication (Kowalski and Horner, 1998). A report published by Bates et al. analyzed the first reduction of 64% in all ME in a hospital for adults, using essential decision support of CPOE, and a reduction of 83% using advanced decision support of CPOE (Bates et al., 1998).

In a well-designed series of studies conducted in Salt Lake city's LDS hospital, researchers verified the significant reduction in antibiotic-associated ME and ADEs due to a computerized clinical decision support program, which reduced the medication cost. From the developer's point of view, effective design and implication of decision support CPOE system are more complex than designing for adults, as the dose depends not only on the weight but also on a few factors. For example, a pediatric computer application should permit simple refreshing of a patient's weight, a day-to-day prerequisite for neonates. Other pathological test values for confirming renal impairment, like varying creatinine levels to higher ranges with child development, require altered checks. These issues recommend that CPOE, with decision support with proper design, may be particularly beneficial for the pediatric use of medications.

15.8.1.2 Computerization of the medication administration record

Coupling computerized medication administration records with CPOE can dispose of numerous transcription errors, a typical kind of medicinal error, and takes into consideration cumulative dose checking, which is especially significant for medications administered based on need.

15.8.1.3 Automated dispensing

Many hospitals generally use automated machines, like robots, to fasten and automate the prescription form filling by using bar codes to recognize medications.

15.8.1.4 Automated drug administration

Administration errors can be reduced using automated pharmacy systems containing computer-controlled devices for packaging, dispensing, distribution, and/or controlling the medications. Barker et al. (Allan and Barker, 1990) 1969 published a study that states the incorporation of a medication profile-linked dispensing envelope system leads to drop down the medication administration error from 13% to 1.9. They reported that an automated dispensing device at the bedside could reduce time and omit errors. The device works on alarming sounds when it is due time for medication and aid with restricted access to particular medicines.

15.8.1.5 Bar coding

Medication administration error rates can also be reduced with the implication of barcoding. But due to the nonuniform approach by pharmaceutical companies, barcoding is not very common in medicines. Due to reduce ME, individual approaches by the hospitals have been made; some worked at relatively modest expense. Identification of drug, dose, time of administration, patient's name, and staff name can be rapidly identified using a barcode. Due to the limited communication skills of pediatric patients, exact matching of the drugs is essential and can be improved by barcoding (Chester and Zilz, 1989).

15.8.1.6 Computerized discharge prescriptions and instructions

Communication errors can be reduced further by using computerized discharge letters for ambulatory patients. AI can also help prescribers to write medical instructions for discharge prescriptions. If an integrated computer system exists, discharge information can be easily shared among the in-patient, out-patient, and emergency departments.

15.8.2 For out-patient setting

The problems associated with ordering medication by a physician for ambulatory patients are different than in-patients. Ambulatory MEs can be reduced by computerized transcription with a direct relay of entered orders to a chosen pharmacy. The use of automated machines like robots could help pharmacists here. At the administering stage, particular information technology interventions are required for pediatrics (Kaushal et al., 2001).

15.8.3 Other recommendations to prevent MEs

15.8.3.1 Clinician and patient education

Clinicians should have easy excess to drug information. Data availability is basic for rarely used, or non-formulary medications since practitioners might be new to their utilization. Sources of information can be tertiary references, online sources of information, newsletters, and/or pharmacist input during patient care. As per the report of Leape et al. for the MEs analysis, around 29% of the 334 errors was due to the dissemination of drug knowledge serving as the most common cause for the same (Leape et al., 1995).

It is assessed that 9 out of 10 adults come up short on abilities to deal with their well-being of health and prevent disease (Kutner et al., 2007). In a 659 public medical clinic patients study, patients with deficient health proficiency abilities were bound to confound (Williams et al., 1995). It has been laid out that the detection of preventable ADEs can be done by advising the patients on their medications. Also, patient mentalities and beliefs toward medications influence medication adherence. Organizations should overcome this gap by bridging the gaps by improving communication and health education.

15.8.3.2 High-risk medications and vulnerable populations

Organizations should identify a list of "high-alert" medications in case any ME is associated with significant harm to the patient (Saedder et al., 2014). Specific consideration should be put on medications administered via the parenteral route. Approaches should be made to address the medication use process related to utilizing these medications and give the essential information about drug information for the appropriate use of medications. The utilization of medication in weak populations should also be addressed. Preparing standard concentrations and restricting formulary is reasonable for all populations yet especially significant in the pediatric population to diminish the probability of mischief coming about because of MEs.

Similarly, recognizing possibly inappropriate medication use in the elderly can limit numerous potentially unwanted drug toxicity (Waller and Maclean, 2003).

15.8.3.3 Formulary management

Formulary management can serve as a potent tool for lowering MEs. Drugs that are old or give a more significant potential for harm versus benefit than comparative/alternative medications should be rethought for formulary inclusion. Numerous preventable ADEs are dosage-related; therefore, consideration should be placed on limiting the dosage of the formulary (Karel et al., 2017).

A summary of factors that contribute to medication and steps that can be implemented to mitigate them has been discussed in Table 15.1.

TABLE 15.1 A summary of factors contributing to medication and steps that can be implemented to mitigate them.

Contributing factors	Prevention strategies
Performance lapse	• Use a peer review process to dissect MEs and address performance issues. • Review health records to identify and address performance lapses.
Lack of knowledge	• Clinician and patient education with tailored attention to specific populations. • Use various methods to relay information throughout the facility. • Incorporate pharmacists into patient care teams.
Lack/failure of safety system	• CPOE. • Barcode medication administration. • Identification of high-risk medications and populations. • Formulary management. • Review health records to identify system failures.

15.8.4 Gathering data

The purposes for gathering data on MEs are essential to detect errors, estimate the frequency of specific errors, assess the effects of changes to the system, and monitor system performance over time. While there are several available approaches to gathering data on MEs, all voluntary reporting is the most common. The voluntary reporting processes generally involve four necessary steps:

i. Error recognition
ii. Assessment of the need to report the error
iii. Incident report preparation
iv. Follow-up response by the party receiving the report

15.9 Recognized medical and ME reporting systems

The most current list of recognized medical and ME reporting systems utilized in the US and internationally (Carothers, 1998) is as follows:

i. State Adverse Event Tracking
ii. FDA
iii. MedWatch
iv. Adverse Event Reporting System
v. Center for Biologics Evaluation and Research
vi. Center for Error and Accident Reporting System
vii. Vaccine Adverse Event Reporting System
viii. Manufacturer and User Device Experience Database
ix. Joint Commission on Accreditation of Healthcare Organizations Sentinel Event Reporting
x. USP-ISMP ME Reporting Program
xi. USP MedMarx
xii. Emergency Care Research Institute Medical Device Safety Reports

15.10 Conclusion

MEs are currently the most critical issue in the healthcare system and profession because of various severe consequences. Prevention of these errors is necessary to save lives, enhance efficiency, and improve the quality of patient care. Various councils and healthcare societies (e.g., NCCMERP and ISMP) give recommendations for preventing these errors and encouraging safe healthcare practices. Computers and Information technology interventions have great potential for reducing the frequency of errors. It includes CPOE, Computerized medication administration records, Automated pharmacy systems, etc.

In India, most of the errors are caused due to the illegibility of prescriptions; computerized prescribing systems are beneficial for preventing these errors. They are complete and legible, standard dosages can be automatically provided, and the doctor prescribing can be identified at any time. Computers are also helpful in gathering data on MEs and therefore detecting and eradicating them.

15.11 List of abbreviations

ADEs adverse drug events
AI artificial intelligence
CPOE Computerized Physician Order Entry
FDA Food and Drug Administration
ISMP Institute for Safe Medication Practices
ME medication errors
NCCMERP National Coordinating Council for ME Reporting and Prevention
US United States
USP United States Pharmacopeia

References

Allan, E.L., Barker, K.N., 1990. Fundamentals of medication error research. Am. J. Hosp. Pharm. 47 (3), 555–571. https://www.ncbi.nlm.nih.gov/pubmed/2180287.

Aronson, J.K., 2009. Medication errors: what they are, how they happen, and how to avoid them. QJM 102 (8), 513–521. https://www.ncbi.nlm.nih.gov/pubmed/19458202.

Aseeri, M., Banasser, G., Baduhduh, O., Baksh, S., Ghalibi, N., 2020. Evaluation of medication error incident reports at a tertiary care hospital. Pharmacy 8 (2).

BBC News, 2006. NHS Drug Error 'crackdown'urged. http://news.bbc.co.uk/1/hi/health/4780487.stm. (Accessed 16 August 2022).

Bates, D.W., Boyle, D.L., Vander Vliet, M.B., Schneider, J., Leape, L., 1995. Relationship between medication errors and adverse drug events. J. Gen. Intern. Med. 10 (4), 199–205.

Bates, D.W., Leape, L.L., Cullen, D.J., Laird, N., Petersen, L.A., Teich, J.M., Burdick, E., Hickey, M., Kleefield, S., Shea, B., Vander Vliet, M., Seger, D.L., 1998. Effect of computerized physician order entry and a team intervention on prevention of serious medication errors. JAMA 280 (15), 1311–1316. https://www.ncbi.nlm.nih.gov/pubmed/9794308.

Billstein-Leber, M., Carrillo, C.J.D., Cassano, A.T., Moline, K., Robertson, J.J., 2018. ASHP guidelines on preventing medication errors in hospitals. Am. J. Health Syst. Pharm. 75 (19), 1493–1517. https://www.ncbi.nlm.nih.gov/pubmed/30257844.

Carothers, N.B., 1998. Medication errors: the problem and its scope. Int. J. Trauma Nurs. 4 (3), 104–108. https://www.ncbi.nlm.nih.gov/pubmed/9855978.

Chester, M.I., Zilz, D.A., 1989. Effects of bar coding on a pharmacy stock replenishment system. Am. J. Hosp. Pharm. 46 (7), 1380–1385. https://www.ncbi.nlm.nih.gov/pubmed/2757044.

Cohen, M., 2002. Institute for safe medication practices. In: Encyclopedia of Clinical Pharmacy. CRC Press. https://doi.org/10.1201/b13789-80.

Cohen, M.R., Smetzer, J.L., Vaida, A.J., 2018. ASHP guidelines on preventing medication errors in hospitals: advancing medication safety to the next level. Am. J. Health Syst. Pharm. 75 (19), 1444–1445.

Cousins, D.D., Heath, W.M., 2008. The national coordinating council for medication error reporting and prevention: promoting patient safety and quality through innovation and leadership. Joint Comm. J. Qual. Patient Saf. 34 (12), 700–702. https://doi.org/10.1016/s1553-7250(08)34091-4.

Crespin, D.J., Modi, A.V., Wei, D., Williams, C.E., Greene, S.B., Pierson, S., Hansen, R.A., 2010. Repeat medication errors in nursing homes: contributing factors and their association with patient harm. Am. J. Geriatr. Pharmacother. 8 (3), 258–270.

Crossman, M., 2009. Technical and environmental impact on medication error in paramedic practice: a review of causes, consequences and strategies for prevention. Australas. J. Paramed. 7 (3).

Dean, B., Barber, N., Schachter, M., 2000. What is a prescribing error? BMJ Qual. Saf. 9 (4), 232–237.
Domb, A.J., Turovsky, L., Nudelman, R., 1994. Chemical interactions between drugs containing reactive amines with hydrolyzable insoluble biopolymers in aqueous solutions. Pharm. Res. (N. Y.) 11 (6), 865–868. https://www.ncbi.nlm.nih.gov/pubmed/7937527.
Donaldson, M.S., Corrigan, J.M., Kohn, L.T., 2000. To Err Is Human: Building a Safer Health System.
Ferner, R.E., Aronson, J.K., 2006. Clarification of terminology in medication errors: definitions and classification. Drug Saf. 29 (11), 1011–1022. https://www.ncbi.nlm.nih.gov/pubmed/17061907.
Flynn, E.A., Barker, K.N., Carnahan, B.J., 2003. National observational study of prescription dispensing accuracy and safety in 50 pharmacies. J. Am. Pharmaceut. Assoc. 43 (2), 191–200. https://www.ncbi.nlm.nih.gov/pubmed/12688437.
Ganeshpurkar, A., Maheshwari, R., Tekade, M., Tekade, R.K., 2018. Concepts of hypothesis testing and types of errors. In: Tekade, R.K. (Ed.), Dosage Form Design Parameters. Academic Press, pp. 257–280. http://www.sciencedirect.com/science/article/pii/B9780128144213000075.
Ghaleb, M.A., Barber, N., Dean Franklin, B., Wong, I.C., 2005. What constitutes a prescribing error in paediatrics? Qual. Saf. Health Care 14 (5), 352–357. https://www.ncbi.nlm.nih.gov/pubmed/16195569.
Gillani, S.W., Gulam, S.M., Thomas, D., Gebreighziabher, F.B., Al-Salloum, J., Assadi, R.A., Sam, K.G., 2021. Role and services of a pharmacist in the prevention of medication errors: a systematic review. Curr. Drug Saf. 16 (3), 322–328.
Hamad, A., Cavell, G., Hinton, J., Wade, P., Whittlesea, C., 2015. A pre-postintervention study to evaluate the impact of dose calculators on the accuracy of gentamicin and vancomycin initial doses. BMJ Open 5 (6), e006610. https://www.ncbi.nlm.nih.gov/pubmed/26044758.
Ibrahim, O.M., Ibrahim, R.M., Meslamani, A.Z.A., Mazrouei, N.A., 2020. Dispensing errors in community pharmacies in the United Arab Emirates: investigating incidence, types, severity, and causes. Pharm. Pract. 18 (4), 2111. https://www.ncbi.nlm.nih.gov/pubmed/33149793.
Isaacs, A.N., Ch'ng, K., Delhiwale, N., Taylor, K., Kent, B., Raymond, A., 2021. Hospital medication errors: a cross-sectional study. Int. J. Qual. Health Care 33 (1).
ISMP, 2021. Error Reporting, Institute of Safe Medication Practices. https://www.ismp.org/report-medication-error. (Accessed 28 May 2021).
Karel, L.I., Delisle, D.R., Anagnostis, E.A., Wordell, C.J., 2017. Implementation of a formulary management process. Am. J. Health Syst. Pharm. 74 (16), 1245–1252. https://www.ncbi.nlm.nih.gov/pubmed/28790076.
Kaushal, R., Barker, K.N., Bates, D.W., 2001. How can information technology improve patient safety and reduce medication errors in children's health care? Arch. Pediatr. Adolesc. Med. 155 (9), 1002–1007.
Kefale, B., Degu, A., Tegegne, G.T., 2020. Medication-related problems and adverse drug reactions in Ethiopia: a systematic review. Pharmacol. Res. Perspect. 8 (5), e00641.
Kohler, D.R., Montello, M., Goldspiel, B.R., DeChristoforo, R., Huntley, C., High, J., Fallavollita Jr., A., Shalabi, A., Meadows, B., Green, L., 2002. ASHP guidelines on preventing medication errors with antineoplastic agents. Am. J. Health Syst. Pharm. 59 (17), 1648–1668.
Koppel, R., Leonard, C.E., Localio, A.R., Cohen, A., Auten, R., Strom, B.L., 2008. Identifying and quantifying medication errors: evaluation of rapidly discontinued medication orders submitted to a computerized physician order entry system. J. Am. Med. Inf. Assoc. 15 (4), 461–465. https://www.ncbi.nlm.nih.gov/pubmed/18436910.
Kowalski, K., Horner, M.D., 1998. A legal nightmare. Denver nurses indicted. MCN Am. J. Matern./Child Nurs. 23 (3), 125–129. https://www.ncbi.nlm.nih.gov/pubmed/9595908.
Kutner, M., Greenberg, E., Jin, Y., Boyle, B., Hsu, Y-c, Dunleavy, E., 2007. Literacy in Everyday Life: Results from the 2003 National Assessment of Adult Literacy. NCES 2007-490. National Center for Education Statistics.
Leape, L., Bates, D., Cullen, D., 1995. Systems analysis of adverse drug evemts, ADE Prevention Study Group. JAMA 27, 218.
Malone, D.C., Abarca, J., Skrepnek, G.H., Murphy, J.E., Armstrong, E.P., Grizzle, A.J., Rehfeld, R.A., Woosley, R.L., 2007. Pharmacist workload and pharmacy characteristics associated with the dispensing of potentially clinically important drug-drug interactions. Med. Care 45 (5), 456–462.
McGovern, K., 1992. 10 golden rules for administering drugs safely. Nursing 22 (3), 49–56. https://www.ncbi.nlm.nih.gov/pubmed/1553091.
Neal, J.M., Neal, E.J., Weinberg, G.L., 2021. American society of regional anesthesia and pain medicine local anesthetic systemic toxicity checklist: 2020 version. Reg. Anesth. Pain Med. 46 (1), 81–82.

Polaka, S., Koppisetti, H.P., Tekade, M., Sharma, M.C., Sengupta, P., Tekade, R.K., 2022a. Drug–drug interactions and their implications on the pharmacokinetics of the drugs. In: Tekade, R.K. (Ed.), Pharmacokinetics and Toxicokinetic Considerations, vol. 2. Academic Press, pp. 291–322. https://www.sciencedirect.com/science/article/pii/B978032398367900007X.

Polaka, S., Rajpoot, K., Tekade, M., Sharma, M.C., Tekade, R.K., 2022b. Food–drug interactions and their implications on oral drug bioavailability. In: Tekade, R.K. (Ed.), Pharmacokinetics and Toxicokinetic Considerations, vol. 2. Academic Press, pp. 263–289. https://www.sciencedirect.com/science/article/pii/B9780323983679000020.

Roy, V., Gupta, P., Srivastava, S., 2006. Medication errors: causes & prevention. Health Adm. 19 (1), 60–64.

Saedder, E.A., Brock, B., Nielsen, L.P., Bonnerup, D.K., Lisby, M., 2014. Identifying high-risk medication: a systematic literature review. Eur. J. Clin. Pharmacol. 70 (6), 637–645. https://www.ncbi.nlm.nih.gov/pubmed/24671697.

Tariq, R.A., Vashisht, R., Sinha, A., Scherbak, Y., 2022. Medication dispensing errors and prevention. In: StatPearls. StatPearls Publishing LLC, Treasure Island (FL). https://pubmed.ncbi.nlm.nih.gov/30085607/.

Vaida, A.J., 2015a. The institute for safe medication practices and poison control centers: collaborating to prevent medication errors and unintentional poisonings. J. Med. Toxicol. 11 (2), 262–264. https://www.ncbi.nlm.nih.gov/pubmed/25840933.

Vaida, A.J., 2015b. The institute for safe medication practices and poison control centers: collaborating to prevent medication errors and unintentional poisonings. J. Med. Toxicol. 2, 262–264. Springer.

Waller, J.L., Maclean, J.R., 2003. Updating the Beers criteria for potentially inappropriate medication use in older adults. Arch. Intern. Med. 163, 2716–2724.

Westbrook, J.I., Rob, M.I., Woods, A., Parry, D., 2011. Errors in the administration of intravenous medications in hospital and the role of correct procedures and nurse experience. BMJ Qual. Saf. 20 (12), 1027–1034. https://www.ncbi.nlm.nih.gov/pubmed/21690248.

Williams, M.V., Parker, R.M., Baker, D.W., Parikh, N.S., Pitkin, K., Coates, W.C., Nurss, J.R., 1995. Inadequate functional health literacy among patients at two public hospitals. JAMA 274 (21), 1677–1682.

Zirpe, K.G., Seta, B., Gholap, S., Aurangabadi, K., Gurav, S.K., Deshmukh, A.M., Wankhede, P., Suryawanshi, P., Vasanth, S., Kurian, M., Philip, E., Jagtap, N., Pandit, E., 2020. Incidence of medication error in critical care unit of a tertiary care hospital: where do we stand? Indian J. Crit. Care Med. 24 (9), 799–803. https://www.ncbi.nlm.nih.gov/pubmed/33132563.

CHAPTER

16

Understanding the bioaccumulation of pharmaceuticals and personal care products

Amarjitsing P. Rajput[1,2], *Madhur Kulkarni*[3], *Prashant L. Pingale*[4], *Muktika Tekade*[5], *Ashok K. Shakya*[6] *and Rakesh Kumar Tekade*[7]

[1]Nanomedicine Laboratory, Department of Biosciences and Bioengineering, Indian Institute of Technology Bombay, Mumbai, Maharashtra, India; [2]Department of Pharmaceutics, Poona College of Pharmacy, Bharti Vidyapeeth Deemed University, Pune, Maharashtra, India; [3]SCES's Indira College of Pharmacy, Pune, Maharashtra, India; [4]Department of Pharmaceutics, GES's Sir Dr. M. S. Gosavi College of Pharmaceutical Education and Research, Nashik, Maharashtra, India; [5]School of Pharmacy, Devi Ahilya Vishwavidyalaya, Indore, Madhya Pradesh, India; [6]Pharmacological and Diagnostic Research Center, Faculty of Pharmacy, Al-Ahliyya Amman University, Amman, Jordan; [7]National Institute of Pharmaceutical Education and Research (NIPER)- Ahmedabad, An Institute of National Importance, Government of India, Department of Pharmaceuticals, Ministry of Chemicals and Fertilizers, Palaj, Gandhinagar, Gujarat, India

16.1 Introduction

During the 19th and 20th centuries, further industrial growth resulted in economic and technological advancement. The development in industrial and technical aspects of various practices and materials resulted in unwanted substances entering the environment without any precautionary measures (Singh et al., 2013). Therefore, in the last century, due to pollution, various complications in patients have been reported, such as 41,996,260 acute (respiratory) infection cases and 3740 deaths in 2018 in India in the National Health Profile. About

Essentials of Pharmatoxicology in Drug Research, Volume 1
https://doi.org/10.1016/B978-0-443-15840-7.00024-5

69% of all communicable disease cases and 23% of such deaths were reported in 2017 (News, November 13, 2019).

Increased industrial development leads to increased ambient metal concentrations liberated into the atmosphere and aggregated in water bodies' soil and sediments (Alonso Castillo et al., 2013; Yi et al., 2011). Some of the most found materials (trace) include cadmium (Cd), arsenic (As), chromium (Cr), zinc (Zn), copper (Cu), mercury (Hg), and lead (Pb) (Chen et al., 2017; Yi et al., 2011). In addition, contaminants of emerging concerns (CECs), mostly pharmaceutical and personal care products (PPCPs), have attained more worries in the last few years because of their probable effects on human health. The United States Environmental Protection Agency (USEPA) describes PPCPs as any substance used in agriculture to enhance growth or health by any individual for personal health or cosmetic purposes (US EPA, 2007).

One of the significant issues of the PPCPs is that they readily dissolve in water and do not undergo evaporation under normal circumstances. This results in easy entry of PPCPs into our water system via different pathways. The production of PPCPs has surpassed 106 tons globally (Richardson et al., 2005), and around 6 million PPCP compounds commercially exist (Ellis, 2006). Although PPCPs are an emerging issue, their impacts have not yet been addressed, they are not known to affect human health. However, pharmaceuticals are made to modify the biological activity and introduce PPCPs into the environment, causing adverse effects due to changes in the physiological and biochemical functions of animals and microbial communities (Spongberg and Witter, 2008).

16.2 Mechanism for the removal of pharmaceuticals and personal care products

The various mechanisms used to remove PPCPs with microorganisms such as bacteria, fungi, or microalgae are the same and consist of biosorption, bioaccumulation, biodegradation, photodegradation, and volatilization (Matamoros et al., 2016). Hena et al. demonstrated the removal of metronidazole using deposition on polymeric (Exo) compounds of *Chlorella vulgaris* (Hena et al., 2020). Similarly, Yu et al. confirmed the assistance of microalgae for the exclusion of micropollutants in the following three stages:

(i) More rapid adsorption is followed by physiochemical connections between the pollutants and the cell wall.
(ii) The passage of molecules through the cell wall is significantly slow.
(iii) Lastly, removal by biodegradation and bioaccumulation of both mechanisms (Yu et al., 2017).

16.2.1 Bioaccumulation

Bioaccumulation (increased concentration of chemicals) is characterized as the aggregation technique of chemical compounds in the body over time. Bioaccumulation is defined by the International Union of Pure and Applied Chemistry (IUPAC) as the direct intake from the atmospheric matrix (known as bioconcentration) and intake from food, the aggregation of biochemical substances in a microorganism (known as biomagnification). Bioaccumulation occurs when the elimination is overcome by intake (Eq. 16.1):

$$\text{Bioaccumulation} = \text{Rate of intake} - \text{Rate of elimination} \tag{16.1}$$

Parameters such as physical, chemical, and biological affect the bioaccumulation and chemical bioavailability of substances. Determining the chemical content at the site of accumulation aids in measuring the amount of bioaccumulation.

16.2.1.1 Bioaccumulation mechanisms

Bioaccumulation uses complex webs of food. The species that remain in the upper part of the chain (food) have more chemical concentrations in their bodies (especially tissues). It all depends on the feeding behaviors, place, and metabolic activities of the species. The bioaccumulated material is metabolized into derivatives relative to the parent compound, which can be considered more lethal; e.g., less-lethal mercury (inorganic) is metabolized into extra-lethal methylmercury. Bioaccumulation relies on the firmness of a chemical's binding inside the cell and half-life compartments (metabolic). It also depends on the reduction, which shows first-order kinetics in general. Distinctive pools are recognized as being swift (a compound disappears in a week/day/hour/minute), slow (in months), and not absorbed from the gut (in animals: days).

16.2.1.1.1 Biomonitoring

Biomonitoring studies are based on the quantity of bioaccumulation calculated by analyzing various biomarkers. Studies are essential for showing the trend and reducing exposure and risk. For example, the number of toxic components in blood, urine, hair, serum, breast milk, or subcutaneous fat. In this case, bioaccumulation of chemicals includes toxic metals (Pb, Cd), polycyclic aromatic hydrocarbons (PAH) metabolites, persistent aromatic contaminants (POP), and volatile organic compounds (VOC). The enhanced concentrations of metals and PAH were observed in young populations and women in industrial zones. The other biomonitoring study showed that the bioaccumulation of toxic metals and Pb was higher in urban residents than in rural locations (Chojnacka and Mikulewicz, 2014).

16.2.2 Bioadsorption

PPCP may impact the healthy lifestyle of human beings. Nonmetabolized materials get released into the atmosphere leading to several adverse effects on the atmosphere, chiefly on the aquatic ecosystem. PPCP is regarded as a secondary pollution-causing agent but can become a primary one because of its bioaccumulation and lasting harmful impacts. Current primary wastewater treatments, such as sedimentation, coagulation, and flocculation, are not suitable or sufficient for removing these contaminants due to their low density and the ability to form an emulsion with other components. Hence, bioabsorption is a potential method because of its easy application, inexpensiveness, and comparatively good effectiveness. It is a passive technique in which extracellular polymer particles (EPS) are dispersed among the liquid component (de Godos et al., 2012). The adsorbent used in this technique is prepared from waste (biological) to make the process cost-effective. Appropriately selecting the adsorbent components to exclude PPCP materials decreases solid waste in the environment (Magesh et al., 2020). The distribution of PPCPs mainly occurs because of ionic or hydrophobic interaction among the exterior (solid) microalgae and pollutants (Fomina and

Gadd, 2014). The bioadsorption of the PPCP depends on its composition, hydrophilic nature, presence of functional groups, and microalgal organisms. Because of functional moieties of carboxyl, hydroxyl, and phosphoryl that participate in electrostatic reactions with charged (positively) PPCP substances, microalgae cell walls and EPS principally hold a negative charge. The ionization or dissociation into the water of PPCPs relies primarily on the water process's pH (de Godos et al., 2012).

The literature has generally proposed that collective processes, where bioadsorption is one of the most widely used mechanisms, eradicate PPCPs. Therefore, the bioadsorption process depends on the microalgae and the micropollutant. One of the best examples in this category is *Chlorella sorokiniana*, which is capable of removing 62% of a mixture of pharmaceutical compounds estrone (E1), β-estradiol (E2), ethynylestradiol (EE2), diclofenac, carbamazepine, ibuprofen, paracetamol, trimethoprim, and metoprolol using combination principles and adsorption results in the removal of 34% materials (de Wilt et al., 2016). Among all previously reported pharmaceuticals, carbamazepine was the greatest adsorbed in microalgal biomass. It resulted in a higher percentage (16.7%) than diclofenac (9.1%) and trimethoprim (7.6%), while the rest exhibited less involvement. Several studies have shown that the adsorption is peculiar to particular species (Hom-Diaz et al., 2015).

16.2.2.1 Bioadsorbent

The bioadsorbent is a compound of biological origin and is valuable for eliminating pollutants from a solution. They contain biomaterials such as agricultural waste, bacteria, algae, and industrial debris. They have been more attractive because they are of renewable origin, cost-effective, biodegradable, and not responsible for generating secondary contaminants (Vijayaraghavan and Yun, 2008). The bioadsorbent is biological and consists of many functional groups that serve as driving forces for the hydrophobic interaction they exhibit during the sorption technique, mostly pH-dependent (Adewuyi and Pereira, 2017; Tadkaew et al., 2011). Several natural compounds act as potential bioadsorbents for the elimination of pollutants in water. They may be inactive or dead microbial biomass and living microorganisms (Adewuyi, 2020).

16.2.2.2 Classification of bioadsorbents

Based on various forms, bioadsorbents are classified into four categories such as

- **(a)** Natural waste
- **(b)** Industrial wastes
- **(c)** Agriculture wastes
- **(d)** Forest wastes (Örnek et al., 2007; Saka et al., 2012)

16.2.2.3 Plant and animal solid waste biosorbent

Plant and animal solid wastes are readily available, cost-effective, and renewable resource compounds. They are generated in vast amounts per year, and their disposal is a major issue (Kulkarni, 2014; Ramachandran et al., 2014). The waste generated from plant sources consists chiefly of cellulose with lignin, sugars, proteins, hemicellulose, and starch, which act as structural materials (Rajapaksha et al., 2015).

16.2.2.4 Microorganisms as biosorbents

Researchers have shown that inactive or dead microbial biomass could passively bind to metal in the initial steps of biosorption technique. Dead microbial biomass has many benefits compared to living microbial biomass: affordability, low toxicity, simple regeneration, ion exchange capability, and a broad range of working pH and temperature. Biosorption consists of microbial biomass and does not depend on the chemical composition of biomass or its physiochemical parameters or matrix chemistry. Biosorption occurs using one or a combination of mechanisms such as complexation, chelation, adsorption, ion exchange, degradation, electrostatic interaction, microprecipitation, coordination, or donor-receptor interaction (Flickinger and Drew, 1999; Vijayaraghavan and Yun, 2008).

16.2.3 Biodegradation

The degradation (metabolic) or disintegration of enzyme-catalyzed products is biodegradation. Typically, microalgae turn the complex parent molecule into a simple molecule. This technique consists of various enzymatic reactions such as hydroxylation, carboxylation, hydrogenation, dehydrogenation, oxidation, reduction, hydrolysis, demethylation, ring cleavage, and glycosylation (Ding et al., 2017; Xiong et al., 2017).

16.2.3.1 Biodegradation of pharmaceuticals and its effect on natural microbiological communities

Natural microbial communities in soil and water are essential parameters in various techniques that mint the excellence of ecosystems and control pollutants released in the atmosphere (de Groot et al., 2002). Microorganisms are utilized in environmental self-purification methods because they can degrade contaminants by metabolic and co-metabolic processes. Biodegradation is the most effective form of removing most xenobiotics, including pharmaceutical products (de Groot et al., 2002; Rodarte-Morales et al., 2012; Topp et al., 2013).

Pharmaceuticals contain hundreds of compounds with different physicochemical characteristics, atmosphere behavior, and biochemical actions (Bottoni et al., 2010). In complex effluents, pharmaceutical products enter the system, so naturally occurring microbial species are exposed to a mixture of active pharmaceutical compounds. For example, certain antibiotics such as sulfamethazine, chlortetracycline, tylosin, other compounds such as paracetamol, diclofenac, ibuprofen, naproxen, clofibric acid, fluoxetine, carbamazepine, and biocides (triclosan and triclocarban) (Bueno et al., 2012; Gavrilescu et al., 2015; Gerbersdorf et al., 2011; Luo et al., 2014; Venkatesan et al., 2012).

16.2.3.2 Nonsteroidal anti-inflammatory compounds

Analgesics are pain-relieving medications made up of narcotic analgesics, nonnarcotic analgesics, and nonsteroidal anti-inflammatory drugs (NSAIDs). NSAIDs obstruct the cyclooxygenase (COX) enzyme, which catalyzes arachidonic acid formation (Vane and Botting, 1996). NSAID consists of naproxen, diclofenac, and ibuprofen, which are widely found in pain killers in surface water from ng/L to μg/L (Gerbersdorf et al., 2011; Luo et al., 2014; Patrolecco et al., 2013).

Naproxen is a hydrophilic pharmaceutical compound primarily seen as a river micro-contaminant (Grenni et al., 2013; Loos et al., 2008; Tixier et al., 2003) as well as aquifer groundwater recharged with recycled water (Rabiet et al., 2006). In earlier literature, naproxen persistence was studied in surface water (Araujo et al., 2011; Grenni et al., 2013; Tixier et al., 2003). The degradation that occurs via a photolytic process is considered a proper abiotic degradation technique, but this technique can break down naproxen completely. The photoproducts were more poisonous than the parent compound (Isidori et al., 2005).

Another study on microorganisms showed that naproxen (100 μg/L starting concentration) was found to be biodegraded by microorganisms (bacteria) from river water, classified as alpha and gamma-proteobacteria (Grenni et al., 2013, 2014).

Similarly, the other classes of pharmaceutical compounds, such as other analgesic and antipyretics, blood lipid regulators, antiepileptics, antidepressants, antibiotics (macrolide sulfonamide, tetracycline), and antiseptic and disinfectants are toxic. Ultraviolet (UV) sunlight irradiation can be absorbed directly and broken down by pollutant compounds containing aromatic rings, π bonds, and other functional groups without microalgae (Barra Caracciolo et al., 2015).

16.2.4 Photo-biodegradation

Most PPCPs have been observed to decompose in sunlight, called photodegradation or photolysis (Hanamoto et al., 2014; Matamoros et al., 2008). This technique is useful, environmental friendly, cost-effective, and easy to scale. The photolysis used in the breakdown of PPCPs present in wastewater is classified into two classes:

(A) Direct photolysis
(B) Indirect photolysis
(A) Direct photolysis

In this process, pollutant compounds containing aromatic rings, π bonds, and other functional groups can directly absorb irradiation in the UV range and undergo breakdown in the absence of microalgae (Challis et al., 2014).

(B) Indirect photolysis

In indirect photolysis, the free radicals such as peroxy (ROO•), oxygen ($^1O_2$) singlet, and hydroxyl (•OH) formed on exposure to the sunlight participate in the process of photolysis. In the presence of UV light, the substances involved in forming free radicals are called photosensitizers. Rontani et al. used Skeletonema costatum to study the indirect mechanisms of photolysis or photo-biodegradation for sterol removal (Rontani et al., 1997).

16.2.5 Volatilization

There are slight differences between volatilization and stripping. In the case of stripping, the elimination of gaseous substances occurs in wastewater treatment plants (WWTPs), while volatilization eliminates volatile substances. In the aerobic chamber or the bioreactor tank, both techniques are more effective and rely on many parameters, such as liquid vapor pressure, Henry coefficient (H), and hydrophobicity (Kow). Materials with an H value of less than 0.005 showed negligible stripping based on Henry's rule (Hena et al., 2021). Suarez et al. studied that in WWTPs except celetolide, which suggested up to 16% removal, the stripping of

PPCPs is negligible. Volatilization is a material-specific process that is more promising than closed photobioreactors in open pond systems (Suarez et al., 2010).

16.2.6 Bioremediation

In addition to all of the above techniques for removing PPCPs, bioremediation is considered a potential method for the breakdown of PPCPs. It is of attention because it is green and sustainable for treating contaminated areas (Azubuike et al., 2016). Moreover, bioremediation is time-consuming and can often not be helpful in managing heavily polluted areas. The critical criteria for selecting acceptable strategies for the remediation of polluted regions are effectiveness, cost-efficiency, accessibility of resources, and duration needed. The use of a single approach is not appropriate for waste treatment. Therefore, both nanomaterials and bioremediation are highly demanded to be competitive and sustainable (Rizwan et al., 2014). Hence, the technique is called nanoremediation.

Nanomaterials have been commonly used in industry, medicine, and atmospheric remediation (Geary et al., 2016). To clean up the atmosphere, various shapes and sizes of nanomaterials can be used (Rizwan et al., 2014). The additional advantage of nanomaterials is that they can penetrate the contaminated environment where microscale size cannot reach.

Titanium oxide nanotubes have been documented to break down pentachlorophenol through photo electrocatalytic reaction (Quan et al., 2005). Remediation of sediments contaminated by nanoscale heavy metal ion compounds has been confirmed. Due to their high reactivity and adsorption capacity, nanoparticles were used as a substitute to treat contaminated sediments (Akcil et al., 2015). Table 16.1 provides brief information regarding various types of plastics.

Jain et al. developed quasi-spherical, symmetrical, polydisperse, well-distributed zinc oxide nanoparticles around 80–120 nm in size. Protein-coated zinc oxide nanoparticles showed elevated photocatalytic properties and showed a 90% breakdown of the methylene blue dye in half an hour. They reported that this photolytic property is due to surface proteins that assist in low-recombination-speed dye adsorption (Jain et al., 2014). Fig. 16.1 represents the mechanisms involved in removing pharmaceuticals and personal care products from microalgae.

16.3 Bioaccumulation

Bioaccumulation is characterized as the net accumulation of all contaminant sources in or on an organism, including water, air, and diet. Bioaccumulation is distinguished as an increase in the concentration of pollutants in aquatic organisms after absorption from the ambient environment. Relative to the environment, bioaccumulation defines the accumulation and enrichment of toxins in organisms (Chojnacka, 2010).

Bioaccumulation evidence allows the risk associated with the use of various chemicals in the surroundings, food, and place of work to be measured and the potential to monitor the usage and emissions of chemicals to be quantitatively defined (Popek, 2017).

TABLE 16.1 Brief information regarding various types of plastics.

Type of plastic	Chemical formula	Reaction starting material	Density	Degradation time (Years)	Major producers	Usage
Polyethylene Terephthalate (PET)	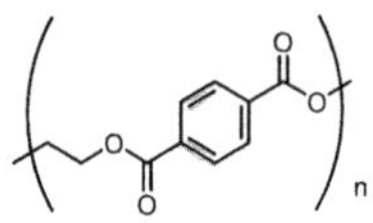 $(C_{10}H_8O4)_n$	Ethylene glycol and terephthalic acid	1.38 g/ cm^3, 20°C	Approx. 450	United States, India, Japan, France, Italy	PET bottles and jars, automotive parts, industrial strapping, fiberfill for winter jackets, construction materials
Polyvinyl Chloride (PVC)	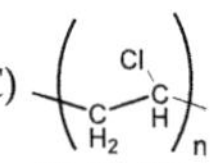 $(C_2H_3Cl)_n$	Chlorine and ethylene	1.38 g/ cm^3	Approx. 100	China, India, Germany, the United States, Japan	Window frames, sewage pipes, medical devices, automotive interiors, resilient flooring, blood storage bags
Polyamide (PA)	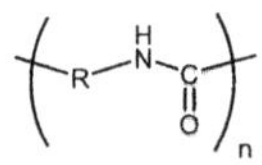 $(RCONH_2)_n$ R = Alkyl group	Diamino	1.14 g/ cm^3	–	Germany, Japan, Italy, China, United States	Electrical connectors, guitar strings and picks, medical implants, tennis racket strings, fishing line
Polypropylene (PP)	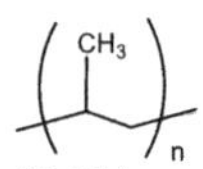 $(C_3H_6)_n$	Propylene gas	1.04 −1.06 g/ cm^3	20–30	Saudi Arabia, Germany, United States, Belgium	Car batteries, clothing and camping equipment, tote bags, ropes, car bumpers
Polystyrene (PS)	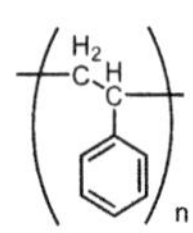 $(C_8H_8)_n$	Styrene	0.96 −1.05 g/ cm^3	Approx. 500	China, Belgium, France, Netherlands	Refrigerators, DVD cases, televisions, egg cartons, disposable eating utensils

TABLE 16.1 Brief information regarding various types of plastics.—cont'd

Type of plastic	Chemical formula	Reaction starting material	Density	Degradation time (Years)	Major producers	Usage
Polyethylene (PE)	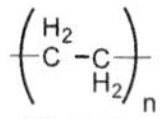 $(C_2H_4)_n$	Ethylene	0.88 −0.96 g/cm^3	Approx. 1000	China, the United States, Russia, South Korea	packaging film, garbage bags, grocery bags, insulation for wires and cables, trays, fruit juice containers, and food packaging products
Polycarbonate	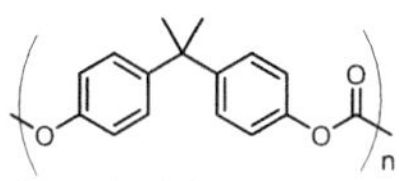 $(C_{16}H_{16}O_4)_n$	Bisphenol A	1.20 −1.22 g/cm^3	Approx. 6.5	USA, Germany, China, South Korea, and Japan	compact disc, safety helmets, bullet-proof glass, car headlamp lenses, baby feeding bottles, roofing, and glazing
Polymethyl methacrylate	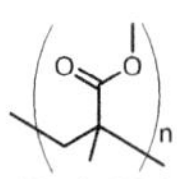 $(C_5O_2H_8)_n$	Methyl methacrylate	1.18 g/cm^3	–	Germany, Taiwan, Saudi Arabia, Japan, South Korea	Aquariums, windows, bone cement, hockey rinks, contact, and intraocular lens, paints
Acrylonitrile butadiene styrene	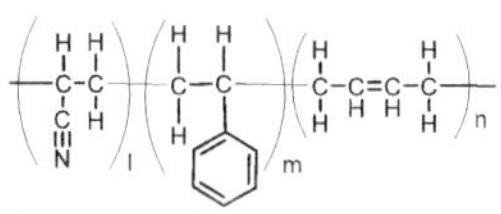 $(C_8H_8.C_4H_6.C_3H_3H)_n$	Acrylonitrile, butadiene, and styrene	1.060 −1.080 g/cm^3	–	South Korea, Japan, China, Taiwan, United States	Pipe, wheel covers, protective head gear, automotive body parts, vacuum construction

16.3.1 Mechanism

Bioaccumulation occurs in living organisms or tissues until the compound concentrates. The effect of atmospheric dispersion can be counteracted by bioaccumulation, and the chemical is redistributed within the biosphere. Bioaccumulation follows the dynamic networks of food. In the tissues of animals, elevated levels of chemicals are present at the topmost of the food chain. It depends on the species' feeding ways, location, and metabolic action (Daley, 2013).

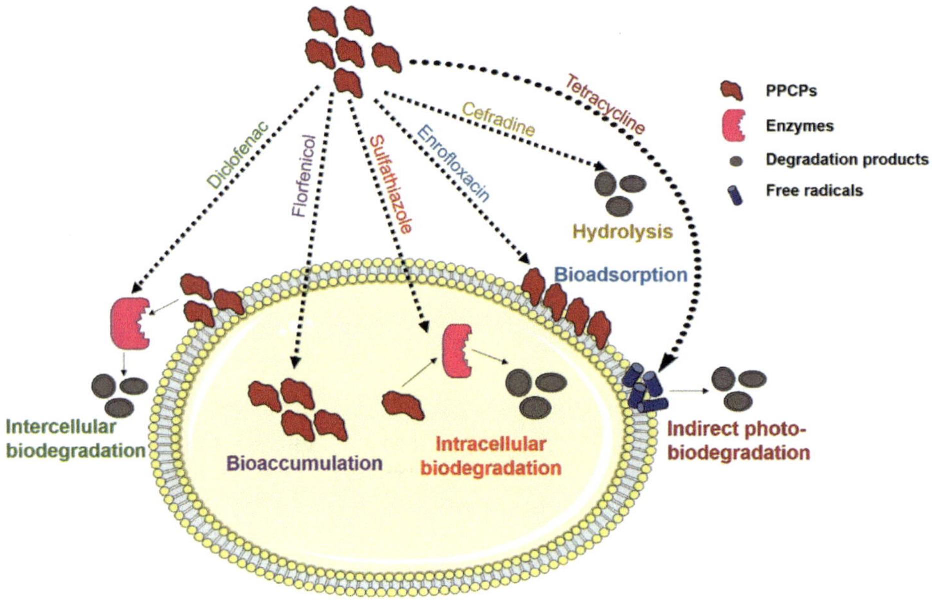

FIGURE 16.1 Mechanisms involved in removal of pharmaceuticals and personal care products by microalgae.

It is based on two ways: the stability of chemical attachment inside cell compartments and metabolic half-life. After exposure to water, food, sediment, and air, bioaccumulation is the product of the absorption, distribution, and removal of a compound in an organism. For bioaccumulation to occur, all sources' absorption rate is greater than the rate of chemical loss of organism tissues. Several highly soluble chemicals like ammonia and inorganic ions are readily bioavailable and quickly enter previous tissues of aquatic organisms (Lushchak et al., 2018).

However, these highly soluble substances are not retained and disappear from the tissues utilizing different processes like active transport, metabolic conversion, or diffusion. The amount of such tissues is the same as or less than its amount in the ambient medium and maintained at a particular level by an organism. Some bioavailable chemicals are not bioaccumulated because of rapid consumption; they are rapidly converted and excreted by the metabolic processes. Bioaccumulation, which typically follows the kinetics of first-order, relies on elimination. There are three ways to differentiate between rapid (a chemical disappears in weeks/days/hours/minutes), sluggish (in months), and nonassimilated from the intestines (in days). Those chemicals that are bioavailable bioaccumulate via passive diffusion or are transported against a concentration gradient through the organism's exterior membrane. As the chemical quantity in the tissues increases, the gradient decreases, and the rate of chemical loss from the tissues via passive diffusion or active transport tends to enhance (Neff, 2002; Wang et al., 2017).

A steady-state marine organism's chemical concentration in the tissues relies on the compound's relative affinity in the organism's tissue for the aqueous phase and some other phases such as tissue water, lipids, solid phase, etc. Bioaccumulation factor (BAF) in all environmental compartments is nothing but equilibrium chemical concentration in marine organism tissues, the ratio of chemical concentration to its equilibrium concentration with the organism. Instead, and more precisely, the bioaccumulation element is the continuation of the total of the constants (chemical absorption rate) from whole species accessible from ecological parts to the sum of the constants (release rate) of the active and passive pathways of the species. For chemicals, large BAFs have more attraction for specific tissue components, such as lipids or the tissue's macromolecules. In tissues, metals bioaccumulate for an animal's lifetime in inactive, nonbioavailable forms; the BAF balance for these metals cannot be estimated (Wang et al., 2017).

16.3.1.1 *Bioaccumulation in the aquatic environment*

Bioaccumulation in the aquatic setting depends on the following factors: biomass per water volume, biomass per chemical concentration, and sampling period. It depends mainly on the climatic conditions of the year, which focuses primarily on the effect of temperature. The solubility of compounds in water determines the quantity of bioaccumulation. In the entry of chemicals into the marine food system, water chemistry plays an important role, such as quantity in water, early tissue amounts in phytoplankton and the primary producers, and higher trophic levels as food consumption (absorption by invertebrates and fish). Animals' gill breathing makes a significant contribution (Fisher, 1995; Neff, 2002).

Bioaccumulation can ensue through uptake from water, crossing chemicals from the cell sheaths, ion channels or pumps, or transport systems. In invertebrates and fish, uptake takes place by food ingestion. Bioaccumulation is caused by the accumulation of chemicals in food and the quantity of food ingested. Two factors can calculate the concentration of chemicals in aquatic organisms; bio-concentration factor (BCF) and bioaccumulation factor (BAF). Both factors demonstrate a chemical's partitioning in steady-state conditions between water and marine species, mostly fish. BCF denotes the levels due to the organism's uptake of the organism from the surrounding water, while BAF also comprises the uptake from food. Therefore, in animals, BCF can be calculated in laboratory experiments, where food intake can be reduced, while BAF is the field ratio (Karlsson et al., 2002; Schäfer et al., 2015).

16.3.1.1.1 Bioaccumulation of pharmaceuticals in the aquatic system

Using an active pharmaceutical ingredient is necessary for the welfare and human health; at the same time, it may pose a threat to the environment if discharged untreated into the ecosystem. Pharmaceuticals and personal care products threaten the environment due to their continuous use, persistent nature, and continuous disposal of these in the environment. These are the micropollutants present in trace quantities and are of great concern as they are persistent. They may cause hazardous effect on the organism through bioaccumulation, biomagnification, and bioconcentration as these are stable and pass through the waste water treatment.

Fonseca and their coworkers (2021) have screened 66 pharmaceutical residues in the surface water, invertebrates, and fishes in the Tejo estuary to evaluate the risk assessment and bioaccumulation of these pharmaceuticals in Europe's largest water reservoir. They identified 16 pharmaceutical residues belonging to 7 different therapeutic classes, with concentrations ranging from 42 to 1762 ng/L. Evaluation of risk assessment via risk quotient predicted a high risk for antibiotics and cardio active drugs. They found that bioaccumulation was species- and compound-specific. It was higher in the species living directly on or above the substrate (e.g., benthic and demersal species). Several reports on the bioaccumulation of pharmaceutical and personal care products emphasize the urgent need for action to manage and treat these micro-pollutants. There are several techniques that emphasize the removal of these pharmaceuticals, which are cost-effective and eco-friendly. Some of the available technologies are phycoremediation. This technology has many benefits, but the only drawback associated with difficulty handling by the industries is a single-stage treatment process. Much of the research is now focused on integrating phycoremediation with other techniques such as activated sludge process (ASP), advanced oxidation process (AOP), up-flow anaerobic sludge blanket reactor (UASBR), UV irradiation, and constructed wetland (CW). There are review articles that highlight the use of this technology in removal of PPCPs (Ricky and Shanthakumar, 2022).

Another method involves the use of microalgae-based treatment of wastewater; this is sustainable and is low-cost, and effective in removing the contaminants (Lindberg et al., 2021). Of the 36 active pharmaceutical ingredients, 16 were removed from HRAPs (North Sweden high-rate algal pond) which was above 50% and seven was from 90% above their initial concentration. Their study highlighted that HRAP treatment removed around 69% of the chemicals. They suggested that the presence of the different APIs in different aqueous phases and biomass may require different approaches, such as removal based on hydrophobicity, bioaccumulation, and bio-sorption.

16.3.1.2 *Bioaccumulation of the terrestrial environment*

In animals, the diet is the critical path to bioaccumulation. Bioaccumulation involves fewer dermal and respiratory ways in a terrestrial environment, excluding dermal exposure in soil species. In animals, the magnitude of the bioaccumulation of chemicals is less than in marine animals. Mammals and birds achieve dynamic equilibrium conditions after a certain amount of time that is nothing but the absorption rate equal to the rate of removal, yielding constant concentrations in tissue. The period needed to achieve balance depends on the chemical, organisms, and food concentration (Gobas et al., 2016; Kelly and Gobas, 2003).

16.3.2 Bioaccumulation testing

Integrated test systems, such as food systems and compartmentalized test systems, i.e., individual organisms; both systems, are both concerned with bioaccumulation testing. Problems relate to individual variables that influence the statistical quantification and interpretation of the effects of bioaccumulation. Bioaccumulation affects size and weight.

Taking into account the trends of bioaccumulation through contamination gradients, the bioaccumulation analysis approach should consist of an assortment of people with the same parameters (age, sex, weight/size, and class). For testing, the selected test chemical and the matrix are linked to the chemical and the quantification limit of the analytical tools, and the amount and intrusiveness of the matrix available.

Testing aims to recognize and remove bases of contact, analyze interval patterns, demonstrate the efficacy of rules, scrutinize the association between exposure and disease or the progress of deformities, and check the relationship between the body's load ingestion habits or work-related exposure.

Establishing standard bioaccumulation testing methods (sample selection and preparation, analysis) is necessary to provide comparable and meaningful outcomes. Chemical bioaccumulation can be regulated by determining the levels in human-sampled matrices, such as milk or adipose tissue. This problem relates to bioaccumulating harmful and persistent chemicals from human foods. Thus, regulating the manufacturing and import of new substances, such as the 8-week bioaccumulation study, should have assessed biodegradability. For example, suppose a material is non-disintegrable and bioaccumulative; such material is prohibited or limited unless no toxicity to humans has been demonstrated in mammal studies.

In static experiments, bioaccumulation testing of inorganic and metalloorganic materials is commonly performed on fish or sediments. The proportion of n-octanol per water in organic compounds is significant and describes the potential for bioaccumulation.

- On rainbow trout or common carp, the tests can be performed, and the period is 1–2 months or till balanced conditions are achieved. The bioconcentration factor is considered as the endpoint of the test in fish tissues. A BCF greater than 1000 is of interest.
- A sediment toxicity study observes the outcome of a chemical on dwelling species, such as Chironomus and Lumbriculus. These studies are carried out to predict sediment exposure for risk assessment (Workgroup, 2000).

16.3.3 Bioaccumulation models

The variables monitoring the environmental partitioning of a contaminant and its passage across the food chain are as intricate as those monitoring its toxicity after an organism consumes it. This chapter discusses various methods that may be valuable tools for bioaccumulation assessment. It is divided into two main parts: the first describing direct bioaccumulation measurement methods and the second describing bioaccumulation model methods. The appropriate approach choice depends on the questions, the type of climate, the organisms, and the troubling pollutants. Due to the qualms related to predictive bioaccumulation and biomagnification models, the European Protection Agency (EPA) desires that direct-field measurements be used to assess the bioaccumulation potential of a chemical. The EPA identified three potential approaches for evaluating bioaccumulation factors (BAFs) in order of preference by the Agency:

(i) A BAF is assessed in the field using animals that live at or nearby the top of the food chain.
(ii) A laboratory-measured BCF represents the disparity between laboratory species and field organisms multiplied by a suitable factor [food chain multiplier, FCM].
(iii) A BCF model of the octanol-water partitioning coefficient of a chemical multiplied by a suitable FCM.

Models such as empirical, generalized, and mechanistic are being developed for chemicals and organisms that are predictive and descriptive. Bioaccumulation modeling is categorized as:

- Dynamic mass balance models
- Steady-state models
- Hybrid models (Gobas et al., 2016; Mackay and Fraser, 2000)

16.3.4 Biomonitoring

The techniques used to determine human exposure or effects of chemicals by testing these chemicals, their metabolites, or reaction products in human specimens are referred to as human biomonitoring. Human biomonitoring requires the analysis of biomarker samples such as blood, urine, saliva, breast milk, sweat, and other samples, such as feces, hair, teeth, and nails, in body fluids. Human biomonitoring involves a practical, readily accessible biological matrix for repetitive processes. Blood and urine samples are the most widely used matrix; nonetheless, toxicological quantification can also be used for hair, exhaled air, teeth, nails, and saliva (Costa and Teixeira, 2014; Schäfer et al., 2015).

The evaluation of toxic ecological waste is traditionally focused on ecological observation, which requires the study of air, soil, water, sediments, and, in many instances, living organisms. But these tests only offer data on the possible toxic effects of chemicals in the atmosphere and organisms. Furthermore, this calculation method does not recognize the dose absorbed or human variability in living organisms. Biomonitoring, which uses living organisms, including humans, to determine the exposure to and effects of environmental pollutants, overcomes this limitation and has become crucial to current awareness of toxic mechanisms, metabolism, and chemical consequences (Bundschuh et al., 2018).

The degree of bioaccumulation was determined by studying various biomarkers, as shown by biomonitoring studies. Studies are necessary to demonstrate patterns and decrease contact and health dangers. Examples include concentrations of toxic elements in blood, serum, urine, hair, nails, breast milk, or subcutaneous fat. The chemicals assessed for bioaccumulation consist of hazardous metals (Pb, Cd), polycyclic aromatic hydrocarbon (PAH) metabolites, persistent organic contaminants (POP), and volatile organic compounds (VOC) (Hansen, 2008).

16.3.5 Bioaccumulation of certain compounds

In recent days, one of the critical issues has been environmental pollution. This is caused by heavy metals resulting from rapid industrialization and urbanization, and since the 1940s, their rates of mobilization and transit in the environment have substantially increased. Living things are seriously at risk from such pollution because of heavy metal exposure over time (Li et al., 2019). Lowering soil fertility was also seen due to the accumulation of metals in the soil that also led to the destruction of the microorganisms in the soil. So, this accumulated metals transfer from soil toward plants, ultimately destroying the food chain (Ali and Khan, 2019). In addition, aquatic life is also in danger due to the effluents containing heavy metals from the industrial area (Okereafor et al., 2020).

In the next section, we have briefly discuss the various metals causing bioaccumulation, such as organic, inorganic, heavy metals, and metal nanoparticles.

16.3.5.1 Organic

It is commonly observed that, compared to the concentrations of these substances in the ecosystem, species may attain high concentrations of such organic pollutants. In this sense, organisms can include plants, invertebrates, and vertebrate species, including fish, mammals, reptiles, and birds. The "climate" involves the air or water in which the species breathe, the air, water, soil, and sediment in which they live and can communicate intimately, and the food they eat. In fat tissue, organic compounds appear to accumulate. The organochlorine chemical is an example. These substances accumulate from food are metabolized and removed (for example, by lactation) by birds and marine mammals, resulting in a body burden. Some characteristics of pure organic compounds behave in indulging high BCF values or more equal distributions within the compartments. There are numerous reasons for increasing BCF elevation, such as lipophilicity, poor solubility in water, small molecular charge and ionization degree, small molecule size, and low biodegradability (Deibel et al., 2007; Gossett et al., 1983).

Organic substances may be metabolized to improve water and urinary excretion solubility, reducing harmfulness. The best counterexample is the transformation of parathion into a paraxon or heptachlor into epoxy, which is more hazardous. The fundamental biochemical transformation steps in microorganisms, plants, and animals are identical and consist of oxidation, reduction, hydrolysis, and conjugation reactions. Plants show slower but complete alterations and store metabolized compounds or their conjugates in the cytoplasm or inside vacuoles (Sehrawat et al., 2021).

16.3.5.2 Inorganic

One of the oldest known toxicants is toxic metals. There is concern about their bioaccumulation in the human body. In the human world, toxic metals are persistent and cannot be produced or removed. Anthropogenic behavior has resulted in increased concentrations of metals, affecting their chemical shape and mobility and resulting in increased bioaccumulation. Toxic metal bioaccumulation is of concern since nonessential toxic metals imitate essential metals and arrive at the path via which vital elements are elated into an organism and interfere with essential cellular purposes. Due to chemical similarities, nonessential features are bioaccumulated (e.g., Cs+ mimics NH_4^+, K^+): solubility and size. The lipophilic properties of organometallic compounds are collected from solution or diet. Their biomagnification relies on lipophilicity/hydrophobicity, indicated as partition coefficient (octanol/water), aqueous phase situation (pH, the existence of complexing agents), and an organism's capability to remove them (Armitage et al., 2017).

Industry-released mercury compounds in surface waters have been observed to be bioaccumulated in fish. Gradually, bioaccumulation occurs in bacteria and plankton from the water. The ingestion of mercury-containing fish resulted in a deficiency in the central nervous system of humans.

16.3.5.3 *Heavy metals*

Most heavy metals in the environment and organisms are found in various organic or inorganic binding partners in ligands. They are defined and differentiated as A-metal cations, B-metal cations, or borderline cations (i.e., cations with features lying between A and B), according to ligand preferences. The electronic sheath of metal cations in type A is not readily deformed, whereas the electronic sheath in type B is more deformable. Metal cations of type B are also more polarizable than metal cations of type A (Wuana and Okieimen, 2011).

16.3.5.4 *Metal nanoparticles*

Nanoparticles (NPs) are a particulate matter between 1 and 100 nm in size in at least one dimension. NPs may be classified as NPs based on carbon (e.g., fullerenes, carbon tubes), inorganic NPs (e.g., metal oxides, metals), or quantum dots (e.g., cadmium selenide). In addition to nanotechnology's rapid development, industries extending from antibacterial activity and cosmetics application to electronics, renewable energy, biological remediation, drug delivery systems, and household and trade applications for NPs have grown tremendously. The enormous production of NPs is focused on these commercially advantageous properties of manufactured NPs, including some of the most commonly used NPs, metal-loaded NPs like titanium dioxide (TiO_2) and silver (Ag) (Khan et al., 2019).

NPs (metal oxide) are widely used nanoparticles in various chemical, material, and biological applications. Because of its capability to block UV radiation, nanosized TiO_2 forms are produced for their application in commercial products like cosmetics, sunscreens, and industrial products such as pigments as paints and lacquers (Musial et al., 2020; Ziental et al., 2020).

16.4 Nanoparticles in the management of bioaccumulation

Ultimately, the nanotechnology industry's rapid growth and advancement have directed the large-scale production of an extensive range of engineered nanomaterials. Because of their unique properties, novel engineered nanomaterials demonstrate excellent performance in mechanical, electrical, electronic, thermal, and optical applications. These are used in consumer products, industries, and pollutant remediation, which are the leading causes of their direct suppliers to the environment (Gadekar et al., 2021; Gorain et al., 2016). Nanomaterials can be unregulated in various environments during their different life stages, including manufacturing, development, transportation, consumer use, waste management facilities, disposal, and landfilling (Dinda, 2018).

One of the main applications of engineered nanomaterials and nanotechnology is diagnosing and treating diseases in humans, plants, and marine animals. Engineered nanomaterials, especially for biomedical applications, have demonstrated their utility and novel approaches (Youngren et al., 2013; Tekade and Chougule, 2013). In recent years, numerous studies have been performed to discuss the fate, toxicity, threat, and safety assessment of nanomaterials in the atmosphere and their impacts on live organisms. Dissolution, agglomeration, sedimentation, chemical transformations, absorption, and transmission into the food system include many interactions of engineered nanomaterials (Nam et al., 2014).

A vital problem in the existing environment is investigating the critical assets and how they affect bioaccumulation, biomagnification, and biotransformation. The absorption of nanomaterials by living organisms can have collective toxic properties, which organisms can counteract benignly by either their storage or excretion. The engineered nanomaterials affect the health of plants and the supply of food. Engineered nanomaterials may impact plant health and food supply. Tenacious lipophilic compounds can aggregate in marine organisms through various pathways: direct absorption from the water through gills or skin (bioconcentration), absorption of particles (suspended) (ingestion), and administration of food (contaminated) (biomagnification). Also, bioaccumulation should be treated as a threat measure in standard ecotoxicity studies without observable acute or chronic effects (Mariano et al., 2020).

16.4.1 Silver nanoparticles

Silver nanoparticles are used mainly in industrial applications and are metal-based. Research into the impact of silver nanoparticles on caudal fin regeneration in zebrafish demonstrates that silver nanoparticles enter fish organelles with mitochondria, nuclei, and blood vessels. During silver nanoparticle exposure, the total silver amount in the gut tissues of the zebrafish is enhanced. In the gills and liver of perch and Japanese medaka, silver nanoparticles were the most significant and were mainly adsorbed and accumulated. The coating of silver nanoparticles at biological interfaces affects behavior and transport, such as fish gill epithelia; silver nanoparticles covered with polyvinylpyrrolidone (PVP) mainly pass through the multilayered multicellular gill epithelium, while citrate-coated silver nanoparticles uptake into individual cells. The degree to which the marine environment will vary the chemical properties of silver nanoparticles; this is what we are considering when researching nanoparticle bioaccumulation (Nam et al., 2014).

16.4.2 Gold nanoparticles

Because of the stability, synthesis, firmness, and incorporation of assets with molecules such as peptides and proteins, gold nanoparticles are particularly helpful for biomedical applications.

Lasagna-Reeves et al. have been experimenting with gold nanoparticles to deliver, study, and cure drugs. They have discovered that the bioaccumulation and toxicity associated with repeated administration of these molecules must be demonstrated. As seen in materials, the potential cause of treatment with gold nanoparticles on organ morphology and cellular dysfunction in hematoxylin/eosin-stained tissues. There was a significant increase in later action in gold levels in all organs tested related to the dose administered (Lasagna-Reeves et al., 2010).

However, blood gold levels have not increased in proportion to the dose, indicating that most gold nanoparticles are absorbed and retained by tissues. On the other hand, since no blood was collected from the lungs, an examination reveals that the contribution of blood was less than 6%, 2%, 3%, 1%, and 7.5%, respectively, of the values recorded in the brain, kidney, liver, spleen, and lung, of the volume obtained in the tissues (Barreto et al., 2019).

Given the comparatively persistent levels of gold in the blood following the administration of gold nanoparticles at different doses, the increased accumulation of gold in the brain indicates that gold nanoparticles may be absorbed unsaturated through the blood-brain barrier. This is imperative for using these nanoparticles for possible therapy and analysis of neurodegenerative diseases. Within the sense of a single trophic level, the localization of nanoparticles has a significant effect on their bioaccumulation capacity. The pharmacokinetics, bioavailability, bioaccumulation, clearance, and harmfulness of nanoparticles depend primarily on the particles' composition, size, and surface characteristics. To achieve the most suitable equilibrium for various applications, these properties may be altered. One of the variables that govern nanoparticles' pharmacological properties is the electrostatic state of the particle (Lopez-Chaves et al., 2018).

16.4.3 Titanium dioxide nanoparticles

Semiconductor solid catalysts such as TiO_2, ZnO, CdS, SnO_2, and WO_3, when illuminated with light radiation of suitable wavelengths, induce the oxidation process. This is termed heterogeneous photocatalysis. TiO_2 shows the most significant potential among the commonly used semiconductor materials. Of the three polymorphs of TiO_2 crystals, viz. anatase, rutile, and brookite, anatase exhibits the highest photocatalytic activity, the most increased longevity, and the fastest action. UV radiation of <380 nm wavelength on the TiO_2 nanoparticles helps overcome the band gap (the energy difference between the valence band and the conduction band) of 3.2 eV. With the incident radiation, the electron gets excited and migrates from the valence band to the conduction band. This causes the generation of electron-hole pairs (e^- and h^+). The hole with its positive charge initiates $-OH$ (hydroxyl) radicals in water. Subsequently, the hydroxyl group reacts with the wastewater contaminants to bring about their degradation. Similarly, the electron trapped on the photocatalyst surface by combining with dissolved molecular oxygen leads to the production of superoxide anion ($-O_2$). $-O_2$ induced chain reaction involves the generation of peroxide radical followed by hydrogen peroxide that ultimately produces OH radicals that can efficiently extract hydrogen from the pharmaceutical contaminant and result in its degradation. The degradation products then release into the bulk fluid (Awfa et al., 2018).

Several reports have given an account of TiO_2-induced photocatalysis of APIs such as diclofenac, ibuprofen, naproxen, paracetamol, antibiotics, and antibacterial like amoxicillin and sulfamethoxazole. The studies have shown variable results regarding API degradation by TiO_2 nanoparticles. The quality of water, pH, temperature, dissolved oxygen, presence of other contaminants and organic matter in the water, the initial load of the contaminant as well as the catalyst, polymorphic form of the catalyst, the source and intensity of UV-visible radiation, duration of the treatment are the key factors that influence the process of degradation and mineralization; TiO_2 anatase polymorph has shown 85% degradation of diclofenac after 4 h of irradiation with UV A radiation (350–400 nm). The pH of the water was 6, and oxygen was purged throughout the experiment (Achilleos et al., 2010). Similarly, the photocatalytic degradation of naproxen (0.8 mM/L) in the presence of 0.1–1 g TiO_2 loading resulted in only 40% naproxen removal, possibly due to lack of higher-energy radiation and lower adsorption by the catalyst and rapid recombination of e^- and h^+ that inhibits further radical production. Therefore, TiO_2 treatment faces specific deficiencies, such as the inability of the efficient catalytic process in visible light, the lower adsorption capacity, and the difficulty recovery from treated water.

Modified TiO_2 nanoparticles have shown better performance for dyes and pharmaceutical removal. Cation or anion doping, coupling with another semiconductor, and co-doping with two different atoms are some modifications to TiO_2 nanoparticles that have brought about efficient catalysis of PPCPs. Doping broadens the light absorption range and enhances the redox potential while inhibiting the recombination of the charge carriers.

TiO_2 nanoparticles doped with a 0.05M concentration of Fe^{+3} could successfully degrade 92% para nitrophenol in 5 h in visible light (Sood et al., 2015). Similarly, Bi–Ni co-doped TiO_2 showed higher photocatalytic degradation of ofloxacin under solar light than neat TiO_2. Up to 86% of ofloxacin at 25 mg L^{-1} concentration was degraded with a dopant concentration of 0.25 wt% and a catalyst dose of 1.5 g L^{-1}. The process was carried out at a pH of 3 for 6 h in the presence of solar light (Bhatia et al., 2016). The potassium peroxodisulfate ($K_2S_2O_8$)-doped TiO_2 photocatalyst at a dose of 2 g of L^{-1} has been shown to degrade 0.1 mM acetaminophen completely within 9 h in the presence of visible light radiation (de Luna et al., 2017). The doping agent, by generating $[SO_4]^-$ radicals, increased the oxidizing potential of TiO_2. Enhancement in the surface charge of TiO_2 due to the presence of $K_2S_2O_8$ helped improve the adsorption and light absorption capacity.

The nanocomposite of the nitrogen and sulfur co-doped carbon quantum dots/TiO2 (N, S-CQDs/TiO2) was incorporated into the polysulfone (PSF) membrane. This membrane exhibited 62.3% degradation of diclofenac of 62.3% in the presence of solar light, while the pure TiO_2 membrane showed barely a degradation of 3.33%. The nanocomposite studded membrane was more hydrophilic, allowing the highest water permeability of 277 L/ m^2.hr.bar (Koe et al., 2020). When coupled with TiO_2 having a higher band gap, an appropriate small bandgap semiconductor allows the efficient transfer of electrons between the two conductors. This prevents the recombination of the charge carriers, thus preserving the catalytic performance of the semiconductor. TiO_2 when coupled with other semiconductors such as CdS, SnO_2, WO_3, or FeO_3. Bi_2S_3 has shown improved catalytic degradation of contaminants under solar radiation.

16.4.4 Zinc oxide nanoparticles

Zinc oxide (ZnO) is a preferred catalyst for the photo-degradation of micro water contaminants. Favorable features of ZnO nanoparticles (ZnONP) are low cost, high capacity to absorb a large quantum of light, and retention of photocatalytic activity in acidic and basic conditions. Particle size close to the nanoscale offers many active sites making ZnONP a potent photocatalyst for degrading organic substrates. ZnONP in the 0.34–1.42 μg L^{-1} range has been routinely used to treat wastewater in Europe from 2008 to 2014 onwards; the treatment concentration has been increased to 1.7–2.1 μg L^{-1}.

Electron-hole pairs are created at the surface of the ZnONP upon irradiation with an appropriate wavelength of UV light. Most of these electron-hole pairs are recombined and become inactive. The remaining free, unpaired electrons and holes initiate redox reactions in the surface-adsorbed microcontaminant, leading to its total photodegradation into simple substances.

There is a positive correlation between the degradation rate, the quantity of the nanoparticles, and the radiation intensity. The pH of the system also has a profound influence on the reaction kinetics. Moreover, doping ZnONP with suitable metals can improve the catalytic performance of the nanoparticles. The reduction in the extent of recombination of an electron-hole pair could be the main reason for the improved rate of harmful organic substrate degradation at the surface of doped ZONP. Doping has been shown to reduce the bandgap energy in doped ZONP, unlike undoped ZONP. The increased surface defects could also be responsible for the enhanced photocatalytic degradation rate in the doped ZONP.

The study by Bhamare and Kulkarni reinforces the advantage of doping ZnONP with a 5% mole ratio of barium metal in improving the degradation rate of zidovudine. Barium-doped ZnONP (BZnONP) led to a higher degradation of zidovudine. Additionally, the alkaline pH of 9 helped to improve the degradation rate due to the abundance of hydroxyl anion at this pH. Hydroxyl ions in the presence of trapped holes get converted to −OH, a precursor responsible for substrate degradation. Treatment of zidovudine-contaminated water with only UV radiation (254 nm), UV + ZnONP, and UV + BZnONP led to a degradation rate constant of 4.26×10^3, 16.91×10^3, and 36.12×10^3 min^{-1} respectively (Bhamare and Kulkarni, 2019). The reaction scheme is given below.

$$\text{BZnONP} + h\gamma \rightarrow \text{BZONPs } (h^+ + e^-) \tag{16.2}$$

where

$h\gamma$ is photo-irradiation,
h^+ is the hole and,
e^- is electron

$$(\text{BZnONP})\ h^+ + H_2O\ H + \cdot OH \tag{16.3}$$

where

−OH is a hydroxyl radical

$$\text{Zidovudine} + \cdot OH \text{ Photodegraded products}$$

$$(\text{BZnONP})\ e^- + \cdot HO_2O_2\ -O_2 \tag{16.4}$$

where

$-O_2$ is a superoxide anion

$$-O_2 + H + \cdot HO_2 \tag{16.5}$$

where,

HO_2 is a peroxide radical

$$HO2 + e- \rightarrow HO_2- \quad (16.6)$$

$$HO_2- + H + H_2O_2 \quad (16.7)$$

$$H_2O_2 + (BZnONP)\ e^- \rightarrow -OH + \cdot OH \quad (16.8)$$

$$\text{Zidovudine} + \cdot OH\ \text{Photodegraded products} \quad (16.9)$$

16.4.5 Copper nanoparticles

Copper nanoparticles can be prepared by natural processes or via chemical synthesis. Historically, copper nanoparticles have been used as coloring agents. They show excellent antibacterial and antimicrobial activity. Apart from these, copper nanoparticles can catalyze redox reactions and hence find application in bioremediation. Copper oxide (CuO) nanoparticles have an excellent ability to remove heavy metals such as arsenic from wastewater. Unlike other metallic nanoparticles, rapid arsenic adsorption by CuO nanoparticles is reasonably independent of water pH and traces of organic contaminants.

Copper nanoparticles (CuNPs) synthesized by the green process have been studied to remove ibuprofen, naproxen, and diclofenac from wastewater samples. The adsorption process was controlled by factors such as temperature, pH, adsorbent concentration, and the duration of contact between the adsorbent and the drug. The maximum removal rates of ibuprofen, naproxen, and diclofenac (74.4%, 86.9%, and 91.4%, respectively) have been observed at an ambient temperature of 25°C, pH of 4.5, a concentration of 10.0 mg Cu NP and 60 min of contact time (Husein et al., 2019).

An aqueous suspension of CuNP prepared using polyethyleneimine as a capping agent comprised a mixture of CuO and Cu_2O (Kalidhasan et al., 2017). Stable nanosuspension induced >99% atrazine degradation in just 1 h. The better performance of CuNPs compared to the commercial nano-copper oxide powder could be attributed to generation of OH radicals. The degradation rate was directly related to the concentration of CuNPs. Furthermore, factors such as neutral pH and the absence of dissolved ionic species in the water favored the degradation process (Abdel-Aziz et al., 2020).

Zero-valent bimetallic iron/copper nanoparticles [nZVI/Cu] synthesized by the green approach have shown excellent caffeine uptake from aqueous solutions. Maximum caffeine removal was observed at a pH of 5, a stirring rate of 100 rpm, and a contact time of 45 min. The rate of caffeine removal ranged between 86% and 33% at different caffeine [5–20 mg L^{-1}]. With the increase in the nanoparticle dose from 0.1 to 0.3 mg $L^{-1,}$ caffeine removal increased by 52%. The presence of nZVI magnetic nanoparticles makes the post-treatment separation easier by applying an external magnetic field. The nZVI/Cu is thus an eco-friendly catalyst offering reusability options for wastewater treatment.

16.4.6 Magnetic nanoparticles

Purported nanoparticles with a high affinity to water pollutants have been successfully employed to maintain and meet high-quality standards in water pollution prevention. Removing these nanoparticles from purified water is an inherent part of a good process design. Particle dispersion recovery by a typical nanofiltration step is feasible but high cost. Coagulation with chemical agents can be tried but is limited due to alteration of water quality parameters and a loss of recyclability of the nanoparticles.

Magnetophoretic is a magnetic separation process of nanoparticles that shows promise as it leads to minimal chemical or physical characteristics alteration. It is cost-efficient, adjustable according to the design process, and leads to the complete recovery of nanoparticles that can be reused during subsequent purification cycles.

Nano adsorbents that demonstrate multiple magnetic response phases are usually rich in iron oxides and zero-valent iron. Iron oxyhydroxides (FeOOH), zerovalent iron (ZVI), and iron oxides (Fe_3O_4, α-Fe_2O_3, γ-Fe_2O_3) are the most preferred iron-rich adsorbents in water purification. Many mechanisms that possibly occur on the surface are postulated as methods of action. The formation of Fe–O bridges between the pollutants and nanoadsorbents increases the reaction's specificity and selectivity. The distinct advantage of iron oxide-based semiconductors is their narrow band gap (2.1 eV), allowing them to utilize solar radiation to bring about degradation (Martínez-Boubeta and Simeonidis, 2019). They also demonstrate a high area-to-volume ratio, fast kinetic reaction property, high reactivity, and strong adsorption. Iron oxide particles are inherently magnetic and hence aggregate rapidly in the presence of an external magnetic field. Their quick separation from the aqueous solution is thus easily possible. This entire process is easily reversed by removing the magnetic field, leading to redistribution. Few iron oxide compounds such as magnetite (Fe_3O_4) or maghemite (γ-Fe_2O_3) demonstrate superparamagnetic properties that aid in rapid dispersion. The iron oxide NPs can be free-floating adsorbents as part of core and shell strategy, multiphase materials, or nanocomposites. A distinct advantage of magnetophoretics is that no secondary harmful compounds are produced, contributing to environmentally friendly regeneration.

Zero-valent metallic iron (ZVI) nanoparticles demonstrate superior magnetization value, leading to easy and efficient recovery. In addition, nanoscale ZVI (nZVI) in a stable, well-dispersed state shows high surface activity and reducing potential. However, surface oxidation and aggregation are the most significant drawbacks of nZVI that are detrimental to their reactivity.

Immobilization on support structures such as mesoporous silica or activated carbon, using anionic dispersants, leaf extracts, or cation resins, helps prevent nZVI passivation. nZVIs manufactured by green synthesis using extracts of grape marc, black tea, and vine leaves have been shown to remove 54%–66% of ibuprofen from water (Machado et al., 2013). Similar remediation efficiency has been observed in decontaminating sandy soils. The application of nZVIs in the adsorption of routinely encountered contaminants like carbamazepine, amoxicillin, and ampicillin has been investigated (Ghauch et al., 2009; Shirazi et al., 2013). The use of adjuvants like polyethylene glycol (PEG) and zeolite as capping agents has notably improved the performance of nZVI by preventing their aggregation. PEG-nZVI could degrade 10% more amoxicillin and 30% more ampicillin than plain nZVI, while nearly 30% higher ampicillin was removed by zeolite-capped nZVI (Ghauch et al., 2009).

16.4.6.1 Magnetite (Fe_3O_4)

Iron oxide nanoparticles are active magnetic nano adsorbents in water purification, with magnetite (Fe_3O_4) being the most widely used. They are cost-effective since iron salts are the starting material used for their synthesis. Magnetite is more stable than nZVI, and has a higher capacity to resist structural and chemical change but has lesser magnetic properties than ZVI. Magnetite nanoparticles have a tremendous affinity for the adsorption of arsenic in the aqueous phase. Magnetite is most commonly used in combination with other remediation materials for easy separation after the treatment.

Aqueous solutions of naproxen, carbamazepine, and bisphenol A were subjected to the action of Fe3O4 nanospheres functionalized with 6-deoxy-6-ethylene diamino-b-cyclodextrin (b-CDen) (b-CDen-MNP) (Ghosh et al., 2013). In this system, b-CDen (prepared by conjugation of beta-cyclodextrin and ethylene diamine) could adsorb organic pollutants through inclusive host-guest interactions. At the same time, Fe_3O_4 nanoparticles provided a means of separating adsorbents after the remediation process. The physicochemical properties, such as pKa, hydrophobicity, etc., of the solution's pollutants and pH are essential factors in the adsorption process. Neutral, unionized states of the contaminants favored their inclusion in the hydrophobic cavities, hence better removal. Drug properties, such as molecular size and geometry, influenced the time required to achieve adsorption equilibrium. With smaller size and planar geometry like bisphenol A and naproxen, faster equilibrium was achieved, unlike the nonplanar drugs like carbamazepine.

Fe_3O_4 nanoparticles help convert persulfate anions ($S_2O_8^{2-}$) into sulfate-free radicals. Organic contaminants are degraded by the intense oxidative action of sulfate radicals (Yan et al., 2011). A combination of 1.20 mM L^{-1} of $S_2O_8^{2-}$ and 2.40 mM L^{-1} of Fe_3O_4 nanoparticles could remove sulfamonomethoxine (0.06 mM L^{-1}) within 15 min of treatment.

Maghemite (γ-Fe_2O_3) has a structurally similar crystalline nature to magnetite. The reduction in the number of iron valencies from 4 to 3 leads to a reduction in magnetic affinity and suppresses the reduction of the maghemite activity. However, this chemistry confers higher stability to these nanoparticles. They have demonstrated excellent adsorption of pollutants having a high affinity for ferric ions, such as organic dyes. Since γ-Fe_2O_3 nanoparticles do not possess strong redox potential, they show limited application in removing PPCPs.

The general formula ascribed to ferrites is MFe_2O_4 (M = Cu, Mn, Co, Mg, or Zn). Their synthesis involves removing and replacing the Fe atom with another bivalent metal in the magnetite crystal.

MFe_2O_4 nanoparticles (M = Co^{+2}, Fe^{+2}, Zn^{+2}, Mn^{+2}) have rapidly degraded about 96% of the 3 antibiotics, including tetracycline, oxytetracycline, and chlortetracycline loaded at 100 μg L^{-1} concentration. Hydrogen bonding and surface complexation were considered the main factors are contributing to the adsorption and degradation of PPCPs (Bao et al., 2013).

Manganese oxide (MnO_2) nanoparticles have demonstrated an appreciable removal of sulfonamides, tetracycline, and endocrine disruptors. Antibiotics like clarithromycin and roxithromycin were rapidly adsorbed onto these nanoparticles, whereas carbamazepine failed to show significant adsorption. The formation mediates the adsorption of pharmaceuticals onto MnO_2. The various properties of PPCPs affect the process of surface complexation, and hence the difference in the adsorption performance is observed (Bernard et al., 1997; Feitosa-Felizzola et al., 2009; He et al., 2012; Remucal and Ginder-Vogel, 2014). The magnetic nanocomposite of Fe_3O_4–Cr_2O_3 has shown UV radiation-induced degradation of 4-chlorophenol and subsequent recovery via magnetic separation (Singh et al., 2017).

16.4.7 Carbon nanoparticles

Carbon-containing adsorbents are preferred for the purification and treatment of water. Of the different materials, such as activated carbon (AC), charcoal, activated sludge, and graphite, AC is the most preferred for water treatment because of its better performance and lower cost.

The typical elemental composition is around 80% carbon, with oxygen and nitrogen accounting for the remaining material. AC is characterized by a highly branched internal structure and high porosity. Micro (<2 nm), meso (2–50 nm), and macro (>50 nm) pores present on AC together attribute a considerable surface area of up to 2500 $m^2\ g^{-1}$ to AC. This results in a large number of binding sites interacting with the adsorbate. Factors like pH, temperature, presence of organic contaminants, and ionic species can influence AC's adsorption capacity to a significant extent. Similarly, the physicochemical properties, such as its particle size and state of ionization, can also affect the adsorption. The larger size of the contaminant has been shown to block the AC pores, ultimately reducing its surface area for adsorption. Adding acidic/basic surface functionality to the AC can improve its specificity and efficiency for removing contaminants. Activated carbon has been shown to remove pharmaceuticals such as sulfamethoxazole, metronidazole, and ibuprofen from aqueous solutions (Ellis, 2006; Mestre et al., 2007). The oxidized ACs have been shown to adsorb 93, 55, 89, and 80 $mg\ g^{-1}$ of atenolol (weakly basic), N, N-diethyl-meta-toluamide (neutral), triclosan (weakly acidic), and naproxen (acidic), respectively (Song et al., 2017).

16.4.8 Carbon nanotubes

With the practical application of AC in wastewater treatment, advanced materials such as carbon nanotubes (CNTs) and graphene with nanoscale particle size ranges are gaining much attention in the management of bioaccumulation. CNTs are capable of adsorbing most of the organic contaminants from water. CNTs are cylindrical structures comprising carbon atoms that are arranged in hexagonal geometry. The ends of the CNTs could be capped with half-fullerene-like structures. The single-walled carbon nanotubes (SWCNT) are made of a monolayer of graphite, also known as graphene, rolled into a tube-like structure. They are usually a nanometer in diameter and several hundred or even thousands of nanometers in length. As the name suggests, multiwalled carbon nanotubes (MWCNTs) consist of several layers of compressed SWCNTs of different diameters concentrically. The MWCNTs can attain diameters up to 100 nm apart from the nano's lengths to the micron range.

Unique tubular structures, superior conductivity, ease of chemical or physical modification, excellent chemical inertness, high surface area, and ability to adsorb a wide range of contaminants are some of the most outstanding merits of CNTs. These properties have been recently exploited for the removal of microcontaminants from wastewater.

CNTs can be employed in powders, sheets, or membranes to remove heavy metals, aromatic compounds, endocrine-disrupting compounds (EDCs), and PPCPs from water. Pollutants can be trapped in the tubes' hollow interiors of the tubes, interstitial channels, and grooves between the concentric tubes. The curved outer surface of the individual tubes is also a prominent area available for adsorption. Though the theoretical specific surface area (SSA) of nanotubes can be as high as 2600 $m^2\ g^{-1}$, the actual surface area is at least 20 times lower. It could be due to tangling, aggregation, and partial closure of tube structures. The factors like purity, surface area, and surface functional groups on CNTs affect their adsorptive potential. Physicochemical characteristics of PPCP, oxygen content, and quality of water samples are crucial parameters affecting the remediation efficiency of the CNTs.

In a study by Wang et al. MWCNT membranes, compared to SWCNT membranes, exhibited lower removal of acetaminophen, triclosan, and ibuprofen, lower specific surface area, and higher surface oxygen content. The extent of removal increased with the increasing number of aromatic rings (acetaminophen = ibuprofen triclosan). The aromatic rings impart hydrophobicity to the drugs, which results in a more significant hydrophobic interaction between the PPCP and CNT. PPCP molecules in neutral rather than ionized states could be removed to a greater extent. The presence of competing natural organic matter reduced the adsorption efficiency of all PPCPs. The elimination of diclofenac and caffeine from surface waters has been studied using a commercially available MWCNT product. With an increase in the quantity from 25 to 100 mg, the adsorption capacity decreased from 3.21 to 1.41 mg g^{-1} for caffeine and from 3.32 to 1.36 mg g^{-1} for diclofenac. An increase in the adsorbent concentration could have led to particle aggregation and overlap of the adsorption sites, thus reducing the effective surface area and the extent of adsorption. Thus, the study highlights the importance of optimizing adsorbent quantities during decontamination (Li et al., 2020).

SWCNTs were synthesized via the thermal decomposition of ferrocene. Their adsorption efficiency was compared with that of the commercially available MWCNTs. The SWCNTs could adsorb nearly 375 mg g^{-1} of benzoic acid from the aqueous solution. This amount was about five times higher than that reported for MWCNTs ($\sim$65 mg g^{-1}). More significant adsorption of benzoic acid on SWCNT materials could be attributed to the higher SSA due to lower diameter and the greater number of binding sites available in the grooves of nanotube clusters. Thus, SWCNT materials provide an attractive option to remove PPCP contaminants (Wang et al., 2015a).

16.4.9 Graphene-based nanoparticles

Graphene is a mechanically robust and optically transparent material belonging to the carbon kin. Graphene can be described as sp^2-hybridized carbons assorted in a 2D honeycomb-like single sheet in its purest form. It provides a vast surface area that is highly hydrophobic. This provides ample sites for bonding with functional groups such as hydroxyls, carboxyls, carbonyls, and epoxy. Such interactions produce graphite oxide or reduced graphite oxides. Graphite oxides (GO) contain large clusters of oxygen functional groups, imparting hydrophilicity to these materials. Partial reduction of GO creates reduced graphite oxides (rGO) that show a much lower oxygen content. The ratio of carbon to oxygen increases from 2:1(GO) to 246:1(rGO). The interest in using graphene-based nanomaterials for PPCP remediation stems from their integral properties of an enormous specific area, ubiquitous sorption loci, low-temperature requirement for creation, smaller intra-particulate diffusion distance, and admirable regenerative and reusable potential. Its massive and delocalized π-electron system boosts bonding attributes with targeted pharmaceuticals. The presence of one or more aromatic rings in most PPCPs makes the π electrons available for π-π interactions with the adsorbent. In addition, Van Der Waal forces, Lewis acid-base interactions, electrostatic attraction between charged drug molecules, and negative surface charges of the carbonaceous material are postulated adsorption mechanisms for the carbon-based nanomaterial. Hydrogen bonding between PPCP and oxygen-containing GO and rGO could provide better adsorption capacity to GO and rGO nanomaterials than graphene.

A large surface area of graphene results in the spontaneous adsorption of pollutants and drugs like aspirin, acetaminophen, and caffeine. Alkali activation of graphene has been shown to enhance its adsorption capacity due to significant surface area improvement. Ciprofloxacin could be removed at 196 mg g^{-1} using activated graphene. Similarly, contact time, pH of the water, and temperature greatly influence the remediation of PPCP using graphene-based nanomaterials. Due to hydrophobic interactions between a neutral drug and the adsorbent, the acidic environment promotes the removal of acidic drugs such as sulfonamides and diclofenac. Several studies involving graphene-related nanomaterial have proven their role in the remediation of pharmaceuticals like tetracycline, oxytetracycline, atenolol, propranolol, caffeine, bisphenol A, gemfibrozil, ibuprofen, triclosan, and carbamazepine (Delhiraja et al., 2019; Khalil et al., 2020).

The nanocomposite of conjugated chitosan GO/poly (acrylic acid) (GO/CSA) has been observed to remove dorzolamide (334 mg g^{-1}), an antiglaucoma drug. The enhanced activity could be attributed to hydrogen bond formation and electrostatic interactions (Kyzas et al., 2014).

Porous membranes comprising polysulfone (PSF) and GO have been able to remove drugs such as rhodamine b, ofloxacin, diclofenac, and Triton X-100 (a surfactant commonly used in PPCP) to >90% after 4 h of treatment. The adsorption efficiencies of these membranes were suggestively higher than those of pure PS membranes. Washing with ethanol rendered the membranes suitable for reuse (Zambianchi et al., 2017). The role of nanoparticles in managing bioaccumulation is shown in Fig. 16.2.

16.4.10 Role of nanocomposites and combination of nanoparticles in water remediation

So far, the individual roles of metallic nanoparticles, heterogeneous nanoparticles, and carbon-based nanoparticles in managing the bioaccumulation of PPCPs have been discussed. A blend of two or more such constituents fabricated through grafting, cross-linking, or simple admixture may impart unique characteristics to the final product and expand the scope and properties. The nanocomposites of the nanomaterials described above have shown removal efficiencies than the separate systems and have gained significant attention in contaminant removal. The following section gives a brief account of the various nanocomposites studied in the bioaccumulation of PPCPs.

16.4.11 Combination of carbon-based adsorbent with semiconductor nanoparticles

Combining TiO_2 or ZnO with carbonaceous materials such as AC, GO, and CNTs has been studied extensively to overcome the disadvantages of using TiO2 or ZnO alone. In the

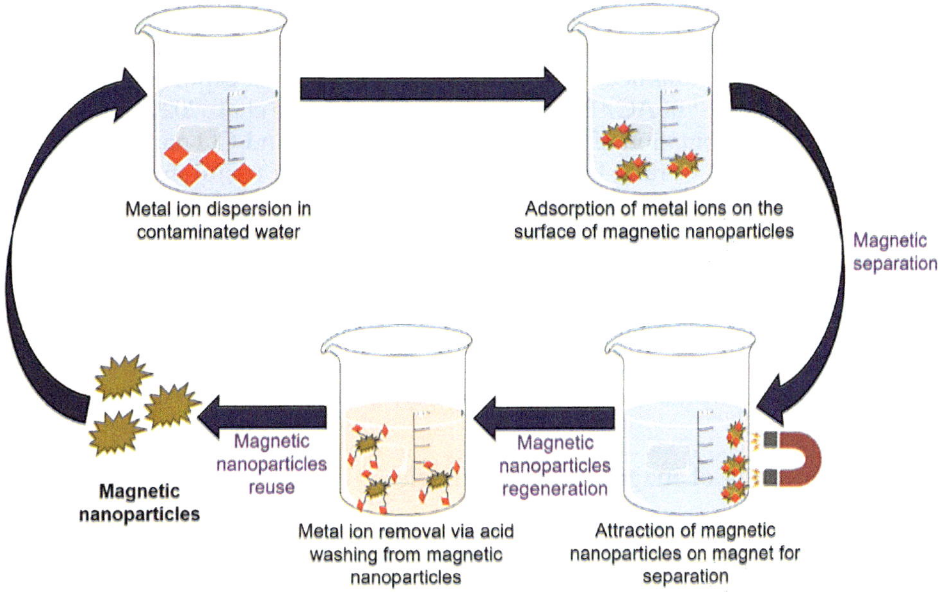

FIGURE 16.2 Role of nanoparticles in management of bioaccumulation.

presence of carbonaceous material, photoexcited electrons in the valence state of TiO_2 transfer to the carbonaceous material. They travel through the hybridized network toward oxygen groups to generate reactive oxygen species such as superoxide ions. The holes (h^+) that remain on the TiO_2 combine with adsorbed water and create hydroxyl radicals. Carbonaceous materials thus help in better and faster redox reactions by preventing the recombination of electrons and holes. There is a distinct reduction in the composite system's bandgap due to the atomic interactions among carbon, oxygen, and titanium. The lower bandgap allows for the catalytic degradation to occur in the presence of lower-energy visible light. The nanocomposites of CNT and TiO_2 and graphene and TiO_2 have shown superior catalytic action in visible radiation. The larger SSA of these nanocomposites further leads to a higher photodegradation rate (Zaib et al., 2013).

A combination of MWCNTs and TiO_2 in the form of membranes has shown excellent adsorption and subsequent degradation of acetaminophen, carbamazepine, and ibuprofen. The pH of drug solutions affected the extent of adsorption. At pH 7 and 11, electrostatic repulsion between the negatively charged surface of MWCNTs and ibuprofen anion significantly reduced the extent of ibuprofen adsorption of the CNT membrane. However, a significant increase in ibuprofen's adsorption was observed when the drug was completely unionized at the solution pH of 4. The MWCNT-TiO_2 membranes could initially remove carbamazepine, ibuprofen, and acetaminophen up to 80%, 45%, and 24%, while their removal efficiency dropped to 55%, 32%, and 19% upon regeneration.

The TiO_2-rGO compound showed significant efficiency in removing sulfamethoxazole, erythromycin, and clarithromycin from the wastewater sample. The addition of TiO_2-rGO composite to the water sample and UV light for 60 min degraded 84 ± 2%erythromycin, 86 ± 5% of clarithromycin, and 87 ± 4% of sulfamethoxazole (Karaolia et al., 2017).

Up to 94% removal of sulfamethazine was observed after 3 h of exposure to solar radiation in the presence of 0.6 g L^{-1} of AC/TiO_2 nanocomposites (Briche et al., 2020; El-Maraghy et al., 2020). Recently, the combination of ZnONP (avg size: 17 nm) and GO nanosheets (avg thickness: 5 nm) in a 0.4: 1 g L^{-1} ratio has been shown to be highly useful in managing bacterial resistance and bioaccumulation of levofloxacin in pharmaceutical wastewater. The photocatalytic degradation of ZnONP-induced levofloxacin and the drug adsorption on a high surface area of GO nanosheets seem to have helped remove more than 99% levofloxacin from pharmaceutical wastewater in just 2 h. The treated water allowed harboring of *Escherichia coli* growth, thus confirming the removal of the antibacterial. Similarly, GO/ZnONP nanocomposites at a dose of 0.02 g have shown up to 98.17% adsorption of methylene blue dye (5 ppm concentration) with a contact time of merely 8.5 min at pH 6 (Hosseini, 2016).

16.4.12 Composites of magnetic nanoparticles

Water remediation using nanomaterials discussed so far involves treating contaminated water with the optimum amounts of nanomaterial for sufficient time and favorable radiation and pH conditions to remove the contaminants to the desired levels.

However, recovery in a large-scale operation can become a challenging and costly, requiring expensive nanofiltration techniques. Magnetophoresis, on the other hand, can tackle the concerns of nanoparticle recovery. This ensures total restoration of nanoparticles, the least contamination of the treated water, affordability, and a wide choice of process designs. When used as actives in contaminants' remediation, nanoparticles like nZVI, magnetite, maghemite, and ferrites easily separate by magnetophoretic. On the other hand, they can also be used as carriers or vehicles for other active nanomaterials during water treatment. Here, they can provide a means of separating the active nanomaterial at the end of the remediation process. Inorganic metal/metal oxide nanoparticles such as TiO_2, Au, or Ag can be coated as a thin layer on the magnetic nanoparticle surface. Inactive organic molecules such as carbon-based nanomaterials, polymers, cyclodextrins, and magnetic nanoparticles are attached through adsorption. nZVI and magnetite are the most commonly used carriers.

The photocatalytic activity of the biogenic Fe_3O_4/Au nanocomposite was studied to remove imatinib and imipenem, commonly found pharmaceuticals, from hospitals' wastewater (Mirsadeghi et al., 2020). The composite could degrade imatinib and imipenem to up to 92% and 96% levels after 5 min of UV light exposure, whereas to 82% and 84% extent upon 60 min of visible light exposure. Fe_3O_4/Au nanocomposite also demonstrated excellent antimicrobial activity against human pathogens *Bacillus subtilis, Staphylococcus aureus, and Escherichia coli.* The design of nanocomposites capable of concurrently removing pharmaceutical and microbial adulterations is essential in hospitals' wastewater treatment environments. rGO–Fe_3O_4 nanocomposite (0.6 g L^{-1}) was studied to extract phenazopyridine residues (10 μ L^{-1}) from wastewater samples. Contact time of 5 min, solution temperature of 25°C, and pH of 6 resulted in 91.4% for removing phenazopyridine in an aqueous solution (Karimi-maleh et al., 2019).

Belachew et al. developed the combination of rGO with magnetite produced a nanohybrid that exhibited capability of removing 95% of crystal violet dye. The system could also extract norfloxacin and ciprofloxacin through π-π and electrostatic interactions (Kahsay et al., 2020; Tang et al., 2013). Magnetically activated carbon composites were prepared by chemical co-precipitation of manganese ferrite nanoparticles ($MnFe_2O_4$) in powdered AC. The maximum adsorption of sulfamethoxazole was found to be 159 mg g^{-1} at a pH of 7. Adsorption remained stable over the pH range of 3-7 and was unaffected in the presence of common ions and humic acids (Wan et al., 2014).

A novel composite of magnesium ferrite and γ-Fe_2O_3 could adsorb 259.1 mg g^{-1} and 200.8 mg g^{-1} of Congo Red and minocycline, respectively, from the wastewater. Hydrogen bond formation and electrostatic attractions were considered adsorption mechanisms for dye and minocycline (Lu et al., 2016).

Nanocomposites of $MnFe_2O_4$ and graphitic carbon (GC), as well as $MnFe_2O_4$ and bentonite (BT), were synthesized to study their PPCP removal efficacy. $MnFe_2O_4$/GC and $MnFe_2O_4$/BT, with a particle size of 50 and 60 nm, respectively, exhibited an excellent adsorption capacity compared to plain $MnFe_2O_4$ nanoparticles. Magnetic studies confirmed the superparamagnetic behavior of $MnFe_2O_4$/GC and $MnFe_2O_4$/BT. Mineralization of ampicillin (AMP) and oxytetracycline (OXT) was achieved under solar light due to shorter band gaps of 2.38 and 2.42 meV $MnFe_2O_4$/GC and $MnFe_2O_4$/BT. Both the nanocomposites could degrade 96% and 83% of AMP within 60 min. OXT was degraded to 99% and 90% in 120 min in the presence of BT- and GC-based nanocomposites, respectively. $MnFe_2O_4$/GC contributed to 100% degradation of AMP within 8 h. In OXT, only 70% of antibiotics were mineralized to CO_2, H_2O, and NO_3^{-2} ions. Magnetically recoverable systems showed appreciable inactivation of antibiotics (Gautam et al., 2017).

About 94% and 93% degradation of ibuprofen and benzophenone were achieved within 5 h by magnetic N$-$$TiO_2$@$SiO_2$@$Fe_3O_4$ nano photocatalyst in visible light radiation. Carbamazepine was degraded to 71% after 9 h. In the N-doped TiO_2 @ SiO_2 @ Fe_3O_4 nano-photocatalyst, Fe_3O_4 formed the core for magnetic separation after water treatment. The photo-dissolution effect was prevented by coating SiO_2 over the TiO_2 layer (Kumar et al., 2019).

16.4.13 Challenges of nanoparticles

Nanotechnology has been a mainstay of research for the past five decades, owing to its tremendous applications in many diverse fields. The studies mentioned above give a detailed account of their potential use in bioaccumulation treatment in various water bodies. Although the merits of nanomaterials are umpteen, the toxicity associated with them cannot be ignored. Many nanometric products are released into lakes, rivers, and oceans. They can cause damage to flora and fauna of the ecosystem, especially the large variety of microbes, benthic animals, and fishes. Their presence in potable water can even cause harm to human beings. In vitro and in vivo studies on inorganic and metallic nanoparticles' safety have highlighted their harmful effects, such as cytotoxicity and genotoxicity via enhanced oxidative stress, inactivating cellular enzymes DNA damage.

Metallic nanoparticles such as silver, iron TiO_2, and ZnO can produce ROS such as $-O_2$ and$^{\cdot}$OH; radicals can increase oxidative stress. Lipid peroxidation, protein carbonylation, and reduction in the levels of a natural antioxidant glutathione are the apparent consequences of increased oxidative stress. At lower concentrations of the nanoparticles and shorter exposure time, antioxidant enzymes such as superoxide dismutase, catalase, glutathione peroxidase, glutathione reductase, and glutathione sulfur transferase increase in response to moderate oxidative stress. However, increased dose and/or duration of nanomaterial exposure suppress these enzymes, ultimately resulting in cytotoxicity and genotoxicity in the organisms. The gills of marine animals are primary nanoparticle targets for the uptake and accumulation. WAG cell lines (prepared from Wallago Attu gill tissue) were subjected to an assessment of ZnONP and TiO_2 nanoparticles. ZnONP was more toxic with an IC50 of 4.92 mg L^{-1} than TiO_2 nanoparticles with an IC50 of 124.5 mg L^{-1}. However, treatment of human skin fibroblasts with these nanoparticles showed a higher IC50 value for ZnONP (2696 $\pm$ 667 ppm) compared to TiO_2 nanoparticles (49.56 $\pm$ 12.89 ppm) (Dubey et al., 2015).

The particle size, surface charge, solubility, chemical composition, aggregation, and oxidation status play a vital role in imparting toxicity to the nanoparticles; simultaneously, the cell type also plays a crucial role in toxic manifestation. Silver nanoparticles have been shown to reduce the antioxidant enzyme activity by inducing reactive oxygen species (ROS) and restraining the metabolism in the benthic species *Corbicula fluminea*. The muscle protein concentration of the Prochilosdis leneatus fish was found to be reduced after exposure to 2.5–25 μg L^{-1} of silver nanoparticles. ZnONP has shown cytotoxicity and genotoxicity among the freshwater molluscan bivalve, *Coelathera aegyptica*, and embryotoxicity in *Amarine medaka* and *Orycias melastigma*. ZnONP at 2 and 4 mg L^{-1} concentrations have shown a remarkable reduction in the aforementioned antioxidant enzymes and enhanced malondianhydride levels (a biomarker of lipid peroxidation) in Nile Tilapia muscles (Abdelazim et al., 2018). CuO nanoparticles in the concentration range of 10–60 μg L^{-1} have been found to reduce the levels of antioxidant enzymes in the cells of Chinook salmon. In comparison, TiO_2 nanoparticles in concentrations of up to 100 mg L^{-1} have shown such results in *Carassius auratus* (goldfish) and *Danio rerio* (zebrafish).

SWCNTs have been found to affect the growth of marine *Artemia salina* (Zhu et al., 2018). The CNTs, when subjected to studies in zebrafish, led to 3- and 6-fold enhancement in dopamine and serotonin levels and substantial reduction in the acetylcholinesterase activity. Such changes in neurotransmitter levels can have a profound impact on animal physiology and behavior. CNTs have also shown high phagocytic activity toward undifferentiated HL 60 cells and promyelocytic cell lines. MWCNTs show specific genotoxicity that affects the gene transcription responsible for apoptosis. They have shown toxic effects on *Dunaliella terriolecta*, phytoplankton. A positive correlation has been observed between the length of CNTs and the damage caused by them (Wei et al., 2010).

GO nanoparticles have shown membrane damage to *Raphdocelis subcapitala* green algae (Nogueira et al., 2015). They also reduce the growth of Scendesmus, a green alga, and *Chlorella Vulgaris*, obliqus microalgae, and reduce the synthesis of chlorophyll a and chlorophyll b in the cells of algae. The burrowing activity of Oligochete, a broad class of terrestrial and aquatic worms, has been shown to diminish upon GO exposure. GO quantum dots have demonstrated embryonic malformation in zebrafish (Wang et al., 2015b). Though graphene-related nanomaterials are extremely useful for managing bioaccumulation, more excellent water solubility as ideal particle size makes their separation difficult after water treatment.

Considering all these studies that show the flip side of nanomaterials' application in bioaccumulation management, one needs to be prudent in selecting the right nanomaterial in the right amounts giving due consideration to the type of water body and its ecosystem. The techniques that can treat the wastewater without discharging the nanomaterials in the water need to be developed to avoid their untoward effects on the ecosystem's flora and fauna. The application of various nanoparticles in the bioaccumulation of PPCPs is shown in Table 16.2.

16.5 Conclusion and prospects

Emerging contaminants such as PPCPs in various water bodies such as wastewater, surface water, groundwater, and drinking water can present severe health and safety concerns to aquatic life and humankind. Hence, removing contaminants from these ecosystems is a significant concern requiring urgent attention. Nanoparticles of metals such as silver, gold, iron, and copper, semiconductor-based nanoparticles like TiO_2 and ZnO, and carbon-based nanomaterials like AC, CNTs, and graphene have been studied extensively to understand their ability and mechanism of PPCP removal. Most have shown their mettle in managing commonly found pharmaceutical contaminants in wastewater like antibiotics, anti-inflammatory, antipyretic, antiepileptic, and antidepressant drugs. Though the individual nanomaterials exhibit good removal potential for PPCPs, the nanocomposites comprising adsorption and photocatalytic functionalities have shown highly improved performance in higher remediation efficiency and greater rate as lower energy requirements. Nanocomposites can trap polar and nonpolar PPCPs from the water with their peculiar surface functions. With all these merits, nanomaterials and nanocomposites discussed in the review are likely to be significant in managing PPCP bioaccumulation in the future. However, many milestones have yet to be crossed before the nanomaterials can become the standard, large-scale remediation technique.

Most of the studies performed hitherto include lab-scale experiments involving synthetic water spiked with the PPCPs under consideration and highly controlled light, oxygen, temperature, and pH conditions. More studies are instead needed to treat wastewater models simulating real-life mechanical, thermal, and chemical conditions. Also, experiments involving the treatment of pilot and large-scale wastewater are necessary to perform. Such studies would manifest the shortcomings of the existing treatment processes and help overcome those with more research and development in this field.

The current scientific literature on bioaccumulation of the PPCPs primarily focuses on the contaminant's disappearance and not on the end products, which could still be more toxic than the original drugs. Complete mineralization of pharmaceuticals to harmless products such as CO_2 and water is the goal of any remediation treatment. More studies need to be planned to investigate whether the materials mentioned earlier attain such goals. The nanomaterials' recovery and recyclability after the water treatment is another challenging area that can pose serious health and safety concerns to the ecosystem. Magnetic nanoparticles as actives or carriers are most recommended due to their amenability to magnetophoresis and

TABLE 16.2 Application of various nanoparticles in bioaccumulation of PPCPs.

Type of nanoparticles (adsorbent)	Contaminants (adsorbate)	pH	Dosage of adsorbent (mg L^{-1})	Conc. of adsorbate (mg L^{-1})	Time for adsorption t-(h)	% Removal	References
Activated carbon	Penicillin G	6	1000	–	–	71%	Aksu and Dede (2005)
	Amoxicillin	4.98	1000	317	0.58	94%	Putra et al. (2009)
Copper nanoparticles	Reactive blue 4 dye	3–4	2000	15	0.25	90%	Marcelo et al. (2018)
	Bromo cresol green dye	4	500	20	1.5	88%	Raju et al. (2017)
	Basic violet16 Basic red 14	7	500	–	0.5	70% 80%	Naghizade Asl et al. (2016)
Ferric oxide nanoparticles	Tetracycline	–	1600	12.5	24	95%	Zhang et al. (2011)
	Oxytetracycline,	7	3000	1	1	96%	Zhang et al. (2017)
	Ceftriaxone	3.1–4	1990	10	1.5	97.18%	Badi et al. (2018)
Graphene-based nanoparticles	Tetracycline	3.6	181	33.33	0.5	50%	Gao et al. (2012)
	Sulfamethoxazole, ciprofloxacin	5.0	100 10	20 10	12 24	47% 34.5%	Chen et al. (2015)
	Ciprofloxacin	7.0	500	150	0.036	84.5%	Yu et al. (2015)
	Ketoprofen, carbamazepine	6.5	–	15 30	2.83 1.6	–	Liu et al. (2014)
Multiwalled carbon nanotubes	Ketoprofen, carbamazepine	6.5	–	15 30	24 48	–	Liu et al. (2014)
	Sulfamethoxazole, thiamphenicol, ibuprofen, diclofenac, carbamazepine	7	427–1556	0.2	12	–	Gao et al. (2012)
	Oxytetracycline, carbamazepine	7	25 50	2.5	24	79% 97%	Oleszczuk et al. (2009)
	Sulfamethazine	5	1000	10	24	90%	Zhang et al. (2016)
Single walled carbon nanotubes	Ketoprofen, carbamazepine	6.5 6.5	–	15 30	48 96	–	Liu et al. (2014)

TABLE 16.2 Application of various nanoparticles in bioaccumulation of PPCPs.—cont'd

Type of nanoparticles (adsorbent)	Contaminants (adsorbate)	pH	Dosage of adsorbent (mg L^{-1})	Conc. of adsorbate (mg L^{-1})	Time for adsorption t-(h)	% Removal	References
Titanium dioxide NP.	Chloramphenicol and tartrazine	6.5	400	20	2	84% 89%	Jodat and Jodat (2014)
	Ibuprofen	6	2000	25	6	78%	Bhatia and Dhir (2016)
	Paracetamol	–	1000	–	1.66	95%	Zhang et al. (2008)
	Oxytetracycline	4.4	500	–	0.66	100%	Pereira et al. (2011)
Zinc oxide nanoparticles	Ciprofloxacin	10	20	5	1	50%	El-Kemary et al. (2010)
	Metronidazole	10	1500	80	–	96.5%	Farzadkia et al. (2014)
	Diclofenac	7	50	1	0.5	68%	Bohdziewicz et al. (2016)

separation ease. However, the possibility of toxicity due to the leaching of metal ions such as Mn and Co cannot be ignored while incorporating ferrite nanomaterials during water purification. Many scientific reports indicate the harmful and detrimental effects of trace nanomaterials on marine and freshwater flora and fauna, not sparing human beings by finding entry into potable water. Hence, it is imperative to study how to separate these photocatalysts and the carbon-based adsorbents from the treated water.

Bioaccumulation of the PPCP and other inorganic and organic pollutants in water bodies, wetlands, and landfills poses a severe threat to the sustainable ecosystem and humankind. Implementing effective remediation measures to deal with these threats is the need of the hour. With continuous research and advancement in nanomaterials, cost-effective, scalable, efficient, and eco-friendly decontamination methods are expected to be evolved and prove beneficial to the pollution-free ecosystem.

16.6 List of abbreviations

$(K_2S_2O_8)^-$ Potassium peroxodisulfate
AC Activated carbon
API Active pharmaceutical ingredient
Au Gold
b-CDen 6-deoxy-6-ethylene diamino-b-cyclodextrin
BAF Bioaccumulation factor
BCF Bioconcentration factors

BT	Bentonite
BZnONP	Barium doped Zinc oxide nanoparticle
CdS	Cadmium sulfide
CECs	Contaminants of emerging concern
CNTs	Carbon nanotubes
COX	Cyclo-oxygenase
Cr_2O_3	Chromium oxide
Cu NPs	Copper oxide nanoparticle
Cu_2O	Cuprous oxide
CuO	Copper oxide
EDCs	Endocrine disrupting compounds
EPA	European protection agency
EPS	Extracellular polymeric particles
FCM	Food chain multiplier
Fe_3O_4	Magnetite
FeOOH	Iron oxy-hydroxides
GC	Graphitic carbon
GO	Graphene oxide
GONS	Graphene oxide nanosheets
IUPAC	International Union of Pure and Applied Chemistry
L	Liter
MNC	Magnetic nanocomposite
$MnFe_2O_4$	Manganese ferrite
MnO_2	Manganese oxide
MWCNTs	Multiwalled carbon nanotubes
N, S-CQDs	Nitrogen and sulfur co-doped carbon quantum dots
ng	Nanogram
NPs	Nanoparticles
NSAIDs	Non-steroidal anti-inflammatory drugs
nZVI/Cu	Zero-valent iron/copper nanoparticles
PA	Polyamide
PAH	Polycyclic aromatic hydrocarbon
PE	Polyethylene
PEG	Polyethylene glycol
PET	Polyethylene terephthalate
POP	Persistent aromatic pollutants
PP	Polypropylene
PPCPs	Pharmaceuticals and personal care products
PS	Polystyrene
PS	Polysulfone
PVC	Polyvinyl alcohol chloride
PVP	Polyvinylpyrrolidone
rGO	Reduced graphite oxides
ROS	Reactive oxygen species
SiO_2	Silicon dioxide
SSA	Specific surface area
SWCNTS	Single-walled carbon nanotubes
TiO_2	Titanium dioxide
USPEA	United States Environmental Protection Agency
UV	Ultraviolet
VOC	Volatile organic compounds
WO_3	Tungsten oxide
WWTPs	Wastewater treatment plants

γ-Fe_2O_3	Maghemite
μg	Microgram
ZnO	Zinc oxide
ZnONP	Zinc oxide nanoparticles
ZVI	Zero-valent metallic iron

References

Abdel-Aziz, H.M., Farag, R.S., Abdel-Gawad, S.A., 2020. Removal of caffeine from aqueous solution by green approach using Ficus Benjamina zero-valent iron/copper nanoparticles. Adsorpt. Sci. Technol. 38, 325–343.

Abdelazim, A.M., Saadeldin, I.M., Swelum, A.A.-A., Afifi, M.M., Alkaladi, A., 2018. Oxidative stress in the muscles of the fish Nile tilapia caused by zinc oxide nanoparticles and its modulation by vitamins C and E. Oxid. Med. Cell. Longev. 2018, 6926712.

Achilleos, A., Hapeshi, E., Xekoukoulotakis, N.P., Mantzavinos, D., Fatta-Kassinos, D., 2010. Factors affecting diclofenac decomposition in water by UV-A/TiO2 photocatalysis. Chem. Eng. J. 161, 53–59.

Adewuyi, A., 2020. Chemically modified biosorbents and their role in the removal of emerging pharmaceutical waste in the water system. Water 12, 1551.

Adewuyi, A., Pereira, F.V., 2017. Underutilized *Luffa cylindrica* sponge: a local bio-adsorbent for the removal of Pb(II) pollutant from water system. Beni-Suef Univ. J. Basic Appl. Sci. 6, 118–126.

Akcil, A., Erust, C., Ozdemiroglu, S., Fonti, V., Beolchini, F., 2015. A review of approaches and techniques used in aquatic contaminated sediments: metal removal and stabilization by chemical and biotechnological processes. J. Clean. Prod. 86, 24–36.

Aksu, Z., Dede, O., 2005. Application of biosorption for penicillin G removal: comparison with activated carbon. Process Biochem. 40, 831–847.

Ali, H., Khan, E., 2019. Trophic transfer, bioaccumulation, and biomagnification of non-essential hazardous heavy metals and metalloids in food chains/webs—concepts and implications for wildlife and human health. Hum. Ecol. Risk Assess. 25, 1353–1376.

Alonso Castillo, M.L., Sánchez Trujillo, I., Vereda Alonso, E., García De Torres, A., Cano Pavón, J.M., 2013. Bioavailability of heavy metals in water and sediments from a typical Mediterranean Bay (Málaga Bay, region of Andalucía, Southern Spain). Mar. Pollut. Bull. 76, 427–434.

Araujo, L., Villa, N., Camargo, N., Bustos, M., García, T., Prieto, A.D.J., 2011. Persistence of gemfibrozil, naproxen and mefenamic acid in natural waters. Environ. Chem. Lett. 9, 13–18.

Armitage, J.M., Erickson, R.J., Luckenbach, T., Ng, C.A., Prosser, R.S., Arnot, J.A., Schirmer, K., Nichols, J.W., 2017. Assessing the bioaccumulation potential of ionizable organic compounds: current knowledge and research priorities. Environ. Toxicol. Chem. 36, 882–897.

Awfa, D., Ateia, M., Fujii, M., Johnson, M.S., Yoshimura, C., 2018. Photodegradation of pharmaceuticals and personal care products in water treatment using carbonaceous-TiO2 composites: a critical review of recent literature. Water Res. 142, 26–45.

Azubuike, C.C., Chikere, C.B., Okpokwasili, G.C., 2016. Bioremediation techniques—classification based on site of application: principles, advantages, limitations and prospects. World J. Microbiol. Biotechnol. 32.

Badi, M.Y., Azari, A., Pasalari, H., Esrafili, A., Farzadkia, M., 2018. Modification of activated carbon with magnetic Fe3O4 nanoparticle composite for removal of ceftriaxone from aquatic solutions. J. Mol. Liq. 261, 146–154.

Bao, X., Qiang, Z., Ling, W., Chang, J.-H., 2013. Sonohydrothermal synthesis of MFe2O4 magnetic nanoparticles for adsorptive removal of tetracyclines from water. Separ. Purif. Technol. 117, 104–110.

Barra Caracciolo, A., Topp, E., Grenni, P., 2015. Pharmaceuticals in the environment: biodegradation and effects on natural microbial communities. A review. J. Pharm. Biomed. Anal. 106, 25–36.

Barreto, A., Luis, L.G., Pinto, E., Almeida, A., Paíga, P., Santos, L.H.M.L.M., Delerue-Matos, C., Trindade, T., Soares, A.M.V.M., Hylland, K., Loureiro, S., Oliveira, M., 2019. Effects and bioaccumulation of gold nanoparticles in the gilthead seabream (*Sparus aurata*)—single and combined exposures with gemfibrozil. Chemosphere 215, 248–260.

Bernard, S., Chazal, P., Mazet, M., 1997. Removal of organic compounds by adsorption on pyrolusite (β-MnO2). Water Res. 31, 1216–1222.

Bhamare, V.S., Kulkarni, R.M., 2019. Photocatalytic degradation of pharmaceutical drug zidovudine by undoped and 5 % barium doped zinc oxide nanoparticles during water treatment: synthesis and characterisation. Int. J. Appl. Pharm. 11, 227–236.

Bhatia, V., Dhir, A., 2016. Transition metal doped TiO2 mediated photocatalytic degradation of anti-inflammatory drug under solar irradiations. J. Environ. Chem. Eng. 4, 1267–1273.

Bhatia, V., Ray, A.K., Dhir, A., 2016. Enhanced photocatalytic degradation of ofloxacin by co-doped titanium dioxide under solar irradiation. Separ. Purif. Technol. 161, 1–7.

Bohdziewicz, J., Kudlek, E., Dudziak, M., 2016. Influence of the catalyst type (TiO2 and ZnO) on the photocatalytic oxidation of pharmaceuticals in the aquatic environment. Desalination Water Treat. 57, 1552–1563.

Bottoni, P., Caroli, S., Caracciolo, A.B., 2010. Pharmaceuticals as priority water contaminants. Toxicol. Environ. Chem. 92, 549–565.

Briche, S., Derqaoui, M., Belaiche, M., EL Mouchtari, E.M., WONG-WAH-Chung, P., Rafqah, S., 2020. Nanocomposite material from TiO2 and activated carbon for the removal of pharmaceutical product sulfamethazine by combined adsorption/photocatalysis in aqueous media. Environ. Sci. Pollut. Res. 27, 25523–25534.

Bueno, M.J.M., Gomez, M.J., Herrera, S., Hernando, M.D., Agüera, A., Fernández-Alba, A.R., 2012. Occurrence and persistence of organic emerging contaminants and priority pollutants in five sewage treatment plants of Spain: two years pilot survey monitoring. Environ. Pollut. 164, 267–273.

Bundschuh, M., Filser, J., Lüderwald, S., Mckee, M.S., Metreveli, G., Schaumann, G.E., Schulz, R., Wagner, S., 2018. Nanoparticles in the environment: where do we come from, where do we go to? Environ. Sci. Eur. 30, 6.

Challis, J.K., Hanson, M.L., Friesen, K.J., Wong, C.S., 2014. A critical assessment of the photodegradation of pharmaceuticals in aquatic environments: defining our current understanding and identifying knowledge gaps. Environ. Sci. Process. Impacts 16, 672–696.

Chen, H., Gao, B., Li, H., 2015. Removal of sulfamethoxazole and ciprofloxacin from aqueous solutions by graphene oxide. J. Hazard. Mater. 282, 201–207.

Chen, Y., Liu, Y., Li, Y., Wu, Y., Chen, Y., Zeng, G., Zhang, J., Li, H., 2017. Influence of biochar on heavy metals and microbial community during composting of river sediment with agricultural wastes. Bioresour. Technol. 243, 347–355.

Chojnacka, K., 2010. Biosorption and bioaccumulation—the prospects for practical applications. Environ. Int. 36, 299–307.

Chojnacka, K., Mikulewicz, M., 2014. Bioaccumulation. In: Wexler, P. (Ed.), Encyclopedia of Toxicology, third ed. Academic Press, Oxford.

Costa, C., Teixeira, J.P., 2014. Biomonitoring. In: Encyclopedia of Toxicology, third ed., vol. 1, pp. 483–484.

Daley, J., 2013. Bioamplification as a Bioaccumulation Mechanism.

De Godos, I., Muñoz, R., Guieysse, B., 2012. Tetracycline removal during wastewater treatment in high-rate algal ponds. J. Hazard. Mater. 229–230, 446–449.

De Groot, R.S., Wilson, M.A., Boumans, R.M.J., 2002. A typology for the classification, description and valuation of ecosystem functions, goods and services. Ecol. Econ. 41, 393–408.

De Luna, M.D.G., Aranzamendez, G.L., Tolosa, N.C., Lu, M.C., 2017. Synthesis of novel potassium peroxodisulfate-modified titanium dioxide for photocatalytic oxidation of acetaminophen under visible light irradiation. Int. J. Environ. Sci. Technol. 14, 973–982.

De Wilt, A., Butkovskyi, A., Tuantet, K., Leal, L.H., Fernandes, T.V., Langenhoff, A., Zeeman, G., 2016. Micropollutant removal in an algal treatment system fed with source separated wastewater streams. J. Hazard. Mater. 304, 84–92.

Deibel, I., Lampe, C., Ulbricht, J., Cnudde, T., Van Dessel, G., 2007. Sustainable management of sediment resources. In: Bortone, P., Palumbo, L. (Eds.), Sediment and Dredged Material Treatment. SedNet.

Delhiraja, K., Vellingiri, K., Boukhvalov, D.W., Philip, L., 2019. Development of highly water stable graphene oxide-based composites for the removal of pharmaceuticals and personal care products. Ind. Eng. Chem. Res. 58, 2899–2913.

Dinda, S.C., 2018. Bioaccumulation and toxic profiling of nanostructured particles and materials. In: Unraveling the Safety Profile of Nanoscale Particles and Materials-From Biomedical to Environmental Applications.

Ding, T., Yang, M., Zhang, J., Yang, B., Lin, K., Li, J., Gan, J., 2017. Toxicity, degradation and metabolic fate of ibuprofen on freshwater diatom Navicula sp. J. Hazard. Mater. 330, 127–134.

Dubey, A., Goswami, M., Yadav, K., Chaudhary, D., 2015. Oxidative stress and nano-toxicity induced by TiO2 and ZnO on WAG cell line. PLoS One 10 e0127493-e0127493.

El-Kemary, M., EL-Shamy, H., EL-Mehasseb, I., 2010. Photocatalytic degradation of ciprofloxacin drug in water using ZnO nanoparticles. J. Lumin. 130, 2327–2331.

El-Maraghy, C.M., EL-Borady, O.M., EL-Naem, O.A., 2020. Effective removal of levofloxacin from pharmaceutical wastewater using synthesized zinc oxid, graphen oxid nanoparticles compared with their combination. Sci. Rep. 10, 5914.

Ellis, J.B., 2006. Pharmaceutical and personal care products (PPCPs) in urban receiving waters. Environ. Pollut. 144, 184–189.

Farzadkia, M., Esrafili, A., Baghapour, M.A., Shahamat, Y.D., Okhovat, N., 2014. Degradation of metronidazole in aqueous solution by nano-ZnO/UV photocatalytic process. Desalination Water Treat. 52, 4947–4952.

Feitosa-Felizzola, J., Hanna, K., Chiron, S., 2009. Adsorption and transformation of selected human-used macrolide antibacterial agents with iron(III) and manganese(IV) oxides. Environ. Pollut. 157, 1317–1322.

Fisher, S.W., 1995. Mechanisms of bioaccumulation in aquatic systems. In: Ware, G.W. (Ed.), Reviews of Environmental Contamination and Toxicology: Continuation of Residue Reviews. Springer, New York, NY. New York.

Flickinger, M.C., Drew, S.W., 1999. Encyclopedia of Bioprocess Technology. John Wiley.

Fomina, M., Gadd, G.M., 2014. Biosorption: current perspectives on concept, definition and application. Bioresour. Technol. 160, 3–14.

Gadekar, V., Borade, Y., Kannaujia, S., Rajpoot, K., Anup, N., Tambe, V., Kalia, K., Tekade, R.K., 2021. Nanomedicines accessible in the market for clinical interventions. J. Control Release 330, 372–397. https://doi.org/10.1016/j.jconrel.2020.12.034. Epub 2020 Dec 25. PMID: 33370576.

Gao, Y., Li, Y., Zhang, L., Huang, H., Hu, J., Shah, S.M., Su, X., 2012. Adsorption and removal of tetracycline antibiotics from aqueous solution by graphene oxide. J. Colloid Interface Sci. 368, 540–546.

Gautam, S., Shandilya, P., Priya, B., Singh, V.P., Raizada, P., Rai, R., Valente, M., Singh, P., 2017. Superparamagnetic MnFe2O4 dispersed over graphitic carbon sand composite and bentonite as magnetically recoverable photocatalyst for antibiotic mineralization. Separ. Purif. Technol. 172, 498–511.

Gavrilescu, M., Demnerová, K., Aamand, J., Agathos, S., Fava, F., 2015. Emerging pollutants in the environment: present and future challenges in biomonitoring, ecological risks and bioremediation. N. Biotechnol. 32, 147–156.

Geary, S.M., Morris, A.S., Salem, A.K., 2016. Assessing the effect of engineered nanomaterials on the environment and human health. J. Allergy Clin. Immunol. 138, 405–408.

Gerbersdorf, S.U., Hollert, H., Brinkmann, M., Wieprecht, S., Schüttrumpf, H., Manz, W., 2011. Anthropogenic pollutants affect ecosystem services of freshwater sediments: the need for a "triad plus x" approach. J. Soils Sediments 11, 1099–1114.

Ghauch, A., Tuqan, A., Abou Assi, H., 2009. Antibiotic removal from water: elimination of amoxicillin and ampicillin by microscale and nanoscale iron particles. Environ. Pollut. 157, 1626–1635.

Ghosh, S., Badruddoza, A.Z., Hidajat, K., Uddin, M., 2013. Adsorptive removal of emerging contaminants from water using superparamagnetic Fe3O4 nanoparticles bearing aminated β-cyclodextrin. J. Environ. Chem. Eng. 1, 122–130.

Gobas, F.A., Burkhard, L.P., Doucette, W.J., Sappington, K.G., Verbruggen, E.M., Hope, B.K., Bonnell, M.A., Arnot, J.A., Tarazona, J.V., 2016. Review of existing terrestrial bioaccumulation models and terrestrial bioaccumulation modeling needs for organic chemicals. Integrated Environ. Assess. Manag. 12, 123–134.

Gorain, B., Choudhury, H., Tekade, R.K., Karan, S., Jaisankar, P., Pal, T.K., 2016. Comparative biodistribution and safety profiling of olmesartan medoxomil oil-in-water oral nanoemulsion. Regul. Toxicol. Pharmacol. 82, 20–31.

Gossett, R.W., Brown, D.A., Young, D.R., 1983. Predicting the bioaccumulation of organic compounds in marine organisms using octanol/water partition coefficients. Mar. Pollut. Bull. 14, 387–392.

Grenni, P., Patrolecco, L., Ademollo, N., Tolomei, A., BARRA Caracciolo, A., 2013. Degradation of Gemfibrozil and Naproxen in a river water ecosystem. Microchem. J. 107, 158–164.

Grenni, P., Patrolecco, L., Ademollo, N., Di Lenola, M., BARRA Caracciolo, A., 2014. Capability of the natural microbial community in a river water ecosystem to degrade the drug naproxen. Environ. Sci. Pollut. Res. 21, 13470–13479.

Hanamoto, S., Kawakami, T., Nakada, N., Yamashita, N., Tanaka, H., 2014. Evaluation of the photolysis of pharmaceuticals within a river by 2 year field observations and toxicity changes by sunlight. Environ. Sci. Process. Impacts 16, 2796–2803.

Hansen, P.-D., 2008. Biosensors and eco-toxicology. Eng. Life Sci. 8, 26–31.

He, Y., Xu, J., Zhang, Y., Guo, C., Li, L., Wang, Y., 2012. Oxidative transformation of carbamazepine by manganese oxides. Environ. Sci. Pollut. Res. 19, 4206–4213.

Hena, S., Gutierrez, L., Croué, J.-P., 2020. Removal of metronidazole from aqueous media by *C. vulgaris*. J. Hazard. Mater. 384, 121400.

Hena, S., Gutierrez, L., Croué, J.-P., 2021. Removal of pharmaceutical and personal care products (PPCPs) from wastewater using microalgae: a review. J. Hazard. Mater. 403, 124041.

Hom-Diaz, A., Llorca, M., Rodríguez-Mozaz, S., Vicent, T., Barceló, D., Blánquez, P., 2015. Microalgae cultivation on wastewater digestate: β-estradiol and 17α-ethynylestradiol degradation and transformation products identification. J. Environ. Manag. 155, 106–113.

Hosseini, S.A., 2016. Graphene oxide/zinc oxide nanocomposite: a superior adsorbent for removal of methylene blue-statistical analysis by response surface methodology (RSM). S. Afr. J. Chem. 69, 105–112.

Husein, D.Z., Hassanien, R., AL-Hakkani, M.F., 2019. Green-synthesized copper nano-adsorbent for the removal of pharmaceutical pollutants from real wastewater samples. Heliyon 5, e02339.

Isidori, M., Lavorgna, M., Nardelli, A., Parrella, A., Previtera, L., Rubino, M., 2005. Ecotoxicity of naproxen and its phototransformation products. Sci. Total Environ. 348, 93–101.

Jain, N., Bhargava, A., Panwar, J., 2014. Enhanced photocatalytic degradation of methylene blue using biologically synthesized "protein-capped" ZnO nanoparticles. Chem. Eng. J. 243, 549–555.

Jodat, A., Jodat, A., 2014. Photocatalytic degradation of chloramphenicol and tartrazine using Ag/TiO2 nanoparticles. Desalination Water Treat. 52, 2668–2677.

Kahsay, M.H., Belachew, N., Tadesse, A., Basavaiah, K., 2020. Magnetite nanoparticle decorated reduced graphene oxide for adsorptive removal of crystal violet and antifungal activities. RSC Adv. 10, 34916–34927.

Kalidhasan, S., Ben-Sasson, M., Dror, I., Carmieli, R., Schuster, E.M., Berkowitz, B., 2017. Oxidation of aqueous organic pollutants using a stable copper nanoparticle suspension. Can. J. Chem. Eng. 95, 343–352.

Karaolia, P., Michael-Kordatou, I., Hapeshi, E., Drosou, C., Bertakis, Y., Christofilos, D., Armatas, G., Sygellou, L., Schwartz, T., Xekoukoulotakis, N., Fatta-Kassinos, D., 2017. Removal of antibiotics, antibiotic-resistant bacteria and their associated genes by graphene-based TiO 2 composite photocatalysts under solar radiation in urban wastewaters. Appl. Catal. B Environ. 224.

Karimi-Maleh, H., Shafieizadeh, M., Taher, M., Opoku, F., Kiarii, E., Govender, P., Ranjbari, S., Rezapour, M., Orooji, Y., 2019. The role of magnetite/graphene oxide nano-composite as a high-efficiency adsorbent for removal of phenazopyridine residues from water samples, an experimental/theoretical investigation. J. Mol. Liq. 298, 112040.

Karlsson, S., Meili, M., Bergstroem, U., 2002. Bioaccumulation Factors in Aquatic Ecosystems A Critical Review. Sweden.

Kelly, B.C., Gobas, F.A.P.C., 2003. An arctic terrestrial food-chain bioaccumulation model for persistent organic pollutants. Environ. Sci. Technol. 37, 2966–2974.

Khalil, A.M., Memon, F.A., Tabish, T.A., Salmon, D., Zhang, S., Butler, D., 2020. Nanostructured porous graphene for efficient removal of emerging contaminants (pharmaceuticals) from water. Chem. Eng. J. 398, 125440.

Khan, I., Saeed, K., Khan, I., 2019. Nanoparticles: properties, applications and toxicities. Arab. J. Chem. 12, 908–931.

Koe, W.S., Chong, W.C., Pang, Y.L., Koo, C.H., Ebrahim, M., Mohammad, A.W., 2020. Novel nitrogen and sulphur co-doped carbon quantum dots/titanium oxide photocatalytic membrane for in-situ degradation and removal of pharmaceutical compound. J. Water Proc. Eng. 33, 101068.

Kulkarni, S.J., 2014. Use of biotechnology for synthesis of various products from different feedstocks-a review. Int. J. Adv. Res. Biotechnol. 2, 01–03.

Kumar, A., Khan, M., Fang, L., Lo, I.M.C., 2019. Visible-light-driven N-TiO2@SiO2@Fe3O4 magnetic nanophotocatalysts: synthesis, characterization, and photocatalytic degradation of PPCPs. J. Hazard. Mater. 370, 108–116.

Kyzas, G.Z., Bikiaris, D.N., Seredych, M., Bandosz, T.J., Deliyanni, E.A., 2014. Removal of dorzolamide from biomedical wastewaters with adsorption onto graphite oxide/poly(acrylic acid) grafted chitosan nanocomposite. Bioresour. Technol. 152, 399–406.

Lasagna-Reeves, C., Gonzalez-Romero, D., Barria, M.A., Olmedo, I., Clos, A., Sadagopa Ramanujam, V.M., Urayama, A., Vergara, L., Kogan, M.J., Soto, C., 2010. Bioaccumulation and toxicity of gold nanoparticles after repeated administration in mice. Biochem. Biophys. Res. Commun. 393, 649–655.

Li, C., Zhou, K., Qin, W., Tian, C., Qi, M., Yan, X., Han, W., 2019. A review on heavy metals contamination in soil: effects, sources, and remediation techniques. Soil Sediment Contam. 28, 380–394.

Li, S., De Silva, T., Arsano, I., Gallaba, D., Karunanithy, R., Wasala, M., Zhang, X., Sivakumar, P., Migone, A., Tsige, M., Ma, X., Talapatra, S., 2020. High adsorption of benzoic acid on single walled carbon nanotube bundles. Sci. Rep. 10, 10013.

Liu, F.-F., Zhao, J., Wang, S., Du, P., Xing, B., 2014. Effects of solution chemistry on adsorption of selected pharmaceuticals and personal care products (PPCPs) by graphenes and carbon nanotubes. Environ. Sci. Technol. 48, 13197–13206.

Loos, R., Gawlik, B.M., Locoro, G., Rimaviciute, E., Contini, S., Bidoglio, G., 2008. EU wide monitoring survey of polar persistent pollutants in European river waters. JRC Sci. Tech. Rep. 1–51.

Lopez-Chaves, C., Soto-Alvaredo, J., Montes-Bayon, M., Bettmer, J., Llopis, J., Sanchez-Gonzalez, C., 2018. Gold nanoparticles: distribution, bioaccumulation and toxicity. In vitro and in vivo studies. Nanomed. Nanotechnol. Biol. Med. 14, 1–12.

Lu, L., Li, J., Yu, J., Song, P., Ng, D.H.L., 2016. A hierarchically porous $MgFe2O4/\gamma$-Fe2O3 magnetic microspheres for efficient removals of dye and pharmaceutical from water. Chem. Eng. J. 283, 524–534.

Luo, Y., Guo, W., Ngo, H.H., Nghiem, L.D., Hai, F.I., Zhang, J., Liang, S., Wang, X.C., 2014. A review on the occurrence of micropollutants in the aquatic environment and their fate and removal during wastewater treatment. Sci. Total Environ. 473–474, 619–641.

Lushchak, V.I., Matviishyn, T.M., Husak, V.V., Storey, J.M., Storey, K.B., 2018. Pesticide toxicity: a mechanistic approach. EXCLI J. 17, 1101–1136.

Machado, S., Stawiński, W., Slonina, P., Pinto, A.R., Grosso, J.P., Nouws, H.P.A., Albergaria, J.T., Delerue-Matos, C., 2013. Application of green zero-valent iron nanoparticles to the remediation of soils contaminated with ibuprofen. Sci. Total Environ. 461–462, 323–329.

Mackay, D., Fraser, A., 2000. Bioaccumulation of persistent organic chemicals: mechanisms and models. Environ. Pollut. 110, 375–391.

Magesh, N., Annam Renita, A., Senthil Kumar, P., 2020. Practice on treating pharmaceutical compounds (antibiotics) present in wastewater using biosorption techniques with different biowaste compounds. A review. Environ. Prog. Sustain. Energy 39, e13429.

Marcelo, C.R., Puiatti, G.A., Nascimento, M.A., Oliveira, A.F., Lopes, R.P., 2018. Degradation of the reactive blue 4 dye in aqueous solution using zero-valent copper nanoparticles. J. Nanomater. 2018, 4642038.

Mariano, S., Panzarini, E., Inverno, M.D., Voulvoulis, N., Dini, L., 2020. Toxicity, bioaccumulation and biotransformation of glucose-capped silver nanoparticles in green microalgae Chlorella vulgaris. Nanomaterials 10, 1377.

Martínez-Boubeta, C., Simeonidis, K., 2019. Magnetic Nanoparticles for Water Purification.

Matamoros, V., Caselles-Osorio, A., García, J., Bayona, J.M., 2008. Behaviour of pharmaceutical products and biodegradation intermediates in horizontal subsurface flow constructed wetland. A microcosm experiment. Sci. Total Environ. 394, 171–176.

Matamoros, V., Uggetti, E., García, J., Bayona, J.M., 2016. Assessment of the mechanisms involved in the removal of emerging contaminants by microalgae from wastewater: a laboratory scale study. J. Hazard. Mater. 301, 197–205.

Mestre, A., Pires, J., Nogueira, J., Carvalho, A., 2007. Activated carbons for the adsorption of ibuprofen. Carbon 45, 1979–1988.

Mirsadeghi, S., Zandavar, H., Yousefi, M., Rajabi, H.R., Pourmortazavi, S.M., 2020. Green-photodegradation of model pharmaceutical contaminations over biogenic Fe3O4/Au nanocomposite and antimicrobial activity. J. Environ. Manag. 270, 110831.

Musial, J., Krakowiak, R., Mlynarczyk, D.T., Goslinski, T., Stanisz, B.J., 2020. Titanium dioxide nanoparticles in food and personal care products—what do we know about their safety? Nanomaterials 10, 1110.

Naghizade Asl, M., Mahmodi, N.M., Teymouri, P., Shahmoradi, B., Rezaee, R., Maleki, A., 2016. Adsorption of organic dyes using copper oxide nanoparticles: isotherm and kinetic studies. Desalination Water Treat. 57, 25278–25287.

Nam, D.-H., Lee, B.-C., Eom, I.-C., Kim, P., Yeo, M.-K., 2014. Uptake and bioaccumulation of titanium- and silver-nanoparticles in aquatic ecosystems. Mol. Cell. Toxicol. 10, 9–17.

Neff, J., 2002. Bioaccumulation Mechanisms.

News, T.O., November 13, 2019. Pneumonia Biggest Killer Infection in India, Pollution Worsening Crisis, Says Report.

Nogueira, P.F.M., Nakabayashi, D., Zucolotto, V., 2015. The effects of graphene oxide on green algae *Raphidocelis subcapitata*. Aquat. Toxicol. 166, 29–35.
Okereafor, U., Makhatha, M., Mekuto, L., UCHE-Okereafor, N., Sebola, T., Mavumengwana, V., 2020. Toxic metal implications on agricultural soils, plants, animals, aquatic life and human health. Int. J. Environ. Res. Publ. Health 17, 2204.
Oleszczuk, P., Pan, B., Xing, B., 2009. Adsorption and desorption of oxytetracycline and carbamazepine by multi-walled carbon nanotubes. Environ. Sci. Technol. 43, 9167–9173.
Örnek, A., Özacar, M., Sengil, I.A., 2007. Adsorption of lead onto formaldehyde or sulphuric acid treated acorn waste: equilibrium and kinetic studies. Biochem. Eng. J. 37, 192–200.
Patrolecco, L., Ademollo, N., Grenni, P., Tolomei, A., BARRA Caracciolo, A., Capri, S., 2013. Simultaneous determination of human pharmaceuticals in water samples by solid phase extraction and HPLC with UV-fluorescence detection. Microchem. J. 107, 165–171.
Pereira, J.H.O.S., Vilar, V.J.P., Borges, M.T., González, O., Esplugas, S., Boaventura, R.A.R., 2011. Photocatalytic degradation of oxytetracycline using TiO2 under natural and simulated solar radiation. Sol. Energy 85, 2732–2740.
Popek, E.P., 2017. Sampling and Analysis of Environmental Chemical Pollutants: A Complete Guide. Elsevier.
Putra, E.K., Pranowo, R., Sunarso, J., Indraswati, N., Ismadji, S., 2009. Performance of activated carbon and bentonite for adsorption of amoxicillin from wastewater: mechanisms, isotherms and kinetics. Water Res. 43, 2419–2430.
Quan, X., Yang, S., Ruan, X., Zhao, H., 2005. Preparation of Titania nanotubes and their environmental applications as electrode. Environ. Sci. Technol. 39, 3770–3775.
Rabiet, M., Togola, A., Brissaud, F., Seidel, J.-L., Budzinski, H., Elbaz-Poulichet, F., 2006. Consequences of treated water recycling as regards pharmaceuticals and drugs in surface and ground waters of a medium-sized Mediterranean catchment. Environ. Sci. Technol. 40, 5282–5288.
Rajapaksha, A.U., Vithanage, M., Ahmad, M., Seo, D.-C., Cho, J.-S., Lee, S.-E., Lee, S.S., Ok, Y.S., 2015. Enhanced sulfamethazine removal by steam-activated invasive plant-derived biochar. J. Hazard. Mater. 290, 43–50.
Raju, C., Nooruddin, S., Babu, K.S., 2017. Studies on leaf extract mediated synthesis of copper nanoparticles for the removal of bromo cresol green dye from synthetic waste waters. IJSETR 6, 1404–1411.
Ramachandran, V., Pujari, N., Matey, T., Kulkarni, S., 2014. Enzymatic hydrolysis of cassava using wheat seedlings. Int. J. Sci. Eng. Technol. Res. 3, 1216–1219.
Remucal, C.K., ginder-Vogel, M., 2014. A critical review of the reactivity of manganese oxides with organic contaminants. Environ. Sci. Process. Impacts 16, 1247–1266.
Richardson, B.J., Lam, P.K.S., Martin, M., 2005. Emerging chemicals of concern: pharmaceuticals and personal care products (PPCPs) in Asia, with particular reference to Southern China. Mar. Pollut. Bull. 50, 913–920.
Rizwan, M., Singh, M., Mitra, C.K., Morve, R.K., 2014. Ecofriendly application of nanomaterials: nanobioremediation. J. Nanoparticles 2014, 431787.
Rodarte-Morales, A.I., Feijoo, G., Moreira, M.T., Lema, J.M., 2012. Biotransformation of three pharmaceutical active compounds by the fungus *Phanerochaete chrysosporium* in a fed batch stirred reactor under air and oxygen supply. Biodegradation 23, 145–156.
Rontani, J.F., Cuny, P., Aubert, C., 1997. Rates and mechanism of light-dependent degradation of sterols in senescent cells of phytoplankton. J. Photochem. Photobiol. Chem. 111, 139–144.
Saka, C., Sahin, Ö., Küçük, M.M., 2012. Applications on agricultural and forest waste adsorbents for the removal of lead (II) from contaminated waters. Int. J. Environ. Sci. Technol. 9, 379–394.
Schäfer, S., Buchmeier, G., Claus, E., Duester, L., Heininger, P., Körner, A., Mayer, P., Paschke, A., Rauert, C., Reifferscheid, G., Rüdel, H., Schlechtriem, C., Schudoma, D., Schröter-Kermani, C., Smedes, F., Steffen, D., Vietoris, F., 2015. Erratum to: bioaccumulation in aquatic systems: methodological approaches, monitoring and assessment. Environ. Sci. Eur. 27, 14.
Sehrawat, A., Phour, M., Kumar, R., Sindhu, S.S., 2021. Bioremediation of pesticides: an eco-friendly approach for environment sustainability. In: Microbial Rejuvenation of Polluted Environment. Springer.
Shirazi, E., Torabian, A., NABI-Bidhendi, G., 2013. Carbamazepine removal from groundwater: effectiveness of the TiO2/Uv, Nanoparticulate zero-valent iron, and Fenton (NZVI/H2O2) processes. CLEAN—Soil Air Water 41, 1062–1072.
Singh, R., Manickam, N., Mudiam, M.K.R., Murthy, R.C., Misra, V., 2013. An integrated (nano-bio) technique for degradation of γ-HCH contaminated soil. J. Hazard. Mater. 258–259, 35–41.

Singh, K.K., Senapati, K.K., Borgohain, C., Sarma, K.C., 2017. Newly developed Fe3O4–Cr2O3 magnetic nanocomposite for photocatalytic decomposition of 4-chlorophenol in water. J. Environ. Sci. 52, 333–340.

Song, J.Y., Bhadra, B.N., Jhung, S.H., 2017. Contribution of H-bond in adsorptive removal of pharmaceutical and personal care products from water using oxidized activated carbon. Microporous Mesoporous Mater. 243, 221–228.

Sood, S., Umar, A., Mehta, S.K., Kansal, S.K., 2015. Highly effective Fe-doped TiO_2 nanoparticles photocatalysts for visible-light driven photocatalytic degradation of toxic organic compounds. J. Colloid Interface Sci. 450, 213–223.

Spongberg, A.L., Witter, J.D., 2008. Pharmaceutical compounds in the wastewater process stream in Northwest Ohio. Sci. Total Environ. 397, 148–157.

Suarez, S., Lema, J.M., Omil, F., 2010. Removal of pharmaceutical and personal care products (PPCPs) under nitrifying and denitrifying conditions. Water Res. 44, 3214–3224.

Tadkaew, N., Hai, F.I., Mcdonald, J.A., Khan, S.J., Nghiem, L.D., 2011. Removal of trace organics by MBR treatment: the role of molecular properties. Water Res. 45, 2439–2451.

Tang, Y., Guo, H., Xiao, L., Yu, S., Gao, N., Wang, Y., 2013. Synthesis of reduced graphene oxide/magnetite composites and investigation of their adsorption performance of fluoroquinolone antibiotics. Colloids Surf. A Physicochem. Eng. Asp. 424, 74–80.

Tekade, R.K., Chougule, M.B., 2013. Formulation development and evaluation of hybrid nanocarrier for cancer therapy: Taguchi orthogonal array based design. BioMed Res. Int.

Tixier, C., Singer, H.P., Oellers, S., Müller, S.R., 2003. Occurrence and fate of carbamazepine, clofibric acid, diclofenac, ibuprofen, ketoprofen, and naproxen in surface waters. Environ. Sci. Technol. 37, 1061–1068.

Topp, E., Chapman, R., Devers-Lamrani, M., Hartmann, A., Marti, R., Martin-Laurent, F., Sabourin, L., Scott, A., Sumarah, M., 2013. Accelerated biodegradation of veterinary antibiotics in agricultural soil following long-term exposure, and isolation of a sulfamethazine-degrading sp. J. Environ. Qual. 42, 173–178.

US EPA, 2007. Contaminants of Emerging Concern Including Pharmaceuticals and Personal Care Products.

Vane, J., Botting, R., 1996. Mechanism of action of anti-inflammatory drugs. Scand. J. Rheumatol. 25, 9–21.

Venkatesan, A.K., Pycke, B.F.G., Barber, L.B., Lee, K.E., Halden, R.U., 2012. Occurrence of triclosan, triclocarban, and its lesser chlorinated congeners in Minnesota freshwater sediments collected near wastewater treatment plants. J. Hazard. Mater. 229–230, 29–35.

Vijayaraghavan, K., Yun, Y.-S., 2008. Bacterial biosorbents and biosorption. Biotechnol. Adv. 26, 266–291.

Wan, J., Deng, H., Shi, J., Zhou, L., Su, T., 2014. Synthesized magnetic manganese ferrite nanoparticles on activated carbon for sulfamethoxazole removal. CLEAN—Soil Air Water 42, 1199–1207.

Wang, Y., Zhu, J., Huang, H., Cho, H.-H., 2015a. Carbon nanotube composite membranes for microfiltration of pharmaceuticals and personal care products: capabilities and potential mechanisms. J. Membr. Sci. 479, 165–174.

Wang, Z.G., Zhou, R., Jiang, D., Song, J.E., Xu, Q., Si, J., Chen, Y.P., Zhou, X., Gan, L., Li, J.Z., Zhang, H., Liu, B., 2015b. Toxicity of graphene quantum dots in zebrafish embryo. Biomed. Environ. Sci. 28, 341–351.

Wang, G., Shi, H., Du, Z., Chen, H., Peng, J., Gao, S., 2017. Bioaccumulation mechanism of organophosphate esters in adult zebrafish (*Danio rerio*). Environ. Pollut. 229, 177–187.

Wei, L., Thakkar, M., Chen, Y., ADDO Ntim, S., Mitra, S., Zhang, X., 2010. Cytotoxicity effects of water dispersed oxidized multiwalled carbon nanotubes on marine alga *Dunaliella tertiolecta*. Aquat. Toxicol (Amsterdam, Netherlands) 100, 194–201.

Workgroup, U.S.E.P.A.B.A., 2000. Bioaccumulation Testing and Interpretation for the Purpose of Sediment Quality Assessment: Status and Needs. US Environmental Protection Agency.

Wuana, R.A., Okieimen, F.E., 2011. Heavy metals in contaminated soils: a review of sources, chemistry, risks and best available strategies for remediation. ISRN Ecol. 2011, 402647.

Xiong, J.-Q., Kurade, M.B., Jeon, B. H., 2017. Biodegradation of levofloxacin by an acclimated freshwater microalga, *Chlorella vulgaris*. Chem. Eng. J. 313, 1251–1257.

Yan, J., Lei, M., Zhu, L., Anjum, M.N., Zou, J., Tang, H., 2011. Degradation of sulfamonomethoxine with Fe3O4 magnetic nanoparticles as heterogeneous activator of persulfate. J. Hazard. Mater. 186, 1398–1404.

Yi, Y., Yang, Z., Zhang, S., 2011. Ecological risk assessment of heavy metals in sediment and human health risk assessment of heavy metals in fishes in the middle and lower reaches of the Yangtze River basin. Environ. Pollut. 159, 2575–2585.

Youngren, S.R., Tekade, R.K., Gustilo, B., Hoffmann, P.R., Chougule, M.B., 2013. STAT6 siRNA matrix-loaded gelatin nanocarriers: formulation, characterization, and ex vivo proof of concept using adenocarcinoma cells. BioMed Res. Int.

Yu, F., Ma, J., Bi, D., 2015. Enhanced adsorptive removal of selected pharmaceutical antibiotics from aqueous solution by activated graphene. Environ. Sci. Pollut. Res. 22, 4715–4724.

Yu, Y., Zhou, Y., Wang, Z., Torres, O.L., Guo, R., Chen, J., 2017. Investigation of the removal mechanism of antibiotic ceftazidime by green algae and subsequent microbic impact assessment. Sci. Rep. 7, 4168–4168.

Zaib, Q., Mansoor, B., Ahmad, F., 2013. Photo-regenerable multi-walled carbon nanotube membranes for the removal of pharmaceutical micropollutants from water. Environ. Sci. Process. Impacts 15, 1582–1589.

Zambianchi, M., Durso, M., Liscio, A., Treossi, E., Bettini, C., Capobianco, M.L., Aluigi, A., Kovtun, A., Ruani, G., Corticelli, F., Brucale, M., Palermo, V., Navacchia, M.L., Melucci, M., 2017. Graphene oxide doped polysulfone membrane adsorbers for the removal of organic contaminants from water. Chem. Eng. J. 326, 130–140.

Zhang, X., Wu, F., Wu, X., Chen, P., Deng, N., 2008. Photodegradation of acetaminophen in TiO(2) suspended solution. J. Hazard. Mater. 157, 300–307.

Zhang, Y., Chen, B., Zhang, L., Huang, J., Chen, F., Yang, Z., Yao, J., Zhang, Z., 2011. Controlled assembly of Fe3O4 magnetic nanoparticles on graphene oxide. Nanoscale 3, 1446–1450.

Zhang, C., Lai, C., Zeng, G., Huang, D., Yang, C., Wang, Y., Zhou, Y., Cheng, M., 2016. Efficacy of carbonaceous nanocomposites for sorbing ionizable antibiotic sulfamethazine from aqueous solution. Water Res. 95, 103–112.

Zhang, Y., Jiao, Z., Hu, Y., Lv, S., Fan, H., Zeng, Y., Hu, J., Wang, M., 2017. Removal of tetracycline and oxytetracycline from water by magnetic Fe 3 O 4@ graphene. Environ. Sci. Pollut. Res. 24, 2987–2995.

Zhu, B., Zhu, S., Li, J., Hui, X., Wang, G.-X., 2018. The developmental toxicity, bioaccumulation and distribution of oxidized single walled carbon nanotubes in *Artemia salina*. Toxicol. Res. 7, 897–906.

Ziental, D., Czarczynska-Goslinska, B., Mlynarczyk, D.T., Glowacka-Sobotta, A., Stanisz, B., Goslinski, T., Sobotta, L., 2020. Titanium dioxide nanoparticles: prospects and applications in medicine. Nanomaterials 10, 387.

More references

Lindberg, R.H., et al., 2021. Fate of active pharmaceutical ingredients in a northern high-rate algal pond fed with municipal wastewater. Chemosphere 271, 129763.

Ricky, R., Shanthakumar, S., 2022. Phycoremediation integrated approach for the removal of pharmaceuticals and personal care products from wastewater—a review. J. Environ. Manag. 302 (Pt A), 113998.

CHAPTER

17

Toxicity of dental materials and ways to screen their biosafety

Prashant L. Pingale[1], *Neetu R. Saudagar*[1], *Amarjitsing P. Rajput*[2], *Kuldeep Rajpoot*[3], *Muktika Tekade*[4], *Anjali Pingale*[5] *and Rakesh Kumar Tekade*[3]

[1]Department of Pharmaceutics, GES's Sir Dr. M. S. Gosavi College of Pharmaceutical Education and Research, Nashik, Maharashtra, India; [2]Department of Pharmaceutics, Poona College of Pharmacy, Bharti Vidyapeeth Deemed University, Pune, Maharashtra, India; [3]National Institute of Pharmaceutical Education and Research (NIPER)- Ahmedabad, An Institute of National Importance, Government of India, Department of Pharmaceuticals, Ministry of Chemicals and Fertilizers, Palaj, Gandhinagar, Gujarat, India; [4]School of Pharmacy, Devi Ahilya Vishwavidyalaya, Indore, Madhya Pradesh, India; [5]Shree Panchavati Education Society's Institute of Pharmacy, Nashik, Maharashtra, India

17.1 Introduction

Dental composites, resins, and implants are just a few materials used in dentistry. The physiochemical characteristics of dental substances, and their biological and toxicological dependability, are essential for their therapeutic usage. Dental materials have been linked to various local and systemic toxicity issues. If these substances are left in the mouth for an extended period, they may cause adverse reactions. Filling materials, restorative substances, intracanal medications, prosthetic components, various types of implants, liners, and root canal irrigants are a few of the components utilized in dentistry. The rising rate of new substances with uses in dentistry has raised awareness of hazards related to biological systems and the tempting limitations of other substances. The biocompatibility of a biomaterial used to replace or fill biological tissue, such as teeth, always showed a serious concern within the healthcare disciplines for patients (Shahi et al., 2019; Tekade and Chougule, 2013).

https://doi.org/10.1016/B978-0-443-15840-7.00005-1

Before applying clinically, a substance must be thoroughly examined for its suitability regarding all possible aspects (Gadekar et al., 2021; Gorain et al., 2016; Muniswamy et al., 2019; Prajapati et al., 2009). Several assays evaluate the biocompatibility of these substances in vitro, in vivo, and in clinical studies (Asati et al., 2022; Rajpoot et al., 2022; Tiwari et al., 2022). In the future, we will further determine if there is any occurrence of chemical cytotoxicity and associated health problems (Gupta et al., 2022a,b). This chapter focuses on the possible toxicity of dental materials and biocompatibility testing. The utilization of healthy and safe substances is critical in restorative procedures. In dentistry, low or nontoxic agents should be used for long-term treatment to overcome some toxicities caused by these agents. Additionally, before clinical use, screening studies should be carried out to identify potential harm (Shahi et al., 2019; Youngren et al., 2013).

17.1.1 Biological interfaces

When a substance is implanted into the body, it forms a static interface that is generally not safe for the patient. It leads to many dynamic interactions between the substance and the body. The body may change the substance in the biological interface formed, which can significantly affect health. However, some determinant of functionality includes (a) the material's location, (b) the length of time it spends in the body, (c) the material's characteristics, and (d) the host's health condition.

17.1.1.1 Types of interactions

Below mentioned are some types of interactions that may occur between dental materials and teeth (Fig. 17.1).

Colonization and biofilm development impact dental elements and denture surfaces, which result in some particular illnesses. To overcome this, two effective methods have been investigated, namely, (a) persistent alteration, this approach uses quaternary ammonium salts, and (b) temporary antimicrobial features generated by utilizing delivery systems. Additionally, several chemical agents were also evaluated in vitro and in vivo to ensure antibacterial and antibiofilm characteristics for the most popular dental materials (Wang et al., 2014; Quintas et al., 2015). On the other hand, ceramics possess the lowest adhesion capacity over all the common dental substances due to their inert surfaces. For example, zirconia dental ceramics have less adhesive properties than metals or natural teeth (Ficai and Ficai, 2017).

17.1.2 Biosafety essentials

Dentists show potential concerns for biosafety in four areas, i.e., the safety of the patient, the safety of the dental staff, regulatory compliance issues, and legal liability. The difficulties of matching animals and user testing for biocompatibility have been demonstrated in several research areas. Inconsistencies associated with these dental biomaterials generate some doubt in the mind of researchers regarding the utility of any test for evaluating them other than the usage test. Scientists and regulatory bodies now also acknowledge the importance of *in vitro* studies and animal testing in the biological analysis of dental substances. The choice to

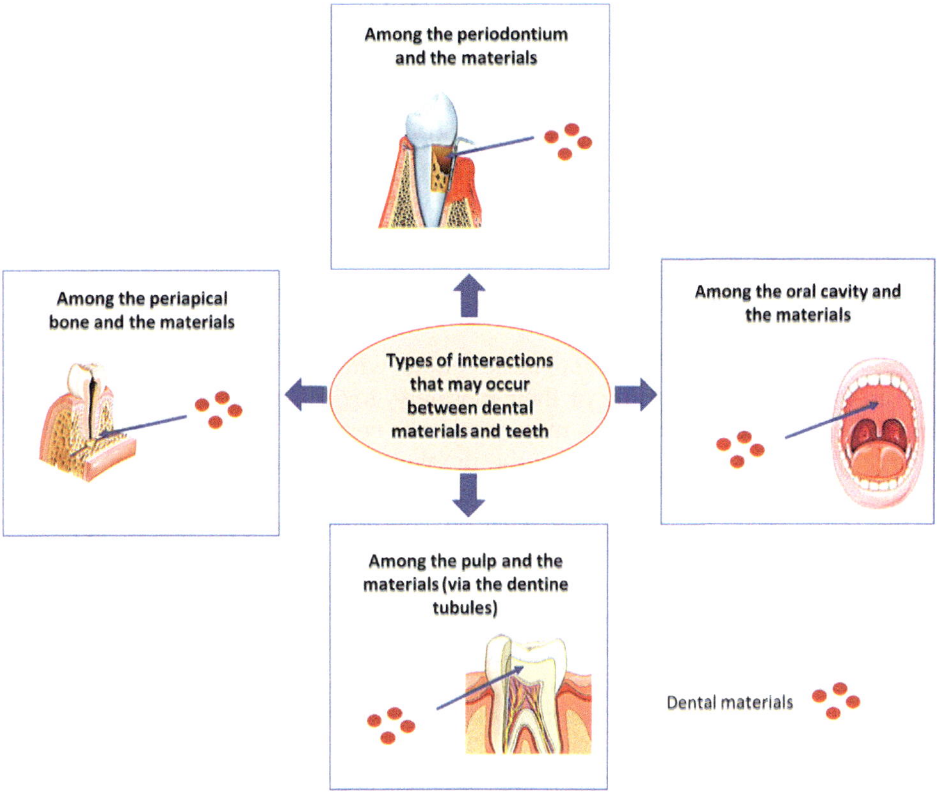

FIGURE 17.1 Some types of interactions that may occur between dental materials and teeth.

employ a novel substance is ultimately a risk versus benefit analysis that dentists must conduct independently. Doctors should look for published data from independent researchers and consider their patients' dental requirements, aesthetic aspirations, health backgrounds, and risk tolerance (Williams, 1987).

Because dental substances come into close touch with live tissues for extended periods, dentists must be aware of the biocompatibility of the substances they employ. Finally, dentists must decide whether the advantages of biomaterials exceed the dangers or not. To eliminate any threat is to deprive the patient of the immense advantages that substances may provide. Taking too much risk might not only keep the patient in endangering but also put the doctor at legal risk. Because many substances have an established background of usage in dental surgery, biocompatibility worries aren't as pressing as other difficulties, including long-term deterioration, mechanical strength problems, and secondary caries preclusion.

Nevertheless, it's crucial to remember that synthetic substances employed in repairing, auguring, and restoring natural tissue structures can cause unfavorable tissue reactions. The problems to be tackled and the methods used may vary as new substances as well as repairing procedures become accessible, and the sophistication of cell-level and subcellular response analyses may grow. Further problems may arise due to the introduction of tissue-engineered therapeutic devices (St John, 2007).

Various sorts of screening assays are now available, which are vital to comprehend the benefits and drawbacks of each so that the right one can be chosen and interpreted correctly. New research in dental substances, gene transfer, treatments related to growth factors, biomaterials, and tissue engineering is under process. These novel treatments enhance the chances of restoring and regenerating oral tissues, but they can also expose patients to new risks. Before being applied in medical practice, most emerging innovations should be proven safe and nonhazardous to people's health (Valderrama et al., 2020).

17.2 Toxicity associated with dental materials

Because dental substances come into close contact with the cavity of the mouth, it is crucial to have an overall understanding of their biosafety, toxicology, and physical and chemical characteristics. Dentists and patients may experience negative responses to dental substances and clinical equipment. An increase in the number of complaints concerning dental treatments and occupational exposure has significantly coincided with the release of novel dental substances and broad knowledge of harmful consequences. Restorative composite substances, orthodontic adhesives and appliances, prosthodontic resins, and impression materials usually contain resin-based compounds with different monomers. Reactions to metals used in extra-oral devices in orthodontics seem relatively frequent, but few reactions have been reported following the use of other alloy systems. A few different responses are caused by toxic or allergic reactions, while others are unclear. Adverse responses to any drug are generally observed first in the environment where the exposure is highest. Fig. 17.2 represents

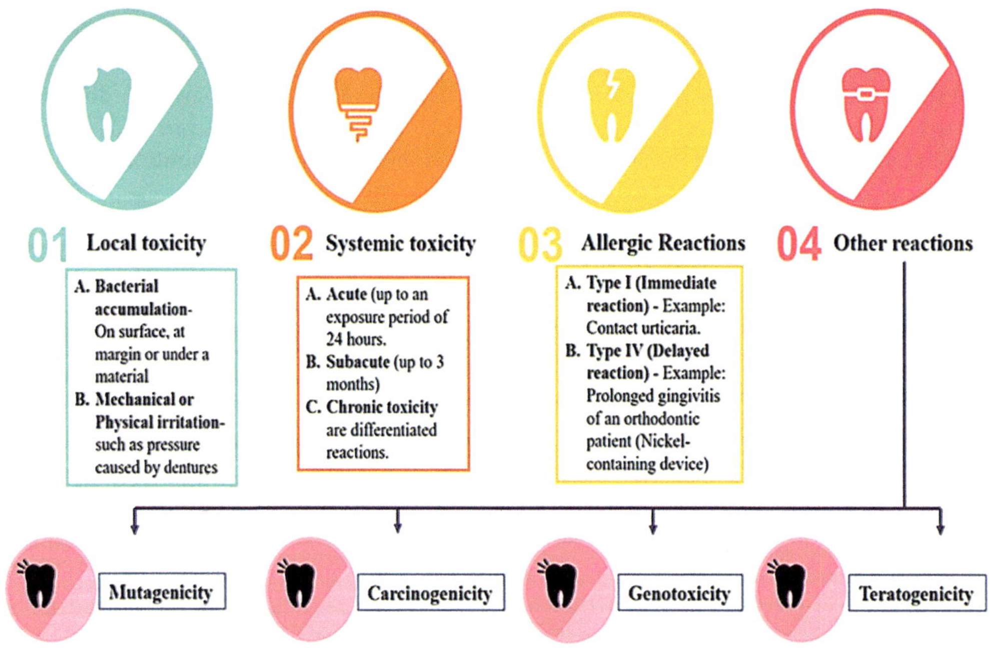

FIGURE 17.2 Representation of toxicities associated with dental compounds.

several toxicities associated with dental compounds. This is also true in dentistry, where certain unpleasant responses may be caused by a lack of understanding of dental substances' poisonous, irritating, and allergic characteristics (Hensten-Pettersen and Jacobsen, 1994).

17.2.1 Local toxicity

Compounds produced by dental medicaments might cause a response (e.g., necrosis or inflammation) to nearby tissues, like the oral mucosa/gingiva, pulp, or alveolar bone (local toxicity). Injury to individual cells, such as in cell cultures, is referred to as cytotoxicity. Necrosis or apoptosis are two processes that cause cells to perish. Moreover, if cell biotransformation is disrupted, proinflammatory mediators may be released. A local tissue response might be caused due to reasons other than chemicals produced by dental materials. The most crucial element that may induce undesired tissue responses can be the presence of microorganisms on the surface, at the edge, or beneath a substance. These processes are the subject of several research in the published literature. Local tissue responses can also be induced by mechanical irritation, such as pressure from dentures. Local responses are relatively common in dental practice; therefore, getting the proper diagnosis is crucial (Garhammer et al., 2001; Schmalz and Arenholt-Bindslev, 2009).

Several adverse clinical responses linked to or supposedly linked to dental cast alloys may exist. Much research has been conducted to determine the frequency of allergies to metals or alloys by confirming a skin test using the appropriate metal salts. Nevertheless, because of the oral mucosa's unique structural and immunological characteristics, these findings cannot simply be applied to dental metals and their usage in the oral cavity (Garhammer et al., 2001).

17.2.2 Systemic toxicity

Nearly most dental substances secrete chemicals inside the mouth cavity. They can permeate the body through various pathways, including saliva ingestion, with subsequent passage via epithelial membranes in the gastric and intestinal systems or lungs. The chemicals might be distributed to various organs via the bloodstream. As a result, it may impact not only the application site but also other places. If the concentration is high enough, there may be an interruption in the functioning of the specific organ at the site of the action (systemic toxicity). Acute (up to a 24 h exposure period), subacute (up to 3 months), and chronic toxicity types are classified depending on the duration of effect. Most case reports show chronic adverse effects of dental compounds. As a result, extra efforts are needed to obtain detailed safety information. Dentists must have thorough knowledge about this topic so that they can provide accurate and appropriate patient information (Schmalz and Arenholt-Bindslev, 2009).

Synthetic implant devices are made up of a wide range of metal polymers, hydrogels, alloys, ceramics, and composites for a wide range of applications as well as characteristics. The implant gadgets are designed to prevent chemical and biological deterioration and little leakage of structural components or additives (excluding medication delivery, sutures, and others that degrade). Chemical and, in certain circumstances, enzymatic activities impact artificial devices, leading to the release of dental biomaterials-linked components. Because no organic fix processes are similar to those found in natural tissues, deterioration (biological material degradation) is a one-way process that causes microscopic and macroscopic surface and mega shifts in gadgets, which the biomechanical and bioelectrical conditions can aid these devices to withstand. Surface modifications, excluding pathologic calcification of a few polymer implants, might not significantly impact the implant's physical strength. Still, released chemicals frequently have biological effects on the surrounding tissues or at other distant sites (Hensten and Jacobsen, 2013).

Toxic chemicals must reach a specific organ with a high susceptibility to a particular toxicant for systemic toxicity. The central nervous system, circulatory system, hematopoietic system, and visceral organs (e.g., liver, kidney, and lungs) are targeted in that sequence. The toxicity is determined by interfering with essential cell processes and is proportional to the dose and length of exposure. Severe side effects may be life-threatening, although most side effects involve localized and reversible cell injury. However, inevitable sublethal consequences might include somatic cell mutations that cause carcinogenesis mutations and reproductive toxicity. The dosage, which is the number of chemicals showing exposure in an organism, is generally stated in mg/kg body weight in the study of essential toxicity. Adverse effects of foreign substances are frequently the consequence of repetitive, chronic exposure to small doses. These can have detrimental effects comparable to a single large dose, providing the repeated doses surpass a specific threshold level. The capability for biotransformation and removal determines this level. Another significant consideration is the potential for synergistic potentiating impacts when many toxicants are exposed simultaneously. Whatever process is at work, systemic toxicity assumes a dose-linked reaction that can be quantified and characterized and interpreted using particular chemical processes (Bidlack, 2002).

17.2.3 Allergic reactions

An allergic reaction might be induced if an organism has already been exposed to a chemical. Four main types of allergic responses may be distinguished, i.e., antibodies (IgE, IgG) mediated types I, II, and III, whereas cells predominantly transmit type IV. Dental substances can induce type I (rapid response) and type IV (slower reaction) allergies (delayed reaction). The dose levels causing allergic reactions are generally significantly lower than those causing toxic reactions. The doses that cause allergic reactions are often far lower than those that cause hazardous reactions. Dental materials can be released into the mouth cavity at high concentrations to cause allergic responses in patients. Allergies to a variety of things might develop at the same time. If an individual has allergies to chemically similar drugs, cross-sensitivity is presumed. Nickel and palladium are two examples of elements that belong to a similar major group in the periodic table. Patients with nickel allergies are also frequently allergic to palladium (Bertolini et al., 2014); therefore, if palladium-containing alloys are utilized for restoration applications, one must keep this in mind. There is also evidence of cross-reactivity with chemically similar methacrylates. Some research articles report allergic effects caused by dental substances (Gottwald et al., 2002). As a result, contact allergies can be divided into three groups: (a) important contact allergens, (b) suspected contact allergens in humans, and (c) less essential contact allergens.

17.2.4 Other reactions

Elements emitted from materials have the potential to induce DNA changes in the genome. Alternatively, controlled cell death can prevent these genetic defects from being passed down to future generations of cells (apoptosis). Nevertheless, this is known as mutagenicity when these genetic damages are transmitted to the following generation. Some of the carcinogenic materials or chemicals that these materials produce can stimulate the growth of cancerous tumors. Some other reactions produced by these materials include mutagenic, carcinogenic, and teratogenic effects.

17.2.4.1 Mutagenicity

The estimation of an accurate proportion of a withdrawal biomaterial of leachable substances into the surroundings is crucial. Deterioration might result in the formation of different mutagenic substances. The physical surrounding and surface properties all impact the biomaterial's carcinogenicity effects. In many cases, the information accessible for evaluation is insufficient, and frequently employed techniques are not verified. Furthermore, wear and corrosion of metal implants generate and release a wide range of degradation products. A constituent can be selectively eliminated or chemically changed, which can result in the modification of the substance's surface. In alloys, the electrochemical characteristics of other metals can significantly impact the release of the specific metal ion. However, most research lacks sufficient data on the possibility of certain chemicals with known mutagenic or carcinogenic properties (McGregor et al., 2000).

17.2.4.2 Carcinogenicity

When an evaluated component of resin composites is introduced into direct contact with fibroblasts, cytotoxicity of newly healed dental substances can be established, and all assessed components of resin composites may induce substantial toxicity. On the other hand, the risk to the tooth pulp is determined by the amounts that infiltrate the dentin and collect in the pulp. Pulpal reactions to acid etching and bonding agents have been seen in a few animal studies indicating a potential danger of pulpal reactions in people. Composite substances may have biological impacts. However, microleakage and bacterial infections make an evaluation of composite effects on the pulp difficult. According to clinical data on the negative impacts of composite filling substances, pulpal and mucosal responses are uncommon. In rare cases, the quantities of specific chemicals in filling senses that professionals and patients are exposed to appear inadequate to induce obvious systemic harmful effects. There is no available information to correlate local concentrations of released chemicals to a significant level that causes hazardous impacts (except methyl methacrylate). Formaldehyde is released from some dental polymers (in vitro), but the levels appear to be low (Gichner, 1985).

17.2.4.3 Genotoxicity

The genotoxic impact of a chemical is defined as the initiation of DNA destruction by the agent. Because of the genetic connection to induce carcinogenic toxicity, it's essential to understand the possible consequences of substances on health (Vasdev et al., 2022). Following national and international norms, medical devices (whether newly created or presently in use) must verify their biosafety and toxicological profile. One of the most severe side effects of chemicals is genotoxicity. Because most dental substances release little quantities of various components into the oral cavity, efforts must be made to minimize the risk of the release of these components (Deliversky et al., 2015; Schmalz and Galler, 2017). Commercial dental bleaching agents have been demonstrated (Ribeiro et al., 2005, 2006). Because bleaching treatments include hydrogen peroxide, the genotoxic impacts of certain dental materials, such as bleaching agents, are apparent. Moreover, the emergence of oxidative damage caused by increased oxidizing chemicals causes DNA destruction and mutations (Ahmadian et al., 2017; Ribeiro et al., 2017).

Furthermore, whitening toothpaste has been shown to cause genetic harm to human gingival cells (Rode et al., 2021). Bisphenol A (a dental restorative substance) has produced DNA adducts in human cells in vitro using the comet assay (Huang et al., 2015, 2016). Micro-nucleated cells in bone marrow rose when experimental animals were exposed to methyl methacrylate, leading to mutagenesis in vivo (Araujo et al., 2013; Li et al., 2012). The preventative function of antioxidants in reducing gene-related abnormalities implies that oxidative risk plays a critical role in dental substances' genotoxicity (Blasiak et al., 2011; Lottner et al., 2013). Endodontic chemicals have also been studied extensively in the context of genotoxicity in various in vitro tests. On the other hand, more dependable use and clinical testing will serve as a road map for future dentistry.

A genotoxin is a chemical or substance that causes DNA or chromosomal damage. However, this form of injury to the germ cell leads to chromosomal alterations. Disruption of DNA in a somatic cell causes a somatic mutation, which can proceed to malignant transformation (Phillips and Arlt, 2009). People exposed to mercury through food, workplace surroundings, or dental restorations showed increased genotoxicity. Mercury might be implicated in four primary mechanisms that produce genotoxicity, including disruption of microtubule development, DNA repair processes, the creation of oxidative damage and free radicals, and direct interactions with DNA molecules (Crespo-Lopez et al., 2009).

Dental amalgam, which contains mercury, is a known clastogen. It was suggested that inorganic mercury acts mainly on cytoskeletal proteins such as kinesin or tubulin, which plays a vital role in chromosomal segregation, resulting in micronuclei formation. In an in vitro study, the genotoxic effect of inorganic mercury was studied using the micronucleus assay. They observed an interaction of inorganic mercury with the microtubule network of cells leading to the induction of micronuclei (Wallin et al., 1977).

Most individuals have a dental filling made of mercury-based amalgam, which was recently launched. These compounds are usually leached into the mouth cavity and cause genotoxic changes in buccal mucosal cells. Dental amalgam is still frequently utilized as a restoration material in underdeveloped nations due to its lower cost and simplicity of handling. The health concerns linked to the ingredients of this restorative substance have long been a source of worry (Mary et al., 2018).

17.2.4.4 Teratogenicity

Four variables significantly influence the teratogenic effect: (a) agent, (b) dose size, (c) stage of embryonic development, and (d) embryo's genetic makeup. However, the first two criteria are fascinating and require more consideration. It's important to note that the mercury emitted by dental amalgam is mostly metallic mercury vapor. Compared to the dosages used in teratological studies, the dose of mercury vapor from dental amalgam fillings is the lowest, on the order of 5 g/day, and is unlikely to surpass the threshold required for a teratogenic impact to arise. These variables may assist in understanding toxicological processes and species variations, and therefore, they must be used when results obtained on the animal are to be extrapolated to humans. According to epidemiological and animal experimental evidence, the emission of metallic mercury vapor from dental amalgam treatment should not produce teratogenic consequences (Larsson, 1992).

Several chemicals (such as thalidomide) induce abnormalities during embryonic growth (teratogenicity). As a result, substances that leak from substances should be assessed for their ability to cause teratogenic effects (Shahi et al., 2019).

17.2.5 Impression material-linked toxicity

All dental impression substances should correctly duplicate oral tissues with accuracy, dimensional stability, elasticity, rip strength, stiffness, detailed reproduction, and biosafety (Barrett et al., 2011; Messer and Wataha, 2002). Studying these substances' cytotoxicity is a crucial step in determining their biosafety. Organizations like the International Organization for Standardization govern in vitro test techniques for evaluating medical gadget substances' acute adverse biological impacts (ISO 10993) (ISO 10993-1, 2018; ISO 10993-5, 2009). In in vitro testing, subconfluent cell monolayers are produced and then exposed to compounds directly or indirectly (Kostoryz et al., 1999; Kopac et al., 2002; Lang and Mertens, 1990). On the other hand, in vitro research on the cell toxicity impacts of impression substances on in vitro cell growth is limited (Chen et al., 2002; Roberta et al., 2003; Liu et al., 2004; Coppi et al., 2007). Polyethers that are elastomers used in impressions have several benefits for clinical usage, but they also have many drawbacks like toxic, and allergic responses (Brunton et al., 2005; Nally and Storrs, 1973; Pameijer, 2017). Vinylpolysiloxanes are the most widely utilized siloxanes; however, studies on their toxicity have shown mixed results since they have been categorized as hazardous in diverse ways (Chen et al., 2002; Roberta et al., 2003). In vitro toxicity grades are determined based on the type of cultures and procedures used for substances' production.

In most cases, impression substances only stay in touch with the oral tissues for a very limited period. The hazard of the tooth imprints material is exceptionally high when a component is held and remains inside this gingival sulcus under the suture during impression formation for implantation or a surgery prosthesis (Garey and Narang, 1976). This also happens in implant dentistry, especially during two-stage implant surgical procedures. Accumulating these pieces can produce severe inflammatory responses (Gunther and Welsh, 1978; Ree, 2001).

The cytotoxicity of imprint dental substances was tested in vitro on Balb/c 3T3 cells (Lang and Mertens, 1990). Human gingival fibroblasts have an increased rate of development, and their response patterns are more similar to that of the mouth cavity. The gingival fibroblasts maintain technical characteristics and could be a fair representation of in vivo circumstances, especially during impression substance retention (Kasten et al., 1982). Consequently, tests revealed that vinylpolysiloxane substances are a little more hazardous than polyether's in their testing circumstances (Boraldi et al., 2009; Roberta et al., 2003).

17.2.6 Three-dimensional (3D) printed resins-linked toxicity

The 3D printing techniques are sophisticated manufacturing techniques that automatically use the virtual model created by computer-aided design to manufacture customized 3D printed items (Rajpoot et al., 2020). Lacking the utilization of molds and tooling fixtures, 3D printing processes may immediately accept Combined Annotation Dependent Depletion (CADD) data and quickly create a new virtual model that can be used to fabricate a full denture resin foundation (Bassoli et al., 2007; Tian et al., 2021).

Additive production technologies, commonly known as 3D printing, allow for the rapid and cost-effective manufacture of standard or personalized components, catalyzing their adoption in innovations and redefining prototype processes in sectors such as construction, consumer products, and aerospace (Tay et al., 2017; Joshi and Sheikh, 2015). The growing use of 3D printing in the biomedical sciences has resulted from the new revelation of biocompatible resins for medicinal equipment and tissue-created structures (Sun, 2021; Gargus et al., 2020). These recent advances prompted a research team to build next-generation fluidic culture methods using 3D printing technology to develop the ex vivo model of the reproductive tract of females (Xiao et al., 2017).

EVATAR (a female reproductive tract on a chip) is a culture method that allows for the protracted culture of various tissues from organs of the female reproductive tract. Beyond standard two-dimensional (2D) static culture approaches, this technology can enhance fundamental biology research, drug development, and reproductive toxicity screening utilizing human cells. However, due to high costs and technological obstacles, the EVATAR system's complexity has been inaccessible to the larger academic community. However, the possible cytotoxicity of frequently employed resins poses a hurdle to 3D printing products. Although biosafety is commonly described as the "capacity of a substance to operate with acceptable body response in a given implementation," there is still a dispute about the word and its definition (Williams, 2020; Ghasemi-Mobarakeh et al., 2019). In reality, "biosafety" is frequently used without qualification and existing efforts to standardize "biosafety" testing. Besides branded "biosafety," leachates from a variety of common plastics and therapeutic devices can potentially harm public health and the environment (Teuten et al., 2009; Rustagi et al., 2011; Lee et al., 2015).

Bisphenol A-induced reproductive toxicity was initially discovered by studying the impacts of plastic leachates on mouse oocyte meiosis (Hunt et al., 2012; Peretz et al., 2014). The majority of the literature has demonstrated the vulnerability of the mammalian oocyte and the larger reproductive system to substitutes for some substances like bisphenols, phthalates, and other endocrine disruptive substances (Vandenberg et al., 2019; Segal and Giudice, 2019; Brehm and Flaws, 2019). A cell's meiotic maturation occurs naturally during ovulation due to an increase in the level of luteinizing hormone, but it may also be produced in vitro by separating the egg from the follicle. As a result, the egg is a highly responsive mammalian cell model. The meiotic maturation biological pathway provides a sensitive and efficient screening test for possible reproductive harm caused by chemicals and substances of interest (Rogers et al., 2021).

17.3 Key mechanisms to detect the adverse reaction of compounds

Noticeably, all dental biomaterials emit chemicals into the oral environment. In this regard, different preclinical biosafety test systems have been developed to determine the possible hazards associated with dental substances. Released chemicals from dental substances have been shown to have potential pathogenic consequences. It is not only necessary for a biomaterial's biosafety that minimum diffusible substances are released when it comes in direct contact with the body. It must also perform the functions for which it is designed.

17.3.1 Metal corrosion

When the environmental pH fluctuates because of acidic materials released from the biotransformation of bacteria and biomedical metallic substances (e.g., titanium), it may face challenging problems. Furthermore, prior research has revealed that saliva pH can drop during an infection or under the impact of several factors including periodontitis, behaviors, systemic illness, and salivary gland radiation. Because of the drop in pH caused by microbes producing metabolites, titanium is reported to be more susceptible to corrosion. The acidic pH was connected to Streptococcus and Lactobacillus mutants. On the other hand, hydrofluoric acid is generated when a large amount of fluoride is present, such as in commercially fluoridated acidic toothpaste and mouthwashes. Titanium shows a strong chemical reactivity and is more prone to corrosion (Souza et al., 2015; Noronha Oliveira et al., 2018; Apaza-Bedoya et al., 2017).

Many types of corrosion have been seen on the surface of dental implants. Due to exposure of the metal surface to cathodic reactants, corrosion occurs, leading to the proliferation of the nucleus of the corroded cell. The formation of voids on the surface, known as pits, is more hazardous than usual corrosion because of the difficulties in detecting, predicting, and designing pits. Pitting corrosion occurs on dental implants made of titanium. Corrosion happens when two metals in an electrolytic solution come into close contact, known as galvanic corrosion. Galvanic corrosion develops on the insides of titanium implants. A kind of localized surface degradation that occurs at the contacting surfaces of implants, abutments, and prosthetic components, resulting in limited oral fluid entry and egress and oxygen depletion, is called crevice corrosion. Because of H+ ions in the media, the physiological fluid becomes acidic in these limited contacting regions by lowering the pH values. As a result of the synergistic impact of corrosion and micro-motions, fretting corrosion results in surface changes. This one is responsible for most metal released in the surrounding tissues (Bhola et al., 2011).

The substance surface and medium can be controlled by using electrochemical methods (in vitro). The capacity of an electron-conducting substance submerged in an ion-conductive electrolyte is measured by using open circuit potential (OCP) and compared to a reference electrode. However, following immersion in artificial saliva, the OCP dropped, although it stabilized after 6 h. On the other hand, electrochemical impedance spectroscopy (EIS) measurements are beneficial for determining the condition of the thin oxide layer produced on the surfaces (Souza et al., 2012). Moreover, EIS tests are used to study the development and growth of the thin oxide layer on the surface and its corrosion kinetics because the corrosion process is determined by capacitance and resistance. For example, the titanium oxide thin film capacitance represents the electric charge stored on the titanium surface submerged in the ion-conductive electrolyte solution. Plasma-mass spectrometry can also determine the number of metal ions emitted (Souza et al., 2020).

Thirty dental restoration samples were tested for corrosion resistance and ion release behavior using three different production systems: (a) computer-aided design and manufacture, (b) conventional casting, and (c) laser sintering. Furthermore, electrochemical corrosion is avoided due to its uniformity as well as corrosion resistance is improved by the lack of flaws and residual tensions. The inclusion of Cr, W, and Nb-rich precipitates in the cast and laser-sintered prostheses is harmful to corrosion resistance. The Cr content on the surface decreases as a result of these precipitates. As a result of the drop in Cr, corrosion and ion release increase (Padrós et al., 2020; Wu et al., 2016).

17.3.2 Surface characteristics and roughness

Because of their biosafety, low heat conductivity, color stability, and aesthetics, dental ceramics are widely used as restoratives. They are also utilized in dentistry because of their high accomplishment and a wide variety of chemical and structural compositions, which have been made possible by recent advances in biomaterial technology. Glassy and crystalline phases are frequent in these substances; generally, heat treatment is performed to give them desired characteristics. Adjustments to fixed prostheses (such as ceramic crowns) are frequently required before and after cementation, typically removing the smooth exterior glazed top layer. In contrast to the smooth glazed surface, the exposed porcelain layer is frequently roughed. Surface roughness (a part of the surface texture) impacts how a substance interacts with its surroundings. Ceramic restorations with a high degree of surface roughness cause more wear on the opposing dentition, impair the restoration's aesthetics, and promote biofilm adherence and development. Surface roughness is typically exacerbated by microscopic imperfections such as cracks, grooves, and abrasion flaws, which are sites of frequent bacteria adherence. Gingivitis and dental caries have been linked to increased biofilm production on tooth surfaces. As a result, material proclivity for biofilm development is an essential factor to consider when choosing restorative materials (Kim et al., 2017).

Most data supporting the therapeutic usage of novel ceramic substances comes from manufacturer information on chemical composition and physical characteristics. There is a scarcity of data on surface features and biofilm development on novel materials, especially regarding the influence of intraoral polishing. Surface roughness can harm ceramic strength because brittle fractures can cause enamel and prosthetic components to break sooner or more catastrophically. Roughened surfaces also increase abrasion to opposing tooth structures. Rough surfaces aid bacterial adherence by creating niches for germs to attach and thrive away from brushing, muscle activity, and salivary flow. Moreover, finishing and polishing treatments are clinically relevant (Kim et al., 2017).

These in vitro and in vivo investigations show the significance of the development of dental plaque. However, rough surfaces will aid plaque development and maturation. Although candida species have been identified on acrylic dentures, denture coating and soaking in disinfectant treatments may be an efficient way to avoid biofilm development. Biofilms on gold and amalgam are thick, but they are not very viable. On the other hand, ceramic biofilms are thin and viable. Biofilms cause surface degradation on composites, which promotes biofilm development (Barfeie et al., 2015; Kraemer Fernandez et al., 2020; Shulev et al., 2016).

17.4 Screening techniques of biosafety

In dentistry and medicine, choosing biosafety materials that may be used along with living tissues and pulp while having low cellular toxicity impacts is critical. Before utilizing them in the clinic, dental materials must pass a series of toxicity and biocompatibility tests. Biocompatibility tests will identify harmful compounds, quantify the number of chemicals produced, and assess how people react to that dosage. Fig. 17.3 highlights screening techniques for safety.

Toxicological studies in the early phases of the substance include systematic techniques to evaluate the bioavailability of newly found compounds. The toxicological profiles of substances are evaluated using International Organization for Standardization (ISO) standards, which are essential in satisfying regulatory requirements for premarketing biosafety evaluations. For example, the ISO 10993 series contains instructions for selecting appropriate procedures for testing the toxicity of medical equipment, including dental substances and methods. At a time, this standard comprises 20 distinct components. However, because of limitations in evaluating material biosafety through preclinical testing, dentists must rely on post-marketing data to identify adverse consequences. In vitro cytotoxicity studies, as with other chemicals, are the initial step in evaluating dental substances. There are certain

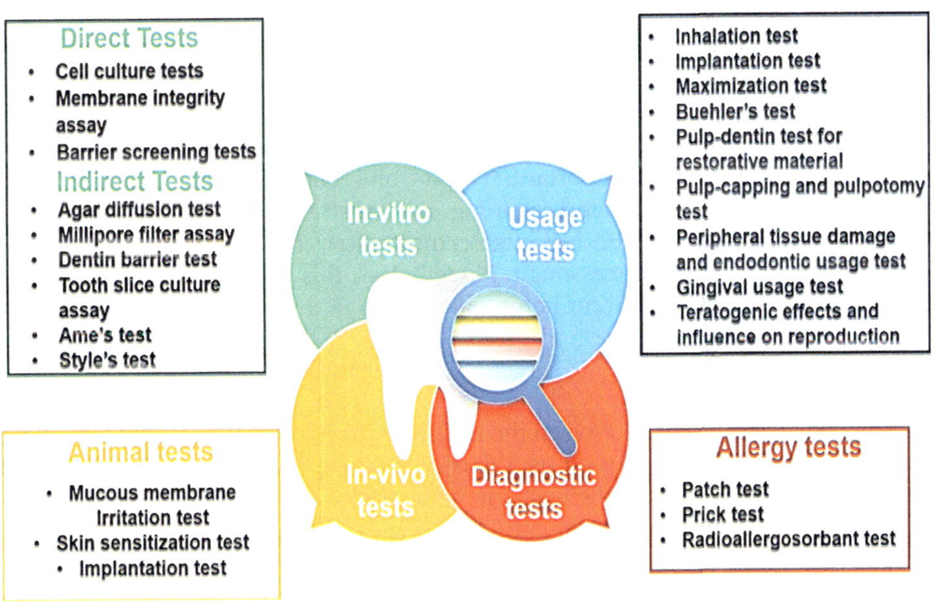

FIGURE 17.3 Schematic representing screening techniques for biosafety.

unique words in biosafety assessment of dental implications, in addition to the use of cell survival tests. As a result, indirect contact tests are created with a barrier between the cells and the tested chemicals. Biological evaluation is heavily reliant on animal testing in the following phases.

17.4.1 In vitro test

These experiments are carried out externally by using a cell system, an enzyme, or another biological system with a substance and its components. The testing techniques that are suggested for in vitro cytotoxicity screening are (a) methods of direct interaction and (b) methods of indirect interaction.

17.4.1.1 Direct interaction tests

Some noteworthy examples of direct interaction tests include (a) cell culture tests, (b) membrane integrity assay, and (c) barrier screening tests.

17.4.1.1.1 Cell culture test

A growing variety of cell culture methods (almost 20) are now accessible in the literature. These tests are performed on human tissues grown in appropriate environments on culture plates. These persistent cell lines have a known and consistent activity that has been extensively understood. The alterations in the cell lines are documented after a careful inspection under the microscope. Dyes are utilized to assess cell destruction by determining the essential amount of stain uptake by cells. The drawbacks of these counts of cells are the difficulty of discriminating between live and deceased cells without causing physical changes. The cell viability count is very subjective, and any artifact exacerbates the situation (Mirbagheri et al., 2019).

17.4.1.1.2 Membrane integrity assay

It is a fluorescent type of assay that determines the permeability of a cell membrane. These tests significantly reduce artifact-related mistakes. The accuracy with which live and dead cells are distinguished is also important. Trypan blue staining, vital red staining, neutral red staining paired with amido black staining, and neutral red staining mixed with amido black staining have been used to investigate the toxicity of various endodontic materials for routine work cell viability assessment. Nonetheless, this test has the drawback of identifying sublethal alterations that occur before alterations in membrane permeability (Bowman et al., 2010).

17.4.1.1.3 Barrier screening test

A dentin layer usually exists between the utilized substance and the pulp tissue. Therefore, in this method, a dentin disc is used as a barrier between the tested substance and the cell culture. If the substance reaches the disc, the toxin-antitoxin (TA)-positive cytotoxic reaction follows (Jiang et al., 2022).

17.4.1.2 *Indirect interaction tests*

On the other hand, indirect tests may include (a) agar diffusion test, (a) millipore filter assay, (c) dentin barrier test, (d) tooth slice culture assay, (e) Ame's test, and (f) Style's test.

17.4.1.2.1 Agar diffusion test

In this test, a coat of agar is layered on a monoculture cell monolayer, also known as the agar overlay. On top of the agar coat, the substance to be tested is put. This method can be used to detect widespread cytotoxicity caused by leachable substances. Red vital stain is the most common dye utilized here. The dye on the cell line shows leaching, indicating that the hazardous chemical has been identified (Camilleri et al., 2020; El Sayed et al., 2021).

17.4.1.2.2 Millipore filter assay

The agar diffusion experiments are pretty similar to this approach. In this assay, a millipore filter is used between the primary cell and the test substance. Any leachable substance can propagate through a 0.45 m filter pore. The used filter paper is rated by ISO, which is usually based on the substance used during the examination.

17.4.1.2.3 Dentin barrier test

This technique closely replicates the oral environment while being an in vitro test. Model cavity technique is another name for it. These tests consider the cytotoxic compounds' distribution via the dentinal tubules (Jiang et al., 2022).

17.4.1.2.4 Tooth slice culture assay

It is feasible to extrapolate a clinical outcome. For animal and human research, the technique is a good substitute. A cellular toxicity influence in pulpal tissue, stem cells, growth-related aspects, and gene treatments can be carefully assessed in contrast to the previously mentioned techniques. Confounding variables that typically skew the results are primarily eliminated using this technique. Additionally, the cost factor has also been significantly decreased (Janjić et al., 2018).

17.4.1.2.5 Ame's test

One of the most often used in vitro assays focuses on discovering environmental chemicals that cause mutations and cancer. This involves the use of microorganisms to discover possible carcinogens without the use of humans. Salmonella mutant strains are generally employed in this study. Moreover, these bacteria show mutations in the enzyme that synthesizes histidine. Histidine, in turn, is vital for protein production. Bacteria are unable to proliferate as well as colonize onto histidine-deficient agar culture. If a mutagenic chemical is present, the bacteria increase rapidly, indicating mutagenicity of the material (Zeiger, 2019; Levy et al., 2019).

17.4.1.2.6 Style's test

The existence of a cancer-causing agent could be detected by adding a chemical into the substance, which, if cancer-causing, transforms it into a quasi-cancerous condition. Outcomes-based only on cytotoxicity testing are difficult to identify. These tests classify substances according to their cytotoxicity under specific conditions (Sakaguchi and Powers, 2012).

17.4.2 In vivo and usage test

The animal study replicates a near-clinical setting, particularly in systemic and cytotoxic studies. Ferrets and dogs are among the animals that have been tested. The ISO 7405 rules divide testing time into short-term and long-term. The researchers choose to split the lap durations into several time intervals ranging from 65 days or more. The expense of choosing a short-term strategy might be a significant stumbling block. Longer durations, on the other hand, provide insight into the healing and regeneration processes.

17.4.2.1 *Inhalation test*

The substance being evaluated is applied as an aerosol. It is sprayed for 30 s around the chest as well as the mouth of the animals. Proceeding, with the substance being sprayed 10 times per 30 min interval. The substance is deemed very hazardous if the animal dies within 3 min. If this is not the case, a long-term follow-up is required before the substance may be classified as safe (Sakaguchi and Powers, 2012).

17.4.2.2 *Implantation test*

In rats, rabbits, and other animals, the substance is implanted subcutaneously or intramuscularly. The time it takes to implant a device might range from many months. Inflammation next to the implanted substance is assessed after a brief implantation test of around 3 weeks. After a long time of implants, connective tissue encapsulation forms, which may be assessed as well. Primates, dogs, pigs, guinea pigs, and other animals might be used to test intraosseous implanted substances. A histological examination of the tissue around the tested substance is possible (Hosseinpour et al., 2022; Kushali et al., 2020).

17.4.2.3 *Maximization test*

A substance known as Complete Freund's Adjuvant (FCA) is utilized in this test. Freund's adjuvant is the most common kind of this substance. FCA has a habit of slowly releasing antigens. After 7 days, the experimental substance is injected intradermally into the animal with FCA and assessed. Similar material is administered topically for the next 2 days on the seventh day. The sensitivity of the tests is improved as a result of this. The skin responses are evaluated after 14 days. When doing this test, use caution since the antigen might cause an unpleasant reaction to the skin, leading to a potential issue if administered in large amounts (Klecak, 2019).

17.4.2.4 *Buehler's test*

The removal of the FCA part is the primary benefit of this test. Because the antigen is no longer present, the experimental animals experience less harm (Frankild et al., 2000). When it comes to restorative substances, compatibility with the pulp is crucial. Test performed in animals or using human teeth will be removed for dental purposes. Upon constructing a Class V cavity, a test substance is placed and maintained in inspection for months. After that, the pulp is histologically examined for symptoms of inflammation and odontoblast response, and the results are microscopically analyzed (Hosseinpour et al., 2022).

17.4.2.5 Pulpotomy material test, as well as pulp-capping

It's a little modified version of the pulp-dentin test. The evaluation of the capping of pulp and pulpotomies can be done if a piece of the pulp is exposed before the substance is implemented (Donnelly et al., 2022).

17.4.2.6 Mucosal damage and mucosa usage test

In this test, inflammatory responses to mucosal membranes and skin abrasions are studied. Photos from before and after surgery are reviewed as biopsy samples for evidence of inflammation.

17.4.2.7 Endodontic usage test and periapical tissue damage test

It mimics the response occurring after traditional endodontic therapy. In this method, normally large animals (such as monkeys) are used as a model. Histological sections of the periapical area are used to assess the condition. Intentional pulp necrosis to mimic a clinical situation is also conducted occasionally. Due to the perplexing ethical problems, research is very scarce. To get a similar result, alternative implant tests might be utilized instead (Hosseinpour et al., 2022).

17.4.2.8 Gingival usage test

Cavity development and subgingival extensions guarantee that the tested substance has a direct touch with the gingiva. In this test, usually assessment is carried out for 7–30 days. The deposition of bacterial plaque, which could contribute to inflammation and obstruct the accurate assessment of substance toxicity, is one of the study's complicating factors. Another crucial factor is whether the margins are under- or over-contoured. However, the situation becomes worse owing to the presence of rough edges. Teratogenic impacts on reproduction are used to determine if a substance might cause harm to fetuses or infants. Any abnormalities in the fetuses and infants are examined microscopically and macroscopically. This can be passed to the following generation to investigate any abnormalities (Suresh et al., 2021; Takenaka et al., 2019).

17.4.3 Diagnostic techniques

It is possible to draw a direct correlation between clinical efficiency and the type of diagnostic tests on patients. While conducting these tests, many legal and ethical issues must be addressed carefully (Momeni-Moghaddam et al., 2022; Kumari et al., 2021). Before commercialization, restorative substances are clinically tested and assessed according to US Public Health Service or Ryge standards. The substances should be checked for an extended time (maybe a year) with a 90% positive outcome.

17.4.3.1 Allergy tests

The evaluation tests for allergy are further subdivided into four categories viz., (a) a patch test (including delayed hypersensitivity reactions), (b) a prick test (including immediate hypersensitivity reaction), (c) an alternative prick test, and (d) radioallergosorbent test.

17.4.3.1.1 Patch test

When a patch is applied to the patient's back, allergens are put on adhesives in moderately large amounts to induce a positive response. These are nonirritating and moderate reactions that are ultimately safe. The patient must take many measures, such as avoiding sun exposure and excessive perspiration. Moreover, symptoms like redness, itching, and blisters are common in this test. After a thorough examination of the skin, the patch is removed after 3 days. However, after 10 days, a second examination should be performed to exclude delayed hypersensitivity reactions. It takes a few days for immunocompetent T cells to show signs of transformation. It is used to detect hypersensitive reactions that are delayed (type IV). As mucosa of the mouth and the skin are significantly similar. During epidermal testing, a similar test is conducted as is performed in the mouth cavity. The allergic response is not always triggered due to variables such as saliva and a small difference in the immunological responses. To solve this issue, you might need to increase the allergen concentration. As a result, the patient's back would be in an optimal, dependable, and exact location. The test should only be carried out when circumstances demand. A prophetic test is one in which a generalized patch test is done despite a previous allergic reaction. If there is any intra-oral evidence of inflammation, the allergy can be verified by removing the suspected allergen and returning the same allergen to explain the previously observed reaction (Japundžić et al., 2018; Kitagawa et al., 2019).

17.4.3.1.2 Prick test

This type of test could be used to identify type I allergic reactions or acute allergic reactions. Allergen is applied to the skin as a drop, and when this is applied it punctures the skin. After 5–30 min, one can observe its effect on the skin as a positive reaction. However, the danger of sensitivity with the prick test is relatively low compared to the patch test (Japundžić et al., 2018).

17.4.3.1.3 Radioallergosorbent test (RAST)

It is used to identify the quick sensitivity of allergens. Allergen is coupled to an insoluble substance, to which the patient's serum is introduced. If the additional serum contains antibodies to the allergen, the allergen elicits a reaction by attaching it to the antibody. After that, a radiolabeled antibody (i.e., IgE) is introduced along with a complex reaction with the previously attached nonsoluble substances. Afterward, nonreacting IgE antibodies are rinsed to remove them. It is a quantitative test in that the associated radioactivity shows the amount of serum IgE released for given allergens (Swetha et al., 2015; Stavreva and Kapusevska, 2019).

17.4.4 Analysis of intraoral alloys

Utilizing analytical procedures (like polish metallic micrograph sections along with dispersive X-ray examination) for removing prostheses using this test is quite simple. When the method has to be expanded to a fixed prosthesis, it becomes complicated. In such cases, a chip test can be utilized, in which the extra coronal surface is brushed with a silicon carbide stone, and the resulting fragments are aggregated on a self-adhesive graphite plate. The carrier of the self-adhesive type however provides electrical conduction. Single alloy components have a precision of up to 1%. As a result, if no past allergic reactions are reported, then a patient with certain metals does not need to undergo an allergic test (Kunrath et al., 2021; Cruz et al., 2018).

17.5 Selection of biosafety screening method

Biosafety testing and assessment of medical equipment are performed to identify the device's potential for causing toxicity when it comes in direct contact with the body. The device substances should not exhibit any local or systemic adverse impacts, or carcinogenic effects, or cause any unfavorable reproductive and developmental consequences (either directly or by the discharge of their constituents) (Montalli et al., 2021).

17.5.1 Testing hierarchy

A distinctive hierarchy governs the patterns of testing. The substance cannot be channeled further to tests with more strength, imitating clinical testing, until unproblematic findings are acquired in the early stages. This testing protocol is performed in accordance with Autian's cumulative measure of biosafety, which he suggested in 1970. The existing literature is evaluated for details on physical, chemical, and biological properties, and investigations on missing dimensions. After completing some fundamental tests, if a change is found in a dental compound that has been used clinically, the substance is considered to have risk. On the other hand, more extensive testing is required if significant changes or new components are introduced (Abebe, 2019).

17.6 Biocompatibility of various dental materials

The requirement for safe analysis and management of dental substances utilized in dentistry has increased in the recent decade. Nevertheless, this work is complicated and time-consuming. Passive dental substances will be steady and durable since they will not remain entrapped in the mouth environment. Dental substances are anticipated to be widely acceptable and will not cause damage to the mouth cavity's surrounding structures (Malli neni et al., 2013; Sefton, 1986).

17.6.1 Bonding agents

Bond abilities to enamel have historically been measured in tensile strength compared to those to dentine are higher. Due to contents (natural and unnatural) having a high moisture level and less content of minerals compared to enamel, bonding to dentine has proven more challenging. Secondary to coating the dentine's surfaces, smear layer debris accumulates inside tubules to create a dentinal plug, which looks impenetrable when seen by electron microscopy. This debris significantly decreases tubular fluid circulation. The existence of this smear layer is critical for regenerative substances' adhesion and biocompatibility (Reichl et al., 2006). A dentine obstacle significantly reduces the cytotoxic impacts of resin materials. In vitro, mixtures of hydroxyethyl methacrylate and additional resins used in dentin bonding agents may produce cytotoxicity (Peliz et al., 2005; Cetinguc et al., 2007). Silane coupling agents are utilized as adhesive boosters between different materials in restorative dentistry and dental technologies (Lung and Matinlinna, 2012; Matinlinna et al., 2006).

17.6.2 Resin-based composites

Patients and the general public are affected by allergic responses to resin-based products (e.g., resin composites). Normally, personnel who are in the dentistry field work with such composites. The sealants' toxicity and efficacy in reducing fissure caries are among the biocompatibility characteristics of these composites. Resin-based composite materials are utilized as luting cement and restorative composites in tooth restoration. These compounds are resin composites of natural and unnatural phases (Goldberg, 2008). A dentine barrier significantly reduces cytotoxicity after 24–48 h of setup. Light-cured resins appear less cytotoxic than chemically treated resins, although this impact dramatically depends on the light's curing effectiveness and the kind of resin system. In vitro, polished composites have significantly lower cytotoxicity. However, some substances remain hazardous even after polishing. In vivo, there is no proof that any commercialized resin has harmful xenoestrogenic impacts (Furuya et al., 2006; Lenie et al., 2008). Other in vivo consequences of liberated composite materials on soft tissues are little understood. Since limited clinical trials have been done, there is some indication that methacrylate-based composite materials may induce substantial frequencies of hypersensitivity. However, allergic responses to acrylic resins have been linked to contact dermatitis.

17.6.3 Dental cast alloys

Non-noble transition metals utilized in the base metal alloys include nickel, molybdenum, and iron. If cells are freed from these alloys, this could perhaps hurt them. Nickel allergy is prevalent, affecting 10%–20% of females and 1% of males (Türkcan and Nalbant, 2015). Considering the liberation of nickel ions from nickel-based alloys is typically more significant than the noble type of alloy, this represents considerable danger. Cast dental alloys made of gold and other noble metal alloys, a variety of materials may be found in restorations, such as platinum, palladium, copper, and silver, either purposefully added or as contaminants. Gold foil is a potent, non-soluble restorative compound with specialized applications. Burning feelings of the oral mucosal membrane in interaction with the gold alloys, lichenoid lesions, and broad systemic responses are all possible side effects of gold foil (Yan Guo et al., 2012).

Moreover, the toxicity of gold has been linked to pulpal irritation, odontoblast damage, and bleeding. Titanium and alloys are preferred choices for implantation because of being nontoxic (because of the thin and compacted oxide coating on the titanium surfaces). They may be surface-modified to enhance osseointegration (a direct structural and functional connection between ordered, living bone, and the surface of a load-carrying implant). It is critical for implant stability and a prerequisite for implant loading and long-term clinical success of endosseous dental implants). Titanium has the unusual ability to attach to live tissues and bones. When metal ions are put on a culture medium, they generally cause an inhibitory zone with diverse species, indicating cytotoxicity or cell injury. Chromium, cobalt, copper, mercury, nickel, tin, and zinc are all used in dentistry as base metal alloys (chromium, cobalt, nickel) and as ingredients in gold dental amalgams (mercury, tin, copper). Because of its outstanding biomechanical characteristics, titanium is also utilized as a crown and a bridge component in prosthodontics (Yan Guo et al., 2012).

17.6.4 Glass ionomer cement

Wilson and Kent were the first to discover glass ionomer cement, which has been utilized in dentistry since around the 1970s. The biocompatibility and long-term stability of this material are critical for its application in neurosurgery. When used as vital components, glass ionomer cement emerges bland to the pulp while employed as a luting agent, which may cause enhanced reactions. After close contact, eugenol liberated from zinc oxide eugenol cement has been shown to fix cells, decrease cell respiration, and decrease nerve transmission in experiments. On the other hand, eugenol is an irritant when it comes to contact with connective tissues. The zinc oxide eugenol cement could provide a transitory barrier against bacterial infection. The studies suggested that in monkey teeth, zinc oxide eugenol cement has been observed to induce just a mild-to-moderate inflammatory response within the initial week in their teeth. When cavities are profound, it changes to a moderate. However, after 8 weeks, it exhibits chronic inflammatory activity with restorative dentine production. For this purpose, it has been employed as a negative control drug in usage tests compared with restorative treatments (Hauman and Love, 2003a,b).

Zinc phosphate cement generates robust to intermediate cytotoxic responses that diminish with time, according to in vitro screening studies. Due to zinc ion leaching and a lower pH, the pulp is protected. In implant studies using zinc phosphate cement injected into rat dental pulp, focal necrotic was found, confirming the cement's cytotoxic impacts while associated with tissues of the pulp. Zinc polyacrylate cement is a kind of polycarboxylate cement that combines the sturdiness of zinc phosphate cement with the adhesion strength and biocompatibility of zinc oxide eugenol cement (Nicholson, 1996).

17.6.5 Liner and varnishes

Cavity liners made of calcium hydroxide occur in various forms, like solutions of saline type ($pH > 12$) and upgraded versions, including zinc oxide, titanium dioxide, and certain resins. In screening tests, the high pH of calcium hydroxide in suspension causes severe cytotoxicity. Nevertheless, some of these components appear to degrade with time, perhaps resulting in a breach between the repair and the cavity wall. Several in vivo experiments using resin-upgraded glass ionomer cement as liners found no pulp degradation. They may also prevent germs from penetrating. However, the stability of these compounds is not as dependable as that of other cavity liners due to the thinness of the film and the development of tiny holes. This liner is likewise fragile and has a low tensile strength (Hilton, 2016).

17.7 Recent advances in toxicity aspects and biosafety related to dental materials

Toxic dental substances elicit toxicity after dentists apply them in patients' mouths for years. Some dental compounds and their toxicities are discussed in Table 17.1.

Some dental filling materials could also exhibit hazardous effects, as described in Fig. 17.4.

If the inclusion of some specific ingredients in the resin composite mixture is omitted, then this could be reasonable. However, it is important to determine precisely what challenges we

TABLE 17.1 Examples of dental compounds and their toxicities.

Dental compounds	Toxicity associated
1. Toxic dental fillings	
a. Dental amalgam fillings (Mercury fillings)	• Mercury toxicity • As the temperature changes, dental amalgam expands and contracts, potentially causing cracks, fracturing, or damage to surrounding teeth.
b. Composite resin fillings	Some resin composite fillings may cause toxicities if they are included (e.g., bisphenol A). Few hazardous chemicals that can enter your body and cause harm are: • Bisphenol A • Bisphenol A–glycidyl methacrylate • Diphenyliodonium chloride • Triphenyl-stibane • Hydroxyethyl methacrylate • Triethylene glycol dimethacrylate.
c. Glass ionomer fillings	Some glass ionomer fillings contain fluoride, which might lead to: • Hypothyroidism • Increased blood pressure and blood calcium • Fluoride accumulation in the pineal gland • Cognitive dysfunction • Insomnia • Fatigue • Muscle weakness • Preeclampsia (which can result in the death of the expecting mother) • Earlier onset puberty • Lower intelligence quotient in infants whose mothers ingested a lethal quantity of fluoride. • Increased risk of attention deficit hyperactivity disorder in children whose mothers ingested a lethal quantity of fluoride • Increased risk of autism in children whose mothers ingested a lethal quantity of fluoride.
d. Resin-ionomer fillings	Depending on the design, the resin-ionomer may include some hazardous substances (e.g., bisphenol A, fluoride, etc.).

TABLE 17.1 Examples of dental compounds and their toxicities.—cont'd

Dental compounds	Toxicity associated
e. Porcelain fused to metal fillings	Heavy metals could leak out from the filling substructure into the mouth cavity when porcelain is bonded to metal, leading to heavy metal poisoning.
2. Toxic dental materials	
a. Metal braces	Teflon may be used as a coating that has been linked to hormone disruption as well as other health issues.
b. Ceramic braces	Ceramic braces are likely to tear off standard tooth structures during removal, and they may still be coated with poisonous Teflon which makes them more expensive than metal braces.
c. Metallic retainers	Heavy metals may leak into your body, causing allergic responses and cytotoxicity. For instance, nickel and chromium appear to be of particular concern.
d. Ceramic retainers	It may contain bisphenol A or bisphenol A-forming chemicals.
e. Fluoride treatments	Fluoride is ineffective in preventing cavities and could cause allergies, lowered intelligence quotient, tiredness, sleeplessness, and other problems.
f. Dental sealants	It might contain toxic bisphenol A
g. Dental bondings	Some dental bonding composites containing bisphenol A might be cytotoxic.
h. Dental implants	Titanium, nickel, and aluminum implants erode and leak heavy metals into your mouth and body. Heavy metal toxicity and allergic responses might occur as a result of this.
i. Crowns	Heavy metals to which the patient is allergic may be present. Although allergic responses are not the same as toxicity, they are unpleasant and should be minimized.

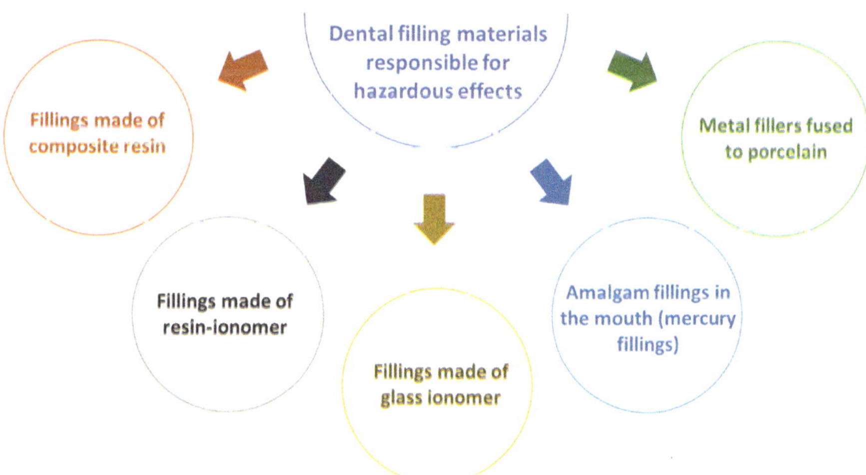

FIGURE 17.4 Dental filling materials responsible for hazardous effects.

can face after their exclusion from the composite resin mixture. Fig. 17.5 highlights some recent advances in dental materials.

17.7.1 Dental amalgam fillings (mercury)

Mercury fillings have been utilized in the United States for over 150 years and are still the most popular dental filling materials. Although the American Dental Association (ADA) asserts that mercury fillings are harmless, other international health organizations agree with the collected data that mercury fillings are poisonous and harmful. It's no surprise that mercury fillings are linked to mercury toxicity. Mercury levels in the skin of dead individuals with mercury fillings showed−−13 times higher than those without mercury fillings. Mercury vapors are emitted most frequently during the insertion and removal of fillings, but they can also be released while eating, cleaning, or crunching the teeth. Furthermore, as temperatures change, dental amalgam expands and contracts, potentially causing fractures, cracking, or damage to surrounding teeth (Parkin Kullmann and Pamphlett, 2018; Keshavarz et al., 2022).

17.7.2 Composite resin fillings

Composite resin fillings are manufactured from various materials (most often plastics). The composition of one batch of composite resin will change from the next. However, some composite resin fillings include bisphenol A or other hazardous chemicals that can leak into the body. Toxic components in composite resin typically permeate into the oral cavity and circulation early on. Manufacturers eventually responded to research and phased out

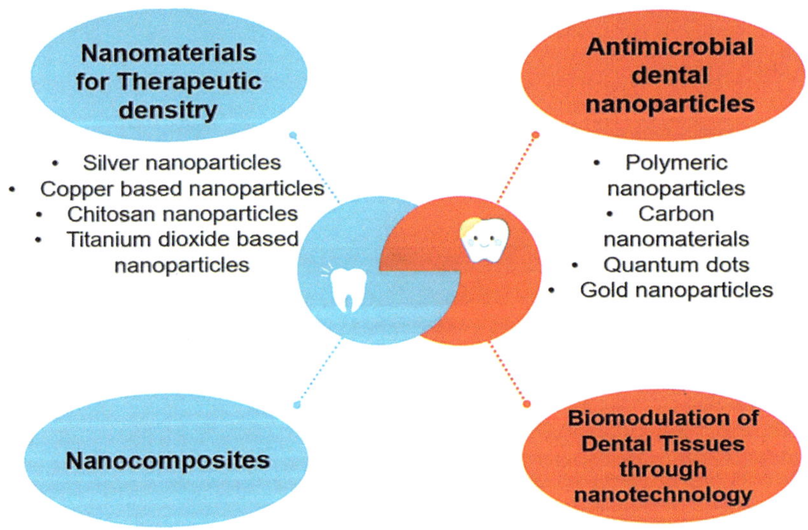

FIGURE 17.5 Recent advances in dental materials.

hazardous composite materials. Biocompatibility is a common feature of modern composite resin (Wang et al., 2021; Lopes-Rocha et al., 2022).

17.7.3 Glass ionomer fillings

Fillings made of glass ionomer cement are tooth-colored and flexible. Sadly, fluoride is present in certain glass ionomer fillings, which many people believe is harmful. Glass ionomer cement was shown to be cytotoxic to human tooth and gum cells in one research. Even though new glass ionomer fillings have increased their efficacy, studies have revealed that the inherent toxicity of glass-ionomer cement is still extremely high (Park and Kang, 2020; Amin et al., 2021).

17.7.4 Resin-ionomer fillings

A hybrid resin-ionomer filling substance may be made by combining composite resin and glass ionomer in different ratios. This combination combines the advantages and disadvantages of composite resin with glass ionomer. Depending on the manufacturer, the resin-ionomer may include bisphenol A, fluoride, or other hazardous substances. On the other hand, many contemporary resin-ionomer fillings incorporate fluoride-free components, including silica, porcelain, and quartz. If a dentist advises you a resin-ionomer filling, you may remain confident that only biosafety materials—no possible poisons are going to occur in your mouth (Dursun et al., 2018; Park and Kang, 2020).

17.7.5 Porcelain fused to metal fillings

Though porcelain is usually considered safe, porcelain-fused-to-metal fillings occasionally produce allergic responses. Porcelain fillings (also called ceramic) are great alternatives to mercury fillings. Porcelain having a natural tooth color is stain-resistant, mercury-free, and free from bisphenol A. Unlike amalgam and other substitutes, porcelain fillings may last up to 20 years. When porcelain is bonded to metal, heavy metals may leach out into your mouth cavity through the filling substructure, causing heavy metal poisoning. Because of the metal substructure, more of the tooth must be taken to put this filling (compared to porcelain) (Clewett, 1995; Mühlemann et al., 2020).

17.8 Conclusion

To protect patients from risk, it is crucial to obtain authentic dental compounds. Before declaring any substance safe, a combination of tests of multi-spectral type should be carried out. Nonetheless, a shorter screening period could be adopted due to ethical and legal considerations. Although, from the dentistry literature, there is no indication that dental alloys are cancerous. On the other hand, research supports the mutagenic ability of metal ions. Mutagenicity can be determined in either bacterial or mammalian cells.

Moreover, in vitro systems' capacity to estimate in vivo mutagenesis or carcinogenesis is presently limited. Surgical and dental substances fail despite current creative metallurgical and technical breakthroughs and significant advances in the design and development of these substances. It is supposed that the corrosion of dental implants may be one of the causes of these problems. The best implant combination can withstand the most severe circumstances that might potentially occur in the mouth. The substances utilized for the implant and implant-borne supra structures must be chosen carefully, and this may be done by assessing their galvanic corrosion tendencies. Implant malfunctions will become an uncommon phenomenon if the processes that enable implant bio acceptance and structural stability are entirely established, provided that they are utilized appropriately and put in the areas for which they are recommended. The mouth cavity is continually exposed to sensitizing chemicals that induce allergic responses, contributing to an annual increase in healthcare costs. Allergies to latex, acrylates, and formaldehyde are dental personnel's most frequent allergic responses. Sodium metabisulphite and nickel produce rapid hypersensitivity reactions, whereas polymethylmethacrylate and latex cause delayed hypersensitivity reactions. Establishing a diagnosis requires a thorough allergy history, clinical examination, and confirmatory testing like patch tests and memory lymphocyte immune-stimulation assay (MELISA). As a result of the rising number of patients with allergies to various substances, practicing dentists should be conscious of documented sensitivities to recognize substances to preclude allergic symptoms in the dental clinic.

The utilization of healthy and safe substances is critical in restorative procedures. In dentistry, using various materials in long-term oral usage necessitates low-toxic substances for patients and health care professionals. Additionally, before clinical use, screening studies should identify any possible damage.

17.9 List of abbreviations

2D two-dimensional
3D three-dimensional
ADA American Dental Association
CADD combined annotation-dependent depletion
EIS electrochemical impedance spectroscopy
EVATAR a female reproductive tract on a chip or the lab model that mimics the female reproductive system
FCA complete Freund's adjuvant
ISO International Organization for Standardization
MELISA memory lymphocyte immune-stimulation assay
MN micronuclei
OCP open circuit potential
RAST radioallergosorbent test
TA toxin-antitoxin

References

Abebe, W., 2019. Review of herbal medications with the potential to cause bleeding: dental implications, and risk prediction and prevention avenues. EPMA J. 10 (1), 51–64.

Ahmadian, E., Eftekhari, A., Babaei, H., Nayebi, A.M., Eghbal, M.A., 2017. Anti-cancer effects of citalopram on hepatocellular carcinoma cells occur via cytochrome C release and the activation of NF-kB. Anti Cancer Agents Med. Chem. 17 (11), 1570–1577. https://www.ncbi.nlm.nih.gov/pubmed/28356024.

Amin, F., Rahman, S., Khurshid, Z., Zafar, M.S., Sefat, F., Kumar, N., 2021. Effect of nanostructures on the properties of glass ionomer dental restoratives/cements: a comprehensive narrative review. Materials 14 (21), 6260.

Apaza-Bedoya, K., Tarce, M., Benfatti, C.A.M., Henriques, B., Mathew, M.T., Teughels, W., Souza, J.C.M., 2017. Synergistic interactions between corrosion and wear at titanium-based dental implant connections: a scoping review. J. Periodontal. Res. 52 (6), 946–954. https://www.ncbi.nlm.nih.gov/pubmed/28612506.

Araujo, A.M., Alves, G.R., Avanco, G.T., Parizi, J.L., Nai, G.A., 2013. Assessment of methyl methacrylate genotoxicity by the micronucleus test. Braz. Oral Res. 27 (1), 31–36. https://www.ncbi.nlm.nih.gov/pubmed/23306624.

Asati, S., Pandey, V., Gour, V., Tiwari, R., Soni, V., Rajpoot, K., Tekade, M., Sharma, M.C., Tekade, R.K., 2022. Toxicity and toxicokinetic considerations in product development and drug research. In: Pharmacokinetics and Toxicokinetic Considerations, vol. 2. Elsevier. https://doi.org/10.1016/b978-0-323-98367-9.00001-9.

Barfeie, A., Wilson, J., Rees, J., 2015. Implant surface characteristics and their effect on osseointegration. Br. Dent. J. 218 (5), E9. https://www.ncbi.nlm.nih.gov/pubmed/25766196.

Barrett, A.A., Anusavice, K.J., Shen, C., 2011. Two-peak fracture stress behavior of surface treated and veneered Y-TZP specimens. Dent. Mater. 27, e53. https://doi.org/10.1016/j.dental.2011.08.526.

Bassoli, E., Gatto, A., Iuliano, L., Grazia Violante, M., 2007. 3D printing technique applied to rapid casting. Rapid Prototyp. J. 13 (3), 148–155. https://doi.org/10.1108/13552540710750898.

Bertolini, M.M., Portela, M.B., Curvelo, J.A., Soares, R.M., Lourenco, E.J., Telles, D.M., 2014. Resins-based denture soft lining materials modified by chlorhexidine salt incorporation: an in vitro analysis of antifungal activity, drug release and hardness. Dent. Mater. 30 (8), 793–798. https://www.ncbi.nlm.nih.gov/pubmed/24933229.

Beyth, N., Yudovin-Farber, I., Perez-Davidi, M., Domb, A.J., Weiss, E.I., 2010. Polyethyleneimine nanoparticles incorporated into resin composite cause cell death and trigger biofilm stress in vivo. Proc. Natl. Acad. Sci. U. S. A. 107 (51), 22038–22043. https://www.ncbi.nlm.nih.gov/pubmed/21131569.

Bhola, R., Bhola, S.M., Mishra, B., Ayers, R., Olson, D.L., Ohno, T., 2011. Cellular response of titanium and its alloys as implants. J. Oral Implantol. 37 (4), 387–399. https://www.ncbi.nlm.nih.gov/pubmed/20557146.

Bidlack, W.R., 2002. Casarett & Doull's toxicology: the basic science of poisons. J. Am. Coll. Nutr. 21 (3), 289–290. https://doi.org/10.1080/07315724.2002.10719223 sixth ed.

Blasiak, J., Kasznicki, J., Drzewoski, J., Pawlowska, E., Szczepanska, J., Reiter, R.J., 2011. Perspectives on the use of melatonin to reduce cytotoxic and genotoxic effects of methacrylate-based dental materials. J. Pineal Res. 51 (2), 157–162. https://www.ncbi.nlm.nih.gov/pubmed/21470304.

Boraldi, F., Coppi, C., Bortolini, S., Consolo, U., Tiozzo, R., 2009. Cytotoxic evaluation of elastomeric dental impression materials on a permanent mouse cell line and on a primary human gingival fibroblast culture. Materials 2 (3), 934–944. https://doi.org/10.3390/ma2030934.

Bowman, A.M., Nesin, O.M., Pakhomova, O.N., Pakhomov, A.G., 2010. Analysis of plasma membrane integrity by fluorescent detection of Tl+ uptake. J. Membr. Biol. 236 (1), 15–26.

Brehm, E., Flaws, J.A., 2019. Transgenerational effects of endocrine-disrupting chemicals on male and female reproduction. Endocrinology 160 (6), 1421–1435. https://www.ncbi.nlm.nih.gov/pubmed/30998239.

Brunton, P.A., Christensen, G.J., Cheung, S.W., Burke, F.J., Wilson, N.H., 2005. Contemporary dental practice in the UK: indirect restorations and fixed prosthodontics. Br. Dent. J. 198 (2), 99–103. Discussion 189. https://www.ncbi.nlm.nih.gov/pubmed/15702109.

Camilleri, J., Moliz, T.A., Bettencourt, A., Costa, J., Martins, F., Rabadijeva, D., Rodriguez, D., Visai, L., Combes, C., Farrugia, C., 2020. Standardization of antimicrobial testing of dental devices. Dent. Mater. 36 (3), e59–e73.

Cetinguc, A., Olmez, S., Vural, N., 2007. HEMA diffusion from dentin bonding agents in young and old primary molars in vitro. Dent. Mater. 23 (3), 302–307. https://www.ncbi.nlm.nih.gov/pubmed/16530820.

Chen, S.Y., Chen, C.C., Kuo, H.W., 2002. Cytotoxicity of dental impression materials. Bull. Environ. Contam. Toxicol. 69 (3), 350–355. https://www.ncbi.nlm.nih.gov/pubmed/12177755.

Clewett, J., 1995. Toxic effects of materials used in dental restorations. Br. Dent. J. 179 (7), 244. https://www.ncbi.nlm.nih.gov/pubmed/7577173.

Coppi, C., Paolinelli Devincenzi, C., Bortolini, S., Consolo, U., Tiozzo, R., 2007. A new generation of sterile and radiopaque impression materials: an in vitro cytotoxicity study. J. Biomater. Appl. 22 (1), 83–95. https://www.ncbi.nlm.nih.gov/pubmed/17065163.

Crespo-Lopez, M.E., Macedo, G.L., Pereira, S.I., Arrifano, G.P., Picanco-Diniz, D.L., do Nascimento, J.L., Herculano, A.M., 2009. Mercury and human genotoxicity: critical considerations and possible molecular mechanisms. Pharmacol. Res. 60 (4), 212–220. https://www.ncbi.nlm.nih.gov/pubmed/19446469.

Cruz, R.S., Lemos, C.A.A., Oliveira, H.F.F., de Souza Batista, V.E., Pellizzer, E.P., Verri, F.R., 2018. Comparison of the use of titanium–zirconium alloy and titanium alloy in dental implants: a systematic review and meta-analysis. J. Oral Implantol. 44 (4), 305–312.

Deliversky, J., Yaneva-Deliverska, M., Lyapina, M., Kisselova, A., 2015. European and international standards on medical devices for dentistry. J. IMAB - Annual Proc. 21 (1), 713–717. https://doi.org/10.5272/jimab.2015211.713.

Donnelly, A., Foschi, F., McCabe, P., Duncan, H.F., 2022. Pulpotomy for treatment of complicated crown fractures in permanent teeth: a systematic review. Int. Endod. J. 55 (4), 290–311.

Dursun, E., Güncü, G.N., Dursun, C.K., Kiremitçi, A., Karabulut, E., Akalın, F.A., 2018. Nanofilled and conventional resin-modified glass ionomer fillings combined with connective tissue grafts for treatment of gingival recessions with non-carious cervical lesions. J. Oral Sci. 60 (3), 344–351.

El Sayed, M., Ghanerad, N., Shabanpour, Z., Shabanpoor, M., Rahimi, F., 2021. Comparing the antifungal effect of sodium hypochlorite gel versus different types of root canal medicaments at different time intervals using the agar diffusion test: an in vitro study. Int. J. Dent. 2021, 6550054.

Ficai, D., Ficai, A., 2017. Prevention of biofilm formation by material modification. In: Biofilms and Implantable Medical Devices. Elsevier. https://doi.org/10.1016/b978-0-08-100382-4.00007-1.

Frankild, S., Volund, A., Wahlberg, J.E., Andersen, K.E., 2000. Comparison of the sensitivities of the Buehler test and the Guinea pig maximization test for predictive testing of contact allergy. Acta Derm. Venereol. 80 (4), 256–262. https://www.ncbi.nlm.nih.gov/pubmed/11028857.

Furuya, M., Adachi, K., Kuwahara, S., Ogawa, K., Tsukamoto, Y., 2006. Inhibition of male chick phenotypes and spermatogenesis by Bisphenol-A. Life Sci. 78 (15), 1767–1776. https://www.ncbi.nlm.nih.gov/pubmed/16297413.

Gadekar, V., Borade, Y., Kannaujia, S., Rajpoot, K., Anup, N., Tambe, V., Kalia, K., Tekade, R.K., 2021. Nanomedicines accessible in the market for clinical interventions. J. Contr. Release 330, 372–397.

Garey, R.C., Narang, R., 1976. An unusual foreign body in the buccal vestibule. Report of a case. Oral Surg. Oral Med. Oral Pathol. 42 (3), 314–315. https://www.ncbi.nlm.nih.gov/pubmed/1067534.

Gargus, E.S., Rogers, H.B., McKinnon, K.E., Edmonds, M.E., Woodruff, T.K., 2020. Engineered reproductive tissues. Nat. Biomed. Eng. 4 (4), 381–393. https://www.ncbi.nlm.nih.gov/pubmed/32251392.

Garhammer, P., Schmalz, G., Hiller, K.A., Reitinger, T., Stolz, W., 2001. Patients with local adverse effects from dental alloys: frequency, complaints, symptoms, allergy. Clin. Oral Invest. 5 (4), 240–249. https://www.ncbi.nlm.nih.gov/pubmed/11800437.

Ghasemi-Mobarakeh, L., Kolahreez, D., Ramakrishna, S., Williams, D., 2019. Key terminology in biomaterials and biocompatibility. Curr. Opin. Biomed. Eng. 10, 45–50. https://doi.org/10.1016/j.cobme.2019.02.004.

Gichner, T., 1985. IARC monographs on the evaluation of the carcinogenic risk of chemicals to humans. Volume 32. Polynuclear aromatic compounds, Part 1, chemical, environmental and experimental data. Biol. Plantarum 27 (1), 33. https://doi.org/10.1007/bf02894630.

Goldberg, M., 2008. In vitro and in vivo studies on the toxicity of dental resin components: a review. Clin. Oral Invest. 12 (1), 1–8. https://www.ncbi.nlm.nih.gov/pubmed/18040729.

Gorain, B., Choudhury, H., Tekade, R.K., Karan, S., Jaisankar, P., Pal, T.K., 2016. Comparative biodistribution and safety profiling of olmesartan medoxomil oil-in-water oral nanoemulsion. Regul. Toxicol. Pharmacol. 82, 20–31.

Gottwald, B., Kupfer, J., Traenckner, I., Ganss, C., Gieler, U., 2002. Psychological, allergic, and toxicological aspects of patients with amalgam-related complaints. Psychother. Psychosom. 71 (4), 223–232. https://www.ncbi.nlm.nih.gov/pubmed/12097788.

Gunther, G., Welsh, S.I., 1978. Evaluation of a rubber-base impression material. J. Prosthet. Dent. 39 (1), 95–99. https://www.ncbi.nlm.nih.gov/pubmed/340664.

Gupta, R., Polaka, S., Rajpoot, K., Tekade, M., Sharma, M.C., Tekade, R.K., 2022a. Importance of toxicity testing in drug discovery and research. In: Pharmacokinetics and Toxicokinetic Considerations, vol. 2. Elsevier. https://doi.org/10.1016/b978-0-323-98367-9.00016-0.

Gupta, R., Rajpoot, K., Tekade, M., Sharma, M.C., Tekade, R.K., 2022b. Methods and models for in vitro toxicity. In: Pharmacokinetics and Toxicokinetic Considerations, vol. 2. Elsevier. https://doi.org/10.1016/b978-0-323-98367-9.00006-8.

Hauman, C.H., Love, R.M., 2003a. Biocompatibility of dental materials used in contemporary endodontic therapy: a review. Part 1. Intracanal drugs and substances. Int. Endod. J. 36 (2), 75–85. https://www.ncbi.nlm.nih.gov/pubmed/12657150.

Hauman, C.H., Love, R.M., 2003b. Biocompatibility of dental materials used in contemporary endodontic therapy: a review. Part 2. Root-canal-filling materials. Int. Endod. J. 36 (3), 147–160. https://www.ncbi.nlm.nih.gov/pubmed/12657140.

Hensten, A., Jacobsen, N., 2013. Systemic toxicity and hypersensitivity. Biomater. Sci. https://doi.org/10.1016/b978-0-08-087780-8.00047-4. Elsevier.

Hensten-Pettersen, A., Jacobsen, N., 1994. Possible side effects related to dental hygienists' treatment. Acta Odontol. Scand. 52 (3), 157–161. https://www.ncbi.nlm.nih.gov/pubmed/8091962.

Hilton, T.J., 2016. Sealers, liners, and bases. J. Esthetic Restor. Dent. 28 (3), 141–143. https://www.ncbi.nlm.nih.gov/pubmed/27178665.

Hosseinpour, S., Gaudin, A., Peters, O.A., 2022. A critical analysis of research methods and experimental models to study biocompatibility of endodontic materials. Int. Endod. J. 55, 346–369.

Huang, F.M., Kuan, Y.H., Lee, S.S., Chang, Y.C., 2015. Cytotoxicity and genotoxicity of triethyleneglycol-dimethacrylate in macrophages involved in DNA damage and caspases activation. Environ. Toxicol. 30 (5), 581–588. https://www.ncbi.nlm.nih.gov/pubmed/24307521.

Huang, F.M., Chang, Y.C., Lee, S.S., Yeh, C.H., Lee, K.G., Huang, Y.C., Chen, C.J., Chen, W.Y., Pan, P.H., Kuan, Y.H., 2016. BisGMA-induced cytotoxicity and genotoxicity in macrophages are attenuated by wogonin via reduction of intrinsic caspase pathway activation. Environ. Toxicol. 31 (2), 176–184. https://www.ncbi.nlm.nih.gov/pubmed/26756871.

Hunt, P.A., Lawson, C., Gieske, M., Murdoch, B., Smith, H., Marre, A., Hassold, T., VandeVoort, C.A., 2012. Bisphenol A alters early oogenesis and follicle formation in the fetal ovary of the rhesus monkey. Proc. Natl. Acad. Sci. U. S. A. 109 (43), 17525–17530. https://www.ncbi.nlm.nih.gov/pubmed/23012422.

ISO 10993-1, 2018. Biological Evaluation of Medical Devices—Part 1: Evaluation and Testing within a Risk Management Process. https://www.iso.org/standard/68936.html.

ISO 10993-5, 2009. Biological Evaluation of Medical Devices—Part 5: Tests for in Vitro Cytotoxicity. BSI British Standards. https://www.iso.org/standard/36406.html.

Janjić, K., Alhujazy, U., Moritz, A., Agis, H., 2018. L-mimosine and hypoxia enhance angiopoietin-like 4 production involving hypoxia-inducible factor-1alpha: insights from monolayer and spheroid cultures of dental pulp-derived cells and tooth slice cultures. Arch. Oral Biol. 85, 172–177.

Japundžić, I., Vodanović, M., Lugović-Mihić, L., 2018. An analysis of skin prick tests to latex and patch tests to rubber additives and other causative factors among dental professionals and students with contact Dermatoses. Int. Arch. Allergy Immunol. 177 (3), 238–244. https://www.karger.com/DOI/10.1159/000490181.

Jiang, R., Xu, Y., Wang, F., Lin, H., 2022. Effectiveness and cytotoxicity of two desensitizing agents: a dentin permeability measurement and dentin barrier testing in vitro study. BMC Oral Health 22 (1), 1–11.

Joshi, S.C., Sheikh, A.A., 2015. 3D printing in aerospace and its long-term sustainability. Virtual Phys. Prototyp. 10 (4), 175–185. https://doi.org/10.1080/17452759.2015.1111519.

Kasten, F.H., Felder, S.M., Gettleman, L., Alchediak, T., 1982. A model culture system with human gingival fibroblasts for evaluating the cytotoxicity of dental materials. In Vitro 18 (7), 650–660. https://www.ncbi.nlm.nih.gov/pubmed/7141449.

Keshavarz, M., Eslami, J., Abedi-Firouzjah, R., Mortazavi, S.A., Abbasi, S., Mortazavi, G., 2022. How Do different physical stressors' affect the mercury release from dental amalgam fillings and microleakage? A systematic review. J. Biomed. Phy. Eng. 12 (3), 227.

Kim, K.H., Loch, C., Waddell, J.N., Tompkins, G., Schwass, D., 2017. Surface characteristics and biofilm development on selected dental ceramic materials. Int. J. Dent. 2017, 7627945. https://www.ncbi.nlm.nih.gov/pubmed/28567055.

Kitagawa, M., Murakami, S., Akashi, Y., Oka, H., Shintani, T., Ogawa, I., Inoue, T., Kurihara, H., 2019. Current status of dental metal allergy in Japan. J. Prosthodont. Res. 63 (3), 309–312.

Klecak, G., 2019. Test methods for allergic contact dermatitis in animals. In: Dermatotoxicology Methods: The Laboratory Worker's Vade Mecum. CRC Press, pp. 121–144.

Kopac, I., Batista, U., Cvetko, E., Marion, L., 2002. Viability of fibroblasts in cell culture after treatment with different chemical retraction agents. J. Oral Rehabil. 29 (1), 98–104. https://www.ncbi.nlm.nih.gov/pubmed/11844038.

Kostoryz, E.L., Tong, P.Y., Chappelow, C.C., Eick, J.D., Glaros, A.G., Yourtee, D.M., 1999. In vitro cytotoxicity of solid epoxy-based dental resins and their components. Dent. Mater. 15 (5), 363–373. https://doi.org/10.1016/s0109-5641(99)00058-5.

Kraemer Fernandez, P., Unkovskiy, A., Benkendorff, V., Klink, A., Spintzyk, S., 2020. Surface characteristics of milled and 3D printed denture base materials following polishing and coating: an in-vitro study. Materials 13 (15), 3305. https://www.ncbi.nlm.nih.gov/pubmed/32722240.

Kumari, M., Rafia, A.K., Shree, R., 2021. Changing Concepts in the Diagnosis of Dental Caries: A Review. Department of Public Health Dentistry, DJ College of Dental Sciences and Research, Modinagar, India, 2642–1623.

Kunrath, M.F., Muradás, T.C., Penha, N., Campos, M.M., 2021. Innovative surfaces and alloys for dental implants: what about biointerface-safety concerns? Dent. Mater. 37 (10), 1447–1462.

Kushali, R., Maiti, S., Rv Geetha, J., 2020. Animal model used in dentistry-A review. Indian J. Forensic Med. Toxicol. 14 (4), 4534–4543.

Lang, H., Mertens, T., 1990. The use of cultures of human osteoblastlike cells as an in vitro test system for dental materials. J. Oral Maxillofac. Surg. 48 (6), 606–611. https://doi.org/10.1016/s0278-2391(10)80475-6.

Larsson, K.S., 1992. Teratological aspects of dental amalgam. Adv. Dent. Res. 6 (1), 114–119. https://www.ncbi.nlm.nih.gov/pubmed/1292450.

Lee, T.W., Tumanov, S., Villas-Boas, S.G., Montgomery, J.M., Birch, N.P., 2015. Chemicals eluting from disposable plastic syringes and syringe filters alter neurite growth, axogenesis and the microtubule cytoskeleton in cultured hippocampal neurons. J. Neurochem. 133 (1), 53–65. https://www.ncbi.nlm.nih.gov/pubmed/25522164.

Lenie, S., Cortvrindt, R., Eichenlaub-Ritter, U., Smitz, J., 2008. Continuous exposure to bisphenol A during in vitro follicular development induces meiotic abnormalities. Mutat. Res. 651 (1–2), 71–81. https://www.ncbi.nlm.nih.gov/pubmed/18093867.

Levy, D.D., Zeiger, E., Escobar, P.A., Hakura, A., Bas-Jan, M., Kato, M., Moore, M.M., Sugiyama, K-i, 2019. Recommended criteria for the evaluation of bacterial mutagenicity data (Ames test). Mutat. Res. Genet. Toxicol. Environ. Mutagen 848, 403074.

Li, Y.C., Kuan, Y.H., Huang, F.M., Chang, Y.C., 2012. The role of DNA damage and caspase activation in cytotoxicity and genotoxicity of macrophages induced by bisphenol-A-glycidyldimethacrylate. Int. Endod. J. 45 (6), 499–507. https://www.ncbi.nlm.nih.gov/pubmed/22242562.

Liu, C.M., Huang, F.M., Yang, L.C., Chou, L.S., Chou, M.Y., Chang, Y.C., 2004. Cytotoxic effects of gingival retraction cords on human gingival fibroblasts in vitro. J. Oral Rehabil. 31 (4), 368–372. https://www.ncbi.nlm.nih.gov/pubmed/15089944.

Lopes-Rocha, L., Hernandez, C., Gonçalves, V., Pinho, T., Tiritan, M.E., 2022. Analytical methods for determination of bpa released from dental resin composites and related materials: a systematic review. Crit. Rev. Anal. Chem. 1–16.

Lottner, S., Shehata, M., Hickel, R., Reichl, F.X., Durner, J., 2013. Effects of antioxidants on DNA-double strand breaks in human gingival fibroblasts exposed to methacrylate based monomers. Dent. Mater. 29 (9), 991–998. https://www.ncbi.nlm.nih.gov/pubmed/23910976.

Lung, C.Y., Matinlinna, J.P., 2012. Aspects of silane coupling agents and surface conditioning in dentistry: an overview. Dent. Mater. 28 (5), 467–477. https://www.ncbi.nlm.nih.gov/pubmed/22425571.

Mallineni, S.K., Nuvvula, S., Matinlinna, J.P., Yiu, C.K., King, N.M., 2013. Biocompatibility of various dental materials in contemporary dentistry: a narrative insight. J. Investig. Clin. Dent. 4 (1), 9–19. https://www.ncbi.nlm.nih.gov/pubmed/23255468.

Mary, S.J., Girish, K.L., Joseph, T.I., Sathyan, P., 2018. Genotoxic effects of silver amalgam and composite restorations: micronuclei-based cohort and case-control study in oral exfoliated cells. Contemp. Clin. Dent. 9 (2), 249–254. https://www.ncbi.nlm.nih.gov/pubmed/29875569.

Matinlinna, J.P., Lassila, L.V., Vallittu, P.K., 2006. Evaluation of five dental silanes on bonding a luting cement onto silica-coated titanium. J. Dent. 34 (9), 721–726. https://www.ncbi.nlm.nih.gov/pubmed/16513239.

McGregor, D.B., Baan, R.A., Partensky, C., Rice, J.M., Wilbourn, J.D., 2000. Evaluation of the carcinogenic risks to humans associated with surgical implants and other foreign bodies—a report of an IARC Monographs Programme Meeting. Eur. J. Cancer 36 (3), 307–313. https://doi.org/10.1016/s0959-8049(99)00312-3.

Messer, R., Wataha, J., 2002. Dental Materials: Biocompatibility. Encyclopedia of Materials: Science and Technology. Elsevier. https://doi.org/10.1016/b0-08-043152-6/01843-x.

Mirbagheri, M., Adibnia, V., Hughes, B.R., Waldman, S.D., Banquy, X., Hwang, D.K., 2019. Advanced cell culture platforms: a growing quest for emulating natural tissues. Mater. Horiz. 6 (1), 45–71. https://doi.org/10.1039/C8MH00803E.

Momeni-Moghaddam, M., Hashemi, C., Fathi, A., Khamesipour, F., 2022. Diagnostic accuracy, available treatment, and diagnostic methods of dental caries in practice: a meta-analysis. Beni-Suef Univ. J. Basic Appl. Sci. 11 (1), 1–11.

Montalli, V.A.M., Garcez, A.S., de Oliveira, L.V.C., Sperandio, M., Napimoga, M.H., Motta, R.H.L., 2021. A novel dental biosafety device to control the spread of potentially contaminated dispersion particles from dental ultrasonic tips. PLoS One 16 (2), e0247029.

Mühlemann, S., Lakha, T., Jung, R.E., Hämmerle, C.H.F., Benic, G.I., 2020. Prosthetic outcomes and clinical performance of CAD-CAM monolithic zirconia versus porcelain-fused-to-metal implant crowns in the molar region: 1-year results of a RCT. Clin. Oral Implants Res. 31 (9), 856–864.

Muniswamy, V.J., Raval, N., Gondaliya, P., Tambe, V., Kalia, K., Tekade, R.K., 2019. 'Dendrimer-Cationized-Albumin' encrusted polymeric nanoparticle improves BBB penetration and anticancer activity of doxorubicin. Int. J. Pharm. 555, 77–99.

Nally, F.F., Storrs, J., 1973. Hypersensitivity to a dental impression material. A case report. Br. Dent. J. 134 (6), 244–246. https://www.ncbi.nlm.nih.gov/pubmed/4269671.

Nicholson, J., 1996. The use of organic compounds of phosphorus in clinical dentistry. Biomaterials 17 (21), 2023–2030. https://doi.org/10.1016/0142-9612(96)00012-9.

Noronha Oliveira, M., Schunemann, W.V.H., Mathew, M.T., Henriques, B., Magini, R.S., Teughels, W., Souza, J.C.M., 2018. Can degradation products released from dental implants affect peri-implant tissues? J. Periodontal. Res. 53 (1), 1–11. https://www.ncbi.nlm.nih.gov/pubmed/28766712.

Padrós, R., Giner-Tarrida, L., Herrero-Climent, M., Punset, M., Gil, F.J., 2020. Corrosion resistance and ion release of dental prosthesis of CoCr obtained by CAD-CAM milling, casting and laser sintering. Metals 10 (6), 827. https://doi.org/10.3390/met10060827.

Pameijer, C.H., 2017. Biocompatibility of luting cements for dental applications. In: Biocompatibility of Dental Biomaterials. Elsevier. https://doi.org/10.1016/b978-0-08-100884-3.00006-0.

Park, E.Y., Kang, S., 2020. Current aspects and prospects of glass ionomer cements for clinical dentistry. Yeungnam Univ. J. Med. 37 (3), 169–178.

Parkin Kullmann, J.A., Pamphlett, R., 2018. A comparison of mercury exposure from seafood consumption and dental amalgam fillings in people with and without amyotrophic lateral sclerosis (ALS): an international online case-control study. Int. J. Environ. Res. Publ. Health 15 (12), 2874.

Peliz, M.I., Duarte Jr., S., Dinelli, W., 2005. Scanning electron microscope analysis of internal adaptation of materials used for pulp protection under composite resin restorations. J. Esthetic Restor. Dent. 17 (2), 118–128. https://www.ncbi.nlm.nih.gov/pubmed/16036128.

Peretz, J., Vrooman, L., Ricke, W.A., Hunt, P.A., Ehrlich, S., Hauser, R., Padmanabhan, V., Taylor, H.S., Swan, S.H., VandeVoort, C.A., Flaws, J.A., 2014. Bisphenol a and reproductive health: update of experimental and human evidence, 2007-2013. Environ. Health Perspect. 122 (8), 775–786. https://www.ncbi.nlm.nih.gov/pubmed/24896072.

Phillips, D.H., Arlt, V.M., 2009. Genotoxicity: damage to DNA and its consequences. Experientia Suppl. https://doi.org/10.1007/978-3-7643-8336-7_4. Birkhäuser Basel.

Prajapati, R.N., Tekade, R.K., Gupta, U., Gajbhiye, V., Jain, N.K., 2009. Dendimer-mediated solubilization, formulation development and in vitro-in vivo assessment of piroxicam. Mol. Pharm. 6, 940–950.

Quintas, V., Prada-Lopez, I., Donos, N., Suarez-Quintanilla, D., Tomas, I., 2015. Antiplaque effect of essential oils and 0.2% chlorhexidine on an in situ model of oral biofilm growth: a randomised clinical trial. PLoS One 10 (2), e0117177. https://www.ncbi.nlm.nih.gov/pubmed/25689859.

Rajpoot, K., Tekade, M., Sharma, M.C., Sreeharsha, N., Arafat, B., Tekade, R.K., 2020. 3D printing as an emerging tool in pharmaceutical product development. In: Tekade, R.K. (Ed.), The Future of Pharmaceutical Product Development and Research. Academic Press, pp. 27–71. http://www.sciencedirect.com/science/article/pii/B9780128144558000025.

Rajpoot, K., Desai, N., Koppisetti, H., Tekade, M., Sharma, M.C., Behera, S.K., Tekade, R.K., 2022. In Silico Methods for the Prediction of Drug Toxicity. Pharmacokinetics and Toxicokinetic Considerations, vol. 2. Elsevier. https://doi.org/10.1016/b978-0-323-98367-9.00012-3.

Ree, M.H., 2001. An unusual swelling following endodontic and prosthodontic treatment of a mandibular molar due to a foreign body reaction. Int. Endod. J. 34 (7), 562–567. https://www.ncbi.nlm.nih.gov/pubmed/11601775.

Reichl, F.X., Simon, S., Esters, M., Seiss, M., Kehe, K., Kleinsasser, N., Hickel, R., 2006. Cytotoxicity of dental composite (co)monomers and the amalgam component Hg(2+) in human gingival fibroblasts. Arch. Toxicol. 80 (8), 465–472. https://www.ncbi.nlm.nih.gov/pubmed/16474958.

Ribeiro, D.A., Marques, M.E., Salvadori, D.M., 2005. Assessment of genetic damage induced by dental bleaching agents on mouse lymphoma cells by single cell gel (comet) assay. J. Oral Rehabil. 32 (10), 766–771. https://www.ncbi.nlm.nih.gov/pubmed/16159356.

Ribeiro, D.A., Marques, M.E., Salvadori, D.M., 2006. Study of DNA damage induced by dental bleaching agents in vitro. Braz. Oral Res. 20 (1), 47–51. https://www.ncbi.nlm.nih.gov/pubmed/16729174.

Ribeiro, D.A., Yujra, V.Q., De Moura, C.F.G., Handan, B.A., Viana, M.D.B., Yamauchi, L.Y., Castelo, P.M., Aguiar Jr., O., 2017. Genotoxicity induced by dental materials: a comprehensive review. Anticancer Res. 37 (8), 4017–4024. https://www.ncbi.nlm.nih.gov/pubmed/28739683.

Roberta, T., Federico, M., Federica, B., Antonietta, C.M., Sergio, B., Ugo, C., 2003. Study of the potential cytotoxicity of dental impression materials. Toxicol. Vitro 17 (5–6), 657–662. https://www.ncbi.nlm.nih.gov/pubmed/14599459.

Rode, S.M., Sato, T.D.P., Matos, F.S., Correia, A.M.O., Camargo, S.E.A., 2021. Toxicity and effect of whitening toothpastes on enamel surface. Braz. Oral Res. 35, e025. https://www.ncbi.nlm.nih.gov/pubmed/33605355.

Rogers, H.B., Zhou, L.T., Kusuhara, A., Zaniker, E., Shafaie, S., Owen, B.C., Duncan, F.E., Woodruff, T.K., 2021. Dental resins used in 3D printing technologies release ovo-toxic leachates. Chemosphere 270, 129003. https://www.ncbi.nlm.nih.gov/pubmed/33515896.

Rustagi, N., Pradhan, S.K., Singh, R., 2011. Public health impact of plastics: an overview. Indian J. Occup. Environ. Med. 15 (3), 100–103. https://www.ncbi.nlm.nih.gov/pubmed/22412286.

Sakaguchi, R.L., Powers, J.M., 2012. Acknowledgments. Craig's Restorative Dental Materials. Elsevier. https://doi.org/10.1016/b978-0-323-08108-5.10022-2.

Schmalz, G., Arenholt-Bindslev, D., 2009. Basic aspects. In: Biocompatibility of Dental Materials. Springer Berlin Heidelberg, pp. 1–12. https://doi.org/10.1007/978-3-540-77782-3_1.

Schmalz, G., Galler, K.M., 2017. Biocompatibility of biomaterials - lessons learned and considerations for the design of novel materials. Dent. Mater. 33 (4), 382–393. https://www.ncbi.nlm.nih.gov/pubmed/28236437.

Sefton, M.V., 1986. Consensus conference on definitions chester, UK march 3–5, 1986. Biomaterials 7 (4), 308–309. https://doi.org/10.1016/0142-9612(86)90057-8.

Segal, T.R., Giudice, L.C., 2019. Before the beginning: environmental exposures and reproductive and obstetrical outcomes. Fertil. Steril. 112 (4), 613–621. https://www.ncbi.nlm.nih.gov/pubmed/31561863.

Shafiee, A., Atala, A., 2016. Printing technologies for medical applications. Trends Mol. Med. 22 (3), 254–265. https://www.ncbi.nlm.nih.gov/pubmed/26856235.

Shahi, S., Ozcan, M., Maleki Dizaj, S., Sharifi, S., Al-Haj Husain, N., Eftekhari, A., Ahmadian, E., 2019. A review on potential toxicity of dental material and screening their biocompatibility. Toxicol. Mech. Methods 29 (5), 368–377. https://www.ncbi.nlm.nih.gov/pubmed/30642212.

Shulev, A., Roussev, I., Karpuzov, S., Stoilov, G., Ignatova, D., See, C., Mitov, G., 2016. Roughness measurement of dental materials. J. Theor. Appl. Mech. 46 (2), 27–36. https://doi.org/10.1515/jtam-2016-0008.

Souza, J.C.M., Barbosa, S.L., Ariza, E., Celis, J.P., Rocha, L.A., 2012. Simultaneous degradation by corrosion and wear of titanium in artificial saliva containing fluorides. Wear 292–293, 82–88. https://doi.org/10.1016/j.wear.2012.05.030.

Souza, J.C.M., Henriques, M., Teughels, W., Ponthiaux, P., Celis, J.-P., Rocha, L.A., 2015. Wear and corrosion interactions on titanium in oral environment: literature review. J. Bio- and Tribo-Corros. 1 (13). https://doi.org/10.1007/s40735-015-0013-0.

Souza, J.C.M., Apaza-Bedoya, K., Benfatti, C.A.M., Silva, F.S., Henriques, B., 2020. A comprehensive review on the corrosion pathways of titanium dental implants and their biological adverse effects. Metals 10 (9), 1272. https://doi.org/10.3390/met10091272.

St John, K.R., 2007. Biocompatibility of dental materials. Dent. Clin. 51 (3), 747–760 viii. https://www.ncbi.nlm.nih.gov/pubmed/17586154.

Stavreva, N., Kapusevska, B., 2019. Biocompatibility and reaction of dental polymers in oral environment. Knowledge-Int. J. 31 (4), 835–839.

Sun, Z., 2021. 3D printing in medical applications. Curr. Med. Imaging. 17 (7), 811–813. https://www.ncbi.nlm.nih.gov/pubmed/34414865.

Sun, X., Cao, Z., Yeh, C.K., Sun, Y., 2013. Antifungal activity, biofilm-controlling effect, and biocompatibility of poly(N-vinyl-2-pyrrolidinone)-grafted denture materials. Colloids Surf. B Biointerfaces 110, 96–104. https://www.ncbi.nlm.nih.gov/pubmed/23708753.

Suresh, S., Arumugham, I.M., Doraikannan, S., Rathinavelu, P.K., Prabakar, J., Balasubramaniam, A., 2021. Comparing the effectiveness of herbal and conventional dentifrices in reducing dental plaque and gingivitis: a systematic review. J. Int. Soc. Prev. Community Dent. 11 (6), 601.

Swetha, B., Mathew, S., Murthy, B.V.S., Shruthi, N., Bhandi, S.H., 2015. Determination of biocompatibility: a review. Int. Dent. Med. J. Adv. Res. 1 (1), 1–6. https://doi.org/10.15713/ins.idmjar.2.

Takenaka, S., Ohsumi, T., Noiri, Y., 2019. Evidence-based strategy for dental biofilms: current evidence of mouthwashes on dental biofilm and gingivitis. Jpn. Dent. Sci. Rev. 55 (1), 33–40.

Tay, Y.W.D., Panda, B., Paul, S.C., Noor Mohamed, N.A., Tan, M.J., Leong, K.F., 2017. 3D printing trends in building and construction industry: a review. Virtual Phys. Prototyp. 12 (3), 261–276. https://doi.org/10.1080/17452759.2017.1326724.

Tekade, R.K., Chougule, M.B., 2013. Formulation development and evaluation of hybrid nanocarrier for cancer therapy: taguchi orthogonal array based design. BioMed Res. Int. 2013, 712678.

Teuten, E.L., Saquing, J.M., Knappe, D.R., Barlaz, M.A., Jonsson, S., Bjorn, A., Rowland, S.J., Thompson, R.C., Galloway, T.S., Yamashita, R., Ochi, D., Watanuki, Y., Moore, C., Viet, P.H., Tana, T.S., Prudente, M., Boonyatumanond, R., Zakaria, M.P., Akkhavong, K., Ogata, Y., Hirai, H., Iwasa, S., Mizukawa, K., Hagino, Y., Imamura, A., Saha, M., Takada, H., 2009. Transport and release of chemicals from plastics to the environment and to wildlife. Philos. Trans. R. Soc. Lond. B Biol. Sci. 364 (1526), 2027–2045. https://www.ncbi.nlm.nih.gov/pubmed/19528054.

Tian, Y., Chen, C., Xu, X., Wang, J., Hou, X., Li, K., Lu, X., Shi, H., Lee, E.S., Jiang, H.B., 2021. A review of 3D printing in dentistry: technologies, affecting factors, and applications. Scanning 2021, 9950131. https://www.ncbi.nlm.nih.gov/pubmed/34367410.

Tiwari, A., Joshi, M., Salvi, N., Gupta, D., Gandhi, S., Rajpoot, K., Tekade, R.K., 2022. Toxicity of pharmaceutical azo dyes. In: Pharmacokinetics and Toxicokinetic Considerations, vol. 2. Elsevier. https://doi.org/10.1016/b978-0-323-98367-9.00004-4.

Türkcan, İ., Nalbant, A.D., 2015. Dental protetik materyallerin biyolojik uyumluluğu ve test yöntemleri. Acta Odontol. Turc. 33 (3), 145–152. https://doi.org/10.17214/aot.05383.

Valderrama, P., Valderrama, A., Baca, P., 2020. Bibliometric analysis and evaluation of the journal medicina oral patologia oral y cirugia bucal (2008–2018). Med. Oral Patol. Oral Cir. Bucal 25 (2), e180–e187. https://www.ncbi.nlm.nih.gov/pubmed/31893475.

Vandenberg, L.N., Hunt, P.A., Gore, A.C., 2019. Endocrine disruptors and the future of toxicology testing - lessons from CLARITY-BPA. Nat. Rev. Endocrinol. 15 (6), 366–374. https://www.ncbi.nlm.nih.gov/pubmed/30842650.

Vasdev, N., Deshpande, M., Katare, P., Makwana, V., Polaka, S., Tekade, M., Sengupta, P., Sharma, M.C., Mishra, D.K., Tekade, R.K., 2022. New emerging technologies for genetic toxicity testing. In: Tekade, R.K. (Ed.), Pharmacokinetics and Toxicokinetic Considerations, vol. 2. Academic Press, pp. 175–219. https://www.sciencedirect.com/science/article/pii/B9780323983679000135.

Wallin, M., Larsson, H., Edstrom, A., 1977. Tubulin sulfhydryl groups and polymerization in vitro. Effects of di- and trivalent cations. Exp. Cell Res. 107 (1), 219–225. https://www.ncbi.nlm.nih.gov/pubmed/558896.

Wang, Z., Shen, Y., Haapasalo, M., 2014. Dental materials with antibiofilm properties. Dent. Mater. 30 (2), e1–e16. https://www.ncbi.nlm.nih.gov/pubmed/24374001.

Wang, Y., Zhu, M., Zhu, X.X., 2021. Functional fillers for dental resin composites. Acta Biomater. 122, 50–65.

Williams, D.R., 1987. Definitions. Animal Feeding Stuffs Legislation of the UK. Elsevier. https://doi.org/10.1016/b978-0-408-03070-0.50007-8.

Williams, D.F., 2020. Assessing the triad of biocompatibility, medical device functionality and biological safety. Med. Devices Sens. 4 (1), e10150. https://doi.org/10.1002/mds3.10150.

Wu, M.K., Song, N., Liu, F., Kou, L., Lu, X.W., Wang, M., Wang, H., Shen, J.F., 2016. Corrosion behaviours of the dental magnetic keeper complexes made by different alloys and methods. Int. J. Oral Sci. 8 (3), 155–163. https://www.ncbi.nlm.nih.gov/pubmed/27388806.

Xiao, S., Coppeta, J.R., Rogers, H.B., Isenberg, B.C., Zhu, J., Olalekan, S.A., McKinnon, K.E., Dokic, D., Rashedi, A.S., Haisenleder, D.J., Malpani, S.S., Arnold-Murray, C.A., Chen, K., Jiang, M., Bai, L., Nguyen, C.T., Zhang, J., Laronda, M.M., Hope, T.J., Maniar, K.P., Pavone, M.E., Avram, M.J., Sefton, E.C., Getsios, S., Burdette, J.E., Kim, J.J., Borenstein, J.T., Woodruff, T.K., 2017. A microfluidic culture model of the human reproductive tract and 28-day menstrual cycle. Nat. Commun. 8, 14584. https://www.ncbi.nlm.nih.gov/pubmed/28350383.

Yan Guo, C., Tin Hong Tang, A., Pekka Matinlinna, J., 2012. Insights into surface treatment methods of titanium dental implants. J. Adhes. Sci. Technol. 26 (1–3), 189–205. https://doi.org/10.1163/016942411x569390.

Youngren, S.R., Tekade, R.K., Gustilo, B., Hoffmann, P.R., Chougule, M.B., 2013. STAT6 siRNA matrix-loaded gelatin nanocarriers: formulation, characterization, and ex vivo proof of concept using adenocarcinoma cells. BioMed Res. Int. 2013, 858946.

Zeiger, E., 2019. The test that changed the world: the Ames test and the regulation of chemicals. Mutat. Res. Genet. Toxicol. Environ. Mutagen 841, 43–48.

CHAPTER

18

Clinical detoxification of the body from chemical toxicants

Muktika Tekade[1], *Prashant L. Pingale*[2], *Sakshi P. Wani*[2], *Kuldeep Rajpoot*[3], *Nagaraja Sreeharsha*[4,5], *Mrudul Deshpande*[3], *Rakesh Kumar Tekade*[3] and *Mukesh C. Sharma*[1]

[1]School of Pharmacy, Devi Ahilya Vishwavidyalaya, Indore, Madhya Pradesh, India; [2]Department of Pharmaceutics, GES's Sir Dr. M. S. Gosavi College of Pharmaceutical Education and Research, Nashik, Maharashtra, India; [3]National Institute of Pharmaceutical Education and Research (NIPER)- Ahmedabad, An Institute of National Importance, Government of India, Department of Pharmaceuticals, Ministry of Chemicals and Fertilizers, Palaj, Gandhinagar, Gujarat, India; [4]Department of Pharmaceutics, Vidya Siri College of Pharmacy, Bengaluru, Karnataka, India; [5]Department of Pharmaceutical Sciences, College of Clinical Pharmacy, King Faisal University, Al-Ahsa, Saudi Arabia

18.1 Introduction

When poisonous compounds are detoxified, they become more soluble and less harmful and are primarily removed through the urine and bile. It is possible to lessen but not wholly remove toxicity. This process of detoxification is known as drug metabolism or biotransformation. The body goes through a series of metabolic processes to change foreign (typically hazardous) substances into less harmful, more easily excretable forms. The physiological or therapeutic removal of hazardous substances from a living entity (including the human body) is known as detoxification or detoxication. This process is mainly carried out by the liver. It can also refer to the time the body takes to return to homeostasis after a period of drug withdrawal that follows a sustained use of an addictive substance. In medicine, toxin decontamination can be used to achieve detoxification. It can be used to describe the time taken during drug withdrawal when an organism regains an equilibrium state following a

https://doi.org/10.1016/B978-0-443-15840-7.00012-9

prolonged usage of an addictive chemical. In medicine, detoxification can be accomplished by removing toxins from the body, the administration of antidotes, as well as techniques like dialysis and chelation therapy (in a few instances) (Pizzorno, 2022; Tambe et al., 2021a). Natural detoxification mechanisms include liver, kidney, and intracellular proteins like Cytochromes P450 (CYP) enzymes usually found in the endoplasmic reticulum or the inner membrane of mitochondria. Dialysis is used to replicate the kidneys' function during renal failure. Moreover, kidney and liver transplantation are also done to treat kidney and liver failure, respectively (Aronica et al., 2022).

For many of the newest detoxification regimens, prescription medications are widely explored as a critical target. Most adverse reactions related to prescription drug fatalities are "poisoning," defined as an overdose or use of incorrect medicine. In a substantial percentage of the documented cases, prescription psychoactive drugs like antidepressants were implicated. Among the deadliest tricyclic antidepressant drugs, imipramine, dosulepin, and amitriptyline are commonly used in overdoses. Detoxification therapies are urgently required due to the toxic effects of prescription medicines such as tricyclic antidepressants and cardioactive steroids, as well as substances of abuse and exposure to environmental toxins. As a kind of detoxification therapy, particles, colloids, antibody fragments, and indirect techniques (e.g., macroemulsions) are now widely studied or used. Adhering to the toxin and lowering its concentration in essential organs, colloids, particles, and protein fragments typically reduce toxicity. The affected organs are directly influenced by indirect techniques like sodium bicarbonate and macroemulsions rather than the toxin (Antonova, 2022; Howell and Chauhan, 2010).

18.2 Hazards/problems associated with chemical toxicants

Only a few of the many substances in the atmosphere are harmful. The majority of hazardous compounds are released during chemical processes. Once they enter the human food chain, they frequently have lethal repercussions. Chemical aspects of the genesis, exposure, and disposal of dangerous compounds are all covered by the science known as chemical toxicology. Any substance whose physiological function damages health is considered a toxic substance. The phrase "toxic" is a relative one that depends on several variables, including the dose, the method of administration, the individual's vulnerability, etc. (Zalat and Abdallah, 2022; Rajpoot et al., 2022c).

The essential elements (e.g., Fe, Cu, Zn, Mo, Co, V, Mn, Na, K, Ca, Mg, and F) are vital to biological systems. They may be hazardous if present in high concentrations. However, certain substances are harmful even at low concentrations. Therefore, these toxic elements should be avoided (e.g., As, Sb, Cd, Hg, Be, Al, and Pb). The atmosphere is full of harmful pollutants (i.e., SO_2, NO_2, and many others). For instance, pesticides and insecticides are considered harmful since they have the potential to damage the land, water, and atmosphere. Like harmful chemicals, radioactive substances also show toxicity to health. Hazardous substances include a variety of organic compounds such as vinyl chloride, polychlorinated biphenyls (PCBs), chlorinated solvents, chlorofluoro chemicals, ethylene dibromide, and ethylene oxide. Some harmful substances have the potential to be teratogenic, mutagenic, and carcinogenic (Gordon, 2003; Mahdiani et al., 2022; Goel et al., 2023). Toxic substances include.

i. Heavy metals such as cadmium, beryllium, lead, arsenic, mercury, white phosphorus, and elemental halogens.
ii. The hazardous inorganic substances include cyanide (both HCN and cyanide salts), CO, nitrogen oxides (NO & NO_2, N_2O), nitrates, hydrogen halides (HF, HCl), interhalogen compounds ($BrCl_2$, ClF_3, BrF_3), and halogen oxides (OF_2, Cl_2O, ClO_2, Cl_2O_7, Br_2O) (Shao et al., 2022).
iii. Silicon inorganic substances, such as quartz, silane, and silicon oxide (McPartland et al., 2022).
iv. Examples of inorganic phosphorus compounds include phosphone, P_2O_5, and $POCl_3$. They produce pulmonary tract irritation, central nervous system depression, tiredness, vomiting, and difficult breathing (Zeng et al., 2022).
v. Inorganic sulfur compounds include H_2S, SO_2, H_2SO_4, S_2F_2, SF_4, S_6, S_2Cl_4, SO_2Cl_2, $SOCl_3$, and CS_2 (Sarkisov et al., 2022).
vi. Organometallic substances include compounds made of organ lead and organotin and carbonyls made of iron pentacarbonyl, nickel tetracarbonyl, and cobalt carbonyl.

18.2.1 Carcinogens

Carcinogens are substances that promote the development of cancer. A biochemical mistake leads to unregulated cell division, which is how cancer develops. However, the environment (such as smoking, eating habits, clothing, etc.) is primarily blamed for cancer development. Moreover, carcinogenic chemicals, radiation, and carcinogenic viruses (such as hepatitis B and the human papilloma virus) also significantly influence. It involves exposure to substances that cause cancer, such as azo dyes (Tiwari et al., 2022), nitrosamines, alkylating agents, and polycyclic aromatic hydrocarbons (PAHs) like -naphthyl amine. In the end, each of these disrupts the DNA of the genetic material. Inhaled carcinogens like PAHs are deposited on meals that have been smoked. The Iranian and Afghani tribes usually eat a lot of smoked meat, with a very high incidence of esophageal cancer. Smoking tobacco produces PAHs, which also contribute to lung cancer in heavy smokers. Chemical preservatives in fast food, food colors, optical brighteners, and crease-resistant substances in the textile sector are all being used more often nowadays, all of which are thought to have harmful effects. Some species are classified as primary or direct-acting carcinogens because they can directly mutate DNA (Raineri, 2001; Goodman et al., 2022). Pre-carcinogens and procarcinogens are those organisms that cannot directly assault DNA but whose metabolic byproducts can commence the carcinogenic action. Epoxidation activates pre-carcinogens, including benzene, PAHs, mycotoxin, etc. (mediated by cytochrome P-450).

18.2.2 Sources of toxic chemicals

Chlorine can be found in drinking water, cleaning chemicals like bleach, "white" wheat, sugar products, and the water we wash, bathe, and swim. Our body absorbs the plastic chemicals found in water bottles, drink and food containers, packaged foods, pacifiers, diapers, some dance and gymnastics clothing, other clothing, dental and sports mouth guards, can linings, lawn furniture, garden hose, vinyl toys and flooring, shower curtains, extension cords, and more. Formaldehyde is a chemical that can be found in diet items, contemporary building materials, nail polish, the majority of vaccinations, carpets, and more. To stay hydrated, check the section on drinking water. Prepared meals, sports drinks, confectionery, children's "fruit" and "juice" items, and many other things, including food dyes and colors. Our processed foods contain pesticides because of fertilizers, herbicides, insect killers, commercial produce, antibacterial hand soaps, hand sanitizers, pet flea collars, garden flowers, lawn & garden items, etc. Fragrances and scents can be found in colognes, perfumes, detergents, bathroom sprays, cleaning products, non-natural skincare products, and many more (Volk et al., 2022; Lin et al., 2022).

18.2.3 Routes of entry

(i) Skin and eye contact

Direct skin or eye contact is the easiest way for chemicals to enter the body. A chemical's contact with the skin might result in a local reaction like a burn or rash or it can enter the bloodstream and have significant adverse health effects. The chemical may then be able to have harmful effects on other biological functions after entering the bloodstream. The state of the skin's health and the characteristics of the chemical affect how well it absorbs substances via intact skin. Skin that is broken, dry, or has wounds provides less resilience. Skin can be easily penetrated by a variety of organic solvents and other fat-soluble chemicals. In some situations, these substances can alter how effectively skin can withstand the absorption of other substances. Skin exposure is indicated by dry, whitened skin, redness, swelling, rashes or blisters, and itching. Contact with hazardous chemicals can result in blindness or severe eye injury. Eye contact is less likely if safety goggles or a face shield are worn. After coming into contact with chemicals, eyes should be immediately and constantly washed with water for at least 15 min (Okoye et al., 2022).

(ii) Inhalational

The respiratory system is the most typical pathway for gases, vapors, particles, and aerosols to enter the body (smoke, mists, and fumes). These substances may be absorbed into the bloodstream or delivered into the lungs, which may have localized effects. Depending on their vapor pressure, solubility, particle size, concentration in the air they are breathed in, and chemical makeup, these substances may be absorbed differently. Higher concentrations in the air result in increased exposure to the lungs and greater absorption into the bloodstream; the vapor pressure gauges a chemical's evaporation rate, amount released into the atmosphere, and maximum allowable air concentration. Headaches increase mucus production, and irritation of the eyes, nose, and throat are all signs of overexposure. Exposure to various compounds, particularly numerous solvents, may have narcotic effects, such as bewilderment, grogginess, drowsiness, or collapse. If exposed, take some immediate precautions like tight containers, enhancing ventilation in some other way, and relocating to a new room area (Pauluhn, 2022).

(iii) Ingestion

Another potential entrance point for hazardous chemicals is the digestive system. Although unusually, a laboratory chemical will be consumed directly, exposure could happen if one consumes contaminated food or drinks, contact lips with contaminated hands, or swallow inhaled particles that have been expelled from the lungs. By abstaining from these activities and washing our hands properly after handling chemicals (even if gloves were worn), we can lessen our risk of exposure. Notably, the antiquated and hazardous practice of mouth pipetting may result in the direct ingestion of chemicals (Ramachandraiah et al., 2022).

(iv) Injection

The most extreme possible approach to chemical exposure is injection. Bypassing the defenses offered by healthy skin, an injection can enable immediate access to the circulation and, in turn, to internal organ systems. Syringe needle mishaps, handling of animals, or occurrences involving pipettes, shattered glass, or other sharp instruments contaminated with hazardous substances can all result in injection. Wash the area with soap and water if an injection happens, and seek medical attention if required (Setiyorini et al., 2022).

18.2.4 Health effects of toxic chemicals on body systems

The health consequences vary based on the hazardous substance type and amount of exposure (concentration and duration). One can ingest a potentially harmful chemical or splash it in the eyes or on the skin. Here are a few possible detrimental health effects:

i. Headache
ii. Ailments of the neurological system
iii. Poisoning
iv. Diseases of the kidney, liver, or lungs
v. Birth flaws
vi. Skin irritations like dermatitis
vii. Dizziness and vomiting

Chemical contaminates can lead to the development of asbestosis, lung cancer, chronic bronchitis, fibrosis, emphysema, and a drop in blood oxygen levels in the respiratory system. Potential pollutants include Asbestos, Radon, Cadmium, Benzene, Carbon Monoxide, and

Soot. Chlorinated hydrocarbon solvents (TCE, PCE, PCT), Cadmium, Lead, Mercury, Uranium, and Lead are a few chemical toxins that can harm the kidneys. Reduced urine production, decreased blood flow to the kidneys, a reduction in kidney function as a blood filter, blocked urine flow, kidney tissue injury, and kidney cancer are all potential health implications for the renal system. Carbon monoxide, carbon disulfide, nitrates, and methylene chloride are a few contaminants.

Furthermore, two possible health effects are heart failure and insufficient oxygen supply by the blood. Immobility, a loss of sensation, disorientation, and a decline in speech, sight, memory, muscular strength, or coordination are some potential health repercussions of the nervous system. Among the pollutants include arsenic, cadmium, carbon monoxide, and cyanide. Some examples of contaminants are nickel, mercury, arsenic, chromium, PCBs, and volatile organic compounds (VOCs). Dermatitis, itching, rash, redness or coloration, and health issues involving various organs and systems are just a few of the potential skin health consequences that pollution may have on humans through their skin (Lin et al., 2022; Bai et al., 2022; Yang et al., 2022). The process of detoxification and elimination is described in Fig. 18.1, while potential stages in the toxicity development after chemical exposure are described in Fig. 18.2.

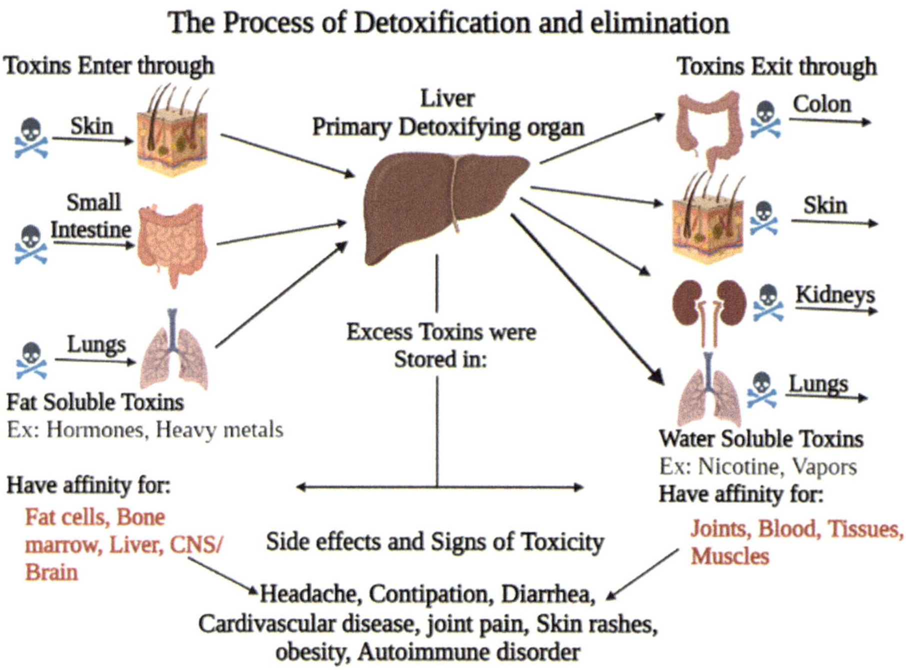

FIGURE 18.1 Process of detoxification and elimination.

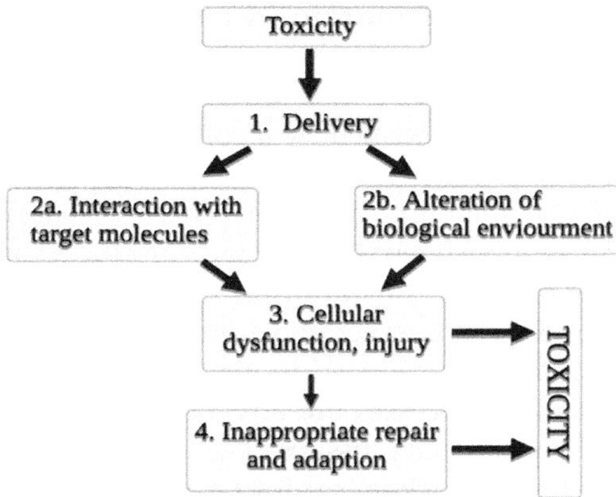

FIGURE 18.2 Potential stages in the development of toxicity after chemical exposure.

18.3 Organs involved in detoxification

Several organs play a crucial role in the detoxification of chemicals, for instance, the liver, kidney, skin, lymphatic system, etc. Organs used in detoxification and their process for detoxification are discussed in Table 18.1.

18.3.1 Lungs

Examples of contaminants include PCBs, nickel, mercury, arsenic, chromium, and VOCs. Irritation, rash, redness or coloring, dermatitis, and health impacts on other organs and

TABLE 18.1 Organs used in detoxification and their process for detoxification.

Organs	Detoxification process
Lungs	Lungs expel carbon dioxide, a consequence of respiration, and exhalation
Skin	Sweating helps the skin get rid of crystal waste
Kidney	The kidneys control aqueous fluid levels and filter excess salts and waste products from cell metabolism
Liver	The liver renders chemicals (including food additives, hazardous minerals, poisonous drugs, and excessive hormones) that we consume inactively and eliminates them
Digestive system	The detoxification mechanism of intestinal epithelial cells acts as a chemical barrier in the gut. Detoxification enzymes break down hazardous xenobiotics, while efflux transporters effectively remove the less-damaging by-products from cells into the intestinal lumen
Lymphatic system	The lymphatic system, a component of the circulatory system, aids in eliminating waste, poisons, and other undesired substances from the body

systems due to contamination through the skin are a few examples of the potential health repercussions of the skin. Cells' ability to modify xenobiotics with which they come into contact makes it easier for lipophilic substances that could otherwise build up in cellular lipids to be cleared from the body. This is accomplished by a collection of enzymes with broad specificities that may either initiate new functional groups (Phase I activities) or couple with internal cell molecules to enhance the solubility in water (Phase II reactions). Hemoproteins (also known as CYP-dependent monooxygenases or P450) produced by CYP genes are thought to play the most significant roles in the biotransformation of xenobiotics among Phase I enzymes. These enzymes (monooxygenases) employ one of the two oxygen atoms to oxidize the substrate, with the other atom being reduced to water by NADPH (Yan et al., 2022).

In general, biotransformation processes are advantageous because they aid in removing foreign substances from the pulmonary tissues (Fig. 18.3). However, sometimes, these enzymes change a normally harmless chemical into a reactive state. Metabolic bioactivation is the process whereby P450-mediated oxidations commonly produce more reactive intermediates. As a result, many substances that cause toxic lung injury are not pneumo-toxic at their core but instead harm target cells after metabolic activation. The activation of benzo(a)pyrene into reactive forms is one well-known example of a chemical abundant in combustion products and cigarette smoke that can bind to DNA and eventually cause cancer (Huang et al., 2021).

The resultant intermediates prefer to exert their toxicity locally rather than in distant tissues because they are incredibly reactive and unstable. The quantity of the reactive agent in the lung, the presence of a sufficient pulmonary detoxication route, and the bioactivation

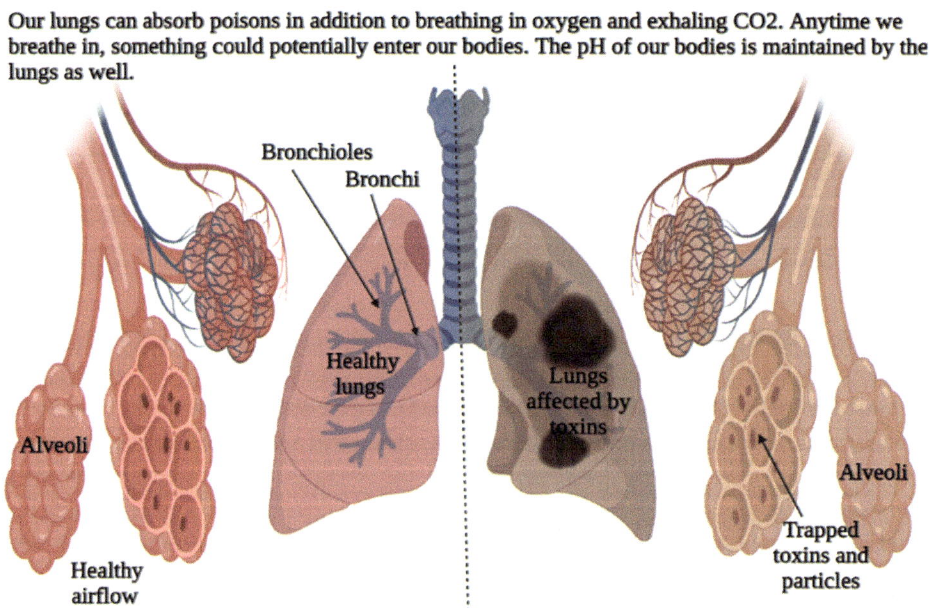

FIGURE 18.3 Entry and exit of toxins in the lungs.

of a more harmful species are three or more elements that ultimately determine the site and significance of the pulmonary damage. Further, metabolic activation followed by the reactive metabolite's improper destiny, i.e., detoxification (commonly carried out by Phase II activities), is usually found responsible for causing toxicity in the target cell. In these situations, the imbalance between activation and detoxification responses manifests as toxicity. The toxicokinetic data gathered from investigations with experimental animals is still extensively used to assess the potential toxicity of novel substances for humans (Rajpoot et al., 2022b; Asati et al., 2022). Moreover, concerns about the reliability of animal data for forecasting lung damage in humans due to bioactivation events due to the well-known species variations in biotransformation enzymes are expressed. Human-relevant in vitro models may be created to better understand the mechanisms of chemically induced lung toxicity in people and, in particular, the role of pulmonary biotransformation enzymes in the bioactivation/detoxication processes (Thimmulappa et al., 2008).

18.3.2 Skin

Skin can age prematurely from toxins like smoke and chemicals from pollution. They might make wrinkles, age spots, and worse color differences. For instance, smokers frequently learn that the chemicals in cigarettes cause the skin's elasticity to be damaged, resulting in drooping or wrinkles. Certain of the largest hazards to skin health and appearance are caused by environmental pollutants. Foods high in processed sugar and unhealthy fats trigger moderate inflammation in some people, which may lead to acne and older-looking skin. Skin is harmed by ultraviolet (UV) rays from the sun and air pollution. This ages it and raises the chance of developing skin cancer.

Interestingly, the skin serves as a natural barrier against contaminants. However, it doesn't significantly remove toxins from the body. Water is expelled by sweat, but hazardous chemicals are not (Fig. 18.4) (Ranouille et al., 2018).

The skin has two main layers, namely the epidermis and dermis. The rigid, lipid-rich stratum corneum of the upper air-exposed epidermis is crucial to the function of the barrier. It primarily comprises stratified, proliferating, and developing keratinocytes, with small amounts of mast cells and Langerhans cells, two important innate immune cells scattered throughout. The dermis beneath provides flexibility and tensile strength. Along with lymphatic and blood vessels, hair follicles and glands are also found in the dermis and indigenous and foreign immune cells. The dermis contains a large number of fibroblasts that are in charge of secreting the extracellular matrix. Ex vivo skin possesses all of these qualities, but its viability is only suitable for 48 h because it lacks a blood supply. A short-term ex vivo skin explant culturing technique was developed to study skin absorption, distribution, metabolism, and excretion for topical and, to a lesser extent, systemic chemical exposure.

(i) Phase I enzymes

A prominent family of enzymes, phase I enzymes in native human skin CYPs, particularly those from the CYP1, CYP2, CYP3, and CYP4 subfamilies, contribute approximately 75% of the total phase I hepatic metabolism by generating reactive intermediates or by triggering the drug molecule with their monooxygenase activity. It has been demonstrated that members of

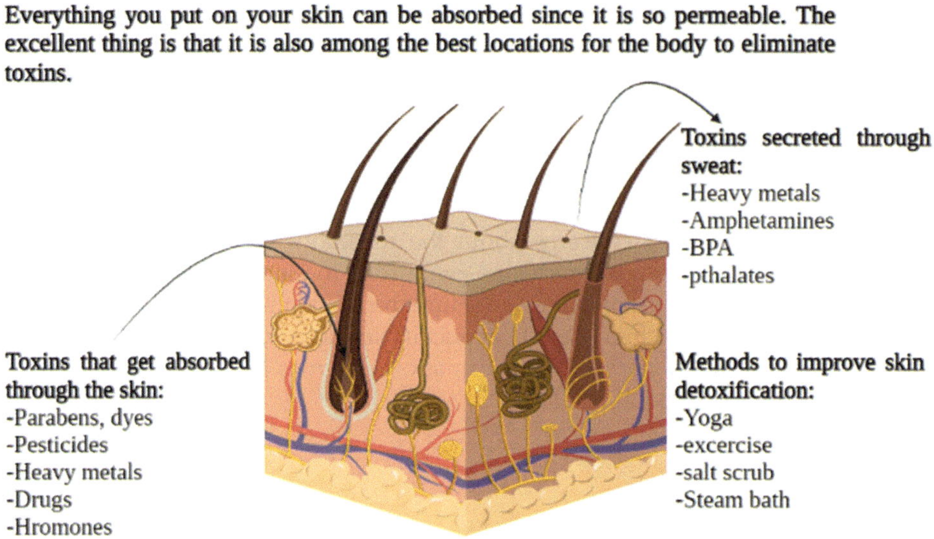

FIGURE 18.4 Entry and exit of toxins throughout the skin.

the CYP1 family manifest themselves in human skin. However, there is disagreement on the CYP1 enzymes' activity when employing several methods, including the well-known 7-ethoxy resorufin O-demethylase (EROD) assay. While some writers report CYP1 enzyme activity as being intermediate, others encountered activity below the assay's threshold limit. Even if the enzyme activity was frequently undetectable or below the detection threshold, messenger RNA (mRNA) for the CYP2 and CYP3 subfamilies has been discovered. It is possible to demonstrate CYP3 activity using the benzyl oxyquinoline (BQ) assay; however, once more, the readings were close to the detection limit. Despite their mRNA levels being demonstrated, the bulk of the other CYP subfamily enzymes, including CYP4, CYP7, CYP8, CYP11, CYP21, CYP26, CYP27, CYP39, and CYP51, have not had their activity examined. Human skin has been found to contain the CYP2S1 mRNA of another CYP enzyme, which is probably implicated in reducing a variety of cancer-causing aromatic amines and heterocyclic hydroxylamine (Chen et al., 2021).

(ii) Phase II enzymes

Phase II metabolizing enzymes frequently activate medicines, cytoprotection against various xenobiotics, and chemical detoxification processes. Some major phase II enzymes are glutathione S-transferase (GST), uridine diphosphate glucuronosyl transferase (UGT), and N-acetyltransferase (NAT). The enzymes of the GST family combine xenobiotics with tripeptide glutathione (GSH), which is present in all living things. One broad-spectrum GST substrate, 1-chloro-2,4-dinitrobenzene, has been used by several investigations to assess the activity of GSTs in diverse human skin sources.

NATs have revealed both O-acetylation-based metabolic activation and N-acetylation-based chemical detoxification. An acetyl group is attached to a substrate by NATs (like aromatic amine, hydrazine, or a sulfonamide) to generate inactive metabolites. In humans, there are several NAT genes. Numerous studies have shown NAT activity in human skin using a variety of substrates, such as procainamide, para-aminobenzoic acid (PABA), N-acetyl-p-phenylenediamine, p-toluidine, and 2,4-toluene diamine. In other trials, natural skin only contained the NAT1 and NAT5 mRNA. The liver's NAT protein level is consistent with this, despite the skin's NAT protein expression being relatively low (0.01%). The enzyme catechol O-methyltransferase catalyzes the transfer of a methyl group to catecholamines (Rysava et al., 2021).

18.3.3 Kidney

The kidneys can carry out large-scale conjugation, hydrolysis, oxidation, and reduction processes. The renal cortex has high concentrations of cytochrome P450 and GST. On the other hand, prostaglandin synthetase is exceptionally active in the renal medulla and is capable of catalyzing the co-oxidation of xenobiotics. Even though these pathways are located in many organs and have higher activities than in the kidney, several necessary mercapturic acids pathway enzymes are present at very high activity in cells of the proximal renal tubule. GSH conjugation is more than just a way to detoxify reactive electrophiles, according to studies done over the past two decades (Ge et al., 2022).

Instead, a branch point occurs when GSH S-conjugates are converted to the matching cysteine S-conjugates. The pyridoxal phosphate-dependent cysteine conjugate beta-lyase can metabolize cysteine S-conjugates by catalyzing either transamination or a beta-elimination process to create unstable thiols, or it can also use them as substrates. These thiols can covalently attach to biological macromolecules and undergo rearrangement to produce strong acylating species that are cytotoxic, mutagenic, and carcinogenic. Two other renal enzymes, cysteine conjugate S-oxidase and L-2-amino (2-hydroxy) acid oxidase, in addition to beta-lyase, can bioactivate xenobiotics to create nephrotoxic species. These mechanisms bioactivate many halogenated alkanes and alkenes. These results demonstrate the high activity of mammalian kidneys in the bioactivation of xenobiotics. Renal metabolism can be a significant factor in determining the risk of chemical harm, even if the characteristics of the relevant enzymes in humans may vary (Gueguen and Frerejacques, 2022; Xu et al., 2021).

18.3.4 Liver

The liver, the largest organ in the body, is crucial to maintaining homeostasis because it regulates metabolism, stores glycogen, detoxifies drugs, produces a variety of serum proteins, and secretes bile. Hepatic cells, especially hepatocytes, can multiply quickly to repair damage in circumstances of acute liver injury. Filtration of the blood, which removes big molecules, including bacteria, bacterial endotoxin, and antigen-antibody complexes, is one of the liver's primary roles. Bile, which means transporting many hazardous compounds into the intestines for disposal, is also produced and secreted by the liver. Phase 1 and phase 2 detoxification are the two stages of the liver's enzymatic breakdown of undesirable substances (Fig. 18.5) (Fan et al., 2021).

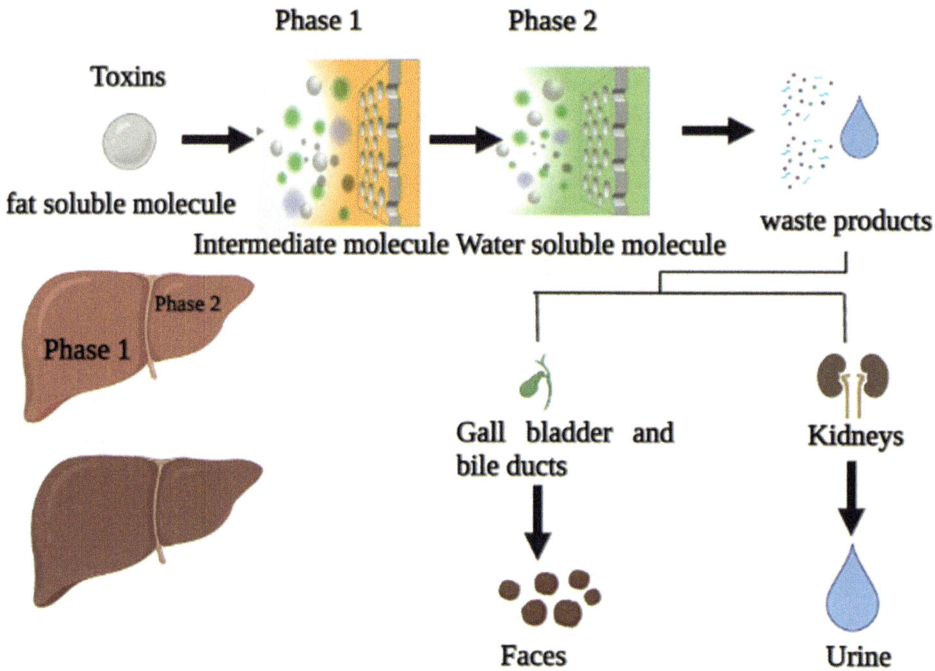

FIGURE 18.5 Liver detoxification.

(i) Phase 1 detoxification

The process of phase 1 detoxification involves the enzymes of the CYP450 family. These phase 1 enzymes either eliminate toxins directly or convert them into active intermediates that are afterward eliminated by phase 2 detoxification mechanisms. Based on a person's genetic make-up, level of exposure to toxins, use of particular medicines, and nutritional state, phase 1 enzyme activity can differ significantly from person to person. Free radical production resulting from phase 1 detoxification is a significant clinical adverse effect. Tissue damage may occur if antioxidant defenses are weak. Antioxidants are crucial, especially those concentrating on the liver (Zhao et al., 2019).

(ii) Phase 2 detoxification

Most compounds digested by phase 1 enzymes are changed into intermediate forms that require phase 2 processing. Typically, these intermediates are chemically more reactive and hazardous in nature. Hence, a quick phase 2 response is crucial and must be applied. These intermediates can significantly harm the body if the phase 2 detoxification processes are not functioning correctly. The six primary stage phase 2 detoxification processes are GSH conjugation, acetylation, amination, methylation, glucuronidation and sulfation. To conjugate oxidized metabolites, these enzyme systems must be particularly reliant upon and sensitive to a sufficient supply of substrates, generally amino acids (Fu et al., 2020).

18.3.4.1 GSH conjugation

GSH conjugation is a crucial phase 2 detoxification procedure. GSH, in addition to performing the conjugation process, is an essential antioxidant in the liver. The GSH-dependent phase 2 function is hampered if the oxidative byproducts of phase 1 deplete GSH. According to certain theories, GSH depletion significantly contributes to oxidative liver damage and the increased morbidity brought on by hepatic hypofunction. Since glutamine, glycine, and cysteine are the three amino acids that make up the tripeptide GSH, sufficient availability of these substrates is crucial. The Brassica family of foods, such as brussels sprouts, broccoli, and cabbage, stimulate this pathway. Particularly effective phase 2 inducers are broccoli sprouts. Sulforaphane, the main compound in broccoli and other brassica vegetables, and Curcuma longa increase GST activity (Jones et al., 2019).

18.3.4.2 Amino acid conjugation

Glycine, as well as, to a lesser extent, taurine, glutamine, arginine, and ornithine, is essential to accomplish phase 2 amino acid conjugation. Individuals on a low-protein diet and regularly exposed to toxins run the risk of poor amino acid conjugation because of a lack of substrates, especially glycine.

18.3.4.3 Methylation

Toxins are coupled with methyl groups through the process of methylation. S-adenosylmethionine (SAMe) serves as the methyl donor. The amino acid methionine is converted into SAMe, a process that calls for the nutrient's choline, vitamin B_6, vitamin B_{12}, and folic acid.

18.3.4.4 Sulfation

Sulfation is the process by which poisons combine with substances containing Sulfur. The amino acids that contain sulfur, especially cysteine and methionine, are essential nutrients for maintaining sulfation. This phase 2 method also requires an adequate amount of molybdenum.

18.3.4.5 Acetylation

Toxins are conjugated with acetyl-CoA through acetylation. Vitamins C, B_1, and B_5 are necessary for acetylation.

18.3.4.6 Glucuronidation

Toxins and glucuronic acid are combined during glucuronidation. This procedure requires sufficient glucuronic acid concentrations. It has been demonstrated that administering green tea improves glucuronidation. Fish oils and the limonene present in citrus fruits, including oranges, lemons, limes, and grapefruits, may also cause glucuronidation.

18.3.4.7 Phase 3 detoxification

The third step in the liver detoxification process involves the involvement of certain antiporter proteins. Toxins are pumped out of the cells during this phase for excretion. This could happen either before or after detoxification. For instance, gastrointestinal tract (GIT) enterocytes express antiporter proteins. The antiporters "pump" certain harmful substances absorbed into the enterocyte back into the lumen, blocking their passage before they can be "deactivated" by CYP450 enzymes. This flawed process allows some poisons to enter the body through the lumen. However, improving the activity of these proteins may reduce exposure to internal toxins and relieve stress on other organ systems involved in detoxification (Wei et al., 2022).

18.3.5 Digestive system

When attempting to lessen a person's buildup of toxins from both external and endogenous sources, the function of the GIT cells must be taken into account. GIT enterocytes are thought to participate in 25% of detoxification processes. To lessen the passage of nonmetabolized xenobiotics into the internal environment, these cells perform phase 1 (by the activity of CYP450 enzymes) and phase 3 (by the action of antiporter proteins) functions (Tawfik et al., 2022; Turner and Bucking, 2019). Most of the poisons we encounter every day enter the body through the foods and beverages we consume. More dangerous compounds can enter the body due to intestinal hyperpermeability, many of which might result in "toxicity" symptoms if they cross a certain threshold. Furthermore, these potentially toxic compounds can bypass the detoxification processes that ordinarily occur within the gut cells due to a leaky gut. A lack of fiber, dysbiosis, and decreased intestinal integrity may all contribute to the reabsorption of toxin metabolites that would otherwise be removed because the GIT is a significant site for their disposal (originating from the liver) (Turner and Bucking, 2019; El-Deeb and Al-Madboly, 2021).

18.3.6 Lymphatic system

One of the essential supporting systems in our body is the lymphatic system. This system assists in the circulation of our interstitial fluid by working in tandem with our immunological and cardiovascular systems. It is regarded as a crucial component of our circulatory system. Up to 700 lymph nodes can be found throughout the body, which is the main "organs" that make up the lymphatic system. To keep everything moving smoothly, there is no pumping mechanism like there is in the heart. Our muscles' action generates pressure that maintains fluid flow. The body's network of tissues and organs, known as the lymphatic system, aids in the elimination of waste materials, poisons, and other undesired substances. It is like the sewer system for the body. Like the blood circulatory system, the lymphatic system is made up of many vessels that branch all around the body (Thomas et al., 2019).

It is a division of the immunological and circulatory systems. Both of them would be unable to function without it. It plays crucial functions like the system returning bodily fluid to the blood from tissues. Plasma leaks out while being transported by blood vessels and feeds cells and tissues throughout the body. Most of this plasma subsequently drains back into the blood arteries, but a small amount is also left behind, along with pathogens, poisons, damaged cells, fat, and waste products (from the job done by the cells). This is what causes lymph to develop (Yiming et al., 2021). Lymph nodes are the sites where lymphocytes are present and filtered and from where lymph circulates across the body. Thus, these white blood cells defend the body against infection. Filtering the fluid, the lymph nodes notify the rest of the immune system about pathogens that they identify. Because of this, the lymphatic system is essential to immunity. In addition, lacteals (specialized lymphatic capillaries of the small intestine) absorb and transport digested lipids. However, in veins, lymphatic flow is observed to be minimal. The immunological and circulatory systems are significantly supported by the lymphatic system (Murota, 2020; Windsor et al., 2022). The best way to help detoxification is to prevent exposure altogether, so think about how much we are exposed to:

i. Pesticides
ii. Heavy smoke
iii. Phthalates
iv. Phthalates
v. Phthalates
vi. Steroids, antibiotics, and analgesics
vii. Heavy metals
viii. Cleaning supplies
ix. Air fresheners
x. Consuming warm items

To promote the detoxification pathways, certain nutrients are essential. These include:

i. Vitamins A, B_2, B_3, B_9, C, and E
ii. Selenium, iron, copper, magnesium, minerals, calcium, and zinc
iii. Artichoke to increase bile flow
iv. Flavonoids
v. Curcumin
vi. Dandelion
vii. Chamomile
viii. Tannins
ix. Milk thistle
x. Antioxidants
xi. Probiotics

18.4 Toxicity testing methods

The acute toxicity of chemical agents can be evaluated by the plethora of developed in vitro cytotoxicity assays. More recently, microorganisms as test organisms have been used for this purpose due to their similar biochemical pathways to higher organisms. Pharmaceutical sciences use a wide variety of in vitro models and in silico methods during studies and analysis (Anadon et al., 2014; Rajpoot et al., 2022a; Tekade et al., 2022). The in vitro toxicity methods can be classified based on specific toxicity and also general toxicity. In vitro assays using bacterial, yeast, protozoan, mammalian, or human cell cultures are widely used to detect various types of toxicity, including dermal toxicity, phototoxicity, ocular toxicity, carcinogenicity, and systemic toxicity (Huggins, 2003; Murthy, 2007). Some of the nonspecific in vitro methods are discussed below.

18.4.1 Perfused cultures

Two-dimensional (2D) cultures are largely based on the static culture environment, where tissue cultures are very often perfused with culture media via pumps. When these cultures are exposed to toxicants, real-time monitoring of cytotoxicity is feasible via the determination of markers in the perfusion flow condition. This method yields essential information regarding the onset-time, duration, and toxicity magnitude, which is problematic to determine in a static culture or under in vivo settings unless and until specific biomarkers indicative of the tissue damage are used (e.g., blood or urine) (Knight, 2008). Because of its increased complexity, perfused cultures cannot find their use in low throughput analysis (Jennings et al., 2004). However, widely used 2D cell cultures cannot provide information on tissue-specific architecture, mechanical and biochemical cues, cell-cell interaction, etc. To overcome these limitations, three-dimensional (3D), perfused cultures are known to bridge the gap between conventional 2D cultures and animal models. By creating several human tissue models in combination with human stem cell technology, we can improve drug efficacy and perform toxicity testing chemical toxicity and can ensure the safety of consumer products and ingredients (Li and Cui, 2014). Table 18.2 lists various types of culture with their advantages and disadvantages.

18.4.2 Test batteries

It has been recognized for a very long time that the ability to identify and characterize the hazardous properties of the numerous chemical toxicants generated as a result of chemical production by the less advanced toxicity testing methods is limited by the laboratory, animal, financial, and expert resources. These constraints are magnified manifold while examining the testing resources during the development of a pharmaceutical or a pesticide product (Bus and Becker, 2009). Due to the massive amount of chemicals generated and the challenge of testing them, the chemical industry has generally applied a tier-based testing system to evaluate toxicants and their by-products (Becker et al., 2007). Even though the test protocols are pretty much similar for testing drugs and pesticides, implementation of the tests is ordered by using triggers to guide decisions on which the test in the full battery of tests is needed (Bus and Becker, 2009). Elsewhere a group detected the rodent carcinogenic ability of around 700 chemicals through a battery of three most common in vitro genotoxicity assays such as Ames *Salmonella typhimurium*, mouse lymphoma assay, and the in vitro micronucleus assay. Although the sensitivity of this technique is high, the specificity is variable. The low specificity is attributed to the decline in the specificity of mammalian cell assay when combined with a battery of tests (Knight, 2008).

18.4.3 Determination of metabolite activity and organ-organ interaction

An important limitation of in vitro cultures is their inability to mimic organ-organ interactions, which is possible in the case of in vivo studies. The substantial formation of hazardous substances by the liver (which may have consequences in distal organs) may result in multiple organ interactions; hence their neutralization is urgently needed as a top priority (Li, 2008). Even though the generation of these reactive metabolites forms a significant portion

TABLE 18.2 Types of culture with their advantages and disadvantages.

Type of culture	Organs from which cells are isolated	Advantages	Disadvantages	References
Organ cultures	Large parts of ganglia, spinal cord, sensory organ (e.g., eye)	1) The concentration of the target calls can be compared with that of the in vivo conditions if the concentration of perfusate is the same as that of the blood stream. 2) Electrophysiological effects can be measured without knowing the target cell type	1) For any individual organ, recordings can be made for only a limited time. 2) Reversibility of the induced effects cannot be beyond this period cannot be determined.	Harry et al. (1998)
Explant/ slice cultures	These are derived from undifferentiated embryonic brain, spinal cord, or sensory organs and thus develop into neuronal and glial cells	It consists of a 3D organization of cells in which the structural and functional characteristics of the organ are retained.	These cultures have difficulty quantifying small changes in differentiation or viability, which depends on the measured parameters.	Harry et al. (1998)
Primary cultures	Brain tissue, neuronal populations of the brain, spinal cord, ganglion, glial cells from rat or mouse cortex, Schwann cells		Uncertainty whether these cultures will reflect the in vivo conditions or not	Harry et al. (1998)
Continuous cell lines	Derived from neuroblastomas, gliomas, or pheochromocytomas	1) Homogenous, and a large number of cells can be quickly grown. 2) The capacity to undergo an unlimited number of cell divisions, altered cell and colony morphology, lack of locomotion, lack of contact inhibition, lack of density-dependent inhibition of cell multiplication, loss of anchorage dependence, and high fibrinolytic activity 3) The phenotype of the cell line, once established, does not change.	1) It's challenging to inhibit cell division experimentally to obtain a stable population of differentiated cell lines. 2) They lack the type of growth conditions seen in vivo	Harry et al. (1998)
Additional culture systems	Cocultures of various cell-types produced in the defined ratio (e.g., The NSC-34 spinal cord neuron x neuroblastoma hybrid cell line has been used to evaluate chemicals that have an in vivo site of action at the motor neuron)	Can be employed to investigate the process of myelin formation in neural cells, fiber outgrowth, synaptogenesis, and other metabolic interactions.	1) As there is an inability to differentiate, the population of cells that can diminish will gradually decrease with subsequent subcultures. 2) Neuronal characteristics tend to get lost from the hybrid cells formed from fusion techniques.	Durham et al. (1993)

of all the toxins, the extent of toxicity imparted due to the metabolic activation is still unknown (Langsch and Nau, 2005).

Therefore, in vitro models like integrated discrete multiple organ co-culture developed by the researcher Li and colleagues in 2008 are particularly notable. These models mainly find their application in determining xenobiotic toxicity and consist of a wells-in-a-well structure. The model houses a system wherein the cells from different organs are co-cultured in distinct inner walls but are interlinked by an overlaying media built into the outer wall. This structure simulates the in vivo milieu, where the organs are physically separated and interconnected by systemic circulation. This model has several applications in the field of toxicology and xenobiotics. Some of the applications include the assessment of multiple organ metabolism, along with the specific drug distribution and toxicity. In addition, the use of human metabolizing cells (i.e., hepatocytes) and the human target organ cultures help to gain the greatest possible human relevance (Knight, 2008).

18.4.4 In vitro models for specific toxicity

(i) Hepatotoxicity

In vitro liver toxicity models commonly use cell lines as they exhibit similar phenotypic and genotypic characteristics of the hepatocytes, along with the presence of the enzymes responsible for the metabolism of toxicants. The best choice for evaluating the toxicological implications and pharmaceutical testing of toxicants is using liver cell lines. Some immortalized cell lines used for in vitro liver toxicity models are HepG2, Hep3B, HBG, and HepaRG (Jain et al., 2018; Guguen-Guillouzo and Guillouzo, 2010). The most commonly used human liver cell lines are HepG2 derived from human hepatocarcinoma (LeCluyse et al., 2012). These have the disadvantage of reduced expression of phase 1 and phase 2 biotransformation enzymes compared to the primary human hepatocytes (LeCluyse et al., 2012; Gerets et al., 2012). More specifically, there is a significant decrease of CYP enzymes up to 50-fold. An alternative to this is the HepaRG cells derived from the same source (Orbach et al., 2017).

The most recent addition to this list of cell lines used for evaluating toxicity is that of induced pluripotent stem cells (LeCluyse et al., 2012). These can be differentiated into hepatocytes by growing them into a medium consisting of supplements like activin a, fibroblast growth factor, insulin, dexamethasone, etc (LeCluyse et al., 2012; Soldatow et al., 2013). Once differentiated into hepatocytes, these IPSCs can be further used in 2D and 3D models (Orbach et al., 2017).

(ii) 2D models for liver toxicity

2D models for liver hepatotoxicity studies involve culturing monolayer hepatocytes in a protein-based substrate. The main advantage of these subcultures is that the liver cells quickly lose their specific function and expression of biotransformation enzymes. Hence these models prove ineffective compared to the native organ, thus resulting in inaccuracy in determining the toxicity. In addition to the hepatocyte monolayer model, the collagen sandwich model, wherein the hepatocyte monolayer is sandwiched between two collagen layers, has shown far greater sensitivity to xenobiotics due to the continued expression of the CYP enzymes (Jemnitz et al., 2008). The disadvantage associated with this model is its inability to show heterotypic cell-cell interactions occurring in the liver (Chatterjee et al., 2014). This disadvantage can be overcome by subculturing these hepatocytes with other cells like endothelial cells, fibroblasts, etc. The expression of hepatic enzymes drastically increases during co-culturing and is, therefore, very useful for toxicity studies (Nelson et al., 2015; Ware et al., 2015).

(iii) 3D models for liver toxicity

The 3D models for liver toxicity demonstrate better properties for toxicity assessment. These maintain the hepatocyte phenotype throughout in addition to expressing the enzymes for biotransformation (LeCluyse et al., 2012; Godoy et al., 2013). These models closely resemble the in vivo characteristics like heterotypic intercellular interactions, stratified structure, hepatocytic tight junctions, polarity induction, kinetic flow, presence of extracellular matrix compounds, etc. The combined benefit of all properties helps prevent dedifferentiation and enhance the sensitivity toward chemicals over an extended period (LeCluyse et al., 2012; Godoy et al., 2013).

One such 3D model is precision-cut liver slices. These are 100−250-micrometer-thick sections of the liver, which can be cultured under in vitro circumstances for 72 hours. This time constrain owing to the limitations in oxygen supply and nutrient diffusion. Moreover, the gene expression varies significantly post-24 h in culture. Diffusion is an important parameter to consider as toxicity and forms a determining factor as chemicals cannot reach all cell populations (Godoy et al., 2013). Spheroids are small cell aggregates prepared by various techniques like the hanging-drop method, cell-seeding on non-adhesive surfaces, and by rotating cell culture approach. These are the most widely used liver 3D-models for liver toxicity and can usually express the biotransformation enzymes over long periods (Godoy et al., 2013; LeCluyse et al., 2012). These are highly advantageous because of their increasing sensitivity to chemicals over time which can be attributed to the growing interactions between cells over time (Bell et al., 2016). The surface used to assemble the model also affects the sensitivity of spheroids to toxicants. A typical example cited is that of the difference between spheroids seeded on Matrigel, which is more responsive to nanoparticle toxicity as compared to those which are seeded on collagen (Sirenko et al., 2016).

18.4.5 Inhalational toxicity

Cell lines are identified as an effective in vitro model for the evaluation of lung toxicity (Jain et al., 2018). Cells that detect pulmonary toxicity have the unique property to model the human epithelial airway and form a valuable approach for investigating the harmful properties of chemical intoxicants. In addition to this, these models use the air-liquid interface and can be used to determine the pathways and mechanisms by which toxicity occurs. To simulate the in vivo conditions, a device that provides adequate exposure to the cultured lung cells is essential. Such an in vitro model is the CULTEX RFS which is suitable for exposing the cells to gases, atomized suspensions, and other volatile compounds, along with micro- and nanosized particles (Aufderheide et al., 2013).

Moreover, the cell culture models using cell lines like calu-3 make it easier to understand the underlying mechanisms after the inhaled toxicants enter the lungs and interact with them due to their simplicity and reproducibility. Despite the existence of these models, enough mechanistic information concerning the transport of these inhalants and their harmful effects (Rim, 2019). In another experiment, bronchial epithelial cells isolated from the lung of a patient with cystic fibrosis were cultured and used in three different approaches. Using chambers to determine amiloride-responsive short circuit currents, continuous perfusion using chambers, and near thin film conditions wherein the airway surface of the inserts is exposed to a small volume (~30 μL) of isosmotic (Rim, 2019; Rasgado-Flores et al., 2013).

These models have found application in phosgene (carbonyl chloride) as a potential inhalational toxicant or the extent of lung toxicity. They are also suitable for the assessment of anti-edemagenic compounds, like corticosteroids or phosphodiesterase inhibitors, for evaluating phosgene therapeutics (Olivera et al., 2017), and this was confirmed by investigating these models for markers of lung cell metabolism and injury in human airway epithelial cells post phosgene inhalation. Though effective, the question of ethics and cost-effectiveness remains a conundrum and has aroused a need for an appropriate model which resembles the in vivo environment (Rim, 2019). The above-mentioned lacuna was overcome by investigating the usefulness of 3D in vitro cultures. They are increasingly used for the determination of nanotoxicology due to their ability to rapidly produce and incorporate engineered nanomaterials into their consumer products. The research which suggests that these nanomaterials can cause genotoxicity, further making them desirable for nano safety screening (Shete et al., 2022; Kalyane et al., 2021; Gadekar et al., 2021). Thus, it was proposed that 3D in vitro models could connect the disconnect between in vitro and in vivo results in nanotoxicology (Rim, 2019).

18.4.6 Neurotoxicity

Detecting neurotoxicity caused by certain chemicals remains a significant challenge due to the complexity associated with the morphological and physiological aspects of the nervous system. Regulatory authorities like the Organisation for Economic Co-operation and Development (OECD) and the US environmental agency use only the in vivo models for adult and developmental neurotoxicity. Despite this fact, in vitro tests are also commonly used to study the potential mechanisms of toxicity rather than its detection and its impact on human health, unlike the in vivo methods, which are generally used in the evaluation of the developing as well as the full-grown nervous system (Bal-Price et al., 2010).

In vitro assays for testing neuronal toxicity are still in the preliminary stages and would need to be formally validated for their neuronal and glial specificity, robustness, and ability to undergo high throughput screening. This calls for a combination of in vitro tests as a standalone or as a part of an integrated test strategy which would, in turn, hasten up the process of testing and delivery of the chemical-induced toxicity (Bal-Price et al., 2010). Until now, the in vitro neurotoxicity assessment has been done based on the test results given by generalized assays like cytotoxicity assays. Hence, these fail to provide endpoints specific to the mechanisms leading to glial and neuronal toxicity. Therefore, these cell viability assays succeeded with critical but general cell function tests like electrical activity, neurotransmission, axonal transport, receptor and channel activation, enzyme activity, synaptogenesis/myelination, excitotoxicity, and neuronal-glial interactions (Clemedson et al., 2007; Bal-Price et al., 2010).

In vitro systems can study the number of biological processes that form the target sites for the intoxicants. These critical processes include a change in size, shape, neurite outgrowth measured by length, expression of microtubule-associated proteins or neurofilament proteins, or alterations in myelin formation, which forms the endpoint for toxicity evaluation. In addition, other more crucial alterations also form functional endpoints like axonal transport, neuronal activity, signal transduction mechanisms, or synaptic transmission. Some in vitro assays can be performed on various levels of complexity, embryonic and somatic stem cell lines, human neural progenitor cells, tumor-derived neural cell lines, etc. A suitable in vitro model for developmental neurotoxicity should target a specific mechanism of toxicity, which studies the relevant biological processes and still simulates the in vivo condition to quite some extent (Gupta et al., 2022c; Rajpoot et al., 2021).

One of the promising models is the human umbilical cord blood-neural stem cell lines which possess various properties like stable growth rate, self-renewability, ability to differentiate into neuronal, astroglial, and oligodendroglia cells (Buzanska et al., 2006). These cell lines can prove to be an important developmental tool for the detection of a whole range of neural growth mechanisms, like cell proliferation, migration, and apoptosis, as well as for late maturation stages like cell type differentiation, synaptogenesis, and neural connectivity (Bużańska et al., 2005). A specific in vitro system with a certain level of complexity is needed to be devised in case the target site of the chemical or the drug and its pharmacological action is known. Such an in vitro method may help investigate the mechanism behind the neurotoxicity induced along with the efficacy and potency of the drug. On the other hand, if the mechanism by which the chemical induces toxicity is unknown, there arises a need to develop a more intricate testing strategy for the detection of neurotoxicity.

18.4.7 Immunotoxicity

Exposure to immunotoxic chemicals in humans occurs through occupational hazards or contaminated food. Various chemicals like polychlorinated bisphenols, chlorinated di benzo-p-doxins, pesticides, heavy metals, therapeutic drugs, and other xenobiotics can produce immunotoxic reactions. These agents suppress the immune system, thus increasing the susceptibility of various bacterial, fungal, and other infectious diseases. In addition, immune system toxicity further leads to immunosuppression, autoimmune diseases, hypersensitivity reactions, etc. Investigating immunotoxicity involves using both in vivo and in vitro toxicity testing methods (Polaka et al., 2022b). However, the in vitro methods have several advantages over the in vivo methods. It begins with a detailed understanding of the mechanistic aspects of the in vitro studies and its species extrapolation to in vivo conditions.

Moreover, in vitro methods help to apply the principle of reduction, refinement, and replacement of animal experiments. In vitro testing can be done through a two-tiered approach. Initially, the first approach is carried out, i.e., the measurement of myelotoxicity. If this test gives a positive result, the compound qualifies as immunotoxic. If this is not the case, it's further tested for lymph toxicity, forming the second tier of the in vitro tests (Lankveld et al., 2010; Gennari et al., 2005).

Although many different types of in vitro assays are available for evaluating immune toxicity, all these assays focus primarily on chemical sensitization for the detection of direct immunotoxicity caused by toxic agents. While in the case of immunostimulation, developmental toxicity, and autoimmunity, in vitro assays haven't yet been explored (Lankveld et al., 2010).

18.4.8 Myelotoxicity

The primary cell types found in the immune system consist of lymphocytes, accessory cells (neutrophils, eosinophils, epithelial cells, macrophages, dendritic cells, natural killer cells, basophils, keratinocytes, etc.) which play a crucial role in providing the body with immunity. All the cells mentioned above ascend from pluripotent stem cells in the bone marrow; hence, the screening for induced toxicity starts from the hemopoietic stem cells. The compounds capable of bringing about immune toxicity will affect these progenitor cells by destroying or damaging the bone marrow, ceasing the formation of immune cells, and in turn, suppressing the immune response. If the compound tests positive for myelotoxicity, it will be designated as immunotoxic, and no further confirmation through other end points is needed (Lankveld et al., 2010).

Myelotoxic assays are performed using methodically authenticated in vitro colony forming granulocyte/macrophage assay (human and mouse origin) to investigate the possible myelotoxicity of therapeutics (Pessina et al., 2001). Apart from granulocytes and macrophages, other hemopoietic cell types like thrombocytes and erythrocytes can also be used to study the malignant effects of xenobiotics through burst forming assay-erythroid and colony forming units -megakaryocyte assay. Although the cost for in vitro assays with the use of human bone marrow systems isn't very effective, the decline has been predicted due to the upcoming use of umbilical cord blood cells, which are well-suited as a dependable source of human myeloid progenitor cells.

18.4.9 Lymphotoxicity

If myelotoxicity-tested compounds give negative results, then they are further tested for lymph toxicity as a confirmatory test, and thus they contribute to the immunosuppression. Testing for lymph toxicity involves several in vitro assays. Before the commencement of these assays, it's essential to check the viability of the lymphocytes to check their functionality. This can be carried out by cytotoxicity assays like 3-(4,5-dimethylthiazol-2-yl)-2,5-diphenyl tetrazolium (MTT), lactate dehydrogenase, or trypan blue assay, which are the most commonly used among others.

(i) Human whole blood cytokine release assay

Cytokines are the first responders to the immune response; therefore, quantitative alterations in the cytokine levels can be used to measure the degree of immunomodulation. This assay is the only assay that is prevalidated for the in vitro immunotoxicology study. This assay is based on a principle similar to the human whole blood test for pyrogen testing. The principle follows that when the whole human blood undergoes treatment with lipopolysaccharide or staphylococcal enterotoxin B, the monocytes and Th2 lymphocytes produce interleukin (IL)-1β and IL-4 production, respectively. This step follows the incubation for

40 h in the presence/absence of immunotoxic/non-immunotoxic compounds. These are quantified in the supernatant half-maximal inhibitory concentration (IC_{50}) for determining the immunotoxic potency (Langezaal et al., 2002).

This assay provides significant advantages in avoiding species differences between humans and animals and applying simple and easy culture techniques. In addition, preparation and culture artifacts can be avoided because of the usage of the primary cells from humans in their innate biological composition. Another advantage of this assay is that both the in vivo and in vitro functions can be monitored using the same model. Other minor obstacles associated with blood accessibility, risk of contaminations, anomalous responses, and donor pooling can be overcome by the recent development of cryopreserved human whole blood. This assay depends upon the IL-4 lymphokine readout, as monocytes do not produce it. It reflects the activation of B cells by Th2 cells, hence allowing the evaluation of the interaction between these two major lymphocyte populations. The differences in cytokine production between donors were attributed to the factors like polymorphisms, number of whole blood cells, cytokine count, and donor age. Nevertheless, these factors didn't affect the IC_{50} values; hence there was no impact on the testing, concluding that the assay is robust.

(ii) Lymphocyte proliferation assay

The primary immune response occurs due to lymphocyte proliferation; hence, the inadequate proliferation of lymphocytes is a suitable indicator of immunosuppression. Proliferation usually takes place in response to mitogens or antigens. T-cell receptor activation, proliferation, cytokine production, and the survival of T-cells occur by anti-CD28. The proliferation levels of B-cell are amplified by mitogen LPS, S. Typhimurium mitogen or the combination of IL-4 and anti-CD40. Literature also reports the use of pokeweed mitogen for enhancing lymphocyte proliferation in some experiments. However, it is rarely used as it lacks specificity, as both B and T cells are stimulated. Cell proliferation assay is commonly used when the incorporation of radiolabeled thymidine has to be done in cellular DNA. Human assays are done on lymphocytes, which are isolated from peripheral blood. These are advantageous compared to rodent assays, as species differences between humans and animals can be circumvented.

On the contrary, human lymphocytes lack uniformity, resulting in reduced reproducibility. Apart from this, the most significant limitation of this assay is the requirement of a radioisotope. To overcome this, several nonradioactive alternatives like flow cytometric assays measuring BrdU incorporation, or adenosine triphosphate (ATP) content, or colorimetric assays like MTT, trypan blue, or Alamar blue have been developed, which have proven to be easy to perform, rapid, sensitive, and applicable to high-throughput screening (HTS) (Lankveld et al., 2010).

(iii) Mixed lymphocyte reaction assay (MLR)

This assay is constructed on the principle of the proliferation of T lymphocytes in response to the allogenic cells. It involves the co-culturing of lymphocyte suspensions from the spleen or lymph nodes along with allogeneic stimulator cells for 4 days. This is followed by the addition of radiolabeled thymidine and measurement of radioactivity within 24 h. The net mixed lymphocyte reaction is calculated as the difference in cell proliferation among lymphocytes co-cultured with the allogeneic cells and syngeneic cells. When this assay is performed on the murine species, splenocytes are the source of both the stimulator as well as responder cells. In the case of rats, MLR lymphocytes from the lymph node are used as responder and stimulator cells. This is because rat splenocytes result in poor lymphocyte proliferation. This assay, widely used across many laboratories for detecting toxic immune effects, hasn't been standardized. Apart from this, it doesn't agree with host resistance assays (Lankveld et al., 2010).

18.5 Excretion of toxicants

Eliminating toxic materials from the body is essential for species' survival (Leblanc, 2004; Gupta et al., 2022a). It's also imperative to determine the potential toxicity of the toxicant. Rapid elimination of the toxic material ensures lesser concentration in the cells and prevents damage to the surrounding critical cells. The terms elimination and excretion can be used interchangeably and refers to the process whereby a particular substance leaves the body. Elimination, though in its broader sense, means the removal of the absorbed xenobiotic utilizing metabolism as well as excretion.

On the other hand, excretion is described as the elimination or removal of the xenobiotic or its metabolites through a specific organ of excretion (Humannutritionblog, 2016; Tambe et al., 2021b; Achanta et al., 2021). Excretion, which is brought about by the principal organs, is termed renal excretion, while that carried out by the other accessory organs is called extra-renal or non-renal excretion (Gupta, 2016). There are several routes by which harmful toxicants can be eliminated from the body. The main organs of excretion include the kidneys, biliary, and lungs.

18.5.1 Urinary excretion

The kidneys are the primary organ for the excretion of foreign compounds and their metabolites from the body (Gupta, 2016). There are two crucial factors that decide whether a particular xenobiotic will get excreted from the kidney or not, and these are the size and water solubility of xenobiotics (Leblanc, 2004; Gupta et al., 2022b).

i. **Size**: Chemicals removed from the reverse filtration process must pass through pores of size 70–100 Å to be removed from the blood. As a rule, chemicals that are less than 65,000 Da can easily undergo reverse filtration (Leblanc, 2004).
ii. **Water solubility**: Substances that are not sufficiently water-soluble will be excreted with the help of transport proteins. These proteins do not allow the water-insoluble toxic chemicals to pass through the pores during reverse filtration. Hence, they must undergo certain metabolic reactions like hydroxylation or oxidation in the liver or elsewhere (Leblanc, 2004).

The mechanisms of renal excretion follow three steps, namely, (a) glomerular filtration, (b) tubular reabsorption, and (c) tubular secretion.

18.5.1.1 *Glomerular filtration*

The blood plasma undergoes passive filtration in the glomerulus due to the blood pressure generated by the heart. This forms the first step of urine formation. Only those molecules which can pass through the glomerular pores (70–100 Å) are seen in the ultrafiltrate. Other molecules bound to any larger molecules won't be able to appear in the ultrafiltrate (Hodgson, 2012). Once the substance has entered the glomeruli, it either remains in the tubular lumen. It gets excreted, or it may undergo passive absorption across tubular cells of the nephron back into the blood circulation. Molecules that are reabsorbed do not appear in the urine at all (Gupta, 2016).

18.5.1.2 *Tubular reabsorption*

This is the second critical stage in the urinary excretion process. This includes the reabsorption of the solutes essential for the usual functioning of the body, like amino acids, glucose, salts, etc., which occurs in the proximal convoluted tubule. Active reabsorption occurs in the case of amino acids, peptides, and glucose, although molecules like water, chlorides, and other ions are absorbed passively (Hodgson, 2012). An important factor that significantly affects reabsorption is the pH of the urine. This prevalently applies to weak electrolytes. In the case of alkaline urine, weak acids are ionized to a greater extent and thus are primarily excreted. While if the urine is acidic, weak acids like glucuronides and sulfate conjugates are less ionized and thus undergo reabsorption (Humannutritionblog, 2016). The reabsorption of toxicants is typically passive and is controlled by the same theories that control their movement across any biomembrane. Hence, lipophilic toxicants will be passively reabsorbed to a more significant extent than the polar ones, thus enhancing the elimination of polar metabolites (Hodgson, 2012).

18.5.1.3 *Tubular secretion*

Tubular secretion is the third and final step of the excretion of solutes by the kidney. Essentially, there are two secretory processes, i.e., one for organic anions and the other for organic cations (Gupta, 2016). The passive secretion takes place to vide the process known as diffusion trapping. The passage of Weak bases and acids that are ionized across the lumen of the tubule depends on the pH of the urine. It may get ionized and thus cannot pass across the lumen wall. The process of diffusion trapping is sensitive to variations in the pH of urine, which plays a vital role in determining the speed of eliminating toxicants. Tubular secretion of organic anions is vital in eliminating pesticides.

18.5.2 Biliary excretion

The liver cleanses the blood of many unwanted substances like endogenous and foreign molecules. It biotransforms them into molecules which are easily eliminated by decreasing their bioreactivity. This mode of excretion is termed biliary excretion. This process occurs through the coordination of three major processes: chemical uptake from the blood, chemical biotransformation, and biliary elimination of chemicals (Leblanc, 2004). As the liver forms a major organ for the metabolism of compounds, the compounds and their metabolites get eliminated directly through the renal system without re-entering the bloodstream. Once a chemical gets cleared off the body by the liver cells through the bile, it finds its way to the intestine. If the drug or chemical possesses properties favorable for intestinal reabsorption, the substance cycles into enterohepatic cycling where the processes of biliary secretion and intestinal reabsorption are repeated until it is completely expelled out of the body by the urinary system (Gupta, 2016).

Enterohepatic cycling forms an important aspect of biliary excretion. An essential prerequisite for the compounds to undergo biliary secretion is their molecular mass, which may occur by passive diffusion or active transport (Hodgson, 2012). This route of excretion is critical for eliminating anions, cations, and non-ionized molecules containing polar and hydrophilic groups. Enterohepatic circulation increases the half-life and thus the adverse events that might occur possibly due to the prolonged accumulation of toxicants in the liver. Apart from this, the liver also has a separate excretion mechanism for metals.

A typical example is that the lead is excreted into the plasma because of a large bile/plasma concentration and an apparent biliary transport maximum (Gupta, 2016). Some poorly ionized substances in plasma very often diffuse through the walls of the capillaries via the intestinal mucosa and finally get eliminated in the feces. Moreover, intestinal excretion is relatively slow and required for only those xenobiotics which undergo slow biotransformation or slow renal and biliary excretion. For the efficient excretion of lipophilic substances, the lipid content of the intestine can be enhanced (Humannutritionblog, 2016).

18.5.3 Respiratory excretion

The lungs play a significant role in eliminating volatile materials like gases (Leblanc, 2004). Volatile toxicants like ethanol and pesticidal fumigants can also undergo respiratory elimination along with the volatile metabolites acetone and carbon dioxide (Hodgson, 2012). Chemical toxicants which have a high vapor pressure can only undergo respiratory elimination. Sufficiently volatile chemicals diffuse across the alveolar membrane, resulting in the removal of toxicants from the blood and, thus, elimination from the air (Humannutritionblog, 2016). The exhalation route has been proven to be an exceptional route of excretion for lipid-soluble substances. The main reason is that the capillary and alveolar membranes are close to each other and allow for normal gaseous exchange due to their thinness (Leblanc, 2004). Other substances excreted by expired air are fluorobenzene, carbon monoxide, and gases having low blood/gas solubility, such as benzene and nitrous oxide, and are excreted rapidly (Gupta, 2016).

18.5.4 Miscellaneous routes of excretion

(i) Sweat

Water-soluble chemicals are usually eliminated through sweat to a significant degree (Leblanc, 2004). An example of the drugs commonly excreted through the sweat is diethyl dithiol iso-phthalate (an anti-leprotic agent), excreted in the sweat in reasonably large amounts. Due to their high permeability, only unionized molecules are readily excreted out of the sweat gland (Gupta, 2016). Apart from this, some metals generally excreted through sweat are nickel, cadmium, copper, iron, lead, and zinc (Humannutritionblog, 2016).

(ii) Milk

Excretion of water-soluble as well as fat-soluble chemicals takes place through the mother's milk due to the rich presence of lipids and lipoprotein (Leblanc, 2004). Due to its lipophilicity, it may contain xenobiotics having various kinds of physicochemical properties, from polar compounds to highly lipophilic substances like dichloro-diphenyl-trichloroethane (DDT), dichloro diphenylethane (DDE), etc (Hodgson, 2012). The biological half-life of the chemical is an essential factor affecting the elimination of toxicants in milk. Chemical toxicants with a shorter biological half-life get excreted to a short extent, while it forms a major excretion mechanism for chemicals with a longer half-life (Hodgson, 2012). Furthermore, compounds are excreted into the milk by simple diffusion due to the acidity of the milk as compared to plasma. Additionally, thiouracil, tetracycline, and erythromycin are generally secreted in milk (Gupta, 2016).

18.6 Detoxification of drugs

18.6.1 Enzymes in xenobiotic metabolism

Detoxification in the body is often carried out through metabolism. The enzymes and transporters involved in this are critical to the detoxification process but may also sometimes lead to bioactivation. These bioactivation products are responsible for the pathogenesis of various diseases like cancers. Xenobiotics can be hydrophilic or lipophilic. However, hydrophilic chemicals are lesser absorbed, and they are more easily excreted. On the other hand, lipophilic drugs are easily absorbed and readily excreted. However, these enzymes exhibit broad substrate specificity. There are reaction-specific enzymes; hence, one type of drug-metabolizing enzyme can catalyze only one reaction (e.g., oxidation) (Chen, 2020).

Functional and enzymes mainly mediate conjugation reactions involved in drug metabolism. The cytochrome P450 and uridine diphosphate (UDP) glucoronyl transferase are the two most important enzymes which bring about the above-mentioned reactions. Functionalization reactions constitute the addition or unmasking of a polar functional group, like a hydroxyl, carboxyl, or amino within the molecule. The conjugation reactions involve an endogenous compound like glucuronic acid, GSH, sulfate, or acetyl, covalently linked to the substrate through a suitable functional group. These reactions are responsible for the elimination of 90% of drugs that are dependent on hepatic clearance. Drug metabolism essentially forms a method of detoxification because, in most cases, the metabolite formed is less biologically active than the parent compound (Rowland et al., 2013). The enzymes catalyzing metabolic reactions occur largely in the hepatocytes and, to a lesser extent, extracellularly. After the detoxification process, the end products are generally hydrophilic and hence do not diffuse across the cellular membranes; instead, they efflux out of the cellular membrane through drug transporters in an active manner (Chen, 2020).

The most common phase I or functionalization reactions are oxidation and hydroxylation; the enzymes catalyzing them are the Cytochrome P450 class. They are the most important and abundantly found intrinsic membrane proteins in the endoplasmic reticulum (Stanley, 2017). Chemically they are monooxygenases and carry out the catalysis of the oxidation reactions. The maximum wavelength for this complex is observed to be 450 nm. The heme group located at the active site of P450 plays a dual role in activating the oxygen molecule to a highly reactive oxygen species and its binding ability to it. The CYP pathways are classified into members like CYP1 and CYP2 based on similar gene sequences and a subfamily member like CYP1A and CYP2D and further differentiated by a number indicating its isoform or individual enzyme, i.e., CYP1A2, CYP2D6 (McDonnell and Dang, 2013).

Structurally, these enzymes contain a heme group that exists in a reduced form as Fe^{2+}. This reduced form gets complexed with carbon monoxide instead of oxygen. This characteristic property helps all the CYP450 enzymes have the ability to monooxygenase any organic chemical moiety (Chen, 2020). To bring about efficient detoxification of the metabolites, the occurrence of the monooxygenation step is essential. Still, many times this leads to the generation of a toxic reactive intermediate which further requires the intermediate to go through phase II reactions (Stanley, 2017).

The CYPs can oxidize any position on the substrate because they can generate highly reactive single oxygen. The oxidized form of Fe^{2+} (i.e., Fe^{3+} in CYP) binds to the substrate to undergo reduction under the action of enzyme NADPH-CYP reductase to form Fe^{2+} (a reduced form). This reduced form has a much higher affinity for the oxygen molecule. After binding the oxygen molecule to the reduced form, the oxygen undergoes reduction once again under the action of the enzyme NADPH-CYP reductase. This follows the oxidation of the substrate as one of the oxygen atoms is activated to single oxygen.

Meanwhile, the other oxygen atom undergoes reduction to form water along with the oxidation of heme, thus completing the catalytic cycle. Other mechanisms for achieving the two reduction steps might also exist, and this typically depends upon the organ system. In the case of mammals, this step is carried out by NADPH-CYP reductase (Chen, 2020).

Flavin-containing monooxygenases (FMO) are another group of enzymes involved in bringing about the detoxification of drugs through metabolism. These enzymes catalyze the oxygenation reactions of heteroatom-containing chemicals. Thus, these enzymes attach oxygen atoms to the nucleophilic compounds, increasing the solubility and thus readily excreted (Eswaramoorthy et al., 2006). Mammalian FMO is an NADP-dependent and oxygen-dependent FAD-containing enzyme system in the microsome, which acts explicitly as sulfur, phosphorus, and nitrogen oxygenase (Strolin Benedetti et al., 2006). The prosthetic group FAD, which forms the structural component of FMO, is an integral part of the protein. In addition to this, it also needs NADPH as a cofactor for its efficient catalytic activity. Preceding its action on the substrate, FMOs exist in the cells in complexation with a reduced form of prosthetic group and NADPH as a co-factor. The oxygenated and reduced forms of the prosthetic group attached to the cofactor and substrate help stabilize interactions with them, ensuring enzyme turnover (Eswaramoorthy et al., 2006).

Apart from these phase 1 enzymes, other oxidases and reductases are also involved in the metabolism of xenobiotics. For example, alcohol dehydrogenases are responsible for catalyzing alcohols to aldehydes through dehydrogenation. These enzymes also further play a role in the reverse reactions in reducing aldehydes and ketones to alcohol. The hydroxyl functional group gets introduced upon these steps, which requires them to undergo phase II reactions. A significant disadvantage of these steps is the formation of reactive free radicle intermediates, which might pose reactivity and toxicity (Chen, 2020).

18.6.2 Phase II metabolizing enzymes

Phase II metabolic reactions form a covalent link between a functional group on the parent compound or on the compound which has already undergone phase 1 metabolic reaction (Iyanagi, 2007). One of the most predominant phase II metabolizing enzymes is the UGTs, which catalyzes the glucuronidation reaction (Rowland et al., 2013). There exist 16 different UGT human enzymes (McCarver and Hines, 2002). The glucuronidation reaction takes place by transferring the glucuronic acid of UDP-glucuronic acid to a functional group like −OH, −SH, $-NH_2$, etc., of a toxicant or xenobiotic (Iyanagi, 2007). This step follows the second-order nucleophilic substitution mechanism, which causes the inversion of configuration at the C_1 atom of glucuronic acid and the conjugate, thus forming a β-D configuration (Rowland et al., 2013). The UGTs bring about the metabolism of many xenobiotics like drugs, chemicals, carcinogens, environmental pollutants, and dietary supplements. It also metabolizes endobiotics like bilirubin, steroid hormones, fat-soluble vitamins, etc. (Jancova et al., 2010).

(i) Sulphotransferases (SULTs)

SULTs carry out sulfation or sulfurization of aliphatic alcohols, phenols, thiols, amines, etc. They require a cofactor, 3′ phosphoadenosine-5′-phosphosulphate (PAPS), to function efficiently (Chen, 2020). These enzymes metabolize endogenous biogenic amines and cause the sulfation of dehydroepiandrosterone and progesterone in the adrenals. SULTs also catalyze synthetic steroids, which might influence the susceptibility of estrogen receptor-positive breast tumors to antiestrogen therapy (Stanley, 2017).

(ii) GSTs

These enzymes form major detoxification enzymes involved in the metabolism of xenobiotics and play an essential role in preventing oxidative stress, thus providing cellular protection (Jancova et al., 2010). These enzymes catalyze thioether conjugation reactions of GSH to substrates containing electrophilic center and bring about the catalysis of reactions like Michael additions, isomerization, and reduction of hyperperoxides in addition to conjugation of many hydrophobic and electrophilic compounds (Jancova et al., 2010). There are a total of 13 different GST subunits which belong to five different classes, i.e., α, μ, π, ϴ, and ζ (McCarver and Hines, 2002).

The mechanism of action of GSTs begins with the activation of GSH to GS^- by the active site of GSTs. This activation assists in the attack of GS^- to the electrophilic atom to form the GSH conjugates (Chen, 2020). The catalyzation reactions mainly occur in the liver and kidney and are mostly cytosolic, along with a broad range of substrate specificity (Stanley, 2017; Chen, 2020). GSTs are also responsible for the detoxification processes of epoxides derived from the PAHs and alpha beta-unsaturated ketones. In addition to this, they detoxify several endogenous compounds, such as prostaglandins and steroids. Hence, altogether GSTs play a significant biological function of defending against the reactive and toxic reactive oxygen species which generally arise as a result of several metabolic processes taking place in the body (Jancova et al., 2010; Kalyane et al., 2022; Polaka et al., 2022a).

The conjugation products formed from these enzymatic reactions are then degraded into N-acetyl cysteine thioethers, also known as mercapturic acid, which is then readily excreted by drug transporters (Chen, 2020; Stanley, 2017). Apart from the enzymes mentioned above, other enzymes like methyl transferases also participate in phase II drug metabolism. This enzyme takes part in catalyzing the methylation of substrates that contain an electron-rich heteroatom. Although methylation doesn't increase the water solubility of the xenobiotic, it increases transport-mediated disposition (Chen, 2020). Other phase II metabolizing enzymes include N-acetyltransferase, epoxide hydrolase, etc., which metabolize and eliminate drugs like isoniazid or toxic and reactive intermediates like epoxides.

(iii) P-glycoprotein (P-gp) in drug detoxification

P-gp and other members of the ABC binding cassette transporter family play a crucial role in expelling the numerous xenobiotic compounds out of the cells. They exhibit different phenotypes due to their expressions to varying extents in several biological aspects such as (a) they cause multi-drug resistance and lead to failure of cancer chemotherapy, (b) they avoid the accumulation of carcinogens and aid in preventing carcinogenesis in healthy tissues, (c) they bring about efficient pharmacokinetics of pharmacological agents in humans, and (d) they protect from environmental toxins in aquatic organisms (i.e., multi-xenobiotic resistance) (Efferth and Volm, 2017; Parikh et al., 2022).

Recent studies have revealed that drug disposition is determined by the carrier-mediated translocation of xenobiotics. The MDR1 gene product of the P-gp is a member of the ATP binding cassette transporters and is initially known for its role in the causation of resistance during the chemotherapy of tumors. The P-gp protein is located in the plasma membrane and functions as a "flippase" or "hydrophobic vacuum cleaner" by translocating its substrates from the inside to the outside. Most P-gp substrates, interestingly, are also substrates of the main drug-metabolizing enzyme, CYP3A4 (Fromm, 2003). The common gene that regulates the expression of both P-gp and CYP3A4 is the pregnane X receptor or xenobiotic receptor. Hence, intestinal efflux pumps like P-gp limit and further regulate the access of drugs to drug-metabolizing enzymes like CYP and prevent them from accumulating in high concentrations in the intestine (Christians, 2004). Even though the CYP3A4-dependent first-pass metabolism takes place in the liver, intestinal CYP3A4 also participates in the first pass metabolism of many orally administered drugs, contributing to their low bioavailability. Quite a few drugs, like cyclosporin A, saquinavir, etc., are known to have a bioavailability of less than 50%, thus indicating both CYP3A4 metabolism as well as P-gp excretion (Chan et al., 2004).

In the case of gut mucosa, the P-gp and cytochrome P-450 enzymes interact with each other in three ways; firstly, drugs that are repeatedly absorbed are pumped out of the enterocytes by P-gp, thus increasing the chances of drugs being metabolized. Secondly, P-gp plays a role in keeping the intracellular concentrations within the range in which the CYP3A metabolizing enzymes are capable. Lastly, P-gp is responsible for transporting the drug metabolites back into the gut lumen (Christians et al., 2005). In addition, P-gp is located in the colon and lung at intermediate levels and in the prostate, skin, spleen, and heart at low levels. It also gets expressed in the brain, choroid plexus, and placenta. The localization of P-gp in the polarised apical membrane of the intestine, liver, and kidney, along with the blood-brain barrier, signifies a normal excretory barrier role for P-gp in bringing about the expulsion of xenobiotics and toxins into the intestinal mucosa, bile, urine, and blood (Chan et al., 2004).

18.7 Conclusion

Detoxification is essentially the method of detoxifying a person safely and effectively from a particular toxicant. Detoxification is used to get rid of or lessen the intensity of withdrawal symptoms that patients experience when they stop taking their medications. The intensity of the symptoms, the length of the withdrawal phase, and the percentage of completed programs should be the primary factors used to evaluate the efficacy of detoxification. Several toxicity methods can be employed to identify specific toxicity. Additionally, not every patient diagnosed with a drug-induced problem will need detoxification. There are several reasons why patients must undergo detoxification, even though addiction may require it at the start of drug rehabilitation therapy. Eventually, the removal of toxins, or "clinical detoxification," is expected to be a key component of medical therapy as increasingly clinical scientists are becoming aware of the realities of toxicant bioaccumulation and its implications on health.

18.8 List of abbreviations

2D two-dimensional
3D three-dimensional
ATP adenosine triphosphate
BQ benzyl oxyquinoline
CYP cytochromes P450
DDE dichlorodiphenylethane
DDT dichloro-diphenyl-trichloroethane
EROD 7-ethoxy resorufin O-demethylase
FMO flavin-containing monooxygenases
GIT gastrointestinal tract
GSH glutathione
GST glutathione S-transferase
GSTs glutathione-S-transferase
HTS high-throughput screening
IC50 half-maximal inhibitory concentration
IL interleukin
iPSCS induced pluripotent stem cells
MLR mixed lymphocyte reaction assay
mRNA messenger RNA
MTT 3-(4,5-dimethylthiazol-2-yl)-2,5-diphenyl tetrazolium bromide
NAT N-acetyltransferase
OECD Organisation for Economic Co-operation and Development
P-gp P-glycoprotein
PABA para-aminobenzoic acid
PAHs polycyclic aromatic hydrocarbons
PAPS 3′-phosphoadenosine-5′-phosphosulphate
PCBs polychlorinated biphenyls
SAMe S-adenosylmethionine
SULTs sulphotransferases
UDP uridine diphosphate
UGT uridine diphosphate glucuronosyl transferase
UV ultraviolet
VOCs volatile organic compounds

References

Achanta, N.S.K., Rajpoot, K., Tekade, R.K., 2021. Drug metabolic kinetics. In: Tekade, R.K. (Ed.), Biopharmaceutics and Pharmacokinetics Considerations. Elsevier, Academic Press, pp. 335–353.

Anadon, A., Martínez, M.A., Castellano, V., Martínez-Larrañaga, M.R., 2014. The role of in vitro methods as alternatives to animals in toxicity testing. Expet Opin. Drug Metabol. Toxicol. 10 (1), 67–79.

Antonova, O.M., 2022. Promising approaches to assessing the public health risk with real ways of entering a toxicant into the body. Povolzhskiy J. Ecol. (4), 371–384. https://doi.org/10.35885/1684-7318-2021-4-371-384.

Aronica, L., Ordovas, J.M., Volkov, A., Lamb, J.J., Stone, P.M., Minich, D., Leary, M., Class, M., Metti, D., Larson, I.A., Contractor, N., Eck, B., Bland, J.S., 2022. Genetic biomarkers of metabolic detoxification for personalized lifestyle medicine. Nutrients 14 (4), 768. https://www.ncbi.nlm.nih.gov/pubmed/35215417.

Asati, S., Pandey, V., Gour, V., Tiwari, R., Soni, V., Rajpoot, K., Tekade, M., Sharma, M.C., Tekade, R.K., 2022. Toxicity and toxicokinetic considerations in product development and drug research. In: Pharmacokinetics and Toxicokinetic Considerations, vol. 2. Elsevier. https://doi.org/10.1016/b978-0-323-98367-9.00001-9.

Aufderheide, M., Halter, B., Mohle, N., Hochrainer, D., 2013. The CULTEX RFS: a comprehensive technical approach for the in vitro exposure of airway epithelial cells to the particulate matter at the air-liquid interface. BioMed Res. Int. 2013, 734137. https://www.ncbi.nlm.nih.gov/pubmed/23509768.

Bai, X., Chen, H., Oliver, B.G., 2022. The health effects of traffic-related air pollution: a review focused the health effects of going green. Chemosphere 289, 133082. https://www.ncbi.nlm.nih.gov/pubmed/34843836.

Bal-Price, A.K., Hogberg, H.T., Buzanska, L., Coecke, S., 2010. Relevance of in vitro neurotoxicity testing for regulatory requirements: challenges to be considered. Neurotoxicol. Teratol. 32 (1), 36–41.

Becker, R.A., Plunkett, L.M., Borzelleca, J.F., Kaplan, A.M., 2007. Tiered toxicity testing: evaluation of toxicity-based decision triggers for human health hazard characterization. Food Chem. Toxicol. 45 (12), 2454–2469. https://www.ncbi.nlm.nih.gov/pubmed/17689851.

Bell, C.C., Hendriks, D.F., Moro, S.M., Ellis, E., Walsh, J., Renblom, A., Puigvert, L.F., Dankers, A.C., Jacobs, F., Snoeys, J., 2016. Characterization of primary human hepatocyte spheroids as a model system for drug-induced liver injury, liver function and disease. Sci. Rep. 6 (1), 1–13.

Bus, J.S., Becker, R.A., 2009. Toxicity testing in the 21st century: a view from the chemical industry. Toxicol. Sci. 112 (2), 297–302. https://www.ncbi.nlm.nih.gov/pubmed/19805406.

Bużańska, L., Habich, A., Jurga, M., Sypecka, J., Domańska-Janik, K., 2005. Human cord blood-derived neural stem cell line—possible implementation in studying neurotoxicity. Toxicol. Vitro 19 (7), 991–999.

Buzanska, L., Jurga, M., Domanska-Janik, K., 2006. Neuronal differentiation of human umbilical cord blood neural stem-like cell line. Neurodegener. Dis. 3 (1–2), 19–26. https://www.ncbi.nlm.nih.gov/pubmed/16909032.

Chan, L.M., Lowes, S., Hirst, B.H., 2004. The ABCs of drug transport in intestine and liver: efflux proteins limiting drug absorption and bioavailability. Eur. J. Pharmaceut. Sci. 21 (1), 25–51. https://www.ncbi.nlm.nih.gov/pubmed/14706810.

Chatterjee, S., Bijsmans, I.T., van Mil, S.W., Augustijns, P., Annaert, P., 2014. Toxicity and intracellular accumulation of bile acids in sandwich-cultured rat hepatocytes: role of glycine conjugates. Toxicol. Vitro 28 (2), 218–230. https://www.ncbi.nlm.nih.gov/pubmed/24211540.

Chen, G., 2020. Xenobiotic metabolism and disposition. In: An Introduction to Interdisciplinary Toxicology. Elsevier, pp. 31–42.

Chen, J., Liu, Y., Zhao, Z., Qiu, J., 2021. Oxidative stress in the skin: impact and related protection. Int. J. Cosmet. Sci. 43 (5), 495–509. https://www.ncbi.nlm.nih.gov/pubmed/34312881.

Christians, U., 2004. Transport proteins and intestinal metabolism: P-glycoprotein and cytochrome P4503A. Ther. Drug Monit. 26 (2), 104–106. https://www.ncbi.nlm.nih.gov/pubmed/15228147.

Christians, U., Schmitz, V., Haschke, M., 2005. Functional interactions between P-glycoprotein and CYP3A in drug metabolism. Expet Opin. Drug Metabol. Toxicol. 1 (4), 641–654.

Clemedson, C., Kolman, A., Forsby, A., 2007. The integrated acute systemic toxicity project (ACuteTox) for the optimisation and validation of alternative in vitro tests. Altern. Lab. Anim. 35 (1), 33–38. https://www.ncbi.nlm.nih.gov/pubmed/17411349.

Durham, H.D., Dahrouge, S., Cashman, N.R., 1993. Evaluation of the spinal cord neuron X neuroblastoma hybrid cell line NSC-34 as a model for neurotoxicity testing. Neurotoxicology 14 (4), 387–395.

Efferth, T., Volm, M., 2017. Multiple resistance to carcinogens and xenobiotics: P-glycoproteins as universal detoxifiers. Arch. Toxicol. 91 (7), 2515–2538.

El-Deeb, N., Al-Madboly, L., 2021. Probiotics and GIT Diseases/Stomach Ulcer. Probiotics, the Natural Microbiota in Living Organisms. CRC Press. https://doi.org/10.1201/9781351027540-3.

Eswaramoorthy, S., Bonanno, J.B., Burley, S.K., Swaminathan, S., 2006. Mechanism of action of a flavin-containing monooxygenase. Proc. Natl. Acad. Sci. U. S. A. 103 (26), 9832–9837. https://www.ncbi.nlm.nih.gov/pubmed/16777962.

Fan, T., Xie, Y., Ma, W., 2021. Research progress on the protection and detoxification of phytochemicals against aflatoxin B1-Induced liver toxicity. Toxicon 195, 58–68. https://www.ncbi.nlm.nih.gov/pubmed/33716068.

Fromm, M.F., 2003. Importance of P-glycoprotein for drug disposition in humans. Eur. J. Clin. Invest. 33 (Suppl. 2), 6–9. https://www.ncbi.nlm.nih.gov/pubmed/14641550.

Fu, H., Qiu, S., Yao, X., Gao, F., Tan, P., Teng, T., Shi, B., 2020. Toxicity of glyphosate in feed for weanling piglets and the mechanism of glyphosate detoxification by the liver nuclear receptor CAR/PXR pathway. J. Hazard Mater. 387, 121707. https://www.ncbi.nlm.nih.gov/pubmed/31776084.

Gadekar, V., Borade, Y., Kannaujia, S., Rajpoot, K., Anup, N., Tambe, V., Kalia, K., Tekade, R.K., 2021. Nanomedicines accessible in the market for clinical interventions. J. Contr. Release 330, 372–397. https://www.ncbi.nlm.nih.gov/pubmed/33370576.

Ge, J., Huang, Y., Lv, M., Zhang, C., Talukder, M., Li, J., Li, J., 2022. Cadmium induced Fak -mediated anoikis activation in kidney via nuclear receptors (AHR/CAR/PXR)-mediated xenobiotic detoxification pathway. J. Inorg. Biochem. 227, 111682. https://www.ncbi.nlm.nih.gov/pubmed/34902763.

Gennari, A., Ban, M., Braun, A., Casati, S., Corsini, E., Dastych, J., Descotes, J., Hartung, T., Hooghe-Peters, R., House, R., 2005. The use of in vitro systems for evaluating immunotoxicity: the report and recommendations of an ECVAM workshop. J. Immunot. 2 (2), 61–83.

Gerets, H., Tilmant, K., Gerin, B., Chanteux, H., Depelchin, B., Dhalluin, S., Atienzar, F., 2012. Characterization of primary human hepatocytes, HepG2 cells, and HepaRG cells at the mRNA level and CYP activity in response to inducers and their predictivity for the detection of human hepatotoxins. Cell Biol. Toxicol. 28 (2), 69–87.

Godoy, P., Hewitt, N.J., Albrecht, U., Andersen, M.E., Ansari, N., Bhattacharya, S., Bode, J.G., Bolleyn, J., Borner, C., Boettger, J., 2013. Recent advances in 2D and 3D in vitro systems using primary hepatocytes, alternative hepatocyte sources and non-parenchymal liver cells and their use in investigating mechanisms of hepatotoxicity, cell signaling and ADME. Arch. Toxicol. 87 (8), 1315–1530.

Goel, H., Goyal, K., Pandey, A.K., Benjamin, M., Khan, F., Pandey, P., Mittan, S., Iqbal, D., Alsaweed, M., Alturaiki, W., Madkhali, Y., Kamal, M.A., Tanwar, P., Upadhyay, T.K., 2023. Elucidations of molecular mechanism and mechanistic effects of environmental toxicants in neurological disorders. CNS Neurol. Disord. Drug Targets 22 (1), 84–97. https://www.ncbi.nlm.nih.gov/pubmed/35352654.

Goodman, S., Chappell, G., Guyton, K.Z., Pogribny, I.P., Rusyn, I., 2022. Epigenetic alterations induced by genotoxic occupational and environmental human chemical carcinogens: an update of a systematic literature review. Mutat. Res. Rev. Mutat. Res. 789, 108408. https://www.ncbi.nlm.nih.gov/pubmed/35690411.

Gordon, C.J., 2003. Role of environmental stress in the physiological response to chemical toxicants. Environ. Res. 92 (1), 1–7. https://www.ncbi.nlm.nih.gov/pubmed/12706749.

Gueguen, Y., Frerejacques, M., 2022. Review of knowledge of uranium-induced kidney toxicity for the development of an adverse outcome pathway to renal impairment. Int. J. Mol. Sci. 23 (8), 4397. https://www.ncbi.nlm.nih.gov/pubmed/35457214.

Guguen-Guillouzo, C., Guillouzo, A., 2010. General review on in vitro hepatocyte models and their applications. Hepatocytes 1–40.

Gupta, P.K., 2016. Fundamentals of Toxicology: Essential Concepts and Applications, vol. 1. Academic Press. https://doi.org/10.1016/C2015-0-01775-0.

Gupta, R., Polaka, S., Rajpoot, K., Tekade, M., Sharma, M.C., Tekade, R.K., 2022a. Importance of toxicity testing in drug discovery and research. In: Pharmacokinetics and Toxicokinetic Considerations, vol. 2. Elsevier. https://doi.org/10.1016/b978-0-323-98367-9.00016-0.

Gupta, R., Rajpoot, K., Tekade, M., Sharma, M.C., Safavi, M., Tekade, R.K., 2022b. Factors influencing drug toxicity. In: Pharmacokinetics and Toxicokinetic Considerations, vol. 2. Elsevier. https://doi.org/10.1016/b978-0-323-98367-9.00014-7.

Gupta, R., Rajpoot, K., Tekade, M., Sharma, M.C., Tekade, R.K., 2022c. Methods and models for in vitro toxicity. In: Pharmacokinetics and Toxicokinetic Considerations, vol. 2. Elsevier. https://doi.org/10.1016/b978-0-323-98367-9.00006-8.

Harry, G.J., Billingsley, M., Bruinink, A., Campbell, I.L., Classen, W., Dorman, D.C., Galli, C., Ray, D., Smith, R.A., Tilson, H.A., 1998. In vitro techniques for the assessment of neurotoxicity. Environ. Health Perspect. 106 (Suppl. 1), 131–158. https://www.ncbi.nlm.nih.gov/pubmed/9539010.

Hodgson, E., 2012. Pesticide Biotransformation and Disposition, vol. 1. Academic Press. https://www.sciencedirect.com/book/9780123854810/pesticide-biotransformation-and-disposition.

Howell, B.A., Chauhan, A., 2010. Current and emerging detoxification therapies for critical care. Materials 3 (4), 2483–2505. https://doi.org/10.3390/ma3042483.

Huang, X.X., Xu, S., Yu, L.J., Zhou, Y.F., Zhou, Y., Liu, Z.H., 2021. Eurotium cristatum fermented loose dark tea ameliorates cigarette smoke-induced lung injury by MAPK pathway and enhances hepatic metabolic detoxification by PXR/AhR pathway in mice. Oxid. Med. Cell. Longev. 2021, 6635080. https://www.ncbi.nlm.nih.gov/pubmed/33777316.

Huggins, J., 2003. Alternatives to animal testing: research, trends, validation, regulatory acceptance. ALTEX 20 (Suppl. 1), 3–61. https://www.ncbi.nlm.nih.gov/pubmed/14671702.

Humannutritionblog, 2016. Excretion of Toxicants. https://humannutritionblog.wordpress.com/2016/01/26/excretion-of-toxicants/. (Accessed 30 September 2022).

Iyanagi, T., 2007. Molecular mechanism of phase I and phase II drug-metabolizing enzymes: implications for detoxification. Int. Rev. Cytol. 260, 35–112. https://www.ncbi.nlm.nih.gov/pubmed/17482904.

Jain, A.K., Singh, D., Dubey, K., Maurya, R., Mittal, S., Pandey, A.K., 2018. Models and methods for in vitro toxicity. In: In Vitro Toxicology. Elsevier, pp. 45–65.

Jancova, P., Anzenbacher, P., Anzenbacherova, E., 2010. Phase II drug metabolizing enzymes. Biomed. Pap. Med. Fac. Univ. Palacky Olomouc Czech Repub. 154 (2), 103–116. https://www.ncbi.nlm.nih.gov/pubmed/20668491.

Jemnitz, K., Veres, Z., Monostory, K., Kobori, L., Vereczkey, L., 2008. Interspecies differences in acetaminophen sensitivity of human, rat, and mouse primary hepatocytes. Toxicol. Vitro 22 (4), 961–967. https://www.ncbi.nlm.nih.gov/pubmed/18346862.

Jennings, P., Koppelstaetter, C., Pfaller, W., Morin, J.P., Hartung, T., Ryan, M.P., 2004. Assessment of a new cell culture perfusion apparatus for in vitro chronic toxicity testing. Part 2: toxicological evaluation. ALTEX 21 (2), 61–66. https://www.ncbi.nlm.nih.gov/pubmed/15195226.

Jones, A.K., Brown, L.D., Rozance, P.J., Serkova, N.J., Hay Jr., W.W., Friedman, J.E., Wesolowski, S.R., 2019. Differential effects of intrauterine growth restriction and a hypersinsulinemic-isoglycemic clamp on metabolic pathways and insulin action in the fetal liver. Am. J. Physiol. Regul. Integr. Comp. Physiol. 316 (5), R427–R440. https://www.ncbi.nlm.nih.gov/pubmed/30758974.

Kalyane, D., Choudhary, D., Polaka, S., Goykar, H., Karanwad, T., Rajpoot, K., Kumar Tekade, R., 2022. Reactive oxygen nano-generators for cancer therapy. Prog. Mater. Sci. 130, 100974. https://www.sciencedirect.com/science/article/pii/S007964252200055X.

Kalyane, D., Kumar, N., Anup, N., Rajpoot, K., Maheshwari, R., Sengupta, P., Kalia, K., Tekade, R.K., 2021. Recent advancements and future submissions of silica core-shell nanoparticles. Int. J. Pharm. 609, 121173. https://www.ncbi.nlm.nih.gov/pubmed/34627997.

Knight, A., 2008. Non-animal methodologies within biomedical research and toxicity testing. ALTEX 25 (3), 213–231. https://www.ncbi.nlm.nih.gov/pubmed/18841317.

Langezaal, I., Hoffmann, S., Hartung, T., Coecke, S., 2002. Evaluation and prevalidation of an immunotoxicity test based on human whole-blood cytokine release. Altern. Lab. Anim. 30 (6), 581–595. https://www.ncbi.nlm.nih.gov/pubmed/12513684.

Langsch, A., Nau, H., 2005. Metabolic activation for in vitro systems in Workshop 5.15 in vitro metabolism: applications in pharmacology and toxicology. ALTEX 22 1 (2), 354–358. https://hugepdf.com/download/download-metabolic-activation-for-in-vitro-systems-workshop-515-in-vitro_pdf.

Lankveld, D.P., Van Loveren, H., Baken, K.A., Vandebriel, R.J., 2010. In vitro testing for direct immunotoxicity: state of the art. Methods Mol. Biol. 598, 401–423. https://www.ncbi.nlm.nih.gov/pubmed/19967527.

Leblanc, G.A., 2004. Elimination of toxicants. A Textbook of Modern Toxicology, p. 203.

LeCluyse, E.L., Witek, R.P., Andersen, M.E., Powers, M.J., 2012. Organotypic liver culture models: meeting current challenges in toxicity testing. Crit. Rev. Toxicol. 42 (6), 501–548. https://www.ncbi.nlm.nih.gov/pubmed/22582993.

Li, A.P., 2008. In vitro evaluation of human xenobiotic toxicity: scientific concepts and the novel integrated discrete multiple cell coculture (IdMOC) technology. ALTEX Alternatives Anim. Experiment. 25 (1), 43–49.

Li, Z., Cui, Z., 2014. Three-dimensional perfused cell culture. Biotechnol. Adv. 32 (2), 243–254. https://www.ncbi.nlm.nih.gov/pubmed/24184152.

Lin, S., Ali, M.U., Zheng, C., Cai, Z., Wong, M.H., 2022. Toxic chemicals from uncontrolled e-waste recycling: exposure, body burden, health impact. J. Hazard Mater. 426, 127792. https://www.ncbi.nlm.nih.gov/pubmed/34802823.

Mahdiani, S., Omidkhoda, N., Heidari, S., Hayes, A.W., Karimi, G., 2022. Protective effect of luteolin against chemical and natural toxicants by targeting NF-kappaB pathway. Biofactors 48 (4), 744–762. https://www.ncbi.nlm.nih.gov/pubmed/35861671.

McCarver, D.G., Hines, R.N., 2002. The ontogeny of human drug-metabolizing enzymes: phase II conjugation enzymes and regulatory mechanisms. J. Pharmacol. Exp. Therapeut. 300 (2), 361–366. https://www.ncbi.nlm.nih.gov/pubmed/11805192.

McDonnell, A.M., Dang, C.H., 2013. Basic review of the cytochrome p450 system. J. Adv. Pract. Oncol. 4 (4), 263–268. https://www.ncbi.nlm.nih.gov/pubmed/25032007.

McPartland, J., Shaffer, R.M., Fox, M.A., Nachman, K.E., Burke, T.A., Denison, R.A., 2022. Charting a path forward: assessing the science of chemical risk evaluations under the toxic substances control act in the context of recent national academies recommendations. Environ. Health Perspect. 130 (2), 25003. https://www.ncbi.nlm.nih.gov/pubmed/35195451.

Murota, K., 2020. Absorption pathway of dietary flavonoids: the potential roles of the lymphatic transport in the intestine. Funct. Foods Health Dis. 10 (7), 274. https://doi.org/10.31989/ffhd.v10i7.723.

Murthy, B., 2007. Relevance of in vitro toxicology studies in risk assessment. ALTEX 24 (3), 174–177. https://www.ncbi.nlm.nih.gov/pubmed/17891324.

Nelson, L.J., Navarro, M., Treskes, P., Samuel, K., Tura-Ceide, O., Morley, S.D., Hayes, P.C., Plevris, J.N., 2015. Acetaminophen cytotoxicity is ameliorated in a human liver organotypic co-culture model. Sci. Rep. 5 (1), 1–12.

Okoye, C.O., Addey, C.I., Oderinde, O., Okoro, J.O., Uwamungu, J.Y., Ikechukwu, C.K., Okeke, E.S., Ejeromedoghene, O., Odii, E.C., 2022. Toxic chemicals and persistent organic pollutants associated with micro- and nanoplastics pollution. Chem. Eng. J. Adv. 11, 100310. https://doi.org/10.1016/j.ceja.2022.100310.

Olivera, D.S., Hoard-Fruchey, H., Sciuto, A.M., 2017. Evaluation of an in vitro screening model to assess phosgene inhalation injury. Toxicol. Mech. Methods 27 (1), 45–51. https://www.ncbi.nlm.nih.gov/pubmed/27696922.

Orbach, S.M., Less, R.R., Kothari, A., Rajagopalan, P., 2017. In vitro intestinal and liver models for toxicity testing. ACS Biomater. Sci. Eng. 3 (9), 1898–1910. https://www.ncbi.nlm.nih.gov/pubmed/33440548.

Parikh, K.J., Christian, J.R., Rajpoot, K., Tekade, R.K., 2022. Environmental and safety aspects of bionanotechnology. In: Pharmacokinetics and Toxicokinetic Considerations, vol. 2. Elsevier. https://doi.org/10.1016/b978-0-323-98367-9.00022-6.

Pauluhn, J., 2022. Derivation of thresholds for inhaled chemically reactive irritants: searching for substance-specific common denominators for read-across prediction. Regul. Toxicol. Pharmacol. 130, 105131. https://www.ncbi.nlm.nih.gov/pubmed/35124139.

Pessina, A., Albella, B., Bueren, J., Brantom, P., Casati, S., Gribaldo, L., Croera, C., Gagliardi, G., Foti, P., Parchment, R., Parent-Massin, D., Sibiril, Y., Van Den Heuvel, R., 2001. Prevalidation of a model for predicting acute neutropenia by colony forming unit granulocyte/macrophage (CFU-GM) assay. Toxicol. Vitro 15 (6), 729–740. https://www.ncbi.nlm.nih.gov/pubmed/11698175.

Pizzorno, J., 2022. Environmental Toxins and Cardiovascular Disease. Nutritional and Integrative Strategies in Cardiovascular Medicine. CRC Press. https://doi.org/10.1201/9781003137849-13.

Polaka, S., Katare, P., Pawar, B., Vasdev, N., Gupta, T., Rajpoot, K., Sengupta, P., Tekade, R.K., 2022a. Emerging ROS-modulating technologies for augmentation of the wound healing process. ACS Omega 7 (35), 30657–30672. https://doi.org/10.1021/acsomega.2c02675.

Polaka, S., Makwana, V., Vasdev, N., Sheth, A., Rajpoot, K., Sengupta, P., Tekade, R.K., 2022b. Engineering immunity via skin-directed drug delivery devices. J. Contr. Release 345, 385–404. https://www.ncbi.nlm.nih.gov/pubmed/35283256.

Raineri, D., 2001. Virtual laboratories enhance traditional undergraduate biology laboratories. Biochem. Mol. Biol. Educ. 29 (4), 160–162. https://doi.org/10.1016/s1470-8175(01)00060-1.

Rajpoot, K., Desai, N., Koppisetti, H., Tekade, M., Sharma, M.C., Behera, S.K., Tekade, R.K., 2022a. In Silico Methods for the Prediction of Drug Toxicity. Pharmacokinetics and Toxicokinetic Considerations, vol. 2. Elsevier. https://doi.org/10.1016/b978-0-323-98367-9.00012-3.

Rajpoot, K., Katare, P., Tekade, M., Sharma, M.C., Polaka, S., Sengupta, P., Tekade, R.K., 2022b. Toxicokinetic and Toxicodynamic Considerations in Drug Research. Pharmacokinetics and Toxicokinetic Considerations, vol. 2. Elsevier. https://doi.org/10.1016/b978-0-323-98367-9.00026-3.

Rajpoot, K., Tekade, M., Sharma, M.C., Arafat, B., Tekade, R.K., 2022c. Principles and concepts in toxicokinetic. In: Pharmacokinetics and Toxicokinetic Considerations, vol. 2. Elsevier. https://doi.org/10.1016/b978-0-323-98367-9.00023-8.

Rajpoot, K., Tekade, R.K., Sharma, M.C., Safavi, M., Tekade, M., 2021. Pharmacokinetics modeling in drug delivery. In: Tekade, R.K. (Ed.), Biopharmaceutics and Pharmacokinetics Considerations. Elsevier, Academic Press, pp. 279–334.

Ramachandraiah, K., Ameer, K., Jiang, G., Hong, G.P., 2022. Micro- and nanoplastic contamination in livestock production: entry pathways, potential effects and analytical challenges. Sci. Total Environ. 844, 157234. https://www.ncbi.nlm.nih.gov/pubmed/35810901.

Ranouille, E., Boutot, C., Bony, E., Bombarde, O., Grosjean, S., Lazewski, A., Berthon, J.-Y., Filaire, E., 2018. Schisandra chinensis protects the skin from global pollution by inflammatory and redox balance pathway modulations: an in vitro study. Cosmetics 5 (2), 36. https://doi.org/10.3390/cosmetics5020036.

Rasgado-Flores, H., Krishna Mandava, V., Siman, H., Van Driessche, W., Pilewski, J.M., Randell, S.H., Bridges, R.J., 2013. Effect of apical hyperosmotic sodium challenge and amiloride on sodium transport in human bronchial epithelial cells from cystic fibrosis donors. Am. J. Physiol. Cell Physiol. 305 (11), C1114–C1122. https://www.ncbi.nlm.nih.gov/pubmed/23986197.

Rim, K.-T., 2019. In vitro models for chemical toxicity: review of their applications and prospects. Toxicol. Environ. Health Sci. 11 (2), 94–103.

Rowland, A., Miners, J.O., Mackenzie, P.I., 2013. The UDP-glucuronosyltransferases: their role in drug metabolism and detoxification. Int. J. Biochem. Cell Biol. 45 (6), 1121–1132.

Rysava, A., Vostalova, J., Rajnochova Svobodova, A., 2021. Effect of ultraviolet radiation on the Nrf2 signaling pathway in skin cells. Int. J. Radiat. Biol. 97 (10), 1383–1403. https://www.ncbi.nlm.nih.gov/pubmed/34338112.

Sarkisov, S.V., Konovalov, V.B., Bondarev, A.V., Lopatin, N.V., El-Salim, S.Z., 2022. Detection of toxic substances in aqueous solutions. In: Paper Presented at the AIP Conference Proceedings 2467, p. 080022. https://doi.org/10.1063/5.0095795.

Setiyorini, Y., Anggraeni, A., Pintowantoro, S., 2022. In-vivo study of nano chitosan as therapeutic agent for toxic metal implant. Results Eng. 13, 100352. https://doi.org/10.1016/j.rineng.2022.100352.

Shao, X., Xu, B., Chen, C., Li, P., Luo, H., 2022. The function and mechanism of lactic acid bacteria in the reduction of toxic substances in food: a review. Crit. Rev. Food Sci. Nutr. 62 (21), 5950–5963. https://www.ncbi.nlm.nih.gov/pubmed/33683156.

Shete, M.B., Patil, T.S., Deshpande, A.S., Saraogi, G., Vasdev, N., Deshpande, M., Rajpoot, K., Tekade, R.K., 2022. Current trends in theranostic nanomedicines. J. Drug Deliv. Sci. Technol. 71, 103280. https://www.sciencedirect.com/science/article/pii/S1773224722001903.

Sirenko, O., Hancock, M.K., Hesley, J., Hong, D., Cohen, A., Gentry, J., Carlson, C.B., Mann, D.A., 2016. Phenotypic characterization of toxic compound effects on liver spheroids derived from iPSC using confocal imaging and three-dimensional image analysis. Assay Drug Dev. Technol. 14 (7), 381–394.

Soldatow, V.Y., Lecluyse, E.L., Griffith, L.G., Rusyn, I., 2013. In vitro models for liver toxicity testing. Toxicol. Res. 2 (1), 23–39. https://www.ncbi.nlm.nih.gov/pubmed/23495363.

Stanley, L., 2017. Drug metabolism. In: Pharmacognosy. Elsevier, pp. 527–545.

Strolin Benedetti, M., Whomsley, R., Baltes, E., 2006. Involvement of enzymes other than CYPs in the oxidative metabolism of xenobiotics. Expet Opin. Drug Metabol. Toxicol. 2 (6), 895–921.

Tambe, V., Pande, S., Gadeval, A., Rajpoot, K., Raval, N., Tekade, R.K., 2021a. Microdialysis: an emerging technique for pharmacokinetic–pharmacodynamic profiling. In: Tekade, R.K. (Ed.), Biopharmaceutics and Pharmacokinetics Considerations, first ed. Elsevier, pp. 601–616. https://doi.org/10.1016/B978-0-12-814425-1.00018-8.

Tambe, V., Sirsat, B., Rajpoot, K., Gadeval, A., Tekade, R.K., 2021b. Pharmacogenomics and drug metabolism. In: Tekade, R.K. (Ed.), Biopharmaceutics and Pharmacokinetics Considerations, vol. 1. Elsevier, Academic Press, pp. 355–385.

Tawfik, N.G., Mohamed, W.R., Mahmoud, H.S., Alqarni, M.A., Naguib, I.A., Fahmy, A.M., Ahmed, O.M., 2022. Isatin counteracts diethylnitrosamine/2-acetylaminofluorene-induced hepatocarcinogenesis in male wistar rats by upregulating anti-inflammatory, antioxidant, and detoxification pathways. Antioxidants 11 (4), 699. https://www.ncbi.nlm.nih.gov/pubmed/35453384.

Tekade, M., Koppisetti, H., Sharma, M.C., Rajpoot, K., Sengupta, P., Kumar, M., Tekade, R.K., 2022. Understanding the concept of signal toxicity and its implications on human health. In: Pharmacokinetics and Toxicokinetic Considerations, vol. 2. Elsevier. https://doi.org/10.1016/b978-0-323-98367-9.00020-2.

Thimmulappa, R.K., Rangasamy, T., Alam, J., Biswal, S., 2008. Dibenzoylmethane activates Nrf2-dependent detoxification pathway and inhibits benzo(a)pyrene induced DNA adducts in lungs. Med. Chem. 4 (5), 473–481. https://www.ncbi.nlm.nih.gov/pubmed/18782044.

Thomas, J.L., Jacob, L., Boisserand, L., 2019. Lymphatic system in central nervous system. Med. Sci. 35 (1), 55–61. https://www.ncbi.nlm.nih.gov/pubmed/30672459.

Tiwari, A., Joshi, M., Salvi, N., Gupta, D., Gandhi, S., Rajpoot, K., Tekade, R.K., 2022. Toxicity of pharmaceutical azo dyes. In: Pharmacokinetics and Toxicokinetic Considerations, vol. 2. Elsevier. https://doi.org/10.1016/b978-0-323-98367-9.00004-4.

Turner, L.A., Bucking, C., 2019. The role of intestinal bacteria in the ammonia detoxification ability of teleost fish. J. Exp. Biol. 222 (Pt 24). https://www.ncbi.nlm.nih.gov/pubmed/31753905.

Volk, H.E., Ames, J.L., Chen, A., Fallin, M.D., Hertz-Picciotto, I., Halladay, A., Hirtz, D., Lavin, A., Ritz, B., Zoeller, T., Swanson, M., 2022. Considering toxic chemicals in the etiology of autism. Pediatrics 149 (1) e2021053012. https://www.ncbi.nlm.nih.gov/pubmed/34972219.

Ware, B.R., Berger, D.R., Khetani, S.R., 2015. Prediction of drug-induced liver injury in micropatterned co-cultures containing iPSC-derived human hepatocytes. Toxicol. Sci. 145 (2), 252–262. https://www.ncbi.nlm.nih.gov/pubmed/25716675.

Wei, Y., Ma, D., Fan, Y., Gao, C., Wang, Q., Yuan, Y., Zhang, Y., Han, J., Hao, Z., 2022. Environmental carbon tetrachloride exposure disrupts the liver structure and metabolic detoxification function in mice via p38MAPK/NF-κB/NLRP3 pathway. Food Agric. Immunol. 33 (1), 235–251. https://doi.org/10.1080/09540105.2022.2060192.

Windsor, J.A., Trevaskis, N.L., Phillips, A.J., 2022. The gut-lymph model gives new treatment strategies for organ failure. JAMA Surg. 157 (6), 540–541. https://www.ncbi.nlm.nih.gov/pubmed/35442412.

Xu, J., Li, S., Jiang, L., Gao, X., Liu, W., Zhu, X., Huang, W., Zhao, H., Wei, Z., Wang, K., Yang, Z., 2021. Baicalin protects against zearalenone-induced chicks liver and kidney injury by inhibiting expression of oxidative stress, inflammatory cytokines and caspase signaling pathway. Int. Immunopharm. 100, 108097. https://www.ncbi.nlm.nih.gov/pubmed/34521024.

Yan, X., Yu, X., Jiang, C., Cao, Y., Zhu, L., Du, C., Jia, Y., 2022. Tonifying-Qi-and-Detoxification Decoction attenuated injuries of colon and lung tissues in ulcerative colitis rat model via regulating NF-kappaB and p38MAPK pathway. Ann. Transl. Med. 10 (8), 455. https://www.ncbi.nlm.nih.gov/pubmed/35571405.

Yang, X., Man, Y.B., Wong, M.H., Owen, R.B., Chow, K.L., 2022. Environmental health impacts of microplastics exposure on structural organization levels in the human body. Sci. Total Environ. 825, 154025. https://www.ncbi.nlm.nih.gov/pubmed/35202683.

Yiming, L., Yanfei, H., Hang, Y., Yimei, C., Guangliang, S., Shu, L., 2021. Cadmium induces apoptosis of pig lymph nodes by regulating the PI3K/AKT/HIF-1alpha pathway. Toxicology 451, 152694. https://www.ncbi.nlm.nih.gov/pubmed/33493553.

Zalat, M.M., Abdallah, A.R., 2022. Occupational reproductive health hazards among university working females. Egypt. J. Occup. Med. 46 (1), 123–140. https://doi.org/10.21608/ejom.2021.87485.1244.

Zeng, J., Wang, T., Cheng, Z., Liu, L., Hu, F., 2022. Ultrahigh adsorption of toxic substances from cigarette smoke using nanocellulose-SiO2 hybrid aerogels. ACS Appl. Polym. Mater. 4 (2), 1173 1182. https://doi.org/10.1021/acsapm.1c01581.

Zhao, M., Zhao, H., Deng, J., Guo, L., Wu, B., 2019. Role of the CLOCK protein in liver detoxification. Br. J. Pharmacol. 176 (24), 4639–4652. https://www.ncbi.nlm.nih.gov/pubmed/31404943.

CHAPTER

19

Molecular mechanisms of the chemopreventive role of dietary phytochemicals

Suryanarayana Polaka[1], *Nupur Vasdev*[1], *Lakshmi Vineela Nalla*[1,2], *Sivarupa Raji*[3], *Muktika Tekade*[4], *Nagendra Singh Chauhan*[5], *Satyajit D. Sarker*[6] *and Rakesh Kumar Tekade*[1]

[1]National Institute of Pharmaceutical Education and Research (NIPER)- Ahmedabad, An Institute of National Importance, Government of India, Department of Pharmaceuticals, Ministry of Chemicals and Fertilizers, Palaj, Gandhinagar, Gujarat, India; [2]Department of Pharmacy, Koneru Lakshmaiah Education Foundation, Vaddeswaram, Andhra Pradesh, India; [3]Redox Biology Lab, National Centre for Cell Science (NCCS), Pune, India; [4]School of Pharmacy, Devi Ahilya Vishwavidyalaya, Indore, Madhya Pradesh, India; [5]Drugs Testing Laboratory Avam Anusandhan Kendra, Raipur, Chhattisgarh, India; [6]Centre for Natural Products Discovery, School of Pharmacy and Biomolecular Sciences, Liverpool John Moores University, Liverpool, United Kingdom

19.1 Introduction

Chemoprevention involves the use of chemotherapeutic agents to prevent or reverse the invasive potential of premalignant cells (Sporn, 1976). Cancer progresses through several phases, the most important of which are initiation, promotion, and metastasis. Most conventional chemotherapeutic agents are used to combat cancer by single target mechanisms. Single target mechanisms are sufficient for curing a few cancers at the initial stages of progression, but cancers like colorectal cancer require two or more hits to eradicate. Multidrug therapy is suggested to target two or more mechanisms involved in cancer progression;

Essentials of Pharmatoxicology in Drug Research, Volume 1
https://doi.org/10.1016/B978-0-443-15840-7.00001-4

however, sophisticated chemotherapeutic drugs have numerous drawbacks, including side effects, cost, a single target mechanism, and drug resistance (Koh et al., 2020).

The recent advancement in cancer therapy mainly focuses on multistage targeting, including initiation, progression, and invasion. Many models for scrutinizing the multistage targeting strategies using therapeutic agents have been successfully introduced into cancer research (Moolgavkar and Luebeck, 2003; Koh et al., 2020). To target cancer progression, it is imperative to understand the biology behind the cancer progression and delineate the pathways leading to the invading ability of cancer cells to other secondary sites of the body.

Alternative strategies are acquiring an interest in recent years of chemotherapy in cancer research. Chemoprevention is one of the effective alternative techniques that has attracted attention since it has been discovered to be possibly engaged in avoiding the occurrence and advancement of malignancies to efficiently target cancer. It has also been revealed that the early stages of cancer are more vulnerable to treatment with cancer drugs and can be successfully targeted to prevent disease relapse. However, in the process of targeting multiple pathways with anticancer drugs, there is a considerable risk of severe side effects of drugs.

Cancer drug development necessitates costly screening procedures to achieve efficacy with minimal side effects, which are time-consuming (Koh et al., 2020). As a result, using dietary phytochemicals as chemopreventive agents has gained significant attention. Phytochemicals have emerged as a potential option for cancer treatment with low side effects. Additionally, phytochemicals have shown their therapeutic effects by targeting many pathological mechanisms at different stages of the disease. For instance, sulforaphane (SFN) inhibits breast cancer progression by causing cell cycle arrest and senescence and acting as an epigenetic modulator in epigenome-targeted cancer therapy (Lewinska et al., 2017). Luteolin, a flavonoid, has multiple anticancer properties in many human cancers such as lung, breast, glioblastoma, prostate, colon, and pancreatic cancers by inhibiting cell proliferation, activation of cell cycle arrest, and by leading to apoptosis of cancer cells (Imran et al., 2019a).

19.2 Importance of plant-derived foods in chemoprevention

The use of phytochemicals has been evolving as an optimistic approach to prevent, inhibit, and cure cancer and postponing its onset more safely and efficiently. They are important because, apart from effective chemopreventive measures, they help reduce the financial and illness load on the already overburdened healthcare system (Dave et al., 2020). Diet has long been recognized as having a positive impact on human diseases. "Let food be the medicine, and medicine be thy nutrition," Hippocrates, a Greek physician, reportedly said. Furthermore, a population meta-analysis data reveals that those who eat five servings of fruits and vegetables had a 50% lower chance of developing most cancer sites than people who eat fewer than two servings. Based on this, the "Five-a-Day for Better Health (1991)" and "Savor the Spectrum (2002)" programs were created in the United States to urge Americans to consume fruits and vegetables to avoid cancer (Surh, 2003a). The healthcare system advises the consumption of more fruits and vegetables in meals for their essential goodness and chemopreventive actions.

Dietary phytochemicals, for instance, lycopene from tomatoes, epigallocatechin-3-gallate from green tea, genistein from soybeans, sulforaphane from broccoli, indole-3-carbinol from cabbage, 6-gingerol from ginger, diallyl sulfide from garlic, caffeic acid phenethyl ester from honey, capsaicin from chili peppers, curcumin from turmeric, resveratrol from grapes, 2-hydroxy flavanone from citrus fruits and vitamin D_3 from mushrooms have been studied for their chemopreventive nature (Chikara et al., 2018; Dave et al., 2020). The chemopreventive phytochemicals named above usually act by affecting multiple signaling and metabolic pathways (Ruiz and Hernández, 2016). Some phytochemicals with promising cancer chemopreventive actions and the pathways they influence will be mentioned in the following sections.

19.3 Mechanisms of chemoprevention

Cancer cells exert multiple mechanisms to create favorable conditions to proliferate and invade other body sites. Simultaneous involvement of different pathological events occurs in the incidence and progression of cancer. Plant-based foods like fruits, vegetables, and whole grains are abundant in phytochemicals and secondary metabolites. They show many beneficial effects in treating different types of cancers by targeting multiple mechanisms of tumorigenesis.

Many epidemiological studies in cancer research support that phytochemicals are promising therapeutic agents to treat diseases like cancer. The phytochemical's chemopreventive role is a complicated control at the cellular and molecular levels, which includes oxidative stress, apoptosis, cell cycle arrest, activation of tumor suppressor genes, metastasis, angiogenesis, etc. (Chikara et al., 2018). Some of the pathways involved are mitogen-activated protein kinase (MAPK), phosphatidylinositol 3-kinase/mammalian target of rapamycin/protein kinase B (PI3K/mTOR/PKB or Akt), and nuclear factor kappa-beta (NF-κβ) pathways. The detailed chemopreventive mechanism of phytochemicals is illustrated in Fig. 19.1.

The phytochemicals mentioned in Table 19.1 interact with specific long noncoding RNAs (LncRNA) as well as affect their expressions in various cancers (Arya and Saldanha, 2019). Resveratrol causes downregulation of LncRNA MALAT1 (Metastasis Associated Lung Adenocarcinoma Transcript 1) as well as diminishes Wnt (Wingless-related integration site)/β-catenin signaling and thereby inhibiting the invasion and metastasis in colon tumor samples from clinical setups. Curcumin causes LncRNA PANDAR (P21-associated ncRNA DNA damage-activated RNA) silencing by switching from senescence to apoptosis in colon tumor samples from clinical setups. Sulforaphane causes reduced expression of LncRNA LINC01116 (long intergenic nonprotein coding RNA 1116) and cellular proliferation in PC-3 prostate cancer cells (Beaver et al., 2017).

Genistein causes a significant reduction in the expression of HOTAIR (HOX antisense intergenic RNA), typically overexpressed in renal and colon cancer. EGCG (epigallocatechin-3-gallate) causes NEAT1 (Nuclear Enriched Abundant Transcript 1) upregulation which decreases drug resistance responses and thus enhances cisplatin treatment sensitivity in NSCLC (nonsmall cell lung carcinoma) as studied in A459, H460, and H1299 NSCLC cell lines. It also favorably enhances cisplatin treatment sensitivity in the case of colon cancer as well.

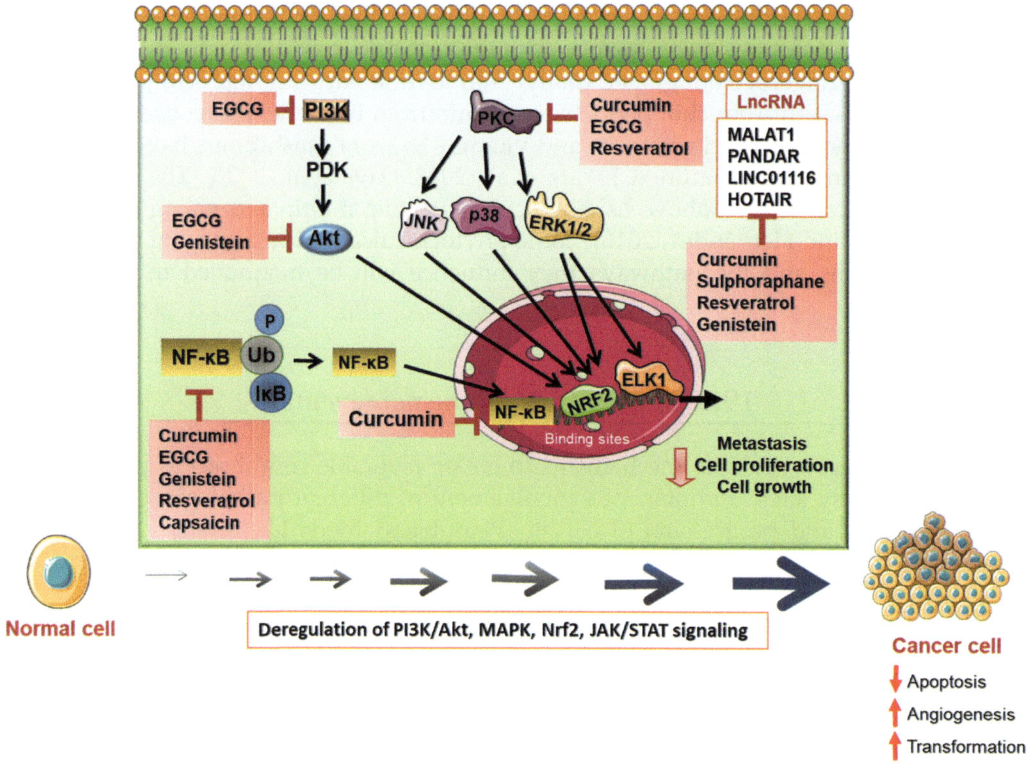

FIGURE 19.1 Effect of phytochemicals on PI3K/Akt, NRF2, ERK1/2, MAPK signaling pathways, and LncRNAs.

19.3.1 Phytochemicals and oxidative stress

Oxidative stress is the triggering event for many pathological mechanisms. Normal levels of reactive oxygen species (ROS) act as signaling molecules and are required for basal cellular functions like cell proliferation, apoptosis, and immune reactions. In contrast, elevated levels of ROS disrupt the DNA sequence and proteins and lipids, if unresolved, may lead to mutations in DNA which eventually causes carcinogenesis. Curcumin's in vitro anticancer potential stems from its ability to decrease oxidative stress in cancer cells by regulating various downstream signaling cascades. ERK1/2, for example, is an essential signaling cascade downstream of ROS implicated in tumor migration and invasion (Wu et al., 2008).

EGCG has been shown to inhibit H_2O_2-mediated cytotoxicity in HepG2 liver cancer cells by increasing cellular GSH levels. Wistar rats were exposed for 30 min to frying oil fumes, a potent environmental toxin linked with lung illnesses, including cancer, which raised ROS levels in the blood as well as ROS and 4HNE levels in the alveolar lavage fluid. Two weeks of pretreatment with green tea extracts dramatically decreased their levels in the lavage fluid (Yang et al., 2009). Resveratrol has been shown to protect PC12 prostate cancer cells against H_2O_2-induced cytotoxicity and oxidative stress by increasing the mRNA and protein levels of HO-1, a critical antioxidant enzyme, through ARE-mediated transcriptional activation of Nrf2 (Chen et al., 2005a).

TABLE 19.1 Different animal models and doses used for in vivo effect of phytochemicals in chemoprevention.

Phytochemical	Chemical nature	Source	Mechanism of chemoprevention	Dose	Species used	References
Epigallocatechin gallate (EGCG)	Catechin	Green tea	Prevent DNA damage, cell signaling pathway alterations, oxidative stress, and mutation	10 mg/kg	Mice	Li et al. (2016)
				0.1, 0.5, or 1.5 mg	Immunodeficient mice	Mah et al. (2014)
				25 mg/kg	Mice	Zhou et al. (2014)
				20 mg/kg	Rat	Darweish et al. (2014)
				5/10/20 mg/kg	Nude mice	Yuan et al. (2007)
Curcumin	Diarylheptanoid	Turmeric (*Curcuma longa*)	Antioxidant	50 mg/kg	Nude mice	Lu et al. (2013)
				0.5% and 1.0% curcumin diet	Mice	Okazaki et al. (2005)
				0.2% or 0.05% pure curcumin	Rat	Ikezaki et al. (2001)
				A diet containing 500 ppm curcumin	Rat	Ushida et al. (2000)
				Diet with 2% curcumin	Mice	Billerey-Larmonier et al. (2008)
[6]-Gingerol	Phenolic compound	Ginger (*Zingiber officinale*)	Suppresses (NF-κB), phosphorylation of IκBα by reducing expression of TNF-α and iNOS	30 mM	Mice	Kim et al. (2007)
				10 mg/kg	Albino mice	Shukla et al. (2007)
				2.5 mM	Mice	Nigam et al. (2009)
				50 mg/kg	Sprague–Dawley rats	Li et al. (2017)
Capsaicin	–	Hot chilli pepper (*Capsicum annum*)	Suppression of NF-κB activation, inhibiting degradation of IκBα, blocking p65 nuclear translocation alleviate activation of AP-1	10 mg/kg	Swiss albino mice	Anandakumar et al. (2013)
				5 mg/kg	Wistar rats	Caetano et al. (2018)
				5 mg/kg	C57BL/6 mice	Venier et al. (2015)

(Continued)

TABLE 19.1 Different animal models and doses used for in vivo effect of phytochemicals in chemoprevention.—cont'd

Phytochemical	Chemical nature	Source	Mechanism of chemoprevention	Dose	Species used	References
Resveratrol	Stilbene	Grapes (*Vitis vinifera*), Japanese knotweed roots (*Polygonum cuspidatum*), berries, red wine, peanuts	CYP450 enzymes modulation, antioxidant, modulation of NF-κB, and inhibition of COX inflammation mediator enzymes	50, 100 or 300 mg/kg	Sprague–Dawley rats	Bishayee and Dhir (2009)
				100 mM	Syrian golden hamsters	Berta et al. (2010)
				1, 5, 10, or 25 mmol	Mice	Jang et al. (1997)
Lycopene	Carotenoid	Tomatoes, red papayas, watermelons, and red carrots	Promote ROS-generating proteins like CLIC-1, ERO-1 and stimulate antioxidants like SOD-1 and glutathione-S-transferase-omega-1	A diet containing 0.005% lycopene	Long-Evans Cinnamon (LEC) rat	Watanabe et al. (2001)
				0.5 and 1.0 mmol/kg	lacZ mouse	Guttenplan et al. (2001)
				70 mg/kg	Wistar rats	Toledo et al. (2003)
Caffeic acid phenethyl ester	Phenylpropane or cinnamic acid derivative	Propolis of honeybee hives extract	Cell transformation by suppressing the 12-*O*-tetradecanoylphorbol-13-acetate	15 mg/kg	Swiss mice	El-Refaei and El-Naa (2010)
				10 mg/kg	C57BL/6 mice	Pramanik et al. (2013)
				20 mg/kg	Wistar rats	Legleu et al. (2004)
Diallyl sulfide	Organo sulfide	Garlic (*Allium sativum)*	Modulate expression of p53mut, p21/Waf1, p53wt and p21/ras	250 μg	Swiss albino mice	Khan et al. (2007)
				1 mg/100 μL of acetone	SENCAR mice	Dwivedi et al. (1993)
				100, 200 and 400 mg/kg	Sprague–Dawley rats	Kim et al. (2014)
Genistein	Isoflavone	Soybeans, fava beans, lupine, psoralea, coffee, kudzu, and flemingia vestita	Inhibits DNA topoisomerase II, augments G2/M and G0/G1 arrest and inhibits Akt signaling pathway and NF-κB	250 mg/kg diet	Sprague–Dawley rats	Lamartiniere et al. (2002)
				250 mg/kg diet	Transgenic adenocarcinoma mouse prostate (TRAMP) mice	Wang et al. (2007)
				750 μg/g of diet	Athymic nude mice	Vantyghem et al. (2005)

TABLE 19.1 Different animal models and doses used for in vivo effect of phytochemicals in chemoprevention.—cont'd

Phytochemical	Chemical nature	Source	Mechanism of chemoprevention	Dose	Species used	References
Sulforaphane	Isothiocyanate	Broccoli, broccoli sprouts, kale, cabbage, cauliflower	Modulation of various events like cell death, susceptibility to carcinogens, angiogenesis, cell cycle, metastasis, and invasion	100 mg/kg	CD-1 mice	Harris et al. (2021)
				150 μmol	Sprague–Dawley rats	Cornblatt et al. (2007)
				200, 500, or 1000 μmol/kg	Fischer 344 rats	Matusheski and Jeffery (2002)
Vitamin D	–	Mushrooms	Modulate proliferation and differentiation-related genes, i.e., tumor-suppressor genes or proto-oncogenes	1000 IU/kg	Male mice	Aslam et al. (2021)
				0.3 μg/100 μL propylene glycol twice a week	Sprague–Dawley rats	Chatterjee et al. (2010)
				400 ng	Male rats	Belleli et al. (1993)

In a rat hepatocarcinogenesis model, resveratrol has upregulated hepatic Nrf2. Similarly, resveratrol has also been shown to suppress hepatic inducible nitric oxide synthase (iNOS), an inflammatory marker, as well as lower the quantity of 3-nitrotyrosine (3-NT)-containing proteins, which are markers of oxidative damage (Bishayee et al., 2010). Sulforaphane has been shown to enhance Nrf2-dependent expression of detoxifying phase I and II drug metabolizing enzymes and phase III transporters in the livers of C57BL/6J mice to protect against ROS-induced DNA and/or protein damage (Hu et al., 2006). Several studies have verified phytochemicals' antioxidant potential; nevertheless, additional research is needed to demonstrate phytochemicals' antioxidant potential and create therapeutically meaningful effects.

19.3.2 Phytochemicals and metastasis

Metastasis is the process of invading cancerous cells from the site of the primary tumor to the secondary site after a series of events such as tumor invasion, angiogenesis, endothelial-mesenchymal transition, etc. Due to complex interactions between tumor cells and their microenvironment at the secondary site, it's very challenging to target metastasized cells with current cancer therapy (Fidler and Kripke, 2015). Evidence from experimental and clinical studies of phytochemicals reveals that phytochemicals prevent metastasis in several cancers by simultaneously targeting different mechanisms.

In a recently published review, Kapinova et al. (2019) summarized the reports of several studies on phytochemicals in metastasis by targeting cell signaling pathways such as PI3K/Akt/mTOR signaling pathway, cysteine-rich angiogenic inducer 61, IL-6/JAK/STAT3 signaling pathway, etc. Imran et al. (2019b) detailed the anticancer property of kaempferol in several types of invasive and aggressive cancers like glioblastoma. Curcumin exhibits an anticarcinogenic effect by inhibiting PI3K phosphorylation, thereby impeding the phosphorylation of mTOR and NF-κB because of overexpression of the PI3K/Akt pathway has been linked to cancer progression (Xu et al., 2020).

Qingdu granule (QDG), traditional Chinese medicine, exerts an anti-angiogenic effect on breast cancer by preventing the NFAT pathway (Zhao et al., 2018). In another study, antitumorigenicity effects of Bupleuri Radix (BR) were investigated in reoccurrence and preventing progression of colonic polyps in colon cancer by inhibiting the angiogenin-2-induced protein kinase B (Ang PKB)/Akt signaling (Gao et al., 2020). Isothiocyanates from cruciferous vegetables have emerged as a strong anticancer agent in preventing bladder cancer by inducing apoptosis which is mediated via Caspase 8 and 9, as well as overexpression of Bax and downregulation of Bcl-2 (Flores-Pérez et al., 2019). However, there is an enormous need to conduct more studies to confirm the antimetastatic potential effects of phytochemicals and to achieve clinically beneficial results.

19.3.3 Phytochemicals and epigenetics

Epigenetic studies including phenotypic changes due to alterations in the genome but not in the sequence of DNA. Epigenetic changes of the genome play a crucial role in genomic instability in cancer etiology, thus leading to the aberrations of the genetic material and thereby causing the activation of oncogenes and silencing of the tumor suppressor genes (Wu et al., 2015). Epigenetic regulation of genes is imperative for a cell's normal functioning. However, aberrant epigenetic changes in the genome have long been documented in multiple cancer research studies. Histone modifications and DNA methylation, two fundamental epigenetic alterations, have been discovered to have a significant impact on many malignancies. Emerging evidence suggests the association between modifications in DNA methylation patterns and cancer pathophysiology (Klutstein et al., 2016).

Several studies have been performed to understand the role of epigenetic modifications in the pathogenesis of different cancers. Natural compounds significantly prevent deleterious epigenetic alterations in genes and can act as anticancer agents. Furthermore, phytochemicals with anticancer activity have a synergistic impact with anticancer medicines and help to reduce the adverse effects of medications.

19.4 Dietary phytochemicals used for chemoprevention

Some specific examples of dietary phytochemicals that have been in use for the purpose of preventing cancers because of their potential cancer chemopreventive role are discussed in the following subsections.

19.4.1 Epigallocatechin gallate (EGCG)

Epigallocatechin-3-gallate (EGCG) is the most abundant catechin in green tea and shows an anticancer effect. EGCG showed its anticancer effect by preventing DNA damage, cell signaling pathway alterations, oxidative stress, and mutation caused by UV radiation and reactive oxygen species (Rizeq et al., 2020; Seeram et al., 2006). Previous literature reported the efficacy of EGCG in inhibiting angiogenesis and tumor proliferation in in vitro and in vivo studies for various cancers like esophagus, head, neck, lung, prostate, breast, and colon cancer (M et al., 2012; Yuan, 2011).

One study investigated the prevention of DNA damage and DNA migration in inner organs and lymphocytes by green tea extract. In this study, low and high dose of green tea extract was consumed, and DNA damage was evaluated by COMET assay in colonocytes, lymphocytes, and hepatocytes. This study suggested that the DNA damage was prevented by the high dose of green tea extract, which is equivalent to 500 mL of green tea consumption per day (Kager et al., 2009). In another study, treating a breast epithelial cell line (MCF10A) with EGCG induces the expression of manganese superoxide dismutase, glutamate-cysteine ligase, and heme oxygenase-1. EGCG treatment also enhances nuclear accumulation, transcriptional activity, and antioxidant response element (ARE) binding of NF-E2 related factor (Nrf2) as Nrf2 controls the ARE-mediated expression of detoxifying enzymes and antioxidants. It also activates extracellular signal-regulated protein kinase1/2 (ERK1/2) and Akt. This study suggested that the EGCG treatment induces the expression of antioxidant enzymes with the help of Nrf2 via ERK1/2 and Akt signaling and prevents the cells from oxidative stress (Na et al., 2008).

19.4.2 Curcumin

Curcumin is a yellow-colored phytochemical that is abundantly present in turmeric (*Curcuma longa*) of the ginger family (Zingiberaceae). Curcumin consists of two phenolic rings (with a methoxyl group and a hydroxyl group attached to each ring) linked by seven carbon chains having α- and β-diketone components. These phenolic rings are mainly responsible for the antioxidant activity, and β-diketone components are responsible for forming chelating complexes with metals to prevent heavy metal poisoning (Priyadarsini, 2012).

Turmeric protects the cells from oxidative stress causing DNA damage and suppresses tumor proliferation. One study revealed the antitumor effects of the topical application of curcumin on female ICR mice (Chun et al., 2003). It was observed that the topical application of 12-O-tetradecanoylphorbol-13-acetate (TPA) induces the mRNA and protein expression of Cox-2. Prior application of curcumin inhibited this TPA-induced Cox-2 expression in a dose-related manner. Decreased Cox-2 expression in the epidermal layer by curcumin treatment was analyzed by immunohistochemical analysis. Activation of NF-κB stimulated by TPA was also attenuated by curcumin treatment (Chun et al., 2003).

Curcumin can also be helpful in the treatment of metabolic diseases like arteriosclerosis, diabetes, metabolic syndrome, and other inflammatory diseases (Ruiz and Hernández, 2016). Curcumin showed its anticancer effect through various pathways. Activating detoxifying enzymes like p21, glutathione-S-transferase was elevated by curcumin-inhibited cell proliferation (Ye et al., 2007). It also inhibits the antiapoptotic proteins like Bcl-xL and Bcl-

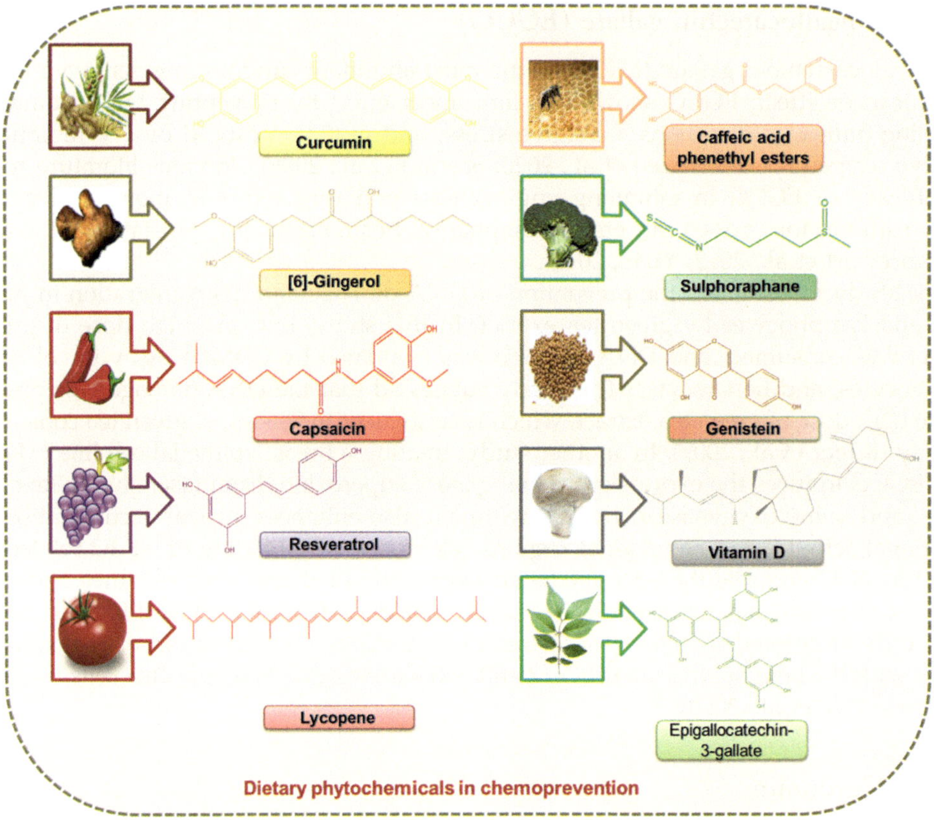

FIGURE 19.2 Various phytochemicals having a role in chemoprevention.

2 and pro-apoptotic proteins like Bim, Noxa, Bak, and Bax expression (Chen et al., 2011). Metastases development was prevented by reducing the expression of matrix metalloproteases and VEGF (Durko and Malecka-Panas, 2014). Fig. 19.2 illustrates various phytochemicals having a role in chemoprevention.

Carroll et al. (2011) reported the phase IIa clinical trial studies of curcumin's effect on preventing adenomas and aberrant crypt foci (ACF) in colorectal carcinogenesis. The authors performed this study with two oral doses, i.e., 2 and 4 gm, for 30 days. In preclinical studies, the decline in 5-hydroxyeicosatetraenoic acid (5-HETE) due to 5-lipoxygenase inhibition and decline in prostaglandin E2 (PGE2) due to cyclooxygenases 1 and 2 inhibition was observed. A nonrandomized, open-label clinical trial was performed on 44 eligible smokers having eight or more ACF in colonoscopy screening. After oral administration of 2 and 4 g doses, the effect of curcumin was evaluated on 5-HETE, PGE2 within ACF, ACF proliferation, and number. The 4 g dose reduced the ACF number by 40%, and no ACF number reduction was observed with the 2 g dose. Post-treatment plasma curcumin/conjugate levels were increased significantly by fivefold with the ACF reduction after a 4 g dose (Carroll et al., 2011).

19.4.3 [6]-Gingerol and capsaicin

[6]-Gingerol, a phenolic compound and the active component of ginger (Zingiber officinale Roscoe), is responsible for the spiciness of ginger. Ginger showed its chemoprotective or anticancer effect in different tumors like ovarian, breast, pancreas, and colon (H et al., 2012). [6]-Gingerol shows anti-inflammatory, antioxidant, and antitumor or chemoprotective effects. [6]-Gingerol suppresses nuclear translocation of nuclear factor-kappa (NF-κB) and phosphorylation of I kappa B alpha (IκBα) by reducing the expression of tumor necrosis factor-alpha (TNF-α) and inducible nitric oxide synthase (iNOS). [6]-Gingerol induces apoptosis and shows antiproliferative action by other mechanisms, like enhancing apoptotic protease-activating factor-1 (Apaf-1), activating caspases, and releasing cytochrome *c* (Oyagbemi et al., 2010).

In another study, the anti-invasive effect of [6]-gingerol and [6]-shogaol was evaluated in hepatoma cells. Phorbol 12-myristate 13-acetate (PMA) enhanced the invasion and migration of Hep3B cells. This study reported the reduction in invasive and migratory ability of PMA-treated and untreated Hep3B cells in a dose-dependent manner with [6]-gingerol and [6]-shogaol treatment. This treatment increases tissue inhibitor metalloproteinase protein (TIMP)-1 expression and decreases the activity of matrix metalloproteinase (MMP)-9 in PMA-treated and untreated cells. This study suggested the anti-invasive role of [6]-gingerol and [6]-shogaol in hepatoma cells by regulating TIMP-1 and MMP-9 (Weng et al., 2010).

Capsaicin is a pungent constituent in the hot chili pepper (*Capsicum annum* L.). Firstly, it was reported as a carcinogen due to its irritant properties, but later this component was observed as a chemoprotective component (Surh, 2003b). After capsaicin treatment, NF-κB activation was suppressed by inhibiting the degradation of IκBα and blocking p65 nuclear translocation in HL-60 cells (human promyelocytic leukemia cells). Capsaicin treatment also alleviates the activation of activator protein-1 (AP-1) induced by TPA (Han et al., 2002). IL-8 expression induced by TNF-α and IL-1β was inhibited due to the inhibition of NF-κB by capsaicin treatment in melanoma cells. Capsaicin showed its effect depending on the dose and treatment duration. Electrophoretic mobility shift assay (EMSA) demonstrated the upregulation of AP-1 and NF-κB by IL-1β treatment, and capsaicin inhibited the NF-κB activation induced by IL-1β, leading to IL-8 expression inhibition. This IL-8 expression downregulation by capsaicin treatment in melanoma cells also inhibits in vitro cell proliferation (Patel et al., 2002).

19.4.4 Resveratrol

Resveratrol is a naturally occurring phytoalexin in various plants, grapes (*Vitis vinifera*), Japanese knotweed roots (*Polygonum cuspidatum*), berries, red wine, and peanuts. The chemical name of resveratrol is trans-3,4,5-trihydroxystilbene. Environmental stress conditions like chemical exposure, UV radiations, and fungal and viral infections stimulate the synthesis of resveratrol in plants as their protective mechanism (Dave et al., 2020). Resveratrol got popular for chemoprevention activity due to the "French paradox" that showed that the mortality rate due to cardiovascular diseases was reduced by red wine consumption even with diet consumption containing rich saturated fat (Scott et al., 2012).

Resveratrol showed chemoprotective activity by various mechanisms like cytochrome P450 family enzymes modulation, antioxidation, modulation of transcription factors like NF-κB, and inhibition of COX inflammation mediator enzymes (Gescher et al., 2013; Ruiz and Hernández, 2016). Resveratrol showed anti-inflammatory effects mediated anti-promotion activity, phase II metabolizing enzymes induced anti-initiation activity, cell differentiation induced anti-progression activity in human promyelocytic leukemia, hydroperoxides, and cyclooxygenase inhibiting functions (H et al., 2012).

As small noncoding RNA, miRNAs have a crucial role in gene silencing and regulation; therefore, the effect of resveratrol on miRNA in cancer was evaluated. It was reported that the miR-34c was downregulated in colon cancer, and tumor proliferation gene repression occurred by restoring this microRNA, leading to reduced malignant growth (Patel et al., 2010; Arya and Saldanha, 2019). The miR-34c level was upregulated by resveratrol treatment to HT-29 and HCT-116 CRC cells, which led to a decline in cellular proliferation (Yang et al., 2015). The effect of resveratrol was evaluated on the $JAK2^{V617F}$ mutant tumor cells having excessive JAK2 pathway activation. It was observed that the resveratrol induces apoptosis and inhibits proliferation in the $JAK2^{V617F}$ mutant cells and the effect of resveratrol on mutant cells was 1.5–6.9 times greater than the other cells. Resveratrol also inhibits the phosphorylation of Tyk2, JAK1, and JAK2 and their downstream mediators, like STAT3 and STAT5. Resveratrol also showed a synergistic effect with another JAK2 inhibitor, ruxolitinib, and eliminated JAK2 mutant tumor cells (Trung et al., 2015).

19.4.5 Lycopene

Lycopene is a naturally occurring carotenoid with red color. It is extracted from various fruits and vegetables like tomatoes, red papayas, watermelons, red carrots, etc., but a high concentration is found in tomatoes (H et al., 2012). Lycopene caused a reduction in intracellular reactive oxygen species by promoting ROS-generating proteins like CLIC-1 and ERO-1 and stimulating antioxidants like superoxide dismutase-1 (SOD-1) and glutathione-S-transferase-omega-1 (Rizeq et al., 2020). Lycopene has 11 conjugated double bonds in the chromatophore, and this conjugated polyene structure is responsible for its antioxidant properties (Clinton, 1998).

Holzapfel et al. (2017) used an intraperitoneal animal model to evaluate the role of lycopene in ovarian cancer prevention and treatment. In preventing ovarian cancer, lycopene decreases the metastatic load, and lycopene reduces the tumor burden for treating recognized tumors. Lycopene also synergized the antitumor effect of carboplatin and paclitaxel. A reduction in the number of proliferating cancer cells was revealed by the immunostaining of metastatic tissues and tumors for Ki67. CA125, an ovarian cancer biomarker expression, was also reduced by the lycopene treatment. Downregulation of various markers like EMT, MMP9, ILK, ITGA, FAK, and ITGB, decreased MAPK activation and reduced integrin α5 protein expression showed antiproliferative and antimetastatic effects. This study revealed the role of lycopene as a preventive and therapeutic agent for ovarian cancer by interfering with the growth and progression mechanism. Table 19.1 demonstrates the different species and doses used in in vivo studies for the chemopreventive role of various phytochemicals.

Another study evaluated the potential of lycopene treatment in preventing the development and progression of colorectal cancer in a mouse xenograft model (Tang et al., 2011).

Development and progression of colon cancer in mice were suppressed and indicated by various methods such as histopathological, bioluminescence, immunohistochemical, and immunofluorescence imaging. Lycopene treatment significantly decreased the β-catenin protein and PCNA nuclear expression in tumor tissues. Lycopene increased the nuclear level of p21(CIP1/WAF1), a cell cycle inhibitor protein, and also increased the E-cadherin adherent molecule. Phosphorylated ERK1/2 proteins, PGE(2), and COX-2 levels were also suppressed for the chemoprotection role of the lycopene in the mouse xenograft model (Tang et al., 2011).

A study aiming at the identification of potential preventive role of lycopene for radiation-induced acute esophageal toxicity in rats revealed that the lycopene administration before and after radiotherapy decreased inflammation, vacuole formation, regeneration-mitosis, intraepithelial degenerative changes-necrosis, and subepithelial bulla formation (Coskun et al., 2017).

19.4.6 Caffeic acid phenethyl ester

Caffeic acid phenethyl ester (CAPE) is a phytochemical obtained from the propolis of honeybee hives extract. 2-phenylethyl (2*E*)-3-(3,4-dihydroxyphenyl) acrylate is the chemical name of CAPE, and it is also known as phenethyl caffeate or phenylethyl caffeate. CAPE is an effective bioactive compound for various conditions like inflammation, oxidative stress, infections, diabetes, anxiety, cancer, and neurodegeneration (Murtaza et al., 2014).

Nomura et al. (2001) reported that caffeic acid phenethyl ester prevents cell proliferation and induces apoptosis in cells for chemoprevention. The mechanism of chemoprevention by CAPE is not well known, but this study suggested that the CAPE causes suppression of cell transformation by suppressing the 12-*O*-tetradecanoylphorbol-13-acetate and also induces cell apoptosis. They evaluated the pathway for apoptosis caused by CAPE and suggested that CAPE can induce apoptosis by either the p-53 dependent pathway or the p-53 independent pathway. Caspase-3 cleavage and DNA fragmentation also happened by CAPE treatment in p-53 deficient and p-53 mutant cell lines (Nomura et al., 2001).

The role of CAPE in the chemoprevention of liver cancer was evaluated and found as a promising chemoprotection compound for liver cancer (Beltrán-Ramírez et al., 2012). In this study, a resistant hepatocyte model of hepatocarcinogenesis was used, and this showed the role of CYP metabolizing enzymes in the chemoprevention by CAPE. CAPE was administered twelve-hour before diethylnitrosamine administration to the male Fischer-344 rats and then sacrificed to identify which CYP enzymes were involved in the neoplastic and preneoplastic lesions prevention. CYP inhibitors SKF525A or α-napthoflavone were also administered to other rats and then sacrificed. Western blotting was used to measure the protein in the microsomes removed from the livers. GGT histochemistry was done for liver histology, and nitrite formation quantified the metabolism of diethylnitrosamine. CYP1A2 and CYP2B1/2 protein levels were decreased due to CAPE, and microsomal assays also confirmed that, like SKF525A, diethylnitrosamine activation was interfered with by CAPE, and inhibition of CYP2B1/2 might be involved in this interference. In conclusion, this study revealed a 43% reduction in tumor appearance by CAPE single-dose administration before diethylnitrosamine (Beltrán-Ramírez et al., 2012).

19.4.7 Diallyl sulfide

Various health benefits of garlic (*Allium sativum*) were reported as a medicinal plant like antimicrobial, lipid-lowering, anticarcinogen, and chemopreventive effects. Organosulfide-based active compounds like diallyl sulfide (DAS) present in garlic are responsible for chemopreventive and antitumor activity. DAS is an organosulfur volatile compound with a characteristic pungent odor. DAS has various therapeutic properties like anti-inflammatory, antioxidant, anticancer, and antimutagenic effects (Agarwal, 1996; Pinto and Rivlin, 2001).

Khan et al. (2007) assessed the chemopreventive role of liposomal DAS for the dimethylbenz(a)anthracene (DMBA) induced skin papilloma. Liposomal formulations were applied topically thrice weekly, 1 h before the DMBA exposure, and treatment was continued for 12 weeks. Tumor nodules number, size, and tumorogenesis incidence parameters were used to assess the efficacy and potential of liposomal DAS. A few markers like p21/Waf1, p52mut, and p53wt were also used to evaluate the efficacy of liposomal DAS. Liposomal DAS formulation reduced the expression of p53mut and increased the expression of p21/Waf1 and p53wt. Reduced number and tumor size were observed, and delayed tumorigenesis onset demonstrated it as an effective treatment for controlling skin papilloma (Khan et al., 2007).

As p21/ras protein, a gene product of H-ras, has a role in the mechanism of chemoprevention in the mouse skin tumor, the effect of DAS on the expression of p21/ras was evaluated (Arora et al., 2006). This study demonstrated the modulation of DMBA-induced p21/ras levels after DAS administration. Cytosolic p21/ras levels were increased by DAS treatment, but the p21/ras levels in membrane fraction were decreased. Skin/tumor immunohistochemical staining demonstrated a 55.82% and 46.86% decline in the expression of p21/ras levels after pre- and post-DAS supplemented groups, respectively. H-ras mRNA level induced by DMBA was also decreased by DAS treatment. This study proposed the modulation of p21/ras protein as an effective mechanism for the suppression of growth and progression of tumors (Arora et al., 2006).

19.4.8 Genistein and sulforaphane

Genistein is a naturally occurring isoflavone that is extracted from various plants like fava beans, lupine, soybeans, Psoralea, coffee, kudzu, and flemingia vestita. Genistein shows various properties like antihelmintic, antioxidant, and antiangiogenic. Genistein inhibits the uncontrolled cell growth of cancer cells by inhibiting various enzymes responsible for cell survival and growth. Genistein inhibited DNA topoisomerase II and showed activity as a tyrosine kinase inhibitor (López-Lázaro and Willmore, 2007). Genistein augments G2/M and G0/G1 arrest. It inhibits the Akt signaling pathway and NF-κB to regulate the cell cycle and apoptosis of several cancer cell lines like breast, prostate, and lung cancer. Genistein increased the expression of pro-apoptotic Bad, Bak, and Bax proteins and decreased the expression of anti-apoptotic Bcl-2 and BcL-XL proteins (Banerjee et al., 2008).

It was observed that the risk of breast cancer was less due to the high level of genistein exposure in the traditional East Asian diets. It may also have a role in preventing inflammatory bowel diseases (IBD). 2,4,6-trinitrobenzene sulfonic acid (TNBS) induced chronic colitis rat model was used to investigate the influence of oral genistein on the inflammatory responses. Myeloperoxidase (MPO) and cyclooxygenase-2 (COX-2), biochemical and molecular inflammatory markers, were evaluated. Sexual organs like seminal vesicles and prostrate wet weight were compared to investigate the effect of genistein treatment. MPO activity was reduced, and COX-2 mRNA and protein expression was also decreased after the genistein treatment. Genistein administration also decreased the wet weight of seminal vesicles and prostates. In conclusion, this study demonstrated the role of oral genistein as an anti-inflammatory agent for TNBS-induced chronic colitis (Seibel et al., 2009).

Another study was performed to evaluate the antitumor effects of the genistein and the mechanism involved in the antitumor effect. MTT assay on HCT-116 cells was used to investigate the influence of genistein on cell proliferation, and flow cytometry was used to measure apoptosis. The effect of genistein on the expression of various markers like Akt, miR-95, and SGK1 was evaluated using real-time PCR, and Western blot evaluated the protein levels of phosphorylated Akt (P-Akt) and total Akt (T-Akt). Cell proliferation was inhibited, and apoptosis was induced in HCT-116 cells after treating the cells with genistein. miR-95, SGK1, and Akt mRNA expression were also downregulated, and Akt phosphorylation was inhibited. Xenograft tumor growth in mice was also inhibited in in vivo studies. Therefore, this study demonstrated the potential role of genistein in inhibiting colorectal cancer (Qin et al., 2015).

Sulforaphane (1-isothiocyanate-(4R)-(methylsulfonyl) butane) is an isothiocyanate phytochemical with anti-carcinogenic properties, and it is found in cruciferous vegetables like kale, cabbage, cauliflower, broccoli, and broccoli sprouts. It aids in the modulation of various cancer processes such as cell death, susceptibility to carcinogens, angiogenesis, cell cycle, metastasis, and invasion (Zhang and Tang, 2007). Epidemiological studies suggested a reduction in the risk of breast cancer by enhanced fluid intake and cruciferous vegetable consumption, especially broccoli. One study showed that two or more servings of broccoli reduced the risk of breast cancer by 39% (Leone et al., 2017). It has antiproliferative, anticancer, and antioxidant properties and has shown a chemopreventive role in various cancers like breast, renal, lung, colon, and prostate cancer (Jiang et al., 2018).

Cornblatt et al. (2007) investigated the chemopreventive effect of sulforaphane on the mammary tissue of animals and humans. A 150 mmol dose was used orally to evaluate the pharmacokinetics and pharmacodynamics of sulforaphane in the rat mammary gland. The quantitative real-time polymerase chain reaction was used to investigate the increased level of cytoprotective heme oxygenase-1 (HO-1) and NAD(P)H: quinine oxidoreductase (NQO1) gene transcripts. A fourfold increase in immunostaining of HO-1 and elevated enzyme activity of NQO1 by threefold demonstrated the potential pharmacodynamic effect of sulforaphane. In the human study, 200 mmol of sulforaphane containing one dose of broccoli sprout was given orally to 8 healthy women, and significant metabolites were observed in the epithelial cells enriched breast tissues. This study revealed the chemopreventive role of broccoli sprouts in women having a risk for breast cancer (Cornblatt et al., 2007).

19.4.9 Vitamin D from mushroom

As vitamin D is generated in the skin of vertebrates by ultraviolet B-light exposure, similarly mushrooms exposed to UV light are an excellent alternative for Vitamin D. It has a role in different cancer like ovarian, breast, pancreatic, and colon cancer. Its role in cancer is still unclear, but vitamin D receptors (VDR) involvement is the most proposed one. It was observed that VDR gene mutation enhanced the breast cancer risk in women, so VDR can be used as a target to prevent or treat breast cancer (Chen et al., 2005b; Garland et al., 2007). Proliferation and differentiation-related genes, i.e., tumor-suppressor genes or proto-oncogenes, are repressed or activated in the tumor and normal tissues by the Vitamin-D treatment. Various encoding genes include transforming growth factor-β (TGF-β) family members, c-MYC, c-FOS, PLCγ, KIP1, WAF1, c-JUN, cyclin C, tenascin, laminin, and fibronectin (Lamprecht and Lipkin, 2003).

A multi-center, placebo-controlled randomized clinical trial was performed on 803 subjects to evaluate the autonomous and joint effects of vitamin D and calcium supplementation on the recurrence of colorectal adenoma. The polymerase chain reaction was used to investigate the Fok 1 and Taq 1 polymorphism in the VDR and serum levels of 1,25-dihydroxy [1,25-(OH)2] vitamin D and 25-hydroxy [25-(OH)] vitamin D. Evaluation of the risk ratio for recurrence of adenoma was done and association of risk recurrence with VDR polymorphism was also investigated. Recurrence of adenoma was not associated with the calcium supplementation in the subjects having baseline or below median 25-(OH) vitamin D levels. Still, the risk reduction was associated with calcium supplementation in subjects with levels above the median. The VDR polymorphism did not influence the recurrence of adenoma, and the association of recurrence with calcium supplementation and vitamin D was also not influenced by the VDR polymorphism. This study revealed that vitamin D and calcium supplementation could decrease the recurrence risk for colorectal adenoma (Grau et al., 2004).

Another study demonstrated the relationship between calcium, vitamin D, and retinol dietary intake to the risk for pancreatic cancer. A prospective study was performed on 75,427 women 38–65 years of age as of 1984 and 46,771 men 40–75 years of age as of 1986, and the incidence of pancreatic cancer was documented through the year 2000. A total of 365 pancreatic cancer cases were reported over 16 years of a prospective study. It was observed that the risk of pancreatic cancer was less in subjects with higher vitamin D intake than in subjects with the lowest vitamin D intake. Men showed a stronger relationship between vitamin D intake to pancreatic cancer than women. This study revealed no association between retinol and calcium intake and the risk of pancreatic cancer. So this study demonstrated the potential role of vitamin D in the chemoprevention of pancreatic cancer (Skinner et al., 2006).

19.5 Future directions

To control and manage cancer, chemoprotective phytochemicals are an efficient, inexpensive, readily acceptable, accessible, and practical alternative. Compared to expensive chemotherapeutics, phytochemicals are an economical approach to prevent cancer. Some phytochemicals showed their chemoprotective role in a cell line or tissues at a specific concentration, but sometimes diet might not be able to provide such concentration. So, bioavailability and pharmacokinetics are critical points to be assessed carefully while performing intervention trials with phytochemicals. With more advanced techniques, the evaluation of SNPs helps in the investigation of a specific gene that is responsible for changes that happen in carcinogenesis. In the future, we can investigate the combination of dietary supplements that can modify the high-risk groups identified by the detection techniques of SNPs (Surh, 2003b).

In the future, the nanotechnology approach can increase the efficiency of the phytochemicals for chemoprotective applications. It will overcome the bioavailability and pharmacokinetics-related challenges. Targeting also can be an effective approach in the near future to increase the efficacy of phytochemicals (Jain et al., 2021). Phytochemicals or dietary supplements showed variation in their action according to the individual genotype, so combining supplements can be a better alternate for chemoprotective roles (Liskova et al., 2020).

In most clinical trials, cancer incidence is selected as the primary endpoint to investigate the role of phytochemicals in cancer prevention. The period from cancer progression to detectable cancer is too long, and no study or trial has the research infrastructure or financial budget to complete the trials for decades. So, by changing how clinical trials are conducted, we can enhance the success rate of the clinical trial. Instead of keeping cancer incidence as the primary endpoint, if the investigator detects the changes that occurred in the gene in cancer progression and taking these biomarkers as endpoints will increase the success rate of clinical trials and also help in the early detection of cancer. Potential biomarkers of carcinogenesis can be easily identified by high throughput screening methods, like transcriptomics, genomics, metabolomics, and proteomics (Kotecha et al., 2016).

19.6 Conclusion

Rising cancer rates and accompanying mortalities have emerged as the most severe challenge in cancer therapy, despite advancements in prognosis, diagnosis, and treatment. The problems connected with chemotherapeutic medications have been worsened by cytotoxicity and nontarget specificity. To counteract the adverse effects of chemotherapy, dietary phytochemicals have emerged as effective pharmacophores in cancer treatments. Using phytochemicals, either alone or in combination, may help in cancer chemoprevention. However, future research should identify the role of phytochemicals in cancer development.

19.7 List of abbreviations

5-HETE 5-hydroxyeicosatetraenoic acid
ACF Aberrant crypt foci
Akt AKT serine/threonine kinase 1
Ang PKB Angiogenin-2-induced protein kinase B
AP-1 Activator protein-1
Apaf-1 Apoptotic protease-activating factor-1
BR Bupleuri Radix
CAPE Caffeic acid phenethyl ester
Cox-2 Cyclooxygenase-2
DAS Diallyl sulfide
DMBA Dimethylbenz(a)anthracene
DNA Deoxyribonucleic acid
EGCG Epigallocatechin-3-gallate
EMSA Electrophoretic mobility shift assay:
EMT Epithelial-to-mesenchymal transition

ERK1/2 Extracellular signal-regulated protein kinase1/2
GGT Gamma-glutamyl transferase
HO-1 Heme oxygenasee-1
HOTAIR HOX antisense intergenic RNA
IBD Inflammatory bowel disease
IL-1β Interleukin 1 beta
IL-6 Interleukin 6
iNOS inducible nitric oxide synthase
IκBα I kappa B alpha
JAK Janus Activated Kinase
LINC01116 Long intergenic nonprotein coding RNA 1116
LncRNA Long non coding RNAs
MALAT1 Metastasis associated lung adenocarcinoma transcript 1
MAPK Mitogen activated protein kinase
miRNA Micro Ribonucleic Acid
MMP-9 Metalloproteinase
MPO Myeloperoxidase
mTOR Mammalian target of rapamycin
MTT 3-(4,5-Dimethylthiazol-2-yl)-2,5-Diphenyltetrazolium Bromide
NEAT1 Nuclear Enriched Abundant Transcript 1
NF- κB Nuclear factor kappa light chain enhancer of activated B cells
NFAT Nuclear factor of activated T-cells
NQO1 NAD(P)H:quinine oxidoreductase
NSCLC Non-small cell lung carcinoma
PANDAR P21-associated ncRNA DNA damage-activated RNA
PCNA Proliferating cell nuclear antigen
PGE2 Prostaglandin E2
PI3K Phosphoinositide 3-kinase
PMA Phorbol 12-myristate 13-acetate
QDG Qingdu granule
ROS Reactive oxygen species
SFN Sulforaphane
SOD-1 Superoxide dismutase-1
STAT3 Signal transducer and activator of transcription 3
TGF-β Transforming growth factor-β
TIMP tissue inhibitor metalloproteinase protein
TNBS 2,4,6-trinitrobenzenesulfonic acid
TNF-α Tumor necrosis factor-alpha
TPA 12-O-tetradecanoylphorbol-13-acetate
UV Ultraviolet
VDR Vitamin D receptors
VEGF Vascular endothelial growth factor
Wnt Wingless-related integration site

References

Agarwal, K., 1996. Therapeutic actions of garlic constituents. Med. Res. Rev. 16, 111–124.

Anandakumar, P., Kamaraj, S., Jagan, S., Ramakrishnan, G., Devaki, T., 2013. Capsaicin provokes apoptosis and restricts benzo(a)pyrene induced lung tumorigenesis in Swiss albino mice. Int. Immunopharm. 17, 254–259.

Arora, A., Kalra, N., Shukla, Y., 2006. Regulation of p21/ras protein expression by diallyl sulfide in DMBA induced neoplastic changes in mouse skin. Cancer Lett. 242, 28–36.

Arya, R., Saldanha, S., 2019. Dietary Phytochemicals, Epigenetics, and Colon Cancer Chemoprevention, pp. 205–229.

Aslam, A., Ahmad, J., Baghdadi, M.A., Idris, S., Almaimani, R., Alsaegh, A., Alhadrami, M., Refaat, B., 2021. Chemopreventive effects of vitamin D3 and its analogue, paricalcitol, in combination with 5-fluorouracil against colorectal cancer: the role of calcium signalling molecules. Biochim. Biophys. Acta (BBA) - Mol. Basis Dis. 1867, 166040.

Banerjee, S., Li, Y., Wang, Z., Sarkar, F., 2008. Multi-targeted therapy of cancer by genistein. Cancer Lett. 269, 226–242.

Beaver, L.M., Kuintzle, R., Buchanan, A., Wiley, M.W., Glasser, S.T., Wong, C.P., Johnson, G.S., Chang, J.H., Löhr, C.V., Williams, D.E., 2017. Long non-coding RNAs and sulforaphane: a target for chemoprevention and suppression of prostate cancer. J. Nutr. Biochem. 42, 72–83.

Belleli, A., Shany, S., Levy, J., Guberman, R., Lamprecht, S., 1993. A protective role of 1,25-dihydroxyvitamin D3 in chemically induced rat colon carcinogenesis. Carcinogenesis 13, 2293–2298.

Beltrán-Ramírez, O., Pérez, R., Sierra-Santoyo, A., Villa-Treviño, S., 2012. Cancer prevention mediated by caffeic acid phenethyl ester involves Cyp2b1/2 modulation in hepatocarcinogenesis. Toxicol. Pathol. 40, 466–472.

Berta, G.N., Salamone, P., Sprio, A.E., DI Scipio, F., Marinos, L.M., Sapino, S., Carlotti, M.E., Cavalli, R., DI Carlo, F., 2010. Chemoprevention of 7,12-dimethylbenz[a]anthracene (DMBA)-induced oral carcinogenesis in hamster cheek pouch by topical application of resveratrol complexed with 2-hydroxypropyl-β-cyclodextrin. Oral Oncol. 46, 42–48.

Billerey-Larmonier, C., Uno, J.K., Larmonier, N., Midura, A.J., Timmermann, B., Ghishan, F.K., Kiela, P.R., 2008. Protective effects of dietary curcumin in mouse model of chemically induced colitis are strain dependent. Inflamm. Bowel Dis. 14, 780–793.

Bishayee, A., Barnes, K.F., Bhatia, D., Darvesh, A.S., Carroll, R.T., 2010. Resveratrol suppresses oxidative stress and inflammatory response in diethylnitrosamine-initiated rat hepatocarcinogenesis. Cancer Prev. Res. 3, 753–763.

Bishayee, A., Dhir, N., 2009. Resveratrol-mediated chemoprevention of diethylnitrosamine-initiated hepatocarcinogenesis: inhibition of cell proliferation and induction of apoptosis. Chem. Biol. Interact. 179, 131–144.

Caetano, B.F.R., Tablas, M.B., Pereira, N.E.F., DE Moura, N.A., Carvalho, R.F., Rodrigues, M.A.M., Barbisan, L.F., 2018. Capsaicin reduces genotoxicity, colonic cell proliferation and preneoplastic lesions induced by 1,2-dimethylhydrazine in rats. Toxicol. Appl. Pharmacol. 338, 93–102.

Carroll, R., Benya, R., Turgeon, D., Vareed, S., Neuman, M., Rodriguez, L., Carpenter, P., Mclaren, C., Meyskens, F., Brenner, D., 2011. Phase IIA clinical trial of curcumin for the prevention of colorectal neoplasia. Cancer Prev. Res. 4, 354–364.

Chatterjee, M., Janarthan, M., Manivannan, R., Rana, A., Chatterjee, M., 2010. Combinatorial effect of fish oil (Maxepa) and 1α,25-dihydroxyvitamin D3 in the chemoprevention of DMBA-induced mammary carcinogenesis in rats. Chem. Biol. Interact. 188, 102–110.

Chen, C.-Y., Jang, J.-H., Li, M.-H., Surh, Y.-J., 2005a. Resveratrol upregulates heme oxygenase-1 expression via activation of NF-E2-related factor 2 in PC12 cells. Biochem. Biophys. Res. Commun. 331, 993–1000.

Chen, C., Liu, Y., Chen, Y., Xu, J., 2011. C086, a novel analog of curcumin, induces growth inhibition and down-regulation of NFκB in colon cancer cells and xenograft tumors. Cancer Biol. Ther. 12, 797–807.

Chen, W., Bertone-Johnson, E., Hunter, D., Willett, W., Hankinson, S., 2005b. Associations between polymorphisms in the vitamin D receptor and breast cancer risk. Cancer Epidemiol. Biomarkers Prev. 14, 2335–2339.

Chikara, S., Nagaprashantha, L.D., Singhal, J., Horne, D., Awasthi, S., Singhal, S.S., 2018. Oxidative stress and dietary phytochemicals: role in cancer chemoprevention and treatment. Cancer Lett. 413, 122–134.

Chun, K.-S., Keum, Y.-S., Han, S., Song, Y.-S., Kim, S.S., Surh, Y.-J., 2003. Curcumin inhibits phorbol ester-induced expression of cyclooxygenase-2 in mouse skin through suppression of extracellular signal-regulated kinase activity and NF KB activation. Carcinogenesis 24, 1515–1524.

Clinton, S., 1998. Lycopene: chemistry, biology, and implications for human health and disease. Nutr. Rev. 56, 35–51.

Cornblatt, B.S., Ye, L., Dinkova-Kostova, A.T., Erb, M., Fahey, J.W., Singh, N.K., Chen, M.-S.A., Stierer, T., Garrett-Mayer, E., Argani, P., Davidson, N.E., Talalay, P., Kensler, T.W., Visvanathan, K., 2007. Preclinical and clinical evaluation of sulforaphane for chemoprevention in the breast. Carcinogenesis 28, 1485–1490.

Coskun, H., Andic, F., Daglioglu, Y., Doran, F., Sahin, K., Tunali, C., Kucuk, O., 2017. Lycopene in the prevention of radiation-induced esophagitis. Nutr. Cancer 69, 1–11.

Darweish, M.M., Abbas, A., Ebrahim, M.A., AL-Gayyar, M.M.H., 2014. Chemopreventive and hepatoprotective effects of Epigallocatechin-gallate against hepatocellular carcinoma: role of heparan sulfate proteoglycans pathway. J. Pharm. Pharmacol. 66, 1032–1045.

Dave, A., Parande, F., Park, E.-J., Pezzuto, J.M., 2020. Phytochemicals and cancer chemoprevention. J. Cancer Metastasis Treatment 2020.

Durko, L., Malecka-Panas, E., 2014. Lifestyle modifications and colorectal cancer. Curr. Color. Cancer Rep. 10, 45–54.

Dwivedi, C., Rohlfs, S., Jarvis, D., Engineer, F., 1993. Chemoprevention of chemically induced skin tumor development by diallyl sulfide and diallyl disulfide. Pharmaceut. Res. 9, 1668–1670.

EL-Refaei, M.F., EL-Naa, M.M., 2010. Inhibitory effect of caffeic acid phenethyl ester on mice bearing tumor involving angiostatic and apoptotic activities. Chem. Biol. Interact. 186, 152–156.

Fidler, I.J., Kripke, M.L., 2015. The challenge of targeting metastasis. Cancer Metastasis Rev. 34, 635–641.

Flores-Pérez, J.A., De La Rosa Oliva, F., Argenes, Y., Meneses-Garcia, A., 2019. Nutrition, cancer and personalized medicine. Adv. Exp. Med. Biol. 1168, 157–168.

Gao, Q., Yu, G., Yu, M., Wang, X., 2020. Bupleuri radix prevents the recurrences of resected colonic polyps by affecting angiogenin-2-induced protein kinase B/Akt signaling. J. Oncol. 2020, 3531652.

Garland, C., Mohr, S., Gorham, E., Grant, W., Garland, F., 2007. Role of ultraviolet B irradiance and vitamin D in prevention of ovarian cancer. Am. J. Prev. Med. 31, 512–514.

Gescher, A., Steward, W., Brown, K., 2013. Resveratrol in the management of human cancer: how strong is the clinical evidence? Ann. N. Y. Acad. Sci. 1290, 12–20.

Grau, M., Baron, J., Sandler, R., Haile, R., Beach, M., Church, T., Heber, D., 2004. Vitamin D, calcium supplementation, and colorectal adenomas: results of a randomized trial. J. Natl. Cancer Inst. 95, 1765–1771.

Guttenplan, J., Chen, M., Kosinska, W., Thompson, S., Zhao, Z., Cohen, L., 2001. Effects of a lycopene-rich diet on spontaneous and benzo[a]pyrene-induced mutagenesis in prostate, colon and lungs of the lacZ mouse. Cancer Lett. 164, 1–6.

Hu, W., Khor, T., Shu, L., Su, Z.-Y., Fuentes, F., Lee, J.H., Kong, A.N., 2012. Plants against cancer: a review on natural phytochemicals in preventing and treating cancers and their drug ability. Anti Cancer Agents Med. Chem. 12 (10).

Han, S.-S., Keum, Y.-S., Chun, K.-S., Surh, Y.-J., 2002. Suppression of phorbol ester-induced NF-kappaB activation by capsaicin in cultured human promyelocytic leukemia cells. Arch Pharm. Res. (Seoul) 25, 475–479.

Harris, C.M., Zamperoni, K.E., Sernoskie, S.C., Chow, N.S.M., Massey, T.E., 2021. Effects of in vivo treatment of mice with sulforaphane on repair of DNA pyridyloxylbutylation. Toxicology 454, 152753.

Holzapfel, N., Shokoohmand, A., Wagner, F., Landgraf, M., Champ, S., Holzapfel, B., Clements, J., Hutmacher, D., Loessner, D., 2017. Lycopene reduces ovarian tumor growth and intraperitoneal metastatic load. Am. J. Cancer Res. 7, 1322–1336.

Hu, R., Xu, C., Shen, G., Jain, M.R., Khor, T.O., Gopalkrishnan, A., Lin, W., Reddy, B., Chan, J.Y., Kong, A.-N., 2006. Gene expression profiles induced by cancer chemopreventive isothiocyanate sulforaphane in the liver of C57BL/6J mice and C57BL/6J/Nrf2 (−/−) mice. Cancer Lett. 243, 170–192.

Ikezaki, S., Nishikawa, A., Furukawa, F., Kudo, K., Nakamura, H., Tamura, K., Mori, H., 2001. Chemopreventive effects of curcumin on glandular stomach carcinogenesis induced by N-methyl-N′-nitro-N-nitrosoguanidine and sodium chloride in rats. Anti-Cancer Res. 21, 3407–3411.

Imran, M., Rauf, A., Abu-Izneid, T., Nadeem, M., Shariati, M.A., Khan, I.A., Imran, A., Orhan, I.E., Rizwan, M., Atif, M., Gondal, T.A., Mubarak, M.S., 2019a. Luteolin, a flavonoid, as an anticancer agent: a review. Biomed. Pharmacother. 112, 108612.

Imran, M., Salehi, B., Sharifi-Rad, J., Aslam Gondal, T., Saeed, F., Imran, A., Shahbaz, M., Tsouh Fokou, P.V., Umair Arshad, M., Khan, H., Guerreiro, S.G., Martins, N., Estevinho, L.M., 2019b. Kaempferol: a key emphasis to its anticancer potential. Molecules 24.

Jain, A., Madu, C., Lu, Y., 2021. Phytochemicals in chemoprevention: a cost-effective complementary approach. J. Cancer 12, 3686–3700.

Jang, M.S., Cai, L., Udeani, G., Slowing, K., Thomas, C.F., Beecher, C., Fong, H., Farnsworth, N.R., Kinghorn, A.D., Mehta, R., Moon, R.C., Pezzuto, J.M., 1997. Cancer chemopreventive activity of resveratrol, a natural product derived from grapes. Science (New York, N.Y.) 275, 218–220.

Jiang, X., Liu, Y., Ma, L., Ji, R., Qu, Y., Xin, Y., Lv, G., 2018. Chemopreventive activity of sulforaphane. Drug Des. Dev. Ther. 12, 2905–2913.

Kager, N., Ferk, F., Kundi, M., Wagner, K.-H., Misik, M., Knasmüller, S., 2009. Prevention of oxidative DNA damage in inner organs and lymphocytes of rats by green tea extract. Eur. J. Nutr. 49, 227–234.

Kapinova, A., Kubatka, P., Liskova, A., Baranenko, D., Kruzliak, P., Matta, M., Büsselberg, D., Malicherova, B., Zulli, A., Kwon, T.K., Jezkova, E., Blahutova, D., Zubor, P., Danko, J., 2019. Controlling metastatic cancer: the role of phytochemicals in cell signaling. J. Cancer Res. Clin. Oncol. 145, 1087–1109.

Khan, A., Shukla, Y., Kalra, N., Alam, M., Ahmad, M.G., Hakim, S.R., Owais, M., 2007. Potential of diallyl sulfide bearing pH-sensitive liposomes in chemoprevention against DMBA-induced skin papilloma. Mol. Med. 13, 443–451.

Kim, J.-K., Kim, Y., Na, K.-M., Surh, Y.-J., Kim, T.-Y., 2007. [6]-Gingerol prevents UVB-induced ROS production and COX-2 expression in vitro and in vivo. Free Radic. Res. 41, 603–614.

Kim, N.H., Lee, S., Kang, M.J., Jeong, H.G., Kang, W., Jeong, T.C., 2014. Protective effects of diallyl sulfide against thioacetamide-induced toxicity: a possible role of cytochrome P450 2E1. Biomol. Therapeut. 22, 149–154.

Klutstein, M., Nejman, D., Greenfield, R., Cedar, H., 2016. DNA methylation in cancer and aging. Cancer Res. 76, 3446–3450.

Koh, Y.C., Ho, C.T., Pan, M.H., 2020. Recent advances in cancer chemoprevention with phytochemicals. J. Food Drug Anal. 28, 14–37.

Kotecha, R., Takami, A., Espinoza, J., 2016. Dietary phytochemicals and cancer chemoprevention: a review of the clinical evidence. Oncotarget 7.

Lamartiniere, C.A., Cotroneo, M.S., Fritz, W.A., Wang, J., Mentor-Marcel, R., Elgavish, A., 2002. Genistein chemoprevention: timing and mechanisms of action in murine mammary and prostate. J. Nutr. 132, 552S–558S.

Lamprecht, S., Lipkin, M., 2003. Chemoprevention of colon cancer by calcium, vitamin D and folate: molecular mechanisms. Nat. Rev. Cancer 3, 601–614.

Legleu, C., Márquez-Rosado, L., Fattel-Fazenda, S., Arce-Popoca, E., Pérez-Carreón, J., Villa-Treviño, S., 2004. Chemoprotective effect of caffeic acid phenethyl ester on promotion in a medium-term rat hepatocarcinogenesis assay. Int. J. Cancer 108, 488–492.

Leone, A., Diorio, G., Sexton, W., Schell, M., Alexandrow, M., Fahey, J.W., Kumar, N.B., 2017. Sulforaphane for the chemoprevention of bladder cancer: molecular mechanism targeted approach. Oncotarget 8 (21).

Lewinska, A., Adamczyk-Grochala, J., Deregowska, A., Wnuk, M., 2017. Sulforaphane-induced cell cycle arrest and senescence are accompanied by DNA hypomethylation and changes in microRNA profile in breast cancer cells. Theranostics 7, 3461–3477.

Li, S., Wu, L., Feng, J., Li, J., Liu, T., Zhang, R., Xu, S., Cheng, K., Zhou, Y., Zhou, S., Kong, R., Chen, K., Wang, F., Xia, Y., Lu, J., Zhou, Y., Dai, W., Guo, C., 2016. In vitro and in vivo study of epigallocatechin-3-gallate-induced apoptosis in aerobic glycolytic hepatocellular carcinoma cells involving inhibition of phosphofructokinase activity. Sci. Rep. 6, 28479.

Li, Y., Xu, B., Xu, M., Chen, D., Xiong, Y., Lian, M., Sun, Y., Tang, Z., Wang, L., Jiang, C., Lin, Y., 2017. 6-Gingerol protects intestinal barrier from ischemia/reperfusion-induced damage via inhibition of p38 MAPK to NF-κB signalling. Pharmacol. Res. 119.

Liskova, A., Stefanicka, P., Samec, M., Karel, Š., Zubor, P., Bielik, T., Biskupska-Bodova, K., Kwon, T.K., Danko, J., Büsselberg, D., Adamek, M., Rodrigo, L., Kruzliak, P., Shleikin, A., Kubatka, P., 2020. Dietary phytochemicals as the potential protectors against carcinogenesis and their role in cancer chemoprevention. Clin. Exp. Med. 20.

López-Lázaro, M., Willmore, E., 2007. Cells lacking DNA topoisomerase IIβ are resistant to genistein. J. Nat. Prod. 70, 763–767.

Lu, W.-D., Qin, Y., Yang, C., Li, L., 2013. Effect of curcumin on human colon cancer multidrug resistance. Clinics 68.

M, A., Sasidharan, S., Gs, S., 2012. Role of nutraceuticals in cancer. Int. J. Pharm. Pharmaceut. Sci. 4, 415–420.

Mah, Y.-J., Song, J.S., Kim, S.-O., Lee, J.-H., Jeon, M., Jung, U.-W., Moon, S.J., Kim, J.-H., Choi, H.-J., 2014. The effect of epigallocatechin-3-gallate (EGCG) on human alveolar bone cells both in vitro and in vivo. Arch. Oral Biol. 59, 539–549.

Matusheski, N., Jeffery, E., 2002. Comparison of the bioactivity of two glucoraphanin hydrolysis products found in broccoli, sulforaphane and sulforaphane nitrile. J. Agric. Food Chem. 49, 5743–5749.

Moolgavkar, S.H., Luebeck, E.G., 2003. Multistage carcinogenesis and the incidence of human cancer. Genes Chromosomes Cancer 38, 302–306.

Murtaza, G., Karim, S., Akram, M., Khan, S., Azhar, S., Mumtaz, A., Bin Asad, M.H., 2014. Caffeic acid phenethyl ester and therapeutic potentials. BioMed Res. Int. 2014, 145342.

Na, H.-K., Kim, E.-H., Jung, J.-H., Lee, H.-H., Hyun, J.-W., Surh, Y.-J., 2008. (−)-Epigallocatechin gallate induces Nrf2-mediated antioxidant enzyme expression via activation of PI3K and ERK in human mammary epithelial cells. Arch. Biochem. Biophys. 476, 171–177.

Nigam, N., George, J., Srivastava, S., Roy, P., Bhui, K., Singh, M., Shukla, Y., 2009. Induction of apoptosis by [6]-gingerol associated with the modulation of p53 and involvement of mitochondrial signaling pathway in B[a]P-induced mouse skin tumorigenesis. Cancer Chemother. Pharmacol. 65, 687–696.

Nomura, M., Kaji, A., Ma, W.-Y., Miyamoto, K.-I., Dong, Z., 2001. Suppression of cell transformation and induction of apoptosis by caffeic acid phenethyl ester. Mol. Carcinog. 31, 83–89.

Okazaki, Y., Iqbal, M., Okada, S., 2005. Suppressive effects of dietary curcumin on the increased activity of renal ornithine decarboxylase in mice treated with a renal carcinogen, ferric nitrilotriacetate. Biochim. Biophys. Acta (BBA) - Mol. Basis Dis. 1740, 357–366.

Oyagbemi, A., Saba, A., Azeez, O., 2010. Molecular targets of [6]-gingerol: its potential roles in cancer chemoprevention. Biofactors 36, 169–178.

Patel, K., Brown, V., Jones, D., Britton, R., Hemingway, D., Miller, A., West, K., Booth, T., Perloff, M., Crowell, J., Brenner, D., Steward, W., Gescher, A., Brown, K., 2010. Clinical pharmacology of resveratrol and its metabolites in colorectal cancer patients. Cancer Res. 70, 7392–7399.

Patel, P., Varney, M., Dave, J., Singh, R., 2002. Regulation of constitutive and induced NF- ?? B activation in malignant melanoma cells by capsaicin modulates interleukin-8 production and cell proliferation. J. Interferon Cytokine Res. 22, 427–435.

Pinto, J., Rivlin, R., 2001. Antiproliferative effects of allium derivatives from garlic. J. Nutr. 131, 1058S–1060S.

Pramanik, K.C., Kudugunti, S.K., Fofaria, N.M., Moridani, M.Y., Srivastava, S.K., 2013. Caffeic acid phenethyl ester suppresses melanoma tumor growth by inhibiting PI3K/AKT/XIAP pathway. Carcinogenesis 34, 2061–2070.

Priyadarsini, I., 2012. Chemical and structural features influencing the biological activity of curcumin. Curr. Pharmaceut. Des. 19.

Qin, J., Chen, J., Zhu, Z., Teng, J., 2015. Genistein inhibits human colorectal cancer growth and suppresses MiR-95, Akt and SGK1. Cell. Physiol. Biochem. 35, 2069–2077.

Rizeq, B., Gupta, I., Ilesanmi, J., Alsafran, M., Rahman, M., Ouhtit, A., 2020. The power of phytochemicals combination in cancer chemoprevention. J. Cancer 11, 4521–4533.

Ruiz, R., Hernández, P., 2016. Cancer chemoprevention by dietary phytochemicals: epidemiological evidence. Maturitas 94.

Scott, E., Steward, W., Gescher, A., Brown, K., 2012. Resveratrol in human cancer chemoprevention - choosing the right' dose. Mol. Nutr. Food Res. 56, 7–13.

Seeram, N., Henning, S., Niu, Y., Lee, R., Scheuller, H., Heber, D., 2006. Catechin and caffeine content of green tea dietary supplements and correlation with antioxidant capacity. J. Agric. Food Chem. 54, 1599–1603.

Seibel, J., Molzberger, A., Hertrampf, T., Laudenbach, U., Diel, P., 2009. Oral treatment with genistein reduces the expression of molecular and biochemical markers of inflammation in a rat model of chronic TNBS-induced colitis. Eur. J. Nutr. 48, 213–220.

Shukla, Y., Prasad, S., Tripathi, C., Singh, M., George, J., Kalra, N., 2007. In vitro and in vivo modulation of testosterone mediated alterations in apoptosis related proteins by [6]-gingerol. Mol. Nutr. Food Res. 51, 1492–1502.

Skinner, H., Michaud, D., Giovannucci, E., Willett, W., Colditz, G., Fuchs, C., 2006. Vitamin D intake and the risk for pancreatic cancer in two cohort studies. Cancer Epidemiol. Biomarkers Prev. 15, 1688–1695.

Sporn, M.B., 1976. Approaches to prevention of epithelial cancer during the preneoplastic period. Cancer Res. 36, 2699–2702.

Surh, Y.-J., 2003a. Cancer chemoprevention with dietary phytochemicals. Nat. Rev. Cancer 3, 768–780.

Surh, Y.J., 2003b. Cancer chemoprevention with dietary phytochemicals. Nat. Rev. Cancer 57, 43–66.

Tang, F.-Y., Pai, M.-H., Wang, X.-D., 2011. Consumption of lycopene inhibits the growth and progression of colon cancer in a mouse Xenograft model. J. Agric. Food Chem. 59, 9011–9021.

Toledo, L.P., Ong, T.P., Pinho, A.L.G., Jordao, A., Vanucchi, H., Salvador Moreno, F., 2003. Inhibitory effects of lutein and lycopene on placental glutathione S-transferase-positive preneoplastic lesions and DNA strand breakage induced in Wistar rats by the resistant hepatocyte model of hepatocarcinogenesis. Nutr. Cancer 47, 62–69.

Trung, L., Espinoza, J., Dao, A., Viet, N., Shimoda, K., Nakao, S., 2015. Resveratrol selectively induces apoptosis in malignant cells with the JAK2V617F mutation by inhibiting the JAK2 pathway. Mol. Nutr. Food Res. 59 n/a-n/a.

Ushida, J., Sugie, S., Kawabata, K., Pham, Q., Tanaka, T., Fujii, K., Takeuchi, H., Ito, Y., Mori, H., 2000. Chemopreventive effect of curcumin on N-Nitrosomethylbenzylamine-induced esophageal carcinogenesis in rats. Cancer Sci. 91, 893–898.

Vantyghem, S., Wilson, S., Postenka, C., AL-Katib, W., Tuck, A., Chambers, A., 2005. Dietary genistein reduces metastasis in a postsurgical orthotopic breast cancer model. Cancer Res. 65, 3396–3403.

Venier, N., Yamamoto, T., Sugar, L., Adomat, H., Fleshner, N., Venkateswaran, V., Klotz, L., 2015. Capsaicin reduces the metastatic burden in the transgenic adenocarcinoma of the mouse prostate model: capsaicin reduces metastasis in TRAMP mice. J. Urol. 193, e549.

Wang, J., Eltoum, I.-E., Lamartiniere, C.A., 2007. Genistein chemoprevention of prostate cancer in TRAMP mice. J. Carcinog. 6, 3.

Watanabe, S., Kitade, Y., Masaki, T., Nishioka, M., Satoh, K., Nishino, H., 2001. Effects of lycopene and Sho-Saiko-to on hepatocarcinogenesis in a rat model of spontaneous liver cancer. Nutr. Cancer 39, 96–101.

Weng, C.-J., Wu, C.-F., Huang, H.-W., Ho, C.-T., Yen, G.-C., 2010. Anti-invasion effects of 6-shogaol and 6-gingerol, two active components in ginger, on human hepatocarcinoma cells. Mol. Nutr. Food Res. 54, 1618–1627.

Wu, W.-S., Wu, J.-R., Hu, C.-T., 2008. Signal cross talks for sustained MAPK activation and cell migration: the potential role of reactive oxygen species. Cancer Metastasis Rev. 27, 303–314.

Wu, Y., Sarkissyan, M., Vadgama, J.V., 2015. Epigenetics in breast and prostate cancer. Methods Mol. Biol. 1238, 425–466.

Xu, F., Na, L., Li, Y., Chen, L., 2020. Roles of the PI3K/AKT/mTOR signalling pathways in neurodegenerative diseases and tumours. Cell Biosci. 10, 54.

Yang, C.-H., Lin, C.-Y., Yang, J.-H., Liou, S.-Y., Li, P.-C., Chien, C.-T., 2009. Supplementary catechins attenuate cooking-oil-fumes-induced oxidative stress in rat lung. Chin. J. Physiol. 52, 151–159.

Yang, S., Li, W., Sun, H., Wu, B., Ji, F., Sun, T., Chang, H., Shen, P., Wang, Y., Zhou, D., 2015. Resveratrol elicits anti-colorectal cancer effect by activating miR-34c-KITLG in vitro and in vivo. BMC Cancer 15, 969.

Ye, S.-F., Hou, Z., Zhong, L.-M., Zhang, Q.-Q., 2007. Effect of curcumin on the induction of glutathione S-transferases and NADP(H): quinone oxidoreductase and its possible mechanism of action. Yao Xue Xue Bao 42, 376–380.

Yuan, J.-M., 2011. Green tea and prevention of esophageal and lung cancers. Mol. Nutr. Food Res. 55, 886–904.

Yuan, J.H., Li, Y.Q., Yang, X.Y., 2007. Inhibition of epigallocatechin gallate on orthotopic colon cancer by upregulating the Nrf2-UGT1A signal pathway in nude mice. Pharmacology 80, 269–278.

Zhang, Y., Tang, L., 2007. Discovery and development of sulforaphane as a cancer chemopreventive phytochemical. Acta Pharmacol. Sin. 28, 1343–1354.

Zhao, X., Liu, J., Feng, L., Ge, S., Yang, S., Chen, C., Li, X., Peng, L., Mu, Y., Wang, Y., Gu, D., Guo, Y., Lin, G., Deng, B., Cheng, Z., Cai, D., 2018. Anti-angiogenic effects of Qingdu granule on breast cancer through inhibiting NFAT signaling pathway. J. Ethnopharmacol. 222, 261–269.

Zhou, J., Farah, B., Sinha, R., Wu, Y., Singh, B., Bay, B.-H., Yang, C., Yen, P., 2014. Epigallocatechin-3-gallate (EGCG), a green tea polyphenol, stimulates hepatic autophagy and lipid clearance. PLoS One 9, e87161.

CHAPTER

20

Toxicity labels

Bhakti Pawar[1], Anoothi Bain[1], Nagaraja Sreeharsha[2,3], Muktika Tekade[4], Nupur Vasdev[1] and Rakesh Kumar Tekade[1]

[1]National Institute of Pharmaceutical Education and Research (NIPER)- Ahmedabad, An Institute of National Importance, Government of India, Department of Pharmaceuticals, Ministry of Chemicals and Fertilizers, Palaj, Gandhinagar, Gujarat, India; [2]Department of Pharmaceutical Sciences, College of Clinical Pharmacy, King Faisal University, Al-Ahsa, Saudi Arabia; [3]Department of Pharmaceutics, Vidya Siri College of Pharmacy, Bengaluru, Karnataka, India; [4]School of Pharmacy, Devi Ahilya Vishwavidyalaya, Indore, Madya Pradesh, India

20.1 Introduction

One of the fundamental concepts in pharmacotoxicology is the evaluation of toxicity, the way a foreign compound enters the body, that is, the exposure route which plays a significant role in defining the efficiency and scope of an effect. Toxicologists are interested in studying the primary mechanism of toxicity, starting from its route of exposure, the dose of an exposed compound, and the level of toxicity achieved. Toxicity can be acute or chronic based on the duration of chemical exposure or any foreign antigen in the body. Acute toxicity can be defined as exposure to chemicals for a shorter period. On the other hand, chronic toxicity can be defined as exposure to chemicals for a more extended period. In 2007, the National research council reported "Toxicity testing in the 21st century" and presented a well-planned strategy to take benefits of state-of-the-art technologies such as in silico techniques for better prediction of toxicity of chemicals which are usually present in the environment and easily exposable to human beings (Krewski et al., 2020).

Exposure to any chemical can be defined as any foreign agent (biological, chemical, or physical) that shows an unwanted effect on the body directly or indirectly. In day-to-day life, with or without intention, human beings are exposed to chemicals, some of which may cause toxicity and can be fatal. "Insecticides rule, 1971" was created by the central government after consultation with Central Insecticides Board to spread awareness about the chemicals handled by researchers or workers in chemical industries (Gupta and Milatovic, 2014).

Essentials of Pharmatoxicology in Drug Research, Volume 1
https://doi.org/10.1016/B978-0-443-15840-7.00023-3

This act suggests the different labeling on containers of chemicals. The label contains information such as manufacturer, brand, antidote, etc.

Additionally, with this information, labeling of different colors is also pasted. These colors indicate toxicity levels, viz. red label, yellow label, blue label, and green label. Similarly, WHO has classified toxicity into four classes: class I (extremely hazardous), class II (highly hazardous), class III (moderately hazardous), and class IV (slightly hazardous). Every person who regularly comes into contact with chemicals will benefit from this classification.

Since 2003, a globally harmonized system (GHS) for categorizing and labeling chemicals has been used. Hazardous chemicals are designated as flammable gas, explosive, flammable liquid, spontaneously combustible, oxidizer, organic peroxide, poison, infectious substance, radioactive, etc. In the case of agrochemicals that the farmers usually handle, they should be aware of these hazardous chemicals and their labeling. This chapter shows the different labels used for specific classes or levels of toxicity in this chapter. Toxicity of any chemical is measured based on its median lethal dose (LD_{50}) value. Lower the LD_{50} value, higher the toxicity (Nidiry, 2021). So, as per their LD_{50} values, chemicals are classified into four different classes: class I-extremely toxic, class II-highly toxic, class III-moderately toxic, and class IV-slightly toxic.

The following section describes the toxicity levels, types of different toxicity labels, and symbols used to indicate the nature of chemicals.

20.1.1 Globally Harmonized System (GHS) of classification and labeling of chemicals

A global system for the uniform classification and labeling of chemicals was developed by the United Nations and is known as the Globally Harmonized System (GHS). On March 26, 2012, the Occupational Safety and Health Administration formally adopted it in the US (OSHA) (Occupational Safety and Health Administration, 2017). In the U.S. Globally Harmonized System of Classification and Labeling of Chemicals (GHS) provided pictograms for different chemicals such as compressed gas, explosives, oxidizers, toxic compounds, exploding bombs, etc., as shown in Fig. 20.1.

- Health hazard: An agent or substance which causes cancer (carcinogen), damage to the respiratory, reproductive system, etc., over a longer period (chronic/health hazard).
- Oxidizer: The chemical (pyrophoric) which facilitates burning and keeps fire for a longer time.
- Exclamation mark: An agent that causes instant skin, eye, or respiratory irritation.
- Flame: A pyrophoric substance that is likely to self-ignite when exposed to air or water or releases flammable gas.
- Compressed gas: Gases such as liquid nitrogen or ammonia are stored under pressure.
- Corrosive: A substance that causes eye or skin irritation when it comes in contact with a corrosive substance.
- Exploding bomb: Substances that are self-reactive (self-explosive) or explode when exposed to air, such as organic peroxides, highly unstable materials, etc.
- Acute toxicity: An agent which causes immediate and severe toxicity, such as poisons, concentrated acids, etc.

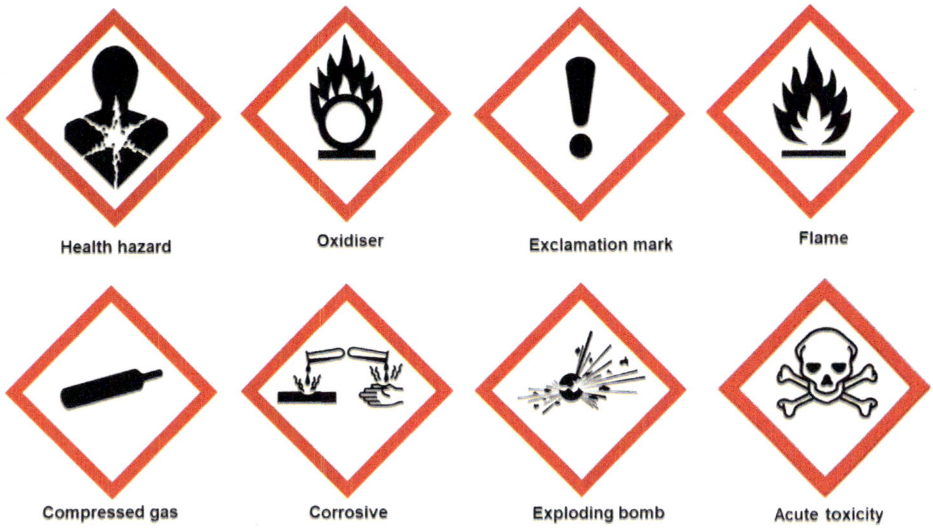

FIGURE 20.1 Representative pictograms showing Globally Harmonized System (GSH) for different chemicals.

20.2 Levels of toxicity

The toxicity of any chemical is its capacity to cause any injury or illness. Usually, toxicity is of two types: acute toxicity and chronic toxicity. In acute toxicity, toxic chemicals are decided by subjecting that chemical to animals for a short duration of action with varying doses. In contrast, chronic toxicity is determined by subjecting the chemicals in different doses to animals for a longer duration of action. In this study, toxicity measurement is done on the basis of the median lethal dose (LD_{50}). The lower the value of LD_{50}, the greater the toxicity to humans and animals (Dar et al., 2020). In the next section, we have discussed the different toxicity levels, such as extremely toxic, highly toxic, moderately toxic, and slightly toxic (Puhalla et al., 2010). Fig. 20.2 indicates different levels and labels of toxicity.

20.2.1 Extremely toxic

The highly toxic chemicals possess oral LD_{50} values of 1–50 mg/kg. These chemicals are generally marked with a red label with a skull and cross bone symbol showing it is poisonous.

20.2.2 Highly toxic

This is the second level of toxicity. Highly toxic chemicals are usually denoted with yellow labels having oral LD_{50} values 51–500 mg/kg. These pesticides or chemicals cause eye and skin disorders. Similar to highly toxic levels, these chemicals are warned with poison tags. Examples of chemicals are quinalphos, carbaryl, etc.

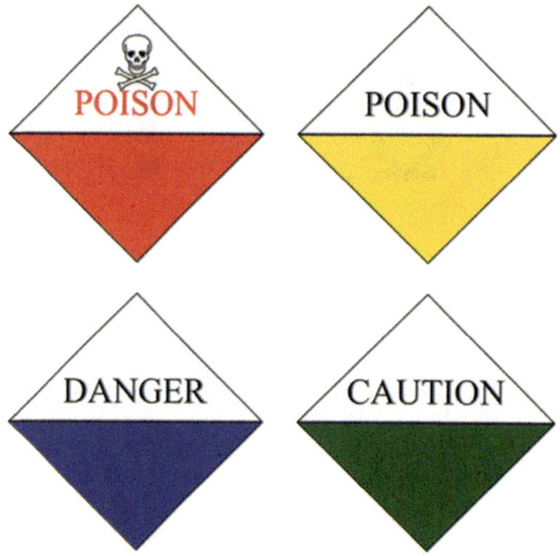

FIGURE 20.2 Labels of toxicity as per Insecticides Rules, 1971.

20.2.3 Moderately toxic

The moderately toxic chemicals are usually represented with a blue label. Their oral lethal dose is 501–5000 mg/kg. These chemicals are dangerous and are warned to keep away from children. Organophosphate, such as Malathion, is a moderately toxic pesticide (Pascale and Laborde, 2020).

20.2.4 Slightly toxic

Slightly or relatively nontoxic is the last level of toxicity in which chemicals possess an oral LD_{50} value of more than 5000 mg/kg. One should handle these chemicals with proper caution. These chemicals are labeled with a blue color code. Even though certain pesticides are just mildly toxic or harmless, all pesticides can be dangerous to humans, animals, other species, and the environment if the product label's instructions are not followed.

20.3 Types of toxicity labels

Toxicity labels that are present on the different pesticides indicate the levels of toxicity. Different colors are used to represent the toxicity labels, such as red, yellow, blue, and green (Friis, 2012). Classification of labels is mainly based on their ability to cause toxicity. The labeling follows a general pattern established by the Insecticides Rules, 1971. It includes information like the brand name, manufacturer's name, antidote name in the condition of accidental ingestion, and so on.

20.3.1 Red label

The chemicals on which red labels are present means this chemical is highly toxic. A prominent label feature is a color mark that uses a color code to signify the material's toxicity (Painkra et al., 2019). "Poison" is written on the chemicals belonging to this label. It is not recommended to inhale or ingest in any form. Examples of pesticides on which red labels are present are monocrotophos, zinc phosphide.

20.3.2 Yellow label

Although it is highly toxic, it is less than the red label. The oral lethal dose for this label is 51–500 mg/kg. When utilizing these pesticides, one must use caution. Example of this label is endosulfan and carbaryl. Similar to the red label, "Poison" is written on this label.

20.3.3 Blue label

The chemicals belonging to this label are moderately toxic. The oral lethal dose for this label is 501–5000 mg/kg. Malathion, glyphosate, thiram, etc., fall under this label. "Danger" is marked on all the chemicals belonging to this class.

20.3.4 Green label

The green label is the last in the list of toxicity labels. The slightly toxic chemicals possess green labels on their covers. The oral lethal dose for this label is above 5000 mg/kg. Clothianidin and mancozeb are examples of chemicals bearing green labels. "Caution" is highlighted on the chemicals possessing this green label (Burton, 2009).

20.4 Chemicals under different types of labels

As per Insecticides Rules, 1971, various chemicals are classified under different labels as mentioned below:

- Red label: monocrotophos (Gupta and Milatovic, 2014), zinc phosphide (Hamade et al., 2021), ethyl mercury acetate, and others.
- Yellow label: endosulfan (Mehta, 2017), carbaryl, quinalphos (Sanganalmath et al., 2019), and others.
- Blue label: malathion, thiram, glyphosate, and others.
- Green label: mancozeb (Dhaneshwar and Hardej, 2021), oxyfluorfen, insecticides, and mosquito repellents.

Here is an example of a GSH toxicity label layout for chemicals falling under different toxicity classes (https://www.bradyid.com/applications/ghs-labeling-requirements, 2022) (Fig. 20.3).

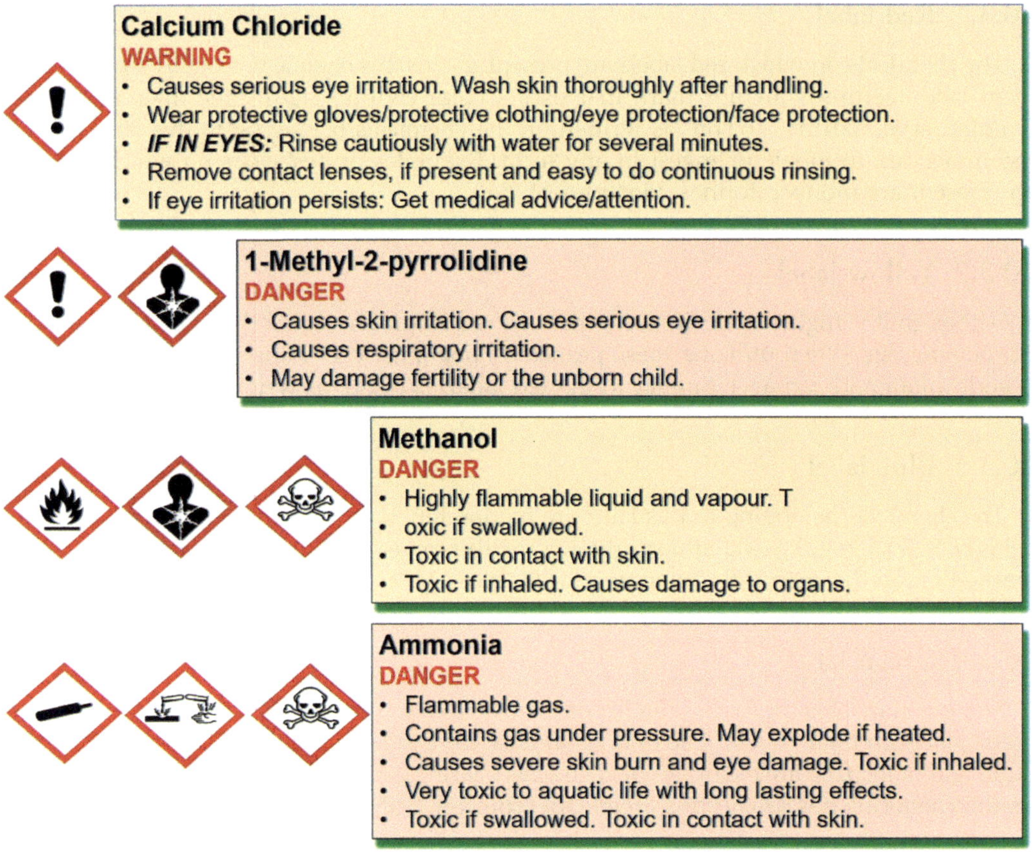

FIGURE 20.3 Globally harmonized system toxicity label layout for different chemicals.

20.4.1 Information required on labels (details and symbols)

A square set at an angle of 45 degrees (diamond shape) must be present on the label in a conspicuous location and take up at least one-sixteenth of its total surface area, as shown in Fig. 20.2. The aforementioned square should be split into two identical triangles, with the symbol and signal word placed in the upper triangle and the color placed in the lower triangle. The upper region of the triangle should contain the signal words such as red label, skull-bone symbol, and POISON shall be written. For the yellow label, the POISON word shall be written without a skull and bone symbol. Next, for the blue label DANGER and the green label, CAUTION must be written (https://shashikallada.com/reading-the-labels-may-save-your-lives-understand-india-toxicity-labels/, 2022). Additionally, in the case of the red label, cautionary warnings must include in the proper locations well outside the triangle, like **"KEEP OUT OF THE REACH OF CHILDREN," "IF SWALLOWED, OR IF SYMPTOMS OF POISONING OCCUR CALL PHYSICIAN IMMEDIATELY**

The label should also contain:

- The name of the manufacturer: If the maker is not the person in whose name the insecticide has been registered under the Act, it must be specified how they are related to the person who manufactures, packs, distribute, or sells the insecticide.
- Brand name: Name of the chemical, act, schedule, or trademark under which the chemical is sold.
- Name of the antidote: In case of overconsumption of chemicals, the antidote name should also be mentioned.
- Registration number of the chemical should also be mentioned on the label.
- Each ingredient's common name accepted by the International Organization for Standardization (ISO) or the Indian Standards Institution must be provided, or in the absence of a common name, the correct chemical name that adheres the closest to the generally accepted rules of chemical nomenclature must be provided.
- Manufacturing batch number.
- Expiry date (the date up to which the chemical should show its safety and efficiency).
- Net content or volume: The net content must be free of any packaging or additional information. The precise declaration of the net content in terms of weight, measure, and the number of activity units, if applicable, must be made. The terms "weight" and "volume" must be used in the metric measurements.
- The label must be attached to the container in such a way that it is usually impossible to separate it (Fig. 20.4).

20.4.2 GSH labels for primary and secondary packaging of chemicals

A globally harmonized system has also given the labeling instructions for the primary and secondary packaging. In the next section, we have briefly discussed the labeling instructions.

20.4.2.1 Toxicity labels for primary packaging

The primary chemical containers you obtain from the manufacturer are bags, barrels, bottles, boxes, cans, cylinders, and drums. According to the GHS label example above, these containers should be labeled with all six labeling components following the GHS regulations. A label with a container from a supplier cannot be taken off, changed, or vandalized. If a new label is required, it must contain the exact details of the old one (Fig. 20.5).

20.4.2.2 Toxicity labels for secondary packaging

Spray bottles, jugs, or jars are examples of secondary containers, which are often smaller than primary containers. Typically, the chemicals in these containers have been transferred from a primary container. The following conditions must be completed before GHS labels for secondary containers can deviate from the labeling requirements: (a) The person who transfers the material uses it during their shift at work. (b) The employee who transferred remains in the work area throughout use. (c) The person who filled the container keeps it in their possession and in the work area.

Occupational Safety and Health Administration (OSHA) did not change the labeling instructions for secondary packaging. Workers can design their field labels by combining the

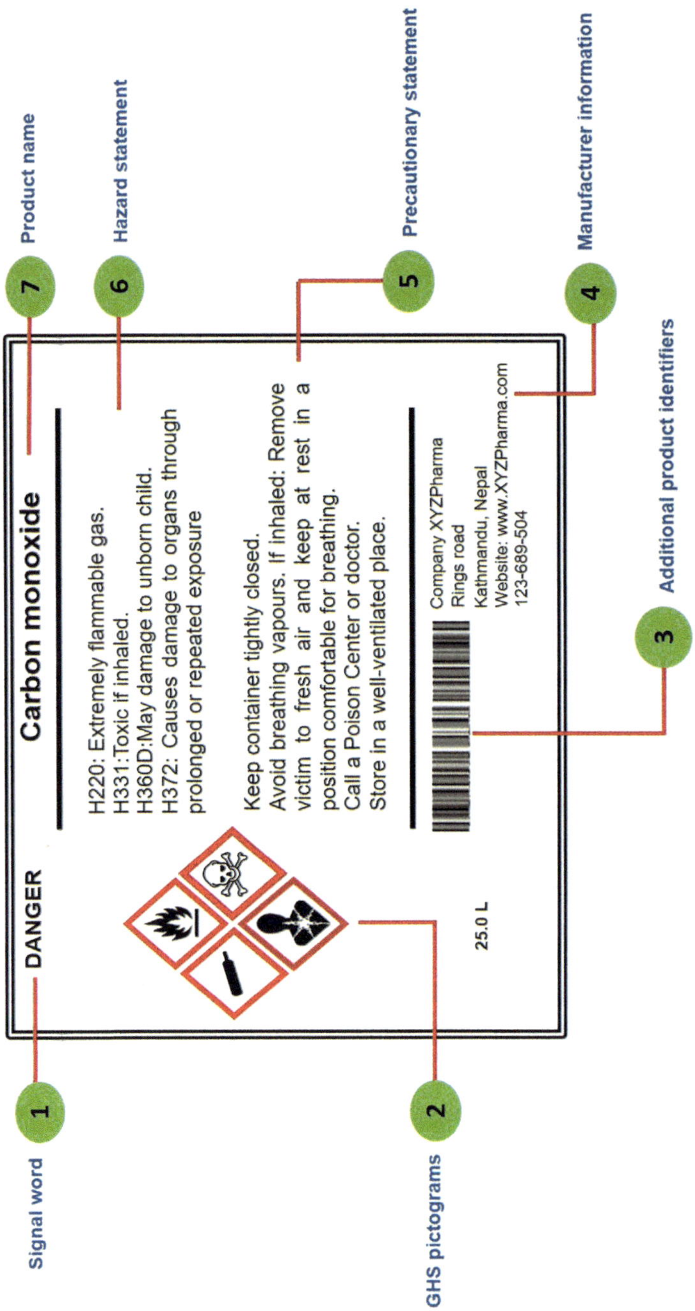

FIGURE 20.4 Representative figure showing each element of toxicity label.

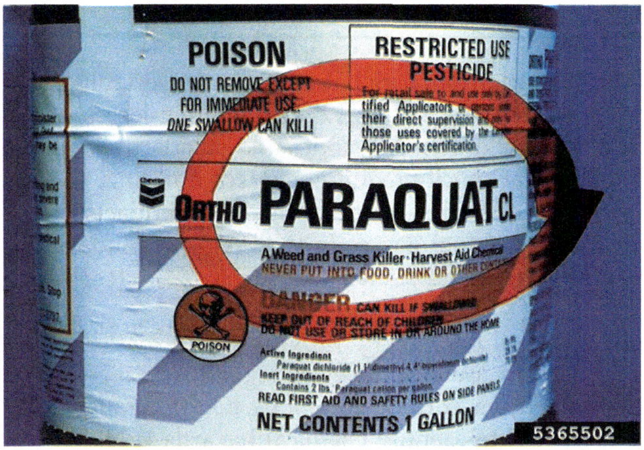

FIGURE 20.5 Example of toxicity label for primary packaging of the container.

components from the GHS label, for example, as shown above, with the data supplied by the manufacturer or by using all of the manufacturer's details. In the next section, we briefly discussed the National Fire Protection Association (NFPA), established mainly to spread awareness about chemical hazards (Fig. 20.6).

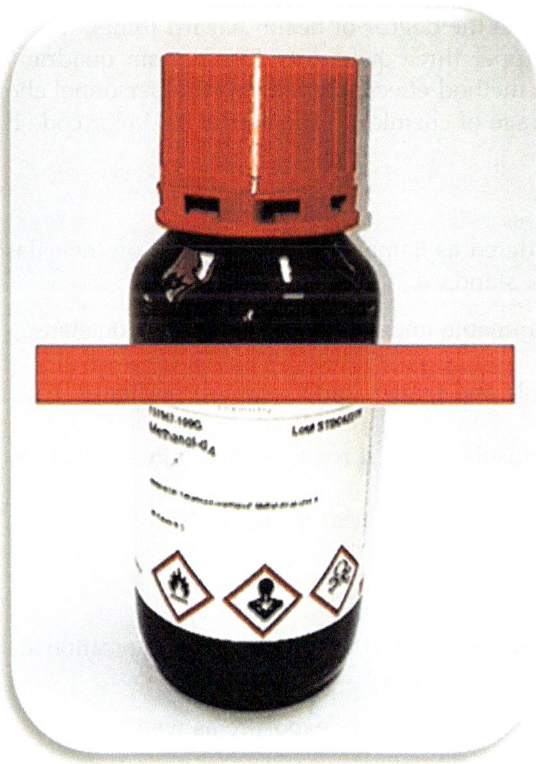

FIGURE 20.6 Representative example of toxicity label for secondary packaging of the container.

20.5 NFPA (National Fire Protection Association)

NFPA operated as a nonprofitable organization on a global scale; it was established in 1896. NFPA seeks to reduce the number of fatalities, injuries, and economic losses due to fire, electrical, and chemical hazards. It is widely known as a codes and standards organization. NFPA created 300 codes and standards that specify requirements for building, processing, design, service, and installations worldwide to lessen the danger and impacts of fire. These codes and standards include the National fuel gas code (NFPA 54), Standards for Portable fire extinguishers (NFPA 10), NFPA diamond standards (NFPA 704), etc. (Pauley, 2017).

NFPA aims to raise awareness about chemical hazards by providing information on the label. All in-plant or in-lab chemical containers must be labeled, tagged, or labeled with the substance's name and any possible dangers, according to OSHA (Occupational Safety and Health Association). Most widely used tool to identify chemical hazards is NFPA Diamond (NFPA, 2005).

20.5.1 NFPA standard

The American National Fire Protection Association created the NFPA ratings. The ratings, as stated by the NFPA 704 standard, are represented by the NFPA diamond. NFPA diamond is also known as "Fire Diamond." The technique employs a color-coded diamond with four quadrants, which includes numbers to indicate the degree of health hazard (blue), flammability (red), and reactivity (yellow) in the upper three quadrants. The bottom quadrant is used to indicate special hazards. The NFPA method effectively informs the personnel about the degree of chemical hazards and the storage of chemicals. The NFPA 704 color code has four divisions which are discussed here.

20.5.1.1 RED: Flammability hazard

Substances that are considered/not considered as flammable liquids based on their flashpoint under OSHA's hazard communication standard.

4. EXTREME—It is considered highly flammable under OSHA communication standards since flash point is below 73°F.
3. SERIOUS—It is considered as flammable and ignites under normal conditions. Flashpoint is 73°F–100°F.
2. MODERATE—It is considered as combustible since it requires moderate heating to ignite. Flashpoint is below 200°F.
1. SLIGHT—Slightly combustible. Must be given prior heat for ignition.
0. MINIMAL—Will not burn under normal conditions.

20.5.1.2 BLUE: Health hazard ratings

Substances considered/not considered toxic under OSHA's hazard Communication standard are based on their combustible property or lethality.

4. EXTREME—Highly toxic. It can be lethal on short-term exposure as well.

3. SERIOUS—Toxic. Exposure may lead to severe injury.
2. HAZARDOUS/MODERATE—Possible residual injury upon prolonged exposure.
1. SLIGHT—May cause slight residual injury or irritation.
0. MINIMAL—Same as that of ordinary material. No precautions are necessary. Same as that of ordinary material.

20.5.1.3 *YELLOW: Reactivity*

Substances considered/not considered as explosives under OSHA's hazard Communication standard are based on chemical reactivity.

4. EXTREME—Explosive at normal temperature.
3. SERIOUS—Reacts explosively with water or can explode with string ignition or shock.
2. HAZARDOUS/MODERATE—Unstable. Capable of reacting vigorously or forming explosive mixtures with water at elevated pressures or temperatures.
1. SLIGHT—Unstable if heated.
0. MINIMAL—Stable. Nonreactive with water.

20.5.1.4 *WHITE: Special hazard/PPE specific symbols*

They indicate the type of personal protective equipment (PPE) that should be used while handling hazards like acid gear, goggles, and a respirator (Head and Wagner, 1995). Chemicals that possess the following properties should be considered as a special hazard.

- Reaction with water
- Potent oxidizing agents
- Corrosive
- Radiation-active substances
- Poison

For example, diesel fuel has an NFPA rating of 0-2-0, i.e., 0 for Health (blue), 2 for Flammability (red), and 0 for Chemical reactivity (yellow).

So, to identify the nature of the chemical hazard and its careful handling, every chemical has its own material safety data sheet. A brief overview of the material safety data sheet is discussed below.

20.6 MSDS (Material Safety Data Sheet)

A material safety data sheet is a technical document that contains information about a potential hazard. It contains information pertaining to:

- Health effects upon product exposure.
- Risk assessment for the product's usage, storage, or handling.
- Precautions for personnel at risk of exposure.
- Emergency protocols.

The MSDS must comply with Workplace Hazardous Materials Information System (WHMIS) regulations on availability, design, and content. It may be written, printed, or expressed in another way.

The objective of MSDS: MSDS is the second component of the WHMIS information system to alert information provided on labels. The third component of the system consists of personnel training on hazards associated with different substances, including instruction on the significance of information included in the Material Safety Data Sheet (2017) (Fig.20.7).

MATERIALS SAFETY DATA SHEET (MSDS) **Ethanol (C_2H_5OH)**	MSDS Number	MSD/A/1
	Version Number	5.0
	Date issued	10 Oct 2022
	Next Review date	October 2024

Company Details		
Name: MSD Alcohols Address :120 Durban,4001, South Africa	Emergency telephone No. Telephone Fax	+27 (31) 579 2005 +27 (31) 579 2005 +27 (31) 579 2006

1. Product & Company Identification	
Trade name- Ethanol (Industrial, Absolute or Anhydrous, Light Spirits, Extra Neutral Potable, Rectified Extra) Chemical Family- Aliphatic Alcohol Chemical Name- Ethanol Synonyms- Ethyl Alcohol	Chemical abstract no.-56-14-3 Molecular Mass - 48.07 NIOSH No.- KQ 8900000 Hazchem code- 2(S) E; 3(S) E UN No. - 1170

2. Composition
Hazardous components: Ethyl Alcohol (75.0 -99.9%) EEC classification :200- 578-6[10] R Phrases- R11

3. Hazard Identification	
Classification of substance 3.1 EU-GHS / CLP Hazard Class and category code(s) EU-DSD / DPD Indication(s) of danger and R phrase(s) 3.2 Label elements EU-GHS / CLP Hazard pictogram(s)/Symbols-	Flammable liquid Flam. Liq. 2 Serious eye Irritation Eye Irrit. 2 Highly flammable R11 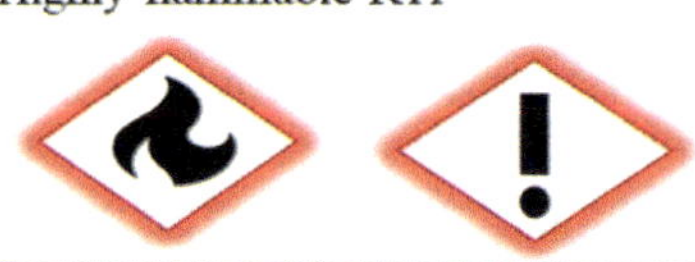

FIGURE 20.7 Example of a material safety data sheet.

20.6.1 MSDS-associated responsibilities

20.6.1.1 Suppliers

- Each controlled product used in a workplace demands the development of MSDS.
- Make sure that the controlled product MSDS should consist of the following:
  - ✓ Data that should be accurate during the product's sale or import.
  - ✓ MSDS should be prepared and dated within 3 years of the date of supply or import. It should be accessible in both official languages.
- Ensure the purchaser provides a copy of the recent MSDS while receiving the controlled product.
- Ensure that the data is exempt from disclosure to any physician who wants it to make a medical diagnosis or prescribe treatment because such information may be confidential (trade secret) (Sugimura, 2002).

20.6.1.2 Employer

- Ensure that the supplier should provide an updated MSDS for a controlled product on receiving in the workplace.
- Examine the date of production of the data sheet received. It must be dated not more than 3 years of the current date.
- Confirming that copies of all data sheets needed are easily accessible at the worksite to:
  - ✓ An employee with possible exposure to the controlled product.
  - ✓ The occupational health committee (OHC).

Note: The MSDSs can be made electronically available by maintaining the terminal in working condition, making the data sheets easily accessible to the employee, and instructing the employee on how to access the computer-stored data.

- The employer can customize data sheets to give more information, provided that the information is identical to that of the original source. Employer should:
  - ✓ Adhere to the safe work practices or preventative measures that the employer specifies.
  - ✓ Follow the preventive measures as instructed by the employer.
  - ✓ Aware of the location of the sheets and how to access information on first aid measures as well as safe use (Tub and Caulk, 2009).

20.6.2 MSDS content

A supplier MSDS must follow sixteen-section formats. It is advised to review the MSDS at least every 3 years. The MSDS should possess the following contents (Lienbenberg, 2020):

I. Product and company identification
   - Product recognition by the supplier label.
   - Information related to chemical names, molecular weight, and molecular formula.
   - Product suppliers, identifiers, manufacturer names, emergency telephone numbers, and addresses should be listed.

II. Hazards identification

- The chemical names and concentrations at which it can be used should be mentioned in MSDS concerning hazardous ingredients.
- CAS number, which helps to provide more information in case the product is identified by multiple names.

III. Data of ingredients
- Chemical characterization of mixtures or substances
- Description of mixtures

IV. First-aid treatments
- Information about first-aid treatment specific to outcomes of acute product exposure.
- Provide information to assist in planning for emergencies.

V. Firefighting measures
- Means of extinction, including the type of fire extinguisher required.
- Personal Protective Equipment (PPE) is required for firefighting.
- Provides information about temperature and storage conditions that might lead to fire catching for chemicals.

VI. Accidental release measures
- Instructions and precautions related to storage, safe use, and handling of the substance.
- Required safety devices or PPE.
- Clean-up procedures for spills.
- Environmental precautions.

VII. Storage and handling
- Preventive measures are to be taken for the handling of the chemical.
- Storage requirements, including compatibility issues.

VIII. Exposure control/PPE
- The concentration of the elements in the working environment should be less than the exposure limits.
- Engineering controls should be there, like proper ventilation, safety showers, and eye baths.
- PPE Kits should be readily available.

IX. Physical and chemical properties
- State of substance, e.g., liquid, solid, gas.
- The product's appearance and odor.
- The specific gravity, evaporation rate, vapor density, freezing, and boiling point.
- The odor threshold—the least airborne concentration of a chemical sensed by smell.
- The pH indicates the irritant or corrosiveness of the product.

X. Stability and reactivity
- The product's chemical stability and its reactivity toward heat, shock, light, moisture, and incompatible materials.
- Storage conditions are based on the instability or reactivity of the product.
- Incompatible products that should not be stored in proximity or mixed.
- Possibility of hazardous reactions and their decomposition products.

XI. Toxicology properties

- Acute and chronic health effects of the product exposure.
- The limits of exposure should be indicated; it defines as the maximum airborne concentration of a hazardous substance (dust, gas, mist, vapor, fume), which is considered safe upon repeated exposure without PPE.

XII. Ecological information
- Persistence and degradability data
- Behavior in environmental systems
- Additional ecological information—The product contains heavy metals. Avoid transferring to the environment. Specific preliminary treatments are necessary.
- Mobility in soil
- A chemical safety assessment (PBT assessment) is required for substances manufactured or imported in amounts of 10 tons or more per year unless exemptions apply.

XIII. Disposal considerations
- Dispose of following appropriate under government regulation.
- For disposal, conform to the applicable laws regarding industrial wastes, such as the "Waste Disposal and Public Cleansing Law" and relevant local by-laws.

XIV. Transport information
- UN number
- Packaging group
- Environmental hazards
- Precautions to be taken

XV. Regulatory information
- MSDS has been prepared according to USA regulations.
- Safety, health, and environmental regulation for the substance or mixtures.
- Carcinogenic profile
- Toxic substance control act.

XVI. Other information (Kit, 2008)
- Date of the latest revision

20.6.3 Marking guide

A four-digit UN number identifies hazardous materials such as explosives, flammable liquids, oxidizers, and some highly poisonous compounds. UN number is set by the United Nations committee of experts on the transport of dangerous goods. The system is designed to reduce the risk of incidents involving dangerous goods.

20.6.3.1 Classification of the UN system

- UN class
- Packaging identification code
- Packaging group level
- Gross mass and specific gravity
- Hydrostatic test procedure
- Year and manufacture
- Identification of the manufacturer or approval agency

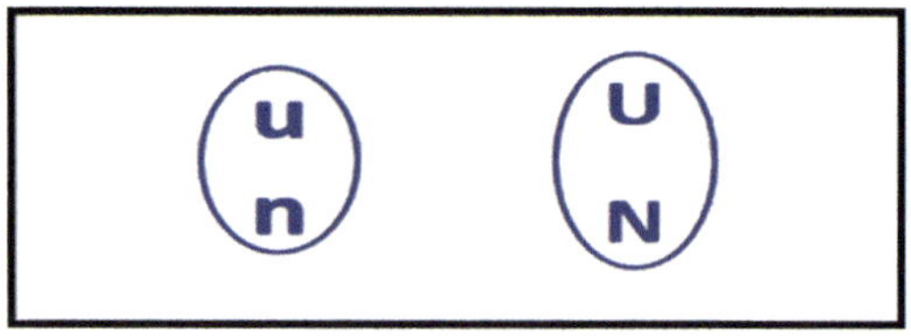

FIGURE 20.8 Symbol of UN indicating certification and testing of packaging material.

20.6.3.1.1 UN symbol

The packaging possessing UN in the circle signifies that it has undergone UN certification and testing. The UN sign can be written as an uppercase "UN" or as a lowercase "u" over a lowercase "n" in a circle, as shown in Fig. 20.8.

The UN packaging codes are a series of letters and numbers found on hazardous material packaging and offer details on various essential characteristics of the chemicals within.

They check that the personnel participating in the shipment of the materials obey the rules. They make it simple to track and search packing codes.

20.6.3.1.1.1 UN packaging groups According to the hazard level, the UN system categorizes chemicals into certain classes or divisions.

Packing group, **X: highly danger**
Packing group, Y: medium danger
Packing group, Z: minor danger

Packaging groups do not imply explosives (Class 1), gases (Class 2), organic oxides (Class 5.2), infectious substances (Class 6.2), and radioactive materials (Class 7). Instead, special transport and packaging provisions for this material are specified. The packaging group for which the package was tested is indicated by the letters X, Y, and Z, as shown in Fig. 20.9.

20.6.3.1.2 Packaging identification code

- It can be an alphanumeric combination suggesting the type of packaging as well as the material of construction, as shown in Table 20.1. e.g., 5H = Bags Plastic.
- It can be an alphanumeric combination additionally suggesting a subcategory within the type of packaging, along with the type of packaging and the material used in the construction of packaging. e.g., 1A1 = nonremoval head steel drum.
- It can be a number-letter-letter-number combination. It includes a number that indicates the type of packaging; the first letter will indicate inner material, the second letter will

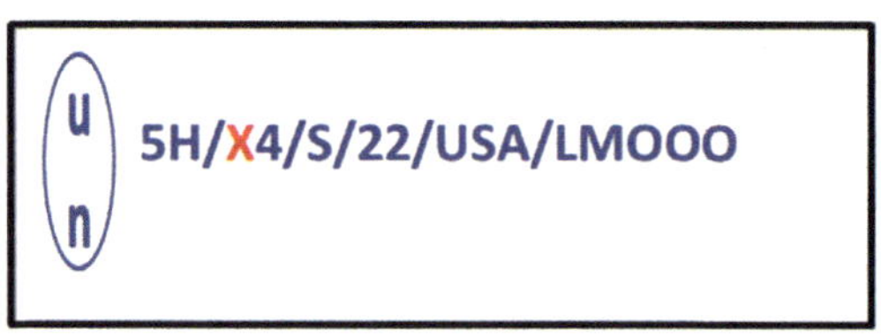

FIGURE 20.9 An example of coding for UN packaging group.

TABLE 20.1 Various codes for the packaging identification.

Type of Container	Container Material	Container packaging head /Material type
1-Drums	**A-Steel**	For drums:
2- Barrels	B-Aluminium	**1- Closed head (Non-Removal Head)**
3-Jerricans	C-Natural woods	2-Open head (Removal Head)
4-Boxes	D-Plywood	For Bags:
5-Bags	F-Reconstituted wood	5M1- Multiwall
6-Composite packaging	G-Fibrewood	5M2- Multiwalled, Water resistant
7-Pressure receptical	**H- Plastic**	
	L-Textile	
	M- Paper	
	N- Metal other than steel/Aluminium	
	P- Glass, Porcelain & Stoneware	

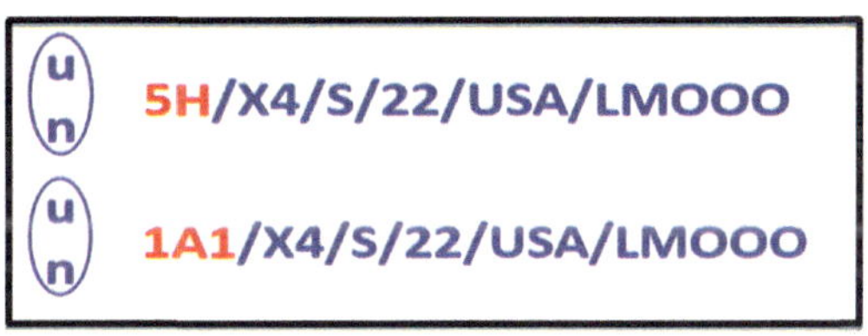

FIGURE 20.10 An example of coding for packaging identification code.

indicate outer material, and the second number indicates the packaging type, as shown in Fig. 20.10.

E.g., 6HA1 = Composite Packaging consists of Plastic inner and Steel outer drum.

20.6.3.1.3 Gross mass and specific gravity

- For combination packaging for all components or composite or single packaging for solids, the mark will specify the maximum gross mass (kilograms) of the package when filled (packaging + contents).

E.g., **4** = Gross mass in kg (for solids).

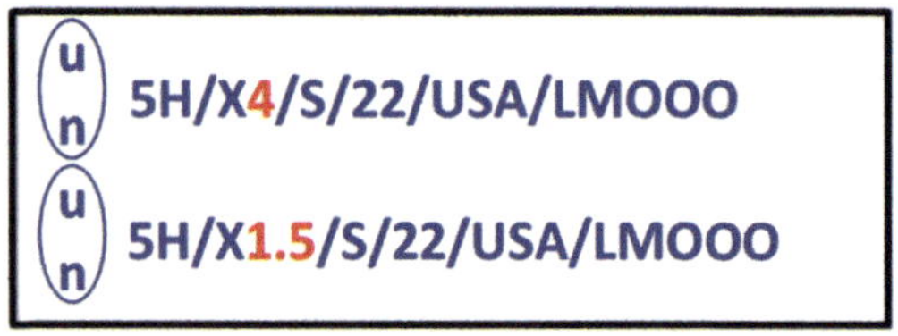

FIGURE 20.11 An example of coding for gross mass and specific gravity code specifically for solid and liquid chemicals.

- The mark must provide the maximum specific gravity permissible for single or composite packaging for liquid hazardous products, as shown in Fig. 20.11.

  E.g., **1.5** = Specific Gravity (for liquids).

20.6.3.1.4 Hydrostatic test pressure

- Solids: The mark shall incorporate a capital **"S"** for single or composite packaging designed to include solids or combination packaging for all ingredients, as shown in Fig. 20.12.
- The mark indicating the hydrostatic pressure conditions used for testing the container must be included for hazardous liquid products in composite or single packaging; the hydrostatic pressure shall be specified in kPa (kilopascals), approximated to the nearest 10 kPa.

20.6.3.1.5 Year and manufacture

- The last two digits of the manufacturing year must be included in the marking (E.g., **22, for 2022**).
- The mark must include the symbol of the nation where the product was manufactured.

E.g.,—The mark **"USA"** must be present if the packaging was developed in the United States (Fig.20.13).

20.6.3.1.6 Identification of the manufacturer or approval agency

- The mark must include the identity of the agency authorizing that the packaging satisfies all of the requisite tests. This might be represented by a name and location, a manufacturer's mark, or a code from the organization that certifies conformity. It is mandatory to register the symbols or code with PHMSA if used (Fig.20.14).

  E.g., LM0000.

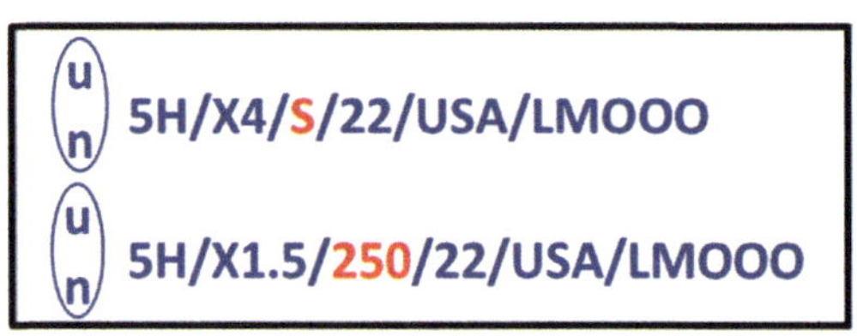

FIGURE 20.12 An example of coding for hydrostatic test pressure.

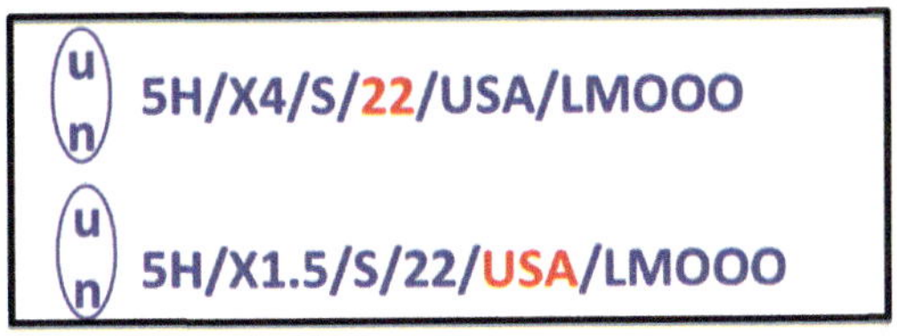

FIGURE 20.13 An example of coding for year and manufacture.

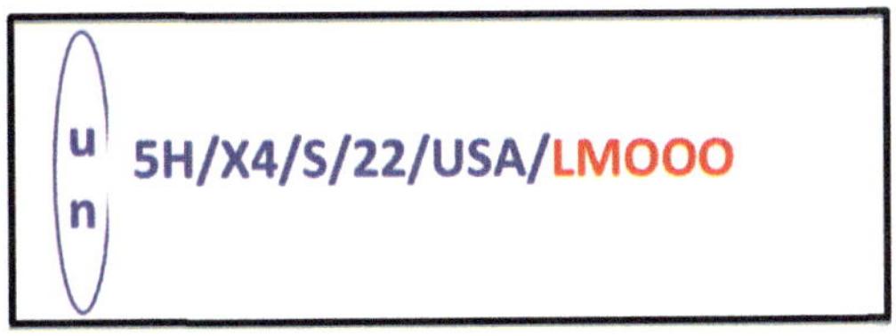

FIGURE 20.14 An example of coding for identification of the manufacturer or approval agency.

20.7 Conclusion

It's long been the chemical industries or any industry handling chemicals in routine life come in contact with hazardous chemicals directly or indirectly. Especially employees working in such area must be aware of the details of hazardous chemicals. To spread awareness about these chemicals, "Insecticides rules, 1971" put forward special labeling to these chemicals known as toxicity labels. These toxicity labels provide every single piece of information about the chemicals. In 2003, Globally Harmonized System (GSH) was established by the United States, and it was accepted for the uniformity in toxicity labels for all chemicals. These labels are presented in a 45 degrees angle triangle shape. It is divided into two parts: the upper part for signal words and the lower part for color indication. These labels are of four types: red, yellow, blue, and green. This label indicates the toxicity levels of chemicals. The chemicals falling under each category of label's has specified the different information required on the toxicity label, such as manufacturer's name, brand name, net content, antidote, etc. are also discussed in this chapter.

To spread awareness about the handling and using such harmful chemicals, there is an urgent need to make more stringent warnings and labels. Moreover, to understand the chemical's flammability level, National Fire Protection Association (NFPA) has a set of color-coded symbols such as red, blue, yellow, and white. To understand every perspective of the chemical material safety data sheet is used. This MSDS provides knowledge about identification, handling, storage, disposal, transport, and associated regulatory guidelines. In addition, the United Nations has also given a marking system for identifying goods while transporting. The United Nations uses the various code system as described above. A detailed information about the careful handling and identification of hazardous chemicals is helpful for people having frequent direct or indirect contact with the chemicals. Furthermore, it is advised that more stringent rules should be established for the appropriate use of the chemicals and their transportation.

20.8 List of abbreviations

GHS Globally Harmonized System
ISO International Organization for Standardization
LD_{50} Median lethal dose
MSDS Material Safety Data Sheet
NFPA National Fire Protection Association
OHC Occupational Health Committee
OSHA Occupational Safety and Health Administration
PPE Personal Protective Equipment
UN United Nations

References

GHS Label Requirements (2022) Elements, Updates & Example, 2022 [Online]. https://www.bradyid.com/applications/ghs-labeling-requirements. (Accessed 20 August 2022).

Burton, L.D.V., 2009. Agriscience Fundamentals and Applications. Cengage Learning.

Dar, S.A., Farook, U.B., Javeed, K., Mir, S.H., Yaqoob, M., Showkat, A., Kundoo, A.A., Hassan, R., Islam, T., 2020. Pesticide legislation, national and international policies to maintain sustainable crop production through insect pollinator intervention. Int. J. Chem. Stud. 8, 34–41.

Dhaneshwar, A., Hardej, D., 2021. Disruption of mitochondrial complexes, cytotoxicity, and apoptosis results from Mancozeb exposure in transformed human colon cells. Environ. Toxicol. Pharmacol. 84, 103614.

Friis, R.H., 2012. The Praeger Handbook of Environmental Health. Praeger.

Gupta, R.C., Milatovic, D., 2014. Chapter 23 - insecticides. In: Gupta, R.C. (Ed.), Biomarkers in Toxicology. Academic Press, Boston.

Hamade, H., Sahin, A., Sukhn, C., EL Tawil, C., Rizk, J., Kazzi, Z., EL Zahran, T., 2021. Human zinc phosphide exposure in Lebanon: a case report and review of the literature. Clin. Pract. Cases Emerg. Med. 5, 50–57.

Head, G.L., Wagner III, B.C., 1995. The NFPA 704 diamond. Prof. Saf. 40, 20.

Kit, C.D.D., 2008. Material safety data sheet (MSDS). Enzyme 110638, 68-1.

Krewski, D., Andersen, M.E., Tyshenko, M.G., Krishnan, K., Hartung, T., Boekelheide, K., Wambaugh, J.F., Jones, D., Whelan, M., Thomas, R., 2020. Toxicity testing in the 21st century: progress in the past decade and future perspectives. Arch. Toxicol. 94, 1–58.

Lienbenberg, D.D., 2020. Ethanol (C2H5OH).

Mehta, K., 2017. Pathological and toxicological profiles of endosulfan and its current status. Int. J. Med. Appl. Sci. 6.

NFPA, 2005. NFPA 654: Standard for the Prevention of Fire and Dust Explosions From the Manufacturing, Processing, and Handling of Combustible Particulate Solids. National Fire Protection Association.

Nidiry, E.S.J., 2021. Pesticides: Myths and Facts. Notion Press.

Occupational Safety and Health Administration, 2017. MSDS Hyper Glossary [Online]. Available. http://www.nfpa.org/.

Painkra, K., Kerketta, A., Jha, M.K., 2019. Chapter-2 tools of IPM and different insecticide act. Recent Trends Entomol. 17.

Pascale, A., Laborde, A., 2020. Impact of pesticide exposure in childhood. Rev. Environ. Health 35, 221–227.

Pauley, 2017. National Fire Protection Association. USA. Available. https://www.nfpa.org/News-and-Research/Publications-and-media/NFPA-Journal-Home.

Puhalla, J.C., Krans, J.V., Goatley, J.M., 2010. Sports Fields: Design, Construction, and Maintenance. Wiley.

Sanganalmath, P.U., Nagaraju, P.M., Sreeramulu, K., 2019. Determination of quinalphos in human whole blood samples by high-performance thin-layer chromatography for forensic applications. J. Chromatogr. A 1594, 181–189.

Reading the Labels May Save Your Lives – Understand India Toxicity Labels, 2022 [Online]. https://shashikallada.com/reading-the-labels-may-save-your-lives-understand-india-toxicity-labels/.

Sugimura, T., 2002. Food and cancer. Toxicology 181, 17–21.

Tub, P., Caulk, T.A., 2009. Material Safety Data Sheet (MSDS).

CHAPTER

21

Toxic potential indicator

Kuldeep Rajpoot[1], Muktika Tekade[2], Bhakti Pawar[1], Nupur Vasdev[1], Tanisha Gupta[1] and Rakesh Kumar Tekade[1]

[1]National Institute of Pharmaceutical Education and Research (NIPER)- Ahmedabad, An Institute of National Importance, Government of India, Department of Pharmaceuticals, Ministry of Chemicals and Fertilizers, Palaj, Gandhinagar, Gujarat, India; [2]School of Pharmacy, Devi Ahilya Vishwavidyalaya, Indore, Madhya Pradesh, India

21.1 Introduction

Living organisms constantly remain in danger when xenobiotics are present in the atmosphere. Nevertheless, to confirm the saturation level of toxicants, this is necessary to identify the organism's level of toxicity and information regarding poisoning causing specific organ changes along with clinical symptoms. It does not only rely on several variables like toxicokinetic and genetic factors but also shows a link between the toxic levels inside the organism (Rajpoot et al., 2022b,c; Tambe et al., 2021d). Furthermore, toxic response is highly challenging to predict. Screening of biomarkers through the application is one way to assess the relationship with xenobiotics and their possible influence on living species (including humans). They might be beneficial to analyze and manage the hazard of long-term consequences linked with exposure to xenobiotics (e.g., heavy metals, halogenated hydrocarbons, and pesticides) (Wołejko et al., 2021). They may be used as exposure indicators and identify harmful reactions and individual susceptibility to environmental compounds (Parikh et al., 2022).

Even though a variety of circumstances, like preexisting medical problems may significantly alter the dosage efficacy and degree of toxicity. Researchers have concentrated their emphasis on the safety of medicines (Gupta et al., 2022b; Kumawat et al., 2020), body temperature (Desai et al., 2021), age (Rajpoot et al., 2021a), diet (Polaka et al., 2022b), enzyme levels (Achanta et al., 2021; Tambe et al., 2021d; Rajpoot et al., 2020a), sleeping pattern (Choudhary et al., 2021; Vasdev et al., 2021), sex (Anup et al., 2021a; Polaka et al., 2022a), etc.

To determine how much of the active substances are needed to produce the desired outcome while minimizing any side effects, a variety of methods, models, and software are utilized (Anup et al., 2021b; Polaka et al., 2021b; Rajpoot et al., 2021b; Tambe et al.,

Essentials of Pharmatoxicology in Drug Research, Volume 1
https://doi.org/10.1016/B978-0-443-15840-7.00009-9

2021a,b,c). Various techniques are also used to confirm medication toxicity, for instance, in vitro toxicity investigation (Gupta et al., 2022c), in vivo animal studies, in silico studies (Rajpoot et al., 2022a), toxicokinetic well as toxicodynamic considerations (Rajpoot et al., 2022b), distinct bioindicators (Tekade et al., 2022), and toxic impacts of additives (Tiwari et al., 2022; Gupta et al., 2022a). It may be possible to lessen the negative effects of any pharmacological substances by improving the pharmacokinetic features of drugs, specifically their absorption, distribution, metabolism, and excretion from the body (Anup et al., 2021c; Padiyar et al., 2020; Polaka et al., 2021a; Rajpoot et al., 2020b, 2021c).

21.2 Toxicity biomarkers

The term "biomarker" refers to a biological reaction to a chemical substance or class of chemical substances that are not the drug agent itself or its metabolites inside the body (internal dose) (Walker et al., 2016). The assessment of a xenobiotic in a living system or specimen, though, is a bioindicator of exposure and might be regarded as a biomarker. Since it detects the dosage of a substance, biological tracking is preferable to environmental surveillance. It is vital to consider interindividual variations in DNA repair, absorption, bioavailability, and excretion. One should also account for intraindividual variations due to physiopathological changes in a particular period. Therefore, to assess exposure to a specific xenobiotic, an individualized biological control is often used (Abouir et al., 2021).

The organism responds as an integrator to exposure as well as some physiological variables that control the absorption of toxic substances. One may infer that a collective cannot be integrated as a homogenous group of people exposed to a xenobiotic with physicochemical characteristics under repeatable and standardized circumstances. In the past 10 years, there has been a noticeable increase in the utilization of biological markers to assess disease susceptibility. The occurrences in the processes contributing to illness are indicated by biomarkers, which are the identifiable endpoints. They are beneficial in assessing progressive disorders where symptoms appear long after exposure to triggering factors. Typical early illness warning signs might not be present in such circumstances. Simultaneously, the condition may be virtually irreversible once it becomes clinically evident (Aaseth et al., 2020). Environmental toxicology and industrial toxicology are the two primary study areas for applying biomarkers in toxicology. Moreover second, it constitutes one of the greatest pertinent and significant subspecialties of medical toxicology (Parikh et al., 2022).

21.3 Different biomarkers acting as biological indicators

21.3.1 Exposure biomarkers

Exposure to biomarkers enable the chemical evaluation of the harmful substances or metabolites in bodily fluids or excretions, for instance, exhaled air, blood, and urine, to determine the internal dosage (Tustin and Cannon, 2022; Hopf and Fustinoni, 2021). The quantity of a substance deposited in one or more bodily compartments, or even the entire body, is called internal dosage. Generally, this is true with cumulatively toxic substances.

For instance, the quantity of polychlorinated biphenyl (PCB) deposited at the primary location is manifested in the blood levels (for instance, fatty tissues). The quantity of substance bound to the target sites usually depends on the internal dosage (Estévez et al., 2019).

According to Bernard and Lauwerys' classification, which is predicated on the direct detection of unaltered chemicals and their metabolites in the biological medium, the exposure biomarkers are divided into two subcategories: (a) selective and (b) nonselective. The nonselective assays are utilized as general indications of chemical exposure. The detection of diazo-positive metabolites in the urine for tracking their exposure to aromatic amines, the measurement of thioethers in the urine, as well as the assessment of urine's mutagenic potential can be an example of nonselective exposure assays. Analytical and toxicokinetic elements of validity must be taken into account when evaluating the utility of a certain exposure biomarker. Standardization is necessary for the best analytical quality, although the particular criteria for certain toxicants differ significantly (Polaka et al., 2021b; Gadekar et al., 2021; Gorain et al., 2016; Muniswamy et al., 2019; Prajapati et al., 2009). Moreover, training and preparation of the person, the sampling process as well as handling, and the assessment process like calibration and quality assurance processes are the main areas of concern. Additionally, the toxicokinetics of a xenobiotic can also be impacted by life activities like reproduction and aging (Rajpoot et al., 2021a; Anup et al., 2021a).

21.3.2 Susceptibility biomarkers

These act as markers for a person's unique receptivity to a xenobiotic's effects or the impacts of a set of similar substances. They might be genetic markers like restriction fragment length polymorphisms, polymorphism of enzyme action, etc., that cause changes in chromosomal integrity (De las Cuevas and Sanz Alvarez, 2017). An organism undergoes a biotransformation phase in two stages after exposure to a xenobiotic. The primary metabolite that is often oxidized and otherwise active forms in the first phase due to the precise action of the microsomal P-450 cytochrome isoenzymes. In phase two, the primary metabolite is changed into a certain new secondary metabolite, which often exists in an inactive form. People with less cytochrome P-450 ability are generally less susceptible to producing principal functioning metabolites. Still, those with poor action levels of second-phase enzymes would produce fewer phase II inert metabolites, which will upsurge the toxic effect.

The polymorphisms of detoxicating systems and polymorphisms of activating system indicators are the two distinct categories of susceptibility biomarkers. Moreover, the activity of cytochrome P-450 isoenzyme is determined by measuring polymorphisms of the activating systems. Numerous xenobiotics are considered toxic and show toxicity due to the involvement of cytochrome P-450 enzymes. The P-450 cytochromes have a broad range of enzyme actions, which are also termed monooxygenase activities. The different cytochrome P-450 enzymes are thought to be encoded by various genes because of the significant disparities in their respective amino acid sequences. It has been supported by nucleotide sequence analyses of numerous genes and the entire amino acid sequences of over 71 distinct types of cytochrome P-450 (Kietzmann, 2001).

21.3.3 Response biomarkers

Response biomarkers are the indicators of metabolic alterations exhibited after xenobiotic exposure in an organism (Fig. 21.1). The perfect biomarkers must identify undesired effects immediately before they become permanent.

21.3.3.1 Organ-specific response biomarkers

21.3.3.1.1 Respiratory system

Low-molecular weight proteins (LMWP) exclusive to the lung have been proposed to function as peripheral indicators of lung damage (El Shafy and El-Sherif, 2019). A lung biomarker can be assessed in different body parts like bronchoalveolar fluid (BAL), serum, and sputum. This biomarker is made up of a microprotein that was first separated from the urine sample

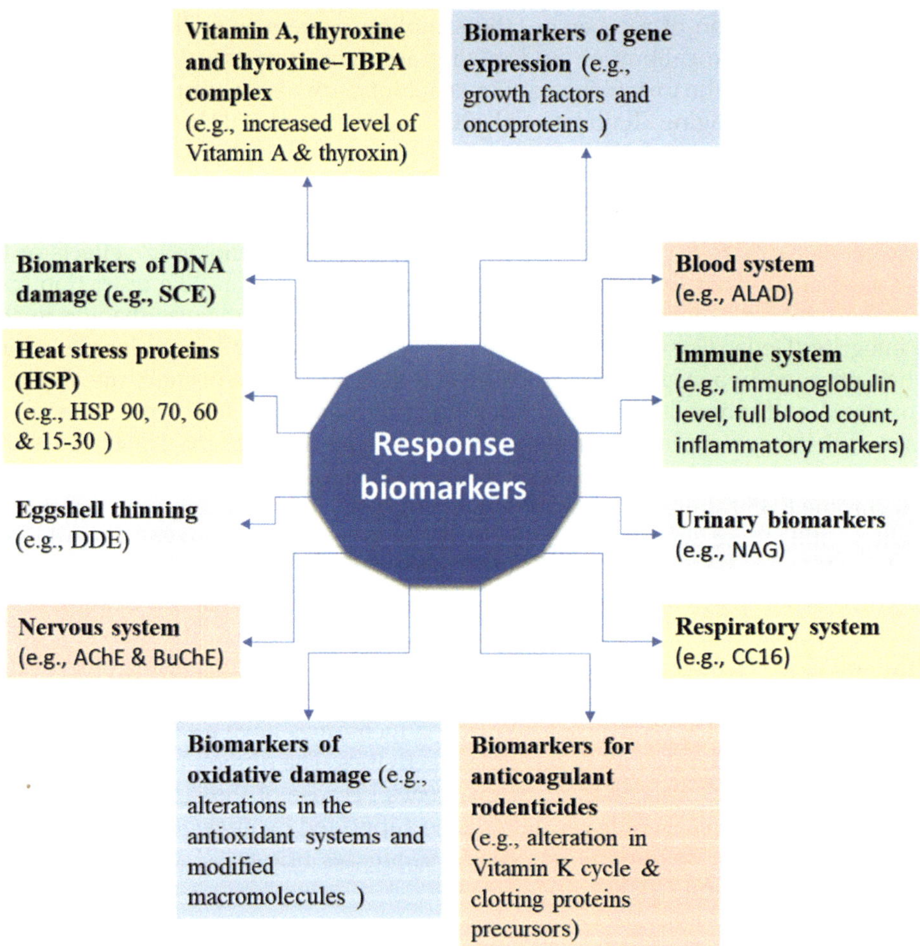

FIGURE 21.1 Types of response biomarkers.

taken from renal tubular dysfunction patients in 1974 under Urine Protein 1. It was later discovered to be the primary secretory substance of the lung Clara cells (nonciliated cells) primarily found in the terminal bronchioles. Furthermore, this homodimer of 15.8 kDa protein is known as Clara cell protein (CC16). Notably, Clara cells have significant xenobiotic metabolizing action and thus are highly vulnerable to toxic lung damage. They also comprise most of the lung cytochrome P-450 action (Oesch et al., 2019; Djidrovski et al., 2022).

The respiratory tract is shielded from unwelcome inflammatory responses caused by CC16. Cytosolic phospholipase A2, a crucial enzyme in inflammatory responses, is inhibited by the CC16. Phospholipase A2 is the rate-limiting enzyme that plays a crucial role in synthesizing arachidonic acid (the building block for creating leukotriene and prostaglandin mediators for inflammation) (Giresha, 2021). However, lung surfactants producing phospholipids may not be digested because of the inhibition of phospholipase A2 by CC16 (Groves et al., 2018; Laucho-Contreras et al., 2018).

The CC16 released by the respiratory tract disperses gradually into the blood plasma through transudation. It is quickly removed by glomerular filtration before getting absorbed and broken down in proximal tubule cells. Findings of Bernard's investigation revealed that the presence of CC16 in different body fluids like serum, sputum, and BAL fluid may be considered a sensitive and relatively accurate marker of acute or ongoing bronchial epithelial damage. Acute or ongoing damage to the bronchoalveolar/blood barrier integrity could be identified by the elevated levels of CC16 in the blood. Sarcoidosis and acute respiratory distress syndrome (ARDS) are also linked to higher blood levels of CC16 (Almuntashiri et al., 2020).

This demonstrates that pathological situations could result in a disturbance of the barrier separating the respiratory epithelium's surface from the vascular compartment, which would disturb the diffusional steadiness among CC16 in the serum as well as the respiratory tract. The substantial upsurge of albumin, 2-microglobulin, and other plasma proteins in BAL fluids, supports the presence of an augmented movement of proteins throughout the blood/bronchoalveolar gap barriers, for instance, in case of acute toxicity in the animals via either inhalation or systemic routes to pneumotoxic compounds (i.e., 1,2-dichloroethylene, naphthalene, 4-ipomeanol, trichloroethylene, 3-methyl furan, etc.). These results show that lung-specific rapidly diffusible proteins could function as peripheral indicators for pneumotoxicity, and thus it is opening another avenue for evaluating lung toxicity (Díaz de León-Martínez et al., 2022).

21.3.3.1.2 Blood system

The response biomarkers linked to alterations in hemoglobin production have received the most attention. Furthermore, the heme biosynthetic route engages the delta-aminolevulinic acid dehydratase (ALAD) enzyme, and therefore, the assay is found to be very precise not only for lead exposure but also for their effects. Investigations carried out on humans as well as on animal models, specifically different species of fish and birds (e.g., ducks, starlings, geese, eagles, etc.), have demonstrated that the suppression of ALAD is a powerful determinant for the influence of lead. The fact is that this biomarker does not need animal sacrifice in ecotoxicology, which is one of its most significant benefits. The impact is gradually reversed, with ALAD readings tuning back to normal only after 4 months (Walker et al., 2016; Melancon et al., 2018).

Porphyrin concentrations are typically observed to be relatively low and heme production is often tightly controlled. However, certain organochlorines (OCs) result in the overproduction of hepatic porphyrins that are heavily carboxylated. Hexachlorobenzene (HCB), as well as PCBs, are the two OCs, which are predominantly responsible for causing porphyria not only in mammals but also in birds (Walker et al., 2016). Exposure to many substances results in the production of hemoglobin adducts like 4-dimethyl-5-OH-pyrido-indole, acrylamide, 3-amino-1,4-aminobiphenyl-2,6-dimethylaniline, ethylene oxide, etc.). Moreover, acrylamide is demonstrated to be a possible carcinogen along with a potential neurotoxic substance that leads to peripheral neuropathy in both people and laboratory animals. The amount of acrylamide that reacts with hemoglobin to form neurotoxic metabolite epoxide, also known as glycidamide, is highly associated with acrylamide translation. Additionally, these adducts may be utilized as potential biomarkers for confirming peripheral neuropathy that occurred due to acrylamide (Kopanska et al., 2018; Bin-Jumah et al., 2021). Owing to the comparatively long lifespan of erythrocytes (around 4 months in humans), these hemoglobin adducts are being exploited beneficially for determining genotoxic agent concentrations in the plasma.

21.3.3.1.3 Nervous system

Neurotoxicity is emerging relatively slower than other disciplines in biological monitoring despite the field's showing clear relevance in toxicology. This slow development is indisputably caused by factors like the nervous system's complexity and unique characteristics and the difficulties in pinpointing the particular targets of neurotoxic activity. Additionally, the remoteness of target tissue restricts the use of neurochemical methods to assess neurotoxicity in humans. The easy and ethical investigation of neurochemical values in peripheral tissues in the patients might also serve as a marker for almost at the same levels as in the nerve tissue, and therefore, it can be an essential method for diagnosing and defining neurotoxicity (Sahu et al., 2022; Edén et al., 2021).

The inactivation of acetylcholinesterase (AChE) exhibited by organophosphorus substances or carbamate insecticides has been observed as most noteworthy and practical for a particular biomarker of neurotoxicity. Even though the enzymatic activity is found in various tissues, inhibition is often detected only in the brain regions and blood plasma. This biomarker is heavily researched in ecotoxicology (e.g., aquatic and bird species, and mammals) and has been applied to human toxicity. Impairment of AChE in the brain can be used as evidence of fatality in birds. However, in other animal studies, like fish, the lethal inhibition varies more widely and can vary from 40 to 80% (Mineau, 2018).

In contrast to that happening in blood with a shorter lifespan, the reduction in AChE action in the brain can last many weeks following the toxic exposure and is sufficiently associated with the result. However, since there is no requirement for animal sacrifice, monitoring blood AchE response offers the benefit of simple sampling (Hill, 1988). Furthermore, butyrylcholinesterase (BuChE) is occasionally assessed in conjunction with AChE. However, its physiological function is uncertain and the level of inhibition is not solely correlated with the toxic impact. A wide range of neurotoxicant xenobiotics targets various other neurotransmission factors. Moreover, fibroblasts, erythrocytes, and lymphocytes are used to test these characteristics (Singh, 2019).

21.3.3.1.4 Urinary biomarkers

Organic solvents (e.g., toluene), halogenated hydrocarbons (e.g., chloroform), heavy metals (for instance, cadmium, mercury, chromium, lead, etc.), as well as medicinal drugs (such as acetaminophen, aminoglycosides, amphotericin B, etc.) are some nephrotoxic substances that have been linked to long-term kidney damage. Nevertheless, owing to its substantial reserve capacity, renal impairment doesn't show any clinical symptoms until it has already caused considerable and irreparable damage. The detection of renal impacts at a phase while they are still adjustable or at least not so progressed as to cause a progressive renal illness demands the utilization of susceptible testing methods (Liu et al., 2020; Xiao et al., 2019).

In real-world situations, it is typically advised to measure at least two plasma-originated proteins within the urine, such as albumin (for the timely identification of a glomerular barrier deformity) and retinol-binding protein (for the advanced screening of proximal destruction) (Kumawat et al., 2020). By monitoring the urine action of kidney-derived enzymes, one can easily determine kidney damage. A potential indicator of nephrotoxicity can be the lysosomal enzyme (i.e., N-acetyl-D-glucosaminidase, NAG). Furthermore, this enzyme has several benefits, like urine consistency and vital kidney function. By testing B isoenzyme, one can determine the diagnostic value of NAG, and thus it could be further increased (Gruba et al., 2022; Okamoto et al., 2021).

Numerous urinary organ damage indicators were assessed by Koutou-Biken Co. in recent research, including creatinine, osmotic pressure, specific gravity, NAG, albumin, protein, glucose, urea nitrogen, uric acid, chloride, phosphate, sodium, potassium, and calcium (Fig. 21.2) (Tominaga et al., 2021). Results showed no significant change in the urine creatinine level (Fig. 21.2A). Following the activity, urine's specific gravity, pH, and osmotic pressure all were reduced (Fig. 21.2B–D). Following exercise, there was an upsurge of albumin, NAG, liver-fatty acid binding protein (L-FABP), intestine-fatty acid binding protein (I-FABP), as well as urine protein (Fig. 21.2E–I). The ideal bile acid-binding protein (I-BABP) level was just below the assay's limit of detection; however, the level of titin N-terminal fragments remained constant (Fig. 21.2J).

Renal antigens—renal constituents found in urine—can be measured using immunochemical techniques, which can also be used to determine the loss of renal tissue. It comprises alanine aminopeptidase, Tamm-Horsfall glycoprotein, carbonic anhydrase, and adenosine deaminase binding protein and has been suggested as a urine indicator of nephrotoxicity (Zheng et al., 2021; Erdbrugger et al., 2021).

21.3.3.1.5 Immune system

Direct influences of xenobiotics potentially modify the development of autoimmunity, disrupt the immune framework, reduce resistance to infections or tumors, or cause hypersensitive responses. While several indicators specifically show immunotoxicity in humans, most information on immunotoxic substances (for instance, dioxin, immunotherapeutic medicines, polychlorinated biphenyls, etc.) is taken through animal studies (e.g., mouse and rat models) (Polaka et al., 2022a; Pollard et al., 2018; Li and Mason, 2020). Antibody-mediated immunity, phenotypic evaluation of lymphocytes through flow cytometry analyses, complete blood count, assessment of nonspecific immunity, cellular immunity assay, as well as estimation

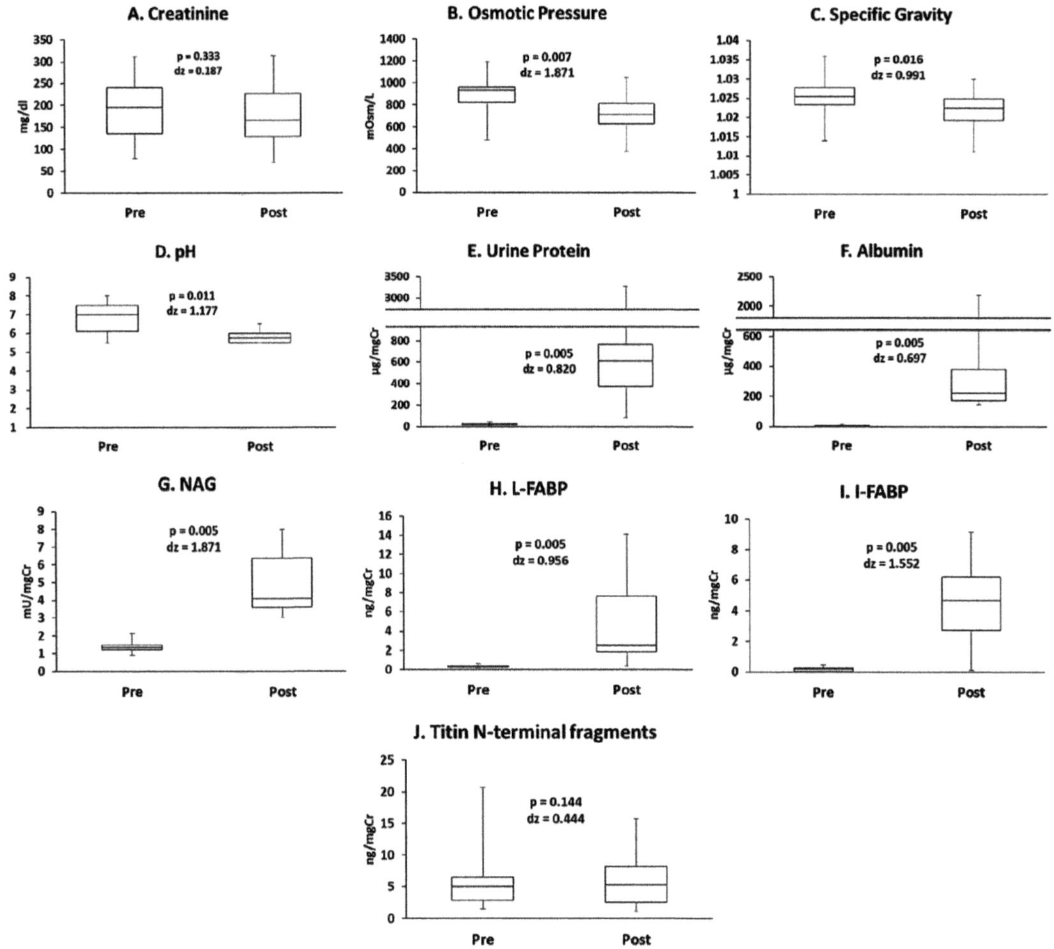

FIGURE 21.2 The concentrations of (A) creatinine, (B) osmotic pressure, (C) specific gravity, (D) pH, (E) urine protein, (F) albumin, (G) NAG, (H) I-FABP, (I) I-FABP, and (J) titin N-terminal fragments. *Adapted from reference Tominaga, T., Ma, S., Sugama, K., Kanda, K., Omae, C., Choi, W., Hashimoto, S., Aoyama, K., Yoshikai, Y., Suzuki, K. 2021. Changes in urinary biomarkers of organ damage, inflammation, oxidative stress, and bone turnover following a 3000-m time trial. Antioxidants 10 (1):79. https://www.ncbi.nlm.nih.gov/pubmed/33435279 under Creative Commons Attribution (CC BY) license Copyright © 2021.*

of antibodies and markers for inducing inflammatory reaction are among the biomarkers suggested for evaluating immunotoxicity in humans. Moreover, biological variables (such as pregnancy condition (Anup et al., 2021a), age of the patient (Rajpoot et al., 2021a), gender (Mishra et al., 2021), etc.), some medicines (like vitamin complexes, nonsteroidal anti-inflammatory drugs, etc.), as well as many other variables, for instance, circadian rhythms (Vasdev et al., 2021; Choudhary et al., 2021), intake of alcohol, stress, dietary uptake, sleep interruptions, disease symptoms (Desai et al., 2021), etc., may potentially impact immunity.

Numerous studies showed that immune checkpoint inhibitors (ICIs) therapy in cancer patients affected the blood levels of soluble immune mediators. A panel of 34 immune soluble molecules (chemokines, soluble immune checkpoints (sICs), adhesion molecules, and cytokines) was analyzed in the sera of 22 nonsmall cell lung cancer (NSCLC) patients obtained before nivolumab therapies (T0) and at first clinical assessment (>T0) to assess the effect of nivolumab therapies on the immune response of NSCLC patients (Zizzari et al., 2020). While no discernible alterations were found for any of the other immune components evaluated, PD1, PDL2, as well as the coinhibitory LAG3 receptor were dynamically altered after nivolumab administration (Fig. 21.3). Following therapy with nivolumab, PD1, as well as its ligand PDL2, drastically dropped, but LAG3 levels rose (Fig. 21.3A). Whenever these data were evaluated because of the clinical outcome, it seemed that PD1 reduction was shown in the responding (R) patient cohort but not in the nonresponding (NR) group (Fig. 21.3B), indicating that this variation is not due to the interaction among soluble PD1 and nivolumab. On the other hand, NR patients had considerably higher LAG3 concentrations. The reaction did not appear to be related to the decrease in PDL2 seen during ICI treatment (Zizzari et al., 2020).

As interferon-gamma (IFN-γ) is a crucial regulator of the stimulation of cell-mediated immunity, researchers looked for immunological stimulation as well as IFN-γ expression in the supernatants of peripheral blood mononuclear cells (PBMC) and tumor co-cultures administered with neutrophil defensins. Results indicated that administration of the coculture using neutrophil defensins increases IFN-γ secretion (Fig. 21.4). Interestingly, the secretion of IFN-γ was not increased when neutrophil defensins were administered to PBMC from healthy donors in the lack of progressed NSCLC cells. This appears to show that neutrophil defensins indirectly stimulate immune response activation. This finding may offer a first clue as to how neutrophil defensins affect the effectiveness of anti-programmed death ligand-1 (anti-PD-L1) immunotherapy (Berghmans et al., 2020).

21.3.3.2 *Miscellaneous response biomarkers*

21.3.3.2.1 Biomarkers of DNA damage

Determining xenobiotic covalent bonds between proteins and other macromolecules is currently made possible by various technical methods. Examples of biomolecules possessing sulfhydryl, amino, or reactive carboxyl groups, which can react with electrophilic substances, include serum albumin and hemoglobin. A possible biomarker for understanding the molecular epidemiology of tumors or cancer is the production of human DNA adducts, which is the covalent alteration of DNA and carcinogen substances. This phenomenon is found to associate with the occurrence of carcinogenic activity (Behl et al., 2021; Stading et al., 2021).

The establishment of adducts is the first step of activities among the initial interaction amid xenobiotic and DNA and the resulting mutation; the second step involves secondary alteration of DNA, like strand rupture or an enhancement in the speed of DNA restoration; and the final step is attained once the structural perturbations of DNA are set and impacted cells frequently exhibit disrupted function. Sister chromatid exchange (SCE) is one of the most frequently utilized procedures to assess chromosomal abnormalities. Ultimately, xenobiotic harm during cell division might result in DNA mutation and subsequent changes to the descent (Walker et al., 2016).

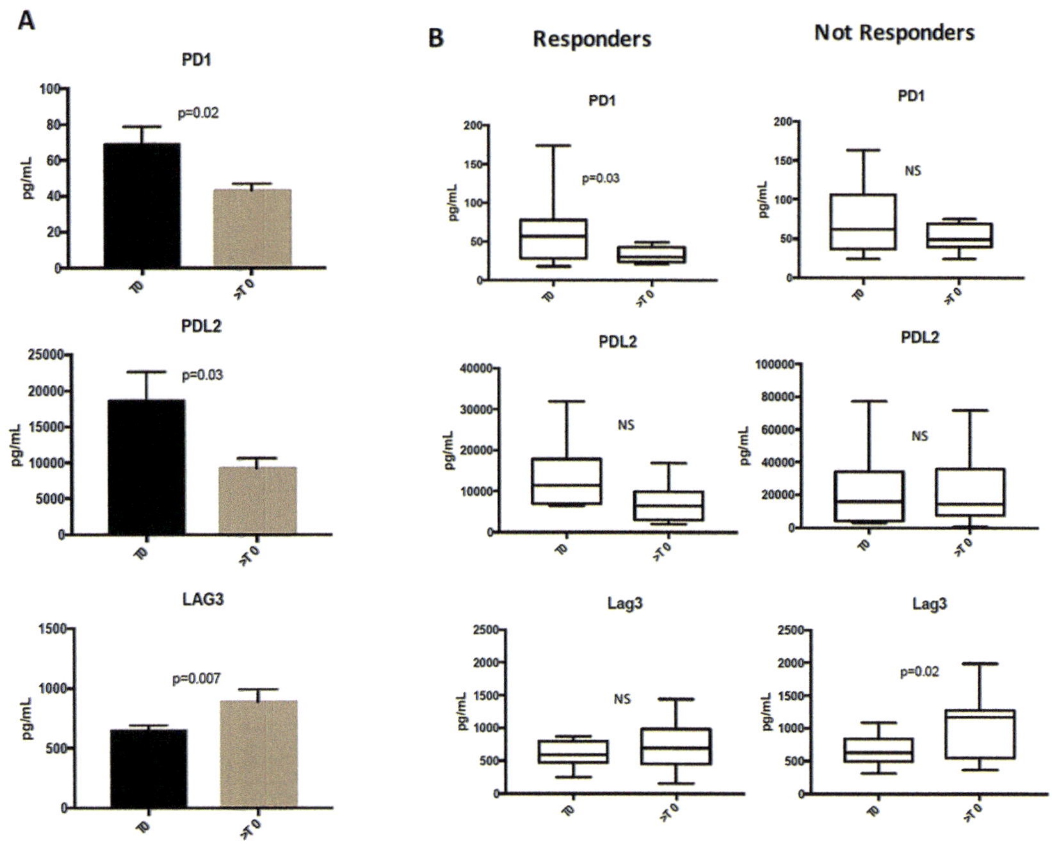

FIGURE 21.3 Changes in sICs in NSCLC patients receiving therapy with Nivolumab. (A) Analysis of the amounts of soluble immune checkpoint-related proteins determined in the whole population of NSCLC patients at the time of the initial clinical assessment (>T0) and before the start of Nivolumab therapy (T0). The Luminex multiplex test was used to evaluate the proteins, and the findings were expressed as the concentration (pg/mL) of sICs found in the patients' sera. (B) Box plots of PD1, PDL2, and LAG3 in patients with R as well as NR during the start of nivolumab treatment (T0) and the initial clinical assessment (>T0). The box's lines display the mean scores. The error bars show the sICs concentration's upper and lower limits (pg/mL). The variances among T0 and >T0 were compared using a student's paired t-test, with p-values below 0.05 regarded as significant. Not significant (NS). *Adapted from reference Zizzari, I.G., Di Filippo, A., Scirocchi, F., Di Pietro, F.R., Rahimi, H., Ugolini, A., Scagnoli, S., Vernocchi, P., Del Chierico, F., Putignani, L., Rughetti, A., Marchetti, P., Nuti, M., Botticelli, A., Napoletano, C. 2020. Soluble immune checkpoints, gut metabolites and performance status as parameters of response to Nivolumab treatment in NSCLC patients. J. Personalized Med. 10 (4):208. https://www.ncbi.nlm.nih.gov/pubmed/33158018 under Creative Commons Attribution (CC BY) license Copyright© 2020.*

21.3.3.2.2 Biomarkers of gene expression

The abnormal manifestation of genes that code for proteins engaged in cellular development is linked to the emergence of numerous cancers connected to xenobiotics. A quantitative variation (increased expression of the protein), as well as a qualitative change, might both be present in this abnormal expression. Even if these indicators are influenced by many harmful

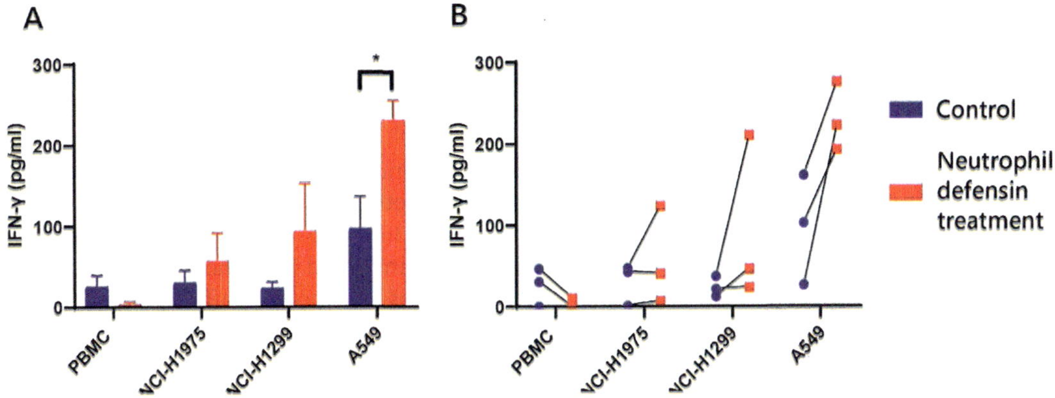

FIGURE 21.4 IFN-γ secretion in the coculture after the treatment of neutrophil defensins 1, 2, and 3. For 3 days, PBMC was either administered alone or in coculture with NSCLC cells (NCI-H1975, NCI-H1299, or A549) using neutrophil defensins 1, 2, and 3 (red, 5 M) or PBS (blue, control). Afterward when supernatants were utilized to calculate the concentration of IFN-γ. (A) Means ± SEM of PBMC from three healthy donors following receiving neutrophil defensin therapy for 66 h. IFN-γ level for A549 significantly rises (*p = 0.05); (B) IFN-γ level rise for every donor separately. *Adapted from reference Berghmans, E., Jacobs, J., Deben, C., Hermans, C., Broeckx, G., Smits, E., Maes, E., Raskin, J., Pauwels, P., Baggerman, G. 2020. Mass spectrometry imaging reveals neutrophil defensins as additional biomarkers for anti-PD-(L)1 immunotherapy response in NSCLC patients. Cancers 12 (4):863. https://www.ncbi.nlm.nih.gov/pubmed/32252405 under Creative Commons Attribution (CC BY) license Copyright© 2020.*

substances, it is crucial to identify any potential confounding variables and evaluate their efficiency, accuracy, and predictive level of tests (Miller et al., 2020; Que et al., 2019). Some gene expression biomarkers can be growth factor receptors, tumor-suppressor gene proteins, oncogene proteins, etc. These bioindicators are being investigated in biological fluids that are readily available, for instance, plasma, BAL, radioimmunoassay (RIA), serum, enzyme-linked immunosorbent assay (ELISA), urine, and immunoblotting.

21.3.3.2.3 Oxidative stress biomarkers

In particular, contaminants derived from free radicals like selenium, polycyclic aromatic hydrocarbons (PAHs), industrial solvents, halogenated aromatic hydrocarbons, heavy metals, and pesticides may result in oxidative stress. Furthermore, antioxidant processes might adapt cellular macromolecules, leading to tissue injury and causing oxidative stress. Therefore, biomarkers can be used for various xenobiotics, altered macromolecules, and alterations to the antioxidant systems. Hence for protection, defense mechanisms comprise catalase, ascorbate, tocopherol, nucleic acids, oxidized/reduced glutathione, superoxide dismutase, glutathione reductase, lipids, and proteins are some examples of macromolecules that can be harmed by free radicals (Othmène et al., 2020; Vona et al., 2019).

21.3.3.2.4 Heat Stress Proteins (HSP)

It is an essential class of ATP-reliant proteins that helps in the folding of forming proteins by limiting their accumulation and chaperoning to regions of membrane translocation. While they grew in reaction to a range of xenobiotics, comprising metals or metalloids (particularly arsenite), oxidizing agents, as well as heavy metals, they were formerly known as heat shock proteins owing to their fast emergence upon heat stress (Sanders, 2018). Four different forms of HSP exist, such as HSP 90, 70, 60, and LMW HSP of 15–30 kDa. However, future research will be crucial for understanding these biomarkers.

21.3.3.2.5 Eggshell thinning

Eggs can fracture if the eggshell is harshly thinned. Hence, thinning of eggs is considered a biomarker in reproductive injury. The dichlorodiphenylethane (DDE) metabolizes dichlorodiphenyltrichloroethane (DDT), which has been most extensively researched in several bird species like eagle and pelican. Although the mechanism involved in pathogenicity is still unidentified, it may be connected to hormonal changes that significantly affect calcium breakdown, which is crucial for developing eggshells. There are two techniques that exist for assessing eggshell thickness. One method uses a micrometer to determine it directly, while another technique allocates shell weight by multiplying the shell's length by the width to achieve a thickness index (Walker et al., 2016).

21.3.3.2.6 Thyroxine–thyroxine-binding prealbumin (TBPA)-retinol-binding protein (RBP) complex

The thyroxine-TBPA-RBP complex is usually formed when thyroxine is attached to transthyretin in the plasma. Thyroxine and several monohydroxy-metabolites of 3, 3r, 4, 4r-tetrachlorobiphenyl (OH-TCBs) produced by the monooxygenase system (cytochrome P-450IA1) fiercely fight for the transthyretin's active site. The presence of such metabolites in the blood results in a rapid depletion of thyroxine and leads to the manifestation of hypothyroidism. Additionally, the attachment of OH-TCBs to transthyretin may result in the conformational shift that lessens the RBP's adhesion to TBPA. Utilizing glomerular filtration, the RBP as well as any connected retinol (i.e., vitamin A) are removed through blood. The results of this attribute include the development of hypovitaminosis A (dermal and epithelial lesions) (Walker, 1995). These results have been demonstrated in lab tests using various animal models like monkeys and mice (Brouwer, 1991). Moreover, the rising concentrations of thyroxine and vitamin A in urine serve as a biomarker of TCB exposure.

21.3.3.2.7 Anticoagulant rodenticides biomarkers

The vitamin K cycle in the vertebrate liver is inhibited by compounds like warfarin as well as second-generation anticoagulant such as flocumafen. These substances work by interfering with vitamin K or its byproducts, and as a result, the vitamin K cycle cannot carboxylate the intermediates of clotting proteins. This causes hemorrhaging, an enhancement in the time for blood clotting, and ultimately death. Measuring variations in the vitamin K cycle or keeping an eye on rises in blood plasma intermediates of these clotting proteins are the two fundamental ways to identify the impact of anticoagulants. In recent times, the advent of ELISA tests has made it possible to identify precursors of clotting proteins in mammals as well as birds (Walker et al., 2016).

21.4 Different techniques used as toxicity indicators

There are different techniques which are widely employed as toxicity indicators (Fig. 21.5). Some of these techniques are discussed in the next sections.

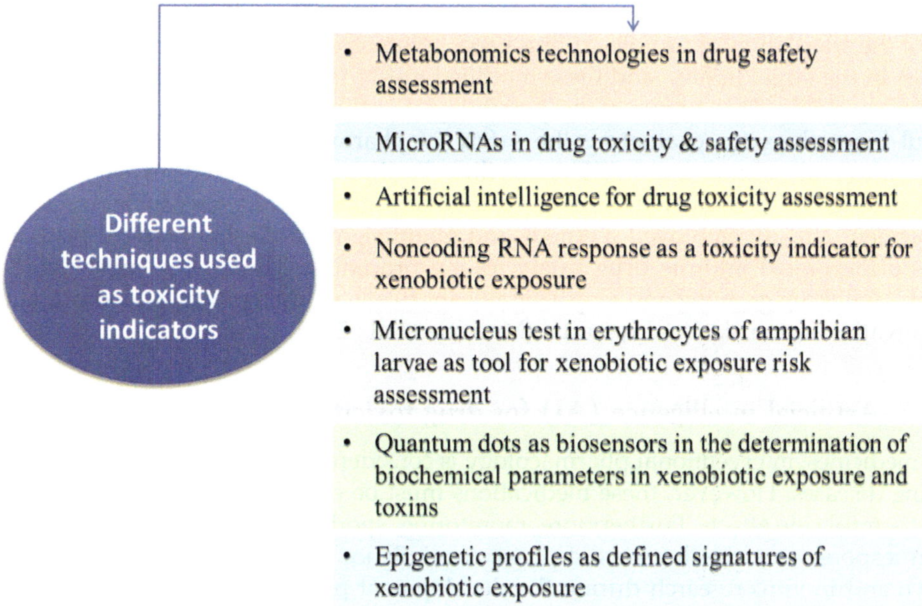

FIGURE 21.5 Schematic describing different techniques employed as toxicity indicators.

21.4.1 Metabonomics technologies in drug safety assessment

As long as the data sources remain rich in molecular research information, some spectroscopic techniques may be employed to produce metabonomic data sets on complicated biological samples. Since mass spectrometry (MS) shows higher sensitivity relative to nuclear magnetic resonance (NMR) spectroscopy, it has been applied in a variety of research, primarily in plant and microbiological applications (Fiehn, 2002). Following chemical derivatization, it has often been connected to either liquid chromatography (LC) or gas chromatography (GC). High-resolution 1H NMR spectroscopy, on the other hand, has been demonstrated to be one of the most potent technologies for biofluids and therefore used proficiently in studying intact tissues for generating a thorough profile of metabolite signals without requiring the use of isolation or derivatization techniques, preselection of assessment parameters, or both (Fiehn, 2002; Tekade et al., 2022).

Typically, biofluid samples are produced for NMR spectroscopy into 96-well plates employing specialized robots such as a Gilson 215 Preparation robot and the Bruker SampleTrack system (Bruker Biospin, Rheinstetten, Germany). Briefly, the flow-injection NMR probe receives a sample injection of around 500 cc (Spraul et al., 1997). By adding a buffer and then centrifuging the sample to eliminate insoluble salts, urine samples can stabilize their pH levels somewhat between samples.

21.4.2 MicroRNAs in drug toxicity and safety assessment

Adverse drug responses pose considerable obstacles to pharmaceutical research and development and place a heavy strain on global public health systems. To find the crucial pathways associated with drug toxicity, the science of toxicology is immensely working on it.

Small, evolutionary conserved endogenous noncoding RNAs called microRNAs (miRNAs) control the translation of protein-coding genes. Numerous toxicants change the amounts of miRNA in the target tissues, and these modified miRNAs can be discovered in readily available bodily fluids. This supports the possibility that these tiny compounds might serve as helpful biomarkers for evaluating the safety of pharmaceuticals, with an initial miRNA response to toxic stimuli and miRNA stability. To find drug-induced toxicity, miRNAs can be promising tools for early detection. Furthermore, the miRNA sequencing approach will complement already employed methods and might significantly improve medication safety if it is incorporated into the drug safety testing procedure. The area of miRNA biomarker research will keep growing and play a significant role in studying human medication toxicity as motivation in translational research (Marrone et al., 2015).

21.4.3 Artificial intelligence (AI) for drug toxicity assessment

In medicines, interventional pharmacology is considered one of the most effective tools for fighting diseases. However, these medications must be constantly checked since they might have harmful side effects. Furthermore, monitoring, spotting, and preventing negative medication responses are the domains of pharmacovigilance science. Safety initiatives start with in vivo and in vitro research during the development phase, extend through clinical trials, and continue postmarketing surveillance of adverse drug reactions in real-world populations. The limitations of these conventional techniques are highlighted by upcoming toxicity and safety problems, such as growing polypharmacy and patient diversity. The vast amount of recently available data presents the possibility of applying AI and machine learning (ML) to advance drug safety science, with a particular focus on ML and deep learning (DL) methodologies (Basile et al., 2019).

It has been demonstrated that AI approaches, particularly in toxicity assessment, are crucial for premarketing medication safety. Assessing the adverse effects (AEs) of chemicals on people, plants, animals, and the environment is critical in defining medication toxicity (Raies and Bajic, 2016). A popularized revamping of neural networks known as ML and DL was spurred by an exponential rise in the computational capacity as well as data accessibility. Furthermore, the researcher examines recent studies using new data sources for preclinical and postmarketing monitoring for pharmacovigilance (PV) that use AI methodologies, including ML and DL (Basile et al., 2019). QSARs, ensemble learning, regression, software, support vector machines (SVMs), and other ML and DL approaches are used to predict and evaluate toxicity.

21.4.4 Noncoding RNA response as a toxicity indicator for xenobiotic exposure

One of the principal risk elements for noncommunicable illnesses, particularly cancer, is human exposure to specific environmental and occupational toxins. As a result, it is essential to employ minor exposure-related unfavorable cellular activity to diagnose diseases early on and to spot any possible risks posed by brand-new, inadequately studied medications and substances. A common characteristic of persistent cellular stress resulting in carcinogenesis is nongenotoxic events brought by exposure to carcinogens or toxicants. Noncoding RNAs (ncRNAs) are used to control these activities on a global scale. The altered expression of ncRNAs caused by cancer-related genotoxic as well as nongenotoxic events may offer a mechanistic explanation for the connection between chemical exposure and carcinogenesis. The remarkable tissue precision, minimal baseline variability, early appearance, as well as stability of ncRNAs in body fluid are advantages of their usages in carcinogenicity analysis, which also implies that incorporating ncRNAs in the evaluation of cancer risk may significantly improve the effectiveness of toxicity and carcinogenicity testing (Marrone et al., 2014).

The evidence after research suggests that aberrations of ncRNAs, particularly miRNAs, play a crucial role in the reactions to carcinogens and toxins and also that miRNAome changes may be early signs of carcinogen/toxin exposure, regardless of the lack of conclusive information to confirm whether or not ncRNA modifications are a significant detrimental response to toxicants or a secondary outcome of the perturbed cellular pathways. Furthermore, miRNA changes have been suggested as potential biomarkers for the detection of carcinogenic substances by several research groups (Hou et al., 2012; Tal and Tanguay, 2012; Gooderham and Koufaris, 2014), as well as advantages of this strategy for safety evaluation have been demonstrated (Koufaris et al., 2012). In particular, a current, in-depth investigation by Koufaris et al. showed that male F344 rats were exposed for 90 days to a variety of liver genotoxic and nongenotoxic carcinogens changed the expression of hepatic miRNAs (Koufaris et al., 2012). More significantly, the hepatic miRNA expression patterns correlated with the carcinogens' mechanisms of action as well as their carcinogenic effects. The extraordinary tissue specificity of miRNAs, uniformity between species and genotypes, as well as stability in a variety of bodily fluids are further advantages of using miRNAs in carcinogen evaluation (Schwarzenbach et al., 2014; Gatti et al., 2011).

This shows that the effectiveness of assessment for carcinogenicity will be significantly improved by including miRNA analysis in cancer risk evaluation. The miRNA biomarkers should be used more frequently in the process of determining cancer risk owing to the following characteristics: (i) relatively early appearance; (ii) target tissue precision; (iii) reduced baseline variability; (iv) existence in biofluids; and (v) suitability to both genotoxic as well as nongenotoxic agents (Marrone et al., 2014).

21.4.5 Micronuclei (MN) test in erythrocytes of amphibian larvae as a tool for xenobiotic exposure risk assessment

A suitable method for assessing short-term environmental mutagenesis is the MN assay, which calculates the genetic susceptibility resulting from xenobiotic exposures. This method is focused on red blood cells, which are nucleated in amphibians—has been widely applied. MN is the consequence of full chromosomes, which have been derived from the central core (aneugenic effect) by inadequate migration or acentric segments of chromosomes (clastogenic effect). As a consequence of the attacks on either chromosomal structure (fragmentation) or centromere kinetochore complexes, failure of the spindle machinery or micronuclei signifies a depletion in chromatin (Bombail et al., 2001; Campana et al., 2003).

The MN test offers certain benefits over other DNA damage detection methods, including quick performance, low cost, lack of complexity, as well as easier and faster preparation and analysis of chromosomal abnormalities (Da Rocha et al., 2009). The genotoxicity of substances has been widely tested using the micronucleus test. With invertebrates, fish, and amphibians, the testing has been effectively utilized as a biological monitor of polluted regions (in situ assay) (Çavas and Ergene-Gözükara, 2005; Klobučar et al., 2003; Wirz et al., 2005) as well as in the assessment of chemicals to detect their genotoxicity following direct or indirect exposure in vivo (Da Rocha et al., 2009; Ossana et al., 2010).

21.4.6 Quantum dots (QDs) as biosensors in the determination of biochemical parameters in xenobiotic exposure and toxins

Establishing flexible analytical techniques that are eco-friendly, easy to use, and reasonably priced is urgently needed to get around the limits of current xenobiotic testing methods. Due to its simple handling and real-time output with great sensitivity and reproducibility, sensor-based evaluation has become an indispensable option in chemical and biological research. Zero-dimensional (0-D) materials, also known as QDs, are innovative in sensing technology. Their size ranges from 1 to 10 nanometers. Due to their superior optical characteristics, QDs have been used for various light-based applications. The size as well as the surface structure of QDs affect their photoluminescence (PL). Since QDs undergo size and surface-level alterations due to the adsorbed ions or molecules, PL intensification or quenching is reflected (Song et al., 2019; Cui et al., 2015; Bera et al., 2010).

The detected PL variations can be used to monitor biological parameters or identify xenobiotics. Plain QDs such as CdTe, carbon, and graphene, as well as core/shell QDs including CdSe/ZnS and CdTe/ZnS, are examples of QD types (Kandasamy, 2019; Molaei, 2020; Iravani and Varma, 2020; Kang and Lee, 2019). Because they can be made from organic carbonaceous materials and are inherently nontoxic (Reshma and Mohanan, 2019), graphene QDs (GQDs) and carbon atom-based QDs (CQDs) have garnered the most attention among the many QD types (Molaei, 2020; Iravani and Varma, 2020; Kang and Lee, 2019).

Most QD-based biosensors are covered with distinct layers of biomolecules, such as enzymes, antibodies, oligosaccharides, macromolecules of amino acids, etc. These biomolecules possess low toxicity as well as excellent biocompatibility (Ma et al., 2018; Wang et al., 2007). QDs are used as biosensors to analyze a wide range of chemical and biological compounds, notably poisons, carcinogens, and biothreat compounds (bacteria and viruses) (Walper et al., 2018). In cellular and tissue imaging studies for biological identification, QDs were also employed (Rosenthal et al., 2002; Dubertret et al., 2002; Wu et al., 2002).

These QD-based sensors are also used to find the tumor and inflammatory biomarkers (Vashist et al., 2006; Lv et al., 2019). The QDs are employed as sensors to assess biochemical key parameters in toxicology, including pH estimation, blood glucose monitoring, identification of biothiols (sulfhydryl molecules), which include amino acids, peptides, proteins, and enzymes, and the evaluation of the well-known neurotransmitter acetylcholine (Ravi and Ganesan, 2021).

21.4.7 Epigenetic profiles as defined signatures of xenobiotic exposure

The phenomenon wherein alterations in gene expression can take place even though a direct impact on the DNA sequence is indeed commonly referred to as epigenetics. These alterations are frequently heritable and are transmitted during cell division across generations

(Thomson et al., 2014). Furthermore, a thorough evaluation of the prospective effects of epigenomics on drug safety sciences was published (LeBaron et al., 2010; Lempiäinen et al., 2012). Briefly stated, without a complete understanding of the medication's mechanism of action, conventional toxicological studies have primarily focused on the phenotypic effects of drug delivery, such as changes in an animal's temperament or the development of tumors. Genotoxicity assessment techniques concentrate on identifying genetic changes brought on by chemical exposure, like chromosomal number changes (aneuploidy or polyploidy) and copy number variations, as well as sequence mutations of genes implicated in carcinogenesis. These genetic assays are typically ineffective at differentiating between genotoxic as well as nongenotoxic substances and are frequently unable to correctly forecast the course of rodent carcinogenesis (Kirkland et al., 2005).

There are several innovative opportunities for improving mechanistic toxicology research at the gene regulation level now that the domain of epigenetic studies is developing at an exponential rate, along with techniques that enable high-resolution genome-wide assessment of multiple epigenetic marks. Incorporated epigenomic and transcriptomic analyses may unveil important details about xenobiotic-induced toxicity processes at some very initial phases of exposure and make it easier to anticipate longer term toxicities like carcinogenesis. This is because epigenetic perturbations can result in both short-term and long-lasting alterations in gene manifestation. Epigenetic endpoints are pretty likely to help improve mechanistic research right now. Before routinely integrating epigenetic endpoints into toxicity assessment methodologies, the information gaps must be filled (Thomson et al., 2014).

21.5 Conclusion

Organisms remain in constant danger when xenobiotics are present in the environment. Nevertheless, to discuss impregnation, it is necessary to identify the organism's toxicity level and the idea that poisoning is associated with certain organ changes and clinical signs. As it relies on many variables like toxicokinetic and genetic variables, toxic levels in the organism, and toxic reactions, it is highly complicated and difficult to predict. Screening via considering biomarkers is a vital tool to assess the association of xenobiotics as well as its possible influence on living species, particularly humans. They could be highly useful to analyze and manage the risk of long-term consequences concomitant to exposure to xenobiotics since they can be used to measure the intake of toxicants, toxic impact, and individual vulnerability to external chemical substances (i.e., insecticides, heavy metals, and halogenated hydrocarbons).

21.6 List of abbreviations

0-D zero-dimensional
AChE acetylcholinesterase
AEs adverse effects
AI artificial intelligence
ALAD delta-aminolevulinic acid dehydratase

anti-PD-L1 anti-programmed death ligand-1
ARDS adult respiratory distress syndrome
BAL bronchoalveolar fluid
BuChE butyrylcholinesterase
CC16 clara cell protein
CQDs carbon atom-based quantum dots
DDE dichlorodiphenylethane
DDT dichlorodiphenyltrichloroethane
DL deep learning
ELISA enzyme-linked immunosorbent assay
GC gas chromatography
GQDs graphene quantum dots
HCB hexachlorobenzene
HSP heat stress proteins
I-BABP ileal bile acid-binding protein
I-FABP intestine-fatty acid binding protein
ICIs immune checkpoint inhibitors
IFN-γ interferon gamma
L-FABP liver-fatty acid binding protein
LC liquid chromatography
LMWP low-molecular weight proteins
miRNAs microRNAs
ML machine learning
MN micronuclei
MS mass spectrometry
NAG N-acetyl-D-glucosaminidase,
ncRNAs non-coding RNAs
NMR nuclear magnetic resonance
NR nonresponding
NS not significant
NSCLC nonsmall cell lung cancer
OCs organochlorines
OH-TCBs monohydroxy-metabolites of 3, 3r, 4, 4r-tetrachlorobiphenyl
PAHs polycyclic aromatic hydrocarbons
PBMC peripheral blood mononuclear cells
PCB polychlorinated biphenyl
PL photoluminescence
PV pharmacovigilance
QDs quantum dots
R responding
RBP retinol-binding protein
RIA radioimmunoassay
SCE sister chromatid exchange
sICs soluble immune checkpoints
SVMs support vector machines
TBPA thyroxine–thyroxine-binding prealbumin

References

Aaseth, J., Buha, A., Wallace, D.R., Bjørklund, G., 2020. Xenobiotics, trace metals and genetics in the pathogenesis of tauopathies. Int. J. Environ. Res. Publ. Health 17 (4), 1269.

Abouir, K., Samer, C.F., Gloor, Y., Desmeules, J.A., Daali, Y., 2021. Reviewing data integrated for PBPK model development to predict metabolic drug-drug interactions: shifting perspectives and emerging trends. Front. Pharmacol. 12, 708299.

Achanta, N.S.K., Rajpoot, K., Tekade, R.K., 2021. Drug metabolic kinetics. In: Tekade, R.K. (Ed.), Biopharmaceutics and Pharmacokinetics Considerations. Elsevier, Academic Press, pp. 335–353.

Almuntashiri, S., Zhu, Y., Han, Y., Wang, X., Somanath, P.R., Zhang, D., 2020. Club cell secreted protein CC16: potential applications in prognosis and therapy for pulmonary diseases. J. Clin. Med. 9 (12), 4039.

Anup, N., Desai, N., Rajpoot, K., Tekade, R.K., 2021a. Kinetics of maternal–fetal drug transfer. In: Tekade, R.K. (Ed.), Biopharmaceutics and Pharmacokinetics Considerations, pp. 145–162. https://doi.org/10.1016/B978-0-12-814425-1.00007-3.

Anup, N., Gadeval, A., Rajpoot, K., Tekade, R.K., 2021b. Software used in ADME computation. In: Tekade, R.K. (Ed.), Biopharmaceutics and Pharmacokinetics Considerations. Elsevier, Academic Press, pp. 699–708.

Anup, N., Rajpoot, K., Tekade, R.K., 2021c. Overview of biopharmaceutics and pharmacokinetics. In: Tekade, R.K. (Ed.), Biopharmaceutics and Pharmacokinetics Considerations, vol. 1. Elsevier, Academic Press, pp. 1–16.

Basile, A.O., Yahi, A., Tatonetti, N.P., 2019. Artificial intelligence for drug toxicity and safety. Trends Pharmacol. Sci. 40 (9), 624–635. https://www.sciencedirect.com/science/article/pii/S0165614719301427.

Behl, T., Rachamalla, M., Najda, A., Sehgal, A., Singh, S., Sharma, N., Bhatia, S., Al-Harrasi, A., Chigurupati, S., Vargas-De-La-Cruz, C., 2021. Applications of adductomics in chemically induced adverse outcomes and major emphasis on DNA adductomics: a pathbreaking tool in biomedical research. Int. J. Mol. Sci. 22 (18), 10141.

Bera, D., Qian, L., Tseng, T.-K., Holloway, P.H., 2010. Quantum dots and their multimodal applications: a review. Materials 3 (4), 2260–2345. https://doi.org/10.3390/ma3042260.

Berghmans, E., Jacobs, J., Deben, C., Hermans, C., Broeckx, G., Smits, E., Maes, E., Raskin, J., Pauwels, P., Baggerman, G., 2020. Mass spectrometry imaging reveals neutrophil defensins as additional biomarkers for anti-PD-(L)1 immunotherapy response in NSCLC patients. Cancers 12 (4), 863. https://www.ncbi.nlm.nih.gov/pubmed/32252405.

Bin-Jumah, M., Abdel-Fattah, A.-F.M., Saied, E.M., El-Seedi, H.R., Abdel-Daim, M.M., 2021. Acrylamide-induced peripheral neuropathy: manifestations, mechanisms, and potential treatment modalities. Environ. Sci. Pollut. Control Ser. 28 (11), 13031–13046.

Bombail, V., Aw, D., Gordon, E., Batty, J., 2001. Application of the comet and micronucleus assays to butterfish (Pholis gunnellus) erythrocytes from the Firth of Forth, Scotland. Chemosphere 44 (3), 383–392. https://doi.org/10.1016/s0045-6535(00)00300-3.

Brouwer, A., 1991. Role of biotransformation in PCB-induced alterations in vitamin A and thyroid hormone metabolism in laboratory and wildlife species. Biochem. Soc. Trans. 19 (3), 731–737. https://doi.org/10.1042/bst0190731.

Campana, M.A., Panzeri, A.M., Moreno, V.J., Dulout, F.N., 2003. Micronuclei induction in *Rana catesbeiana* tadpoles by the pyrethroid insecticide lambda-cyhalothrin. Genet. Mol. Biol. 26 (1), 99–103. https://doi.org/10.1590/s1415-47572003000100016.

Çavas, T., Ergene-Gözükara, S., 2005. Micronucleus test in fish cells: a bioassay for in situ monitoring of genotoxic pollution in the marine environment. Environ. Mol. Mutagen. 46 (1), 64–70. https://doi.org/10.1002/em.20130.

Choudhary, D., Goykar, H., Rajpoot, K., Tekade, R.K., 2021. Chronopharmacokinetics. In: Tekade, R.K. (Ed.), Biopharmaceutics and Pharmacokinetics Considerations. Elsevier, Academic Press, pp. 163–194.

Cui, L., He, X.-P., Chen, G.-R., 2015. Recent progress in quantum dot based sensors. RSC Adv. 5 (34), 26644–26653. https://doi.org/10.1039/c5ra01950h.

Da Rocha, C.A.M., Dos Santos, R.A., Bahia, M.D.O., Da Cunha, L.A., Ribeiro, H.F., Burbano, R.M.R., 2009. The micronucleus assay in fish species as an important tool for xenobiotic exposure risk assessment—a brief review and an example using neotropical fish exposed to methylmercury. Rev. Fish. Sci. 17 (4), 478–484. https://doi.org/10.1080/10641260903067852.

De las Cuevas, C., Sanz Alvarez, E.J., 2017. Road safety and behavioural toxicity due to psychotropic drugs. Health Sci. 22 (4), 379–382. https://doi.org/10.21840/siic/153618.

Desai, N., Koppisetti, H., Rajpoot, K., Tekade, M., Sharma, M.C., Tekade, R.K., 2021. Influence of fever on pharmacokinetics of drugs. In: Tekade, R.K. (Ed.), Biopharmaceutics and Pharmacokinetics Considerations, first ed. Elsevier, pp. 451–463. https://doi.org/10.1016/B978-0-12-814425-1.00011-5.

Díaz de León-Martínez, L., Grimaldo-Galeana, J.M., Alcántara-Quintana, L.E., Díaz-Barriga, F., Pérez-Vázquez, F.J., Flores-Ramírez, R., 2022. Evaluation of cytokines in exhaled breath condensate in an occupationally exposed population to pneumotoxic pollutants. Environ. Sci. Pollut. Control Ser. 1–13. https://link.springer.com/article/10.1007/s11356-022-20101-8.

Djidrovski, I., Georgiou, M., Tasinato, E., Leonard, M.O., Van den Bor, J., Lako, M., Armstrong, L., 2022. Direct transcriptomic comparison of xenobiotic metabolism and toxicity pathway induction of airway epithelium models at an air–liquid interface generated from induced pluripotent stem cells and primary bronchial epithelial cells. Cell Biol. Toxicol. 1–18.

Dubertret, B., Skourides, P., Norris, D.J., Noireaux, V., Brivanlou, A.H., Libchaber, A., 2002. In vivo imaging of quantum dots encapsulated in phospholipid micelles. Science 298 (5599), 1759–1762. https://doi.org/10.1126/science.1077194.

Edén, A., Simrén, J., Price, R.W., Zetterberg, H., Gisslén, M., 2021. Neurochemical biomarkers to study CNS effects of COVID-19: a narrative review and synthesis. J. Neurochem. 159 (1), 61–77.

El Shafy, W.S., El-Sherif, G.H., 2019. Serum clara cell protein (cc16) in relation to pulmonary functions among workers exposed to naphthalene in pvc manufacture. Egyptian J. Occup. Med. 43 (2), 175–188.

Erdbrugger, U., Blijdorp, C.J., Bijnsdorp, I.V., Borras, F.E., Burger, D., Bussolati, B., Byrd, J.B., Clayton, A., Dear, J.W., Falcon-Perez, J.M., Grange, C., Hill, A.F., Holthofer, H., Hoorn, E.J., Jenster, G., Jimenez, C.R., Junker, K., Klein, J., Knepper, M.A., Koritzinsky, E.H., Luther, J.M., Lenassi, M., Leivo, J., Mertens, I., Musante, L., Oeyen, E., Puhka, M., van Royen, M.E., Sanchez, C., Soekmadji, C., Thongboonkerd, V., van Steijn, V., Verhaegh, G., Webber, J.P., Witwer, K., Yuen, P.S.T., Zheng, L., Llorente, A., Martens-Uzunova, E.S., 2021. Urinary extracellular vesicles: a position paper by the urine task force of the International Society for extracellular vesicles. J. Extracell. Vesicles 10 (7), e12093. https://www.ncbi.nlm.nih.gov/pubmed/34035881.

Estévez, J., Vilanova, E., Sogorb, M.A., 2019. Biomarkers for testing toxicity and monitoring exposure to xenobiotics. In: Biomarkers in Toxicology. Elsevier, pp. 1165–1174.

Fiehn, O., 2002. Metabolomics—the link between genotypes and phenotypes. Funct. Genom. https://doi.org/10.1007/978-94-010-0448-0_11.

Gadekar, V., Borade, Y., Kannaujia, S., Rajpoot, K., Anup, N., Tambe, V., Kalia, K., Tekade, R.K., 2021. Nanomedicines accessible in the market for clinical interventions. J. Control Release 330, 372–397.

Gatti, D.M., Lu, L., Williams, R.W., Sun, W., Wright, F.A., Threadgill, D.W., Rusyn, I., 2011. MicroRNA expression in the livers of inbred mice. Mutat. Res. 714 (1–2), 126–133. https://pubmed.ncbi.nlm.nih.gov/21616085. https://www.ncbi.nlm.nih.gov/pmc/articles/PMC3166582/.

Giresha, A.S., 2021. Secretory phospholipase A2 group IIA: a potential therapeutic target in inflammation. Curr. Res. Trends Med. Sci. Technol. 34.

Gooderham, N.J., Koufaris, C., 2014. Using microRNA profiles to predict and evaluate hepatic carcinogenic potential. Toxicol. Lett. 228 (2), 127–132. https://doi.org/10.1016/j.toxlet.2014.04.015.

Gorain, B., Choudhury, H., Tekade, R.K., Karan, S., Jaisankar, P., Pal, T.K., 2016. Comparative biodistribution and safety profiling of olmesartan medoxomil oil-in-water oral nanoemulsion. Regul. Toxicol. Pharmacol. 82, 20–31.

Groves, A.M., Williams, J.P., Hernady, E., Reed, C., Fenton, B., Love, T., Finkelstein, J.N., Johnston, C.J., 2018. A potential biomarker for predicting the risk of radiation-induced fibrosis in the lung. Radiat. Res. 190 (5), 513–525.

Gruba, N., Stachurski, L., Lesner, A., 2022. Chemical tools to monitor bladder cancer progression. Biomarkers 1–41.

Gupta, R., Polaka, S., Rajpoot, K., Tekade, M., Sharma, M.C., Tekade, R.K., 2022a. Importance of toxicity testing in drug discovery and research. In: Pharmacokinetics and Toxicokinetic Considerations, vol. 2. Elsevier. https://doi.org/10.1016/b978-0-323-98367-9.00016-0.

Gupta, R., Rajpoot, K., Tekade, M., Sharma, M.C., Safavi, M., Tekade, R.K., 2022b. Factors influencing drug toxicity. In: Pharmacokinetics and Toxicokinetic Considerations, vol. 2. Elsevier. https://doi.org/10.1016/b978-0-323-98367-9.00014-7.

Gupta, R., Rajpoot, K., Tekade, M., Sharma, M.C., Tekade, R.K., 2022c. Methods and models for in vitro toxicity. In: Pharmacokinetics and Toxicokinetic Considerations, vol. 2. Elsevier. https://doi.org/10.1016/b978-0-323-98367-9.00006-8.

Hill, E.F., 1988. Brain cholinesterase activity of apparently normal wild birds. J. Wildl. Dis. 24 (1), 51–61. https://doi.org/10.7589/0090-3558-24.1.51.

Hopf, N.B., Fustinoni, S., 2021. Biological monitoring of exposure to industrial chemicals. In: Patty's Industrial Hygiene, Evaluation and Control, vol. 3.

Hou, L., Zhang, X., Wang, D., Baccarelli, A., 2012. Environmental chemical exposures and human epigenetics. Int. J. Epidemiol. 41 (1), 79–105. https://pubmed.ncbi.nlm.nih.gov/22253299. https://www.ncbi.nlm.nih.gov/pmc/articles/PMC3304523/.

Iravani, S., Varma, R.S., 2020. Green synthesis, biomedical and biotechnological applications of carbon and graphene quantum dots. A review. Environ. Chem. Lett. 1–25. https://pubmed.ncbi.nlm.nih.gov/32206050. https://www.ncbi.nlm.nih.gov/pmc/articles/PMC7088420/.

Kandasamy, G., 2019. Recent advancements in doped/co-doped carbon quantum dots for multi-potential applications. Chimia 5 (2), 24. https://doi.org/10.3390/c5020024.

Kang, Z., Lee, S.-T., 2019. Carbon dots: advances in nanocarbon applications. Nanoscale 11 (41), 19214–19224. https://doi.org/10.1039/c9nr05647e.

Kietzmann, M., 2001. Toxicology—principles and applications. In: Niesink, R.J.M., De Vries, J., Hollinger, M.A. (Eds.), Toxicon, vol. 39, pp. 1612–1613. https://doi.org/10.1016/s0041-0101(01)00112-x.

Kirkland, D., Aardema, M., Henderson, L., Müller, L., 2005. Evaluation of the ability of a battery of three in vitro genotoxicity tests to discriminate rodent carcinogens and non-carcinogens: I. Sensitivity, specificity and relative predictivity. Mutat. Res. 584 (1), 1–256. https://www.sciencedirect.com/science/article/pii/S1383571805000835.

Klobučar, G.I.V., Pavlica, M., Erben, R., Papeš, D., 2003. Application of the micronucleus and comet assays to mussel *Dreissena polymorpha* haemocytes for genotoxicity monitoring of freshwater environments. Aquat. Toxicol. 64 (1), 15–23. https://doi.org/10.1016/s0166-445x(03)00009-2.

Kopanska, M., Muchacka, R., Czech, J., Batoryna, M., Formicki, G., 2018. Acrylamide toxicity and cholinergic nervous system. J. Physiol. Pharmacol. 69 (6), 847–858.

Koufaris, C., Wright, J., Currie, R.A., Gooderham, N.J., 2012. Hepatic MicroRNA profiles offer predictive and mechanistic insights after exposure to genotoxic and epigenetic hepatocarcinogens. Toxicol. Sci. 128 (2), 532–543. https://doi.org/10.1093/toxsci/kfs170.

Kumawat, A., Raval, N., Reddy, G., Rajpoot, K., Tekade, R.K., 2020. Gene delivery to tackle diabetic nephropathy. In: Tekade, R.K. (Ed.), The Future of Pharmaceutical Product Development and Research, vol. 1. Academic Press, pp. 515–537. http://www.sciencedirect.com/science/article/pii/B9780128144558000153.

Laucho-Contreras, M.E., Polverino, F., Rojas-Quintero, J., Wang, X., Owen, C.A., 2018. Club cell protein 16 (Cc16) deficiency increases inflamm-aging in the lungs of mice. Physiol. Rep. 6 (15), e13797.

LeBaron, M.J., Rasoulpour, R.J., Klapacz, J., Ellis-Hutchings, R.G., Hollnagel, H.M., Gollapudi, B.B., 2010. Epigenetics and chemical safety assessment. Mutat. Res. Rev. Mutat. Res. 705 (2), 83–95. https://www.sciencedirect.com/science/article/pii/S1383574210000487.

Lempiäinen, H., Luisier, R., Müller, A., Marc, P., Heard, D., Bolognani, F., Moulin, P., Couttet, P., Grenet, O., Marlowe, J., Moggs, J., Terranova, R., 2012. Epigenomics – impact for drug safety sciences. Toxicol. Epigenet. 365–385. https://doi.org/10.1002/9781118349045.ch19.

Li, Y.Q., Mason, A.L., 2020. Environmental exposure and risk in autoimmune liver diseases. In: Autoimmune Liver Disease: Management and Clinical Practice, pp. 83–102.

Liu, K.-Z., Tian, G., Ko, A.C.T., Geissler, M., Brassard, D., Veres, T., 2020. Detection of renal biomarkers in chronic kidney disease using microfluidics: progress, challenges and opportunities. Biomed. Microdevices 22 (2), 1–18.

Lv, Y., Wang, F., Li, N., Wu, R., Li, J., Shen, H., Li, L.S., Guo, F., 2019. Development of dual quantum dots-based fluorescence-linked immunosorbent assay for simultaneous detection on inflammation biomarkers. Sensor. Actuator. B Chem. 301, 127118. https://doi.org/10.1016/j.snb.2019.127118.

Ma, F., Li, C.-C., Zhang, C.-Y., 2018. Development of quantum dot-based biosensors: principles and applications. J. Mater. Chem. B 6 (39), 6173–6190. https://doi.org/10.1039/c8tb01869c.

Marrone, A.K., Beland, F.A., Pogribny, I.P., 2014. Non-coding RNA response to xenobiotic exposure: an indicator of toxicity and carcinogenicity. Expet Opin. Drug Metabol. Toxicol. 10 (10), 1409–1422. https://doi.org/10.1517/17425255.2014.954312.

Marrone, A.K., Beland, F.A., Pogribny, I.P., 2015. The role for microRNAs in drug toxicity and in safety assessment. Expet Opin. Drug Metabol. Toxicol. 11 (4), 601–611. https://doi.org/10.1517/17425255.2015.1021687.

Melancon, M.J., Alscher, R., William, B., George, K., Lee, R.F., Sikka, H.C., Spies, R.B., 2018. Metabolic products as biomarkers. Biomarkers. https://doi.org/10.1201/9781351070270-3.

Miller, R.E., Leary, A., Scott, C.L., Serra, V., Lord, C.J., Bowtell, D., Chang, D.K., Garsed, D.W., Jonkers, J., Ledermann, J.A., 2020. ESMO recommendations on predictive biomarker testing for homologous recombination deficiency and PARP inhibitor benefit in ovarian cancer. Ann. Oncol. 31 (12), 1606–1622.

Mineau, P., 2018. Obsolete: cholinesterase-inhibiting insecticides and birds. In: Reference Module in Earth Systems and Environmental Sciences. Elsevier. https://doi.org/10.1016/b978-0-12-409548-9.09887-0.

Mishra, A., Rajpoot, K., Agrawal, O.P., Tekade, R.K., 2021. Implications for sex-related issues in clinical pharmacology and biopharmaceutics. In: Tekade, R.K. (Ed.), Biopharmaceutics and Pharmacokinetics Considerations. Elsevier, Academic Press, pp. 465–485.

Molaei, M.J., 2020. Principles, mechanisms, and application of carbon quantum dots in sensors: a review. Anal. Methods 12 (10), 1266–1287. https://doi.org/10.1039/c9ay02696g.

Muniswamy, V.J., Raval, N., Gondaliya, P., Tambe, V., Kalia, K., Tekade, R.K., 2019. Dendrimer-Cationized-Albumin'encrusted polymeric nanoparticle improves BBB penetration and anticancer activity of doxorubicin. Int. J. Pharm. 555, 77–99.

Oesch, F., Fabian, E., Landsiedel, R., 2019. Xenobiotica-metabolizing enzymes in the lung of experimental animals, man and in human lung models. Arch. Toxicol. 93 (12), 3419–3489.

Okamoto, M., Ichii, O., Mie, K., Nishida, H., Akiyoshi, H., 2021. Altered clinicopathology and renal pathology in dogs treated with a clinical dose of cisplatin. Jpn. J. Vet. Res. 69 (2), 109–124.

Ossana, N.A., Castañé, P.M., Poletta, G.L., Mudry, M.D., Salibián, A., 2010. Toxicity of waterborne copper in premetamorphic tadpoles of Lithobates catesbeianus (Shaw, 1802). Bull. Environ. Contam. Toxicol. 84 (6), 712–715. https://doi.org/10.1007/s00128-010-0014-0.

Othmène, Y.B., Hamdi, H., Amara, I., Abid-Essefi, S., 2020. Tebuconazole induced oxidative stress and histopathological alterations in adult rat heart. Pestic. Biochem. Physiol. 170, 104671.

Padiyar, A., Agrawal, O.P., Rajpoot, K., Tekade, R.K., 2020. Hydrotropy, mixed hydrotropy, and mixed solvency as trending concept for solubilization of lipophilic drugs. In: Tekade, R.K. (Ed.), The Future of Pharmaceutical Product Development and Research. Academic Press, pp. 145–178. http://www.sciencedirect.com/science/article/pii/B9780128144558000050.

Parikh, K.J., Christian, J.R., Rajpoot, K., Tekade, R.K., 2022. Environmental and safety aspects of bionanotechnology. In: Pharmacokinetics and Toxicokinetic Considerations, vol. 2. Elsevier. https://doi.org/10.1016/b978-0-323-98367-9.00022-6.

Polaka, S., Desai, N., Kshirsagar, B., Rajpoot, K., Tekade, R.K., 2021a. Revamping the pharmacokinetics of poorly soluble drugs using different formulations. In: Tekade, R.K. (Ed.), Biopharmaceutics and Pharmacokinetics Considerations, first ed. Elsevier, pp. 387–413. https://doi.org/10.1016/B978-0-12-814425-1.00005-X.

Polaka, S., Makwana, V., Vasdev, N., Sheth, A., Rajpoot, K., Sengupta, P., Tekade, R.K., 2022a. Engineering immunity via skin-directed drug delivery devices. J. Contr. Release 345, 385–404. https://www.ncbi.nlm.nih.gov/pubmed/35283256.

Polaka, S., Rajpoot, K., Tekade, M., Sharma, M.C., Tekade, R.K., 2022b. Food–drug interactions and their implications on oral drug bioavailability. In: Pharmacokinetics and Toxicokinetic Considerations, vol. 2. Elsevier. https://doi.org/10.1016/b978-0-323-98367-9.00002-0.

Polaka, S., Swetha, K.L., Dittakavi, S., Rajpoot, K., Tekade, R.K., 2021b. Bioanalytical method development and validation for establishing bioavailability and bioequivalence. In: Tekade, R.K. (Ed.), Biopharmaceutics and Pharmacokinetics Considerations. Elsevier, pp. 487–516. https://doi.org/10.1016/B978-0-12-814425-1.00001-2.

Pollard, K.M., Christy, J.M., Cauvi, D.M., Kono, D.H., 2018. Environmental xenobiotic exposure and autoimmunity. Curr. Opin. Toxicol. 10, 15–22.

Prajapati, R.N., Tekade, R.K., Gupta, U., Gajbhiye, V., Jain, N.K., 2009. Dendimer-mediated solubilization, formulation development and in vitro–in vivo assessment of piroxicam. Mol. Pharm. 6 (3), 940–950.

Que, S.-J., Chen, Q.-Y., Liu, Z.-Y., Wang, J.-B., Lin, J.-X., Lu, J., Cao, L.-L., Lin, M., Tu, R.-H., Huang, Z.-N., 2019. Application of preoperative artificial neural network based on blood biomarkers and clinicopathological parameters for predicting long-term survival of patients with gastric cancer. World J. Gastroenterol. 25 (43), 6451.

Raies, A.B., Bajic, V.B., 2016. In silico toxicology: computational methods for the prediction of chemical toxicity. WIREs Comput. Mol. Sci. 6 (2), 147–172. https://doi.org/10.1002/wcms.1240.

Rajpoot, K., Desai, N., Koppisetti, H., Tekade, M., Sharma, M.C., Behera, S.K., Tekade, R.K., 2022a. In silico methods for the prediction of drug toxicity. In: Pharmacokinetics and Toxicokinetic Considerations, vol. 2. Elsevier. https://doi.org/10.1016/b978-0-323-98367-9.00012-3.

Rajpoot, K., Katare, P., Tekade, M., Sharma, M.C., Polaka, S., Sengupta, P., Tekade, R.K., 2022b. Toxicokinetic and toxicodynamic considerations in drug research. In: Pharmacokinetics and Toxicokinetic Considerations, vol. 2. Elsevier. https://doi.org/10.1016/b978-0-323-98367-9.00026-3.

Rajpoot, K., Tekade, M., Sharma, M.C., Arafat, B., Tekade, R.K., 2022c. Principles and concepts in toxicokinetic. In: Pharmacokinetics and Toxicokinetic Considerations, vol. 2. Elsevier. https://doi.org/10.1016/b978-0-323-98367-9.00023-8.

Rajpoot, K., Tekade, M., Sharma, M.C., Sreeharsha, N., Sharma, A., Tekade, R.K., 2020a. Recombinant blood products and therapeutic enzymes: an update. In: Tekade, R.K. (Ed.), The Future of Pharmaceutical Product Development and Research. Academic Press, pp. 447–482. http://www.sciencedirect.com/science/article/pii/B978012814455800013X.

Rajpoot, K., Tekade, M., Sreeharsha, N., Sharma, M.C., Tekade, R.K., 2020b. Recent advancements in solubilization of hydrophobic drugs. In: Tekade, R.K. (Ed.), The Future of Pharmaceutical Product Development and Research. Academic Press, pp. 109–144. http://www.sciencedirect.com/science/article/pii/B9780128144558000049.

Rajpoot, K., Tekade, R.K., Chatterjee, B., Sharma, M.C., Tekade, M., 2021a. Biopharmaceutical considerations in the pediatric and geriatric formulation development. In: Tekade, R.K. (Ed.), Biopharmaceutics and Pharmacokinetics Considerations, vol. 1. Elsevier, Academic Press, pp. 109–144.

Rajpoot, K., Tekade, R.K., Sharma, M.C., Safavi, M., Tekade, M., 2021b. Pharmacokinetics modeling in drug delivery. In: Tekade, R.K. (Ed.), Biopharmaceutics and Pharmacokinetics Considerations. Elsevier, Academic Press, pp. 279–334.

Rajpoot, K., Tekade, R.K., Sharma, M.C., Tekade, M., 2021c. Pharmacokinetics and biopharmaceutics: "a leader or attendant". In: Tekade, R.K. (Ed.), Biopharmaceutics and Pharmacokinetics Considerations. Elsevier, Academic Press, pp. 17–27.

Ravi, P., Ganesan, M., 2021. Quantum dots as biosensors in the determination of biochemical parameters in xenobiotic exposure and toxins. Anal. Sci. 37 (5), 661–671. https://www.ncbi.nlm.nih.gov/pubmed/33390416.

Reshma, V.G., Mohanan, P.V., 2019. Quantum dots: applications and safety consequences. J. Lumin. 205, 287–298. https://doi.org/10.1016/j.jlumin.2018.09.015.

Rosenthal, S.J., Tomlinson, I., Adkins, E.M., Schroeter, S., Adams, S., Swafford, L., McBride, J., Wang, Y., DeFelice, L.J., Blakely, R.D., 2002. Targeting cell surface receptors with ligand-conjugated nanocrystals. J. Am. Chem. Soc. 124 (17), 4586–4594. https://doi.org/10.1021/ja003486s.

Sahu, R., Mehan, S., Kumar, S., Prajapati, A., Alshammari, A., Alharbi, M., Assiri, M.A., Narula, A.S., 2022. Effect of alpha-mangostin in the prevention of behavioural and neurochemical defects in methylmercury-induced neurotoxicity in experimental rats. Toxicol. Rep. 9, 977–998.

Sanders, B., 2018. Stress proteins: potential as multitiered biomarkers. Biomarkers Environ. Contaminat. https://doi.org/10.1201/9781351070263-12.

Schwarzenbach, H., Nishida, N., Calin, G.A., Pantel, K., 2014. Clinical relevance of circulating cell-free microRNAs in cancer. Nat. Rev. Clin. Oncol. 11 (3), 145–156. https://doi.org/10.1038/nrclinonc.2014.5.

Singh, S., 2019. Zinc oxide nanoparticles impacts: cytotoxicity, genotoxicity, developmental toxicity, and neurotoxicity. Toxicol. Mech. Methods 29 (4), 300–311.

Song, H., Su, Y., Zhang, L., Lv, Y., 2019. Quantum dots-based chemiluminescence probes: an overview. Luminescence 34 (6), 530–543. https://doi.org/10.1002/bio.3633.

Spraul, M., Hofmann, M., Ackermann, M., Shockcor, J.P., Lindon, J.C., Nicholls, A.W., Nicholson, J.K., Damment, S.J.P., Haselden, J.N., 1997. Flow injection proton nuclear magnetic resonance spectroscopy combined with pattern recognition methods: implications for rapid structural studies and high throughput biochemical screening. Anal. Commun. 34 (11), 339–341. https://doi.org/10.1039/a705551j.

Stading, R., Gastelum, G., Chu, C., Jiang, W., Moorthy, B., 2021. Molecular Mechanisms of Pulmonary Carcinogenesis by Polycyclic Aromatic Hydrocarbons (PAHs): Implications for Human Lung Cancer, vol. 2021. Elsevier, pp. 3–16.

Tal, T.L., Tanguay, R.L., 2012. Non-coding RNAs–novel targets in neurotoxicity. Neurotoxicology 33 (3), 530–544. https://pubmed.ncbi.nlm.nih.gov/22394481. https://www.ncbi.nlm.nih.gov/pmc/articles/PMC3462486/.

Tambe, V., Desai, N., Rajpoot, K., Tekade, R.K., 2021a. "Organ-on-a-chip"-based physiologically relevant pharmacokinetic models. In: Tekade, R.K. (Ed.), Biopharmaceutics and Pharmacokinetics Considerations, first ed. Elsevier, pp. 643–673. https://doi.org/10.1016/B978-0-12-814425-1.00024-3.

Tambe, V., Kathar, U., Raval, N., Rajpoot, K., Shilpi, S., Khatri, K., Tekade, R.K., 2021b. Positron emission tomography as a noninvasive tool in pharmacokinetic studies. In: Tekade, R.K. (Ed.), Biopharmaceutics and Pharmacokinetics Considerations. Elsevier, Academic Press, pp. 617–641.

Tambe, V., Pande, S., Gadeval, A., Rajpoot, K., Raval, N., Tekade, R.K., 2021c. Microdialysis: an emerging technique for pharmacokinetic–pharmacodynamic profiling. In: Tekade, R.K. (Ed.), Biopharmaceutics and Pharmacokinetics Considerations, first ed. Elsevier, pp. 601–616. https://doi.org/10.1016/B978-0-12-814425-1.00018-8.

Tambe, V., Sirsat, B., Rajpoot, K., Gadeval, A., Tekade, R.K., 2021d. Pharmacogenomics and drug metabolism. In: Tekade, R.K. (Ed.), Biopharmaceutics and Pharmacokinetics Considerations, vol. 1. Elsevier, Academic Press, pp. 355–385.

Tekade, M., Koppisetti, H., Sharma, M.C., Rajpoot, K., Sengupta, P., Kumar, M., Tekade, R.K., 2022. Understanding the concept of signal toxicity and its implications on human health. In: Pharmacokinetics and Toxicokinetic Considerations, vol. 2. Elsevier. https://doi.org/10.1016/b978-0-323-98367-9.00020-2.

Thomson, J.P., Moggs, J.G., Wolf, C.R., Meehan, R.R., 2014. Epigenetic profiles as defined signatures of xenobiotic exposure. Mutat. Res. 764–765, 3–9. https://www.sciencedirect.com/science/article/pii/S1383571813002313.

Tiwari, A., Joshi, M., Salvi, N., Gupta, D., Gandhi, S., Rajpoot, K., Tekade, R.K., 2022. Toxicity of pharmaceutical azo dyes. In: Pharmacokinetics and Toxicokinetic Considerations, vol. 2. Elsevier. https://doi.org/10.1016/b978-0-323-98367-9.00004-4.

Tominaga, T., Ma, S., Sugama, K., Kanda, K., Omae, C., Choi, W., Hashimoto, S., Aoyama, K., Yoshikai, Y., Suzuki, K., 2021. Changes in urinary biomarkers of organ damage, inflammation, oxidative stress, and bone turnover following a 3000-m time trial. Antioxidants 10 (1), 79. https://www.ncbi.nlm.nih.gov/pubmed/33435279.

Tustin, A.W., Cannon, D.L., 2022. Analysis of biomonitoring data to assess employer compliance with OSHA's permissible exposure limits for air contaminants. Am. J. Ind. Med. 65 (2), 81–91.

Vasdev, N., Rajpoot, K., Tekade, R.K., 2021. Molecular mechanisms of circadian rhythm and its influence on the pharmacokinetics of drugs. In: Tekade, R.K. (Ed.), Biopharmaceutics and Pharmacokinetics Considerations. Elsevier, Academic Press, pp. 415–449.

Vashist, S.K., Tewari, R., Bajpai, R.P., Bharadwaj, L.M., Raiteri, R., 2006. Binding of mouse immunoglobulin G to polylysine-coated glass substrate for immunodiagnosis. In: Paper Presented at the Proceedings of SPIE. https://doi.org/10.1117/12.695554.

Vona, R., Gambardella, L., Cittadini, C., Straface, E., Pietraforte, D., 2019. Biomarkers of oxidative stress in metabolic syndrome and associated diseases. Oxid. Med. Cell. Longev. 19. https://doi.org/10.1155/2019/8267234.

Walker, C.H., 1995. Biochemical biomarkers in ecotoxicology—some recent developments. Sci. Total Environ. 171 (1–3), 189–195. https://doi.org/10.1016/0048-9697(95)04720-6.

Walker, C.H., Sibly, R.M., Sibly, R.M., Peakall, D.B., 2016. Principles of Ecotoxicology. CRC Press. https://doi.org/10.1201/b11767.

Walper, S.A., Lasarte Aragonés, G., Sapsford, K.E., Brown, C.W., Rowland, C.E., Breger, J.C., Medintz, I.L., 2018. Detecting biothreat agents: from current diagnostics to developing sensor technologies. ACS Sens. 3 (10), 1894–2024. https://doi.org/10.1021/acssensors.8b00420.

Wang, X., Ruedas-Rama, M.J., Hall, E.A.H., 2007. The emerging use of quantum dots in analysis. Anal. Lett. 40 (8), 1497–1520. https://doi.org/10.1080/00032710701381044.

Wirz, M.V.M.A., Saldiva, P.H., Freire-Maia, D.V., 2005. Micronucleus test for monitoring genotoxicity of polluted river water in *Rana catesbeiana* tadpoles. Bull. Environ. Contam. Toxicol. 75 (6), 1220–1227. https://doi.org/10.1007/s00128-005-0879-5.

Wołejko, E., Jabłońska-Trypuć, A., Butarewicz, A., Wydro, U., 2021. Heavy metals, hydrocarbons, radioactive materials, xenobiotics, pesticides, hazardous chemicals, explosives, pharmaceutical waste and dyes bioremediation. In: Rhizomicrobiome Dynamics in Bioremediation, pp. 269–298.

Wu, X., Liu, H., Liu, J., Haley, K.N., Treadway, J.A., Larson, J.P., Ge, N., Peale, F., Bruchez, M.P., 2002. Immunofluorescent labeling of cancer marker Her2 and other cellular targets with semiconductor quantum dots. Nat. Biotechnol. 21 (1), 41–46. https://doi.org/10.1038/nbt764.

Xiao, J., Ding, R., Xu, X., Guan, H., Feng, X., Sun, T., Zhu, S., Ye, Z., 2019. Comparison and development of machine learning tools in the prediction of chronic kidney disease progression. J. Transl. Med. 17 (1), 1–13.

Zheng, Z., Geng, J., Jiang, Y., Zhang, M., Yang, R., Ge, G., Xu, H., Zhang, X., 2021. Kidney diseases. In: Clinical Molecular Diagnostics. Springer, pp. 553–582.

Zizzari, I.G., Di Filippo, A., Scirocchi, F., Di Pietro, F.R., Rahimi, H., Ugolini, A., Scagnoli, S., Vernocchi, P., Del Chierico, F., Putignani, L., Rughetti, A., Marchetti, P., Nuti, M., Botticelli, A., Napoletano, C., 2020. Soluble immune checkpoints, gut metabolites and performance status as parameters of response to nivolumab treatment in NSCLC patients. J. Personalized Med. 10 (4), 208. https://www.ncbi.nlm.nih.gov/pubmed/33158018.

CHAPTER

22

Concept of pharmacotherapy and managed care in clinical interventions

Vishakha Tambe, Kuldeep Rajpoot, Nimeet Desai and Rakesh Kumar Tekade

National Institute of Pharmaceutical Education and Research (NIPER)- Ahmedabad, An Institute of National Importance, Government of India, Department of Pharmaceuticals, Ministry of Chemicals and Fertilizers, Palaj, Gandhinagar, Gujarat, India

22.1 Introduction

Managed care has been considered one of the leading models for healthcare, especially in developed countries like the United States, over the last two decades. It can be described as a healthcare delivery system that provides health benefits and additional services through contracted arrangements between state agencies and managed care organizations (MCOs). Stakeholders can reduce operational costs involved in patient care and therapeutic interventions by contracting with various types of MCOs to deliver healthcare services to their beneficiaries and manage the utilization of health services (Rodwin, 2010). It is widely prevalent in employer-sponsored health insurance and government-sponsored health benefits. Thus, there is an immense need to understand the role of managed care in the healthcare system and its considerable impact on pharmacotherapy management (Happe et al., 2014). In the United States, around 58% of the hospitals (accounting for about 70% of total bed strength) are community-based nonprofit organizations (Joshi and Krishnan, 2017). In these hospitals, roughly 40% of the physicians operate as single practitioners, and around 60% work in a group of two or more physicians. Thus, the fast growth of managed care results in rising demand for primary care providers. These primary care providers account for almost 40% of physicians in the United States. Fig. 22.1 depicts the overview of healthcare in some of the developed countries.

Essentials of Pharmatoxicology in Drug Research, Volume 1
https://doi.org/10.1016/B978-0-443-15840-7.00017-8

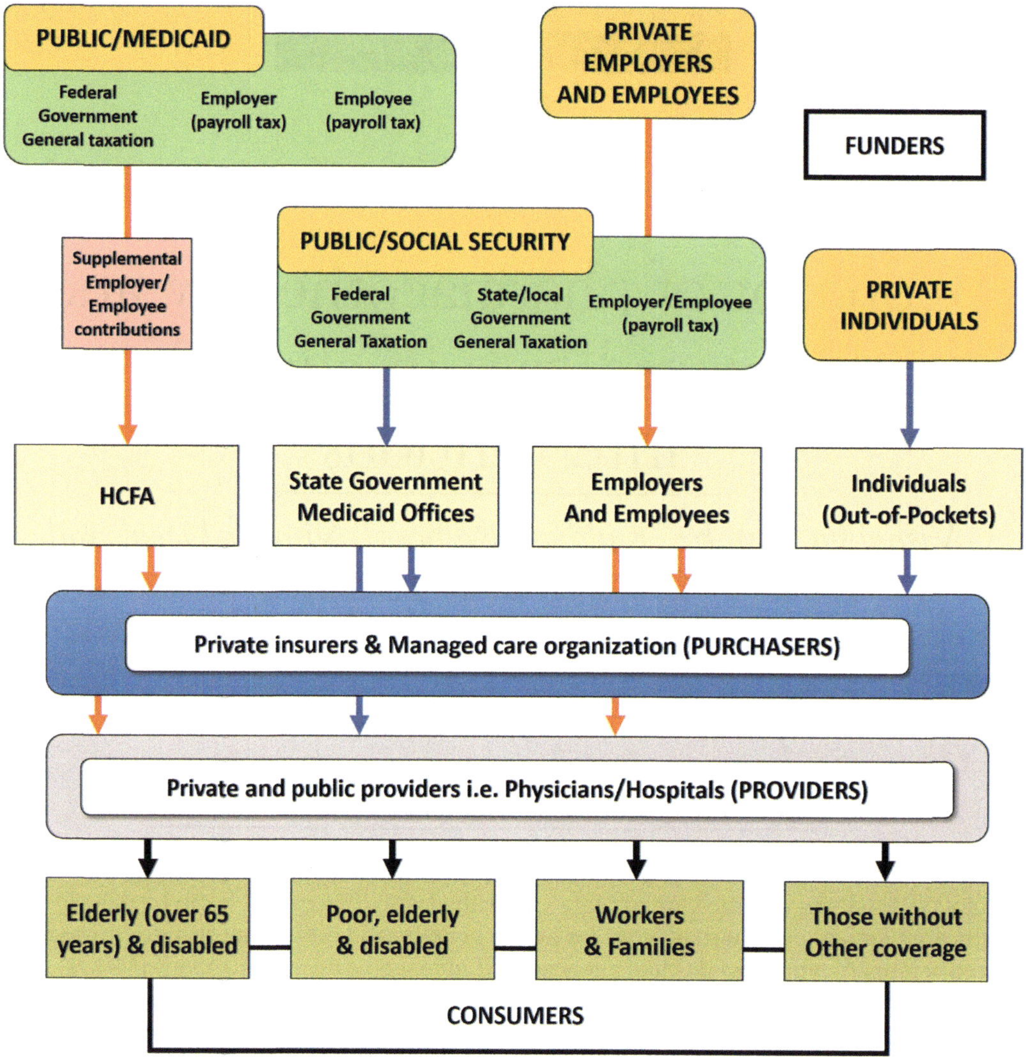

FIGURE 22.1 **Overview of the healthcare system in the USA.** The schematic chart depicts funders, purchasers, and care providers as separate entities. MCOs served as both purchasers and providers of care. It illustrates that all the people are enrolled in either one or the other type of health plan.

22.2 Traditional managed care

Traditional managed care involves the purchaser's contracts with specific providers to provide a predefined package of services with a fixed fee per person or service. Fig. 22.2 depicts transactions between the patient and provider, but the patient or his employer pays a premium to the insurance company. Furthermore, from the schematic, it is clear that the patient

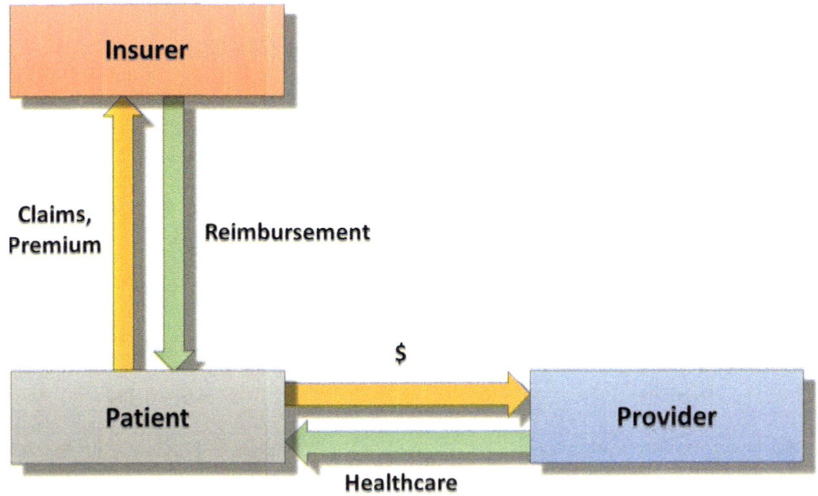

FIGURE 22.2 **Traditional care model.** The schematic depicts the relationship between the patient, provider, and insurer. Herein patient pays the premium to the insurer. On receipt of healthcare service from the provider, he claims the reimbursement equivalent to the amount he has already paid to the provider.

will submit the claims to the insurance company to get reimbursement for the same amount they gave to the provider. It involves health maintenance organizations (HMOs), wherein HMOs first confirm whether members are ill or not. Besides, traditional managed care includes an option of discount on the fee for services availed by members from selected providers. Furthermore, it also involves direct access to products that offer an opportunity to allow patients to self-refer to specialists (Harrington, 2019).

22.3 Knowing managed care pharmacy (MCP)

The MCP is described as a collection of actions meant to lower the price of supplying "for-profit health care" and "American health insurance" while enhancing the standard of managed care techniques. Briefly, patients select healthcare providers, and after getting any health services, providers will generate a bill to the private Insurer. Private insurers will reimburse these providers on a per-case basis or a price for service. However, this is associated with certain drawbacks in certain circumstances. The patient has to pay directly to the provider and then request compensation from the insurance with a total payment of less than the charges. The primary characteristic of the managed care model is the contractual connection between the Insurer and the providers. Also, they show dominance over the patient-provider interaction. Fig. 22.3 depicts the vicious relationship between patients, providers, and MCOs. The ultimate goal of MCOs is to reduce costs without loss in quality of care (Shmueli et al., 2015).

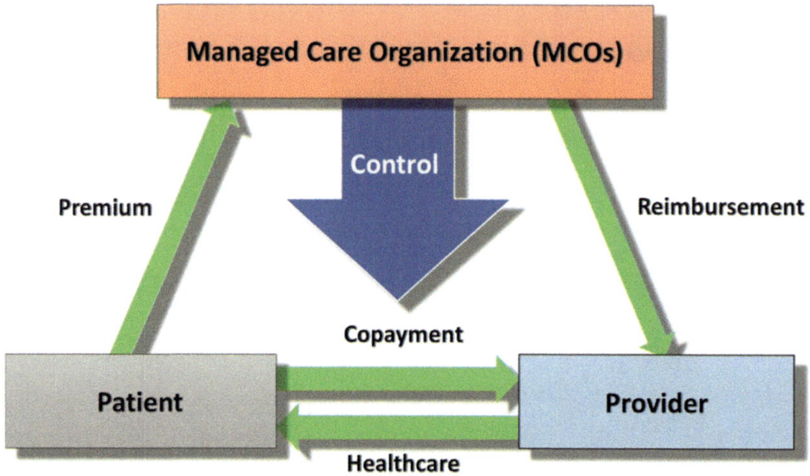

FIGURE 22.3 **Managed care model.** Schematic depicts the relationship between the patient, MCOs, and provider. The patient pays the premium to MCOs, and these MCOs reimburse the provider for providing healthcare services to the patients. However, the patient also pays for co-payments to the provider.

22.4 Managed care principles

The ultimate aim of managed care principles is to offer high-quality and cost-efficient healthcare facilities to society. In this regard, MCOs contribute by providing such managed care principles to society by having a robust healthcare system. Firstly, it involves in monitoring and coordinating primary care through tertiary services. Secondly, it supports by providing incentives to promote the cost-effective use of services. Thirdly, it emphasizes on prevention of diseases and health education. Fourthly, by encouraging care provision by appropriate settings and suitable providers (Kongstvedt, 2013).

22.5 Types of MCOs

22.5.1 HMOs

HMOs are defined as an organization that provides comprehensive healthcare for prepaid payment. These HMOs are the most common examples of managed care in the USA (Ganther and Doucette, 2002). The HMOs legislation was founded in 1973 to encourage the formation and growth of HMOs. However, it was observed that due to an increase in health expenditure, the number of HMOs rapidly increased in the late 1980 as well as 1990. HMOs include three models such as staff model, group model, and network model (Fig. 22.4).

In 1993, a healthcare plan was created between physicians and insurance agents. The plan stated that the physician would be paid 0.05 dollars per worker per day to provide work-related healthcare to workers. In this context, industrialist Henry Kaiser asked the physicians to provide similar plans to his workers, leading to the initiation of Kaiser Permanente or the Harvard community health plan. It consists of mutual exclusivity between the physicians and

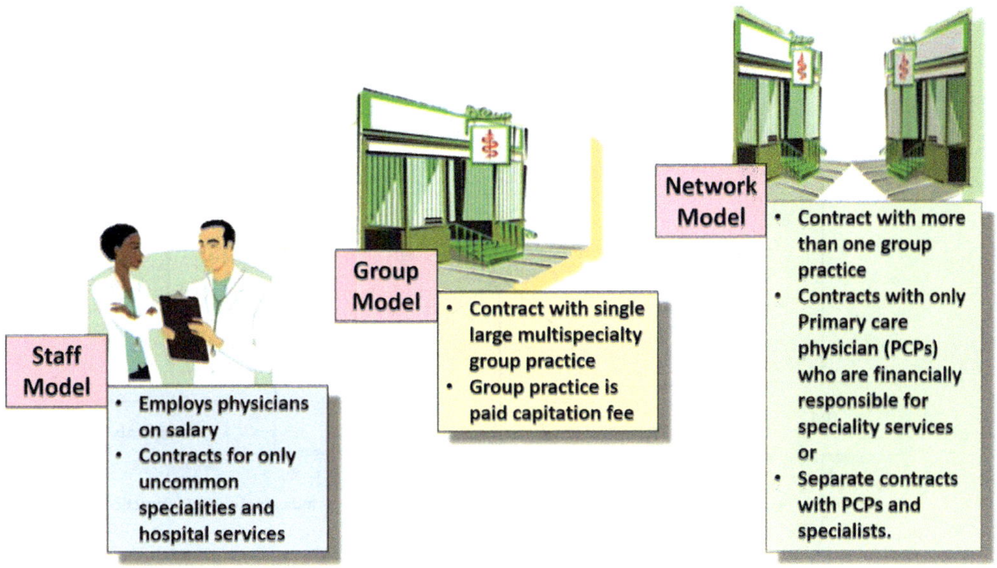

FIGURE 22.4 **HMOs models.** This diagram depicts the least standard staff model, group model, and network model and their characteristics.

the health plans. Kaiser Permanente's model involves linking the insurance function to an integrated system of hospitals and physicians. Physicians who have an exclusive contract with the health plan are either employed by the health plans or members of a medical organization. Furthermore, this health plan enters into agreements with public or private healthcare vendors to offer a specified range of services at prepaid per capita prices on a member- or month-by-member basis. Thus, in such a model, systems receive capitation payment from the funder (Meredith et al., 1999).

In the case of physicians, they can obtain a capitated payment, or particular physicians may get either a salary or both salary as well as incentive payment. On the other hand, hospitals are paid based on per case, per diem, or even fee for service basis, or in another case wherein the physician specialists and hospitals are involved, they may receive a global budget. This type of model governance is shared among physicians or administrators. In contrast, decision-making is a collective effort with physicians and health plan which manages administrative and insurance functions (Glied, 2000).

Main attribute of HMO is that they don't cover services offered by providers outside of their provider network. They share the supplier's risks as well as access to the services that can go via a gatekeeper (Cutler et al., 2000).

22.5.2 Independent practice associations (IPAs)

IPAs involve a legal entity that agreements with a physicians' group to offer the facility to the HMO's members. Moreover, these physicians can also provide care to non-HMO patients; however, in this case, physicians are remunerated based on capitation. In other words,

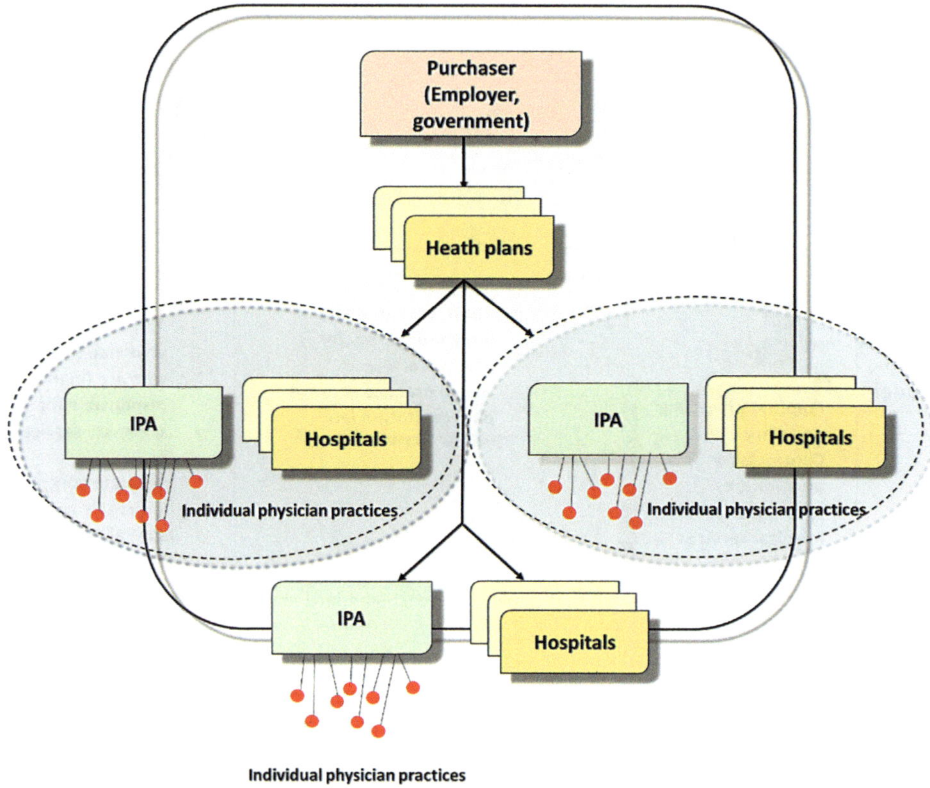

FIGURE 22.5 **Flowchart indicating horizontally integrated managed care systems.** The chart demonstrates a provider network wherein physicians practice in their individual settings; however, they are paid through associations. The IPAs further link with the hospitals and individual physicians belonging to several IPAs and thus have enough health plans contract to sustain the physician's practice.

regardless of whether a patient wants treatment, a predetermined sum is allotted to that doctor or group of doctors for every enrolled patient (Murphy et al., 1998). The governing body of IPAs chooses the appropriate methods of practice (Fig. 22.5). Typically, the agreement is not limited and enables physicians to sign agreements with different HMOs individually or as a group. IPA participants frequently treat fee-for-service individuals who are not enrolled for managed care.

22.5.3 Preferred provider organizations (PPOs)

PPOs are defined as an arrangement wherein a designated group of customers receives services from hospitals and physicians under a contract with a subsidized charge for service. It provides a way for providers to contract with the PPOs. PPOs are the least restrictive MCO.

PPOs make revenue by billing the insurance company an entry charge to utilize their service. The group offers designated experts a significant discount off their standard prices

(Hester et al., 1987). In regards to utilizing such a plan, a PPO often does not include a co-payment but instead provides a minimum and a coinsurance feature, in contrast to an HMO plan, which typically includes a small payment given at the time of treatment. Before receiving any rewards, the deductible amount to be paid in advance. The coinsurance advantages start to affect once the deductible is met. For example, if the PPO plan has an 80% coinsurance rate and a $1000 deductible, the customer is responsible for paying the full $1000 of the permitted provider cost. The patient will be responsible for the final 20% of the other expenses once the insurance has covered 80% of them. The doctor writes off charges over the permitted sum as a discount rather than being paid for by the patient or their insurance (Heymann et al., 2006). PPOs are the most affordable forms of coverage since the patient is responsible for paying the majority of the initial dollars of coverage. In the United States, it was reported that PPO plans were enhanced from 27% (in 1993) to 34% (in 1998) (Wouters and Hester, 1988).

22.5.4 Point of service (POS)

The POS uses some of the features of the above-listed plans. Patients' or consumers' dissatisfaction with restrictions in HMOs has led to the growth of POS plans. They are also called open-ended HMOs. These plans have higher levels of a patient's financial participation and offer more flexibility than the HMOs. Contrary to HMOs, patients can get coverage through doctors even beyond the plan in POS plans. Employer-sponsored medical insurance with POS policies increased from 7% in 1993% to 22% in 1998 (Dixon, 2002).

22.5.5 Private fee for service (PFFS)

PFFS involves two types of insurance, namely indemnity (service fee) and managed care. A classic type of health insurance is a service fee, which is paid by the insurance company to medical staff in terms of salaries for each service rendered to an insured patient. In addition, the fee for service covers basics like hospital rooms, hospital services, cost of surgery both in and out of the hospital, supplies, and care, as well as doctor visits and primary medical protection such as severe illnesses require prolonged treatment with rehabilitation (if required) (Wright et al., 1984)

22.5.6 Managed care in indemnity insurance plans

An indemnity health insurance plan differs from the services offered by HMOs and PPOs because it allows the patient to obtain medical care where they choose by providing compensation for a portion of all associated costs. They allow patients to self-refer to a specialist without requiring a referral to get compensated (Davidson et al., 2003). Precertification of nonemergency hospitalizations as well as utilization reviews are two managed care elements that are increasingly included in indemnity health insurance policies. Sometimes, these are referred to as managed indemnity plans (Perneger et al., 1995).

22.6 Pharmacotherapy management

Pharmacotherapy management is a measure taken by the MCOs other than prescribing to control the use of drugs within the desired organization by affecting physicians' prescribing and pharmacists' dispensing decisions. It involves the following tools.

22.6.1 Networks and tools in pharmacotherapy

Provider networks, if established in a better way, can help in controlling the costs of pharmacotherapy. Moreover, pharmacies are the best providers of pharmacotherapy management. MCOs intend to have a cost-effective pharmacy network so that sufficient pharmacies can remain available to cater to the needs of the patients. MCOs can establish the provider network of pharmacies in three steps. Firstly, by developing an in-house pharmacy owned by MCOs, which will act as a starting point for their pharmacy networks, and then if required, further chains of pharmacies can be added to it. Secondly, by establishing a direct contract with the pharmacy providers' network. The last step is forming a contract with the pharmacy benefits manager (PBM) (Ali and Mantrala, 2010).

PBMs are widely known as organizations specializing in managing the pharmacy provider network and providing better pharmacotherapy management services. In technical terms, when anyone hires a PBM, it is known as a carveout of pharmacy benefits. Pharmacies develop a contract with MCOs or PBM, as depicted in Fig. 22.6, under an assignment stating that the pharmacy will not bill the patients higher than the sum described in the contract.

In the case of a drug product having a generic equivalent, the maximum allowable cost (MAC) plus dispensing fee is set in the contract. However, the MAC of a product is determined by the pharmacy cost that it generally pays for the specific drug product. Pharmacy services are offered at a reduced cost by pharmacies that have an agreement with an MCO or PBM. Additionally, prescription medicine reimbursement often happens at a typical wholesale price. This product price is also kept cheaper than what the drugstore charges other consumers (Berndt and Newhouse, 2010). The difference between these two charges depends on the negotiating stance that the MCOs have to obtain discounts. Thus, often in the provider network, the pharmacies have to make the tough decision of either signing a contract with heavy discounts or losing their percentage of a business. Conversely, MCOs must have enough pharmacies in the network to provide essential patient access. However, this will limit the discounts these MCOs can extract from the pharmacy providers.

22.6.2 Risks allocation and promotion scheme

Prescription drugs are included in the complete capitation rate for essential care physicians. However, sharing of risks virtue of capitation is not done separately for prescription drugs. Promotion schemes, including incentives for providers to control the utilization of prescription drugs, may be implemented (Furrow, 1996). If the expenses for a prescription drug are kept below a lower margin of specified values, then they will only receive withheld payment. Multiple incidences of physicians being penalized for violating pharmacy prescribing policies and fraudulent activities are reported (Qureshi et al., 2011). It also involves bonuses

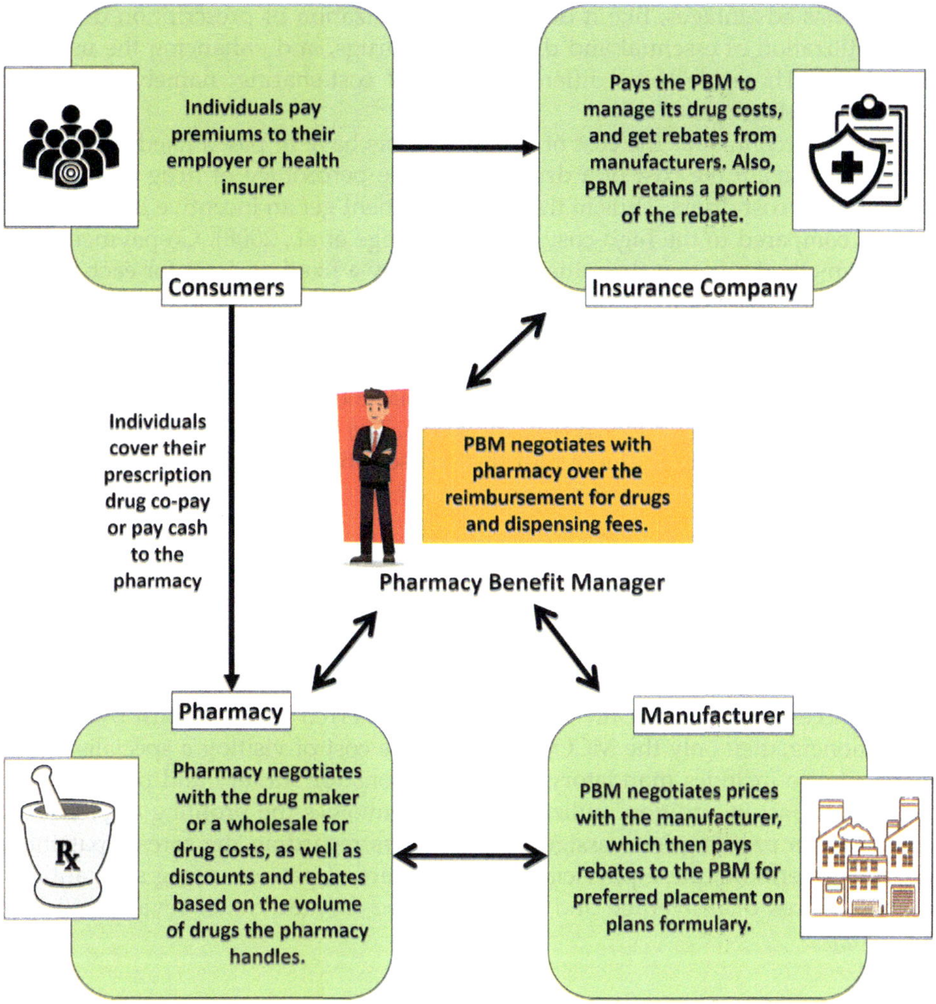

FIGURE 22.6 **Role of pharmacy benefits manager.** The figure depicts the different roles of PBM concerning insurance companies, drug manufacturers, and pharmacies. Further, it displays the interplay among consumers, pharmacies, insurance companies, and manufacturers to provide patients with cost-effective and quality health care collectively.

to physicians if they can lower prescription medication expenditure levels or follow pharmacy prescribing guidelines.

22.6.3 The notion of cost-sharing

Cost-sharing is another management tool used by MCOs. The purpose of cost-sharing results in lowering the expenditures on prescription drugs by the MCOs and a decrease in the number and the cost of prescription medicines employed by the patients. Further, cost-sharing has advantages, like it decreases the utilization of prescription drugs, discouraging the utilization of essential and discretionary drugs, and enhancing the use of specific types of drugs. There are three different modes of cost-sharing, namely coinsurance, co-payment, and deductibles.

Coinsurance accounts for the cost of drugs. Patients have to pay a fixed percentage of the cost of drugs. Thus, if the cost of a drug is high, the percentage of drug costs will be high compared to low-cost drugs. Thus in this method patient get an incentive if he opts for lower costs drugs compared to the high-cost drugs (Lee Page et al., 2008). Co-payment involves a cost-sharing method wherein the patients have to pay a fixed amount for each prescription. Generally, the co-payment for generic drugs is lower than for branded drugs. Three tiers co-payment plan wherein the lowest co-payment is for generic prescription drugs, followed by brand name drugs, and the highest co-payment is for nonformulary brand name drugs. The main disadvantage of the co-payment method is that there is no direct relation between the amount that patients pay and the costs of the drugs. The deductibles cost-sharing method involves patients paying a fixed amount for their prescription drugs before their managed care plans do so. They are often used with co-payment or coinsurance (Grootendorst and Hoar, 2007).

22.6.4 Utilization management

Utilization management is one of the methods used by MCOs to control costs. In this tool, the patient needs to have a primary care physician called a gatekeeper through whom the patient will access healthcare. Only if the patient is referred to a specialist by their primary care practitioners, then only the MCOs will cover the cost of visiting a specialist. Utilization management also includes mandatory second opinions for surgery and prior authorization for hospitalizations. In addition, utilization review involves the profiling of physicians. The goal of physician profiling is to assign all particulars regarding the care of patients to one physician. Furthermore, these physicians can take care of patients using substantially more or lesser resources than average and are considered for additional review (Wickizer and Lessler, 2002).

22.6.5 Formulary management

Formulary management involves establishing and maintaining the formulary of all the specific drug products which have been permitted for use within the MCOs. The drugs in the formulary are generally covered as per the managed care plan. It has been used as a tool in utilization management in 92.2% of HMOs or 71.6% of PPOs having drug formulary. The objective of a formulary is to confirm medically appropriate and cost-effective drug products and treatments that can benefit a certain patient population's health. A formulary can significantly lower drug prices by advising doctors and pharmacists to adopt less costly, equally efficient drugs (Studdert et al., 2019).

Formulary management is regulated by two bodies, namely the pharmacy and therapeutics committee of the MCOs (Fig. 22.7). It comprises physicians, pharmacists, and administrators. The committee validates the therapeutic effect of drugs by reviewing different aspects such as effectiveness, toxicity, or cost differences of a similar class of pharmaceutical

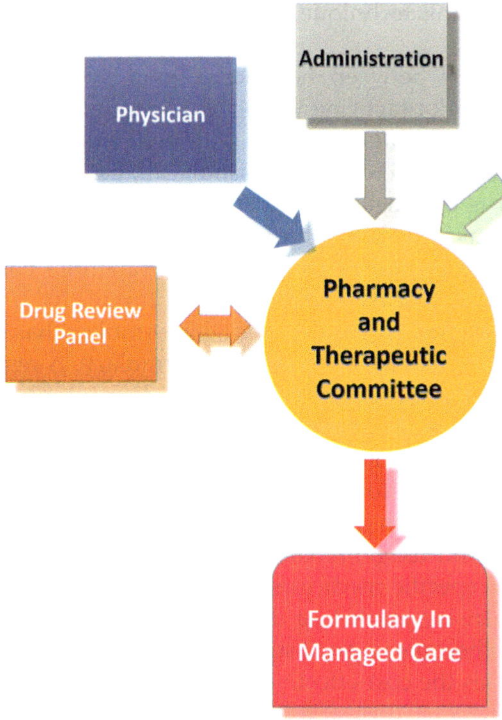

FIGURE 22.7 **Formulary management.** Physicians, administration, and pharmacists from the pharmacy and therapeutics committees (PTC) decide and manage the formulary in managed care. Opinions and reviews from the drug review panel and safety committee are considered by PTC of MCOs.

medications (Kongstvedt, 2013). After reviewing, the optimal drug products are listed in the formulary. This review is performed annually or biannually to update the drug products in the formulary. In addition, information such as any adverse drug reaction (ADR), new information about the drug, or rapid increase in drug expenditure or usage is also mentioned in this review. It also performs the function of educating practitioners on the usage of drugs within the MCOs.

Drug inventory management is compared by considering two important factors: monetary accounting and medical decision-making. Moreover, when several generic alternatives exist for a given product, the medication inventory management strategy is applied. It is based on the assumption that all substances in a class are similar in terms of safety, efficacy, and bioequivalence. The cost assessment method is predicated on the assumption that similar drugs are equivalent in terms of safety, effectiveness, bioequivalence, and related costs. This model applies to drug-driven costs, including administration costs, packaging designs, as well as therapeutic regimens. The objective of cost accounting is to select products with minimal acquisition and drug-driven costs. Clinical decision analysis qualifies the agent based on a broader scope of safety, efficacy, and bioequivalence, along with considering the overall therapeutic results of the decision (Wang et al., 2004). The goals involve comparing and selecting therapeutic options, decreasing the overall cost of therapy, and optimizing the therapeutic outcomes cost-effectively. In addition, this technique also quantifies the outcomes along with the costs of therapy.

Collaborative working relationships between healthcare employees, defining medical workers and physician provider network practicing within MCO, and viewing the pharmacy and therapeutics committee as a medical staff committee are three critical elements required for maintaining the formulary. There are two essential formularies, i.e., open and closed. An open formulary consists of a few lists of drugs with little or no restrictions in prescribing. It includes 3000 drugs and dosage forms. The closed formulary includes a limited set of drugs that qualifies the inclusion criteria set by the pharmacy and therapeutics committee. They have fewer than 1000 drugs and dosage forms (Ganther and Doucette, 2002).

In addition, depending upon restriction on prescription, the formulary has been classified into two types (a) restrictive formulary and (b) nonrestrictive formulary. A restrictive formulary involves only drugs included in the formulary that needs to be prescribed unless documentation for nonformulary medicines is offered to the pharmacy and therapeutics committee. On the other hand, in a nonrestrictive formulary, physicians are encouraged to prescribe drugs from the formulary, but nonformulary drugs can be prescribed with relative ease. One can choose the formulary restriction to balance concerns against costs with the quality of care. In this era of modernization usage, rebates have increased for pharmaceuticals. These create incentives to prescribe specific medicines. Nowadays, the success of the drug is also determined by the comprehensive marketing demands it caters. If the drug is listed in any healthcare plans or policies, it becomes a great success. This has led to the development of pharmacoeconomics, which studies the cost-effectiveness of drugs (Robinson et al., 2001).

22.6.6 Practice guidelines

Practice guidelines are the developed statements that assist the practitioner in providing care for specific clinical interventions. They are made separately for each clinical condition as well as they are reliant on recent clinical evidence. The main goals include the most cost-effective therapies that should be confirmed and used within the MCOs. In addition, more expensive and least effective therapy should be avoided. However, the success of this tool will be depended upon how the practitioners accept and implement these guidelines. More or less, these guidelines should be simple and concise because if they are brief, then physicians will be reluctant to read those guidelines. Thus, practice guidelines offer a comprehensive template for curing individuals with specific clinical interventions (Shekelle, 2018).

However, in the case of critical conditions, some specific guidelines must be provided that can be achieved with critical pathways. It consists of a detailed plan for treating illnesses or processes employed and for a particular diagnostic purpose. It describes the application and timings of complete activities needed for patient care by optimizing cost-effectiveness and improving patient outcomes. Furthermore, critical pathways are the extra effort made other than the practice guidelines due to their comprehensive nature. Critical pathways enhance communication and coordination among practitioners treating a particular patient.

Another tool is step therapy, which consists of protocols prohibiting pharmaceutical use until cheaper substitutes have been explored first (Borum, 1996). Step therapy promotes the employment of older, more affordable drugs with a long history of clinical efficacy over utilizing newer ones that frequently have a lesser history of clinical efficacy and greater costs. It mainly focuses on first trying low-cost drugs, followed by an expensive drug if needed. In 1988, in the USA, step therapy procedures were implemented at 68.5% of HMOs. This technique does not remove decision-making authority from practitioners but provides information and guidelines which lead to the best utilization of the available therapy (Fischer and Avorn, 2017).

22.6.7 Quality improvement

The main objective of quality improvement (QI) is to keep an eye on as well as enhance the care provided to MCO beneficiaries. This can be achieved by quality programs that have a systemwide perspective and structure-process-outcome approach. Structure refers to capital resources, for instance, types of equipment and facilities, personnel like physicians, pharmacists, and organizations of resources such as separate clinics and departments. The process includes any activity occurring during the delivery of care, like support activities, the person performing the care activity, and the place and time where the care activities are performed. Outcomes include the result of healthcare service and its impact on a patient. Various MCOs develop their criteria in these areas as a part of the quality improvement process (Shmueli et al., 2015).

Quality assurance (QA) is defined as a systematic method where various issues related to the delivery of health care are determined, solutions to these problems are devised and implemented, and follow-up checking is carried out. Thus, QA contributes to the quality improvement process in MCOs. Another tool to improve the quality of drug utilization within the MCOs is drug utilization review (DUR). This continuing program reviews, analyses, and interprets patterns of drugs to use against predetermined standards. Patients or prescribers correct any drug-related problem found during the review process. DUR also serves as a tool to monitor the frequency of the refills of dangerous drugs by patients, and it monitors the prescribing patterns of physicians for expensive antibiotics (Edmunds et al., 1997). One such study was carried out for the health of North Carolina in the USA. Wherein they develop a flowchart described in Fig. 22.8 to devise aims, goals, and the objective to provide quality healthcare through North Carolina Medicaid Managed Care.

22.6.8 Educational activities

Another tool for pharmacotherapy within an MCO is to instruct practitioners and patients about various methods of managing care. Educational activity by MCOs may be prospective or retrospective. The prospective educational activity includes communicating the anticipated information before treatment decisions. This will guide the patient on the treatment choices and enable him to select the appropriate one to avoid problems. The retrospective educational activity includes information provided after evaluating treatment choices, for instance, DUR evaluation. These educational activities by MCOs can correct wrong therapy choices (Ganther and Doucette, 2002).

Methods for educating patients or practitioners involve one-to-one discussions, printed materials, oral presentations, seminars, lectures, or symposia. Newsletters addressing specific new treatments or new drugs for a particular disease can be used for educating practitioners and patients. If communication is needed in a focused manner, then booklets or brochures

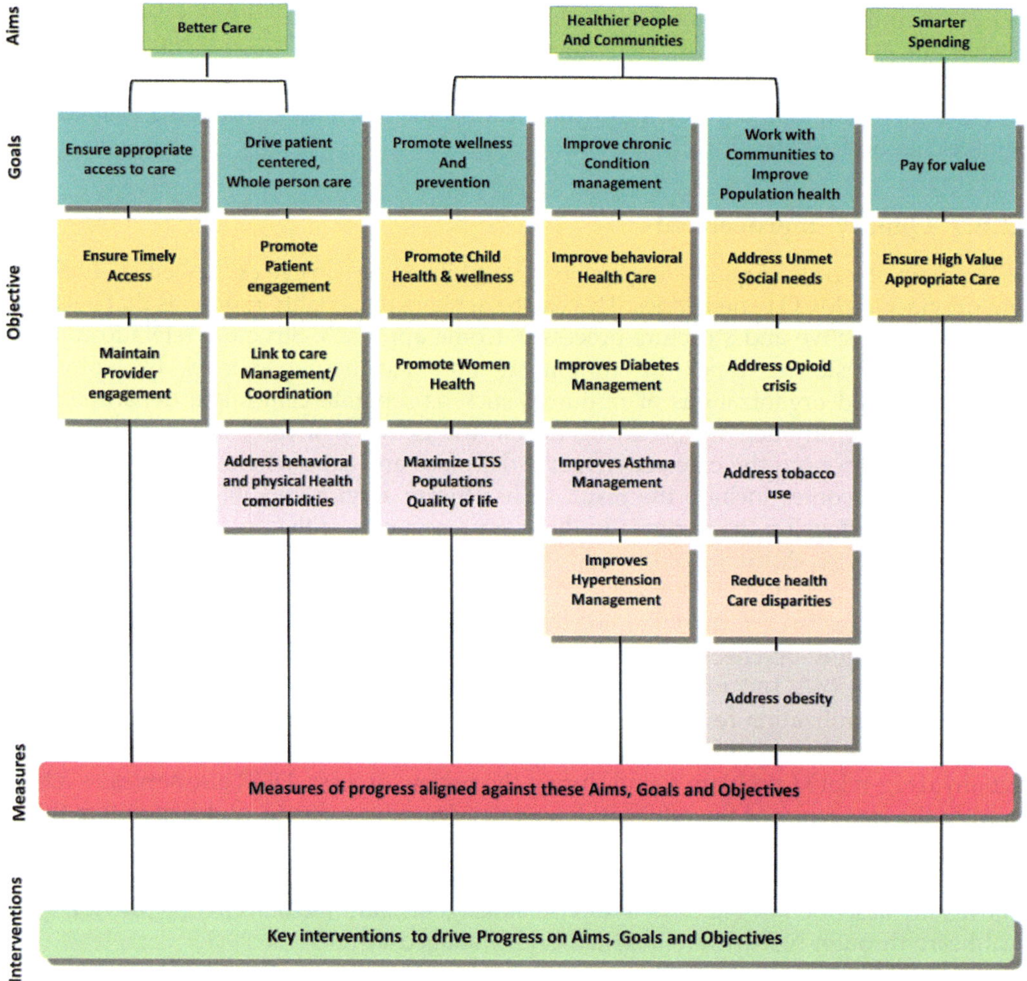

FIGURE 22.8 **North Carolinians Medicaid quality strategy, aims, goals, and objectives.** Schematic depicts a department goal to improve the health of North Carolinians through an innovative, whole-person-centered, and well-coordinated system of care and measurement of quality, which addresses both medical and nonmedical drivers of health.

can be used. On the other hand, oral lectures or symposia facilitate two-way interaction on the topic, thus further adding to better clarity and utilization of the information. Another way is a one-to-one dialogue with practitioners about the correct therapy choices. Such discussion focusing on pharmacotherapy is called academic detailing. It involves physicians or pharmacists meeting the prescriber to improve pharmacotherapy by offering information on prescribing patterns (Glied, 2000).

Another one-to-one presentation with prescribers (mainly a physician who prescribes more particular antibiotics) can help the other practitioners to gather information about the accepted use of widely prescribed antibiotics.

22.6.9 Computerized monitoring

Another tool in pharmacotherapy management is computerized monitoring, wherein the ADRs of drugs are recorded and stored in the computer. In this method, the quality of treatment can be monitored using inbuilt computer systems for low-dose potent drugs (Teagarden et al., 2000). Multiple cases of successful implementation of a computer-assisted monitoring system for detecting undesired drug reactions in clinical settings are reported. These systems use integrated patient information containing details from the pharmacy, microbiology division, radiology service, and other resources. This system's predetermined criteria, such as medication dose reduction, antidote prescriptions, or abnormal laboratory readings, might serve as "trigger signals" for possible ADR detection (Chen et al., 2020; Hoang et al., 2018).

22.6.10 Handling lawsuit

This is also an important tool to be considered in pharmacotherapy management. Lawsuits can be filed if the claim made by MCO is not fulfilled. Many commercial players use litigation against suppliers to overcome alleged fraud or abuse (Friedman et al., 2014).

22.7 Disease management with pharmacotherapy as a primary focus

22.7.1 Attention-deficit/hyperactivity disorder

Psychostimulants are the first-line therapy drug for attention-deficit/hyperactivity disorder (ADHD). There are many benefits of ADHD management along with managed care, which not only leads to an improvement in the symptoms but also improves the quality of life of patients and their families. In addition, it further reduces costs for purchasers and payers. Furthermore, ADR monitoring, education of patients or parents, and regular follow-up by the MCOs can lead to better pharmacotherapy management for ADDH. After considering the rising costs associated with pharmacotherapy of ADDH, it indicates that plans have invested a significant amount in treating the disorder. However, to obtain good returns, stakeholders must promote good outcomes. Thus, monitoring the patient's adherence to medication, educating of patient and parent, and follow-up MCOs can help enhance the patient's quality of life. They can tell the patient how to deal with anxiety and other side effects of the medications. Thus, interventions, as described above by MCOs, can help to treat the patient with ADHD, which benefits the purchasers and payers (Dopheide, 2009).

22.7.2 Chronic constipation

Chronic constipation affects 12%–19% of Americans, especially women and children. In a study, Eoff and limbo have reported how all providers can work collectively to improve the quality of care and enhance health outcomes. Many agents available to treat chronic constipation are over-the-counter drugs, although their efficacy has not been extensively tested. Many prescription agents are available in the market, but the MCOs restrict their usage for patients due to their higher cost. This restriction keeps those patients void of the treatment who fail to respond to traditional treatment. Many providers are treating patients empirically due to the lack of evidence-based algorithms. Thus, practitioners can provide proper assistance to patients by seeking recommendations. Additionally, they can holistically consider the above consideration that can provide information about the treatment options (Eoff and Lembo, 2008).

22.7.3 Asthma

Asthma is a chronic disease affecting children as well as adults. In a research analysis, Donahue et al. carried out pharmacotherapy and healthcare utilization by selecting children aged between 3 and 15 years. Further, they included children diagnosed with asthma in the previous year and were compared in the year 1996–1997 at MCOs. After extracting data from three MCOs, they finally concluded that the pattern of asthma therapy did not reflect the recommendations of the guidelines. Despite good utilization of health services, there exists a lot of variation in asthma therapy among healthcare organizations. It was reported that controlling medications need not be used by all children who could benefit them (Donahue et al., 2000).

22.7.4 Diabetes

Diabetes patient counseling, as well as training, are advised as a crucial component of an all-illness care plan. It comprises instruction and training from a qualified practitioner to help diabetic patients successfully manage their disease independently. Sullivan et al. performed an insurance claims database's historical cohort investigation of individual insurance claims information to evaluate the clinical and cost outcomes of managed care patients with type 2 diabetes. The database analysis findings imply that certain patients with type 2 diabetes mellitus are far more prone than others to get counsel and education, impacting clinical outcomes, medical resources, and financial consequences. Diabetes counseling and education were more common among younger patients, women, and those with higher levels of comorbidity and medications at baseline. Patients given counseling and education along with pharmacotherapy were substantially more likely than individuals who did not get the treatment to achieve glycemic control (Sullivan et al., 2013).

22.7.5 Hypertension

A significant risk element for heart failure (HF) or cardiovascular disease progression is elevated blood pressure, often known as hypertension (HTN). The chance of getting a cardiovascular disease is nearly double in people with diabetes and HTN. The renin-angiotensin-aldosterone system (RAAS) can be hindered by either blocking the transformation of angiotensin I to angiotensin II with ACE inhibitors or by explicitly inhibiting the attachment of angiotensin II to the AT1 receptor subtype with Angiotensin II receptor blockers (ARB), has been linked to the pathogenic mechanisms of HTN as well as the advancement of HF (Shah and Stafford, 2017). In managed care, Jackson IV et al. planned research to evaluate blood pressure monitoring and medication treatment for individuals with concomitant HF and HTN. The research reveals that one out of every three hypertensive patients having

HF was not getting either an ACE inhibitor or an ARB. However, more than two-thirds of the studied group did not have their blood pressure managed to target. ACE inhibitor usage was the most common form of pharmacotherapy. The study's findings show a gap in the management of HTN among individuals suffering from HF and HTN, necessitating the implementation of training initiatives by MCOs to enhance the therapy of hypertensive patients (Jackson et al., 2004).

22.8 Role of pharmacist in MCP

22.8.1 Drug information

Drug information pharmacists help in MCP by fostering rational drug therapy through input on pharmacy and therapeutics committees (Fig. 22.9). They also work with clinical pharmacists to provide the practitioners or physicians with information necessary for optimal drug therapy in particular patients. All these data collected by drug information pharmacists are stored in computer technology which can be assessed with permission. Their role mainly involves responding to drug information requests, reviewing generic drug products, and conducting postmarket surveillance (McCloskey and Vogenberg, 1998).

22.8.2 Industry relations

Pharmacists can develop relations with the pharmaceutical industry to develop MCOs. Health economics and outcomes research carried out by industry can help evolve MCOs by devising better insurance plans and patient benefits (McDermott et al., 2008).

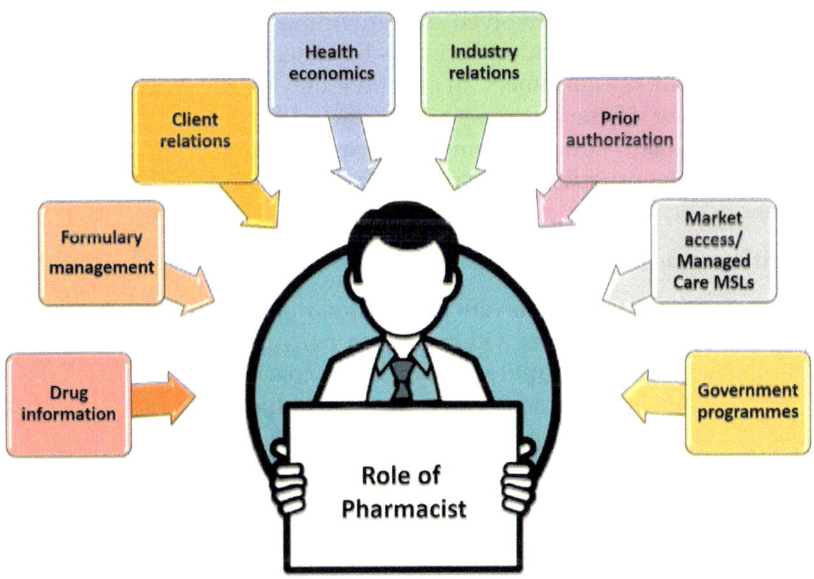
Health economics
Industry relations
Client relations
Prior authorization
Formulary management
Market access/ Managed Care MSLs
Drug information
Government programmes
Role of Pharmacist

FIGURE 22.9 **Role of pharmacists in MCOs.** The figure depicts the different roles of pharmacists in MCOs.

22.8.3 Prior authorization

Prior authorization requires that your physician obtains approval from your healthcare provider before prescribing a specific medication for you or performing a particular operation. Prior authorization involves some necessary steps, such as the physician ordering lab tests; after this, the lab receives orders and starts the prior authorization (MacKinnon & Kumar, 2001). In brief, the people from the lab will check whether prior authorization requirements have been made as per different health plans that consist of different rules. Afterward, they will contact the required health plan, and a form specific to the plan will be retrieved. Prior authorization is faxed out after attaching medical documents. In case it gets approved, it is sent to the insurance agent who reviews it. If rejected, one must appeal again (Balkrishnan et al., 2007).

22.8.4 Client relations

An efficient connection between the patient and health care professional is needed to manage optimal medication. The new role of pharmacists has evolved from the conventional dispensing of drugs to more enormous liabilities of pharmaceutical care, where factors influencing client relationships can impact the development of MCOs. Pharmacists must build good relations with the client by providing sufficient knowledge about the prescribed drugs and guiding them on the dosage regimen. Patient satisfaction is a significant sign of the eminence of health care services as well as a predictor of adherence to the medication regimen and desired therapy outcome (Shrank and Avorn, 2007).

22.8.5 Industry: market access/managed care MSLs

Pharmacists are constantly involved in providing scientific and medical supports, including designs and communication of results from health outcome studies. They maintain good relationships with key customers. In addition, they are also involved in effective teaching and understanding of the customers. Medical science liaison (MSL) calls on various healthcare professionals to educate them on the uses, merits, and scientific data related to the products their firms produce (Kientop, 2010).

22.8.6 Health economics

Pharmacists play a vital role in health economics, mainly by participating in making decisions about the use of medicines. Other studies performed by pharmacists include cost-minimization analyses and cost-utility analyses. Pharmacists, with their unique knowledge of medicines along with pharmacoeconomic analysis, influence the expenditure and distribution of resources on medicines. The pharmacist helps MCOs save costs by using approved formulary to dispense less expensive but equally effective products, by therapeutic interchange or substitution with generics, and by implementing schemes for prior authorization to regulate the use and cost of particular items. Knowledge of health economics and political insights is necessary for a modern healthcare setup to manage expenditure and resource allocation (Schweitzer and Lu, 2018).

22.8.7 Formulary management

Pharmacists are essential to formulary management. Many of the aspects of formulary management are performed by pharmacists, like maintaining the inventory of drug products and dispensing them properly with directions for use. It is often essential to make the right decision at the right time to efficiently manage the formulary. Hence, they are also involved in distributing the formulary effectively and efficiently. However, in several of the MCOs, it is the pharmacy department that is in charge of controlling the use of formulary (Goldberg, 1997).

22.8.8 Government programs

Pharmacists have a significant role in quality assurance programs of the government to enhance patient safety and service. Public health has always been associated with government initiatives as well as services for the underprivileged. Still, a more fitting meaning to the term "public health" would be "fulfilling society's interest in assuring conditions in which people can be healthy." This necessitates pharmacists adopt a population-based approach to avoid illness and enhance general health to promote long and fruitful lives (Farris and Johnson, 2010). They are constantly involved in medication management programs funded by the government to improve patient health and other programs such as fraud, waste, and abuse programs to decrease medication misuse and drug diversion (Hokenstad et al., 2009). They are also involved in drug benefit programs to ensure broad patient outreach and access to needed medications. Thus, pharmacists connect the dots between the prescribers and significantly impact the clinical and economic effects of drugs in highly dynamic MCOs.

22.8.9 Current trends and problems in managed care

An increase in managed care in Medicaid involves impoverished or medically indigent beneficiaries or Medicare, including individuals aged 65 or higher or disabled. In the case of the Medicaid program, providers must be present in locations easily assessed by the poor or medically needy people.

However, enrollment in these programs has created additional issues for MCOs. A concern is that enrollees in Medicaid and Medicare programs have more health problems than the enroller in MCOs, either individually or through employers. Thus, the previous use of more prescription drugs compared to the latter and thus offer more challenges in pharmacotherapy than the latter (Ganther and Doucette, 2002). Thus, MCOs have to broaden their provider network. Another challenge is that MCOs, to control costs, have restricted the use of providers. Thus, due to limited choices, patients remain unhappy. A further concern is assessing the quality of care provided by MCOs. This led to the development of the Health Plan Employer Data and information set (HEDIS), a standard set of quality metrics applied when contrasting healthcare programs. The measure they laid down allows the employer and employee to assess different plans. However, there are only a few HEDIS indicators for medication use currently. Although the usage of less restrictive plans (e.g., PPOs and POS plans) is increased, these plans bear a higher premium and more patient charges. This trend is creating another concern among patients about allowing less restriction but at higher prices (Glied, 2000).

The trade-off between controlling costs as well as maintaining patient gratification is a concern, which is associated with pharmacotherapy. Moreover, in the United States, prescription drug costs have dramatically increased in the last 10 years. Also, the introduction of newer and expensive prescription drugs along with new expensive therapy for common ailments can devastate the drug budget of MCOs for the year.

Thus, the MCOs must have a mechanism for examining costs across different categories. In addition, the MCOs can consider how to enhance access to nonformulary medication if needed by the patients (Eichenholz, 2002).

22.8.10 Worries about managed care in the public sector

Launching managed care in the public sector is reorganizing the public sector. With the aid of MCOs, most purchasers can achieve specific goals like managing the price of therapy and increasing the efficiency, quality, and accessibility of care. Managed care tool usage will lead to an improved combination of functions of the distinct public and private systems of care. Most public sectors face difficulty in managing mental health care and substance misuse. Thus, care for these can be enhanced with better usage of MCOs. Some health plans need updating concerning special facilities for mental health and substance abuse care. Furthermore, prepaid capitated financing features of managed care plans are not widely trusted due to promising financial incentives to reduce care and increase the benefits (Kongstvedt, 2013).

22.8.11 Ethical issues in managed healthcare

Some ethical concerns are also associated with the quality of care, for instance, confidentiality. The physician, who is the primary care provider, requires prior authorization; in this regard, it demands the sharing of medical information. In MCOs, this information can be transferred from one provider to another. Hence, patients, especially those with mental health, may be concerned with confidentiality-related issues due to stigmatism by society (Boyle and Callahan, 1995). Thus, limitations on who can provide or obtain information, as well as its usage, must be imposed by MCOs. The second issue is patient autonomy, and it is the right of individuals to have the freedom to choose among options. MCOs limit the choice for patients with respect to providers and what services are available. The third issue is the practitioners-patient relationship, and practitioners should disclose and always suggest ways to holistically improve patient care (Cooper and Gottlieb, 2000).

22.8.12 Effect of managed care on prescription medicine use

Managed care has an impact on prescription drug use. Some health plans prescribe a particular class of drugs. There exists a significant difference between the health services utilization patterns of patients enrolled in health maintenance organizations and those receiving care under fee-for-service. Considering that less than 7% of US healthcare costs are spent on medicines, there is no empirical data on how HMOs affect the usage of prescription medications. To determine the annual prescriptions filled by the individual, by drug type, and by the health plan, Weiner et al. reviewed a sizable information. It was shown that prescription is very susceptible to variance in practice patterns that may be difficult to justify

(Weiner et al., 1991). As most HMOs place controls on physician prescribing and pharmacist dispensing, further trends in prescription drug usage and pharmacotherapy management can be predicted. As the financial access of the patients to pharmaceuticals improve, MCO can lead to the expansion of marketed innovative drugs (Kongstvedt, 2013).

22.9 Conclusion

MCOs are growing as there is an immense need to provide healthcare facilities at an affordable cost. With the rapidly increasing cost of healthcare, the insurer will find ways to control its growth. As more consumers develop a liking for the less restrictive plans, it is certainly expected that POS and PPO plans will see a surge in use compared to the other plans. But still, the MCOs will be seen relying on and utilizing pharmacotherapy management tools to combat their challenges. In some countries, MCOs strive to deliver quality healthcare at an affordable cost. However, on the other side, MCOs are linked to a wholly commercialized, profit-driven, or competitive paradigm. Introducing private health insurance and adopting managed care methods in Asia's growing nations will play a significant role in providing patient incentives and limiting unnecessary demands through a provider. Performance monitoring, reducing clinical variation, managing chronic diseases, and measuring the outcomes are some of the debatable components present in various health policies of different countries.

22.10 List of abbreviations

ADHD attention-deficit/hyperactivity disorder
ADR adverse drug reaction
DUR drug utilization review
HEDIS health plan employer data and information set
HMOs health maintenance organizations
IPAs independent practice associations
MAC maximum allowable cost
MCOs managed care organizations
MCP managed care pharmacy
PBM pharmacy benefits manager
PFFS private fee for service
POS point of service
PPOs preferred provider organization
PTC pharmacy and therapeutics committees
QA quality assurance
QI quality improvement

References

Ali, O.G., Mantrala, M., 2010. Pharma rebates, pharmacy benefit managers and employer outcomes. Health Care Manag. Sci. 13 (4), 281–293. https://www.ncbi.nlm.nih.gov/pubmed/20963550.

Balkrishnan, R., Joish, V.N., Bhosle, M.J., Rasu, R.S., Nahata, M.C., 2007. Prior authorization of newer insomnia medications in managed care: is it cost saving? J. Clin. Sleep Med. 3 (04), 393–398.

Berndt, E.R., Newhouse, J.P., 2010. Pricing and reimbursement in US pharmaceutical markets. National Bureau of Economic Research.

Borum, R., 1996. Improving the clinical practice of violence risk assessment. Technology, guidelines, and training. Am. Psychol. 51 (9), 945–956. https://www.ncbi.nlm.nih.gov/pubmed/8819363.

Boyle, P.J., Callahan, D., 1995. Managed care in mental health: the ethical issues. Health Aff. 14 (3), 7–22 discussion 23–33. https://www.ncbi.nlm.nih.gov/pubmed/7498905.

Chen, C., Jia, W., Guo, D., Zhu, M., Xu, Y., Wang, X., Wang, D., Wang, W., Tang, Z., 2020. Development of a computer-assisted adverse drug events alarm and assessment system for hospital inpatients in China. Ther. Innov. Regul. Sci. 54 (1), 32–41. https://www.ncbi.nlm.nih.gov/pubmed/32008241.

Cooper, C.C., Gottlieb, M.C., 2000. Ethical issues with managed care: challenges facing counseling psychology. Counsel. Psychol. 28 (2), 179–236.

Cutler, D.M., McClellan, M., Newhouse, J.P., 2000. How does managed care do it? Rand J. Econ. 526–548.

Davidson, S.M., Davidson, H., Miracle-McMahill, H., Oakes, J.M., Crawford, S., Blumenthal, D., Valentine, D.P., 2003. Utilization of services by chronically ill people in managed care and indemnity plans: implications for quality. Inquiry 40 (1), 57–70. https://www.ncbi.nlm.nih.gov/pubmed/12836908.

Dixon, A., 2002. Are medical savings accounts a viable option for funding health care? Croat. Med. J. 43 (4), 408–416. https://www.ncbi.nlm.nih.gov/pubmed/12187518.

Donahue, J.G., Fuhlbrigge, A.L., Finkelstein, J.A., Fagan, J., Livingston, J.M., Lozano, P., Platt, R., Weiss, S.T., Weiss, K.B., 2000. Asthma pharmacotherapy and utilization by children in 3 managed care organizations. The pediatric Asthma Care Patient Outcomes Research team. J. Allergy Clin. Immunol. 106 (6), 1108–1114. https://www.ncbi.nlm.nih.gov/pubmed/11112894.

Dopheide, J.A., 2009. The role of pharmacotherapy and managed care pharmacy interventions in the treatment of ADHD. Am. J. Manag. Care 15 (5 Suppl. l), S141–S150. https://www.ncbi.nlm.nih.gov/pubmed/19601689.

Edmunds, M., Frank, R., Hogan, M., McCarty, D., Robinson-Beale, R., Weisner, C., 1997. Managing Managed Care: Quality Improvement in Behavioral Health. National Academies Press.

Eichenholz, J., 2002. Trends in managed care pharmacy: responding to changing environments. J. Manag. Care Pharm. 8 (2), 102–107.

Eoff, J.C., Lembo, A.J., 2008. Optimal treatment of chronic constipation in managed care: review and roundtable discussion. Acad. Managed Care Pharmacy.

Farris, K.B., Johnson, K.A., 2010. Pharmacists in public health: it's a good start. J. Am. Pharmaceut. Assoc. (2003) 50 (2), 128–130. https://www.ncbi.nlm.nih.gov/pubmed/20199951.

Fischer, M.A., Avorn, J., 2017. Step therapy-clinical algorithms, legislation, and optimal prescribing. JAMA 317 (8), 801–802. https://www.ncbi.nlm.nih.gov/pubmed/28166322.

Friedman, J., Collura, E., Ryan, N.M., Bowen, J.D., 2014. A crystal ball: managed care litigation in light of the patient protection and affordable care act. Health Law 27, 1.

Furrow, B.R., 1996. Managed care organizations and patient injury: rethinking liability. Georgia Law Rev. 31, 419.

Ganther, J.M., Doucette, W.R., 2002. Managed care and pharmacotherapy management. In: Modern Pharmaceutics. CRC Press, pp. 1195–1214.

Glied, S., 2000. Managed care. In: Handbook of Health Economics, vol 1. Elsevier, pp. 707–753.

Goldberg, R., 1997. Managing the pharmacy benefit: the formulary system. J. Manag. Care Pharm. 3 (5), 565–573.

Grootendorst, P., Hoar, J., 2007. Effect of co-payments on drug use in the presence of annual payment limits. Am. J. Manag. Care 13 (part 2), 328–334.

Happe, L.E., Clark, D., Holliday, E., Young, T., 2014. A systematic literature review assessing the directional impact of managed care formulary restrictions on medication adherence, clinical outcomes, economic outcomes, and health care resource utilization. J. Manag. Care Spec. Pharm. 20 (7), 677–684. https://www.ncbi.nlm.nih.gov/pubmed/24967521.

Harrington, C., 2019. Social health maintenance organizations: an innovative financing and service delivery model. Caregiving Systems: Informal and Formal Helpers.

Hester, J.A., Wouters, A., Wright, N., 1987. Evaluation of a preferred provider organization. Milbank Q. 65 (4), 575–613. https://www.ncbi.nlm.nih.gov/pubmed/3132599.

Heymann, A.D., Chodick, G., Halkin, H., Karasik, A., Shalev, V., Shemer, J., Kokia, E., 2006. The implementation of managed care for diabetes using medical informatics in a large Preferred Provider Organization. Diabetes Res. Clin. Pract. 71 (3), 290–298.

Hoang, T., Liu, J., Roughead, E., Pratt, N., Li, J., 2018. Supervised signal detection for adverse drug reactions in medication dispensing data. Comput. Methods Progr. Biomed. 161, 25–38. https://www.ncbi.nlm.nih.gov/pubmed/29852965.

Hokenstad, A., Shineman, M., Auerbach, R., 2009. An Overview of Medicaid Long-Term Care Programs in New York. Medicaid Institute at United Hospital Fund.

Jackson IV, J.H., French, F., Ronen, R., Mullany, L., Lennert, B., Jhaveri, V., 2004. Assessment of drug therapy management and the prevalence of heart failure in a managed care population with hypertension. J. Manag. Care Pharm. 10 (6), 513–520.

Joshi, S., Krishnan, R., 2017. Economic Models of Hospital Behavior.

Kientop, D., 2010. Integrating medical science liaisons into key account management. J. Med. Market. 10 (1), 45–51.

Kongstvedt, P.R., 2013. Essentials of Managed Health Care. Jones & Bartlett Publishers.

Lee Page, R., Barton, P., Nair, K., 2008. Effect of cost-sharing for prescription medications on health outcomes in older adults: a critical review of the literature and potential implications for managed care. Consult. Pharm. 23 (1), 44–54.

MacKinnon, N., Kumar, R., 2001. Prior authorization programs: a critical review of the literature. J. Manag. Care Pharm. 7 (4), 297–303.

McCloskey, W.W., Vogenberg, F.R., 1998. Drug information resources in managed care organizations. Am. J. Health Syst. Pharm. 55 (19), 2007–2009. https://www.ncbi.nlm.nih.gov/pubmed/9784788.

McDermott, K.J., Holland, E.T., Navarro, R.P., 2008. Role of the pharmaceutical company in managed care. Managed Care Pharmacy Practice.

Meredith, L.S., Rubenstein, L.V., Rost, K., Ford, D.E., Gordon, N., Nutting, P., Camp, P., Wells, K.B., 1999. Treating depression in staff-model versus network-model managed care organizations. J. Gen. Intern. Med. 14 (1), 39–48. https://www.ncbi.nlm.nih.gov/pubmed/9893090.

Murphy, M.J., DeBernardo, C.R., Shoemaker, W.E., 1998. Impact of managed care on independent practice and professional ethics: a survey of independent practitioners. Prof. Psychol. Res. Pract. 29 (1), 43–51. https://www.ncbi.nlm.nih.gov/pubmed/11660484.

Perneger, T.V., Allaz, A.-F., Etter, J.-F., Rougemont, A., 1995. Mental health and choice between managed care and indemnity health insurance. Am. J. Psychiatr. 152, 1020–1055.

Qureshi, Z.P., Liu, Y., Sartor, O., Chu, Y.H., Bennett, C.L., 2011. Enforcement actions involving Medicaid fraud and abuse, 1996–2009. Arch. Intern. Med. 171 (8), 785–787. https://www.ncbi.nlm.nih.gov/pubmed/21518950.

Robinson, G., Chimento, L., Bush, S., Papay, J., 2001. Comprehensive mental health insurance benefits: case studies. In: DHHS Pub No SMA 01-341. Center for Mental Health Services, Rockville, MD, pp. 1–80. https://www.ce-credit.com/articles/100177/MentalHealthInsuranceBenefitsCase100177.pdf.

Rodwin, M.A., 2010. The metamorphosis of managed care: implications for health reform internationally. J. Law Med. Ethics 38 (2), 352–364. https://www.ncbi.nlm.nih.gov/pubmed/20579232.

Schweitzer, S.O., Lu, Z.J., 2018. Pharmaceutical Economics and Policy: Perspectives, Promises, and Problems. Oxford University Press.

Shah, S.J., Stafford, R.S., 2017. Current trends of hypertension treatment in the United States. Am. J. Hypertens. 30 (10), 1008–1014. https://www.ncbi.nlm.nih.gov/pubmed/28531239.

Shekelle, P.G., 2018. Clinical practice guidelines: what's next? JAMA 320 (8), 757–758. https://www.ncbi.nlm.nih.gov/pubmed/30098168.

Shmueli, A., Stam, P., Wasem, J., Trottmann, M., 2015. Managed care in four managed competition OECD health systems. Health Pol. 119 (7), 860–873. https://www.ncbi.nlm.nih.gov/pubmed/25776034.

Shrank, W.H., Avorn, J., 2007. Educating patients about their medications: the potential and limitations of written drug information. Health Aff. 26 (3), 731–740.

Studdert, A.L., Gong, C.L., Srinivas, S., Chin, A.L., Deresinski, S., 2019. Application of pharmacoeconomics to formulary management in a health system setting. Am. J. Health Syst. Pharm. 76 (6), 381–386. https://www.ncbi.nlm.nih.gov/pubmed/31361838.

Sullivan, S.D., Dalal, M.R., Burke, J.P., 2013. The impact of diabetes counseling and education: clinical and cost outcomes from a large population of US managed care patients with type 2 diabetes. Diabetes Educat. 39 (4), 523–531. https://www.ncbi.nlm.nih.gov/pubmed/23640302.

Teagarden, J.R., Clotz, M., Angaran, D., Kenreigh, C., 2000. Computer implemented patient medication review system and process for the managed care, health care and/or pharmacy industry. Google Patents.

Wang, Z., Salmon, J.W., Walton, S.M., 2004. Cost-effectiveness analysis and the formulary decision-making process. J. Manag. Care Pharm. 10 (1), 48–59. https://www.ncbi.nlm.nih.gov/pubmed/14720105.

Weiner, J.P., Lyles, A., Steinwachs, D.M., Hall, K.C., 1991. Impact of managed care on prescription drug use. Health Aff. 10 (1), 140–154.

Wickizer, T.M., Lessler, D., 2002. Utilization management: issues, effects, and future prospects. Annu. Rev. Publ. Health 23 (1), 233–254. https://www.ncbi.nlm.nih.gov/pubmed/11910062.

Wouters, A.V., Hester, J., 1988. Patient choice of providers in a preferred provider organization. Med. Care 26 (3), 240–255. https://www.ncbi.nlm.nih.gov/pubmed/3127640.

Wright, C.H., Gardin, T.H., Wright, C.L., 1984. Obstetric care in a health maintenance organization and a private fee-for-service practice: a comparative analysis. Am. J. Obstet. Gynecol. 149 (8), 848–856. https://www.ncbi.nlm.nih.gov/pubmed/6465249.

CHAPTER

23

Understanding the connection between dietary supplementation and inadvertent doping

Manish Kumar Sharma[1,2], *Hari Priya Koppisetti*[1], *Priyanka Lohar*[1], *Rahul Maheshwari*[3], *Pinaki Sengupta*[1] *and Rakesh Kumar Tekade*[1]

[1]National Institute of Pharmaceutical Education and Research (NIPER)- Ahmedabad, An Institute of National Importance, Government of India, Department of Pharmaceuticals, Ministry of Chemicals and Fertilizers, Palaj, Gandhinagar, Gujarat, India; [2]College of Pharmacy, Pharmacy Practice, and Science, University of Nebraska Medical Center, NE, United States; [3]School of Pharmacy and Technology Management, SVKM' NMIMS, Hyderabad, Telangana, India

23.1 Doping: things to know!

Sports play a crucial role in physical as well as mental well-being. It promotes international appreciation and association. The usage of doping products or unethical practices affects not only the health of athletes but also the sport's image. Doping cheats the fans of their belief, and therefore, it is incumbent on every sports body to ensure that there is no cheating in sports for fair play and clean competition. According to World Anti-Dopping Agency (WADA), doping is defined as an act of violation of any of the rules set out in the anti-doping code, which ranges from the possession, use, and trafficking of illegal substances to engaging in behavior associated with illicit substances, and refusing or tampering with sample collection for drug testing (WADA, 2009; Hughes, 2015).

Anti-doping authorities mention that athletes using endurance-enhancing drugs will be considered faulted against the "spirit of sport." Sports organizations of every country are coordinating strict regulation and implementation of WADA rules for all levels of games and promoting equal opportunity for athletes in the drug-free sports movement, showing

Essentials of Pharmatoxicology in Drug Research, Volume 1
https://doi.org/10.1016/B978-0-443-15840-7.00021-X

an exemplary effect on the public for several decades. Every athlete is tested for doping before the game. If someone fails the test or is found tampering with the samples collecting samples for the dope test or refusing a control, the act resembles an athlete's behavior against the spirit of sport. As an outcome, the prohibited substances list and methods have been developed under the WADA doping code to keep alive the spirit of sports as clean and fair as possible throughout the world (Brand et al., 2014). The sample testing protocol for the dope test by the National dope testing laboratory is mentioned in Fig. 23.1.

Doping can be intentional or unintentional. The unintentional doping results from nutritional supplements that do not entirely disclose the substances included in them and will

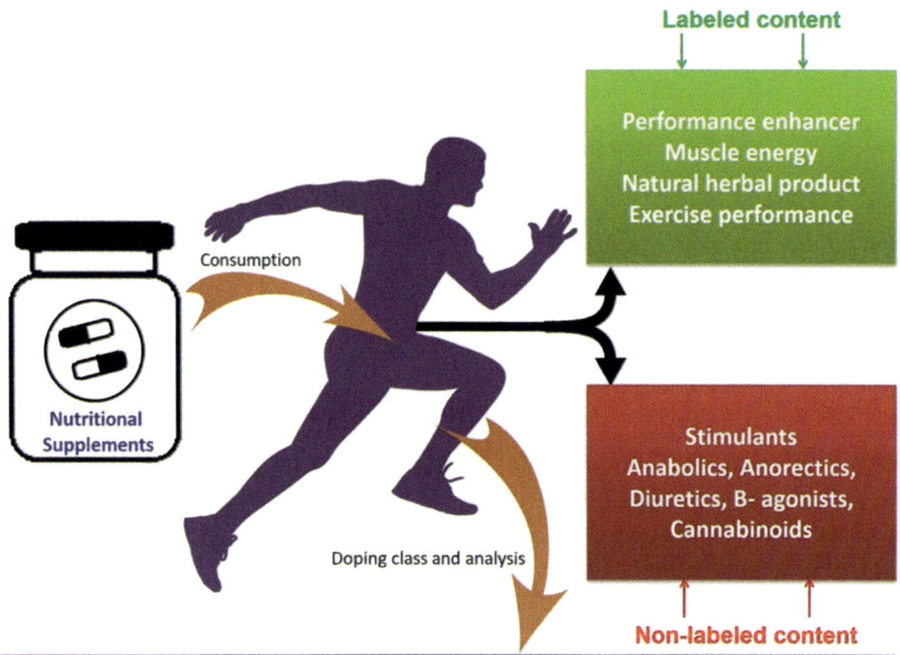

Sample ports	Screening	
Urine	**In and out of competition** S1 Anabolic agents S2 Peptide hormones, growth factors, and related substances S3 Beta-2 agonists S4 Hormone antagonists and modulators S5 Diuretics and other masking agents M1 Enhancements of oxygen transfer	**In competition** S6 Stimulants S7 Narcotics S8 Cannabinoids S9 Glucocorticosteroids P1 Alcohol P2 Beta-blockers
Blood	Erythropoietin Stimulating Agents (ESAs) and its analogs Human growth hormone; Blood parameters; Blood transfusion; Haemoglobin based oxygen carriers	

FIGURE 23.1 **Nutritional supplements as a source of positive doping.** Bottom Insat is showing sample ports for the dope test. Out-of-competition testing is done for the training period and off-season, whereas, in-competition testing is done during the selection trial, state-level championship, national competition, and international competition.

be detected in the test. To identify these hidden or unlabeled substances in dietary supplements, qualitative and quantitative tests are performed. Most of the encountered hidden substances in supplements were found in a random sampling of available marketed products such as anabolic steroids, stimulants, and other prohibited substances like glucocorticoids, beta-2 agonists, peptides, and growth hormones. These banned substances have been controversial for deliberately taking dietary supplements in high-competition sports (Mathews, 2018). These supplements are freely available in the market as well as on various online platforms. They lack the stringent quality controls test and certification of intense performance products. Moreover, the safety, efficacy, and potency of these supplements have not been thoroughly investigated by controlled clinical studies and remain, for the most part, anecdotal.

These unlabeled substances could be the main reason for doping violations, whether intentional or unintentional, leading to athlete sanctions or penalties. Thus, a wide range of available marketed supplements has created a lot of confusion and ambiguity regarding quality, and safety and increased the risk of positive doping due to the maximum use of nutritional supplements among high-profile athletes (Committee, 1999).

To maintain the spirit of sports throughout the world, WADA mandate anti-doping violation rules to strengthen the National Anti-Doping Control Authority to prevent the use of banned substances, trafficking of illegal substances, awareness about the marketed nutrition supplements, labeled or unlabeled substance and also refusing or tampering with sample collection which attributed against the WADA anti-doping code. However, it is tough and challenging to define where allowed nutritional supplements end and doping starts. Thus, many sports organizations are following the mission of WADA anti-doping rules and codes to promote, coordinate, and monitor at the international level (WADA, 2009). To accomplish this mission and fill up the voids, the International Association of Sports Federation was the first international governing body to take the initiative and strictly handle this situation. In the beginning, stages of fighting against doping, they had to rely on the athlete's word due to the lack of advanced scientific procedures and testing of a banned substance to tighten the rules and guidelines.

This chapter showcases the use of dietary supplements and associated risks as they may contain prohibited substances as enlisted by WADA. This chapter also provides a roadmap guide to the athletes who often consume nutritional supplements and are unaware of the hidden, unlabeled substances, which leads to their failure in dope tests and sentence the penalty even though it was unintentional.

23.2 A historical perspective of doping and anti-doping

It all began in ancient times when Greeks and Romans consumed brandy and wine as a part of their sports diet to overcome fatigue or recover from injury and enhance their energy. Later consumption of fig fruits, bufetone, mushroom, and coca leaves was observed in players' sports diets to enhance their performance (Yesalis and Bahrke, 2002). Earlier in the 19th century, certain performance-enhancing compounds were mixed and given to athletes; their performance was improved to an extreme level that they could perform in ultramarathons. Later in the 20th century, a few anabolic steroids and stimulants were identified to enhance performance. Military soldiers in the Second World War were supplied with these enhancers in their diet to improve their energy during warfare, which was later followed by some sportspersons, which was against sports ethical values (Holt et al., 2009). The first documented doping case was identified in 1904 at St. Louis, the summer Olympics. An American marathoner was recognized to consume stimulants that are strychnine, brandy, and some egg-white before the marathon (Kremenik et al., 2006).

The term doping originated from the word "dop," which implies stimulants in Africa's local language. It is also claimed that it originated from an American expression, "dope," slang of opium, as opium was the first well-known stimulant used to enhance horse performance in sports (Holt et al., 2009). Until 1900, Federation Internationale de Football Association (FIFA) thought doping was found outside of football. In contrast, the International Amateur Athletic Foundation (IAAF) considers it one of the major concerns of every athlete's significant problems. These two federations led to the establishment of a new organization, WADA, by the International Olympic Committee (IOC). According to WADA, the international level's mission is to monitor, promote, delegate, and commission work in different countries to regional and national anti-doping organizations (RADOs and NADOs) and mandate them to work with the World Anti-Doping Code (Wagner, 2011).

In parallel to governmental and sports authority activities, Anti-Doping Commission in 1966 started drug testing, facilitated enlightenment through campaigns against doping, stimulated the International Federations to remit doping rules, and restricted positive athletes from participating in Olympic Games. Consequently, the first doping test initiative in the early 1960s, the development of anti-doping rules, was made by the Union Cycliste Internationale (UCI) in the same period, which was also broadly revised by the IOC and currently by the WADA mission code. These rules have a stringent penalties and include numerous approved and non-approved drug substances and prohibited methods (Committee, 1999).

Unfortunately, that time in the early 1960s, the analytical testing method was not sensitive enough to identify and quantify the lower-level limit of a banned substance in a positive sample, and at the same time, a medical committee of the IOC foundation established in 1967 faced challenges in doping control testing of samples with detailed measurement of the banned substance. Furthermore, doping tests were integrated into the Olympic rules for the first time in the following same year when the IOC published the first list of prohibited substances for doping classes, including stimulants, narcotics, antidepressant drugs, and tranquilizers, and sanctions were also described for the usage of banned substances (Thieme and Hemmersbach, 2009).

WADA is working as an independent agency entrusted with harmonizing the anti-doping program. To promote and educate awareness on doping, the Ministry of sports governing bodies in each country have endorsed WADA and its programs coordinating with United Nations Education Science and Cultural Organization (UNESCO). This program consisted of mainly five documents, for instance, the WADA Code, the Standard International Testing, the International Standard for accredited Laboratories, the International Standard for Therapeutic Use Exemptions form, and substance and method prohibited at all times (In and Out-competitions). This approach was uniform for the international federations and national anti-doping agencies for applying anti-doping rules and codes to implement effectively. To maintain the international standards for laboratories, a testing system was established for the expectations of quality criteria and competence among laboratories across the countries recognized by WADA inspection, including accreditation under ISO/IEC 17025.

Currently, many sports organizations like IOC, International Federations (IFs), and National Federation are also taking active participation in to fight against doping in sports using banned exercise-enhancing drugs and have stringent rules and penalties for people who are caught using them during and out of competitions (Kamber, 2011).

23.3 Intended and un-intended doping practices

The sudden growth in business for dietary supplements available through the clandestine market led to the question of the quality of manufacturing practice. Doping can be intentional or unintentional. Unintentional doping can happen by using a nutritional supplement that is not precisely labeled with ingredients in supplements and cross-contamination of illegal, banned substances, which may cause positive dope tests in and out of competition in sports (Chan et al., 2016). This is due to the lack of stringent quality policy of the Dietary Supplement and Health Education Act. On the other hand, the quality of dietary supplements is usually not inspected by regulatory agencies in most countries, and traveling athletes may also buy the supplements unavailable in their home countries. Moreover, the internet selling "shoddy source," i.e., clandestine market, made these products available freely by the open-source to grab sports persons' attention for using these supplements, effectively deviating most of the country quality controls policy (Baron et al., 2007).

In some circumstances, the athlete may assume that protein or nutrition supplements will help recover from injury during training or reduce illness or infection. In this context, some athletes commonly may be guilty of deliberate cheating or unintentional ingestion of prohibited substances in noncertified protein supplements. Some cases may show unintended doping. In maximum cases of unintentional doping, test results have demonstrated a lack of sound knowledge, particularly from the intake of newly available supplement products, which might have a chance of unknown substances considered in S_0 (nonapproved substance prohibited list). It is indeed a fact that nonlabeled ingredients may contain banned substances. For instance, MaHuang herbal products/extracts contain the chemical ephedrine, which comes under the prohibited list's S_6 stimulant category. Several examples of headlines in newspapers and sports magazines reported a positive doping case. Some sportspersons feel cheated by failing the dope test due to the regular use of supplements that out numbered as fraudulently uncertified products by manufacturer default (Martínez-Sanz et al., 2017).

Intentional doping is significantly observed in sports by many athletes fascinated by an advertisement of online products to improve their stamina, physical exercise, and endurance. They believe a regular diet will not affect their exercise tolerance to gain cut and throat competition. It could not be possible to improve their performance for consistent results. Moreover, the pressure is also often enforced on athletes exposed to the intake of supplements in critical situations without evaluating the potential benefits and pushing themselves to the risks associated with deliberately taking hidden banned substances (Martínez-Sanz et al., 2017).

Dascombe et al. surveyed a few athletes to check the nutritional supplements in their daily diet. It was found that among 72 athletes tested, 63 were using at least one dietary supplement in their day-to-day life (Dascombe et al., 2010). It is not always that every dietary supplement contains prohibited substances. Some nutritional supplements are to supply the proper intake of daily vitamins and proteins to the body. But due to the increased interest in sports people and increased sponsors, sports have become more of a business than an ethical game. To maintain consistency in performance, some athletes deliberately may consume the supplements even after knowing about the prohibited contents in the product, thinking in a way that it would not be detected or will not remain in their system and washes out from the body by the time of doping test (Vlad et al., 2018).

Furthermore, social cultures and physical demands with fitness tests in different sports may encourage varying nutritional supplement levels. To achieve good results in their performance, they consume dietary supplements keeping their health and career at risk without confirmation and authenticity of nutritional supplements. Several intended or unintended doping incidents in a different way may influence youth and junior athletes regarding the prevalent use of dietary supplements (Mangan and Dyreson, 2013).

Contrary to intended and unintended doping cases of nutritional supplements, high-profile athletes usually justify their comments for default of manufacturing practice regarding the unlabeled or hidden substance. As advised by coaches, friends, or fast recovery from injury, etc., are commonly given reasons during the doping control panel hearing time. But the purpose of nutrition supplements, if recommended, is to compensate for athletic injury, promoting health benefits suffering from a deficiency of essential nutrients in the body (Martínez-Sanz et al., 2017).

23.4 Nutritional supplements as a source of positive doping

The nutrition supplements could be categorized into classes according to their intended use and target functions. In US Congress, according to Dietary Supplements Health and Education Act (DSHEA), dietary supplements are defined as a product that contains one or more dietary ingredients, including a vitamin, a mineral, a herb or other botanical, an amino acid, a dietary substance for use to supplement the diet by increasing the total dietary intake, or a concentrate, metabolite, constituent, extract, or combination of any of the ingredients mentioned above (Health, 1994).

However, it is challenging to generalize the range of dietary supplements used by athletes because of the high risks of contamination of hidden substances, which are promoted based on enhancing exercise and intense performance benefits. Food supplements are not considered medication and are not subject to regulatory and quality controls in the manufacturing process. Thus, they increase the probability of contamination with undeclared substances prohibited in the sport at all times.

Due to the hidden or unlabeled prohibited substances, the risk factors for health increase. Anabolic supplements are recommended to be trained harder, enhance exercise performance, and achieve a competitive edge for the well-trained elite and recreational athletes suffering from a deficiency of essential nutrients in the body (Maughan et al., 2007). If they are deemed mandatory, athletes should avoid buying products labeled in foreign languages, purchased through third parties, or over shoddy sources without knowing their origin and level of confidence, increasing the chances of buying "contaminated" supplements. It is important to notice for an athlete that till now, no supplement industry could give a hundred percent assurance that its products are entirely free from contaminants. Even product quality tests have gone through standardized testing laboratories to confirm the 100% purity test of products (Baume et al., 2006).

23.4.1 Nutritional supplements for enhancing physical performance

Dietary supplements consist of biologically active substances such as amino acids, vitamins, minerals, enzymes, and many other substances like omega fatty acids derived from plant or animal origin and various ergogenic compounds. An athlete must know these labeled substances present in dietary supplements like Ma Huang or contaminated with prohormones (natural anabolic androgenic steroids), which are not precisely declared on the ingredient label list supplements. The summary of these ingredients in different kinds of nutritional supplements with the intended use and function is given in Table 23.1 (Maughan, 2002).

Protein supplements composed of different amino acids (essential or nonessential) are often recommended to athletes in some circumstances to increase muscle mass and nitrogen

TABLE 23.1 Labeled ingredients in marketed nutritional supplements.

Labeled ingredients	Intended use (function)	Ref.
Essential amino acids, protein hydrolysate; protein powder; β-hydroxy β-methyl butyric acid (HMB), individual amino acids like glutamine, BCAA; leucine, lysine, arginine, and ornithine	Muscle growth and repair	Rathmacher et al. (2017), Beelen et al. (2008), Fild (1991)
Caffeine, carnitine pyruvate; MaHuang	Fat reduction	Saper et al. (2004)
Carbohydrates, caffeine, bicarbonate, creatine	Exercise metabolism	Romijn et al. (1993), Söderlund et al. (1994)
Protein, carbohydrate bars, whole protein powders, protein isolates, and hydrolysate; ginseng	Promoting recovery	Mech (2013)
Glucosamine; chondroitin sulfate	Joint health	Kelly (1998)
Vitamins; minerals; evening primrose oil	General health	Belay et al. (1993)
Echinacea; zinc; glutamine; lycopene; pycnogenol, antioxidants	Immune function	Hicks (2012)
Taurine; caffeine; guarana	CNS stimulation	Pennay et al. (2011)
Sports bars, carbohydrate gels, fluid, and electrolytes, sports drinks	Meal/ replacement liquid meals	Sarkar (2010)

retention, decrease protein catabolism during prolonged exercise, and synthesize muscle glycogen. It also improves hemoglobin synthesis, myoglobin, oxidative enzymes, and mitochondrial oxidative capacity during aerobic exercise. Thus, dietary supplements' significance depends on a mixture of 20 essential amino acids to induce ergogenic potential and enhance exercise endurance activity to promote physically weak individual candidates in elite sports (Maughan, 2005; Williams, 2005). These essential and nonessential amino acids indirectly have an impact on the body. They are preferably used for the secretion of anabolic hormones for performance enhancement, modifying fuel during intense exercise, preventing adverse effects of overtraining, and preventing mental fatigue (Eslami et al., 2009; Pipe and Ayotte, 2002).

Apart from amino acids, many-body elements which are known to play a crucial role, such as iron, magnesium, bicarbonate, caffeine, carnitine, creatine, pyruvate, hornet juice, guarana ribose, etc., are the ingredients formulated in protein supplements. This wide variety of supplements offers a choice for athlete body requirements and claims to improve exercise performance by boosting up intense energy supply to the body, contributing potential benefits in some critical situations, and synergistic effects like reducing mental fatigue. A detailed summary of different amino acids in supplements, their use, and their side effects on the body is given in Table 23.2. The most acceptable way to select supplements is to have additional benefits over a balanced diet. Still, athletes must be aware of the allowed legal use of dietary supplements, which, if overlooked, may result in individuals at risk, as well as may be disqualified from competitions.

23.4.2 Potential health issues and side effects of consuming banned substances present in the nutritional supplements

Potential health issues related to dietary supplements are significant problems concerning the product's efficacy and safety, as DHEA has no control and stringent rules for manufacturing practice and quality compliance certification. This is the main drawback of dietary supplements freely available in the market. This creates confusion for sportspersons whether they can be taken or not, and if accepted, what the risk factors may be associated (Duiven and de Hon, 2018).

Furthermore, these adulterated products containing banned or illegal substances are frequently available in the market without knowledge of ingredients interaction or counteraction, which might cause a higher risk of heath. This freedom of manufacturing company and distribution throughout the world made it easy access for athletes to use them even though they are not aware and educated about the severe side effects and toxic compounds that accumulate in the body, which may spoil their professional career for an extended period (Corrigan and Kazlauskas, 2003). These hidden/banned drug substances might subsequently cause potential adverse outcomes, such as renal failure, increased blood pressure, psychiatric symptoms, cardiovascular disease, aggression, and even death (Greydanus and Patel, 2002). A summary of a nonlabeled substance contaminated or adulterated or banned drugs in nutrition supplements available in the market may have a potential health issue and side effects given in Table 23.3.

TABLE 23.2 Amino acids in the nutritional supplements and their reported health risk.

Amino acid	Use and effect on the body	Health risk and side effects	Ref.
Tryptophan	Increase serotonin production to high tolerance to pain during intensive exercise.	Influences the brain's serotonin levels	Fernstrom and Wurtman (1971)
Branched-chain amino acids (BCAA)	Reduce central nervous system fatigue and boost exercise performance in prolonged aerobic endurance events by increasing the BCAA: fTRYP ratio and mitigating serotonin synthesis.	Decrease levels of the neurotransmitters	Blomstrand (2006)
Glutamine	Energy fuel for the immune system, such as macrophages and lymphocyte cells, may be decreased during prolonged exercise related to overtraining.	Decrease intestinal permeability	Newsholme and Calder (1997)
Aspartates (K and Mg)	Acts as an ergogenic substance that possibly enhances fatty acid metabolism and muscle glycogen utilization by mitigating ammonia accumulation during exercise.	Epileptic seizures and declined vision	Williams (1995)
Arginine	A potent endogenous vasodilator is used as a substrate for nitric oxide (NO) synthesis to help blood flow and endurance capacity.	Gastrointestinal discomfort	Maiorana et al. (2003)
Ornithine, lysine, and arginine	To increase human growth hormone (HGH) production and increase lean muscle mass and muscle strength.	Bloating, abdominal pain, diarrhea, and gout	Fild (1991)
Tyrosine	Precursor for the synthesis of catecholamine hormones and neurotransmitters, mainly epinephrine, norepinephrine, and dopamine.	Optimal physical performance	Lehnert and Wurtman (1993)
Taurine	Influence cardiac parameters like increased stroke volume, heart contraction during recovery after exercise, and several metabolic processes such as antioxidant activity.	Bipolar disorder and DNA damage	Butler et al. (2017)

A survey report showed that athletes might take without following a systemic way by using them to gain any short-term benefits by taking a high dose that increases the tolerance to extend a more intense training schedule. These supplements show positive and negative side effects, as shown in Fig. 23.2 (Ronis et al., 2018; Maughan, 2005). Nevertheless, most of the supplement's biomedical side effects or interactions and flexibility in regulatory authority that demands essential scientific human studies under standardized conditions before the product is available for public use are deficient. Thus, according to the WADA code, if any prohibited substances or method which is potentially harmful to the health of athletes or capable of enhancing their performance is found in the body at the time of testing, then the athlete is responsible or liable to penalties regardless of their intentional or unintentional intake of supplements (Maughan, 2005).

TABLE 23.3 Potential health issues and side effects of consuming banned substances present in the nutritional supplements.

Banned substances in nutritional supplements	Reported health issues and side effects	Ref.
Ephedrine (Herbal Ma Huang and Guarana)	Hypertension, stroke, memory loss, palpitation, and anxiety	Dhar et al. (2005)
Anabolic-androgenic steroids	**Cardiovascular:** Hypertrophy of heart muscle, lipid metabolism negative changes in the body. **Endocrine (MAN):** Reduce spermatogenesis, impotence, testicular shrinkage **(Women):** Abnormality in menstrual cycles, masculinization, and virilization. **Skeletal:** Premature closure of the growth of long bones and enhanced tendon ruptures.	Saartok et al. (1984), Karila et al. (2004), Luke et al. (1990)
Narcotics	Euphoria, feeling of invincibility, increased pain threshold, and overdose lead to respiratory depression and death.	Emran et al. (2014)
Stimulants	Reduced fatigue, aggressiveness, anxiety, insomnia, alterations in hemodynamics (increased heart rate and blood pressure), increased risk of stroke, heart attack, and sudden death.	Avois et al. (2006)
β-2-Agonists	Increased muscle mass while decreasing body fat, nausea, nervousness, increased heart rate, blood pressure, headache, and tremor	Clarkson and Thompson (1997)

23.5 Anti-doping organizations for nutritional supplement alert

The WADA anti-Doping code in the practice of doping is to be condemned utterly; any person accepting or offering to supply prohibited substances is strictly prohibited from entering any sports federation to play at the national or international level or Olympic games. According to WADA code 1999, the use of any prohibited substance by an athlete which is harmful to health or capable of increasing their exercise endurance or the presence of a banned substance in the athlete's body indicates the obvious reckless sign of the use of these substances among WADA prohibited substance (Maughan et al., 2007). The WADA code's main objective deals with detecting and preventing doping in athletes and has established a strict principal liability policy that applies to even unintentional doping risk of the athlete and is solely responsible for any substance found in their body irrespective of how it got there. The athlete is, therefore, technically guilty (WADA, 2009).

Different countries' national anti-doping organizations (NADOs) like USADA, ASADA, and NADA INDIA are formed to implement the WADA code. They provide monthly and quarterly updates, alerts, and warnings on the webpage about using food supplements/products with the synthetic compound that may lead to a positive test for various stimulants, anabolic agents, etc., prohibited at all times. Besides these official sites of doping control

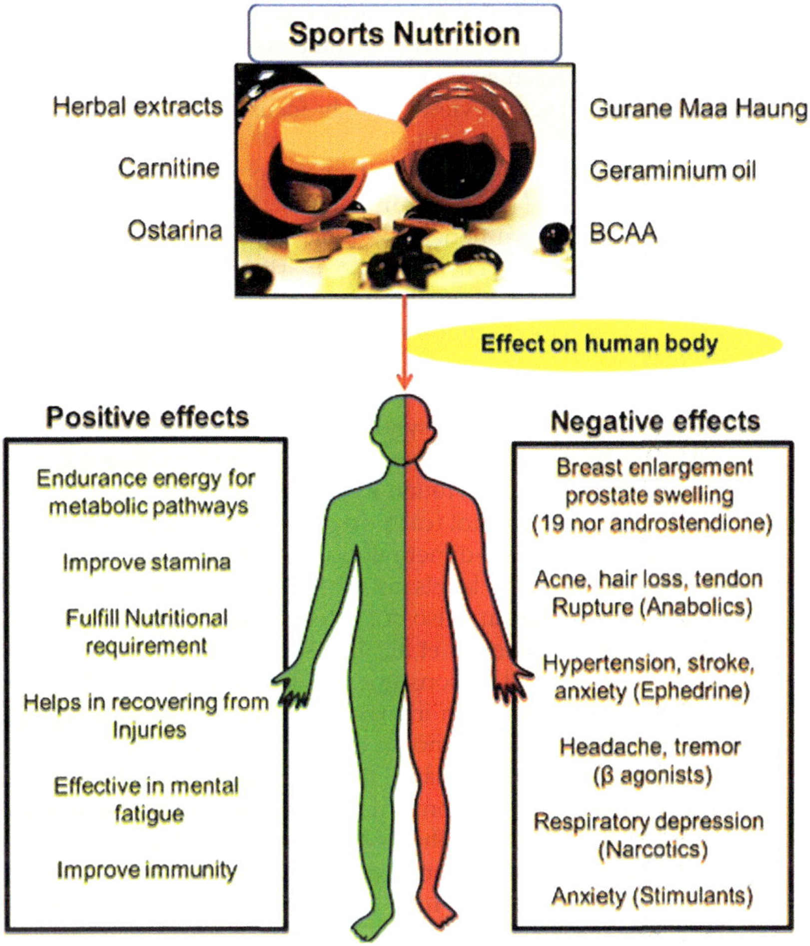

FIGURE 23.2 Different positive and negative effects of using nutritional supplements.

authorities, other means to check the safety of ergo nutritional supplements unofficially and without being endorsed by the WADA or the respective country's NADO to confirm whether the most commonly prescribed and over-the-counter medicines are prohibited are also available (Houlihan, 2002).

Adverse analytical finding reports addressed by different doping control organization, as well as WADA annual report, shows that most of the athlete caught positive for doping are due to the use of protein powders and nutritional supplements that include anabolic steroids (prohormones), stimulants, antidepressants, diuretics and laxatives, appetite suppressors in weight loss, phosphodiesterase type-5 enzyme (PDE-5) inhibitors contaminated in food/or in sexual performance enhancement supplements, except for PDE-5 inhibitor category hidden substances are not yet enlisted in WADA prohibited list (Tokish et al., 2004).

Moreover, suppose anyone can freely manufacture supplements without proper knowledge or training. In that case, it can be indicated that manufacturers may not be aware of the ingredients in the formula. Even some may try to make components appear natural by using herbal medicine names. These reviews mainly focus on the valid point to be kept in mind by sports persons when they encounter a label as "all-natural." Hence, "all-natural" does not always contain naturally derived substances. Some companies may intentionally mislead consumers by the label of contents. In contrast, these ingredients reality is found as some adulterant or counterfeit components in their supplements.

For instance, some herbal supplement company marketed their products as All-natural Weight loss pills, but these products in quality tests confirmed the presence of sibutramine, a prohibited substance (S_6 specified stimulant) among WADA prohibited list (Kim et al., 2010; Koehler et al., 2007).

Similarly, other companies may market herbal sex-enhancement pills, but when tested, these pills frequently contain powerful and synthetic Viagra-like drugs like sildenafil, Flibanserin, etc. (Campbell et al., 2013). Numerous supplement samples enlisted in the ingredients as "geranium oil" on the label, but it was found in quality tests as methylhexanamine. A synthetically produced substance, a stimulant (categorized in S_6 stimulant) prohibited was found in 1, 3-dimethyylamylamine, and 1, 3-dimethylbutylamine (or DMBA) as an active ingredient, is often listed on supplement labels as AMP Citrate. Similar chemical names N, alpha-diethyl-benzene ethane amine, are also not listed on the supplement's ingredient label, which links to methamphetamine (Cohen et al., 2018).

Thus, the athletes are advised not to consume any herbal supplement assuming it to be completely natural. For example, as given in article 4.2.2 of the world anti-doping code for specified stimulants, Citrus aurantium, known as orange peel or bitter orange, produces the prohibited substance octopamine. Similarly, the ephedra plant has been banned as it produces ephedrine and pseudoephedrine; Cannabis sativa produces prohibited tetrahydrocannabinol, and Tinospora crops produce prohibited higenamine (β2-agonist) (Klaschka, 2015). Few examples of manufacturers that have marketed seemingly low-risk supplements, herbal products, vitamins, and electrolytes that may contain dangerous and prohibited anabolic agents and warnings risks of athletes are presented in Table 23.4. Moreover, an athlete must be alert about other general words highlighted in bold letters or given the label content of products "To be safe for use." Therefore, it becomes necessary for an athlete to be responsible and alert to exercise caution, avoid mistakes, and identify the risks associated with supplement use.

If detected in an athlete sample, these substances tested positive in any quantity subject to threshold limits except higenamine and octopamine like ephedrine, methyl ephedrine, and pseudoephedrine. These substances, in combination with a diuretic or masking agent, will be considered as an adverse analytical finding (AAF) unless the athlete has an approved therapeutic use exemption (TUE) concerning that substance (Sjöqvist et al., 2008). Although an athlete desires to take natural herbal products, they must consult a nutrition specialist to understand what compounds are produced by the plant and their potential interactions. Hence, it must be explicit that athletes think that taking herbal supplements naturally contains compounds that could interact with each other or with medications (Millman and Ross, 2003).

According to FDA views, many safe and healthy supplement ingredients are not naturally derived or harvested. For example, the FDA allows some nutrients to be synthesized in a

TABLE 23.4 Inadvertent doping (intentional/unintentional consumption) of herbal nutritional supplements.

Labeled claim of herbal nutritional supplements	Nonlabeled contents on the label	Prohibited doping list category	Reported health issues and adverse effects	Ref.
Weight loss pill	Sibutramine	Specified Stimulant(S_6)	Dry mouth, constipation	Lean (1997)
Geranium oil	Methylhexanamine (1,3-dimethylamyl amine, dimethyl amyl amine, and 1,3-dimethyl butyl amine or DMBA)	Specified stimulant (S_6)	Increase heart pressure	Archer et al. (2015)
Cannabis sativa plant	THC	Cannabinoids (S_8)	Decreased concentration levels, reduced short-term memory	Makela et al. (2006)
Ephedra plant	Ephedrine (greater than 10 micrograms per milliliter) and pseudoephedrine (greater than 15 μg per milliliter)	Specified stimulant (S6)	Hypertension, stroke, memory loss and palpitation, and anxiety	Dhar et al. (2005)
Citrus aurantium (orange peel or bitter orange)	Octopamine (β,4-dihydroxyphenethylamine)	Specified stimulant (S_6)	CNS effects, epigastric difficulty in micturition with urinary retention	Singh et al. (2012)
Tinosporacripsa (Nandina domestica, Demethyl-Coclaurine, norcoclaurine, Tinospora crispa, Aconitum japonicum, Gnetum)	Higenamine (OxyShred, Alpha T2, PES Amphamine advanced)	β_2 agonist (S_3)	Tachycardia, palpitations, and hypertension	Zhang et al. (2017)
Ostarine, MK-2866, enobasarm,(2S)-3-(4-cyano phenoxy)-N-[4-cyano-3 (trifluoro methyl) phenyl]-2-hydroxy-2 methyl propan amide	Selective androgen receptor modulator (SARM) GTx-024	Other anabolic agents (S_1)	Kidney and liver dysfunction	Zilbermint and Dobs (2009)
Anorexic agents	Phentermine and fenfluramine	Nonspecified stimulant (S_6)	Stimulant effect on CNS	Connolly et al. (1997)
Branched amino acid hydroxymethyl butyrate	19-Norandrostenedione	Anabolic-androgenic steroids (S_1)	Gynecomastia and prostate swelling	Kamber et al. (2001)
Guarana supplement	Androstenedione, norandrostenedione	Anabolic-androgenic steroids (S_1)	Gynecomastia and prostate swelling	Brown et al. (2006)
Iron tablet	19- Norandrostenedione (prohormones)	Anabolic-androgenic steroids (S_1)	Acne, hair loss, breast tissue enlargement (gynecomastia) in men, and prostate swelling in men	Yau et al. (2013)

factory and sold in supplements, such as vitamin C. This means that athletes/coaches/accredited sports nutritional dieticians should not put too much stake in something being "natural" or think it is inherently better just because it's natural (de Hon and Coumans, 2007). FDA highlighted tainted supplements containing hazardous and unlabeled ingredients given with product name and product category of supplements are shown in Table 23.5. Some supplements are marketed as "for treatment or arrhythmia" or "heart stabilizing" or some similar words are most likely to contaminate with beta-blockers which are prohibited in following particular sports such as archery, shooting, billiards (all disciplines), skiing/snowboarding in ski jumping, freestyle, automobile, golf, and snowboard halfpipe/big air.

23.6 Nutritional supplements contaminated with illegal and botanical substances under WADA prohibited list

In 2003, the IOC Nutrition Working Group advised athletes to be careful against the indiscriminate use of dietary supplements that provide essential nutrients, which may help when food intake or food choices are restricted. Still, achieving adequate nutrient intake is usually only a short-term option. Many supplements are available in the market, but data ensure products' safety for use, and dope-free certification is unavailable (Burke, 2003). Recently, the definition of doping has been modified according to WADA's updated list. For many years, its meaning may be pharmacologically understood as attempts to enhance

TABLE 23.5 FDA highlighted tainted nutritional supplements containing hazardous and unlabeled ingredients.

Product name	Hidden ingredients unlabeled ingredients	Product category
Black Gold X Advanced	Sibutramine	Weight loss
3rd Degree	Sibutramine	Weight loss
Black Label X	Sildenafil	Sexual enhancement
Libimax Nature and Health Co.	Tadalafil	Sexual enhancement
JianbuHuqian Wan	Dexamethasone, chlorpheniramine, furosemide	N/A
Slim Xtreme Herbal	Sibutramine	Weight loss
Asihuri Plus Forte	Dexamethasone, pphenylbutazone	N/A
Que She	Fenfluramine; propranolol; sibutramine; ephedrine	Weight loss
1, 4AD, M1, 4AD and 3-AD	Steroid	Muscle building
Testra-Flex Novedex XT	Steroid	Muscle building
Halodrol liquid gels	Steroid	Muscle building

Source: Data obtained from www.accessdata.fda.gov.

performance (mainly strength and endurance) in sport by illegal marketing and ingestion of supplements, regardless of its motivation (e.g., unbounded expectations, collective chauvinism, or substantial financial interest), which led to the increase in doping phenomenon for many years (Jones, 2014). However, a new sample contaminated with nutritional supplements is rarely accepted to reduce a sanction. The result of the particular competition is permanently nullified with 2–4 years of suspension as a penalty. It has become a scrupulous division between nutritional supplements and banned drug substances that could potentially produce positive results and be dangerous to the athlete (Atienza-Macías, 2015).

23.6.1 Cross-contamination of nutritional supplements with illegal, banned adulterated substances

Intake of nutritional supplements to become challenging, and moving to higher levels of competition by adopting all possible ways to cut-throat competition throughout the world has become a trend in sports. In literature, a sports journal, papers, and survey reports state that cannabinoids (marijuana, hashish, cocaine) and other social/psychotic drug consumption have increased. The prohibited substance business is flourishing, which has become a problem not only in society but in sports. Survey reports of sports institutes and nutritional expert comments that millions of men and women are currently using potent, nonapproved, and prohibited substances widely sold over the counter as supplements are adulterated.

There are certain potential health risks of dietary supplements adulterated by the illegal adulteration of supplements, despite knowing the prevalence of common adverse effects. Such substances are more commonly used in high-elite sports like weight and powerlifting (Tokish et al., 2004). However, using these substances knowingly or unknowingly affects their long-term health with various side effects and possibly abuse or dependence (Van der Merwe and Grobbelaar, 2004). Many athletes usually are more prone to admit to either striking their spouse or using illicit drugs (e.g., cocaine or marijuana) than they would admit to doping. Therefore, when assessing the incidence and prevalence of doping, the data's accuracy must be thoroughly scrutinized (Yager and O'Dea, 2014).

Several authors (Geyer and others, 2004; Pipe and Ayotte, 2002; Maughan, 2005; van der Merwe and Grobbelaar, 2005) in their work have reported adulteration of dietary supplements with unlawful substances, which gives a detailed explanation of substances that may lead to a positive anti-doping test (Geyer et al., 2004; Pipe and Ayotte, 2002; Van der Merwe and Grobbelaar, 2005). Over the past years, unscrupulous manufacturing practices adulterating illegal substances in supplements have happened to get fraudulent profit without proper labeling ingredients to deceive consumers and attempt to conceal their acceptance from regulators, which may impose potential threats to doping consequences in sports (Temple, 2012).

Also, the flexibility in norms for Dietary Supplements and Health Education Act relaxed in manufacturing practice for any manufacturer of supplements to maintain expected quality standards and approval of products license. As cross-contamination of nutritional supplements has been identified, various prohormones and androgenic steroids, androstenedione and dehydroepiandrosterone, testosterone, and nandrolone, ephedrine freely available over the counter without a prescription for a young athlete (Martínez-Sanz et al., 2017).

Certain products are advertised as "no hormonal" supplements and promoted in the market. When tested for quality, certain products show 19-nor steroids containing steroids or precursor products (like creatine, vitamin complex, various minerals, carnitine, Tribulus terrestris, chrysin, and herbal extracts). This malfunction is being practiced in different countries to attract sports personnel to maximize enhanced performance (Parr et al., 2007). Moreover, few contaminated supplements have shown harmful impurities like lead, zinc, arsenic, broken glass, animal feces, etc. These impurities produce an array of toxic substances in the body that potentially harm human health (Raman et al., 2004; Korfali et al., 2013).

A recently published article reported that certain energy drinks contain taurine and caffeine that resemble those without them in the market. They attribute to ergogenic effects favorably influencing the cardiac parameters, i.e., increased stroke volume during recovery after exercise. Another potential source of inadvertent doping is guarana drinks in the European market. Surprisingly deliberately added caffeine could lead to a positive dope test (Salinero et al., 2014). Similarly, so many foods/herbal products are available that contain guarana, carnitine, choline, cayenne powder, vitamin B_6, and other substances described as 'plus much more, which are initially contaminated with androstenedione and nor-androstenedione (approximately 6.3 mg/gm) (Corrigan and Kazlauskas, 2003).

However, analogs of illegal or trafficking substances that are not enrolled on the prohibited list but are undergoing clinical trials and pharmacological studies and not yet reported might have a chance to misuse counterfeit drugs as the questionable quality of supplements. Hence, every year, WADA regularly updates the prohibited list of drug substances and adapts changes in the practical use of doping substances in sports (Kazlauskas, 2008).

23.6.2 Herbal food supplements as a source of positive doping

Many botanical ingredients and herbal extracts are often promoted in the market with several names like hormone regulation, weight loss/burning fat, metabolite activating agents, increasing energy levels, and muscle strengthening. Several commercial products like "SportPharm" and "AdvoCare" containing various herbals, like thermadrene, MaHuang, Guarana, Caffeine, Purple Willow Bark, Cayenne pepper, and ginger root, increase mental vigilance, increase fat-burning metabolism, and improves muscle performance (Williams, 2006). Detailed information on the effects of these herbal constituents is shown in Fig. 23.3 (Sellami et al., 2018).

Furthermore, the proportion of all botanical supplements with a finding result of ephedrine and its analog (pseudoephedrine, methyl ephedrine), methylenedioxy methamphetamine, or β-methyl phenethylamine, methylhexanamine (geranium oil), higenamine (norcoclaurine), and formation of different anabolic steroids as a stimulant in low or above the threshold limit of a prohibited substance is identified (Mathews, 2018). However, information on the most used botanical supplement screening is still limited, and scientific data reports have been entirely lacking regarding severe toxicity. In contrast, other evidence related to information from studies of isolated tissues exposed to physiological amounts of supplements is unknown for the substance's safety and efficacy.

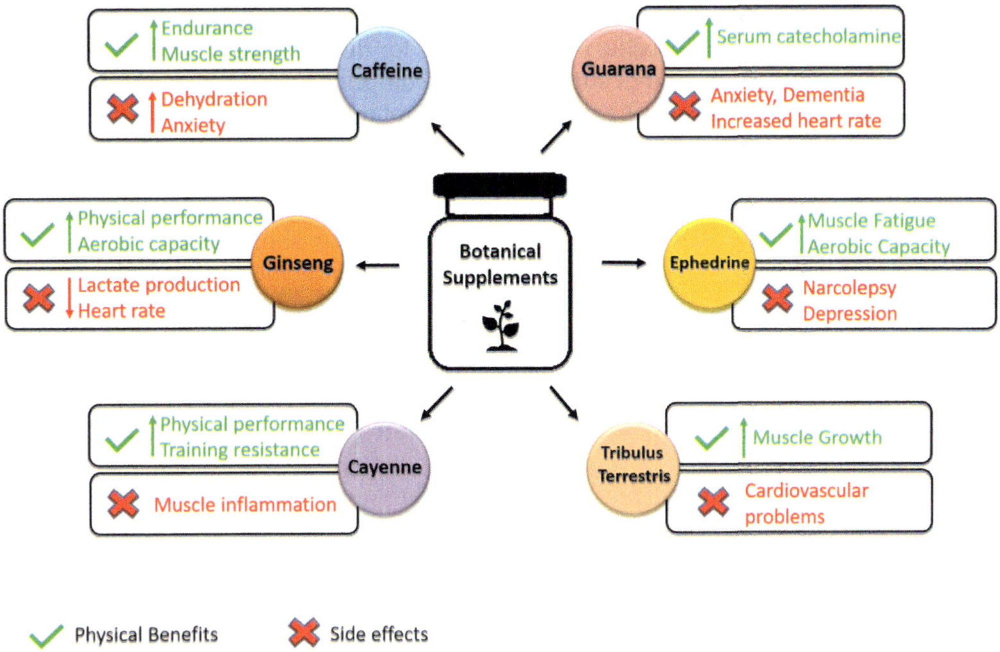

FIGURE 23.3 Description of prohibited substances found in herbal supplements with their physical benefits and side effects.

23.7 Nutritional supplementation habits of elite athletes

According to the IOC consensus statement on sports nutrition, the natural supplement habit of an elite athlete is not just to compensate for the requirement of low food and inadequate diet but also to contemplate the prevalent use of supplements in terms of their safety, efficacy, cost, and the potential issue for a positive doping test (Burke, 2003). Nowadays, sports competitions at different levels of games will become tough and move to higher levels. Each athlete wants to reach the top position, explore themselves to stay at higher positions, and then adopt all possible means of securing fruitful professional careers. Many potential factors affect the use of supplements: rewards for victory, strength, publicity, quick recovery from injury, more challenging training, and lack of knowledge concerning unlabeled banned substance risk.

A relatively low-quality assessment of an athlete's diet is not enough to meet their fitness goals and compete in the games. In such cases, supplements must be taken under the supervision of an accredited sports dietitian or qualified sports nutritionist for the daily routine of practice to stay healthy and fit. Nutritional experts and coaches can advise the athlete to regularly use multivitamins and mineral supplements when the body is restricted to reduce body fat or to prevent weight gain, to meet nutrition requirements (Dunn et al., 2007).

Some athletes are very scrupulous with their body image and feel low compared to others and believe that taking supplements will improve their body appearance and physical performance. These marketed products may be essential in fulfilling the desired physical constitution and maintaining specific restrictive diets for their stamina and exercise tolerance capacity (Williams, 2005). Although supplement consumption prevalence varies with gender, educational background, dietary habits, training adaptation, and competition level among the athlete, it was evident that higher proportions of supplementation occur in the high-profile elite athlete (Maughan et al., 2004).

In a national survey report on US college athletes, the proportion of different ingredients in supplements consumed was found to be energy drinks and shots (28.6%), protein amino products (41.7%), amino acids (12.1%), multivitamins with caffeine (5.7%), and minor quantities of beta-hydroxy-beta-methyl butyrate (HMB; 0.2%), dehydroepiandrosterone (DHEA; 0.1%), and an unspecified mixture of "testosterone boosters" (1.6%). So, nutritional experts' role has become necessary to alert about supplements, especially those that may have fascinated advertisements to enhance intense performance (Green et al., 2001).

Currently, the complexity of the manufacturer quality of supplements/herbal products is also a serious concern. To solve this problem, each country's sports authority must appoint qualified and experienced nutritional professionals for young athletes' counseling and guidance to consume supplements in the proper systemic way (de Hon and Coumans, 2007). Consequently, doping prevention education programs should be conducted to supplement risk levels. They must articulate directions, coordinate with sports institute centers, and communicate between doping agencies and other countries to protect athletes. The athlete cannot discriminate between scientific evidence reports and supplement suppliers' effective advertising policy due to a lack of scientific communication. As a result, this novel idea of educating the athlete helps protect against potential health issues and positive testing (Wippert and Fließer, 2016).

23.8 Recent inadvertent doping cases from nutritional supplements

When an athlete's official testing was initiated by the doping control authority worldwide, plenty of doping cases were reported in newspapers and magazines between the 19th and half of the 20th century. From a published literature on positive doping cases in media in the recent times, most of the athlete samples found in adverse analytical findings as positive results were using supplements somewhere contaminated/adulterant with banned substance procured through shoddy sources via clandestine market illegal trafficking of the drugs (Committee, 1999).

A national survey report highlighted that the following intense performance enhancement products' proportional ratio was high among men than women, except for unlikely energy drinks and shots. The maximum cases are observed among the affirmative situation in sports with a higher percentage of using performance enhancers in hockey, wrestling, powerlifting, and baseball among the men, whereas swimming, ice hockey, and volleyball among the women (Green et al., 2001).

Therefore, it has become a controversial issue for the intake of supplements whether and whose company-certified supplements must be used to reduce the risk associated with using them. Many journal articles, newspaper blogs, and magazines report positive doping due to the consumption of hidden substances like steroid precursors (androstenedione, Nandrolone, methadone), methylhexanamine stimulant phentermine, and sibutramine, fenfluramine in natural products for weight loss as well as anorexic agents. Surprisingly, Athletes claim that during the hearing, to justify their statements against violation of doping rules, they had never used a banned substance and unknown to the misleading inferior labeling ingredient in allowable supplements (Mazzoni et al., 2011).

In the 2008 summer Olympics held in Beijing, an American, Jessica Hardy, deliberately took legally sold supplements. She failed the dope test as trace amounts of clenbuterol were identified in the sample after rigorous testing analysis and claimed while hearing that her sample tested positive due to the nutritional supplement, "Arginine Extreme" manufactured by AdvoCare as a health and wellness product (Wendt, 2009).

Another case of LA Shawn Merritt, who has also requested in his hearing positive dope test link to Extenz product (Gandert, 2012). In a similar doping case in Track and Field, on July 19, 2011, USA athlete Michael Rodgers of Hutto, Texas, tested positive in a urine sample for a prohibited substance methylhexanamine (dimethyl pentylamine), a stimulant. Rodgers requested a hearing and provided independent corroborating proof that his sample tested positive for using the supplement known as JACK 3D lists 1, 3-dimethylamylamine HCl on its label in front of the independent American Arbitration Association (AAA) panel. Four of the 47 currently sanctioned cases on athletes in Australia were caught in a positive sample of methylhexanamine, which belongs to a stimulant category contaminated in some pre-workout supplements.

Besides, another five sanctions were for some "fat burner" capsules that added oxilofrine drug substance. One sanction was for sibutramine, mixed in weight loss supplements used as an appetite suppressant. Several cyclists tested positive in the nutritional supplement "Diet Full" from "Twin Lab," athermogenic herbal preparation containing ephedrine. Seven professional tennis players tested positive for the nandrolone metabolite nor-androsterone attributed to the use of a nutritional supplement distributed among those players by ATP-accredited physicians. As a result, all seven athletes were acquitted of a doping offense. Similarly, stories can be attributed to a female marathon runner who used contaminated nutritional supplements and tested positive for anorexic agents (Maughan et al., 2007).

Moreover, WADA and NADO and their doping control agency promote the doping awareness education program regarding the prevalence of supplement use during the training camps. During these camps, the organizer presented case studies to demonstrate how the athletes fall into the trap leading to a consequential positive dope test.

23.9 Sociomedical aspects of doping

Social media is a multi-communication platform where a person can directly interact with the public. With the tremendous increase in social media platforms like Facebook, Instagram, YouTube, etc., sportsmen's influence on the public has also increased. In an article published by Western Carolina University, social media platform is defined as a platform that allows the individual to (i) construct their profile for direct communication with the public, (ii) the list of users with whom they share information, which socializes and creates a profile in a domain. This platform played a crucial role in seeking motivation and getting inspired to show their talent (McFarland and Ployhart, 2015).

As every source in nature comes with a pay, extensive use of social media platforms led to publicizing information related to the professional and personal life of public deities. This resulted in spreading every detail, whether positive or negative, influencing their fame (Maughan et al., 2007). This platform is even a basis for marketing the companies of their products. Even individual sports persons wear the costumes or advertise certain nutrition supplements, leading to an increased market share of that particular product as fans without proper knowledge buy those products. This also influences young athletes to use nutrition supplements to enhance performance because fans see athletes as icons for inspiration and feel proud of their country (McCrory, 2007).

By the increase in demand for nutrition supplements by a sportsperson in high-level competition, the economic growth curve of the companies increased as well as doping cases are observed continuously in all category events, that is, junior, senior-level, and even in particular unexpected sports like archery, shooting, skiing/snowboarding, billiards, golf, and automobile. Hence, an authorized agency's importance in fighting against doping increased and strengthened the WADA code to keep alive sports spirit and fair competition. Because according to WADA strict liability code, the athlete is liable for whatever is present in his/her body at the time of testing, the manufacturer's error or any excuse regarding supplement quality will not make a defense against the disqualification or suspension to participate different level of sports events (Lippi et al., 2004, 2007).

In addition to doping's social aspect, an adaptation of social drugs like cannabis, cocaine, and marijuana makes the athlete harder to bear the mental pressure to use illicit aids. Even sound and high-tech media have raised public awareness of this addiction problem of illegal drug use in the sports profession. Most sportspersons continuously seek a large variety of dietary supplements, performance-enhancing ergogenic substances, social drugs, and alcohol consumption to improve their stamina and exercise tolerance (McCrory, 2007). The country's sports authority is concerned with this serious issue and made its annual plan to take initiatives in education and awareness programs addressing "No doping," especially for youth and junior athletes (Laure et al., 2003; Kayser et al., 2007).

23.10 Quality control and testing of nutritional supplements

Nowadays, most athletes are exposed to deliberate intake of hidden substances in supplements that are banned at all times in sports, such as anabolic steroids, stimulants, and other prohibited substances like glucocorticoids, beta-2 agonist, peptides, and growth prohormones have been a controversial issue in high competition profile sports (Duclos, 2010).

To overcome this fraudulent manufacturing practice in adulterated supplement products, previously high-performance liquid chromatography (HPLC), supercritical fluid chromatography(SFC), and capillary electrophoresis were used to screen essential drugs (Sefiha and Reichman, 2017). Gas chromatography evolved to be an efficient way to analyze the banned substances even in minute concentration as time passed. Gas chromatography and mass spectrometry give efficient quantitative detail regarding the drugs that could be rarely studied.

During Athens Olympics 2004, 3617 samples were analyzed using LC-MS (ion trap). Of that, 23 prohibited drugs have been identified with more doping cases than in previous Olympics (Tsivou et al., 2006). With emerging techniques like Liquid Chromatography Quadrupole Time-Of-Flight (LC-QTOF/Orbitrap), the HRMS technique has played a vital role in restricting the limit of these banned substances and provided the best choice in terms of accurate mass determination technique to accomplish the manifest of WADA mission to control the presence of illegal adulteration and contamination of prohibited substance in dietary supplements.

23.11 Conclusion

Sports are known for their fair and clean competition, as this impacts society and country pride worldwide. But as the years passed, due to increasing competition and pressure, athlete's usage of nutrient supplements to enhance their performance without proper knowledge of risk factors has also increased. The athlete's dope control declaration form about the medicines and supplements taken within a week of the competition revealed that most cases were related to dietary supplements used for fitness and daily body requirements.

Various governing and international organizations are crucial in controlling doping in sports. These organizing bodies and WADA promote education programs, scientific research, anti-doping capacity, and investigations to harmonize the anti-doping policies worldwide. This review gives an insight into various aspects of doping, intentional or unintentional, and social aspects. A section on recent doping cases has also been highlighted where banned substances were found adulterated in various nutritional supplements, even manufactured as botanical or natural products.

Hence, as an authoritative organization, WADA has formed stringent rules and initiated various awareness programs to prevent all these malpractices. Indeed, this effective prevention program is an effective strategy to screen banned substances in nutritional supplements to improve surveillance and maintain the spirit of sport. Furthermore, screening techniques to explore the qualitative and quantitative aspects of nutritional supplements and knowledge about those prohibited substances identified smoothens the sports and the sportsmen's spirit.

23.12 Abbreviations

ASADA Australian sports anti-doping authority
DSHEA Dietary supplements health, and education act
FDA Food and drug administration
FIFA Federation internationale de football association
IAAF International association of athletics federations
IEC International elector-technical commission
IF'S Internal federations
IOC International operational committee
ISO International organization for standardization
NADA National anti-doping agency
NADO National anti-doping organization

PDE-5 Phosphodiesterase type-5 enzyme inhibitors
QC Quality control
RADO Regional national anti-doping organization
USADA United States anti-doping authority
WADA World anti-doping agency

References

Archer, J., Dargan, P.I., Lostia, A.M., van der Walt, J., Henderson, K., Drake, N., Sharma, S., Wood, D.M., Walker, C.J., Kicman, A.T., 2015. Running an unknown risk: a marathon death associated with the use of 1, 3-dimethylamylamine (DMAA). Drug Test. Anal. 7, 433.

Atienza-Macías, E., 2015. 2015 WADA code comes into effect: significant changes in the Spanish legal arena. Int. Sports Law J. 15, 49–54.

Avois, L., Robinson, N., Saudan, C., Baume, N., Mangin, P., Saugy, M., 2006. Central nervous system stimulants and sport practice. Br. J. Sports Med. 40, i16–i20.

Baron, D.A., Martin, D.M., Magd, S.A., 2007. Doping in sports and its spread to at-risk populations: an international review. World J. Psychiatry 6, 118.

Baume, N., Mahler, N., Kamber, M., Mangin, P., Saugy, M., 2006. Research of stimulants and anabolic steroids in dietary supplements. J. Med. Sci. Sports 16, 41–48.

Beelen, M., Tieland, M., Gijsen, A.P., Vandereyt, H., Kies, A.K., Kuipers, H., Saris, W.H.M., Koopman, R., Van Loon, L.J.C., 2008. Coingestion of carbohydrate and protein hydrolysate stimulates muscle protein synthesis during exercise in young men, with No further increase during subsequent overnight recovery. J. Nutr. 138, 2198–2204.

Belay, A., Ota, Y., Miyakawa, K., Shimamatsu, H., 1993. Current knowledge on potential health benefits of Spirulina. J. Appl. Phycol. 5, 235–241.

Blomstrand, E., 2006. A role for branched-chain amino acids in reducing central fatigue. J. Nutr. 136, 544S–547S.

Brand, R., Heck, P., Ziegler, M., 2014. Illegal performance enhancing drugs and doping in sport: a picture-based brief implicit association test for measuring athletes' attitudes. Subst. Abuse Treat. Prev. Policy 9, 1–11.

Brown, G.A., Vukovich, M., King, D.S., 2006. Testosterone prohormone supplements. Med. Sci. Sports Exerc. 38, 1451–1461.

Burke, L.M., 2003. The IOC consensus on sports nutrition 2003: new guidelines for nutrition for athletes. Int. J. Sport Nutr. Exerc. Metab. 13, 549–552.

Butler, T.L., Cyr, J.S., Johnson, C.A., 2017. Compositions and methods for improving cardiovascular function. Google Patents.

Campbell, N., Clark, J.P., Stecher, V.J., Thomas, J.W., Callanan, A.C., Donnelly, B.F., Goldstein, I., Kaminetsky, J.C., 2013. Adulteration of purported herbal and natural sexual performance enhancement dietary supplements with synthetic phosphodiesterase type 5 inhibitors. J. Sex Med. 10, 1842–1849.

Chan, D.K.C., Ntoumanis, N., Gucciardi, D.F., Donovan, R.J., Dimmock, J.A., Hardcastle, S.J., Hagger, M.S., 2016. What if it really was an accident? The psychology of unintentional doping. BMJ 50, 898–899.

Clarkson, P.M., Thompson, H.S., 1997. Drugs and sport. Sports Med. 24, 366–384.

Cohen, P.A., Travis, J.C., Keizers, P.H., Deuster, P., Venhuis, B., 2018. Four experimental stimulants found in sports and weight loss supplements: 2-amino-6-methylheptane (octodrine), 1, 4-dimethylamylamine (1, 4-DMAA), 1, 3-dimethylamylamine (1, 3-DMAA) and 1, 3-dimethylbutylamine (1, 3-DMBA). Clin. Toxicol. 56, 421–426.

Committee, I.O., 1999. Olympic Movement Anti-doping Code. International Olympic Committee.

Connolly, H.M., Crary, J.L., Mcgoon, M.D., Hensrud, D.D., Edwards, B.S., Edwards, W.D., Schaff, H.V., 1997. Valvular heart disease associated with fenfluramine–phentermine. N. Engl. J. Med. 337, 581–588.

Corrigan, B., Kazlauskas, R., 2003. Medication use in athletes selected for doping control at the Sydney Olympics (2000). Clin. J. Sport Med. 13, 33–40.

Dascombe, B., Karunaratna, M., Cartoon, J., Fergie, B., Goodman, C., 2010. Nutritional supplementation habits and perceptions of elite athletes within a state-based sporting institute. J. Sci. Med. Sports 13, 274–280.

De Hon, O., Coumans, B., 2007. The continuing story of nutritional supplements and doping infractions, 41, 800–805.

Dhar, R., Stout, C.W., Link, M.S., Homoud, M.K., Weinstock, J., ESTES III, N.M., 2005. Cardiovascular toxicities of performance-enhancing substances in sports. In: Mayo Clinic Proceedings. Elsevier, pp. 1307–1315.

Duclos, M., 2010. Glucocorticoids: a doping agent? Endocrinol. Metab. Clin. 39, 107–126.

Duiven, E., De Hon, O., 2018. INDR commentary, Erik Duiven, Olivier de Hon & Laila Spruijt.

Dunn, D., Turner, L.W., Denny, G., 2007. Nutrition knowledge and attitudes of college athletes. Sports J. 10.

Emran, M.A., Hossain, S.S., Salek, A., Khan, M.M., Ahmed, S.M., Khandaker, M.N., Islam, M.T., 2014. Drug abuse in sports and doping. Bangladesh Med. J. 43, 46–50.

Eslami, S., Karandish, M., Marandi, S., Zand-Moghaddam, A., 2009. The study of whey protein supplementation on plasma essential amino acids concentrations after resistance exercise in healthy young athletes. J. Biol. Sci. 9, 145–151.

Fernstrom, J.D., Wurtman, R., 1971. Brain serotonin content: physiological dependence on plasma tryptophan levels. Science 173, 149–152.

Fild, D.S., 1991. The effects of oral arginine supplementation on growth hormone, arginine, and somatomedin levels during energy restriction in male weight lifters. Virginia Tech.

Gandert, D., 2012. The Battle over the Osaka Rule, pp. 109–119.

Geyer, H., Parr, M., Mareck, U., Reinhart, U., Schrader, Y., Schänzer, W., 2004. Analysis of non-hormonal nutritional supplements for anabolic-androgenic steroids-results of an international study. Int. J. Sports Med. 25, 124–129.

Green, G.A., Uryasz, F.D., Petr, T.A., Bray, C.D., 2001. NCAA study of substance use and abuse habits of college student-athletes. Clin. J. Sports Med. 11, 51–56.

Greydanus, D.E., Patel, D.R., 2002. Sports doping in the adolescent athlete: the hope, hype, and hyperbole. Pediat. Clin. 49, 829–855.

Health, N.I.O., 1994. Dietary Supplement Health and Education Act of 1994; Public Law 103-417, 103rd Congress.

Hicks, J.J.C.O.C., 2012. The Use of Nutrition and Dietary Supplements as Complimentary Care in Children with Cancer, vol. 12.

Holt, R.I., Erotokritou-Mulligan, I., Sönksen, P.H., 2009. The history of doping and growth hormone abuse in sport. Growth Horm. IGF Res. 19, 320–326.

Houlihan, B., 2002. Managing compliance in international anti-doping policy: the world anti-doping code. Eur. Sport Manag. Q. 2, 188–208.

Hughes, D., 2015. The world anti-doping code in sport: update for 2015. Aust. Prescr. 38, 167.

Jones, K., 2014. Lunch and learn: WADA Code 2015–the key changes. Int. Sports Law J. 14, 143–147.

Kamber, M., Baume, N., Saugy, M., Rivier, L., 2001. Nutritional supplements as a source for positive doping cases? Int. J. Sport Nutr. Exerc. Metab. 11, 258–263.

Kamber, M., 2011. Development of the role of National Anti-Doping Organisations in the fight against doping: from past to future. Forensic Sci. Int. 213, 3–9.

Karila, T., Hovatta, O., Seppälä, T., 2004. Concomitant abuse of anabolic androgenic steroids and human chorionic gonadotrophin impairs spermatogenesis in power athletes. Int. J. Sports Med. 25, 257–263.

Kayser, B., Mauron, A., Miah, A., 2007. Current anti-doping policy: a critical appraisal. The Ethics of Sports Technologies and Human Enhancement, 8, pp. 1–10.

Kazlauskas, R., 2008. WADA list. Rec. Adv. Doping Anal. 16, 21–32.

Kelly, G.S., 1998. The role of glucosamine sulfate and chondroitin sulfates in the treatment of degenerative joint disease. Altern. Med. Rev. 3, 27–39.

Kim, J., Chun, Y.-S., Kang, S.-K., Cho, H. C., 2010. The Use of Herbal/Traditional Products Supplementation and Doping Tests in Elite Athletes, vol. 22.

Klaschka, U., 2015. Naturally toxic: natural substances used in personal care products. Environ. Sci. Eur. 27, 1.

Koehler, K., Geyer, H., Guddat, S., Orlovius, A., Parr, M., Thevis, M., Mester, J., Schänzer, W., 2007. Sibutramine found in Chinese herbal slimming tea and capsules. Recent Advances in Doping Analysis, p. 367.

Korfali, S.I., Hawi, T., Mroueh, M., 2013. Evaluation of heavy metals content in dietary supplements in Lebanon. Chem. Cent. J. 7, 10.

Kremenik, M., Onodera, S., Nagao, M., Yuzuki, O., Yonetani, S., 2006. A historical timeline of doping in the Olympics (Part 1 1896–1968). Kawasaki Med. Welf. J. 12, 19–28.

Laure, P., Binsinger, C., Lecerf, T., 2003. General practitioners and doping in sport: attitudes and experience. Br. J. Sports Med. 37, 335–338.

Lean, M., 1997. Sibutramine—a review of clinical efficacy. Int. J. Obes. 21, S30.

Lehnert, H., Wurtman, R., 1993. Amino acid control of neurotransmitter synthesis and release: physiological and clinical implications. Psychother. Psychosom. 60, 18–32.

Lippi, G., Franchini, M., Guidi, G.C., 2007. Tour de chaos. British Association of Sport and Excercise Medicine.

Lippi, G., Mattiuzzi, C., Guidi, G., 2004. Prevention of doping in sports: epidemiological issues and ethical implications. Epidemiol. Prev. 28, 178–183.

Luke, J.L., Farb, A., Virmani, R., Sample, R.B., 1990. Sudden cardiac death during exercise in a weight lifter using anabolic androgenic steroids: pathological and toxicological findings. J. Forensic Sci. 35, 1441–1447.

Mahipal, D., Sharma, A.K. Doping in sports: a review. 2, 51–58.

Maiorana, A., O'driscoll, G., Taylor, R., Green, D., 2003. Exercise and the nitric oxide vasodilator system. Sports Med. 33, 1013–1035.

Makela, P., Wakeley, J., Gijsman, H., Robson, P.J., Bhagwagar, Z., Rogers, R.D., 2006. Low doses of Δ-9 tetrahydrocannabinol (THC) have divergent effects on short-term spatial memory in young, healthy adults. Neuropsychopharmacology 31, 462–470.

Mangan, J.A., Dyreson, M., 2013. Olympic Legacies: Intended and Unintended: Political, Cultural, Economic and Educational. Routledge.

Martínez-Sanz, J.M., Sospedra, I., Ortiz, C.M., Baladía, E., Gil-Izquierdo, A., Ortiz-Moncada, R., 2017. Intended or unintended doping? A review of the presence of doping substances in dietary supplements used in sports. Nutrients 9, 1093.

Mathews, N.M., 2018. Prohibited contaminants in dietary supplements. Sports Health 10, 19–30.

Maughan, R.J., Depiesse, F., Geyer, H., 2007. The use of dietary supplements by athletes. J. Sports Sci. 25, S103–S113.

Maughan, R.J., King, D.S., Lea, T., 2004. Dietary supplements. J. Sports Sci. 22, 95–113.

Maughan, R., 2002. The scope of nutritional supplement use in sport. Health and Doping Risks of Nutritional Supplements and Social Drugs, pp. 7–9.

Maughan, R.J., 2005. Contamination of dietary supplements and positive drug tests in sport, 23, 883–889.

Mazzoni, I., Barroso, O., Rabin, O., 2011. The list of prohibited substances and methods in sport: structure and review process by the world anti-doping agency. J. Anal. Toxicol. 35, 608–612.

Mccrory, P., 2007. The drug wars. Br. J. Sports Med. 41, 1-1.

Mcfarland, L.A., Ployhart, R.E., 2015. Social media: a contextual framework to guide research and practice. J. Appl. Psychol. 100, 1653.

Mech, G., 2013. Dietary supplement with protein activator. Google Patents.

Millman, R.B., Ross, E.J., 2003. Steroid and nutritional supplement use in professional athletes. Am. J. Addict. 12, S48–S54.

Newsholme, E.A., Calder, P.C., 1997. The proposed role of glutamine in some cells of the immune system and speculative consequences for the whole animal. Nutrition 13, 728–730.

Parr, M.K., Geyer, H., Hoffmann, B., Köhler, K., Mareck, U., Schänzer, W., 2007. High amounts of 17-methylated anabolic-androgenic steroids in effervescent tablets on the dietary supplement market. Biomed. Chromatogr. 21, 164–168.

Pennay, A., Lubman, D.I., Miller, P.J.A.F.P., 2011. Combining energy drinks and alcohol: a recipe for trouble? Aust. Fam. Physician 40, 104.

Pipe, A., Ayotte, C., 2002. Nutritional supplements and doping. Clin. J. Sport Med. 12, 245–249.

Raman, P., Patino, L.C., Nair, M.G., 2004. Evaluation of metal and microbial contamination in botanical supplements. J. Agric. Food Chem. 52, 7822–7827.

Rathmacher, J., Fuller, J., Baier, S., Nissen, S., Abumrad, N., 2017. Nutritional intervention for improving muscular function and strength. Google Patents.

Romijn, J., Coyle, E., Sidossis, L., Gastaldelli, A., Horowitz, J., Endert, E., Wolfe, R., 1993. Regulation of endogenous fat and carbohydrate metabolism in relation to exercise intensity and duration. Am. J. Physiol. Endocrinol. Metab. 265, E380–E391.

Ronis, M.J., Pedersen, K.B., Watt, J., 2018. Adverse effects of nutraceuticals and dietary supplements. Annu. Rev. Pharmacol. Toxicol. 58, 583–601.

Saartok, T., Dahlberg, E., Gustafsson, J.-Å., 1984. Relative binding affinity of anabolic-androgenic steroids: comparison of the binding to the androgen receptors in skeletal muscle and in prostate, as well as to sex hormone-binding globulin. Endocrinology 114, 2100–2106.

Salinero, J.J., Lara, B., Abian-Vicen, J., Gonzalez-Millán, C., Areces, F., Gallo-Salazar, C., Ruiz-Vicente, D., del Coso, J., 2014. The use of energy drinks in sport: perceived ergogenicity and side effects in male and female athletes. Br. J. Nutr. 112, 1494–1502.

Saper, R.B., Eisenberg, D.M., Phillips, R.S., 2004. Common dietary supplements for weight loss. Am. Fam. Physician 70, 1731–1738.

Sarkar, J., 2010. Sports Nutrition: Maximising Performances.

Sefiha, O., Reichman, N., 2017. Social media and the doping of sport surveillance. Sociol. Compass 11, e12509.

Sellami, M., Slimeni, O., Pokrywka, A., Kuvačić, G., Hayes, L.D., Milic, M., Padulo, J., 2018. Herbal medicine for sports: a review. J. Int. Soc. Sports Nutr. 15, 14.

Singh, D., Gupta, R., Saraf, S.A., 2012. Herbs–are they safe enough? An overview. Crit. Rev. Food Sci. Nutr. 52, 876–898.

Sjöqvist, F., Garle, M., Rane, A., 2008. Use of doping agents, particularly anabolic steroids, in sports and society. Lancet 371, 1872–1882.

Söderlund, K., Balsom, P., Ekblom, B., 1994. Creatine supplementation and high intensity exercise: influence on performance and muscle metabolism. Clin. Sci. Mol. Med. 87, 120–121.

Temple, N.J., 2012. The Marketing of Dietary Supplements: Profit before Health. Nutritional Health. Springer.

Thieme, D., Hemmersbach, P., 2009. Doping in Sports. Springer Science & Business Media.

Tokish, J.M., Kocher, M.S., Hawkins, R., 2004. Ergogenic aids: a review of basic science, performance, side effects, and status in sports. Am. J. Sports Med. 32, 1543–1553.

Tsivou, M., Kioukia-Fougia, N., Lyris, E., Aggelis, Y., Fragkaki, A., Kiousi, X., Simitsek, P., Dimopoulou, H., Leontiou, I.-P., Stamou, M., 2006. An overview of the doping control analysis during the Olympic Games of 2004 in Athens, Greece. Anal. Chim. Acta 555, 1–13.

van der Merwe, P., Grobbelaar, E., 2004. Inadvertent doping through nutritional supplements is a reality. S. Afr. Med. J. 16, 3–7.

van der Merwe, P., Grobbelaar, E., 2005. Unintentional doping through the use of contaminated nutritional supplements. S. Afr. Med. J. 95.

Vlad, R.A., Hancu, G., Popescu, G.C., Lungu, I.A., 2018. Doping in sports, a never-ending story? Adv. Pharm. Bull. 8, 529.

WADA. 2009. https://www.wada-ama.org/en Accessed October 5, 2020.

Wagner, U., 2011. Towards the construction of the world anti-doping agency: analyzing the approaches of FIFA and the IAAF to doping in sport. Eur. Sport Manag. Q. 11, 445–470.

Wendt, J.T., 2009. Reflecting on Beijing-a time of transition in the war on Doping. Ent. Sports Law. 26.

Williams, M.H., 1995. Nutritional ergogenics in athletics. Int. J. Sports Sci. 13, S63–S74.

Williams, M., 2005. Dietary supplements and sports performance: amino acids. J. Int. Soc. Sports Nutr. 2, 63.

Williams, M., 2006. Dietary supplements and sports performance: herbals. J. Int. Soc. Sports Nutr. 3, 1.

Wippert, P.-M., Fließer, M., 2016. National doping prevention guidelines: intent, efficacy and lessons learned-A 4-year evaluation. Subst. Abuse Treat. Prev. Policy 11, 1–7.

Yager, Z., O'dea, J.A., 2014. Relationships between body image, nutritional supplement use, and attitudes towards doping in sport among adolescent boys: implications for prevention programs. J. Int. Soc. Sports Nutr. 11, 1–8.

Yau, A.A., Decort, R.M., Ng, S.B., Lemar Jr., H.J., 2013. Use and abuse of anabolic-androgenic steroids and androgen precursors. Endocrine Secrets, pp. 415–420.

Yesalis, C.E., Bahrke, M.S., 2002. History of doping in sport. Int. Sports Stud. 24, 42–76.

Zhang, N., Lian, Z., Peng, X., Li, Z., Zhu, H.J.J.O.E., 2017. Applications of Higenamine in pharmacology and medicine. J. Ethnopharmacol. 196, 242–252.

Zilbermint, M.F., Dobs, A.S.J.F.O., 2009. Nonsteroidal selective androgen receptor modulator Ostarine in cancer cachexia. Future Oncol. 5, 1211–1220.

CHAPTER

24

Cells and tissue-based models as a rational substitute in toxicity testing

Mamata Panchal[1], *Vinayak Pawar*[1], *Mahi Mhatre*[1], *Shweta Ingole*[1], *Suryanarayana Polaka*[1], *Muktika Tekade*[2], *Kuldeep Rajpoot*[1] *and Rakesh Kumar Tekade*[1]

[1]National Institute of Pharmaceutical Education and Research (NIPER)- Ahmedabad, An Institute of National Importance, Government of India, Department of Pharmaceuticals, Ministry of Chemicals and Fertilizers, Palaj, Gandhinagar, Gujarat, India; [2]School of Pharmacy, Devi Ahilya Vishwavidyalaya, Indore, Madhya Pradesh, India

24.1 Introduction

In the early 1950s, scientists began using in vitro cell culture techniques to test the cellular toxicity of various drugs by using different cells, which could determine the cell toxic dose of the tested drugs (Rim, 2019). Research on experimental animal models has traditionally been conducted as an alternative to humans to understand how the body's cells, organs, and systems function and regulate and how disorders might result in pathological situations (Rim, 2019). Currently, toxicity testing of drugs, biomaterial, and environmental material exposure is conducted using human-derived cell or tissue-based assays (Langhans, 2018). Almost all assays might be modified for use in different bioactivity test applications. For instance, various medical research sectors have effectively used cell lines for toxicity assessment. In particular, animal cell culture have been used to develop several areas of contemporary virology (Dolskiy et al., 2020).

Tissue-based in vitro models can be used in various ways for preclinical drug testing. Optimizing the method's endpoints and cell selection is one such tactic. For instance, the first technique that uses advanced endpoints is now employed to identify the local eye toxicity of compounds in human corneal cells. The second tactic to cover the majority of fundamental cell operations is to use various cell types. A third tactic is to conduct a more fundamental analysis of the underlying processes of toxicity or bioactivity. Appropriate in vitro models could be created once these pathways are identified.

Essentials of Pharmatoxicology in Drug Research, Volume 1
https://doi.org/10.1016/B978-0-443-15840-7.00018-X

A fourth strategy, in contrast, disregards whether the hazardous mechanisms being screened for are known or not. The test can be employed if its endpoint correlates well with in vivo toxicity (Yang and Xiong, 2012).

Optimizing the pharmacokinetics properties of the drug, particularly absorption, distribution, metabolism, and excretion of drug from the body, might reduce the harmful consequences of any pharmaceutical substances (Anup et al., 2021c; Padiyar et al., 2020; Polaka et al., 2021; Rajpoot et al. 2020b, 2021c). In recent studies, researchers have focused on the safe delivery of pharmaceuticals, even though a range of factors that may considerably impact the medication's effectiveness and induce toxicity like preexisting medical conditions (Gupta et al., 2022b; Kumawat et al., 2020), body temperature (Desai et al., 2021), age of patient (Rajpoot et al., 2021a), diet (Polaka et al., 2022e), enzyme levels in the body (Achanta et al., 2021; Tambe et al., 2021c; Rajpoot et al., 2020a), sleeping pattern (Choudhary et al., 2021; Vasdev et al., 2021), patients sex (Anup et al., 2021a; Polaka et al., 2022c), etc.

Additionally, a variety of methods have been utilized to understand the impact of chemical agents on the body, such as in vitro toxicity investigation (Gupta et al., 2022c; Polaka et al., 2022f; Vasdev et al., 2022), in vivo animal studies, in silico studies (Rajpoot et al., 2022a), etc. Furthermore, scientists are also understanding the toxic impacts of additives (Tiwari et al., 2022; Gupta et al., 2022a; Pandey et al., 2022; Polaka et al. 2022a,d), toxicokinetic and toxicodynamic effects of drugs (Rajpoot et al., 2022b; Polaka et al., 2022b), and role of distinct bioindicators in toxicity studies (Tekade et al., 2022).

In the laboratory, tissue-based models (in vitro) are common and widely used to screen and classify chemicals, especially in drug testing at preclinical stages. Moreover, in silico toxicology models also offer an alternative to computational analysis, simulation, and prediction of the toxicity of new drugs/agents (Rajpoot et al., 2022a). Studies have advocated that not merely active agents but other elements of formulations, such as azo dyes, may also show significant toxicity (Tiwari et al., 2022; Tekade et al., 2022). Toxic responses may include mutagenicity (Honma, 2020), general cytotoxicity (Pandey et al., 2020; Rajpoot and Jain, 2019), carcinogenicity (Tiwari et al., 2022; Cohen et al., 2019), and genotoxicity (Bolt, 2003; Corvi and Madia, 2017).

24.2 Relevance of 3R principles in animal research

Animal models are beneficial for research on human diseases, but still, there are some restrictions on their use. For instance, more ethical concerns have arisen in recent years regarding using living organisms in research (Bédard et al., 2020). Scholars Russell and Burch from Universities Federation for Animal Welfare (UFAW) released the Principles of Humane Experimental Technique in 1959 to treat laboratory animals with greater care. This book outlined the principles of the 3Rs: reduction, replacement, and refinement (Hubrecht and Carter, 2019). The principles were defined as "(a) a reduction in the number of animals used in studies, (b) avoiding or replacing the use of animals in areas where they otherwise would have been used, (c) application of methods that cause animals significantly less suffering and pain" (Bédard et al., 2020; Clark 2018).

24.2.1 Reduction

In the United States, 780,070 animals were used for research in 2018. Many animals, like mice and rats, are not included in this number mainly because the Animal Welfare Act does not protect them (Bédard et al., 2020). The Animal Welfare Act does not protect 93% of the animals that are utilized in research. In 2018, it was anticipated that 11–23 million animals would be used for research. This was a slight rise over 2017; however, animal research has declined by more than half since 1985. The use of animals in scientific research has been reduced in recent years for a variety of reasons, including ethical considerations relating to the potential for animals to suffer from pain and discomfort during procedures (Council, 2009) but also the potential problems with these models (Bédard et al., 2020).

Legislation requiring compliance with the 3Rs has also necessitated a reduction in animal testing. Since 2006, animal testing has been regulated under registration, evaluation, authorization, and restriction of chemicals (REACH) in the European Union (EU). Its primary objective is to reduce animal testing as much as possible while simultaneously promoting the use of nonanimal alternative approaches. Several in vitro techniques have been created to reduce the usage of animals, particularly for toxicological testing. For example, an alternative to in vivo Draize rabbit eye and skin irritation testing was set up utilizing 3D reconstructed human cornea-like epithelium and epidermis models (Lee et al., 2017).

24.2.2 Replacement

In vitro models that are more accurate and inventive should take the role of animal models in various instances. First, numerous ethical issues exist with using animals in research (Mather, 2019). The translation of outcomes from animal models to people has been questioned for a long time. In certain circumstances, animal studies do not reliably predict human responses, similar to past toxicity trials that failed to accurately predict human toxicity (Olson et al., 2000). Animal models have improved over the years; however, there are still unpredictable aspects of animals (Greek and Menache, 2013). Animal models must successfully bridge the translational gap between preclinical and clinical research (Greek and Menache, 2013).

Additionally, animal model-based research has been criticized for having poor reproducibility, particularly in preclinical research (Collins and Tabak 2014). Some consider this method inefficient due to the likely absence of relevant animal testing data (Barnard and Kaufman, 1997; Sápi 2017). For instance, in the 1990s, the chimpanzee was thought to be a good model for developing a human immunodeficiency virus (HIV) vaccine. Some vaccinations showed promise in primate studies, but when they were tested on humans, the outcomes were very different. The immune system of a chimpanzee is not the same as that of a human. As a result, there is still no vaccine to protect against HIV (Bailey, 2008). The economy is another reason why there is a need to switch to different in vitro models. The costs associated with housing and animal breeding for scientific research are significant and must be considered (Chu et al., 2010; Meigs et al., 2018). Moreover, animal protocols are notorious for being time-consuming and need experienced professionals to carry out specific experiments (Doke and Dhawale, 2015).

24.2.3 Refinement

The term "refinement" refers to approaches that increase the welfare of study animals while also reducing the amount of pain, suffering, discomfort, or long-term harm that may be experienced by the animals used in the research. Animals are capable of feeling pain and mental distress. For example, to obtain measurable data, a research team in 2010 linked the degree of pain that mice were experiencing with their facial expressions (Langford et al., 2010). Distress and discomfort imposed on animals during experiments may result in variable results and demand repeating similar procedures and increasing the number of animals (Bédard et al., 2020). The main objective of the refinement is to improve the methodology used on animals by minimizing, eliminating, or relieving their discomfort or distress and so enhancing their well-being by employing noninvasive or painless procedures, organizing the protocol to reduce stress, and improving the conditions for transit, breeding, and housing (Bédard et al., 2020).

24.3 Cell-based toxicity testing methods

Cytotoxicity is the molecule's capacity to cause cell death. Necrosis is often measured using in vitro cytotoxicity testing. In contrast, apoptosis is a similarly significant approach for inducing cell death that necessitates other techniques. In-depth research on the processes underlying hazardous effects on cells, such as necrosis, apoptosis, or other events, may be found in studies on the dose- and time-dependent effects on cells as well as the observation of impacts on the cell cycle, including their reversibility. However, several circumstances, including fever, patient age, health conditions (such as pregnancy and diabetes), etc (Desai et al., 2021; Choudhary et al., 2021; Anup et al. 2021a,c), might affect a drug's pharmacokinetics as well as its toxicity impact (Gupta et al. 2022a,b; Asati et al., 2022).

In a study, the cytotoxicity of the mycotoxins ceauvericin and ochratoxin A (OTA) alone as well as in combination on HepG2 cells for 24, 48, and 72 h was examined using the 3-(4,5-dimethylthiazol-2-yl)-2,5 diphenyl tetrazolium bromide (MTT) test. The goal of the test was to calculate the inhibition of the cell population to half-maximal inhibitory concentration (IC_{50}). Studies revealed that beauvericin (BEA) was more toxic than OTA according to the IC_{50} values, while each therapy was assessed separately (Fig. 24.1A and B). Nevertheless, a dose-dependent pattern of toxicity in the IC_{50} values was attained for combinations of both mycotoxins (Fig. 24.1C). BEA showed the most toxic impact after 72 h (Juan-Garcia et al., 2019).

To identify basal cytotoxicity, such as the inherent capacity of a substance to induce cell death as a result of causing harm to fundamental cellular activities, in vitro cytotoxicity assays are helpful and essential. To offer relevant data on factors like genotoxicity and the generation of mutations, including programmed cell death, cytotoxicity studies are often required to determine the concentration range for additional and more extensive in vitro testing (He et al., 2021; Huang et al., 2022). It is feasible to assess quantitatively the reactions of a single chemical in several systems or many compounds in various systems by determining the dosage where 50% cell toxicity occurs. Fig. 24.2 describes some endpoints/parameters employed in cellular toxicity testing.

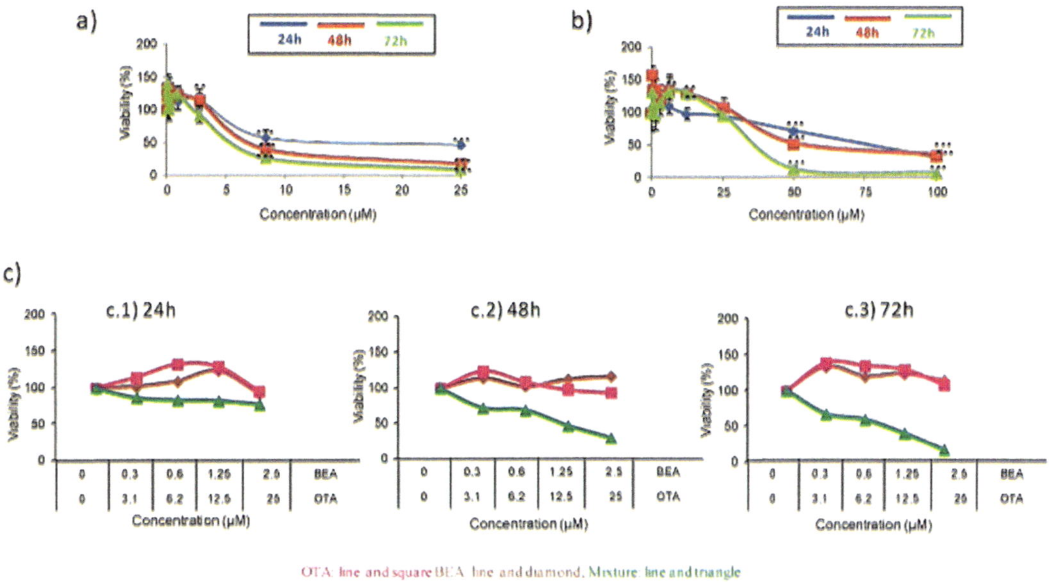

FIGURE 24.1 BEA's cytotoxicity (A), OTA cytotoxicity (B), and BEA + OTA cytotoxicity (C) on HepG2 cells after treatment with mycotoxin for 24, 48, and 72 h. *$P \leq .05$ (Juan-Garcia et al., 2019).

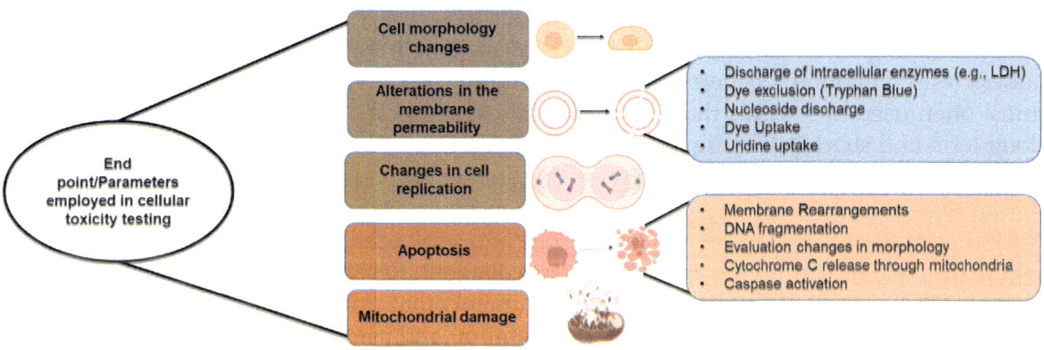

FIGURE 24.2 Endpoint/parameters employed in cellular toxicity testing.

It has frequently been argued that cell or tissue cultures would make an appropriate testing medium for drugs in pharmacology. Organ culture (Jia and Zhao, 2022), sphere culture (Pisciotta et al., 2018), suspension culture (Kumar et al., 2019), clone culture on soft agar (Borrego et al., 2019), and monolayer cell culture (Yan et al., 2019) are a few examples of the culture techniques. Organ culture offers a model for drug evaluation that is closer to an in vivo environment, but because of the size variation of organ implants as well as the heterogeneity of the cells inside the explants during subsequent trials, such type of model is not considered suitable for efficacious quantitative investigations (Jia and Zhao, 2022).

The tumor cells can be grown in spheres culture, which resembles tumor nodules in vivo and thus can be utilized to explore how three-dimensional relationships affect medication sensitivity (Pisciotta et al., 2018). Suspension culture is helpful for chemosensitivity investigations and is practical for radionuclide research because it inhibits the proliferation of connective tissue cells that are a source of "cell pollution" (fibroblast). Besides cells with low proliferative capability, clone culture on soft agar is ideal for cells with a strong capacity for self-renewal (i.e., tumor cells) (Borrego et al., 2019). For testing cell line cytotoxicity as well as the chemosensitivity of different tumor biopsy samples, monolayer cell culture works best (Yan et al., 2019).

Cell culture systems are essential for cytotoxicity testing as well as metabolism research, including biotransformation, interactions with endogenous metabolites, binding to cells, and activation of metabolism. Some examples of cell lines that are used more often include diploid human fibroblast cell lines (such as WI-38) and tumor cell lines (e.g., HeLa). When investigating the mechanism of toxicity of a chemical, when it becomes crucial to consider the unique characteristics of specialized cell types, it is common to employ primary cell cultures of the target organ or tissue in combination with cell lines of the exact origin.

24.3.1 Cell culture method

Four types of culture methods are commonly employed in toxicity studies. Among these, the first one is used in toxicity testing. In this method, organ tissues and primary cells are used as test subjects. The cultivation of organisms is beyond the scope of the topics covered in this chapter. Nevertheless, information about these processes may be obtained elsewhere (Wickramasinghe, 1996). The second one is spheroid cultures, which are generally utilized to assess test compounds' penetration ability. The third one is suspension cultures which are most often used in systems that use tumor biopsy material. However, they may be used in long-term and short-term drug sensitivity investigations. The fourth one is the most common culture technique used in cytotoxicity testing is monolayer culture. This approach provides the most versatility regarding drug exposure, recovery, and measurement.

The primary purpose of the cell cytotoxicity and proliferation tests is to screen the response of the cells to a medication or any other chemical agent. Researchers use a variety of assays to evaluate the efficacy of newly discovered treatments that primarily target cancer cells (Adan et al., 2016). Methods for detecting cell proliferation and cytotoxicity are categorized according to their prevalence and importance.

24.3.1.1 Dye exclusion

Dye exclusion methods differentiate between living and dead cells (e.g., Trypan blue, eosin, Congo red, erythrosine B assays) (Strober, 2001).

24.3.1.2 MTT assay

The principle of colorimetric assays is the measurement of a biochemical marker to evaluate the metabolic activity of the cells (e.g., MTT assay, MTS assay, XTT assay, WST-1 assay, WST-8 assay, LDH assay, SRB assay, NRU assay, and crystal violet assay). MTT assay depends on the conversion of MTT to insoluble formazan (purple color) crystals by mitochondrial NAD(p) H-dependent oxidoreductase enzymes produced from live cells (Fig. 24.3) (van Meerloo

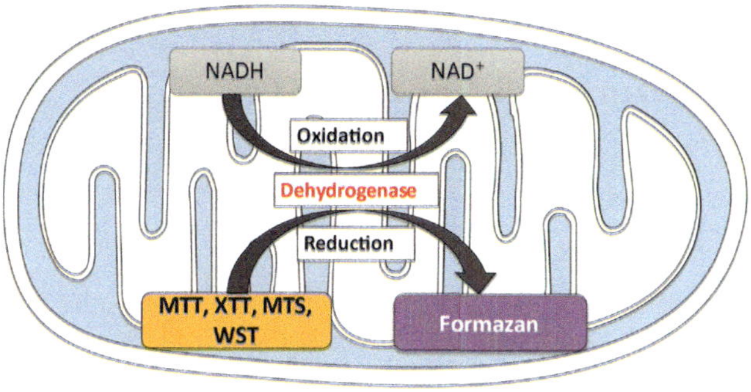

FIGURE 24.3 MTT, XTT, MTS, WST assay.

et al., 2011). It determines cell viability by determining the mitochondrial function of cells, which is proportional to the quantity of formazan crystals (van Meerloo et al., 2011).

24.3.1.3 XTT assay

It is a colorimetric method based on the tetrazolium salt 2,3-bis (2-methoxy-4-nitro 5-sulphophenyl)-5-carboxanilide-2H-tetrazolium, monosodium salt (XTT). This assay is based on the ability to reduce tetrazolium salt XTT to orange-colored formazan compounds by using active metabolic cells (Cory et al., 1991; Kuhn et al., 2003; van Meerloo et al., 2011).

24.3.1.4 WST-1 and WST-8 assay

Mitochondrial dehydrogenase enzymes are responsible for transforming the tetrazolium salt 2-(4-iodophenyl)-3-(4-nitrophenyl)-5-(2,4-disulfophenyl)-2H-tetrazolium monosodium salt (WST)-1 into a highly water-soluble formazan, which is the basic concept behind this assay. In this assay, the color change is directly proportional to the amount of mitochondrial dehydrogenase in the cell culture (Berridge and Tan, 1993).

24.3.1.5 Lactate dehydrogenase (LDH) assay

LDH catalyzes the transformation of lactate to pyruvate by reducing NAD+ to NADH. This is followed by the reduction of a tetrazolium salt (i.e., Iodo-nitro-tetrazolium, INT) to a red formazan by diaphorase enzymes utilizing produced NADH (Fig. 24.4) (Sumantran, 2011; Wolterbeek and van der Meer, 2005).

24.3.1.6 AlamarBlue (AB) assay

AB assay is also known as resazurin reduction assay. The AB assay is based on converting the blue nonfluorescent dye resazurin, which is converted to the pink fluorescent resorufin by mitochondrial enzymes (Fig. 24.5) (Al-Nasiry et al., 2007).

24.3.1.7 Adenosine 5′-triphosphate (ATP) assay

The ATP assay relies on bioluminescent detection to measure ATP concentrations. A specific quantity of light is produced due to the reaction between the natural firefly enzyme luciferase and added amount of luciferin and the cellular ATP (Fig. 24.6). This reaction may be

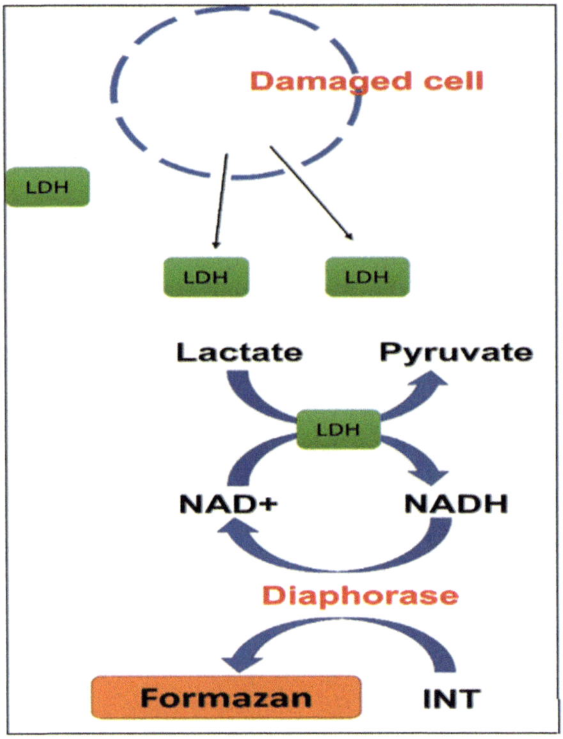

FIGURE 24.4 LDH release assay.

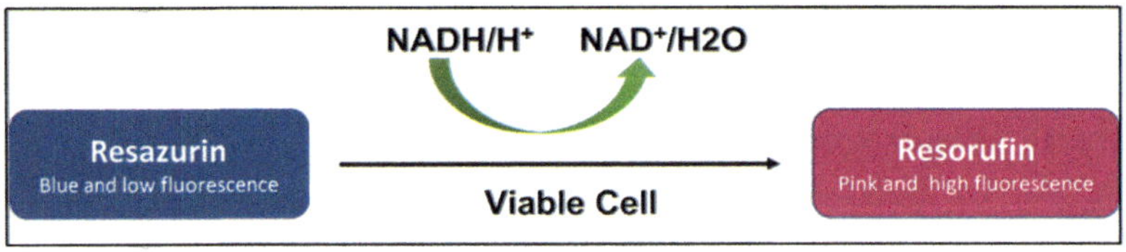

FIGURE 24.5 AB assay.

quantified using a luminometer. The viability of a cell directly relates to the quantity of luminescent light (Crouch et al., 1993; Voigt, 2005).

The results of the cell culture-based toxicity endpoint are summarized in Table 24.1.

24.4 Plant-based toxicity testing methods

All living species on earth could be impacted by human activity. Examining the environmental risk and ecotoxicological potential of pesticide pollution, industrial waste, and other chemicals has become vital. External forces have the potential to harm biological

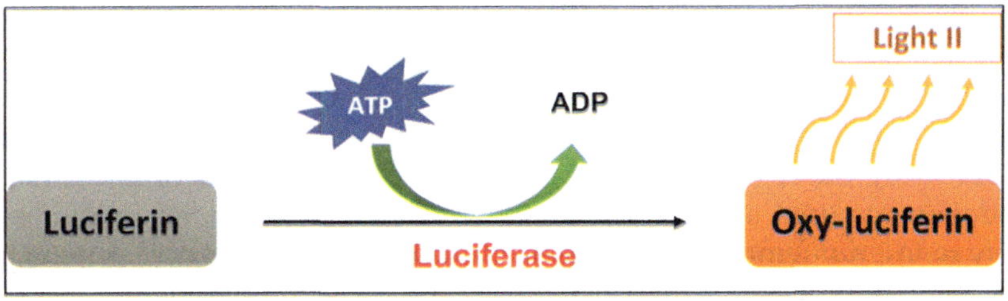

FIGURE 24.6 ATP assay.

TABLE 24.1 Mammalian cell culture-based materials toxicity assessment.

Test substance	Cell line	Endpoint detection	Outcomes	References
Antibody-drug conjugate (ADC)	Human cell lines (MCF7 and N87 cells)	MTT assay (reduction of yellow tetrazolium salts to purple formazan)	Helps to evaluate and assess the bystander impact of ADCs in vitro in a co-culture setup.	Wu and Shah (2020)
Geigerin	Murine myoblast cell line (C2C12)	LDH assay (the reduction of a tetrazolium salt to a red formazan)	Cytotoxic effect was proportional to the concentration.	Botha et al. (2017)
Doxorubicin (DOX)	Lung cancer cell line (H460 and A549)	XTT assay (reduction of the tetrazolium salt XTT to orange-colored formazan)	Compared to the blank NPs and the free DOX, the DOX NPs demonstrated a significantly greater level of cytotoxicity at the maximum dose evaluated for both cell lines.	Azarmi et al. (2006)

communities and cause the extinction of species. The plant-based bioassay is an appropriate method for estimating environmental consequences for ecosystems and, in some situations, for animals and humans (Oprea et al., 2007). Plant-based toxicity tests have been used as a substitute for animal assays in investigating environmental contaminant concentrations, evaluating phytotoxicity, assessing the biotransformation of xenobiotics, and estimating bioaccumulation.

Typically, aquatic plants like algae and duckweed or terrestrial plants (particularly crop plants) have been utilized in toxicity testing. A more exhaustive phytotoxicity database built from investigations including a wide range of plant species and test compounds shows that plant and animal sensitivity is chemical and species-dependent and unpredictable (Lytle and Lytle, 2001). Recent years have seen a notable increase in using plant-based bioassays in toxicological and ecotoxicological evaluation techniques. Due to their relative ease, sensitivity, and cost-effectiveness, as well as a strong association with other toxicity tests, they are widely used (Siddiqui et al., 2011).

The European Chemicals Agency (ECHA) made a conclusion based on the scientific evidence presented by Organization for Economic Co-operation and Development (OECD) TG 208 and ISO TG 22030, two guidelines relevant to evaluating effects on terrestrial plants. The OECD Guideline 208, which was released in 1984, might be seen as the initial step toward standardizing the regulatory setting for toxicity assessments of terrestrial plants. The recommendation required at least three species. The 2006 amended guideline maintained the necessity to test numerous species but clarified that the number of species to be examined depends on regulatory needs. Afterward, during the revision of guideline 208, guideline 227 was created to investigate spray impacts on plants/leaves.

In addition, the ISO guidelines include a screening method for a single species (ISO 17126:2005; ISO/DIS 29200) and a chronic toxicity guideline for two plants specie (ISO 22030). In addition to this, it also has testing alternatives for evaluating the inhibition of root growth (ISO 11269-1), as well as the emergence and early growth (ISO11269-2) (Tarazona et al., 2013).

In toxicity testing, various crop plants like Zea mays, Sorghum bicolor, and *Triticum aestivum*, and Cucumis sativus have been used (An, 2006). The toxic effect of pharmaceuticals has been carried out on macrophytes species. Allium cepa species is commonly used for assessing the genotoxic potential of the toxicant. Metals, herbicides, insecticides, and chemicals found in crude oil are detected by using algae in bioassays. Test species such as Chlorella fusca and Selensastrum cupricornutum have been employed as indicator species (Tothill and Turner, 1996). In upcoming sections, a detailed view of the plant tissue-based toxicity evaluation method is given.

Aquatic and terrestrial plants are essential components of a healthy ecosystem. Herbicides, pesticides, metals, pharmaceuticals, industrial waters, and waste waters potentially affect various plants in the ecosystem. Aquatic biota is primarily exposed to wastewater during their life cycle. These toxicants may be hazardous to plant species throughout their lifespan. The toxic effect of these substances is investigated through the characterization of various growth parameters such as seed germination, root elongation, biomass production chlorophyll and carotenoid content, protein, and enzyme activity. All these assays are discussed briefly in the below section and depicted in Fig. 24.7.

24.4.1 Vegetative vigor test

The purpose of the vegetative vigor test is to assess any potential effects a drug may have on the vigor of terrestrial plants. The test evaluates possible impacts on plants after the test chemical is deposited on the leaf and above-ground parts of plants. At various time intervals, the plants are compared to untreated control plants for biomass content and adverse aesthetic effects like chlorosis, death, and atypical plant development (OECD-227 2003).

24.4.2 Lemna test

Duckweed (Lemna minor L.) is an aquatic plant that may selectively accumulate particular chemicals and function as a biological monitor. As a result, duckweed is employed in water quality studies to detect heavy metals and other water pollutants. To assess the toxicity, plants are exposed to a toxic substance over time, and the potential growth inhibition and

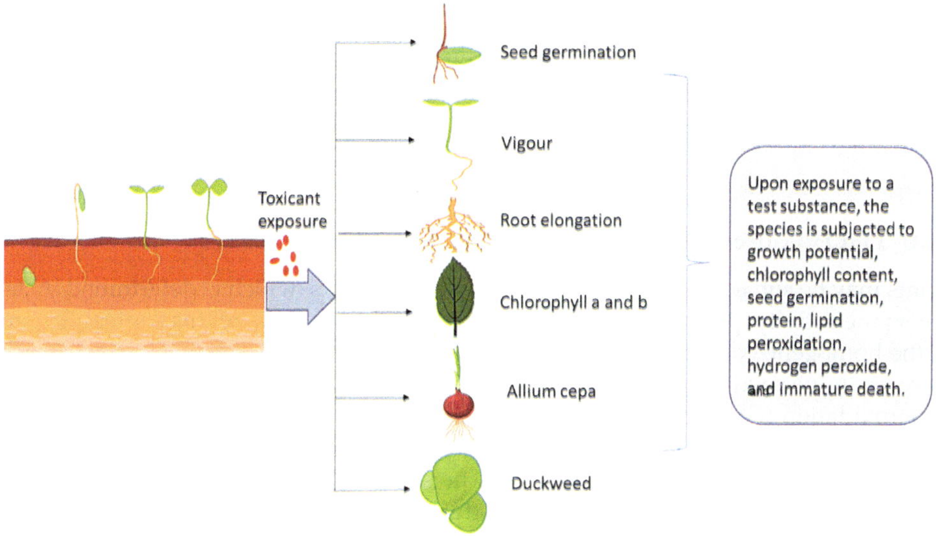

FIGURE 24.7 Principles of plant tissue-based toxicity assay.

the results are evaluated together to determine the levels of chlorophyll and carotenoids as well as the activity of enzymes (e.g., peroxidase) (Radić et al., 2011).

24.4.3 Seed germination and root elongation test

Germinating plant seeds are susceptible to environmental stress. This test can potentially analyze liquid and solid phase studies, making it versatile. The germination capacity of toxicant-treated seed is examined in test settings. To determine the toxicity of the test drug, relative seed germination, relative radicle growth, seed germination index, and seed germination are investigated (Luo et al., 2018; Wang, 1991). Root elongation test for toxicity testing is based on the ability of the toxicant to inhibit the root elongation when it is incubated for a particular period (Di Salvatore et al., 2008).

24.4.4 Allium cepa test

Allium cepa is usually used to characterize the genotoxicity of the toxin. It has been utilized to evaluate many chemical agents, contributing to its expanding use in environmental monitoring. It can identify DNA damage, such as chromosomal abnormalities and mitotic cycle disruptions. The mitotic index and several nuclear abnormalities are used to assess cytotoxicity and analyze micronucleus to determine the mutagenicity of various substances. Furthermore, the Allium cepa test system provides critical information for assessing the action mechanisms of a substance's effects on genetic material (Leme and Marin-Morales, 2009).

24.4.5 Chlorophyll pigment assay

The content of chlorophyll a and chlorophyll b upon treatment with toxic substances gets reduced. In this, the chlorophyll, after exposure to the toxicant, is extracted from the species, and its content is measured to investigate the toxicity profile of the sample (Thwala et al., 2021).

24.4.6 H_2O_2 content, lipid peroxidation, and enzyme assays

Plants may be subjected to oxidative stress from toxicants, which is determined by test species' enzyme activity, protein content, and H_2O_2 content. To analyze this content, supernatant from the homogenized test species is extracted and subjected to catalase, superoxide dismutase, ascorbate peroxidase, and guaiacol peroxidase activities well as for H_2O_2 content and lipid peroxidation (Gutiérrez-Martínez et al., 2020).

To establish a connection between the toxicity of environmental contaminants and harmful ecological impacts, tests on plants are used. The selection of the species takes place based on the sensitivity of test material, lifecycle characteristics, taxonomic distribution, ecological relevance of plants, and the feasibility of the plant to test conditions. The plant must withstand laboratory testing, with repeatable results within and between labs. The most common species of higher plants used to assess environmental pollution are Vicia faba, tradescantia, Allium cepa nicotiana tabacum, *Crepis capillaris*, Hordeum vulgare, and Zea mays (Leme and Marin-Morales, 2009). Algae and macrophytes are also used in biomonitoring and phytotoxicity studies (Lytle and Lytle, 2001).

The physical and chemical properties of test substances are also considered during toxicity testing. Toxicity testing of the complex mixture also can be done. Still, the test substance purity, solubility behavior, partition coefficient, chemical stability, and biodegradability help in the designing of the method of toxicity testing. Test substances are applied in the carrier to get access by the plants (OECD-208 2003).

To ensure that test results and the responses of the test plants have not altered considerably over time, reference chemicals used in the toxicity assessment and tested at regular intervals (Environmental, 1998). The control group is also included to verify that observed effects may be attributable to the presence of the test chemical alone. The ideal control group would share every characteristic with the experimental group except for the exposure to the experimental chemical.

To determine whether or not the test material has a hazardous impact, it is first exposed to plants and then either directly mixed into the soil (OECD-208 2003), sprayed on the plants that are growing (Riemens et al., 2009), or exposed with filter paper that has been soaked in solutions of the test substance (Stefanello et al., 2019). In addition, it is cultivated by supplying a growth medium for a predetermined amount of time. After the words, the plant is analyzed using several factors, as was already said, to figure out if the test chemical could be toxic.

24.4.7 Case studies

The impact of exposure mediums and silver nanoparticle (NPs) size on the toxicological behavior of NPs on higher plants, Salvinia minima, has been studied by Thwala and coworkers (Thwala et al., 2021). In this study, they investigated two sizes of silver NPs (AgNPs) (i.e., 10 and 40 nm) in three exposure media such as moderately hard water, moderately hard water with increased calcium (Ca^{2+}), and moderately hard water with organic matter. They concluded that the toxicity pattern was connected to the increased dissolution of AgNPs having the smallest particle size. AgNPs reduced plant growth and chlorophyll pigments a and b.

Alkimin has estimated the toxicity potential of paracetamol, chlorpromazine, and paracetamol on macrophyte species of Lemna minor and Lemna gibba (Alkimin et al., 2019). After exposure to the toxicant for 96 h, species were analyzed for pigments, enzymatic activity, and chlorophyll fluorescence. According to the findings of this study, higher doses of the medicines under test had substantial effects on both Lemna species in terms of the various endpoints examined.

Toxicity evaluation of the electroplating sludge has been investigated using a plant-based approach (Orescanin et al., 2018). Herein they used Hordeum vulgare L species. They treated this species with different sludge concentrations before and after its treatment and assessed for germination index, root elongation, and seed germination ability. They have verified the effectiveness of the employed approach for detoxifying electroplating sludge by comparing the findings from treated and untreated sludge.

Allium cepa and seed germination tests have been designed and standardized by researchers for the routine monitoring of diverse water bodies in India as well as to assess the toxicity of crucial water pollutants using these tests (Siddiqui et al., 2011). Knauer et al. and colleagues have developed herbicide toxicity testing using Elodea canadensis Michx. and Myriophyllum spicatum L (Knauer et al., 2006). They were provided Elendt-M4 as a growth medium. Following that, they placed cuttings of the species in an artificial M4 medium to evaluate their toxicity potential. They were measured for biomass, root growth, and the length of the leading and secondary shoots after a certain amount of time they were planted. The research employed using plant-based toxicity assay is depicted in Table 24.2.

24.5 Yeast-based toxicity testing methods

Over the decades, invertebrate and vertebrate species have been employed to evaluate acute and chronic toxicity. Moreover, these tests are time-consuming and take many days to finish. Furthermore, it might be challenging to interpret entire species toxicity test data regarding toxicity processes (Haubenstricker et al., 1990). Toxicity assessment using animal models has constraints that make it tough to deal with the growing number of potentially harmful compounds in the environment and pharmaceutical sector (North and Vulpe, 2010; Dos Santos et al., 2012). Since eukaryotes are simple to maintain and cultivate under controlled circumstances, they can avoid the variability problems associated with even more complex biological systems. Yeasts are an example of a eukaryote that may provide an excellent model for testing toxicity (Esteve et al., 2009).

In molecular and cell biology fields, the eukaryotic model organism *S. cerevisiae* (*Saccharomyces cerevisiae*) is well-established and often utilized. Yeast has several natural qualities that

TABLE 24.2 Plant-based toxicity assessment.

Test substance	Species	Endpoint detection	Outcomes	References
Electroplating sludge	Hordeum vulgare L	• Seed germination • Root elongation • Germination index	H. Vulgare L. showed even greater sensitivity compared to the human cells to assess the toxic material is electroplating sludge.	Orescanin et al. (2018)
Tepraloxydim	E. crus-galli, E. repens, P. annua and P. milliaceum.	• Seed production • Seedling emergence • Visual symptoms • Biomass	Impact on the biomass of greenhouse and field-grown plants was discovered to be correlated at different effect levels.	Riemens et al. (2009)
Heavy metals, phenolics, and industrial waste-water	Brassica spp., Cucumis spp., Panicum spp., and Phaseolus spp.	• Allium cepa test • Seed germination test	Significant amounts of chromosomal abnormalities were recorded with both the industrial waste water and the XAD concentrated river water samples by the A. cepa test.	Siddiqui et al. (2011)
Chlorpromazine, paracetamol, and diclofenac	Lemna minor and Lemna gibba.	• Lemna spp. assay • Pigments analyses • Biochemical marker—catalase activity • Protein determination	Macrophyte-based tests (nonstandard endpoints) are more sensible and provide additional information about the chemical contamination effects in plants.	Alkimin et al. (2019)
Textile sludge compost	Soybean and wheat	• Seed germination assay • Plant growth bioassays	Textile sludge compost presented great phytotoxicity under hydroponics conditions, and the soybean and wheat were sensitive for evaluating organic wastes in plant growth bioassays.	Araújo and Monteiro (2005)
Herbicides	Elodea canadensis Michx. Myriophyllum spicatum L	• Primary and secondary shoot length • Biomass and root formation	Growth in total plant length and growth in biomass of the two species have the potential as measures of toxicity.	Knauer et al. (2006)
AgNPs	Salvinia minima	• Plant growth • Chlorophyll production	AgNPs reduced plant growth and the production of chlorophyll pigments a and b.	Thwala et al. (2021)

make it an excellent model system. This model is fast and exhibits efficient growth as a nonpathogenic unicellular microorganism. Further, genetic manipulation is easy to make in yeast cells. A wide range of experimental methods and biological materials are readily available for genome-wide association studies. For instance, *Saccharomyces cerevisiae* has promising functional conservation as in the human genome and other higher eukaryotic genomes.

Also, it has the unique benefit of having functional data accessible for almost all genes (Dos Santos et al., 2012).

The yeast *Saccharomyces cerevisiae* is a beneficial model organism for studies of cellular responses to various types of stress. Upon exposure of a toxicant to the yeast cells, various colorimetric, bioluminance, and fluorescence assays have examined cell viability. The toxic effect of a test substance does not always result in the death of yeast cells. It may alter the morphology and metabolic conditions of yeast cells. It may be recognized by monitoring the metabolic activity, enzyme activity, mitochondrial membrane potential, and ATP content of exposed cells (Kwolek-Mirek and Zadrag-Tecza, 2014).

24.5.1 Yeast culture method

A specific methodology for yeast-based toxicity assays has not been reported. It may vary from endpoint detection. Based on the requirements, we should choose an appropriate strain of yeast cells. Afterward, yeast culture should be maintained in a feasible growth medium to facilitate the growth of yeast cells. The yeast extract peptone dextrose is mostly used as a growth medium containing glucose (2%, w/v), peptone (1%, w/v), yeast extract (0.5%, w/v), and agar (2%, w/v). Additionally, it must be incubated in a suitable growth medium according to the study's requirements. During the exponential growth phase, harvest the yeast cells, centrifuge them, wash them, resuspend them in ice-cold deionized water, and incubate the test substance at various concentrations with yeast culture. Add the assay reagent as per the research requirement. Detect the endpoint at various time intervals to assess its viability and proliferation. Calculate the IC_{50} value. As per IC_{50}, assess the toxicity potential of the test substance (Ribeiro et al., 2000; Bitton et al., 1984). The methodology of yeast-based toxicity assay is illustrated in Fig. 24.8.

24.5.2 Case studies

Saccharomyces cerevisiae (strain RXII) was employed to assess the octanol/water partition coefficients associated with toxic effects by measuring cell proliferation photometrically at 530 nm (Stadtlander and Lawohnus, 1990). Researchers looked at the wild diploid variant of baker's yeast for rapid toxicity testing, focusing on the respiratory activity. The biological sensor was a strain of *Saccharomyces cerevisiae* called C 276 a/a. Using a dissolved oxygen electrode, this method looks for any changes in the rate of respiration in yeast cells that are still whole (Haubenstricker et al., 1990).

Studies have also been done on the yeast Pichia pastoris as a eukaryotic model to examine the cytotoxicity and photo-induced toxic effects of carbon dots (CDs). The pyrolysis procedure was used to make CDs from citric acid. Relative yeast cell growth was measured in the presence of various CDs concentrations to determine toxicity. Spectrophotometry was utilized to observe the interaction between CDs and yeast cells and the possibility of CDs adhering to the cell surface. Moreover, scanning electron microscopy (SEM) was used to study the morphological alterations of yeast treated with CDs. Since light is an essential environmental component, its effect on CD toxicity was also investigated. Finally, intercellular reactive oxygen species (ROS) generation-induced CDs were investigated. According to the

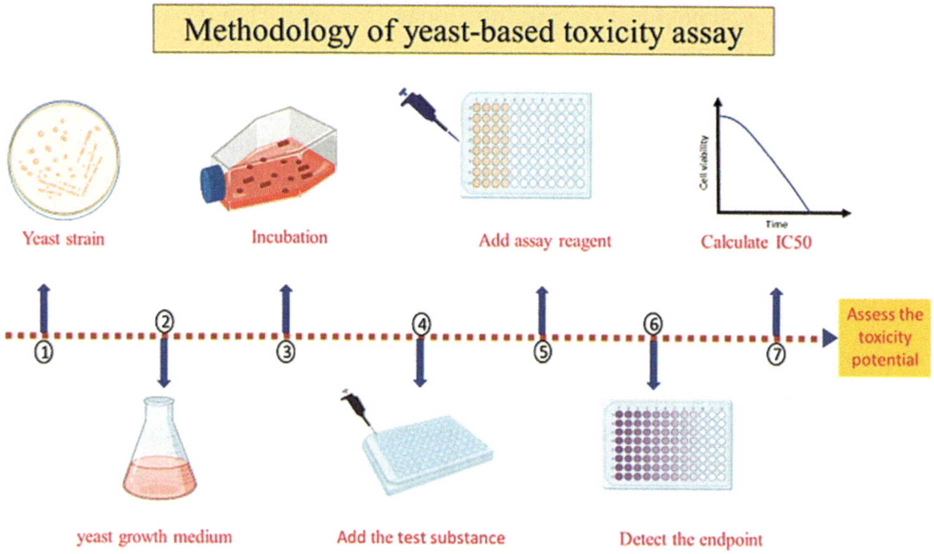

FIGURE 24.8 Methodology of the yeast-based assay.

results, it has been concluded that CDs showed dose-dependent toxic effects on yeast cells. The contact between CDs and the yeast cell surface was verified by the CDs binding curve. SEM scans revealed that the CDs led to yeast cell surface hole development, cell shrinkage, and moderate cell deformation. Additionally, it was shown that CDs might induce ROS dose-dependently. Results demonstrated that light exposure (a crucial environmental element) improved the inhibition of CD growth and ROS production effects (Bagheri et al., 2018).

24.6 In-silico-based toxicity testing methods

The preclinical toxicity investigations of drugs to determine harmful consequences and endpoints involve both economic and ethical constraints. Because of many obstacles, such as lack of time, money, and ethical issues over animal testing, it is not practical to test all these compounds in a laboratory environment. The EU enacted REACH in 2007 to investigate chemicals internationally, including the phased registration and evaluation of all current compounds made and imported lacking safety information (Rim, 2020). In silico toxicology is one of the alternative options to animal testing that complement in vivo and in vitro toxicity evaluations to limit animal testing, save costs and time, and enhance toxicity prediction and safety evaluation (Parthasarathi and Dhawan, 2018). It is possible to conduct preliminary screening using computational toxicity prediction methods, which may then be used to guide additional toxicity testing and the selection of compounds. As a result, in silico toxicity is rapidly developing as an essential platform for predicting the potential toxicity that may be detrimental to animals, humans, and the environment (Raies and Bajic, 2016; Zhang et al., 2014; Bhat and Chatterjee, 2021).

The application of interdisciplinary knowledge gained from advances in chemistry, molecular biology, and computational science by computational toxicology is a step that can be taken to alleviate the challenges that have been outlined. This knowledge can be used to maximize the effectiveness with which the toxicity profile can be determined. Increasing performance and productivity in this field would result in less uncertainty in safeguarding human health by more accurately identifying the risks of the many toxicants that must be addressed (Kavlock et al., 2008).

In silico toxicity assessment involves analysis, simulation, visualization, or predictions of the toxicity of compounds using computer methods. In silico toxicology seeks to enhance current toxicity assessments by predicting toxicity, prioritizing compounds, guiding toxicity studies, and reducing late-stage drug design failures. Thus, various models are generated to predict toxicity outcomes (Raies and Bajic, 2016; Anup et al., 2021b). In silico toxicology refers to a wide range of computational methods consisting of (a) databases used to store information about compounds, their toxic effects, and chemical characteristics such as ToxRefDB (Watford et al., 2019) and aggregated computational toxicology resource (AcTOR) (Judson et al., 2008), (b) simulation tools for use in the forms of molecular dynamics and systems biology, (c) software designed to generate molecular descriptors, (d) computer modeling methods, (e) expert systems, and (f) visualization tools (Dhanya et al., 2018).

In silico toxicity assessment aims to predict chemical toxicity using computational modeling, quantitative structure-activity relationships (QSAR), and algorithms with toxicity data (Rim, 2020). It is widely agreed that in silico approaches will be utilized for the categorization and labeling of new chemicals, risk evaluation of new and existing chemicals, and prioritizing existing substances for additional testing or assessment (Cronin, 2006). With the aid of in silico toxicity testing, pertinent information can be retrieved, and/or chemical effects can be predicted. The various tools used in the in silico evaluation are described in the below paragraphs.

In computational modeling, machine learning techniques like the support vector machine (SVM), artificial neural network (ANN), and random forest (RF) are crucial (Kar and Leszczynski, 2019). Structural alerts are utilized in toxicity assessment to identify the structural fragments or toxicophore associated with toxicity. On the other hand, rule-based models are also there, which are of two types, i.e., induction-based rules (IBRs) and human-based rules (HBRs). IBRs are derived computationally, whereas HBRs are derived from subject matter experts' human expertise or literature (Venkatapathy and Wang, 2013; Roncaglioni et al., 2013). The docking approach is also utilized for evaluating the interaction between two molecular structures (Kar and Leszczynski, 2019). Expert systems are more practical alternatives to QSAR models for the estimation of toxicity because they need inputs for structure, endpoint, and environment compartment. Moreover, the AIM, Toxtree, OCED Tool Box, Derek Nexus, AMBIT, DSSTox, CASE, HazardExpert, PASS, cat-SAR, Toxmatch, and Ambit-Discovery are the most favorable expert systems for toxicity predictions (Roy and Kar, 2016).

Computer simulation is a process of creating a mathematical model of a specific event, which involves describing as precisely as possible each of the individual physical or biological process's fundamental elements. So long as the framework is similar to relevant biochemical and physiological structures and systems (in vivo), this computed behavior will be the same as expected (in vivo) (Kavlock et al., 2008; Clewell III & Andersen, 1989).

The process of in silico toxicity evaluation includes many steps that lead to the endpoint detection of risk or hazard assessment. As previously mentioned, there are many in silico tools employed in toxicity. Based on the kind of toxicological effect and the mechanism of the toxicant, in silico approaches are chosen for the toxicity evaluation. The data required for the in silico evaluation must be obtained by searching the data that is currently accessible on that specific molecule. A model for the assessment of toxicity is created with the help of molecular descriptor evaluation. With that endpoint is detected based on the in silico predictions. The methodology of in silico toxicity testing is represented in Fig. 24.9.

In silico chemical safety assessment can consider many different kinds of data. Data from toxicological tests that have already been done is one of the most critical data sources for modeling. This kind of information could be public or private business information, including physicochemical and toxicological information. In the past, these data were the most critical part of in silico modeling, which is still crucial for figuring out how safe chemicals are (Pawar et al., 2019). A molecular descriptor's evaluation is necessary since it determines a molecule's structural or physicochemical characteristics or components. Molecular descriptors of a chemical and its toxicological outcome have a mathematical resemblance to the predictive toxicology model. Atomic or molecular properties can be used to translate a physicochemical and structural property into molecular descriptors. This lays the groundwork for "in silico" predictive toxicology (Parthasarathi and Dhawan, 2018).

The model validation usually occurs at various phases utilizing the data set splitting. Since experimental data for compounds included in the validation set were not yet available at the first modeling stage, chemicals from the test sets were explicitly used to evaluate the models calibrated on the training samples. Internal cross-validation was utilized to optimize model parameters throughout the modeling phase (Ballabio et al., 2019). Determining a model's applicability domain is crucial. The applicability domain of a QSAR is the physicochemical, structural, or biological space, knowledge, or information on which the model was trained to forecast new compounds (Raunio, 2011). Appropriate application of the model to test

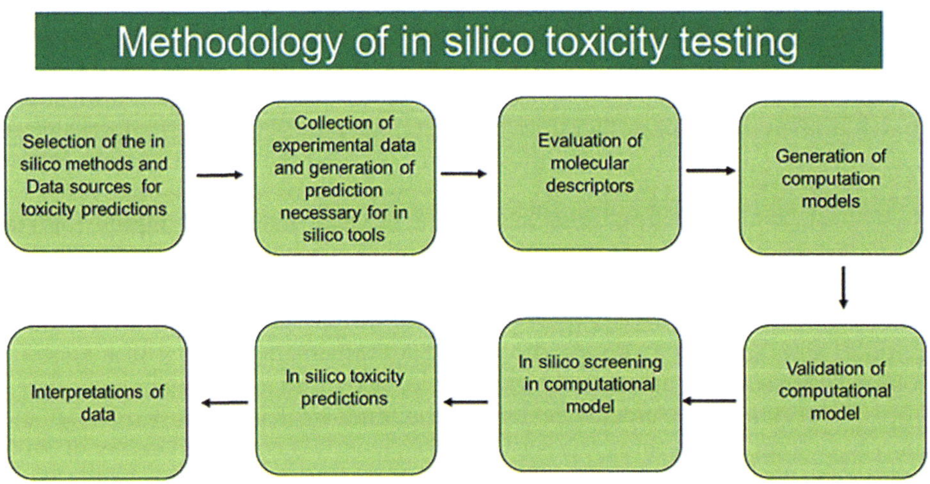

FIGURE 24.9 Methodology of in silico toxicity testing.

compounds is carried out. It is also essential to provide a thorough justification for the model results. Models ought to offer a level of confidence in their predictions. A prediction's level of confidence should be provided by models. Users can use this to decide whether or not to accept the model predictions (Raies and Bajic, 2016).

Due to the quick predictions made and the constrained physical resources required, in silico approaches would seem to be the best option for screening chemicals with unknown hazardous potential. However, because of the intricacy and frequently significant variability of the data itself, in silico modeling of toxicity data is incredibly difficult. The complexity of the biological response and the scarcity of publicly accessible mechanistic data are the main reasons why in silico techniques have so far had trouble producing predictions that apply to in vivo situations (Gleeson et al., 2012). The precautions that are needed to be taken into consideration are discussed in the below paragraph.

The central aspect of computational chemistry is that related compounds behave similarly. However, it is well recognized that this is not always the case. Molecules with relatively little differences exhibit significantly divergent biological functions. Finding a precise correlation between structure and observed toxicity is much more complicated if the harmful event is caused by numerous processes, each of which depends on a compound's molecular structure differently (Gleeson et al., 2012). Limiting variables for predictive QSAR modeling include the certainty and accessibility of the high-quality experimental evidence used to construct the training data set and the familiarity of the QSAR model's end users with the specifics of the phenomenon being modeled. When erroneous information is used to build a model for toxicity research, the resulting inaccuracy is amplified (Valerio, 2009). An essential component of in silico evaluation is the development of a model for toxicity assessment. However, the prediction is invalid if a drug undergoing in silico screening does not fall under the applicability domain (Ballabio et al., 2019).

The researchers have investigated the toxicity profile of SARS-CoV-2 inhibitors by using in silico tools. They predicted the toxicity profile of 19 experimental compounds using web-based servers and applications. These compounds were monitored for hepatotoxicity, carcinogenicity, cardiotoxicity, mutagenicity, and acute oral toxicity testing. Based on the displayed toxicity endpoint, compounds were classified into three categories. This study data suggested 10 compounds (10/19) belong to category 1 (i.e., least likely toxic). Five compounds (5/19) make up category 2, which was primarily classified based on its high degree of resemblance to or the existence of structural alerts. Three compounds (3/19) were lastly placed in category 3 (Bhat and Chatterjee, 2021). However, one compound (1/19) was not classified owing to inadequate data to predict hepatotoxicity. An overview of this research is depicted in Fig. 24.10.

24.6.1 Case studies

Zhu et al. investigated in silico the genotoxicity of descarboxyl levofloxacin (an impurity in levofloxacin). They have used a commercial structure-activity relationship software package as an in silico tool. Molecular structures are entered into the program in MDL MOL format. The results showed a structural alert (quinoline) in this impurity. In vitro genotoxicity assays concluded that descarboxyl levofloxacin could be controlled as a nongenotoxic impurity (Zhu et al., 2014). Zhang et al. reported the evaluation of developmental toxicity employing

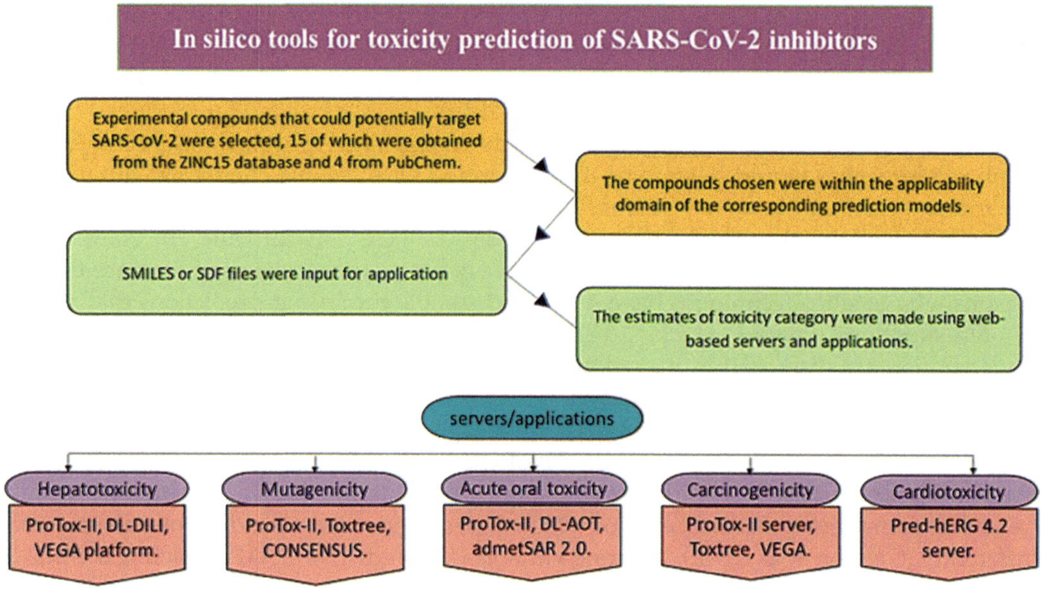

FIGURE 24.10 In silico tools for toxicity prediction of SARS-CoV-2 inhibitors.

methodologies from machine learning. In this study, binary classification systems for developmental toxicity were created using seven machine learning techniques, including naïve Bayes, k-nearest neighbor, support vector machines, recursive partitioning, random forest, C4.5 decision trees, and Adaboost. With this research, they have created an interpretable and practical developmental toxicology prediction model (Zhang et al., 2020).

The online server's admetSAR, ADMETlab, ProTox, ADVERPred, Pred-hERG, and Vienna LiverTox were used to conduct a thorough in silico toxicity evaluation of salubrinal and its analogs that had a cinnamic acid residue or quinoline ring. Salubrinal and its analogs were expected to have immunotoxic, cardiotoxic, and hepatotoxic effects. Using the homologous modeling method, models of the primary expected anti-targets hERG, bile salt export pump, multidrug resistance proteins 3, multidrug resistance proteins 4, and aryl hydrocarbon receptor were built. The resulting models were used to conduct molecular docking investigations. All targets underwent molecular docking using AutoDock Vina, a feature of the PyRx 0.8 software. The compounds were evaluated for their potential to inhibit targets following the findings of molecular docking (Zadorozhnii et al., 2020).

24.7 Chip technology in toxicity testing

24.7.1 DNA chip in toxicity testing

The expression of various genes may be used to describe how cells and organisms adapt to a disease state, toxicant exposure, or cellular metabolism (Lettieri, 2006). The development of technological tools for analyzing genetic data is accelerating. These tools include bioinformatics, DNA sequencing, and hybridization-based methods for detecting DNA and RNA. The development of DNA chips is also referred to as the DNA microarray technique. With miniaturization and multiplexation techniques, this technology enables examining thousands of genes in a single experimental run while using a smaller number of biological samples (Wilson and Nock, 2003). Long DNA molecules are immobilized on the chips (which are typically constructed of semiconductor materials like silicon and germanium) with the aid of high-speed robots and subsequent hybridization of these molecules and samples (Gabig-Cimińska and Wegrzyn, 2001). Typically, the complementary target DNA (cDNA) is radio-labeled, and the cDNA clones are spotted on nylon or nitrocellulose filter membranes. The target cDNAs are then hybridized in parallel or sequentially, and the data is obtained using a phosphoimager (Zarbl, 2001). Identifying single nucleotide polymorphisms (SNPs), genes for tumor suppressors, genes undergoing mutation, cancer biomarkers, the discovery of the toxicity's molecular causes, and drug development are all applications of microarray (Govindarajan et al., 2012).

The traditional methods for determining a substance's toxicity include rodent toxicity testing and testing for carcinogenicity. However, alternative in vitro tests such as the Ames test, cell transformation assays, and human cell mutation assays are gradually replacing animal models. The issue with these tests is that they produce complicated endpoints far from the initial exposure. Except for acute cell necrosis, every toxic agent has the potential to change the genetic makeup of the exposed cell, and gene expression, therefore, continues to be the first detectable biological reaction following exposure to a toxin. This property of the toxin has assisted researchers in identifying a particular toxicity signature concerning a certain kind of toxin (Zarbl, 2001). Thus, the creation of these signatures using microarray techniques may facilitate quicker toxicant screening for substances that are unknown or believed to be toxic (Lettieri, 2006). Therefore, using array technology in toxicology testing may enable the identification of physiologically significant toxicity thresholds (Zarbl, 2001).

Combining bioassay and gene screening using microarray methods enables low toxicant dosages, and minimal animal use since even a tiny amount of a toxicant can induce a change in gene expression. The link between chronic and acute toxicity may be determined by determining the subsequent effects of the toxicant and analyzing its gene expression profile and exposure (Nuwaysir et al., 1999). To comprehend how hazardous compounds affect human health negatively and from a regulatory standpoint, it is vital to understand their processes. As hundreds of genes are monitored by DNA chips, researchers may quickly pinpoint several harmful biochemical pathways. As a result, this will assist in understanding how cellular pathways are impacted by chemical agents, which will then aid in gaining mechanistic data (Hamadeh et al., 2001).

Chemical toxicity assessments may now be completed more quickly and effectively thanks to DNA chip technology, which has made it possible to monitor the genes implicated in toxicity and the pharmacologically active genes concurrently. Microarray technology is used in the domains of bioinformatics, pharmacogenomics, and genomics, which in combination have created the field of toxicogenomics (Sahu and Kishor, 2014). The use of microarrays to determine the signature of the toxicant and the expression of the gene patterns that are distinctive to a particular toxicant has greatly revolutionized toxicogenomics, which has caused a paradigm change in toxicology (Boverhof and Zacharewski, 2006).

To evaluate the chemical's toxicologic profile based on its gene expression patterns, DNA microarrays are utilized as quick screening methods (Pennie et al., 2001). There must be some degree of resemblance or a generalized pattern belonging to a class of toxicants to analyze the effect and verify the expression of the genes and how they regulate the various molecular mechanisms on exposure to the toxicant (Afshari et al., 1999). Different statistical methodologies and algorithms are required to assist in creating and designing mini arrays that would provide customized toxicity endpoints to discover the toxicity pattern of a particular chemical (Pennie et al., 2000).

Since mRNA copies are created during the transcription phase, which ultimately results in the production of proteins during the translation phase, mRNA serves as a substitute marker of gene expression. Thus, the genetic information may be evaluated by examining various mRNA expressions. Since mRNA is quickly degraded, turning it into stable cDNA makes it stable. The fundamental idea underlying DNA chips is the attachment of molecules with complementary sequences to one another. Because hydrogen bonds develop between the complementary base pairs of the nucleotide, the sequences of nucleic acids are linked explicitly with their complementary strands. Endonuclease-acted DNA sample molecules that are fluorescent, thanks to fluorochrome dyes like Cy5 and Cy3, are reacted with the probes of the DNA chips. Due to their fluorescence, the target DNA fragments that hybridize because they are complementary to the probe DNA are detected, while the uncomplimentary pairs are washed off. The chip's surface may be analyzed quantitatively and qualitatively using autoradiography, laser scanning, enzyme detection methods, and fluorescence detection techniques. As a result, this approach is recognized as quick, precise, and sensitive (Govindarajan et al., 2012).

Based on the deviation from unity created as a drop (<1) or an increase (>1) in the fluorescence data, the difference in the amount of expression between the reference and test samples is detected. The database with all the information about the gene's identification is then combined with this data. Concerning the reference condition, a particular set of changes characterized by the experimental condition's signature may be identified. Then, these signals may be contrasted using various visual techniques and tools for data mining and statistics (Zarbl, 2001). Lower confidence levels combined with biological and hybridization duplicates are an excellent method for identifying substantial changes in gene expression (Hamadeh et al., 2001).

The two primary high-density DNA microarrays are cDNA arrays and oligonucleotide arrays. The former is based on photolithography, which produces short oligonucleotides of 20 bases or less (Singh-Gasson et al., 1999). The cDNA arrays are created by the robotic arms depositing PCR fragments that range in size from 0.5 to 2 kb. On a single chip, around 25,000 cDNA spots may be arrayed (Guerreiro et al., 2003). In the microarray approach, either completely sequenced cDNA with known function or partly sequenced cDNA obtained from expressed sequence tags (ESTs) and corresponding to the mRNAs of unknown genes may be employed. It is possible to compare two different tissues (i.e., untreated and exposed cells) or diseased and healthy tissue cells. Their photos are scanned, superimposed, and their intensities are compared (Lobenhofer et al., 2001). Therefore, it is known that DNA chips can reduce the expense and time required to locate the altered expression of the genetic pattern caused by the toxin and get rid of such substances. It not only aids in determining the mechanism of action but also identifies the numerous off-target effects of the substance, aiding in the regulatory assessment of the substance. Fig. 24.11 demonstrates the principle of the DNA chip.

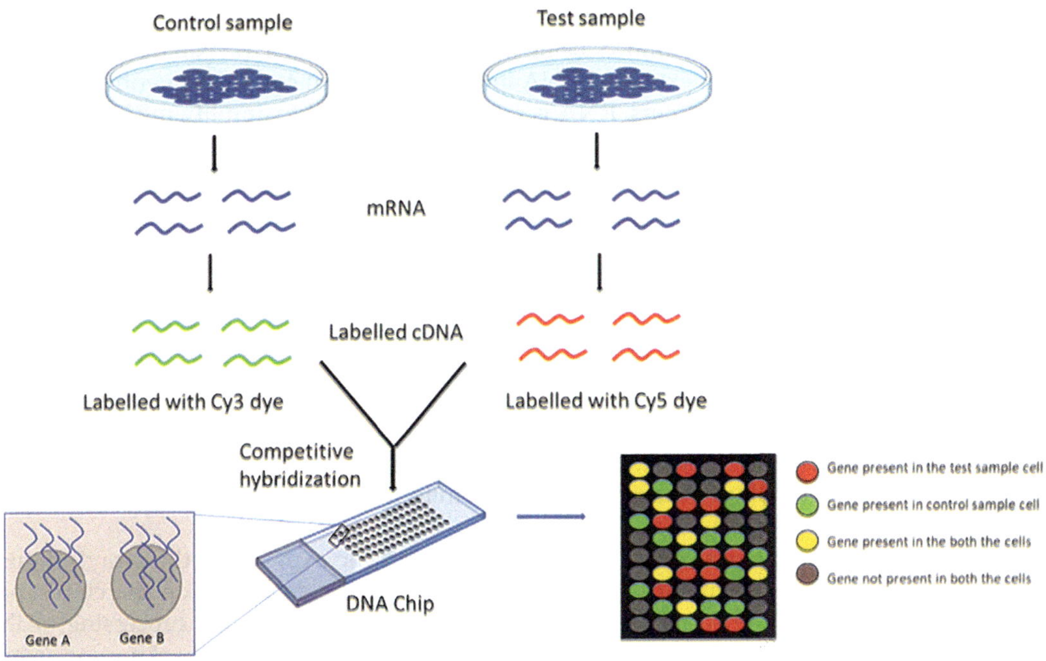

FIGURE 24.11 Principle of DNA chips.

The animal is administered with the substance of interest, then its tissue is extracted, and subsequent gene expression changes are examined using the microarray approach. Following excitation by the laser to the microarray, fluorescent signal intensities of the sample are analyzed, and the data produced is compared to the control samples to obtain a quantitative value of the change detected in the gene expression levels (Guerreiro et al., 2003).

With the use of high-speed robotic printers, cDNAs belonging to the specific gene sequence are spotted on the glass slide in the configuration required by the researcher. The cDNA is attached to the glass slide surface either by electrostatic interaction or by covalent linkage. After spotting the DNA, the chip is dried, treated with ultraviolet (UV) to cross-link, and a block treatment is given. Nonspecific binding by the cDNA to the chip during the hybridization process is prevented by the blocking procedure, while firm attachment of the cDNA to the chip is achieved with the help of UV cross-linkage. To increase the detection sensitivity, optimizing the signal-to-noise ratio by blocking is necessary, as it helps minimize the background noise. Gene expression variations as modest as a 1.2-fold increase or reduction can be detected by optimizing the measurements of the microarray procedure (Hamadeh et al., 2001).

Although the needed amount may vary based on various methods, it should typically be more than 1 μg. The microarray approach can only be carried out when there is a sufficient amount of RNA present. The RNA that has been extracted from the sample material has to be purified, the quality of which can be determined using capillary electrophoresis and the amount of which may be determined using either NanoPhotomer or NanoDrop. Reverse transcriptase may convert this extracted RNA into cDNA, which can subsequently be amplified using PCR. With polyT primers, RNA is reverse-transcribed to amplify mRNA. However, any RNA can be amplified using random primers. The deoxycytidine triphosphate (dCTP) or deoxyuridine triphosphate (dUTP) nucleotide is often changed by adding a chromophore. This is employed to use the reverse transcriptase process to transform the extracted RNA into fluorescently tagged targets. When they are stimulated by lasers and linked to the RNAs being compared, the fluorescent tags Cy5 and Cy3 show distinct emission colors or wavelengths. For Cy5 and Cy3, separate laser excitations are carried out at 632 and 532 nm, respectively. Data collected by scanning the microarray chips are transformed into 16-bit TFF pictures corresponding to each fluorophore. Following image conversion, two pictures are superimposed on top of one another, and with the use of specialist image processing software, each image is given a color intensity. As a result, the cDNA signals are shown in shades of green and red (Hamadeh et al., 2001). With the probe and target hybridization, which uses targets that have been silver, fluorophore, or chemiluminescence tagged, gene expression may be quantified (Khelurkar et al., 2017).

To determine the biological relevance of variations in gene expression, the array's digital picture is processed and then subjected to analysis. Localizing each spot on the chip separately and establishing the spot's border are the initial steps in the data processing of the raw material. After measuring the fluorescence intensity of each spot, the background intensity of the microarray is removed from the signal intensity, and the signal is then normalized (Li et al., 2002). The RNA must be of high quality, there must be little cross-hybridization, and the signal-to-noise ratio must be at its ideal for the hybridization to be successful and the analysis that follows. Although the RNA level is monitored by DNA chips or DNA microarray technology, the information translated into a functioning protein cannot be validated (Hamadeh et al., 2001).

24.7.2 Case studies

Using a DNA microarray technique, Turkez et al. investigated the impact of boron carbide NPs on human primary alveolar epithelial cells. It is well known that nozzles, low-wear bearings, cutting tools, and ballistic armor include boron carbide molecules. When it comes to medicinal applications, it is used in boron neutron capture therapy (BNCT), which is used to cure cancer. Using transmission electron microscopy (TEM), SEM, and X-ray diffraction (XRD) techniques, the author examined the properties of the created NPs. Following the characterization, they were added to the HPAEpiC cell line for 72 h at various concentrations.

To comprehend the connections between the NPs and their impacted gene pathways, a database for annotation, visualization, and integrated (DAVI) analysis was carried out. The quality of the extracted RNA was first assessed before amplification was carried out to carry out the microarray procedure. Twenty genes were found to be downregulated, while the remaining 12 genes were found to be upregulated among the 32 expression changes that were examined using this approach. The TGF-β pathway is the process of amino acid production, and developmental processes accounted for most of the expression alterations.

The downregulated genes were demonstrated to have a favorable effect on drug resistance and tumor progression. In contrast, the upregulated genes were revealed to be essential for stopping the cell growth cycle. Given the minimal toxicity profile of boron carbide NPs as determined by the microarray approach, it is, therefore, possible to conclude from this work that they may be employed as a safe nanomaterial (Turkez et al., 2019).

Hou et al. used the microarray approach to investigate the harmful effects of zinc oxide NPs on the zebrafish cell cycle. The research concluded that exposure to NPs reduced zebrafish growth and development. A total of 4170 differentially expressed genes were examined using the microarray method. These genes' gene ontologies revealed 63 enriched terms for cellular components, 166 enriched terms for biological processes, and 64 enriched terms for molecular processes. The toxicity of zinc oxide NPs was observed by determining the function of intracellular organelles in cell component processes, the function of cell metabolism in biological processes, and the function of transferase activity in molecular processes. Further, the results of the Kyoto encyclopedia of genes and genomes (KEGG) pathway analysis revealed that the cell cycle and DNA replication were most significantly impacted by the toxicity of zinc oxide NPs. Due to the inhibition of cyclin-dependent kinase, microsome maintenance, and cyclin expression, the DNA replication phases were disorganized during various cell cycle phases. The findings of the quantitative real-time polymerase chain reaction (RT-qPCR) were used to validate further the microarray results (Hou et al., 2019). Using microarray technology, Sheng et al. investigated the biological route of titanium dioxide NPs to determine the toxicity they caused in the spleen. Different NPs concentrations were administered intra-gastrically to mice over 90 days for the study.

Further analysis of the altered gene expression in the injured mouse spleen revealed that exposure to the NPs caused immune system malfunction, increased spleen indexes, a significant infiltration of macrophagic cells, and spleen death. The genes that were seen to be altered were all involved in signal transduction, cell division, stress responses, inflammatory responses, ion transport, and apoptosis. Of these genes, 744 genes were downregulated, and 450 were upregulated. Lbp, Cd86, Cd14, Mt1, Cyp2e1, Cd80, Il7r, and Fcnb were also shown to be some of the possible biomarkers of spleen toxicity that developed following exposure to titanium NPs. Therefore, specific biomarkers associated with spleen toxicity were discovered using DNA chip technology, and molecular pathways causing splenic damage were also evaluated (Sheng et al., 2014). Table 24.3 summarizes the DNA chip technology for testing the materials.

24.7.3 Microfluidic chips in toxicity testing

With biochemical analysis, the mechanism behind many life processes may be established for biological study. Animal models used today are expensive, time-consuming, and fraught with ethical dilemmas. Because human pathology is a complicated process, it is difficult to comprehend its mechanism. As a result, microfluidics has now established itself as a crucial instrument for study (Jiang et al., 2013). Microfabrication technique with enhanced surface chemistry, made feasible by the microfluidic system, may successfully recreate tissue microenvironment at the cellular level (Jiang et al., 2013). The benefits of microfluidics include its ability to operate at the microscale level, the ease with which different detection techniques

TABLE 24.3 Summary of research utilizing DNA chip technology to test toxicity.

The sample analyzed/ toxicant	Target/cell line used	Bead chips/ microarray used	Assay	Readout systems	Informatics	References
Boron carbide NPs	Human primary alveolar epithelial cells	Human HT-12 v 4.0 expression bead chips	MTT, LDH, and NR assays	Illumina bead array reader	DAVI analysis, cytotoxicity analysis	Turkez et al. (2019)
Titanium dioxide NPs	Spleen of mouse	Illumina human HT-12 v 3.0 bead vhips	Quantitative real-time PCR and enzyme-linked immunosorbent assay (ELISA)	Illumina bead array reader	Genome studio software version 2009	Sheng et al. (2014)
T-2 toxin and deoxynivalenol (DON)	Human chondrocytes	Affymetrix human gene chip	RT-qPCR	Affymetrix® GeneChip® command Console® (AGCC) software	Gene ontology analysis, KEGG pathway analysis	Yang et al. (2020)
Silica NPs and benzo[*a*]pyrene	Zebrafish embryos	Zebrafish gene 1.0 ST array	MTT assay	Affymetrix® expression console software	Gene ontology (GO) analysis, STC and STC-GO analysis, pathway analysis, signal-net analysis	Asweto et al. (2018)
Copper oxide NPs	Rat lungs	SurePrint G3 Rat 8 × 60 K microarrays	ELISA	Software feature extraction 10.7.3	Gene ontology analysis, pathway analysis	Gosens et al. (2021)

may be included, and its flexibility in terms of design (Wu et al., 2016). Due to its high level of automation, use of fewer samples, quick turnaround times for analysis, provision of miniaturization-based in vitro testing, and microfluidics outperform conventional approaches. Thus, a single microfluidic chip can detect, process, and react with various substances.

As two-dimensional (2D) cell cultures cannot anticipate cellular activities due to insufficient cellular microenvironments, they are replaced by three-dimensional (3D) cell cultures, adding tissue complexity and enabling the investigation of cell interactions. However, even in this setting, it is challenging to accurately analyze the function of the transport system and cell genetics. Microfluidic technologies have enabled it to overcome this drawback (Aziz et al., 2017). The microchannel is utilized in microfluidics because of its large surface area, high mass transfer, and compact size. This allows for reduced reagent usage, quick reactions, quick fixing rates, and adjustable volumes (Whitesides, 2006). Microfluidic systems like "cell on a chip" and "organ on a chip" have both been created. The cell on the chip uses various cytotoxicity data from human and animal research that helps screen the chemical's toxicological data. These technologies are made of either a cell chamber or a simple channel with tested and cultivated cell monolayers. Different kidney, lung, liver, central nervous system, bone marrow, and intestinal chips have been designed for organ-on-a-chip systems. These organ systems support the development of 3D microarchitecture, provide the system with a sophisticated biochemical and organ-specific milieu, and enable beneficial tissue-tissue interactions. As a result, they more closely resemble in vivo circumstances than the single monolayer of primary cells (Dai et al., 2016).

"Organs on chips" have perfused microchannels that make it easier to in vitro simulate organ-level architecture and functions. This approach impacts the pathophysiology and development of human tissue because it can offer pertinent mechanical cues, high-resolution imaging, and independent access to the vascular compartment, parenchymal compartment, and tissue's apical lumina. By utilizing stem cell biology, tissue engineering, and microfluidic methods, organs-on-chips technology is revolutionizing drug research, its screening, and preclinical testing (Jalili-Firoozinezhad et al., 2021). Only substances that pass safety and performance tests move on to clinical trials. Thus, it's critical to assess a compound's toxicity in preclinical research to provide information about the safety and dosage of a given medicine (Wu et al., 2010). Thus, microfluidic chips help create a noninvasive imaging-based test to assess the drug's toxicity by tracking and analyzing multiple toxicity markers and cellular processes (Cui and Wang, 2019).

It is crucial to carry out both in vitro and in vivo toxicity tests to assess the safety of the chemical compounds being created. Traditional 2D culture models can be used to evaluate a compound's toxicity and effectiveness, but they cannot adequately simulate physiological settings and hence cannot demonstrate tissue-to-tissue interactions. Additionally, they might be time-consuming and expensive automation methods. Therefore, microfluidic chips facilitate quicker evaluation and provide high throughput parallel examination of the materials. They are also cost-effective for submitting toxicity data to regulatory filings (McCormick et al., 2017).

Using the fundamental governing equations, the field of fluid mechanics known as microfluidics investigates fluid flow physics. A microfluidic system primarily has laminar fluid flow. To create a master mold, materials like silicon, glass, or plastic are frequently utilized (Balijepalli and Sivaramakrishan, 2017). The array of microchannels on the thin plastic or glass chip used in microfluidic devices, sometimes referred to as miniature labs, measures several centimeters in width and 100 μm in length (Li, 2010). By puncturing the chips with holes, syringe adapters, or output and input tubing on the microchannel network, the interface between the micro and the macro world is created. Through these, the gases or liquids are introduced into and evacuated from the system using external active systems like peristaltic pumps, syringe pumps, and pressure controllers or by various passive methods like hydrostatic pressure (Casquillas et al., 2018). The wells at the ends of the microchannel branches serve as a reservoir for different reagents and samples to be added to them.

Furthermore, by concurrently applying various voltages to various wells, they attach the electrodes to the liquid and subsequently regulate the flow of the liquid. This procedure aids in directing and managing the solution's flow in a specific direction without interfering with the stationary solutions in other wells. The essential features of microfluidics are dispensing a particular amount of solution from one microchannel to another and combining various solutions. These tasks may be accomplished with electrophoresis and electroosmotic flow (Li, 2010).

Organ-on-chip microfluidics technology enables the mimicking of the natural physiology and diverse mechanical forces that exist in the human body. The chips are lined with a monolayer of human cells, and the tiny fluidic channels replicate blood and air flow precisely as they do in the human body. This enables the chips to simulate various human physiological circumstances, such as muscular contractions or breathing motions. The transparency of the chips makes it possible to observe the molecular and cellular behavior, responses, and activities of the organ. Microfluidics, living cell tissues, drug delivery stimulation, and sensing and analysis components are the chips' primary important constituents (Mandenius, 2018). The target cells are delivered to the predetermined area via the microfluidic component, which is automated and has a mechanism for supplying culture fluid and releasing waste liquid throughout the culturing process (Kwon and Oh, 2018). The live tissue cell component can be aligned in either a 2D or 3D configuration. In the latter, the hydrogel scaffold gives the structure strength and aids in preventing mechanical damage to the structure (Tibbe et al., 2018).

Chemical and physical signals, such as electrical stimulation, are necessary for the maturation of the myocardial tissue to imitate the physiological microenvironment and so enhance the function and tissue maturation of the system. For the complete assessment, the metabolic status at characteristic locations must be read using microsensors (Wu et al., 2020). Appropriate biomarkers must be used for toxicity testing since increased biomarker expression will cause the limit of detection to be lowered (Cong et al., 2020). Fig. 24.12 illustrates the fabrication process of a microfluidic chip and lung-on-chip microfluidic device.

24.7.3.1 Case studies

Bircsak et al. used microfluidic technology by designing a 3D microfluidic liver. Hepatocytes generated from aggregates of induced pluripotent stem cells were cocultured with endothelial cells and THP-1 monoblasts, which were developed into macrophages. The system was fully automated to seed, dose, collect, replace, and simultaneously add different test reagents to the medium. The vitality of the cells for 15 days was determined using various image-based analytic techniques, and albumin and urea secretions were examined. By introducing them at a concentration of 50 μM for 72 h, the toxicity of around 159 compounds was examined, along with their Toxicological Prioritization ratings (Bircsak et al., 2021).

Khalid et al. developed a multi-organ on-chip platform for lung cancer to measure the transepithelial electrical resistance (TEER) impedance and assess the cytotoxicity of docetaxel and doxorubicin. The 3D-printed digital microscope and indium tin oxide electrodes allowed for the visual monitoring of the system. An optical pH sensor was used to assess the pH of the media. Real-time biosensor data was gathered when NCI–H1437 lung cancer cells were planted on the microfluidic glass chip. The live/dead test and the cell index were used to assess the TEER impedance response. Utilizing imaging software, the vitality of the cells was quantified, and the results were then compared to the impedimetric cell index. According to the statistics, it was found that docetaxel has a lower toxicity index than doxorubicin (Khalid et al., 2020).

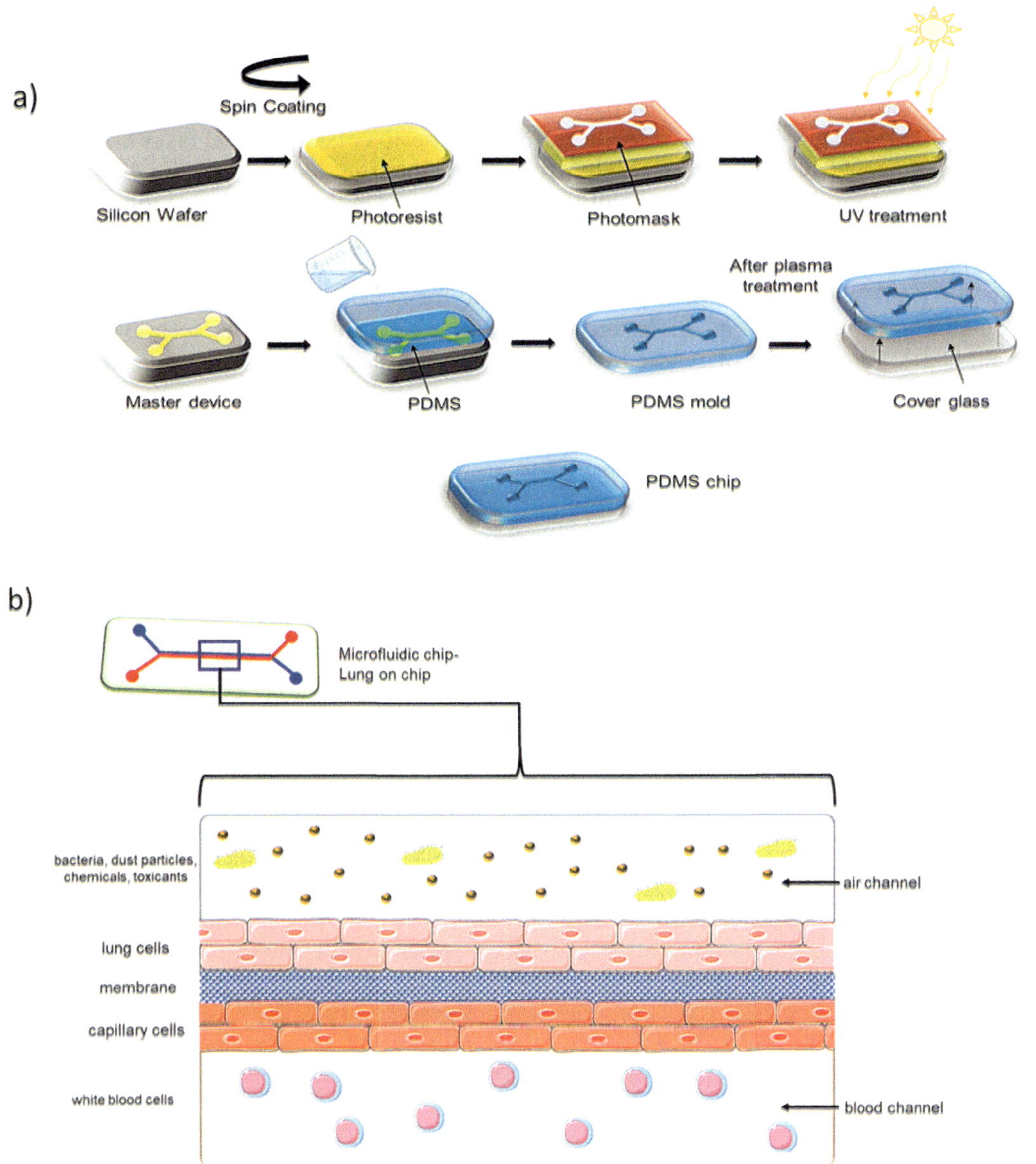

FIGURE 24.12 (A) Fabrication of microfluidic chip and (B) lung-on-chip model of the microfluidic chip. A membrane sits between air and the blood channel, through which the compartments can interact like the physiological process in the body.

Different respiratory conditions, including pneumonia, asthma, upper respiratory infections, and chronic obstructive pulmonary disease, are linked to a toxin called PM2.5. PM2.5's propensity to collect in the lung's alveoli and its capacity to enter the circulatory system through the alveolar-capillary exchange (ACE) mechanism is responsible for its toxicity. An ACE chip was therefore created by Guan et al. to evaluate the toxicity of the PM2.5 chemical. The ACE chip comprised of human umbilical vein endothelial cells (HUVEC) and A549 human alveolar basal epithelial cells were seeded in the polydimethylsiloxane (PDMS) chamber, which aided in simulating the alveolar epithelial layer and vascular endothelial layer. The microporous polycarbonate membrane that divided the two compartments allowed for the exchange of soluble materials between them. To define the mechanism of oxidative damage and endoplasmic reticulum stress in apoptosis induced by exposure to PM2.5, the chip was used to act as a model of the blood and air barriers. It was discovered that PEAK-eIF2 signaling is primarily responsible for causing the toxic effects. Hence, the toxic mechanism route was discovered with the aid of microfluidic technology (Guan et al., 2021). A summary of research utilizing microfluidic chip technology to test toxicity is described in Table 24.4.

TABLE 24.4 Summary of research utilizing microfluidic chip technology to test toxicity.

Target model	Cell types	Cocultured cells	Fabrication methods	Assays	References
Liver chip	iPSC iCell 2.0 hepatocytes	Differentiated THP-1, HMEC-1 endothelial cells	OrganoPlate 2-lane	Secretome measurements, ell viability assessment, immunofluorescent staining	Bircsak et al. (2021)
Lung cancer chip	Lung cancer NCI–H1437 cells	RPMI 1640 cell culture medium supplemented with 10% FBS v/v and 1% v/v pen/strep antibiotic solution	Fabricated using two soda lime glass layers- 3D printing to discharge the biocompatible silicone elastomer	Impedimetric cell index and live/dead assay	Khalid et al. (2020)
Alveolar-capillary exchange (ACE) chip	Alveolar epithelial cells and vascular endothelial cells	Vascular endothelial cells	Two PDMS layers were combined by electrostatic adsorption.	Immunolabeling for phosphorylated histone H3 (PHH3), apoptosis assay, ROS assay, cytokine analysis	Guan et al. (2021)
CNS chip	Cells from hippocampi of 18 or 21-day-old fetal rats	E18 dissociated cells, poly-L-lysine, neurobasal medium	Photolithography based on SU-8 photoresist	Calcium imaging, TEM and thioflavin-T characterization, toxicity analysis by dye method	Ruiz et al. (2014)
Ovarian follicle chip	Intact multilayered ovarian follicles were isolated from rats	Inhibitor, DOX, cultural medium, PP1, 2APB, AZD1208	Two plates of polymethyl methacrylate substrate and three layers of polydimethylsiloxane (PDMS)	Diameter measurement and hormone test, PCR, TUNEL assay	Aziz et al. (2020)

Over the previous few decades, nothing has changed concerning the fundamental technique of general toxicity. Clinical chemistry, hematological, and histological data have been primarily used to assess toxicity in animal models as indications of organ dysfunction (Bojarski and Witeska, 2020; Uzoekwe et al., 2020). A harmful chemical's impact on gene expression reflects its impact on a biological system at the cellular level. As a result, it is possible to learn important information about a substance's potential toxicity until a hazardous or pathological reaction develops by measuring the transcription (i.e., mRNA) as well as translation (i.e., protein) products for gene regulation (Huang et al., 2018; Balasubramanian et al., 2020).

Together with the ever-growing power of bioinformatics, the quick advancement of genomic (DNA sequence), transcriptomic (gene expression), as well as proteomic (the investigation of proteins expressed by a genome, tissue, or cell) techniques offers a rare opportunity to serve as the foundation for enhanced hazard identification for further predictive safety assessment (Manzoni et al., 2018; Stenton et al., 2020). Some currently available methods for studying gene expression at the transcription level are discussed in Fig. 24.13.

Two-dimensional gel electrophoresis, which separates proteins using isoelectric focusing in the first dimension and sodium dodecyl sulfate-polyacrylamide gel electrophoresis (SDS-PAGE) based on the molecular weight in the second dimension, is an extremely sensitive method of monitoring for toxicity as well as probing toxic mechanisms (Borna et al., 2019; Baillie, 2020). The ability to detect variations in biochemical pathways via observed changes in sets of genes/proteins that might have been linked to the toxicity provides the means to describe the expression of thousands of messengers RNAs as well as proteins and can be

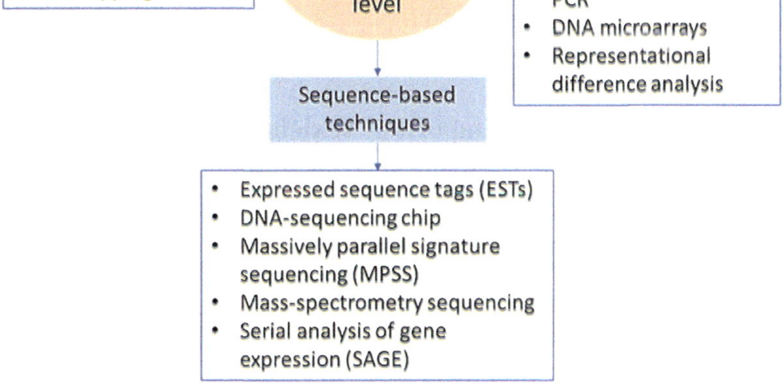

FIGURE 24.13 The available transcript level methods for the study of gene expression.

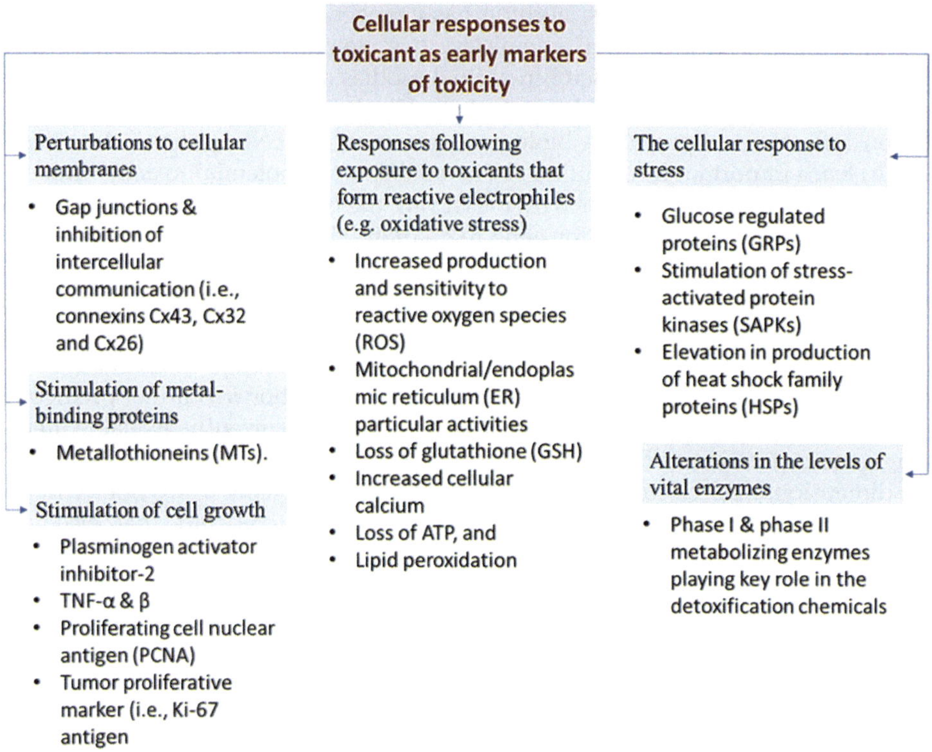

FIGURE 24.14 Some critical cellular responses employed as early markers of toxicity to toxicant exposure.

obtained by analyzing gene/protein expression upon exposure of a biological test system to a chemical present under untreated conditions.

Over the past few years, an enormous quantity of research has led to an explosion in knowledge about the mechanisms behind toxicity and the development of brand-new techniques for investigating biological reactions to toxic stress. Some vital cellular responses to toxicant exposure are described in Fig. 24.14. These cellular responses could potentially be used as early toxicity markers.

24.8 Some important toxicity endpoints

24.8.1 Toxicokinetic study

The metabolism as well as the removal of xenobiotics inside a body as a result of dosage and time are described by toxicokinetic modeling (Asati et al., 2022; Gupta et al., 2022c; Tambe et al., 2021a). Compartmental models that are based on data and those that are based on physiological principles make up the two primary categories of toxicokinetic models. To get essential data in this field, in vitro methods might be applied. In vitro studies can be used to determine one representative model, the physiologically based toxicokinetic (PB-TK) model, as well as the tissue-blood partition coefficients, the kinetics of every active transport method, and the kinetics of metabolism through the liver or any organ able for biotransforming the substance (Rajpoot et al. 2021b, 2022b; Achanta et al., 2021; Tambe et al., 2021b). The determination of concentration/time effects in various tissues results from toxicokinetic models. An estimate of the substance's acute systemic toxicity may be made using this information and the data on baseline cytotoxicity (Rajpoot et al., 2022c).

24.8.2 Genotoxicity

Additionally, three levels of mutation (i.e., gene, chromosomal, and genomic mutations) can be evaluated for genotoxicity using the in vitro system to detect probable carcinogens (Kohl et al., 2020; White et al., 2019). The following are confirmed as the commonly accepted goals of testing chemicals for genotoxicity i.e., (a) identifying germ cell mutagens due to their potential role in the etiology of heritable genetic defects in humans and (b) identifying somatic cell mutagens due to their role in neoplastic transformation (Kirsch-Volders et al., 2019). The OECD protocols, which modified six prior standards and established a new one in 1997, are advised for usage in terms of test methodologies.

All such guidelines offer guidance for both the in vivo testing (such as micronuclei as well as chromosomal aberrations in rodent bone marrow, rat liver unscheduled DNA synthesis and chromosomal aberrations in spermatogonia) and the in vitro screening tests (such as gene mutations in bacteria and mammalian cells, chromosomal aberrations in vitro) (OECD, 2016a,b,c,d, 2022). Genetic toxicity can also be ascertained using a variety of practical approaches that have been established. An alternative to the in vitro chromosomal aberration assay presently being studied for inclusion in test cells is the in vitro micronucleus test procedure (Cayir et al., 2020; Sommer et al., 2020).

Large-scale production of titanium dioxide (TiO_2) NPs is done for various uses. The reliability of TiO_2 NPs in the perspective of deliberate and accidental human exposure, occupational exposure, as well as environmental exposure expresses concern due to their widespread use. In a study, the micronucleus (MN) assay was used to evaluate the genotoxicity of TiO_2 NPs (Fig. 24.15) using different cell lines, namely human lung epithelial cell line (A549), human liver cell line (HepG2), human glial cell line (A172), and human neuronal cell line (SH-SY5Y). Neither of the cell lines demonstrated appreciable improvements in MN frequencies under the studied circumstances (Brandao et al., 2020).

Chromosome loss, as well as nondisjunction-specific probes based on fluorescence in situ hybridization (FISH) (Albertini and Kaden, 2020), enable quick scoring of aneuploidy in a range of cell types, particularly human cells. Mammalian cell tests must be regularly carried out following the most recent standard methods for identifying fundamental chromosomal abnormalities by metaphase analyses or gene mutation (at tk, HPRT, or other loci) (White et al., 2019). As shown in Fig. 24.16A, certain typical processes can be used to assess a compound's non-genotoxic carcinogenicity. In addition, some potential short-term tests are also designed for nongenotoxic carcinogens (Fig. 24.16B).

Generally, no technique is sufficient to identify even a considerable proportion of nongenotoxic carcinogens. Nevertheless, it could be able to pinpoint critical toxicological reactions that give a prominent indicator of carcinogenicity by concentrating on those pathways that seem to affect people.

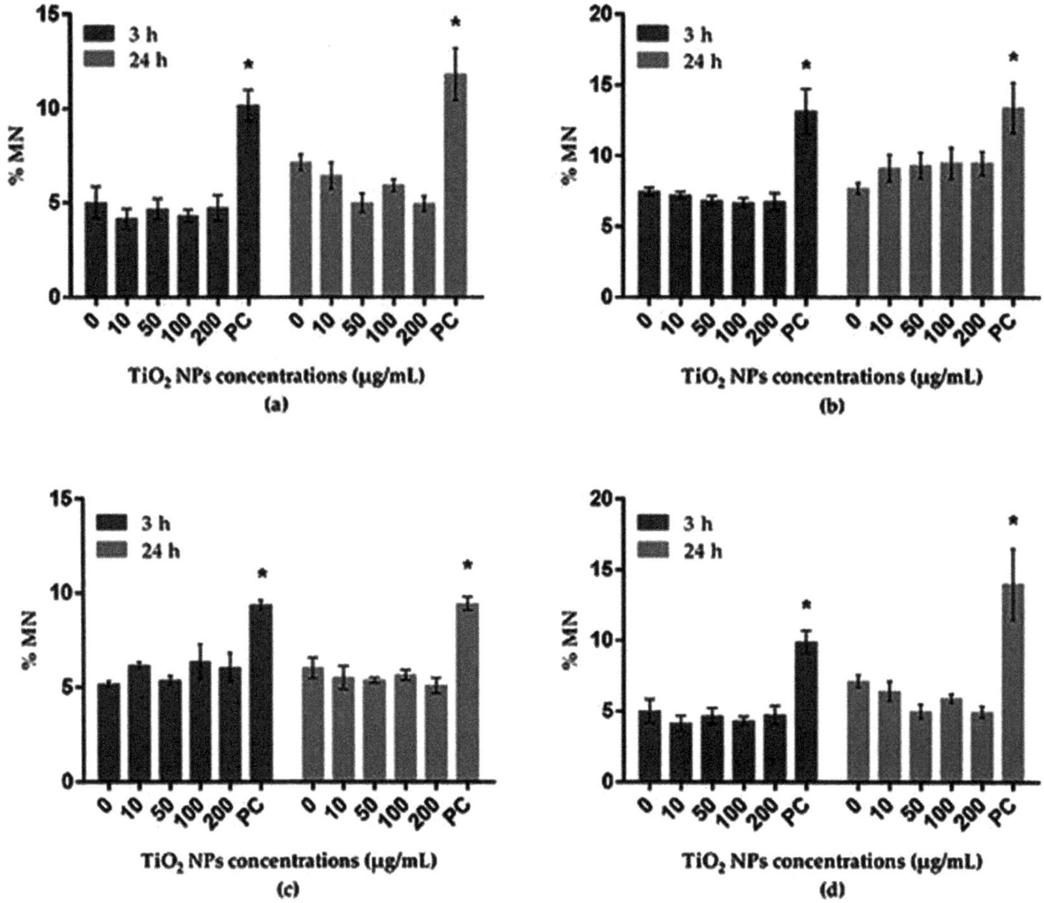

FIGURE 24.15 MN frequency was confirmed using flow cytometry in A549 (A), HepG2 (B), A172 (C), and SH-SY5Y (D) after exposure to TiO_2 NPs. PC, positive control (*$P \leq .05$) (Brandao et al., 2020).

24.8.3 Developmental toxicity

Investigations on male and female fertility, as well as developmental toxicity, are included in the area of reproductive toxicology, with a focus on investigations on embryotoxicity and teratogenicity (Li et al., 2022). Over 30 distinct culture techniques have been suggested as assays for developmental toxicity over the past decades. Different types of culture systems frequently employed for toxicity assessment are described in Fig. 24.17.

24.8.4 Cell lines and embryonic stem cells (ESCs)

In the 1980s, many well-established cell lines were utilized for screening of drugs. These include neuroblastoma cells, mice ovarian tumor cells, & human embryonic palate mesenchymal cells. The findings reveal a significant percentage of false positives results. Using

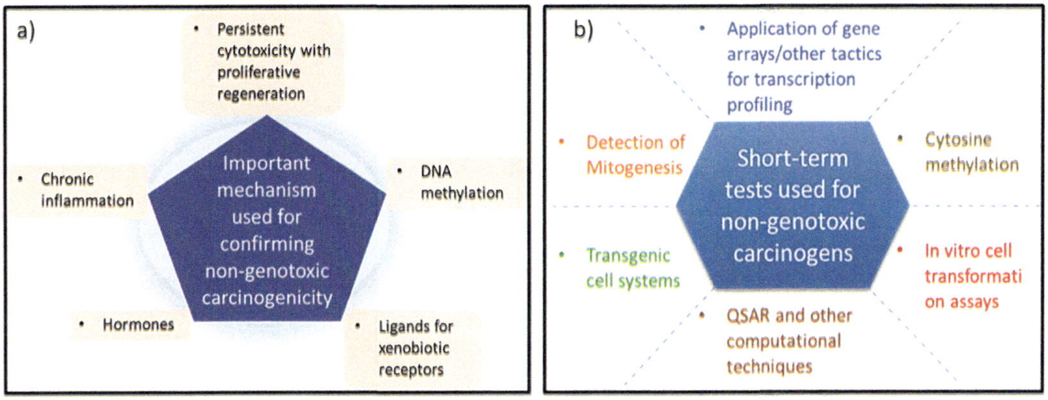

FIGURE 24.16 (A) Mechanisms used for determining non-genotoxic carcinogenicity. (B) List of short-term tests used for identification of non-genotoxic carcinogens.

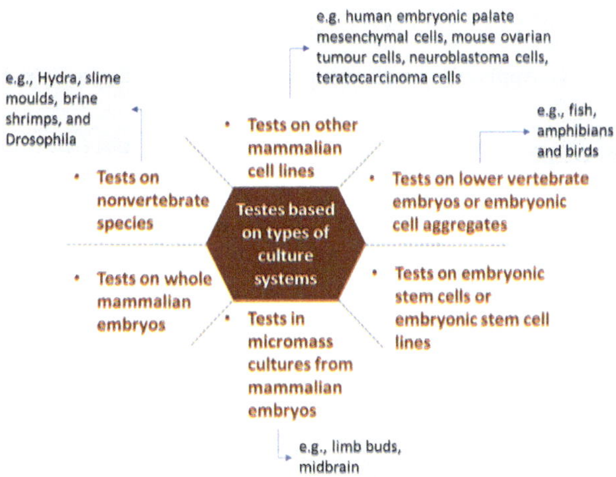

FIGURE 24.17 Different types of toxicity testing culture systems.

omnipotent embryonic stem cell lines yields more favorable outcomes (Charitos et al., 2021; Gorantla et al., 2021). For example, blastocyst totipotent ESCs can be grown under circumstances that allow the cells to develop into various types, including muscle and hemopoietic cells. The two essential characteristics of embryotoxicity—inhibition of differentiation and/or increased susceptibility to cytotoxic effects in embryonic cells than over adult tissues—can be identified using these culture methods (Ahmed et al., 2021; Kim et al., 2019).

The outcomes of this kind of assay were equivalent to those of testing the embryotoxicity of rats' entire embryo cultures. The development of transgenic cells with specific mutations and reporter components using ESCs might make it possible to create tests with easy-to-use outcomes that can be applied to automated assay methods. Furthermore, recent research shows great promise in isolating multipotent (or even totipotent) stem cells using adult tissues.

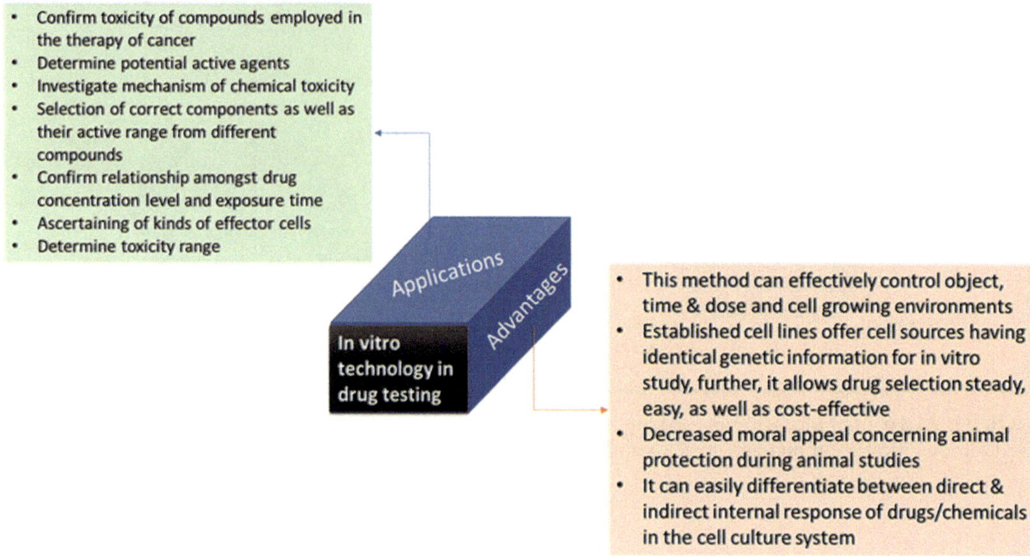

FIGURE 24.18 Applications and advantages of in vitro technology in drug testing.

For instance, hematopoietic stem cells may develop from neural tissue stem cells, and vice versa (Ottoboni et al., 2020).

Additionally, testing methods for identifying developmental toxicity employing aggregate and micro mass cultures, lesser-order species' embryos, as well as entire mammalian and avian embryo cultures have also been reported and are often employed. They make it possible to identify dysmorphogenesis in several distinct organs and to compare the particular consequences of dysmorphogenesis with broader negative effects on development and differentiation. Additionally, they make it possible to rate the efficacy of compounds with structural similarities. These methods' drawbacks include the possibility that they can be expensive, mainly cover a small portion of organogenesis, are highly technical, and are pretty sophisticated. Additionally, in vitro culture detection systems are better suited for teratogenic, carcinogenic, and mutagenic substances as well as anticancer medications (Mattes, 2020).

In vitro culture technique has established itself as a standard method for assessing cytotoxicity and efficacy internationally (Riss et al., 2019), even if the efficacy, adverse response, and safety assessment of the medicine need certain animal trials. As a result, in vitro testing for drugs is being used more and more often. Fig. 24.18 describes the applications and advantages of in vitro technology in drug testing.

24.9 Conclusions

Determining how different medications affect cells in vitro at different doses is not entirely applicable to in vivo conditions. The in vivo developing environment is far more complex than the in vitro culture conditions, which is one of the drawbacks of in vitro testing. In addition to having a fully functional regulatory system, in vivo trials can also change metabolism and pharmacological biochemistry (via the liver, kidneys, and various organs, etc.) and have an immunological impact. Further, monomer drugs (other than compound medications) and Chinese patent medicines can be tested for cytotoxicity and activity utilizing an in vitro technique. Compared to the water-insoluble drug, which may require a suitable solvent to dissolve it, and a control group in the study designed to conquer the influence of the solvent itself on the cell, the medication soluble in water is easy to test. Because the in vitro technique is best suited for studying acute toxicity, developing the culture system is necessary for studying persistent effects.

24.10 List of abbreviations

2D two-dimensional
3D three-dimensional
A172 human glial cell line
A549 human lung epithelial cell line
AB alamarblue
ACE alveolar-capillary exchange
AcTOR aggregated computational toxicology resource
ADC antibody drug conjugate
AGCC affymetrix GeneChip Command Console
AgNPs silver NPs
ANN artificial neural network
ATP adenosine 5′-triphosphate
BEA beauvericin
BNCT boron neutron capture therapy
cDNA complementary DNA
CDs carbon dots
DAVI database for annotation, visualization, and integrated
dCTP deoxycytidine triphosphate
DON deoxynivalenol
DOX doxorubicin
dUTP deoxyuridine triphosphate
ECHA European Chemicals Agency
ELISA enzyme-linked immunosorbent assay
ESCs embryonic stem cells
ESTs expressed sequence tags
EU European Union
FISH fluorescence in situ hybridization
GO gene ontology
HBRs human-based rules
HepG2 human liver cell line
HIV human immunodeficiency virus
HUVEC human umbilical vein endothelial cells
IBRs induction-based rules
IC50 half-maximal inhibitory concentration
KEGG kyoto encyclopedia of genes and genomes
LDH lactate dehydrogenase
MN micronucleus

MTT 3-(4,5- dimethylthiazol-2-yl)-2,5 diphenyl tetrazolium bromide
NPs nanoparticles
OECD Organization for Economic Co-operation and Development
OTA ochratoxin A
PB-TK physiologically based toxicokinetic
PDMS polydimethylsiloxane
QSAR quantitative structure-activity relationships
REACH registration, evaluation, authorization and restriction of chemicals
RF random forest
ROS reactive oxygen species
RT-qPCR quantitative real time polymerase chain reaction
SDS-PAGE sodium dodecyl sulfate-polyacrylamide gel electrophoresis
SEM scanning electron microscopy
SH-SY5Y human neuronal cell line
SNPs single nucleotide polymorphisms
SVM support vector machine
TEER trans-epithelial electrical resistance
TEM transmission electron microscopy
TiO_2 titanium dioxide
UFAW Universities Federation for Animal Welfare
UV ultra-violet
WST 2-(4-iodophenyl)-3-(4-nitrophenyl)-5-(2,4-disulfophenyl)-2Htetrazolium monosodium salt
XRD X-ray diffraction
XTT 2,3-bis (2-methoxy-4-nitro 5-sulphophenyl)-5-carboxanilide-2H-tetrazolium, monosodium salt

References

Achanta, N.S.K., Rajpoot, K., Tekade, R.K., 2021. Drug metabolic kinetics. In: Tekade, R.K. (Ed.), Biopharmaceutics and Pharmacokinetics Considerations. Elsevier, Academic Press, pp. 335–353.

Adan, A., Kiraz, Y., Baran, Y., 2016. Cell proliferation and cytotoxicity assays. Curr. Pharmaceut. Biotechnol. 17 (14), 1213–1221. https://www.ncbi.nlm.nih.gov/pubmed/27604355.

Afshari, C.A., Nuwaysir, E.F., Barrett, J.C., 1999. Application of complementary DNA microarray technology to carcinogen identification, toxicology, and drug safety evaluation. Cancer Res. 59 (19), 4759–4760. https://www.ncbi.nlm.nih.gov/pubmed/10519378.

Ahmed, U., Ahmed, R., Masoud, M.S., Tariq, M., Ashfaq, U.A., Augustine, R., Hasan, A., 2021. Stem cells based in vitro models: trends and prospects in biomaterials cytotoxicity studies. Biomed. Mater. 16 (4), 042003. https://www.ncbi.nlm.nih.gov/pubmed/33686970.

Al-Nasiry, S., Geusens, N., Hanssens, M., Luyten, C., Pijnenborg, R., 2007. The use of Alamar Blue assay for quantitative analysis of viability, migration and invasion of choriocarcinoma cells. Hum. Reprod. 22 (5), 1304–1309. https://www.ncbi.nlm.nih.gov/pubmed/17307808.

Albertini, R.J., Kaden, D.A., 2020. Mutagenicity monitoring in humans: global versus specific origin of mutations. Mutat. Res. Rev. Mutat. Res. 786, 108341. https://www.ncbi.nlm.nih.gov/pubmed/33339577.

Alkimin, G.D., Daniel, D., Frankenbach, S., Serodio, J., Soares, A., Barata, C., Nunes, B., 2019. Evaluation of pharmaceutical toxic effects of non-standard endpoints on the macrophyte species Lemna minor and Lemna gibba. Sci. Total Environ. 657, 926–937. https://www.ncbi.nlm.nih.gov/pubmed/30677958.

An, Y.-J., 2006. Assessment of comparative toxicities of lead and copper using plant assay. Chemosphere 62 (8), 1359–1365.

Anup, N., Desai, N., Rajpoot, K., Tekade, R.K., 2021a. Kinetics of maternal–fetal drug transfer. In: Tekade, R.K. (Ed.), Biopharmaceutics and Pharmacokinetics Considerations, pp. 145–162. https://doi.org/10.1016/B978-0-12-814425-1.00007-3.

Anup, N., Gadeval, A., Rajpoot, K., Tekade, R.K., 2021b. Software used in ADME computation. In: Tekade, R.K. (Ed.), Biopharmaceutics and Pharmacokinetics Considerations. Elsevier, Academic Press, pp. 699–708.

Anup, N., Rajpoot, K., Tekade, R.K., 2021c. Overview of biopharmaceutics and pharmacokinetics. In: Tekade, R.K. (Ed.), Biopharmaceutics and Pharmacokinetics Considerations, vol. 1. Elsevier, Academic Press, pp. 1−16.

Araújo, A.S.F., Monteiro, R.T.R., 2005. Plant bioassays to assess toxicity of textile sludge compost. Sci. Agric. 62, 286−290.

Asati, S., Pandey, V., Gour, V., Tiwari, R., Soni, V., Rajpoot, K., Tekade, M., Sharma, M.C., Tekade, R.K., 2022. Toxicity and toxicokinetic considerations in product development and drug research. In: Pharmacokinetics and Toxicokinetic Considerations, vol. 2. Elsevier. https://doi.org/10.1016/b978-0-323-98367-9.00001-9.

Asweto, C.O., Hu, H., Liang, S., Wang, L., Liu, M., Yang, H., Duan, J., Sun, Z., 2018. Gene profiles to characterize the combined toxicity induced by low level co-exposure of silica nanoparticles and benzo[a]pyrene using whole genome microarrays in zebrafish embryos. Ecotoxicol. Environ. Saf. 163, 47−55. https://www.ncbi.nlm.nih.gov/pubmed/30036756.

Azarmi, S., Tao, X., Chen, H., Wang, Z., Finlay, W.H., Lobenberg, R., Roa, W.H., 2006. Formulation and cytotoxicity of doxorubicin nanoparticles carried by dry powder aerosol particles. Int. J. Pharm. 319 (1−2), 155−161. https://www.ncbi.nlm.nih.gov/pubmed/16713150.

Aziz, A.U., Geng, C., Fu, M., Yu, X., Qin, K., Liu, B., 2017. The role of microfluidics for organ on chip simulations. Bioengineering 4 (2). https://doi.org/10.3390/bioengineering4020039.

Aziz, A.U.R., Yu, X., Jiang, Q., Zhao, Y., Deng, S., Qin, K., Wang, H., Liu, B., 2020. Doxorubicin-induced toxicity to 3D-cultured rat ovarian follicles on a microfluidic chip. Toxicol. Vitro 62, 104677. https://www.ncbi.nlm.nih.gov/pubmed/31629067.

Bagheri, Z., Ehtesabi, H., Hallaji, Z., Latifi, H., Behroodi, E., 2018. Investigation the cytotoxicity and photo-induced toxicity of carbon dot on yeast cell. Ecotoxicol. Environ. Saf. 161, 245−250. https://www.ncbi.nlm.nih.gov/pubmed/29886311.

Bailey, J., 2008. An assessment of the role of chimpanzees in AIDS vaccine research. Altern. Lab. Anim. ATLA 36 (4), 381−428. https://www.ncbi.nlm.nih.gov/pubmed/18826331.

Baillie, T.A., 2020. Drug−protein adducts: past, present, and future. Med. Chem. Res. 29 (7), 1093−1104.

Balasubramanian, S., Gunasekaran, K., Sasidharan, S., Jeyamanickavel Mathan, V., Perumal, E., 2020. MicroRNAs and xenobiotic toxicity: an overview. Toxicol. Rep. 7, 583−595. https://www.ncbi.nlm.nih.gov/pubmed/32426239.

Balijepalli, A., Sivaramakrishan, V., 2017. Organs-on-chips: research and commercial perspectives. Drug Discov. Today 22 (2), 397−403. https://www.ncbi.nlm.nih.gov/pubmed/27866008.

Ballabio, D., Grisoni, F., Consonni, V., Todeschini, R., 2019. Integrated QSAR models to predict acute oral systemic toxicity. Mol. Inform. 38 (8−9), e1800124. https://www.ncbi.nlm.nih.gov/pubmed/30549437.

Barnard, N.D., Kaufman, S.R.J.S.A., 1997. Anim. Res. Wasteful Misleading 276 (2), 80−82.

Bédard, P., Gauvin, S., Ferland, K., Caneparo, C., Pellerin, È., Chabaud, S., Bolduc, S.J.B., 2020. Innovative human three-dimensional tissue-engineered models as an alternative to animal testing. Bioengineering 7 (3), 115.

Berridge, M.V., Tan, A.S., 1993. Characterization of the cellular reduction of 3-(4,5-dimethylthiazol-2-yl)-2,5-diphenyltetrazolium bromide (MTT): subcellular localization, substrate dependence, and involvement of mitochondrial electron transport in MTT reduction. Arch. Biochem. Biophys. 303 (2), 474−482. https://www.ncbi.nlm.nih.gov/pubmed/8390225.

Bhat, V., Chatterjee, J., 2021. The use of in silico tools for the toxicity prediction of potential inhibitors of SARS CoV-2. Alternatives to laboratory animals. ATLA 49 (1−2), 22−32. https://www.ncbi.nlm.nih.gov/pubmed/33845649.

Bircsak, K.M., DeBiasio, R., Miedel, M., Alsebahi, A., Reddinger, R., Saleh, A., Shun, T., Vernetti, L.A., Gough, A., 2021. A 3D microfluidic liver model for high throughput compound toxicity screening in the OrganoPlate(R). Toxicology 450, 152667. https://www.ncbi.nlm.nih.gov/pubmed/33359578.

Bitton, G., Koopman, B., Wang, H.D., 1984. Baker's yeast assay procedure for testing heavy metal toxicity. Bull. Environ. Contam. Toxicol. 32 (1), 80−84. https://www.ncbi.nlm.nih.gov/pubmed/6365213.

Bojarski, B., Witeska, M., 2020. Blood biomarkers of herbicide, insecticide, and fungicide toxicity to fish-a review. Environ. Sci. Pollut. Res. Int. 27 (16), 19236−19250. https://www.ncbi.nlm.nih.gov/pubmed/32248419.

Bolt, H.M., 2003. Genotoxicity–threshold or not? Introduction of cases of industrial chemicals. Toxicol. Lett. 140−141, 43−51. https://www.ncbi.nlm.nih.gov/pubmed/12676450.

Borna, H., Hosseini Qale Noe, S.H., Harchegani, A.B., Talatappe, N.R., Ghatrehsamani, M., Ghanei, M., Shahriary, A., 2019. A review on proteomics analysis to reveal biological pathways and predictive proteins in sulfur mustard exposed patients: roles of inflammation and oxidative stress. Inhal. Toxicol. 31 (1), 3−11. https://www.ncbi.nlm.nih.gov/pubmed/31010353.

Borrego, S.L., Lin, D.-W., Kaiser, P., 2019. Isolation and characterization of methionine-independent clones from methionine-dependent cancer cells. In: Methionine Dependence of Cancer and Aging. Springer, pp. 37–48.

Botha, C.J., Clift, S.J., Ferreira, G.C.H., Masango, M.G., 2017. Geigerin-induced cytotoxicity in a murine myoblast cell line (C2C12). Onderstepoort J. Vet. Res. 84 (1), e1–e7. https://www.ncbi.nlm.nih.gov/pubmed/29113440.

Boverhof, D.R., Zacharewski, T.R., 2006. Toxicogenomics in risk assessment: applications and needs. Toxicol. Sci. Off. J. Soc. Toxicol. 89 (2), 352–360. https://www.ncbi.nlm.nih.gov/pubmed/16221963.

Brandao, F., Fernandez-Bertolez, N., Rosario, F., Bessa, M.J., Fraga, S., Pasaro, E., Teixeira, J.P., Laffon, B., Valdiglesias, V., Costa, C., 2020. Genotoxicity of TiO2 nanoparticles in four different human cell lines (A549, HEPG2, A172 and SH-SY5Y). Nanomaterials 10 (3), 412. https://www.ncbi.nlm.nih.gov/pubmed/32120981.

Casquillas, G.V., Houssin, T., Durieux, L., 2018. Microfluidics and microfluidic devices: a review. Elveflow Microfluidic Instruments RSS. https://www.elveflow.com/microfluidic-reviews/general-microfluidics/microfluidics-and-microfluidic-device-a-review/.

Cayir, A., Cobanoglu, H., Coskun, M., 2020. Assessment of the genotoxic potential of a migraine-specific drug by comet and cytokinesis-block micronucleus assays. Expet Opin. Drug Metabol. Toxicol. 16 (5), 441–446. https://www.ncbi.nlm.nih.gov/pubmed/32275455.

Charitos, I.A., Ballini, A., Cantore, S., Boccellino, M., Di Domenico, M., Borsani, E., Nocini, R., Di Cosola, M., Santacroce, L., Bottalico, L., 2021. Stem cells: a historical review about biological, religious, and ethical issues. Stem Cell. Int. 2021, 9978837.

Choudhary, D., Goykar, H., Rajpoot, K., Tekade, R.K., 2021. Chronopharmacokinetics. In: Tekade, R.K. (Ed.), Biopharmaceutics and Pharmacokinetics Considerations. Elsevier, Academic Press, pp. 163–194.

Chu, C.R., Szczodry, M., Bruno, S., 2010. Animal models for cartilage regeneration and repair. Tissue Eng. B Rev. 16 (1), 105–115. https://www.ncbi.nlm.nih.gov/pubmed/19831641.

Clark, J.M.J.B.J.N., 2018. The 3Rs in research: a contemporary approach to replacement, reduction and refinement, 120 (s1), S1–S7.

Clewell III, H.J., Andersen, M.E., 1989. Improving toxicology testing protocols using computer simulations. Toxicol. Lett. 49 (2–3), 139–158.

Cohen, S.M., Boobis, A.R., Dellarco, V.L., Doe, J.E., Fenner-Crisp, P.A., Moretto, A., Pastoor, T.P., Schoeny, R.S., Seed, J.G., Wolf, D.C., 2019. Chemical carcinogenicity revisited 3: risk assessment of carcinogenic potential based on the current state of knowledge of carcinogenesis in humans. Regul. Toxicol. Pharmacol. 103, 100–105. https://www.ncbi.nlm.nih.gov/pubmed/30634021.

Collins, F.S., Tabak, L.A., 2014. Policy: NIH plans to enhance reproducibility. Nature 505 (7485), 612–613. https://www.ncbi.nlm.nih.gov/pubmed/24482835.

Cong, Y., Han, X., Wang, Y., Chen, Z., Lu, Y., Liu, T., Wu, Z., Jin, Y., Luo, Y., Zhang, X., 2020. Drug toxicity evaluation based on organ-on-a-chip technology: a review. Micromachines 11 (4), 381. https://www.ncbi.nlm.nih.gov/pubmed/32260191.

Corvi, R., Madia, F., 2017. In vitro genotoxicity testing-Can the performance be enhanced? Food Chem. Toxicol. 106 (Pt B), 600–608. https://www.ncbi.nlm.nih.gov/pubmed/27554597.

Cory, A.H., Owen, T.C., Barltrop, J.A., Cory, J.G., 1991. Use of an aqueous soluble tetrazolium/formazan assay for cell growth assays in culture. Cancer Commun. 3 (7), 207–212. https://www.ncbi.nlm.nih.gov/pubmed/1867954.

Council, N.R., 2009. Pain in research animals: general principles and considerations. In: Recognition and Alleviation of Pain in Laboratory Animals. National Academies Press (US).

Cronin, M., 2006. The use of in silico technologies to predict toxicity and fate: implementation and acceptance. ALTEX Alternativen zu Tierexperimenten 23 (Suppl. 1), 365–368.

Crouch, S.P., Kozlowski, R., Slater, K.J., Fletcher, J., 1993. The use of ATP bioluminescence as a measure of cell proliferation and cytotoxicity. J. Immunol. Methods 160 (1), 81–88. https://www.ncbi.nlm.nih.gov/pubmed/7680699.

Cui, P., Wang, S., 2019. Application of microfluidic chip technology in pharmaceutical analysis: a review. J. Pharm. Anal. 9 (4), 238–247. https://www.ncbi.nlm.nih.gov/pubmed/31452961.

Dai, J., Hamon, M., Jambovane, S., 2016. Microfluidics for antibiotic susceptibility and toxicity testing. Bioengineering 3 (4). https://doi.org/10.3390/bioengineering3040025.

Desai, N., Koppisetti, H., Rajpoot, K., Tekade, M., Sharma, M.C., Tekade, R.K., 2021. Influence of fever on pharmacokinetics of drugs. In: Tekade, R.K. (Ed.), Biopharmaceutics and Pharmacokinetics Considerations, I edn. Elsevier, pp. 451–463. https://doi.org/10.1016/B978-0-12-814425-1.00011-5.

Dhanya, S., Lal, K., Reena, S., 2018. Silico toxicology-a tool for early safety evaluation of drug. J. Bioinform. Genomics. Proteomics 3, 1030–1041.

Di Salvatore, M., Carafa, A., Carratù, G., 2008. Assessment of heavy metals phytotoxicity using seed germination and root elongation tests: a comparison of two growth substrates. Chemosphere 73 (9), 1461–1464.

Doke, S.K., Dhawale, S.C., 2015. Alternatives to animal testing: a review. Saudi Pharmaceut. J. 23 (3), 223–229. https://www.ncbi.nlm.nih.gov/pubmed/26106269.

Dolskiy, A.A., Grishchenko, I.V., Yudkin, D.V., 2020. Cell cultures for virology: usability, advantages, and prospects. Int. J. Mol. Sci. 21 (21), 7978. https://www.ncbi.nlm.nih.gov/pubmed/33121109.

Dos Santos, S.C., Teixeira, M.C., Cabrito, T.R., Sá-Correia, I., 2012. Yeast toxicogenomics: genome-wide responses to chemical stresses with impact in environmental health, pharmacology, and biotechnology. Front. Genet. 3, 63.

Environmental, A., 1998. Development of plant toxicity tests for assessment of contaminated soils—document prepared for method development and application section. Environ. Technol. Centre Environ. Canada. https://www.canada.ca/en/environment-climate-change/services/wildlife-research-landscape-science/biological-test-method-publications/terrestrial-plants-contaminants-soil/references.html.

Esteve, K., Poupot, C., Dabert, P., Mietton-Peuchot, M., Milisic, V., 2009. A Saccharomyces cerevisiae-based bioassay for assessing pesticide toxicity. J. Ind. Microbiol. Biotechnol. 36 (12), 1529–1534. https://www.ncbi.nlm.nih.gov/pubmed/19856193.

Gabig-Cimińska, M., Wegrzyn, G.J.A., 2001. An introduction to DNA chips: principles, technology, applications and analysis. Acta Biochim. Pol. 48, 615–622.

Gleeson, M.P., Modi, S., Bender, A., Robinson, R.L., Kirchmair, J., Promkatkaew, M., Hannongbua, S., Glen, R.C., 2012. The challenges involved in modeling toxicity data in silico: a review. Curr. Pharmaceut. Des. 18 (9), 1266–1291. https://www.ncbi.nlm.nih.gov/pubmed/22316153.

Gorantla, V.R., Bhat, A., Ghosh, A.R., Bolla, S.R., Bhojaraj, S., Mohan, S.K., Veeraraghavan, V.P., Chidambaram, S.B., Essa, M.M., Qoronfleh, M.W., 2021. Stem cells therapy: a ray of hope for Huntington disease. Int. J. Nutr. Pharmacol. Neurol. Dis. 11 (2), 95.

Gosens, I., Costa, P.M., Olsson, M., Stone, V., Costa, A.L., Brunelli, A., Badetti, E., Bonetto, A., Bokkers, B.G.H., de Jong, W.H., Williams, A., Halappanavar, S., Fadeel, B., Cassee, F.R., 2021. Pulmonary toxicity and gene expression changes after short-term inhalation exposure to surface-modified copper oxide nanoparticles. NanoImpact 22, 100313. https://www.ncbi.nlm.nih.gov/pubmed/35559970.

Govindarajan, R., Duraiyan, J., Kaliyappan, K., Palanisamy, M., 2012. Microarray and its applications. J. Pharm. BioAllied Sci. 4 (Suppl. 2), S310–S312. https://www.ncbi.nlm.nih.gov/pubmed/23066278.

Greek, R., Menache, A., 2013. Systematic reviews of animal models: methodology versus epistemology. Int. J. Med. Sci. 10 (3), 206–221. https://www.ncbi.nlm.nih.gov/pubmed/23372426.

Guan, M., Tang, S., Chang, H., Chen, Y., Chen, F., Mu, Y., Zhao, D., Fan, W., Tian, H., Darland, D.C., Zhang, Y., 2021. Development of alveolar-capillary-exchange (ACE) chip and its application for assessment of PM2.5-induced toxicity. Ecotoxicol. Environ. Saf. 223, 112601. https://www.ncbi.nlm.nih.gov/pubmed/34385060.

Guerreiro, N., Staedtler, F., Grenet, O., Kehren, J., Chibout, S.D., 2003. Toxicogenomics in drug development. Toxicol. Pathol. 31 (5), 471–479. https://www.ncbi.nlm.nih.gov/pubmed/14692614.

Gupta, R., Polaka, S., Rajpoot, K., Tekade, M., Sharma, M.C., Tekade, R.K., 2022a. Importance of toxicity testing in drug discovery and research. In: Pharmacokinetics and Toxicokinetic Considerations, vol. 2. Elsevier. https://doi.org/10.1016/b978-0-323-98367-9.00016-0.

Gupta, R., Rajpoot, K., Tekade, M., Sharma, M.C., Safavi, M., Tekade, R.K., 2022b. Factors influencing drug toxicity. In: Pharmacokinetics and Toxicokinetic Considerations, vol. 2. Elsevier. https://doi.org/10.1016/b978-0-323-98367-9.00014-7.

Gupta, R., Rajpoot, K., Tekade, M., Sharma, M.C., Tekade, R.K., 2022c. Methods and models for in vitro toxicity. In: Pharmacokinetics and Toxicokinetic Considerations, vol. 2. Elsevier. https://doi.org/10.1016/b978-0-323-98367-9.00006-8.

Gutiérrez-Martínez, P.B., Torres-Morán, M.I., Romero-Puertas, M.C., Casas-Solís, J., Zarazúa-Villaseñor, P., Sandoval-Pinto, E., Ramírez-Hernández, B.C., 2020. Assessment of antioxidant enzymes in leaves and roots of Phaseolus vulgaris plants under cadmium stress. Biotecnia 22 (2), 110–118.

Hamadeh, H.K., Bushel, P., Paules, R., Afshari, C.A., 2001. Discovery in toxicology: mediation by gene expression array technology. J. Biochem. Mol. Toxicol. 15 (5), 231–242. https://www.ncbi.nlm.nih.gov/pubmed/11835620.

Haubenstricker, M.E., Meier, P.G., Mancy, K.H., Brabec, M.J., 1990. Rapid toxicity testing based on yeast respiratory activity. Bull. Environ. Contam. Toxicol. 44 (5), 669–674. https://www.ncbi.nlm.nih.gov/pubmed/2188688.

He, Y., Zhu, L., Ma, J., Lin, G., 2021. Metabolism-mediated cytotoxicity and genotoxicity of pyrrolizidine alkaloids. Arch. Toxicol. 95 (6), 1917–1942. https://www.ncbi.nlm.nih.gov/pubmed/34003343.

Honma, M., 2020. An assessment of mutagenicity of chemical substances by (quantitative) structure-activity relationship. Gene Environ. 42 (1), 23. https://www.ncbi.nlm.nih.gov/pubmed/32626544.

Hou, J., Liu, H., Zhang, S., Liu, X., Hayat, T., Alsaedi, A., Wang, X., 2019. Mechanism of toxic effects of Nano-ZnO on cell cycle of zebrafish (*Danio rerio*). Chemosphere 229, 206–213. https://www.ncbi.nlm.nih.gov/pubmed/31078877.

Huang, J., Chang, Z., Lu, Q., Chen, X., Najafi, M., 2022. Nobiletin as an inducer of programmed cell death in cancer: a review. Apoptosis 27 (5–6), 297–310.

Huang, Q., Liu, Y., Dong, S., 2018. Emerging roles of long non-coding RNAs in the toxicology of environmental chemicals. J. Appl. Toxicol. 38 (7), 934–943. https://www.ncbi.nlm.nih.gov/pubmed/29388697.

Hubrecht, R.C., Carter, E., 2019. The 3Rs and Humane experimental technique: implementing change. Animals (Basel) 9 (10), 754. https://www.ncbi.nlm.nih.gov/pubmed/31575048.

Jalili-Firoozinezhad, S., Miranda, C.C., Cabral, J.M.S., 2021. Modeling the human body on microfluidic chips. Trends Biotechnol. 39 (8), 838–852. https://www.ncbi.nlm.nih.gov/pubmed/33581889.

Jia, S., Zhao, F., 2022. Ex vivo development of the entire mouse fetal reproductive tract by using microdissection and membrane-based organ culture techniques. Differentiation 123, 42–49. https://www.ncbi.nlm.nih.gov/pubmed/35030420.

Jiang, B., Zheng, W., Zhang, W., Jiang, X., 2013. Organs on microfluidic chips: a mini review. Sci. China Chem. 57 (3), 356–364. https://doi.org/10.1007/s11426-013-4971-0.

Juan-Garcia, A., Tolosa, J., Juan, C., Ruiz, M.J., 2019. Cytotoxicity, genotoxicity and disturbance of cell cycle in HepG2 cells exposed to OTA and BEA: single and combined actions. Toxins 11 (6), 341. https://www.ncbi.nlm.nih.gov/pubmed/31208011.

Judson, R., Richard, A., Dix, D., Houck, K., Elloumi, F., Martin, M., Cathey, T., Transue, T.R., Spencer, R., Wolf, M., 2008. ACToR–Aggregated computational toxicology resource. Toxicol. Appl. Pharmacol. 233 (1), 7–13. https://www.ncbi.nlm.nih.gov/pubmed/18671997.

Kar, S., Leszczynski, J., 2019. Exploration of computational approaches to predict the toxicity of chemical mixtures. Toxics 7 (1), 15. https://www.ncbi.nlm.nih.gov/pubmed/30893892.

Kavlock, R.J., Ankley, G., Blancato, J., Breen, M., Conolly, R., Dix, D., Houck, K., Hubal, E., Judson, R., Rabinowitz, J., Richard, A., Setzer, R.W., Shah, I., Villeneuve, D., Weber, E., 2008. Computational toxicology–a state of the science mini review. Toxicol. Sci. Off. J. Soc. Toxicol. 103 (1), 14–27. https://www.ncbi.nlm.nih.gov/pubmed/18065772.

Khalid, M.A.U., Kim, Y.S., Ali, M., Lee, B.G., Cho, Y.-J., Choi, K.H., 2020. A lung cancer-on-chip platform with integrated biosensors for physiological monitoring and toxicity assessment. Biochem. Eng. J. 155, 107469. https://www.sciencedirect.com/science/article/pii/S1369703X19304085.

Khelurkar, V., Ingle, K., Padole, D., 2017. DNA Microarray: Basic Principle and It's Applications, pp. 488–490.

Kim, T.-W., Che, J.-H., Yun, J.-W., 2019. Use of stem cells as alternative methods to animal experimentation in predictive toxicology. Regul. Toxicol. Pharmacol. 105, 15–29.

Kirsch-Volders, M., Pacchierotti, F., Parry, E.M., Russo, A., Eichenlaub-Ritter, U., Adler, I.D., 2019. Risks of aneuploidy induction from chemical exposure: twenty years of collaborative research in Europe from basic science to regulatory implications. Mutat. Res. Rev. Mutat. Res. 779, 126–147. https://www.ncbi.nlm.nih.gov/pubmed/31097149.

Knauer, K., Vervliet-Scheebaum, M., Dark, R.J., Maund, S.J., 2006. Methods for assessing the toxicity of herbicides to submersed aquatic plants. Pest Manag. Sci. 62 (8), 715–722. https://www.ncbi.nlm.nih.gov/pubmed/16703656.

Kohl, Y., Runden-Pran, E., Mariussen, E., Hesler, M., El Yamani, N., Longhin, E.M., Dusinska, M., 2020. Genotoxicity of nanomaterials: advanced in vitro models and high throughput methods for human hazard assessment-a review. Nanomaterials 10 (10), 1911. https://www.ncbi.nlm.nih.gov/pubmed/32992722.

Kuhn, D.M., Balkis, M., Chandra, J., Mukherjee, P.K., Ghannoum, M.A., 2003. Uses and limitations of the XTT assay in studies of Candida growth and metabolism. J. Clin. Microbiol. 41 (1), 506–508. https://www.ncbi.nlm.nih.gov/pubmed/12517908.

Kumar, S.V., Er, P.X., Lawlor, K.T., Motazedian, A., Scurr, M., Ghobrial, I., Combes, A.N., Zappia, L., Oshlack, A., Stanley, E.G., Little, M.H., 2019. Kidney micro-organoids in suspension culture as a scalable source of human pluripotent stem cell-derived kidney cells. Development 146 (5), dev172361. https://www.ncbi.nlm.nih.gov/pubmed/30846463.

Kumawat, A., Raval, N., Reddy, G., Rajpoot, K., Tekade, R.K., 2020. Gene delivery to tackle diabetic nephropathy. In: Tekade, R.K. (Ed.), The Future of Pharmaceutical Product Development and Research, vol. 1. Academic Press, pp. 515–537. http://www.sciencedirect.com/science/article/pii/B9780128144558000153.

Kwolek-Mirek, M., Zadrag-Tecza, R., 2014. Comparison of methods used for assessing the viability and vitality of yeast cells. FEMS Yeast Res. 14 (7), 1068–1079.

Kwon, J.-S., Oh, J.H., 2018. Microfluidic technology for cell manipulation. Appl. Sci. 8 (6). https://doi.org/10.3390/app8060992.

Langford, D.J., Bailey, A.L., Chanda, M.L., Clarke, S.E., Drummond, T.E., Echols, S., Glick, S., Ingrao, J., Klassen-Ross, T., Lacroix-Fralish, M.L., Matsumiya, L., Sorge, R.E., Sotocinal, S.G., Tabaka, J.M., Wong, D., van den Maagdenberg, A.M., Ferrari, M.D., Craig, K.D., Mogil, J.S., 2010. Coding of facial expressions of pain in the laboratory mouse. Nat. Methods 7 (6), 447–449. https://www.ncbi.nlm.nih.gov/pubmed/20453868.

Langhans, S.A., 2018. Three-dimensional in vitro cell culture models in drug discovery and drug repositioning. Front. Pharmacol. 9, 6. https://www.ncbi.nlm.nih.gov/pubmed/29410625.

Lee, M., Hwang, J.H., Lim, K.M., 2017. Alternatives to in vivo draize rabbit eye and skin irritation tests with a focus on 3D reconstructed human cornea-like epithelium and epidermis models. Toxicol. Res. 33 (3), 191–203. https://www.ncbi.nlm.nih.gov/pubmed/28744350.

Leme, D.M., Marin-Morales, M.A., 2009. Allium cepa test in environmental monitoring: a review on its application. Mutat. Res. 682 (1), 71–81. https://www.ncbi.nlm.nih.gov/pubmed/19577002.

Lettieri, T., 2006. Recent applications of DNA microarray technology to toxicology and ecotoxicology. Environ. Health Perspect. 114 (1), 4–9. https://www.ncbi.nlm.nih.gov/pubmed/16393650.

Li, D., 2010. Microfluidic lab-on-a-chip devices for biomedical applications. In: Kakaç, S., Kosoy, B., Li, D., Pramuanjaroenkij, A. (Eds.), Microfluidics Based Microsystems, Dordrecht. Springer Netherlands, pp. 377–397.

Li, M., Gong, J., Gao, L., Zou, T., Kang, J., Xu, H., 2022. Advanced human developmental toxicity and teratogenicity assessment using human organoid models. Ecotoxicol. Environ. Saf. 235, 113429.

Li, X., Gu, W., Mohan, S., Baylink, D.J., 2002. DNA microarrays: their use and misuse. Microcirculation 9 (1), 13–22. https://www.ncbi.nlm.nih.gov/pubmed/11896556.

Lobenhofer, E.K., Bushel, P.R., Afshari, C.A., Hamadeh, H.K., 2001. Progress in the application of DNA microarrays. Environ. Health Perspect. 109 (9), 881–891. https://www.ncbi.nlm.nih.gov/pubmed/11673116.

Luo, Y., Liang, J., Zeng, G., Chen, M., Mo, D., Li, G., Zhang, D., 2018. Seed germination test for toxicity evaluation of compost: its roles, problems and prospects. Waste Manag. 71, 109–114. https://www.ncbi.nlm.nih.gov/pubmed/29030118.

Lytle, J.S., Lytle, T.F., 2001. Use of plants for toxicity assessment of estuarine ecosystems. Environ. Toxicol. Chem. Int. J. 20 (1), 68–83.

Mandenius, C.-F., 2018. Conceptual design of micro-bioreactors and organ-on-chips for studies of cell cultures. Bioengineering 5 (3). https://doi.org/10.3390/bioengineering5030056.

Manzoni, C., Kia, D.A., Vandrovcova, J., Hardy, J., Wood, N.W., Lewis, P.A., Ferrari, R., 2018. Genome, transcriptome and proteome: the rise of omics data and their integration in biomedical sciences. Briefings Bioinf. 19 (2), 286–302.

Mather, J.A.J.A., 2019. Ethics and care: for animals, not just mammals, 9 (12), 1018.

Mattes, W.B., 2020. In vitro to in vivo translation. Curr. Opin. Toxicol. 23–24, 114–118. https://www.sciencedirect.com/science/article/pii/S2468202020300528.

McCormick, S.C., Kriel, F.H., Ivask, A., Tong, Z., Lombi, E., Voelcker, N.H., Priest, C., 2017. The use of microfluidics in cytotoxicity and nanotoxicity experiments. Micromachines 8 (4). https://doi.org/10.3390/mi8040124.

Meigs, L., Smirnova, L., Rovida, C., Leist, M., Hartung, T.J.A.-A., 2018. Animal testing and its alternatives—the most important omics is economics, 35 (3), 275–305.

North, M., Vulpe, C.D., 2010. Functional toxicogenomics: mechanism-centered toxicology. Int. J. Mol. Sci. 11 (12), 4796–4813. https://www.ncbi.nlm.nih.gov/pubmed/21614174.

Nuwaysir, E.F., Bittner, M., Trent, J., Barrett, J.C., Afshari, C.A., 1999. Microarrays and toxicology: the advent of toxicogenomics. Mol. Carcinog. 24 (3), 153–159. https://www.ncbi.nlm.nih.gov/pubmed/10204799.

OECD-208, 2003. OECD 208 guideline for the testing of chemicals proposal for updating guideline 208 terrestrial plant test: 208: seedling emergence and seedling growth test. TEST 227, 1–19.

OECD-227, 2003. OECD Guideline for the Testing of Chemicals Proposal for a New Guideline 227 Terrestrial Plant Test: Vegetative Vigour Test. OECD Guideline for the Testing of Chemicals. https://www.google.co.in/url?sa=t&rct=j&q=&esrc=s&source=web&cd=&cad=rja&uact=8&ved=2ahUKEwiL7qnUzf_6AhV-8zgGHa9fCWUQFnoECBUQAQ&url=https%3A%2F%2Fwww.oecd.org%2Fchemicalsafety%2Ftesting%2F11988186.pdf&usg=AOvVaw3fcRi95He-4VZyynVNOCFL.

OECD, 2016a. Test No. 474: Mammalian Erythrocyte Micronucleus Test. OECD Guidelines for the Testing of Chemicals, Section 4. https://www.oecd-ilibrary.org/content/publication/9789264264762-en.

OECD, 2016b. Test No. 487: In Vitro Mammalian Cell Micronucleus Test. OECD Guidelines for the Testing of Chemicals, Section 4. https://www.oecd-ilibrary.org/content/publication/9789264264861-en.

OECD, 2016c. Test No. 489: In Vivo Mammalian Alkaline Comet Assay. OECD Guidelines for the Testing of Chemicals, Section 4. https://www.oecd-ilibrary.org/content/publication/9789264264885-en.

OECD, 2016d. Test No. 490: In Vitro Mammalian Cell Gene Mutation Tests Using the Thymidine Kinase Gene. OECD Guidelines for the Testing of Chemicals, Section 4. https://www.oecd-ilibrary.org/content/publication/9789264264908-en.

OECD, 2022. Test No. 488: Transgenic Rodent Somatic and Germ Cell Gene Mutation Assays. OECD Guidelines for the Testing of Chemicals, Section 4. https://www.oecd-ilibrary.org/content/publication/9789264203907-en.

Olson, H., Betton, G., Robinson, D., Thomas, K., Monro, A., Kolaja, G., Lilly, P., Sanders, J., Sipes, G., Bracken, W., Dorato, M., Van Deun, K., Smith, P., Berger, B., Heller, A., 2000. Concordance of the toxicity of pharmaceuticals in humans and in animals. Regul. Toxicol. Pharmacol. 32 (1), 56–67. https://www.ncbi.nlm.nih.gov/pubmed/11029269.

Oprea, A., Tanase, C., Teach, C.-A., 2007. Use of vascular plants for toxicity assessments. Cellul. Chem. Technol. 41 (7), 437.

Orescanin, V., Durgo, K., Mikelic, I.L., Halkijevic, I., Kuspilic, M., 2018. Toxicity assessment of untreated/treated electroplating sludge using human and plant bioassay. J. Environ. Sci. Health Part A 53 (10), 925–930.

Ottoboni, L., von Wunster, B., Martino, G., 2020. Therapeutic plasticity of neural stem cells. Front. Neurol. 11, 148. https://www.ncbi.nlm.nih.gov/pubmed/32265815.

Padiyar, A., Agrawal, O.P., Rajpoot, K., Tekade, R.K., 2020. Hydrotropy, mixed hydrotropy, and mixed solvency as trending concept for solubilization of lipophilic drugs. In: Tekade, R.K. (Ed.), The Future of Pharmaceutical Product Development and Research. Academic Press, pp. 145–178. http://www.sciencedirect.com/science/article/pii/B9780128144558000050.

Pandey, A.N., Rajpoot, K., Jain, S.K., 2020. Using 5-fluorouracil-encored PLGA nanoparticles for the treatment of colorectal cancer: the in-vitro characterization and cytotoxicity studies. Nanomed. J. 7 (3), 211–224.

Pandey, V., Polaka, S., Nalla, L.V., Tekade, M., Sharma, M.C., Tekade, R.K., 2022. Excipient toxicity and safety. In: Pharmacokinetics and Toxicokinetic Considerations. Elsevier, pp. 487–511.

Parthasarathi, R., Dhawan, A., 2018. In silico approaches for predictive toxicology. In: In Vitro Toxicology. Elsevier, pp. 91–109.

Pawar, G., Madden, J.C., Ebbrell, D., Firman, J.W., Cronin, M.T.D., 2019. In silico toxicology data resources to support read-across and (Q)SAR. Front. Pharmacol. 10, 561. https://www.ncbi.nlm.nih.gov/pubmed/31244651.

Pennie, W.D., Tugwood, J.D., Oliver, G.J., Kimber, I., 2000. The principles and practice of toxigenomics: applications and opportunities. Toxicol. Sci. Off. J. Soc. Toxicol. 54 (2), 277–283. https://www.ncbi.nlm.nih.gov/pubmed/10774809.

Pennie, W.D., Woodyatt, N.J., Aldridge, T.C., Orphanides, G., 2001. Application of genomics to the definition of the molecular basis for toxicity. Toxicol. Lett. 120 (1–3), 353–358. https://www.ncbi.nlm.nih.gov/pubmed/11323194.

Pisciotta, A., Bertoni, L., Riccio, M., Mapelli, J., Bigiani, A., La Noce, M., Orciani, M., de Pol, A., Carnevale, G., 2018. Use of a 3D floating sphere culture system to maintain the neural crest-related properties of human dental pulp stem cells. Front. Physiol. 9, 547. https://www.frontiersin.org/article/10.3389/fphys.2018.00547.

Polaka, S., Desai, N., Kshirsagar, B., Rajpoot, K., Tekade, R.K., 2021. Revamping the pharmacokinetics of poorly soluble drugs using different formulations. In: Tekade, R.K. (Ed.), Biopharmaceutics and Pharmacokinetics Considerations, 1st ed. Elsevier, pp. 387–413. https://doi.org/10.1016/B978-0-12-814425-1.00005-X.

Polaka, S., Gomte, S.S., Pandey, V., Tella, J.D., Tekade, M., Sharma, M.C., Molugulu, N., Tekade, R.K., 2022a. Pharmaceutical excipients: special focus on adverse interactions. In: Pharmacokinetics and Toxicokinetic Considerations. Elsevier, pp. 513–542.

Polaka, S., Koppisetti, H., Pande, S., Tekade, M., Sharma, M.C., Tekade, R.K., 2022b. Zebrafish models for toxicological screening. In: Pharmacokinetics and Toxicokinetic Considerations. Elsevier, pp. 221–240.

Polaka, S., Makwana, V., Vasdev, N., Sheth, A., Rajpoot, K., Sengupta, P., Tekade, R.K., 2022c. Engineering immunity via skin-directed drug delivery devices. J. Contr. Release 345, 385–404. https://www.ncbi.nlm.nih.gov/pubmed/35283256.

Polaka, S., Pawar, B., Tekade, M., Satvase, R., Manchikalapudi, A.L., Sharma, M.C., Pandey, V., Jhariya, A.N., Tekade, R.K., 2022d. Emerging role of novel excipients in drug product development and their safety concerns. In: Pharmacokinetics and Toxicokinetic Considerations. Elsevier, pp. 543–567.

Polaka, S., Rajpoot, K., Tekade, M., Sharma, M.C., Tekade, R.K., 2022e. Food–drug interactions and their implications on oral drug bioavailability. In: Pharmacokinetics and Toxicokinetic Considerations, vol. 2. Elsevier. https://doi.org/10.1016/b978-0-323-98367-9.00002-0.

Polaka, S., Vasdev, N., Raji, S., Makwana, V., Rajput, A., Kulkarni, M., Tekade, M., Pingale, P., Sharma, M.C., Tekade, R.K.J.P., Considerations, T., 2022f. Toxicogenomics in drug safety assessment. In: Pharmacokinetics and Toxicokinetic Considerations, pp. 73–98.

Radić, S., Stipaničev, D., Cvjetko, P., Rajčić, M.M., Širac, S., Pevalek-Kozlina, B., Pavlica, M., 2011. Duckweed Lemna minor as a tool for testing toxicity and genotoxicity of surface waters. Ecotoxicol. Environ. Saf. 74 (2), 182–187.

Raies, A.B., Bajic, V.B., 2016. In silico toxicology: computational methods for the prediction of chemical toxicity. Wiley Interdiscip. Rev. Comput. Mol. Sci. 6 (2), 147–172. https://www.ncbi.nlm.nih.gov/pubmed/27066112.

Rajpoot, K., Desai, N., Koppisetti, H., Tekade, M., Sharma, M.C., Behera, S.K., Tekade, R.K., 2022a. In silico methods for the prediction of drug toxicity. In: Pharmacokinetics and Toxicokinetic Considerations, vol. 2. Elsevier. https://doi.org/10.1016/b978-0-323-98367-9.00012-3.

Rajpoot, K., Jain, S.K., 2019. Irinotecan hydrochloride trihydrate loaded folic acid-tailored solid lipid nanoparticles for targeting colorectal cancer: development, characterization, and in vitro cytotoxicity study using HT-29 cells. J. Microencapsul. 36 (7), 659–676. https://www.ncbi.nlm.nih.gov/pubmed/31495238.

Rajpoot, K., Katare, P., Tekade, M., Sharma, M.C., Polaka, S., Sengupta, P., Tekade, R.K., 2022b. Toxicokinetic and toxicodynamic considerations in drug research. In: Pharmacokinetics and Toxicokinetic Considerations, vol. 2. Elsevier. https://doi.org/10.1016/b978-0-323-98367-9.00026-3.

Rajpoot, K., Tekade, M., Sharma, M.C., Arafat, B., Tekade, R.K., 2022c. Principles and concepts in toxicokinetic. In: Pharmacokinetics and Toxicokinetic Considerations, vol. 2. Elsevier. https://doi.org/10.1016/b978-0-323-98367-9.00023-8.

Rajpoot, K., Tekade, M., Sharma, M.C., Sreeharsha, N., Sharma, A., Tekade, R.K., 2020a. Recombinant blood products and therapeutic enzymes: an update. In: Tekade, R.K. (Ed.), The Future of Pharmaceutical Product Development and Research. Academic Press, pp. 447–482. http://www.sciencedirect.com/science/article/pii/B978012814455800013X.

Rajpoot, K., Tekade, M., Sreeharsha, N., Sharma, M.C., Tekade, R.K., 2020b. Recent advancements in solubilization of hydrophobic drugs. In: Tekade, R.K. (Ed.), The Future of Pharmaceutical Product Development and Research. Academic Press, pp. 109–144. http://www.sciencedirect.com/science/article/pii/B9780128144558000049.

Rajpoot, K., Tekade, R.K., Chatterjee, B., Sharma, M.C., Tekade, M., 2021a. Biopharmaceutical considerations in the pediatric and geriatric formulation development. In: Tekade, R.K. (Ed.), Biopharmaceutics and Pharmacokinetics Considerations, vol. 1. Elsevier, Academic Press, pp. 109–144.

Rajpoot, K., Tekade, R.K., Sharma, M.C., Safavi, M., Tekade, M., 2021b. Pharmacokinetics modeling in drug delivery. In: Tekade, R.K. (Ed.), Biopharmaceutics and Pharmacokinetics Considerations. Elsevier, Academic Press, pp. 279–334.

Rajpoot, K., Tekade, R.K., Sharma, M.C., Tekade, M., 2021c. Pharmacokinetics and biopharmaceutics: "a leader or attendant". In: Tekade, R.K. (Ed.), Biopharmaceutics and Pharmacokinetics Considerations. Elsevier, Academic Press, pp. 17–27.

Raunio, H., 2011. In silico toxicology—non-testing methods. Front. Pharmacol. 2, 33.

Ribeiro, I., Veríssimo, I., Moniz, L., Cardoso, H., Sousa, M., Soares, A., Leão, C., 2000. Yeasts as a model for assessing the toxicity of the fungicides Penconazol, Cymoxanil and Dichlofluanid. Chemosphere 41 (10), 1637–1642.

Riemens, M.M., Dueck, T., Kempenaar, C., Lotz, L.A., Kropff, M.J., 2009. Sublethal effects of herbicides on the biomass and seed production of terrestrial non-crop plant species, influenced by environment, development stage and assessment date. Environ. Pollut. 157 (8–9), 2306–2313. https://www.ncbi.nlm.nih.gov/pubmed/19395134.

Rim, K.-T., 2019. In vitro models for chemical toxicity: review of their applications and prospects. Toxicol. Environ. Health Sci. 11 (2), 94–103. https://doi.org/10.1007/s13530-019-0402-8.

Rim, K.T., 2020. In silico prediction of toxicity and its applications for chemicals at work. Toxicol. Environ. Health Sci. 12 (3), 191–202. https://www.ncbi.nlm.nih.gov/pubmed/32421081.

Riss, T., Niles, A., Moravec, R., Karassina, N., Vidugiriene, J., 2019. Cytotoxicity assays: in vitro methods to measure dead cells. Assay Guidance Manual [Internet]. https://www.ncbi.nlm.nih.gov/books/NBK540958/.

Roncaglioni, A., Toropov, A.A., Toropova, A.P., Benfenati, E., 2013. In silico methods to predict drug toxicity. Curr. Opin. Pharmacol. 13 (5), 802–806. https://www.ncbi.nlm.nih.gov/pubmed/23797035.

Roy, K., Kar, S., 2016. In silico models for ecotoxicity of pharmaceuticals. In: Silico Methods for Predicting Drug Toxicity. Springer, pp. 237–304.

Ruiz, A., Joshi, P., Mastrangelo, R., Francolini, M., Verderio, C., Matteoli, M., 2014. Testing Abeta toxicity on primary CNS cultures using drug-screening microfluidic chips. Lab Chip 14 (15), 2860–2866. https://www.ncbi.nlm.nih.gov/pubmed/24914747.

Sahu, R.K., Kishor, K., 2014. Evaluating toxicity mechanisms using DNA. Lab. Anim. 43 (8), 269. https://doi.org/10.1038/laban.582.

Sápi, J., 2017. Animal experiments in cancer research: wasteful or unavoidable?. In: 2017 IEEE 30th Neumann Colloquium (NC). IEEE, pp. 000157–000162.

Sheng, L., Wang, L., Sang, X., Zhao, X., Hong, J., Cheng, S., Yu, X., Liu, D., Xu, B., Hu, R., Sun, Q., Cheng, J., Cheng, Z., Gui, S., Hong, F., 2014. Nano-sized titanium dioxide-induced splenic toxicity: a biological pathway explored using microarray technology. J. Hazard Mater. 278, 180–188. https://www.ncbi.nlm.nih.gov/pubmed/24968254.

Siddiqui, A.H., Tabrez, S., Ahmad, M., 2011. Validation of plant based bioassays for the toxicity testing of Indian waters. Environ. Monit. Assess. 179 (1–4), 241–253. https://www.ncbi.nlm.nih.gov/pubmed/21042847.

Singh-Gasson, S., Green, R.D., Yue, Y., Nelson, C., Blattner, F., Sussman, M.R., Cerrina, F., 1999. Maskless fabrication of light-directed oligonucleotide microarrays using a digital micromirror array. Nat. Biotechnol. 17 (10), 974–978. https://www.ncbi.nlm.nih.gov/pubmed/10504697.

Sommer, S., Buraczewska, I., Kruszewski, M., 2020. Micronucleus assay: the state of art, and future directions. Int. J. Mol. Sci. 21 (4), 1534. https://www.ncbi.nlm.nih.gov/pubmed/32102335.

Stadtlander, K., Lawohnus, H., 1990. Yeast cells as a test system for evaluating the toxicity of chemicals. Altern. Lab. Anim. 17 (3), 203–206.

Stefanello, R., Viana, B.B., das Neves, L.A.S., 2019. Cadmium toxicity on seed germination and initial growth of chia. Acta Sci. Biol Sci. 41, e42174.

Stenton, S.L., Kremer, L.S., Kopajtich, R., Ludwig, C., Prokisch, H., 2020. The diagnosis of inborn errors of metabolism by an integrative "multi-omics" approach: a perspective encompassing genomics, transcriptomics, and proteomics. J. Inherit. Metab. Dis. 43 (1), 25–35. https://www.ncbi.nlm.nih.gov/pubmed/31119744.

Strober, W., 2001. Trypan blue exclusion test of cell viability. Curr. Protoc. Immunol. Appendix 3: Appendix 3B. https://www.ncbi.nlm.nih.gov/pubmed/18432654.

Sumantran, V.N., 2011. Cellular chemosensitivity assays: an overview. Methods Mol. Biol. 731, 219–236. https://www.ncbi.nlm.nih.gov/pubmed/21516411.

Tambe, V., Desai, N., Rajpoot, K., Tekade, R.K., 2021a. "Organ-on-a-chip"-based physiologically relevant pharmacokinetic models. In: Tekade, R.K. (Ed.), Biopharmaceutics and Pharmacokinetics Considerations, I edn. Elsevier, pp. 643–673. https://doi.org/10.1016/B978-0-12-814425-1.00024-3.

Tambe, V., Shukla, H., Rajpoot, K., Pandey, M.M., Tekade, R.K., 2021b. Pharmacokinetics aspects of biotechnological products. In: Tekade, R.K. (Ed.), Biopharmaceutics and Pharmacokinetics Considerations. Elsevier, Academic Press, pp. 539–565.

Tambe, V., Sirsat, B., Rajpoot, K., Gadeval, A., Tekade, R.K., 2021c. Pharmacogenomics and drug metabolism. In: Tekade, R.K. (Ed.), Biopharmaceutics and Pharmacokinetics Considerations, vol. 1. Elsevier, Academic Press, pp. 355–385.

Tarazona, J.V., Cesnaitis, R., Herranz-Montes, F.J., Versonnen, B., 2013. Identification of chemical hazards for terrestrial plants in the regulatory context: comparison of OECD and ISO guidelines. Chemosphere 93 (10), 2578–2584. https://www.ncbi.nlm.nih.gov/pubmed/24206832.

Tekade, M., Koppisetti, H., Sharma, M.C., Rajpoot, K., Sengupta, P., Kumar, M., Tekade, R.K., 2022. Understanding the concept of signal toxicity and its implications on human health. In: Pharmacokinetics and Toxicokinetic Considerations, vol. 2. Elsevier. https://doi.org/10.1016/b978-0-323-98367-9.00020-2.

Thwala, M., Klaine, S., Musee, N., 2021. Exposure media and nanoparticle size influence on the fate, bioaccumulation, and toxicity of silver nanoparticles to higher plant Salvinia minima. Molecules 26 (8), 2305. https://www.ncbi.nlm.nih.gov/pubmed/33923373.

Tibbe, M.P., Leferink, A.M., van den Berg, A., Eijkel, J.C.T., Segerink, L.I., 2018. Microfluidic gel patterning method by use of a temporary membrane for organ-on-chip applications. Adv. Mater. Technol. 3 (3), 1700200. https://doi.org/10.1002/admt.201700200.

Tiwari, A., Joshi, M., Salvi, N., Gupta, D., Gandhi, S., Rajpoot, K., Tekade, R.K., 2022. Toxicity of pharmaceutical azo dyes. In: Pharmacokinetics and Toxicokinetic Considerations, vol. 2. Elsevier. https://doi.org/10.1016/b978-0-323-98367-9.00004-4.

Tothill, I., Turner, A., 1996. Developments in bioassay methods for toxicity testing in water treatment. TrAC, Trends Anal. Chem. 15 (5), 178–188.

Turkez, H., Arslan, M.E., Sonmez, E., Geyikoglu, F., Acikyildiz, M., Tatar, A., 2019. Microarray assisted toxicological investigations of boron carbide nanoparticles on human primary alveolar epithelial cells. Chem. Biol. Interact. 300, 131–137. https://www.ncbi.nlm.nih.gov/pubmed/30684454.

Uzoekwe, N.M., Ejidike, I.P., Ukhun, M.E., 2020. An investigation into the biochemical, hematological, and histopathological effects of glyphaea brevis extracts in albino rats: toxicological appraisal. Int. J. Med. Rev. 7 (4), 146–156.

Valerio Jr., L.G., 2009. In silico toxicology for the pharmaceutical sciences. Toxicol. Appl. Pharmacol. 241 (3), 356–370. https://www.ncbi.nlm.nih.gov/pubmed/19716836.

van Meerloo, J., Kaspers, G.J., Cloos, J., 2011. Cell sensitivity assays: the MTT assay. Methods Mol. Biol. 731, 237–245. https://www.ncbi.nlm.nih.gov/pubmed/21516412.

Vasdev, N., Deshpande, M., Katare, P., Makwana, V., Polaka, S., Tekade, M., Sengupta, P., Sharma, M.C., Mishra, D.K., Tekade, R.K.J.P., Considerations, T., 2022. New emerging technologies for genetic toxicity testing, pp. 175–219.

Vasdev, N., Rajpoot, K., Tekade, R.K., 2021. Molecular mechanisms of circadian rhythm and its influence on the pharmacokinetics of drugs. In: Tekade, R.K. (Ed.), Biopharmaceutics and Pharmacokinetics Considerations. Elsevier, Academic Press, pp. 415–449.

Venkatapathy, R., Wang, N.C., 2013. Developmental toxicity prediction. Methods Mol. Biol. 930, 305–340. https://www.ncbi.nlm.nih.gov/pubmed/23086848.

Voigt, W., 2005. Sulforhodamine B assay and chemosensitivity. Methods Mol. Med. 110, 39–48. https://www.ncbi.nlm.nih.gov/pubmed/15901925.

Wang, W., 1991. Literature review on higher plants for toxicity testing. Water Air Soil Pollut. 59 (3), 381–400.

Watford, S., Ly Pham, L., Wignall, J., Shin, R., Martin, M.T., Friedman, K.P., 2019. ToxRefDB version 2.0: improved utility for predictive and retrospective toxicology analyses. Reprod. Toxicol. 89, 145–158. https://www.ncbi.nlm.nih.gov/pubmed/31340180.

White, P.A., Luijten, M., Mishima, M., Cox, J.A., Hanna, J.N., Maertens, R.M., Zwart, E.P., 2019. In vitro mammalian cell mutation assays based on transgenic reporters: a report of the International Workshop on Genotoxicity Testing (IWGT). Mutat. Res. Genet. Toxicol. Environ. Mutagen 847, 403039. https://www.ncbi.nlm.nih.gov/pubmed/31699347.

Whitesides, G.M., 2006. The origins and the future of microfluidics. Nature 442 (7101), 368–373. https://www.ncbi.nlm.nih.gov/pubmed/16871203.

Wickramasinghe, S.N., 1996. Culture of animal cells. A manual of basic technique, 3rd ed. R. Ian Freshney, Wiley-Liss, Inc, New York. xxiv + 486 pages (1994). Cell Biochem. Funct. 14 (1), 75–76. https://doi.org/10.1002/cbf.646.

Wilson, D.S., Nock, S., 2003. Recent developments in protein microarray technology. Angew Chem. Int. Ed. Engl. 42 (5), 494–500. https://www.ncbi.nlm.nih.gov/pubmed/12569479.

Wolterbeek, H.T., van der Meer, A.J., 2005. Optimization, application, and interpretation of lactate dehydrogenase measurements in microwell determination of cell number and toxicity. Assay Drug Dev. Technol. 3 (6), 675–682. https://www.ncbi.nlm.nih.gov/pubmed/16438662.

Wu, J., He, Z., Chen, Q., Lin, J.-M., 2016. Biochemical analysis on microfluidic chips. TrAC Trends Anal. Chem. 80, 213–231. https://www.sciencedirect.com/science/article/pii/S016599361530145X.

Wu, M.H., Huang, S.B., Lee, G.B., 2010. Microfluidic cell culture systems for drug research. Lab Chip 10 (8), 939–956. https://www.ncbi.nlm.nih.gov/pubmed/20358102.

Wu, Q., Liu, J., Wang, X., Feng, L., Wu, J., Zhu, X., Wen, W., Gong, X., 2020. Organ-on-a-chip: recent breakthroughs and future prospects. Biomed. Eng. Online 19 (1), 9. https://www.ncbi.nlm.nih.gov/pubmed/32050989.

Wu, S., Shah, D.K., 2020. Determination of ADC cytotoxicity in immortalized human cell lines. Methods Mol. Biol. 2078, 329–340. https://www.ncbi.nlm.nih.gov/pubmed/31643068.

Yan, X., Zhou, L., Wu, Z., Wang, X., Chen, X., Yang, F., Guo, Y., Wu, M., Chen, Y., Li, W., Wang, J., Du, Y., 2019. High throughput scaffold-based 3D micro-tumor array for efficient drug screening and chemosensitivity testing. Biomaterials 198, 167–179. https://www.ncbi.nlm.nih.gov/pubmed/29807624.

Yang, L., Wang, S., Zhao, G., Wang, X., Guo, X., 2020. Comparison of the toxic mechanism of T-2 toxin and deoxynivalenol on human chondrocytes by microarray and bioinformatics analysis. Toxicol. Lett. 321, 61–68. https://www.ncbi.nlm.nih.gov/pubmed/31863870.

Yang, Z., Xiong, H.-R., 2012. In vitro, tissue-based models as a replacement for animal models in testing of drugs at the preclinical stages. In: Ceccherini-Nelli, L., Matteoli, B. (Eds.), Biomedical Tissue Culture. InTech. https://doi.org/10.5772/52300.

Zadorozhnii, P.V., Kiselev, V.V., Kharchenko, A.V., 2020. In silico toxicity evaluation of Salubrinal and its analogues. Eur. J. Pharmaceut. Sci. 155, 105538. https://www.ncbi.nlm.nih.gov/pubmed/32889087.

Zarbl, H., 2001. DNA microarrays: an overview of technologies and applications to toxicology. Curr. Protoc. Toxicol. Chapter 1 (1). Unit1 4. https://www.ncbi.nlm.nih.gov/pubmed/23045022.

Zhang, H., Mao, J., Qi, H.-Z., Ding, L., 2020. In silico prediction of drug-induced developmental toxicity by using machine learning approaches. Mol. Divers. 24 (4), 1281–1290.

Zhang, L., McHale, C.M., Greene, N., Snyder, R.D., Rich, I.N., Aardema, M.J., Roy, S., Pfuhler, S., Venkatactahalam, S., 2014. Emerging approaches in predictive toxicology. Environ. Mol. Mutagen. 55 (9), 679–688. https://www.ncbi.nlm.nih.gov/pubmed/25044351.

Zhu, Q., Li, T., Wei, X., Li, J., Wang, W., 2014. In silico and in vitro genotoxicity evaluation of descarboxyl levofloxacin, an impurity in levofloxacin. Drug Chem. Toxicol. 37 (3), 311–315. https://www.ncbi.nlm.nih.gov/pubmed/24224725.

CHAPTER

25

Regulatory agencies for toxicological studies

Kuldeep Rajpoot[1], *Anand More*[1], *Yogesh Wankhede*[1], *Shyam Gomte*[1], *Muktika Tekade*[2], *Tanisha Gupta*[1], *Bhakti Pawar*[1], *Sanyam Gandhi*[3] *and Rakesh Kumar Tekade*[1]

[1]National Institute of Pharmaceutical Education and Research (NIPER)- Ahmedabad, An Institute of National Importance, Government of India, Department of Pharmaceuticals, Ministry of Chemicals and Fertilizers, Palaj, Gandhinagar, Gujarat, India; [2]School of Pharmacy, Devi Ahilya Vishwavidyalaya, Indore, Madhya Pradesh, India; [3]Takeda Pharmaceuticals, Cambridge, MA, United States

25.1 Introduction

Worldwide, the usage of personal care products and active medicinal components is expanding daily. As a result, these substances have emerged as pollutants of rising concern that pose risks and are hazardous to both aquatic and terrestrial life. Regulatory bodies have developed multiple guidelines and regulations worldwide for the risk assessment of medicines and personal care items to the ecosystem (Kar et al., 2020).

This interaction between regulation and toxicology defines the concept of regulatory toxicology. The likelihood that exposure to a chemical might endanger humans, the level of risk involved, and the expense and consequences of regulation may all be considered. The regulation of chemical hazards is the responsibility of regulatory organizations in the United States, including the Occupational Safety and Health Administration (OSHA), the Environmental Protection Agency (EPA), the Consumer Product Safety Commission (CSPC), and the Food and Drug Administration (FDA). Various bodies have created testing criteria for performing toxicological research in this regard. For instance, US FDA has ascertained that the analysis of testing drugs must be carried out in preclinical examinations to defend human subjects in consequent clinical trials (Persad, 2020).

https://doi.org/10.1016/B978-0-443-15840-7.00015-4

Recently, the use of information through new approach methodologies (NAMs) has been suggested by several organizations, including governmental regulatory bodies in the US and overseas, for enhancing and speeding up chemical evaluations (Harrill et al., 2019). Human medicines are challenged through nonclinical testing to see whether they are safe for use in clinical studies on humans and to commercialize novel medications. The conventional approach has been described in various US FDA and International Council for Harmonization (ICH) guidance documents and consists of in vitro assays and entire animal testing techniques. However, there is no actual figure or type of nonclinical research requisite for safety evaluations because there is inherent versatility for every new molecule. Multiple NAMs for nonclinical assessment have emerged recently because of scientific advancements, and they are being employed in many stages of drug discovery. Conventional nonclinical assessment techniques can anticipate clinical results, but advancements in these techniques to boost clinical outcome predictability are encouraged and found essential (Avila et al., 2020).

The Center for Drug Evaluation and Research (CDER) of the FDA is dedicated to researching the use of NAMs to enhance regulatory effectiveness and hasten the discovery of new drugs. They invite discussions with stakeholders concerning NAMs. The goal of CDER is to ensure that safe and efficient medications are available so that people's health in the US may improve. This contains information on the pharmacology and the pharmacokinetic disposition of the medication or biologic drug, including its absorption, distribution, metabolism, and excretion (ADME) and toxicology (acute, subacute, or chronic, developmental, and reproductive toxicology, carcinogenicity, and "special" toxicology, as needed). This nonclinical material addresses crucial topics of interest to drug researchers at pivotal periods in pharmaceutical research processes (Avila et al., 2020).

Genetic alterations that might take place in somatic and/or germ cells after exposure to a chemical agent are the result of genetic toxicology, also known as "genotoxicity" Chemical substances can affect DNA via direct or indirect contact, as well as the effects of the genetic changes can cause mutations and/or cell death in people with exposed cells. Impacted somatic cells could, for instance, lead to the emergence of cancer or neurodegenerative conditions. Conversely, if the damage is to the germ cells, it may show up as heritable alterations or reproductive problems that might lead to genetic illnesses (OECD, 2015).

25.2 Historical rules for drug safety testing

The Council Directives and Council Recommendations 1983, 1984 of the European Commission (EC) are quoted in place of other national or international regulatory standards when promoting new proprietary medicines in the European region. In principle, to the extent that specific regulations do not replace them, they also include the safety testing of chemicals created by biotechnology. The main objectives of EC safety regulation concerning biotechnology are to ensure the development of all new types of new therapies.

There are two choices until precise guidelines for biotechnological goods become readily accessible. Before marketing, most toxicological analyses outlined in the book (Notes for Guidance in Council Directive 1983 and Proposal for a Council Recommendation 1984) should be conducted, with the obvious exception of those studies which are evidently inappropriate. However, several regulatory authorities appear to be against this practice. The second is to conduct individual case-by-case investigations. Member states are attempting to safeguard their agencies or assist industry by writing or preparing national rules before the EC has prepared "Points to Consider" or "Notes for Guidance" (France, United Kingdom). Other nations, including the United States, Japan, and Sweden, did likewise in the past. According to scientists, these nations either follow the two choices mentioned above or don't have a stance (Bass and Scheibner, 1987).

Regulation authorities and the industry have steadily developed guidelines on the quality attributes of biotechnological products, and it is still controllable. The requirements for pharmacological testing are clearly stated, and it is evident how to conduct thorough clinical trials with the correct design and implementation, including monitoring. Toxicological research and guidance, which are essential for patient care as well as the registrability of the medicine, is, nevertheless, yet in its infancy. It should be acknowledged that monitoring at the toxicological stage can only be as accurate and exact as the scientific state of the art will permit; in contrast, the developing state of the art depends on the research and development of enterprises. Antineoplastic drugs are present in several biopharmaceuticals. To minimize conflict between the therapy's method used for cytostatic and the comprehensive safety technique used for biotechnological goods, one would be well recommended to modify toxicological screening for these medications to the stated purpose and then determine extra requirements. Regulating preclinical and clinical needs for antineoplastics has regrettably not been well-developed, documented, or internationally standardized (Bass and Scheibner, 1987).

The following are the additional major international institutions that publish documentation on toxicity and nonclinical development:

- The Agency for Toxic Substances and Disease Registry (ATSDR)
- European Chemicals Agency
- The Canadian Centre for Occupational Health and Safety
- Dutch Expert Committee on Occupational Standards (DECOS)
- European Centre for Ecotoxicology and Toxicology of Chemicals
- UK Health and Safety Executive (HSE)
- International Agency for the Research of Cancer
- International Programme on Chemical Safety
- The Japanese Association of Industrial Health
- MAK Commission (German Research Foundation)
- The Nordic Expert Group
- Scientific Committee on Occupational Exposure Limits (SCOEL)—EC

25.3 Guidelines issued by regulatory agencies for drug safety

25.3.1 ICH safety guidelines

To identify possible dangers against carcinogenicity and genotoxicity, ICH has developed different safety guidelines (Some important ICH guidelines issued for drug safety are described in Fig. 25.1). A nonclinical testing technique for determining the QT interval

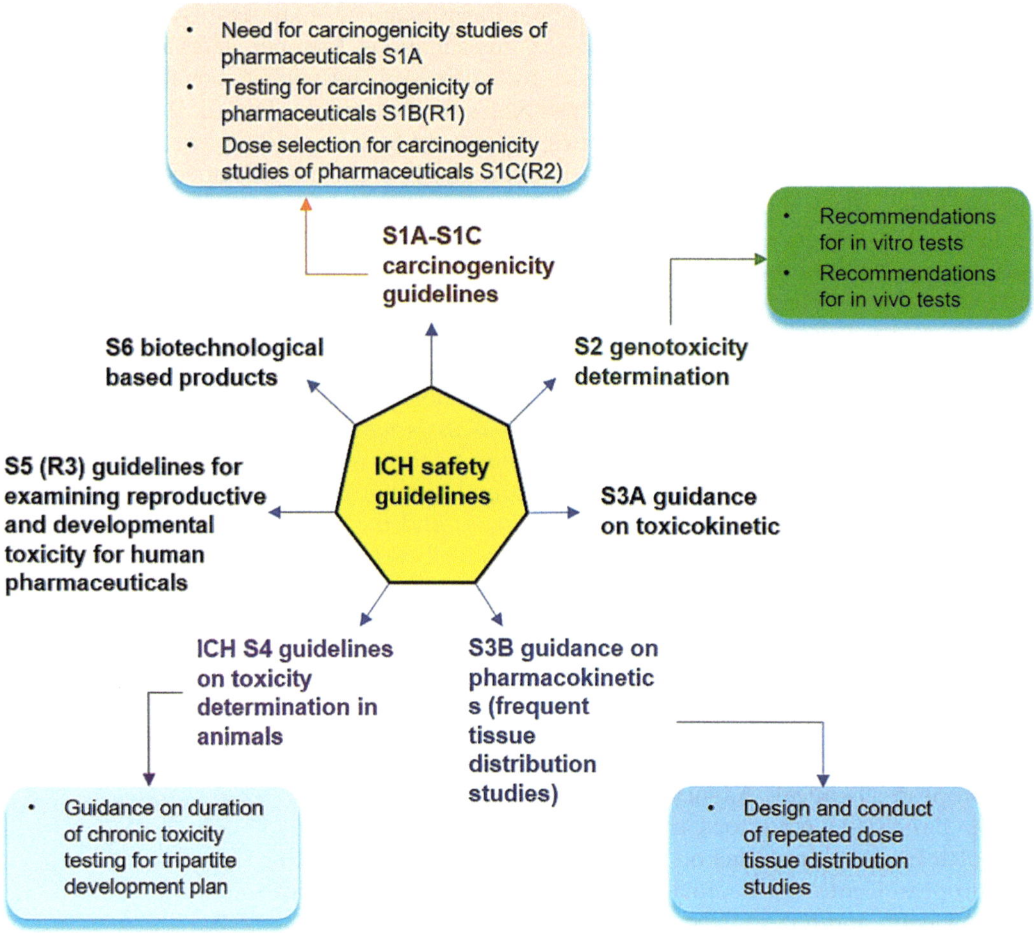

FIGURE 25.1 Some important ICH guidelines issued for drug safety.

prolongation liability, the leading factor in drug discontinuation in recent decades, has recently made significant progress.

25.3.1.1 S1A-S1C carcinogenicity guidelines

25.3.1.1.1 Need for carcinogenicity studies of pharmaceuticals S1A

Identifying a tumorigenic capability in animals and evaluating the pertinent danger in humans are the goals of carcinogenicity research. Carcinogenicity tests may be required if there is any significant worry predicated upon laboratory research, animal toxicity research, or information from human subjects (ICH Expert Working Group, 1995). To prevent the needless utilization of animals in experimentation and ensure uniformity in regulatory analyses of applications throughout the world, the S1A-S1C carcinogenicity guideline aims to specify the circumstances within which carcinogenicity investigations should be carried out. It is anticipated that all this research will be conducted following the most recently recognized scientific norms.

The maximal patient medication time and any apparent cause for risk resulting from previous investigations serve as the essential criteria in determining the necessity of carcinogenicity research. Other variables could also be considered, including the target patient group, previously determined carcinogenic risk, systemic exposure level, resemblance to endogenous chemicals, the proper research design, or the time of research execution for clinical development (ICH Expert Working Group, 1995). For carcinogenicity screening, there are several points to consider:

- **i.** The extent of systemic exposure
- **ii.** Genotoxicity
- **iii.** Duration and exposure
- **iv.** Cause for concern
- **v.** Route of exposure
- **vi.** Indication and patient population
- **vii.** Endogenous peptides, protein compounds, or analogs of those substances

There is much discussion on the applicability of the findings from research on the carcinogenicity of animals to the evaluation of human safety. More studies into the method of action might be required to validate the presence or absence of human carcinogenicity. Mechanistic investigations help determine if tumor discoveries in animals impact human safety.

25.3.1.1.2 Testing for the carcinogenicity of pharmaceuticals S1B(R1)

The recommendation covers all pharmaceutical substances that, as stated in Guideline S1A, require testing for carcinogenicity. Refer to Guideline S6 for medications generated from biotechnology. Only after gathering specific key data, such as the outcomes of genetic toxicology research findings (Guidelines S2A and S2B), destined patient populations, clinical dosage regimens (Guideline S1A), pharmacodynamics in animals as well as people (selectivity, dose-response) (Guideline S1C), and repeated-dose toxicology research, can a test plan for a drug's carcinogenic potential be established. Repeated-dose toxicology research in any species, such as non-rodents, could reveal that the particular substance exhibits immunosuppressive qualities, hormonal action, or other behavior that is thought to be a potential risk for living beings. This data should be considered when designing any additional research to evaluate the carcinogenicity of the chemical (ICH Expert Working Group, 2022). Based on the following factors, the species chosen for long-term carcinogenicity research must be acceptable:

- **i.** Repeated-dose toxicology
- **ii.** Pharmacology
- **iii.** Toxicokinetic
- **iv.** Metabolism
- **v.** Administrative route (e.g., lesser popular ways of drug administration)

i. Further, in vivo carcinogenicity testing might be either (a) or (b) (ICH Expert Working Group, 2022): (a) In vivo rodent test systems for short- or medium-term studies. The utilization of in vivo models that can shed light on carcinogenic outcomes ought to be the primary priority of potentials. These might comprise rodent models of carcinogenesis employing transgenic or neonatal rodents or initiation-promotion models in rodents. (b) It is still permitted to do a long-term carcinogenicity investigation in a different species of rodent. Further, mechanistic investigations can help explain tumor data from carcinogenicity research and shed light on how relevant they are to identifying risk factors for humans. The following aspects should be analyzed during drug discoveries:
   i. Cellular changes
   ii. Factors to consider for further genotoxicity testing
   iii. Biochemical measurements
   iv. Modified protocols

25.3.1.1.2.1 The following general factors should be considered when selecting an acceptable species for long-term carcinogenicity testing In the lack of any other substantial evidence, several general factors led to the selection of rats as the preferred species for long-term carcinogenicity studies and including.

i. Practicality
ii. Data from surveys on prescription drugs
iii. Metabolic disposition
iv. Potential to research mechanisms
v. Examination of several species
vi. Exceptions

25.3.1.1.3 Dose development as per S1C(R2)

As per ICH guidelines, the development of a process established to standardize scientifically based standards for high-dosage selection to attain international harmonization of demands for high-dose choice for carcinogenicity research of pharmaceuticals to create a rational basis for high-dose choice. Many characteristics of pharmaceutical substances set them apart from other environmental contaminants and can support a recommendation that may differ from other guidelines in specific ways (ICH Expert Working Group, 2008). A flexible strategy for dosage assessment is required due to the variety of the chemical and pharmacological properties of pharmaceutically manufactured drugs and the diversity of carcinogenesis pathways. The study suggests that any of the many methods may be helpful for dosage selection (Fig. 25.2), and it should offer a more logical method for dose identification for pharmaceutical carcinogenicity research (ICH Expert Working Group, 2008). The S1C(R2) guidelines provide direction in challenging and complicated areas, acknowledging the significance of revising the specific provisions as depicted in Fig. 25.3 as new information becomes available (ICH Expert Working Group, 2008).

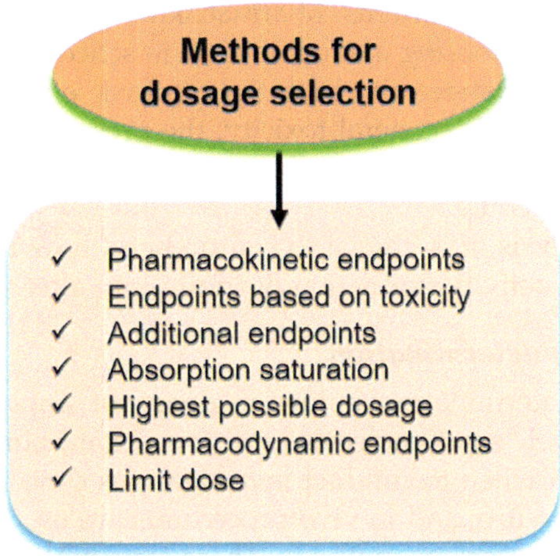

FIGURE 25.2 Methods for dosage selection.

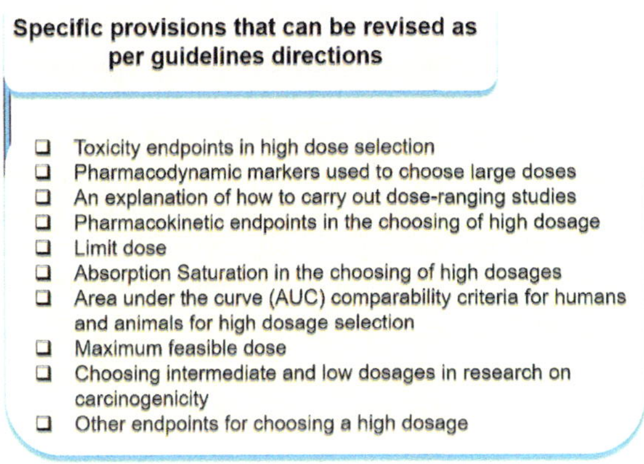

FIGURE 25.3 Some specific provisions that can be revised as per guidelines directions.

Regardless of the endpoint employed, general criteria for executing dose-ranging experiments are made when choosing the high dosage for carcinogenicity research (ICH Expert Working Group, 2008).

i. In practice, where possible, utilizing animal models with rapid tumor development is used in carcinogenicity investigations. It is desirable to study mouse species/strains having metabolic characteristics that are as compared to those of humans as feasible.
ii. All selected animal models to be examined in the carcinogenicity testing must undergo dose-ranging experiments in both males and females.
iii. Most of the time, the decision about dosing is made from 3 months of investigations utilizing the same route and technique employed in the bioassay.

iv. Clinical usage, vulnerability patterns, pharmacokinetics, and practical concerns should all be considered when choosing a suitable dosage schedule and regimen.
v. Ideally, it is essential to characterize both the cytotoxic effect as well as any dose-limiting effects. Additionally, general toxicity, the presence of preneoplastic lesions and/or tissue-specific proliferative impacts, and abnormalities in endocrine balance should be taken into account.
vi. For proper study analysis, it is crucial to comprehend how metabolite profiles or metabolizing enzyme activity (induction or inhibition) alter.

25.3.1.2 S2 genotoxicity determination

The S2 genotoxicity determination guideline does not apply to biologics and thus is focused on evaluating novel "small molecule" medicinal compounds. The ICH M3 (R2) guidance offers suggestions on when to conduct investigations concerning clinical development. Genotoxicity assays are in vitro, and in vivo procedures are used to identify substances that cause genetic harm through various methods. These tests make it possible to identify DNA breakage and its repair risks. Fixing DNA damage caused by genotoxicity is usually seen as crucial for heritable implications or in the multistep development of malignancy, a complicated process wherein genetic alterations could play a role a minor role (ICH Expert Working Group, 2011).

The genotoxic risk of medications must be thoroughly evaluated before registration. Numerous studies have demonstrated that many mutagenic substances in the Ames test are carcinogenic in rodents. In vitro mammalian testing boost susceptibility to detecting rodent carcinogens and widen the range of genetic alterations identified. However, they also reduce prediction specificity, i.e., raise the frequency of favorable outcomes that do not match rodent carcinogenicity. Though no test can detect all genotoxic pathways critical to carcinogenesis, a battery technique is still appropriate. The following are a standard test battery's general features (ICH Expert Working Group, 2011):

i. Testing for mutagenicity in bacteria using a reverse gene mutation method. It was used to identify most genotoxic rodent and human carcinogens as well as critical genetic alterations.
ii. In vitro and/or in vivo testing of genotoxicity in mammalian cells is also essential.

Two possibilities for the common battery that are thought to be equally appropriate are discussed in Fig. 25.4 (ICH Expert Working Group, 2011).

The following circumstances demand modification of the typical test battery:

i. Exploratory clinical investigations
ii. Restrictions on the application of in vivo testing
iii. Substances with structural clues to their potential for genotoxicity
iv. Evaluating substances that are harmful to bacteria

25.3.1.2.1 Suggested in vitro studies

25.3.1.2.1.1 Test repetition and interpretation Research involving innovative methodologies or unanticipated results must have reproducible research outcomes, although regular drug

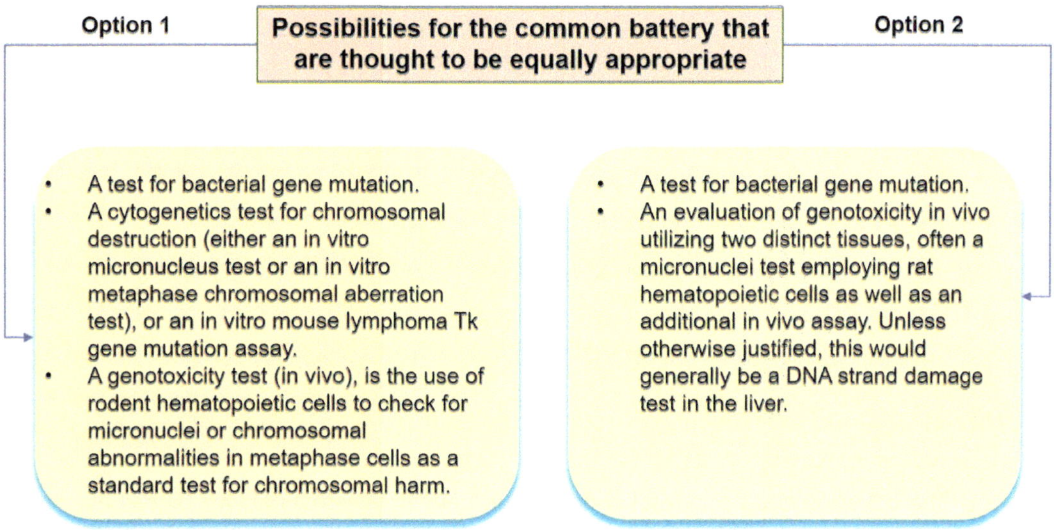

FIGURE 25.4 Two possibilities for the common battery that are considered equally appropriate.

testing using well-accepted genotoxicity assays frequently does not need replication. Repeating an assay that is obviously positive or negative is typically not necessary since it is adequately well-described and has appropriate in-process parameters (ICH Expert Working Group, 2011).

25.3.1.2.1.2 The recommended protocol for the bacterial mutation assay

A. Choosing the highest dosage level comprises:

- **a.** Maximum dose level

  When cytotoxicity or solubility is not concerned, a maximum dosage level of 5000 μg/plate (or 5 μL/plate for liquid test material) is advised.
- **b.** Limit of solubility
- **c.** All minimum possible precipitation should be evaluated, even in the highest or low dose if any sign of cytotoxicity is observed.
- **d.** Limit related to cytotoxicity

  All dosages evaluated in the Ames test should provide indications of considerable toxicity but not over the maximum dose of 5000 μg/plate. Decreasing revertants with reducing background grass are potential signs of toxicity.

B. Study Design/Test Protocol

Bacteria strains listed in Fig. 25.5 are among those that the Organisation for Economic Co-operation and Development (OECD) recommends for detecting base replacement and frameshift mutations.

25.3.1.2.1.3 Factors to consider to perform an assay on mammalian cells

A. Selection of Top Concentration

- **a.** Maximum concentration

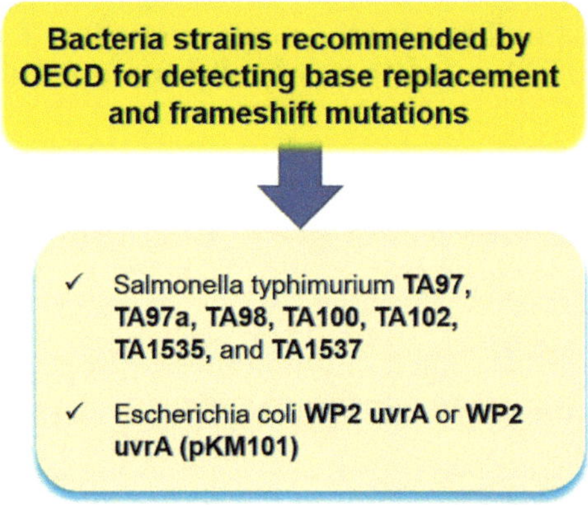

FIGURE 25.5 Bacteria strains recommended by OECD for detecting base replacement and frameshift mutations.

The recommended maximal concentration is 1 mM or 0.5 mg/mL, whichever is lesser unless cytotoxicity or solubility in a solvent or culture medium limits the concentration.

b. Limit of solubility

If cytotoxicity is not the determining factor, whereas solubility is, the highest concentration ought to be the minimum concentration during which minimum precipitate is evident in cultures, assuming that scoring is not affected. Observing precipitation that remains or manifests throughout culture and evaluating it visually or using techniques such as light microscopy (after the course of therapy).

c. Cytotoxicity

In vitro, cytogenetic experiments for metaphase chromosomal abnormalities or micronuclei must only be subjected to cytotoxicity, resulting in a 50% decrease in cell growth or less. In the mouse lymphoma assay (MLA) case, the relative total growth (RTG) must range from 20% to 10% at the maximum dosage, indicating 80%–90% cytotoxicity.

B. Study Design/Test Protocols

The test procedure for the in vitro cytogenetic assessment of chromosomal disruption in metaphase cells must comprise the execution of assays with and without metabolization and adequate positive and negative controls. The assay materials may be used for 3–6 h of therapy, with sampling occurring 1.5 normal cell cycles after the initiation of the therapy. Suppose either the short therapies with metabolization or the short therapies without metabolization provide negative or inconclusive findings. In that case, continued therapy without metabolization should be conducted up to the sampling duration of around 1.5 normal cell cycles. The in vitro micronucleus assay uses similar concepts, but samples are taken 1.5 to 2 normal cell cycles after therapy, allowing time for cells to undertake mitosis and reach the subsequent interphase (ICH Expert Working Group, 2011).

C. Positive Controls

Although concurrent positive controls are crucial, in vitro mammalian cell assessments for genetic toxicity are adequately standardized that utilization of positive controls is typically limited to a positive control to metabolic activation (when this is accomplished simultaneously with the nonactivated test) to show the processes of the metabolic activation system and the sensitivity of the test system (ICH Expert Working Group, 2011).

25.3.1.2.2 Recommendations for in vivo tests

On the following essential subjects, guidelines for in vivo testing are given (ICH Expert Working Group, 2011):

i. Tests to identify chromosomal damage in living organisms
ii. Additional in vivo genotoxicity assessments
iii. Choosing a dose for in vivo tests
iv. Administration route
v. Target tissue exposure must be shown for negative in vivo test findings
vi. Using positive controls in in vivo research
vii. Number of animals examined
viii. Timing of sampling for in vivo tests
ix. In vivo genotoxicity testing on male and female rodents

25.3.1.3 S3A guidance on toxicokinetic

Toxicokinetics is the process of producing pharmacokinetic data to evaluate systemic exposure, either as a crucial part of nonclinical toxicity investigations or in specially tailored supporting studies. The understanding of toxicological results as well as their applicability to clinical safety problems, might well be aided by these findings (ICH Expert Working Group, 1994a). Toxicokinetics' main goal is to explain the systemic toxicity attained in animals and how it relates to the dosage level and the length of the toxicity research. On the other hand, supplementary goals include (a) to correlate the exposure attained in toxicity tests with toxicological results to help to determine how relevant these results are for clinical safety; (b) to provide evidence to justify the selection of the animal and a treatment plan in nonclinical toxicity studies; and (c) to give details that, together with the toxicity data, assist in the development of future nonclinical toxicity research. The following are general guidelines for toxicokinetic studies (ICH Expert Working Group, 1994a):

i. Measurement of exposure
ii. Assessing the degree of exposure in toxicity testing
iii. The rationale for sampling time points
iv. Right dose
v. Administration route
vi. Analytical techniques
vii. Complicating variables in the assessment of exposure
viii. Reporting

ix. Data assessment using statistics
x. Identifying metabolites

Particular considerations mentioned in Fig. 25.6 relate to various aspects of toxicity testing and are based on the toxicokinetics principles mentioned above. If required, the exposure assessment or profiling incidence can be increased or decreased (ICH Expert Working Group, 1994a).

25.3.1.4 S3B guidance on pharmacokinetics (frequent tissue distribution studies)

The evaluation of pharmacology and toxicological findings requires a thorough understanding of a compound's absorption, distribution, metabolism, and elimination. The design of toxicological and pharmacology investigations and the interpretation of their findings may benefit from the knowledge of the pharmacokinetic factors in tissues, particularly concerning probable sites of action (ICH Expert Working Group, 1994b). Instances where repeated dosage tissue distribution investigations must be taken into consideration (ICH Expert Working Group, 1994b).

i. Repeated dose tissue distribution analyses could be necessary. In contrast, research suggested by single dose tissue distribution that the apparent half-life of the experimental substance (and/or metabolites) in organs or tissues substantially surpasses the apparent half-life of the elimination phase in plasma and is much more than twice the dosing interval in the toxicity testing.
ii. Repeated dose tissue distribution investigations must be considered when steady-state values of a chemical or metabolite in the blood are noticeably more significant than those expected by single-dose pharmacokinetic or toxicokinetic research.
iii. Repeated dose tissue distribution research findings could help analyze results when histopathological alterations that are crucial for the safety assessment of the test compound are identified that cannot be described by short-term toxicity testing, single dose tissue distribution research findings, or pharmacological studies. Such research must concentrate on the organs or tissues where the lesions are detected.
iv. Repeated dosage tissue distribution experiments could be necessary for targeted therapy.

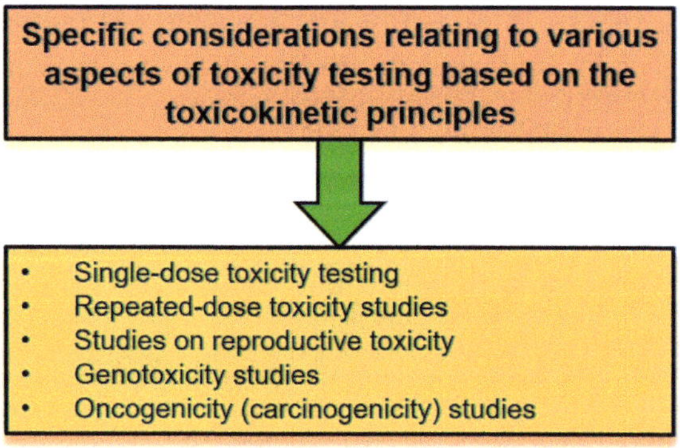

FIGURE 25.6 Specific considerations relating to various aspects of toxicity testing based on the toxicokinetic principles.

25.3.1.4.1 Design and conduct of repeated dose tissue distribution studies

Goals of repeated dose tissue distribution research can be attained using radiolabeled chemicals or equivalent techniques with enough sensitivity and specificity. To resolve the problems that prompted consideration of the repeated dosage tissue distribution studies, the appropriate dose level(s) and species must be selected. In repeated dosage tissue distribution investigations, the treatment period should be chosen based on prior pharmacokinetic and toxicokinetic research data. However, a minimum timeframe for a dosage regimen is often thought to be 1 week. When the substance and/or its metabolites' blood/plasma concentrations do not attain a steady state, an extended period must be preferred. Doses administered over 3 weeks are often inappropriate (ICH Expert Working Group, 1994b).

25.3.1.5 ICH S4 guidelines on toxicity determination in animals

The ICH S4 guideline outlines the factors that should be considered when testing for chronic toxicity in rats and other animals as part of a medication's safety assessment. An applicant could provide a rationale for a different strategy because the guideline is not legally binding. This guideline was developed for the production of pharmaceuticals (ICH Expert Working Group, 1998).

25.3.1.5.1 Guidance on the duration of chronic toxicity testing for the tripartite development plan

Due to the thorough examination and assessment of the data in non-rats indicated above and the successes of ICH1 for evaluation in rodents, to prevent duplication and to adhere to a single development strategy for chronic toxicity testing of novel pharmaceuticals, the research listed below are accepted for submission in these areas: (a) Rodents: an investigation lasting 6 months; (b) Non-rodents: an investigation lasting 9 months (ICH Expert Working Group, 1998).

25.3.1.6 S5 (R3) guidelines for examining reproductive and developmental toxicity of human pharmaceuticals

The S5 (R3) guideline document aims to encourage harmonization and suggest worldwide standards for evaluating nonclinical developmental and reproductive toxicity (DART) tests needed to assist human clinical trials, including pharmaceutical marketing approval. The guidance provides various methodologies and research designs to complement existing data to detect, analyze, or communicate risk. Additionally, general ideas and suggestions are given that must be considered while evaluating the study results. This is an update to the 1993-published ICH guideline "S5 Detection of Toxicity to Reproduction for Medicinal Products." This update extends the utilization of exposure margins in dosage level choice, includes a section on hazard analysis, aligns the guideline with existing ICH recommendations, and broadens the scope to cover vaccinations, including biopharmaceuticals.

Additionally, it gives choices for delaying developing toxicity investigations and outlines the eligibility of alternate assays and probable application scenarios (ICH Expert Working Group, 2020). The purpose of DART research is to identify possible effects of the drug on mammalian reproduction that are important for evaluating human hazards. The series of investigations should, where necessary, include assessments to identify overt and covert adverse effects. Fig. 25.7 describes reproductive phases that are often evaluated (ICH Expert Working Group, 2020).

Further, the following are the key elements to take into account when creating an entire integrated testing approach to assess impacts on development and reproduction are (ICH Expert Working Group, 2020):

i. The intended patient group and usage circumstances (specifically in connection to reproduction capability and the severity of illness)
ii. The drug's formulation and the route(s) of administration
iii. Relevant toxicity information (this may also comprise structure-activity relationships, in vitro, ex vivo, and nonmammalian study data), pharmacokinetics, pharmacodynamics, and pharmacological resemblance to other drug formulations
iv. General biological characteristics of the drug target or recognized functions in development or reproduction.

25.3.1.7 S6 biotechnological-based products

Beginning in the 1980s, the first biopharmaceuticals (drugs produced from biotechnology) were introduced. Afterward, the first marketing authorizations were provided. The regulatory requirements for drugs produced from biotechnology have typically been similar in (ICH Expert Working Group, 1997). To promote clinical development or marketing authorization, all countries have implemented a versatile, case-by-case, science-based methodology for

FIGURE 25.7 Frequently evaluated reproductive phases.

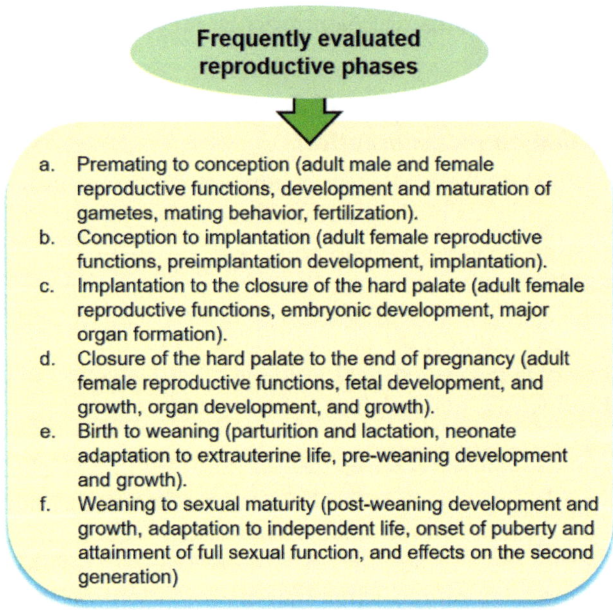

preclinical safety analysis. Here is a requirement for consensus and effective dialogue between the countries in this fast-expanding scientific field. Preclinical safety evaluation's main objectives include the following (ICH Expert Working Group, 1997):

i. To determine a safe starting dosage and dose escalation strategies for people
ii. To determine possible damaging organ targets and determine if such toxicity is treatable
iii. To define safety metrics for clinical assessment. The preclinical risk information used to assist the development of biopharmaceuticals will be of higher quality and consistency if the guidelines outlined in this document are followed.

Preclinical hazard investigations aim to determine pharmacological and toxicological consequences during clinical development as well as before the start of human investigations. Research conducted both in vitro and in vivo may help describe this phenomenon. Less thorough toxicity testing may be required for biopharmaceuticals structurally and pharmacologically identical to a drug with significant clinical usage (ICH Expert Working Group, 1997). Preclinical safety assessment should take into account:

i. Choosing the appropriate animal species
ii. Physical condition
iii. Delivery method
iv. Age
v. Dosage
vi. Administration method
vii. Therapy regimen
viii. Stability of the test substance under actual usage circumstances.

Traditional methodologies for toxicity assessment of pharmaceuticals might not be relevant for these substances because of the unique pathophysiology of these species. Some particular factors could include (ICH Expert Working Group, 1997):

i. Study on local tolerance
ii. Tests on the toxicity of single dosage
iii. Pharmacology safety
iv. Genotoxicity testing
v. Research on immune toxicity
vi. Research on the toxicity of development and reproductive function
vii. Toxicity studies at repeated doses
viii. Carcinogenicity studies

25.3.2 OECD guidelines for examining pesticides and chemicals

A set of OECD rules governs the process of assessing the safety of environmental chemicals in the European Union as well as several other nations (OECD Chemicals Testing

Guidelines, 2012). On the other hand, these recommendations contain several methodological aspects to those used in pharmaceutical analysis. However, there are distinctions in the way hazard evaluation is done for the different types of chemicals (Buschmann, 2013). The evaluation of possible toxicity to reproduction and development must be considered per the OECD criteria (Fig. 25.8) (OECD, 2001a, 1983, 2001b, 1995, 1996, 2007).

25.3.3 Registration, Evaluation, and Authorization of Chemicals (REACH)

REACH is an organization responsible for regulating chemicals used in the European Union by industries. Reach and evaluate chemical properties for humans and the environment. There are a few internal departments in the REACH, like the Risk Assessment Committee and Socioeconomic committee, which regulate many requirements of chemicals and its substitute.

25.3.4 European Chemicals Bureau (ECB)

ECB is based in Italy and provides guidance for chemicals very specific to toxicity. It is a legal reference point for categories based on the toxic effects. It also guides to the

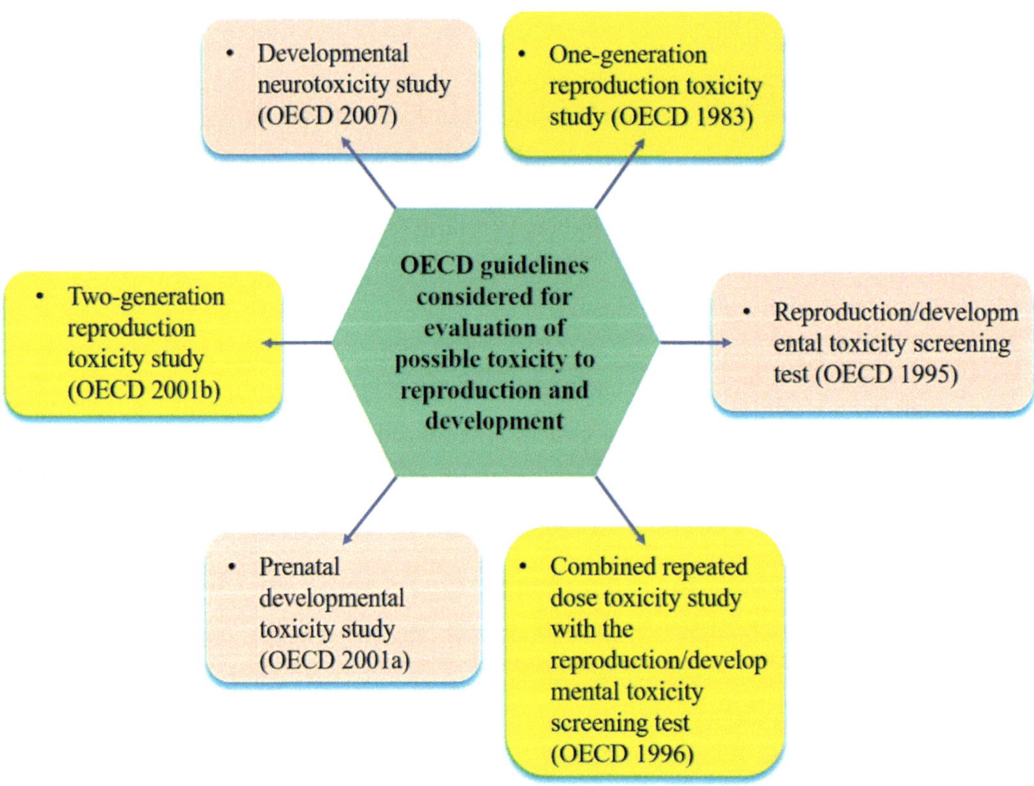

FIGURE 25.8 OECD guidelines considered for evaluation of possible toxicity to reproduction and development.

development of analytical methods for testing. It notifies all the member states of Europe about international trade.

25.4 In vitro analysis of toxicology

The earliest in vitro techniques in regulatory toxicity testing included in vitro mutagenicity testing, which was employed approximately 20 years ago. Numerous validation tests of different in vitro techniques were conducted between 1985 and 1995 for their ability to change the Draize eye irritation testing for objectives of animal protection and improved science. Even though four in vitro techniques, including the bovine corneal permeability and opacity assay (BCOP), the isolated rabbit eye (IRE), and the hen's egg test chorioallantoic membrane (HET-CAM), have been given, these severe eye irritants and related acquired acknowledge were foundation for OECD. Similarly, skin corrosivity and phototoxicity are endorsed as test methods B in Europe for regulatory purposes i.e., B. 40 and B. 41 of Directive 67/548/EEC's Annex V (Liebsch and Spielmann, 2002; Barile, 2010). Several instances of regulatory approval as well as subsequent validation of in vitro toxicity studies are (Liebsch and Spielmann, 2002):

i. Validation of the 3T3 NRU in vitro phototoxicity test
ii. Validation of two in vitro skin corrosivity tests
iii. Validation of the Epiderm human skin model for corrosivity testing
iv. ECVAM validation study of three in vitro embryotoxicity tests
v. Validation of the local lymph node assay (LLNA) for sensitizing properties
vi. Regulatory acceptance of four alternatives to the Draize eye irritation test

25.5 Regulatory perspectives of application of latest techniques in toxicology

Incorporating new methods that involve constant communication among scientists from the FDA, academia, and corporate. Recent scientific advancements must be adopted to enhance the safety evaluation of novel pharmaceuticals and boost the responsiveness and predictiveness of models. The FDA's Critical Path Initiative went into considerable speed about the necessity to enhance safety evaluation and the tools to do this. The Critical Path Initiative specifically targeted areas of immunological toxicity, including liver and cardiovascular safety assessment (Leighton, 2005).

A combination of techniques employed in addition to or in place of the typical toxicological tests carried out to assist an Investigational New Drug (IND) application or New Drug Application (NDA) is referred to as innovative technologies utilized in the regulatory area. Common toxicological investigations of varying durations, pharmacological safety investigations, genotoxicity research, and reproduction system-related toxic studies analyses are all included in the standard package. The employment of the latest biomarkers, trans-infected cells, genetically modified animals, and "omics" technologies are some of the newer and developing technologies being used to regulate new medications (proteomics, metabonomics, toxicogenomics, etc.). Various levels of regulatory development and adoption are present for these technologies. For instance, regulatory bodies now permit the utilization of model organisms to substitute a 2-year carcinogenicity testing.

On the other hand, the "omics" technologies are not adequately developed to obtain regulatory clearance as substitutes. However, these tests are essential early in the drug development process and might be helpful as add-ons to traditional research. Together with conventional toxicological tests, information from these experiments has been utilized to answer particular mechanistic problems (Leighton, 2005).

The Pharmacology Toxicology Coordinating Committee (PTCC) is the primary decision-making authority for scientific assessments as well as decisions addressing pharmacology and toxicology concerns impacting numerous divisions under the CDER. The group leaders of CDER's operating divisions constitute this committee. The PTCC has established various working groups and subcommittees to help with technical issues. Every novel or developing technology would eventually be assessed by one of the PTCC's working groups or subcommittees (Leighton, 2005).

25.6 Amendments in the test guidelines for reproduction and developmental toxicity studies

Regularly, OECD Guidelines for Testing of Chemicals are updated in the era of technological advancements. The first version of Test Guideline (TG) 421 was approved in 1995, using a "Preliminary Reproduction Toxicity Screening Test" methodology. Initial data on potential impacts on reproduction and development can be gathered by using a screening test protocol, either in the preliminary stages of evaluating the toxicity of substances. In addition, it can be employed as one of several preliminary tests on already-existing compounds for which no or little toxicological information exists. So this is important that such guidelines should be updated regularly as day-by-day science is emerging (Saghir et al., 2016). In 1998, the new USEPA rules were made available for public use. This included the risk of developmental harm in fetuses and infants, studies on reproduction and conceiving, and research on neurotoxicity in the developing brain (Kimmel and Makris, 2001). In 2008, the TG 407, known as the "Repeated Dose 28-Day Oral Toxicity Study in Rodents," was improved by adding criteria that can determine the endocrine activity of test compounds. This update to TG 421 was to incorporate endpoints related to endocrine disruptors into the screening of Test Groups (OECD, 2016).

25.6.1 Developmental toxicity study for prenatal

In this area of most common species are rabbits and rats, which will be exposed to the substance during the pregnancy or at least from the time of implantation (which typically occurs around day 6) until the day before delivery. For maternal animals, the recording of clinical indicators and body weights throughout the dosage period is required, they are then sacrificed the day before they give birth, and their bodies are checked for gross signs of disease. Fetuses are removed from the uterus of a pregnant woman, after which they are weighed and checked for problems in their visceral, skeletal, and exterior structures (Rao and Dong, 2013). The first edition of this Test Guideline (TG 414) was released to the public in 1981. It was updated and altered in 2001 based on the recommendations made by an OECD Expert Group on the Evaluation of Toxicity to Reproduction and Development. The TG 414 underwent yet another round of revisions in 2018 to incorporate other endpoints, which increased the likelihood of identifying substances that affect endocrine function. The TG 414 will be updated in 2018 to incorporate rat-specific requirements, and as a result, this modification is only relevant to rats, not rabbits (Kimmel and Makris, 2001; OECD, 2018a).

(i) To account for the likelihood of late gestational developmental effects, the dosage duration was extended to at least encompass the period starting from the time of implantation and continuing until the end of gestation. According to the guideline, if preliminary examinations do not show a significant risk of miscarriage or fetal loss before implantation, then the therapy can be prolonged so that it covers the entirety of the gestational period, beginning with fertilization and continuing up to around 1 day before the day of predicted termination. (ii) The procedures that enable skeletal assessment of cartilage and bone are recommended as the preferred option. In most instances, this is accomplished by applying a twofold stain on fetal skeletons using alizarin red S and alcian blue. However, any approach that permits a comprehensive study of both is permissible. (iii) The minimum number of rabbit dams that are required has been raised to at least 20 for each dosage group. These measures are taken so that effects in research with rabbits can be detected with a higher degree of statistical certainty. (iv) Fetal rabbits' head examinations are further developed to include an internal inspection such that the brain, nasal airway, and eye may all be evaluated more thoroughly (Kimmel and Makris, 2001; OECD, 2018a).

25.6.2 Fertility and reproduction study

Typically, male and female animals (rats) are exposed 10 times earlier to coupling as part of the procedure for studies on fertility and reproduction throughout pregnancy and the mating cycle for females. Breastfeeding mothers and certain male/female F1 offspring continue to be exposed for 10 weeks following weaning. It is a widespread practice to breed F1 males and females and to keep the F1 females exposed during their pregnancies and while nursing. It is possible to get a second litter every generation for research purposes. As an illustration, the developmental neurotoxicity study might be repeated with a second F2 litter, or a conventional fetal assessment comparable to that used in the prenatal study could be performed. In the 1998 updates, this study was expanded to include several outcomes of reproductive toxicity (Kimmel and Makris, 2001; Saghir et al., 2016).

(i) The reproductive cycle of F1 and P females is monitored for 3 weeks before and during the mating process. At the time of termination, the sperm of the F1 and P males are examined for their quality in terms of their number, morphology, and motility. (ii) F1 and F2 generations are analyzed for their reproductive maturity by measuring the time between the vaginal entrance and preputial detachment. Anogenital distance is evaluated in newborn F2 pups to see if there is a medicine-related impact on the F1 sex ratio or sexual maturity. (iii) Weights and histological analyses of reproductive and other organs from animals over generations are performed. In addition, the weights of the brain, thymus, and spleen are measured on F1 and

F2 pups sacrificed when they are weaned. (iv) Primordial follicles in the ovaries of F1 females are subjected to quantitative analysis. These amendments were made as this study is the only study where F1 offspring are subjected to their parents before conception, during lactation, and pregnancy (Kimmel and Makris, 2001; Rao and Dong, 2013).

25.6.3 Developmental neurotoxicity study

It is recognized that various substances have been used to develop neurotoxic effects in humans and other species. To analyze the hazardous properties of a chemical agent or mixture, it may be essential to confirm its potential for developmental neurotoxicity. It is possible to examine developmental neurotoxicity in three separate ways: as a stand-alone study, as part of a more considerable reproductive toxicity investigation, as part of an adult neurotoxicity study, or prenatal developmental toxicity study. In 1995, an OECD Working Group on Reproduction and Developmental Toxicity met in Copenhagen to consider the necessity of revising the existing OECD Test Guidelines for reproduction and developmental toxicity and creating new Guidelines for endpoints not previously addressed. Based on a US EPA guideline that has subsequently been changed, the Working Group suggested creating a Test Guideline for developmental neurotoxicity (OECD, 2007).

In October 2000, an OECD Expert Consultation Meeting and an ILSI Risk Science Institute Workshop were held simultaneously, and in 2005, an Expert Consultation Meeting took place in Tokyo. These sessions were organized to examine the scientific and technological concerns associated with the current Test Guideline, and the recommendations from these meetings were included in creating this Test Guideline (TG 426). According to OECD guidelines (TG 426), the test material is given to the animals during pregnancy and lactation. During fetal development and the first few months after birth, the offspring are exposed to the chemical through the mother's circulation and/or milk. Dams are examined to evaluate the impact on pregnant and lactating females and to give comparison data where offspring are chosen randomly from litters for neurotoxicity testing.

The assessment involves observations to find severe behavioral and neurologic anomalies, evaluations of motor activity, motor and sensory function, learning, and memory, and assessments of physical development, behavioral ontogeny, and the assessment of neuropathology and brain weights during neonatal development and maturity (OECD, 2007). Extra animals from each group may be utilized for specialized neurobehavioral, neuropathological, neurochemical, or electrophysiological procedures to enhance the data gained from the tests specified in this guideline when the test technique is undertaken as independent research. TG 426 recommends that rat is commonly employed as a test subject; however other species might be utilized if necessary. The guideline's gestational and postnatal days only apply to selected rat strains. The test and control groups contain a significant number of females (pregnant) to be subjected to the test substance to ensure sufficient offspring are produced to evaluate neurotoxicity. This TG suggested 20 liters for each dose level; if the maximum number of litters per group is attained, replicate and staggered-group dosing strategies are allowed. To achieve a consistent litter size throughout all litters, the size of each litter should be changed on or before postnatal day four by removing excess pups at random. The litter size should not be larger than the typical litter size for the type of rodents employed. There should be almost equal numbers of male and female puppies in the litter (OECD, 2007).

25.6.4 OECD efforts

OECD has spent considerable time updating and harmonizing its toxicological testing guidelines with the USEPA's regulations by its Chemicals Programme. Over the previous few years, there have been numerous updates made to OECD Guidelines 414 (prenatal developmental toxicity research), 421 (Reproduction/Developmental Toxicity Screening Test), and 443 (Extended One-Generation Reproductive Toxicity Study) that helps to practice revised guidelines for particular test study. Additionally, in 2007 OECD gave a TG 426 (Developmental Neurotoxicity Study) that studied the effects of repeated exposure to a chemical during gestation and early postnatal development is called developmental neurotoxicity (OECD, 2007). In 1995, OECD panel recommended several changes, such as postnatal dosing duration extension, the degree of reflex maturity before weaning, progressive morphometric assessment of progeny's brains, and a more refined approach to allocating animals for experiments (Kimmel and Makris, 2001).

25.6.5 Food and Drug Administration (FDA) guidelines

The revised draft from the Food Safety and Nutrition FDA explains how to test food-related color additives. It also guides neurotoxic, reproductive, and developmental toxicity; however, there is no particular methodology specified. Rather, a tiered testing strategy comprising a preliminary screening study preceded by advanced neurotoxicity testing was mentioned. Based on advancements in safety and risk assessment and an increasing understanding of the pharmacokinetics and metabolism of food constituents, it became clear that the 1982 document must be updated and revised. In 1993, Redbook II was made available for public feedback in draft form. Changes to the reproduction and developmental toxicity guidelines were made after a thorough review of the literature and feedback from the public (Kimmel and Makris, 2001).

The exposure period for pregnant animals in developmental toxicity research typically spans from the day of implantation up until the day before the expected day of delivery. The pregnant females are sacrificed just before the day of anticipated delivery, analyzing the uterine contents, and extracting the fetuses. The fetuses are monitored, stored, and checked for anomalies in the skeleton and soft tissues. The goal of developmental toxicity testing is to determine how an experimental chemical would affect a fetus if the mother or father were exposed to it before or during pregnancy. The adverse effects serve as endpoints for evaluating the hazardous potential of chemical substances. The test for developmental toxicity may be conducted separately or as a component of multigenerational reproduction research. If the study is conducted in conjunction with a reproduction experiment, the teratological effects might be evaluated on either the first or second generation. However, it is typically performed on the last litter of a generation to optimize the animal's exposure to the test substance (FDA US, 2000; OECD, 2018b).

25.7 Amendments in the risk assessment and regulatory requirements

Over the past few years, numerous amendments have taken place to support the USEPA's guidance. Like the US Congress approved the Food Quality Protection Act (FQPA) in 1996, which named pesticides in the diets of infants and children, highlighting issues for earlier methods of addressing pediatric health concerns (Naidenko, 2020). The FQPA is a revision to the FIFRA and the FFDCA, two laws that regulate pesticides and food and cosmetics, respectively. The FQPA required attention to pesticide exposures and their potential effects on children's health. Specifically, it noted "an extra tenfold margin of safety for pesticide chemical residue" and other potential risk factors. The administrator can distinguish the therapeutic window for pesticide residue if accurate data is available. Executive Order No. 13045, which was passed into Law by Clinton in 1997, and the FDA Modernization Act, which did pass by the US Congress in 1997, were two other examples of government decisions that helped bring attention to the issue of the health of children (Cecot et al., 2022). Four areas were chosen as priorities in an executive order: cancer, asthma, injuries, and developmental disorders. Research and community engagement are two main ways that progress is being made in these four areas. The Food and Drug Administration Modernization Act of 1997 was yet another landmark legislation that primarily impacted young people by requiring the FDA to publish many registered medicine for children's health that might make them healthier (Naidenko, 2020; Kimmel and Makris, 2001).

25.7.1 Toxicology data requirements and Office of Pesticide Programs (OPP) 10X Policy

Since the FQPA law was passed in 1996, steps have been taken to put it into effect, as it needed to be used immediately after being passed. At first, only temporary rules were made, and in February 1998, the USEPA set up an office-wide group called the "10X Task Force" to figure out the right set of information about exposure and toxicity for children that is needed to make decisions under FQPA. The Toxicology Working Group is one of the groups that make up this task force especially talked extensively about the idea of a "core toxicology database" that lists the kinds of information that would be required to figure out how dangerous conventional food-use pesticides might be for babies and kids (Makris and Journal, 1999). OPP accepted most of the Toxicology Working Group's suggestions in a draught 10X policy given to the FIFRA SAP in May 1999. According to the guideline, each pesticide's toxicological database must be analyzed using multiple factors. For example, accessibility of toxicology studies, including supporting data. The toxicology data set comprises chronic, subchronic, acute, carcinogenicity, metabolism, and developmental toxicity studies.

In addition, OPP proposed neurotoxicity and immunotoxicity-related studies in adult rats. The draught policy report also had suggestions about how to evaluate each database to figure out how worried people should be about prenatal and postnatal toxicity, including the study of pre and postnatal toxicity, the dose-response aspect of the experimental animal data; and how the animal data applies to people. The Toxicology Working Group concluded that inadequate data on neurotoxic agents and their related side effect is available. Hence, they recommended that neurotoxicity studies should be a priority for all kinds of food usage. These recommendations were proposed by OPP in its draft policy, USEPA 199a (Assessment, 2002; Naidenko, 2020).

25.7.2 OPP data call-in (DCI) for organophosphate insecticides

In the draught 10X policy document, OPP said it planned to use its FIFRA DCI authority to evaluate developmental neurotoxicity for food-use pesticides in a more significant way. Pesticides were selected based on certain criteria. This criterion includes organophosphates, carbamates (inhibit cholinesterase), pyrethrins, organochlorines, organotins, mectins, and arsenicals (Fang et al., 2019). The first set of DCIs for 34 organophosphorus (OP) pesticides with tolerances came out on September 10, 1999. They asked for specific changes to be made in the guideline to address the concerns raised, such as the need to keep giving the drug until postnatal day 21 and comparing how cholinesterase inhibition (or other biomarkers) affects the behavior of adults and children. These changes to the standard design of the OPPTS 870.6300 guideline study are meant to (i) promote the creation of individualized developmental neurotoxicity protocols that make use of other available data on the chemical and chemical class to make the study as good as possible at finding treatment-related effects. In compliance with the goals of the Food Quality Protection Act, we must collect information to examine the relative vulnerability of infants, mothers, and other adults (FQPA); (ii) maximize exposure to investigate potential developmental neurotoxic effects under as many situations as possible; in compliance with the goals of the Food Quality Protection Act, we must collect information to examine the relative vulnerability of infants, mothers, and other adults (FQPA) (Kimmel and Makris, 2001; Naidenko, 2020).

25.7.3 Office of Prevention, Pesticides, and Toxic Substances (OPPTS) voluntary children's testing program

In reaction to Vice President Gore's introduction of the Chemical Right-to-Know Initiative on April 21, 1998, the United States Environmental Protection Agency (EPA) Office of Pollution Prevention and Toxics (OPPT) suggested that (Makris and Journal, 1999), studies of prenatal toxicity, neurotoxicity in the development stage and reproductive toxicity in multiple generations, should be performed as first-tier toxicity tests for evaluation of substances governed by Toxic Substances Control Act (TSCA) to make sure that sufficient data is available to evaluate potential toxicity to infants and children (Kimmel and Makris, 2001). A proposal titled Framework for a Voluntary Children's Chemical Evaluation Program discusses the current state of this initiative (Reiss et al., 2003).

25.7.4 Review of the reference dose (RfD) and reference concentration (RfC) process

In response to concerns voiced by the USEPA 10X Task Force, the agency's Risk Assessment Forum convened a technical panel at the outset of 1999 to examine these concerns in greater depth. The RfD Technical Panel's mission was to analyze the RfD/RfC procedure as a whole, paying particular attention to how well it takes into account vulnerable populations, children's health risks were included too. Consideration was to be given to the 10X Task Force's recommendations for additional testing in the pediatric population, including when such testing should be required, how the results of such tests should be interpreted, and what data should be used to determine risk (Makris and Journal, 1999; Kimmel and Makris, 2001). The goal was to provide a concise summary of potential new scientific challenges to the procedure.

In parallel to the present chronic RfD and RfC, the RfD Technical Panel recommends setting benchmarks for acute, long, and short settings (Rice, 2004). The method used to evaluate the information required to determine various length reference values consisted of looking over the existing testing instructions from three angles:

(i) The scope of exposure and outcome studies across different periods of life.
(ii) What structural and functional endpoints are considered for the human body as a whole and specific organ systems, including nervous, CVS, immune, and reproductive.
(iii) How long subjects are exposed and what effects are measured across different test methods.

This data can be established for reference values. Existing testing criteria for children's health concerns have significant limitations, such as inadequate knowledge of developmental exposures (long-term effects, including diabetes, cancer, or neurotoxicity) and peripubertal exposure effects (Kimmel and Makris, 2001). The pharmacodynamic and kinetic data for distinct stages of life across different age groups can be utilized to determine whether additional testing or assessment may be necessary across age groups and drive interpretation and study designs. The utilization of knowledge which is increasingly available with the advent of genomes, proteomics, etc. provides a specific difficulty for application in the risk assessment process, not just for specific compounds but for numerous agents or mixtures (Ohanian et al., 2002; Rice, 2004; Assessment, 2002).

25.8 Regulatory needs for nanomedicines

It is commonly acknowledged that the use of nanotechnology in medicine has the promise to spur the biomedical revolution (Ditani et al., 2021; Gadekar et al., 2021; Kalyane et al., 2021). Nanomedicines may detect, heal, and control biological systems by taking advantage of their unique physicochemical qualities to treat disorders for which there are now no or just inadequate diagnostic and therapeutic tools accessible (Gadekar et al., 2021; Gorain et al., 2016; Muniswamy et al., 2019; Prajapati et al., 2009; Youngren et al., 2013; Tekade and Chougule, 2013).

Because they are a new product category in the healthcare industry, nanomedicines must abide by the strict guidelines of the medical product regulation or other relevant legal frameworks, such as the medical device regulations. Nanomaterials may need more quality and safety screening than conventional goods owing to their size-related physicochemical features as well as the resultant biological impacts (Sadrieh and Tyner, 2010; Tyner et al., 2015). Critical quality attributes (CQAs) and extra toxicological evaluations must be considered and converted into standardized, regulatory-accepted test techniques and assessment processes for properly examining and monitoring nanomedicines (Bremer-Hoffmann et al., 2018).

However, there are difficulties in regulating such goods that go along with the potential of nanotechnologies in the medical field. To assist regulatory judgment and enable an easy transition to therapeutic interventions, adequate information about their safety, stability, including effectiveness must be acquired. Standardized techniques should be availed. The finding has shown that there are significant local variations in the regulation of nanomedicines, and it has also verified the necessity of harmonizing the informational needs of the unique characteristics of nanomaterials. In particular, the study confirmed a variety of crucial physicochemical characteristics which have previously been put out in scholarly papers as pertinent for regulatory decision-making. Furthermore, the survey has shown that regulatory agencies are interested in a capability for independent nanomedicine characterization that may assist regulators in assessing these platforms and evaluating the effectiveness of both innovative and current test techniques for use in the domain of nanomedicine (Bremer-Hoffmann et al., 2018).

Although the promise of nanotechnology in the healthcare profession is still being fully realized, there are still no reliable datasets from which it is possible to make inferences about informational needs. Competent authorities have begun publishing preliminary reflection papers to offer early guidance on the regulatory data requisites that could be demanded during the various approval steps of pioneering products to foresee regulatory requirements (Committee for Medicinal Products for Human Use) (European Medicines Agency, 2013a,b,c, 2015; US Food Drug Administration, 2015).

25.9 Advanced Therapy Medicinal Products (ATMPs)

ATMPs can be classified broadly into Cell-Based Medicinal Products (CBMPs) and Gene Therapy Medicinal Products (GTMPs). ATMPs is a very complex drug product and is registered only with a centralized process by European Medicinal Agency (EMA). These are complex products compared to conventional medicinal products; all regulatory agencies have more stringent requirements because they include vector insertion and stem cell therapies with more toxicity. In general, ATMPs are single-dose therapy but have long lasting therapeutic effects on patients, so ATMPs require more extended observation studies compared to single-dosage nonclinical studies. Toxicity may appear in weeks or even in months.

"Guideline on non-clinical testing for inadvertent germline transmission of gene transfer vectors" explains pharmacokinetics studies related to GTMPs (EMEA, 2009; EC, 2007). In these cases, biodistribution, expression of the transgene, and observation of genetic change in the body are very important for nonclinical and toxicological studies. Depending on the type of transduction of stem cells, type of toxicology study may vary. For example, if GTMP expresses any growth factor, then tumorigenicity is required. Tumorigenicity should be carefully addressed in nonclinical studies because reports suggest that cells may arise due manufacturing process.

25.10 Conclusion

Toxicology and the introduction of regulations are interrelated. Many government programs use toxicology research findings to promote the regulation of chemicals and other toxic drugs. While some government programs have more formal means of fostering high toxicological research, others use more informal techniques. This interaction between regulation and toxicology defines the concept of regulatory toxicology. The likelihood that exposure to a chemical might endanger humans, the level of risk involved and the expense and consequences of regulation may all be considered. The regulation of chemical hazards is the responsibility of regulatory organizations in the United States, including the OSHA, EPA, CSPC, and FDA. Various bodies have created testing criteria for performing toxicological research in this regard. For instance, this has ascertained that drugs' analysis must be conducted in preclinical examinations to defend human subjects in consequent clinical trials.

25.11 List of abbreviations

ADME	Absorption, Distribution, Metabolism, and Excretion
ATMPs	Advanced Therapy Medicinal Products
ATSDR	Agency for Toxic Substances and Disease Registry
BCOP	Bovine Corneal Permeability, and Opacity Assay
CBMPs	Cell-Based Medicinal Products
CDER	Centre for Drug Evaluation and Research
CQAs	Critical Quality Attributes
CSPC	Consumer Product Safety Commission
DART	Developmental and Reproductive Toxicity
DCI	Data-Call-In
DECOS	Dutch Expert Committee on Occupational Standards
EC	European Commission
ECB	European Chemical Bureau
ECVAM	European Centre for the Validation of Alternative Methods
EMA	European Medicinal Agency
EPA	Environmental Protection Agency
FDA	Food and Drug Administration
FQPA	Food Quality Protection Act
GTMPs	Gene Therapy Medicinal Products
HET-CAM	Hen's Egg Test Chorioallantoic Membrane
HSE	Health and Safety Executive
ICH	International Council for Harmonization
IND	Investigational New Drug
IRE	Isolated Rabbit Eye
LLNA	Local Lymph Node Assay
MLA	mouse lymphoma assay
NAMs	New Approach Methodologies
NDA	New Drug Application
OECD	Organization for Economic Co-operation and Development
OSHA	Occupational Safety and Health Administration
OP	organophosphorus
OPP	Office of Pesticide Programs
OPPT	Office of Pollution Prevention and Toxics

OPPTS	Office of Prevention, Pesticides, and Toxic Substances
PTCC	Pharmacology Toxicology Coordinating Committee
REACH	Registration, Evaluation, and Authorization of Chemicals
RfC	reference concentration
RfD	review of the reference dose
RTG	relative total growth
SCOEL	Scientific Committee on Occupational Exposure Limits
TG	Test Guideline
TSCA	Toxic Substances Control Act

References

Assessment, C.R., 2002. Determination of the Appropriate FQPA Safety.

Avila, A.M., Bebenek, I., Bonzo, J.A., Bourcier, T., Davis Bruno, K.L., Carlson, D.B., Dubinion, J., Elayan, I., Harrouk, W., Lee, S.-L., Mendrick, D.L., Merrill, J.C., Peretz, J., Place, E., Saulnier, M., Wange, R.L., Yao, J., Zhao, D., Brown, P.C., 2020. An FDA/CDER perspective on non-clinical testing strategies: classical toxicology approaches and new approach methodologies (NAMs). Regul. Toxicol. Pharmacol. 114, 104662. https://www.sciencedirect.com/science/article/pii/S027323002030088X.

Barile, F.A., 2010. Validating and troubleshooting ocular in vitro toxicology tests. J. Pharmacol. Toxicol. Methods 61 (2), 136–145.

Bass, R., Scheibner, E., 1987. Toxicological evaluation of biotechnology products: a regulatory viewpoint. In: Chambers, C.M., Chambers, P.L., Davies, D.S. (Eds.), Mechanisms and Models in Toxicology. Springer Berlin Heidelberg, Berlin, Heidelberg, pp. 182–190.

Bremer-Hoffmann, S., Halamoda-Kenzaoui, B., Borgos, S.E., 2018. Identification of regulatory needs for nanomedicines. J. Interdisc. Nanomed. 3 (1), 4–15. https://doi.org/10.1002/jin2.34.

Buschmann, J., 2013. The OECD guidelines for the testing of chemicals and pesticides. In: Barrow, P.C. (Ed.), Teratogenicity Testing: Methods and Protocols. Humana Press, Totowa, NJ, pp. 37–56. https://doi.org/10.1007/978-1-62703-131-8_4.

Cecot, C., Hahn, R.W., 2022. Incorporating equity concerns in regulation. In: George Mason Law & Economics Research Paper.

Ditani, A.S., Mallick, P.P., Anup, N., Tambe, V., Polaka, S., Sengupta, P., Rajpoot, K., Tekade, R.K., 2021. Biosimilars accessible in the market for the treatment of cancer. J. Contr. Release 336, 112–129. https://www.ncbi.nlm.nih.gov/pubmed/34126171.

EC, 2007. Regulation (EC) No 1394/2007 of the European Parliament and of the Council on advanced therapy medicinal products and amending Directive 2001/83/EC and Regulation (EC) No 726/2004. Off. J. Eur. Union 324, 121–137.

EMEA, 2009. Guideline on Non-Clinical Testing for Inadvertent Germline Transmission of Gene Transfer Vectors (EMEA/CHMP/273974/2005). http://www.ema.europa.eu/docs/en_GB/document_library/Scientific_guideline/2009/10/WC500003982.pdf.

European Medicines Agency, 2013a. Committee for Medicinal Products for Human Use- Reflection Paper on Surface Coatings: General Issues for Consideration Regarding Parenteral Administration of Coated Nanomedicine Products. EMA/325027/2013. https://www.ema.europa.eu/en/documents/scientific-guideline/reflection-paper-surface-coatings-general-issues-consideration-regarding-parenteral-administration_en.pdf.

European Medicines Agency, 2013b. Committee for Medicinal Products for Human Use-Joint MHLW/EMA Reflection Paper on the Development of Block Copolymer Micelle Medicinal Products. EMA/CHMP/13099/2013. https://www.ema.europa.eu/en/documents/scientific-guideline/draft-joint-ministry-health-labour-welfare/european-medicines-agency-reflection-paper-development-block-copolymer-micelle-medicinal-products_en.pdf.

European Medicines Agency, 2013c. Committee for Medicinal Products for Human Use-Reflection Paper on the Data Tequirements for Intravenous Liposomal Products Developed with Reference to an Innovator Liposomal Product-Final. EMA/CHMP/806058/2009/Rev.02. http://www.ema.europa.eu/docs/en_GB/document_library/Scientific_guideline/2013/03/WC500140351.pdf.

European Medicines Agency, 2015. Committee for Medicinal Products for Human Use-Reflection Paper on the Data Requirements for Intravenous Iron-Based Nano-Colloidal Products Developed with Reference to an Innovator

Medicinal Product. EMA/CHMP/SWP/620008/2012. https://www.ema.europa.eu/en/documents/scientific-guideline/reflection-paper-data-requirements-intravenous-iron-based-nano-colloidal-products-developed_en.pdf.

Fang, Y., Shi, W.-Q., Wu, J.-T., Li, Y.-Y., Xue, J.-B., Zhang, Y.J.P., VECTORS, 2019. Resistance to pyrethroid and organophosphate insecticides, and the geographical distribution and polymorphisms of target-site mutations in voltage-gated sodium channel and acetylcholinesterase 1 genes in Anopheles Sinensis populations in Shanghai, China, 12, 1–13.

FDA US, 2000. Toxicological principles for the safety assessment of food ingredients. Redbook 1–286. https://www.fda.gov/files/food/published/Toxicological-Principles-for-the-Safety-Assessment-of-Food-Ingredients.pdf. (Accessed 17 August 2022).

Gadekar, V., Borade, Y., Kannaujia, S., Rajpoot, K., Anup, N., Tambe, V., Kalia, K., Tekade, R.K., 2021. Nanomedicines accessible in the market for clinical interventions. J. Contr. Release 330, 372–397. https://www.ncbi.nlm.nih.gov/pubmed/33370576.

Gorain, B., Choudhury, H., Tekade, R.K., Karan, S., Jaisankar, P., Pal, T.K., 2016. Comparative biodistribution and safety profiling of olmesartan medoxomil oil-in-water oral nanoemulsion. Regul. Toxicol. Pharmacol. 82, 20–31.

Harrill, J., Shah, I., Setzer, R.W., Haggard, D., Auerbach, S., Judson, R., Thomas, R.S., 2019. Considerations for strategic use of high-throughput transcriptomics chemical screening data in regulatory decisions. Curr. Opin. Toxicol. 15, 64–75. https://www.sciencedirect.com/science/article/pii/S2468202019300129.

ICH Expert Working Group, 1994a. ICH Harmonised Tripartite Guideline - Note for Guidance on Toxicokinetics: The Assessment of Systemic Exposure in Toxicity Studies S3A. International Council for Harmonisation of Technical Requirements for Pharmaceuticals for Human Use. https://database.ich.org/sites/default/files/S3A_Guideline.pdf. (Accessed 18 August 2022).

ICH Expert Working Group, 1994b. ICH Harmonised Tripartite Guideline Pharmacokinetics: Guidance for Repeated Dose Tissue Distribution Studies S3B. International Council for Harmonisation of Technical Requirements for Pharmaceuticals for Human Use. https://database.ich.org/sites/default/files/S3B_Guideline.pdf. (Accessed 18 August 2022).

ICH Expert Working Group, 1995. ICH Harmonised Tripartite Guideline: Guideline on the Need for Carcinogenicity Studies of Pharmaceuticals S1A. International Council for Harmonisation of Technical Requirements for Pharmaceuticals for Human Use. https://database.ich.org/sites/default/files/S1A%20Guideline.pdf. (Accessed 17 August 2022).

ICH Expert Working Group, 1997. ICH Harmonised Tripartite Guideline Preclinical Safety Evaluation of Biotechnology-Derived Pharmaceuticals S6(R1). International Council for Harmonisation of Technical Requirements for Pharmaceuticals for Human Use. https://database.ich.org/sites/default/files/S6_R1_Guideline_0.pdf. (Accessed 18 August 2022).

ICH Expert Working Group, 1998. ICH Harmonised Tripartite Guideline Duration of Chronic Toxicity Testing in Animals (Rodent and Non Rodent Toxicity Testing) S4. International Council for Harmonisation of Technical Requirements for Pharmaceuticals for Human Use. https://database.ich.org/sites/default/files/S4_Guideline.pdf. (Accessed 18 August 2022).

ICH Expert Working Group, 2008. ICH Harmonised Tripartite Guideline Dose Selection for Carcinogenicity Studies of Pharmaceuticals S1C(R2). International Council for Harmonisation of Technical Requirements for Pharmaceuticals for Human Use. https://database.ich.org/sites/default/files/S1C%28R2%29%20Guideline.pdf. (Accessed 17 August 2022).

ICH Expert Working Group, 2011. ICH Harmonised Tripartite Guideline Guidance on Genotoxicity Testing and Data Interpretation for Pharmaceuticals Intended for Human Use S2(R1). International Council for Harmonisation of Technical Requirements for Pharmaceuticals for Human Use. https://database.ich.org/sites/default/files/S2%28R1%29%20Guideline.pdf. (Accessed 18 August 2022).

ICH Expert Working Group, 2020. ICH Harmonised Guideline Detection of Reproductive and Developmental Toxicity for Human Pharmaceuticals S5(R3). International Council for Harmonisation of Technical Requirements for Pharmaceuticals for Human Use. https://database.ich.org/sites/default/files/S5-R3_Step4_Guideline_2020_0218_1.pdf. (Accessed 18 August 2022).

ICH Expert Working Group, 2022. ICH Harmonised Guideline Testing for Carcinogenicity of Pharmaceuticals S1B(R1). International Council for Harmonisation of Technical Requirements for Pharmaceuticals for Human Use. https://database.ich.org/sites/default/files/S1B-R1_FinalGuideline_2022_0719.pdf. (Accessed 17 August 2022).

Kalyane, D., Kumar, N., Anup, N., Rajpoot, K., Maheshwari, R., Sengupta, P., Kalia, K., Tekade, R.K., 2021. Recent advancements and future submissions of silica core-shell nanoparticles. Int. J. Pharm. 609, 121173. https://www.ncbi.nlm.nih.gov/pubmed/34627997.

Kar, S., Sanderson, H., Roy, K., Benfenati, E., Leszczynski, J., 2020. Ecotoxicological assessment of pharmaceuticals and personal care products using predictive toxicology approaches. Green Chem. 22 (5), 1458–1516. https://doi.org/10.1039/C9GC03265G.

Kimmel, C.A., Makris, S.L., 2001. Recent developments in regulatory requirements for developmental toxicology. Toxicol. Lett. 120, 73–82.

Leighton, J.K., 2005. Application of emerging technologies in toxicology and safety assessment: regulatory perspectives. Int. J. Toxicol. 24 (3), 153–155. https://doi.org/10.1080/10915810590948352.

Liebsch, M., Spielmann, H., 2002. Currently available in vitro methods used in the regulatory toxicology. Toxicol. Lett. 127 (1), 127–134. https://www.sciencedirect.com/science/article/pii/S0378427401004921.

Makris, S.L., 1999. The FQPA 10X safety factor: how traditional risk assessment practices play a role in its application. Human & Ecol. Risk Assess. Inter. J. 5, 1003–1012.

Muniswamy, V.J., Raval, N., Gondaliya, P., Tambe, V., Kalia, K., Tekade, R.K., 2019. 'Dendrimer-Cationized-Albumin' encrusted polymeric nanoparticle improves BBB penetration and anticancer activity of doxorubicin. Int. J. Pharm. 555, 77–99.

Naidenko, O.V., 2020. Application of the food quality protection act children's health safety factor in the US EPA pesticide risk assessments. Environ. Health 19, 1–15.

OECD, 1983. Test Guideline 415. OECD Guideline for Testing of Chemicals. One-Generation Reproduction Toxicity Study. http://www.oecd-ilibrary.org/environment/test-no-415-one-generation-reproduction-toxicity-study_9789264070844-en. (Accessed 18 August 2022).

OECD, 1995. Test Guideline 421. OECD Guideline for Testing of Chemicals. Reproduction/developmental Toxicity Screening Test. http://www.oecd-ilibrary.org/environment/test-no-421-reproduction-developmental-toxicity-screening-test_9789264070967-en. (Accessed 18 August 2022).

OECD, 1996. Test Guideline 422. OECD Guideline for Testing of Chemicals. Combine Repeated Dose Toxicity Study with the Reproduction/developmental Toxicity Screening Test. http://www.oecd-ilibrary.org/environment/test-no-422-combined-repeated-dose-toxicity-study-with-the-reproduction-developmental-toxicity-screening-test_9789264070981-en. (Accessed 18 August 2022).

OECD, 2001a. Test Guideline 414. OECD Guideline for Testing of Chemicals. Prenatal Developmental Toxicity Study. http://www.oecd-ilibrary.org/environment/test-no-414-prenatal-development-toxicity-study_9789264070820-en. (Accessed 18 August 2022).

OECD, 2001b. Test Guideline 416. OECD Guideline for Testing of Chemicals. Two-Generation Reproduction Toxicity Study. http://www.oecd-ilibrary.org/environment/test-no-416-two-generation-reproduction-toxicity_9789264070868-en. (Accessed 18 August 2022).

OECD, 2007. Test Guideline 426. OECD Guideline for Testing of Chemicals. Developmental Neurotoxicity Study. http://www.oecd-ilibrary.org/environment/test-no-426-developmental-neurotoxicity-study_9789264067394-en. (Accessed 18 August 2022).

OECD Chemicals Testing Guidelines, 2012. http://www.oecd.org/department/0,3355,en_2649_34377_1_1_1_1_1,00.html. (Accessed 18 August 2022).

OECD, 2015. Guidance Document on Revisions to OECD Genetic Toxicology Test Guidelines. https://www.oecd.org/env/ehs/testing/Draft%20Guidance%20Document%20on%20OECD%20Genetic%20Toxicology%20Test%20Guidelines.pdf.

OECD, 2016. Test No. 421: Reproduction/Developmental Toxicity Screening Test.

OECD, 2018a. Test No. 414: Prenatal Developmental Toxicity Study.

OECD, 2018b. Test No. 443: Extended One-Generation Reproductive Toxicity Study.

Ohanian, E., ORME-Zavaleta, J., Rice, D., Seed, J., Tilson, H., Vu, V., 2002. A Review of the Reference Dose and Reference Concentration Processes.

Persad, A.S., 2020. Chapter 47 - regulatory toxicology. In: Wexler, P. (Ed.), Information Resources in Toxicology, fifth ed. Academic Press, pp. 503–507 https://www.sciencedirect.com/science/article/pii/B9780128137246000475.

Prajapati, R.N., Tekade, R.K., Gupta, U., Gajbhiye, V., Jain, N.K., 2009. Dendimer-mediated solubilization, formulation development and in vitro-in vivo assessment of piroxicam. Mol. Pharm. 6, 940–950.

Rao, K., Dong, J., 2013. Non-clinical reproductive toxicity testing requirements for drugs, pesticides, and industrial chemicals in India and China. Teratogen. Testing Methods Prot. 13–30.

Reiss, R., Anderson, E.L., Lape, J., 2003. A framework and case study for exposure assessment in the Voluntary Children's Chemical Evaluation Program. Risk Anal Inter. J. 23, 1069–1084.

Rice, D.C., 2004. The US EPA reference dose for methylmercury: sources of uncertainty. Environ. Res. 95, 406–413.

Sadrieh, N., Tyner, K.M., 2010. Nanotechnology and therapeutic delivery: a drug regulation perspective. Ther. Deliv. 1 (1), 83–89.

Saghir, S.A., Dorato, M.A., 2016. Reproductive and developmental toxicity testing: examination of the extended one-generation reproductive toxicity study guideline. Regul. Toxicol. & Pharmacol. 79, 110–117.

Tekade, R.K., Chougule, M.B., 2013. Formulation development and evaluation of hybrid nanocarrier for cancer therapy: taguchi orthogonal array based design. BioMed Res. Int. 2013, 712678.

Tyner, K.M., Zou, P., Yang, X., Zhang, H., Cruz, C.N., Lee, S.L., 2015. Product quality for nanomaterials: current U.S. experience and perspective. Wiley Interdiscip. Rev. Nanomed. Nanobiotechnol. 7 (5), 640–654.

US Food Drug Administration, 2015. Liposome Drug Products-Guidance for Industry. FDA-2016-D-2817. Center for Drug Evaluation and Research. https://www.fda.gov/media/70837/download. (Accessed 18 August 2022).

Youngren, S.R., Tekade, R.K., Gustilo, B., Hoffmann, P.R., Chougule, M.B., 2013. STAT6 siRNA matrix-loaded gelatin nanocarriers: formulation, characterization, and ex vivo proof of concept using adenocarcinoma cells. BioMed Res. Int. 2013, 858946.

Further reading

Encha Europa. https://echa.europa.eu/regulations/reach/understanding-reach.

CHAPTER

26

Key challenges for toxicologists in the 21st century

Havish Shukla[1], *Muktika Tekade*[2], *Bhakti Pawar*[1], *Kuldeep Rajpoot*[1] *and Rakesh Kumar Tekade*[1]

[1]National Institute of Pharmaceutical Education and Research (NIPER)- Ahmedabad, An Institute of National Importance, Government of India, Department of Pharmaceuticals, Ministry of Chemicals and Fertilizers, Palaj, Gandhinagar, Gujarat, India; [2]School of Pharmacy, Devi Ahilya Vishwavidyalaya, Indore, Madhya Pradesh, India

26.1 Introduction

The science of toxicity deals with testing chemical products, pesticides, medicines, and toxicants for their potential to cause harmful and adverse health effects. Environmental toxicology, forensic toxicology, and economic toxicology are the three major branches of toxicology (Wexler et al., 2005). Environmental toxicity mainly deals with occupational health and industrial hygiene, while forensic toxicology deals with the deleterious effect of poisons and psychoactive substances (Chung and Choe, 2019). Economic toxicity covers the study of the harmful effects of substances related to economics. In addition, food toxicology and drug toxicology are the two subdivisions of economic toxicology, as food and drugs are directly related to the economics of the country. Risk assessment pattern and nature of toxicity testing depend upon the substance under investigation (Council, 2006). Pharmaceutical drugs require extensive testing as compared to food materials.

Toxicologists are the researchers who identify the potential of a compound to cause toxicity upon exposure. Therefore, toxicologists play a vital role in the protection of human health from different harmful substances. The science of toxicology has been a topic of interest since ancient times. This is because health has always been an important concern for humankind. Paracelsus (a physician from the 16th century) is considered the father of toxicology (Borzelleca, 2000). Compared to ancient times, today's science of toxicology has evolved a lot. However, toxicologists are facing many challenges that remain unresolved over the period of time and still need resolution (Smith, 2001). In the 21st century, toxicologists face a new set of

https://doi.org/10.1016/B978-0-443-15840-7.00019-1

challenges due to advancement in modern biology and biotechnology. Advancements in toxicogenomics and system biology introduced nonanimal-based approaches for toxicity testing (Smith, 2006). Apart from advances in system biology, advances in nanoscience present a new challenge among toxicologists due to the unique characteristics of nanomaterial. Public concern and information regarding the effects of chemical exposure have increased due to access to information via the internet. So, there is pressure among toxicologists to properly present information in risk communication (Lilienblum and Lilienblum, 2020).

26.2 Challenges and limitations of animal-based toxicity testing

Since the 18th century, animals have been used to study the effect of poisons on the body fluids and tissues of the animal (Smith, 2006). Various types of animals, for instance, rodents, dogs, and non-human primates, are used for the toxicity study of chemical agents. Animal tests are conducted to predict the potential of the chemical agent to cause various adverse effects on human health, but several challenges are associated with animal-based toxicity testing (Worth, 2019).

Extrapolation of animal toxicity data to humans is a crucial challenge for the toxicologist (Smith, 2001). Extrapolation of animal toxicity data involves the application of uncertain factors as well as many assumptions owing to high-dose exposure to a small number of animals in toxicological studies. In toxicity testing, animals are usually exposed to the highest dose level, also termed the maximum tolerated dose (MTD) (Chevret, 2014). Sometimes, animals exhibit adverse effects when they are exposed to a chemical agent. However, there may be the possibility that these chemical agents do not show any adverse effects in humans. This is because MTD used in animal testing is usually much higher than typical human exposure, and this higher dose may be responsible for causing toxic responses in the animals, which might not occur at human dose. Therefore, it presents a big challenge to toxicologists to determine the relevant MTD that should be exposed to animals (Smith, 2001).

Not limited to this, sometimes the use of animals in toxicity testing raises ethical issues, which result in the restricted use of animals in toxicological studies. Hence, extrapolation of toxicology data from a few animals of a specific strain to a large human population with very different genetic backgrounds is also a big challenge for toxicologists (Smith, 2001; Tambe et al., 2021f). Animal-based toxicity testing procedures are not only expensive but also time-consuming, and therefore, only a few specific agents are selected for testing purposes, and a large number of compounds remain untested. Animal-based toxicological studies are wholly based on the animal biological system. Hence, the relevancy of these animal-based toxicity tests to human biology is a big question mark (Worth, 2019; Andersen and Krewski, 2009). As a result, the development of human-specific animal-based toxicity testing procedures is a big challenge to the toxicologist.

26.3 Nonanimal-based toxicity testing methods

Traditionally, animals are used to check the toxicity potential of chemical agents. Still, their restricted use owing to growing ethical concerns and the lack of relevancy of these tests to human biology demands some other alternative approaches for carrying out efficient toxicological studies. In this regard, to overcome disadvantages associated with animal-based toxicity testing, some other alternative approaches, like in vitro cell culture methods and in silico methods, have come into the picture due to the advancement of technology in the 21st century (Sun et al., 2012; Pamies and Hartung, 2017). A comparison of animal-based and nonanimal-based toxicity is discussed in Fig. 26.1.

26.3.1 Advancement of technology in the 21st century

Advances in emerging technologies like biotechnology, omics technologies, molecular biology, and computational biology can predict the toxicity of chemicals by minimizing or replacing the use of animals (Krewski et al., 2020; Worth, 2019). Emerging technology, such as computational biology, can predict the toxicity of chemical agents by analyzing its data after toxicological studies. Advances in biotechnology and molecular biology make toxicity testing cheaper and quicker by evaluating risk assessment of chemical agents using in silico methods and physiologically relevant high-throughput in vitro screening. Advances

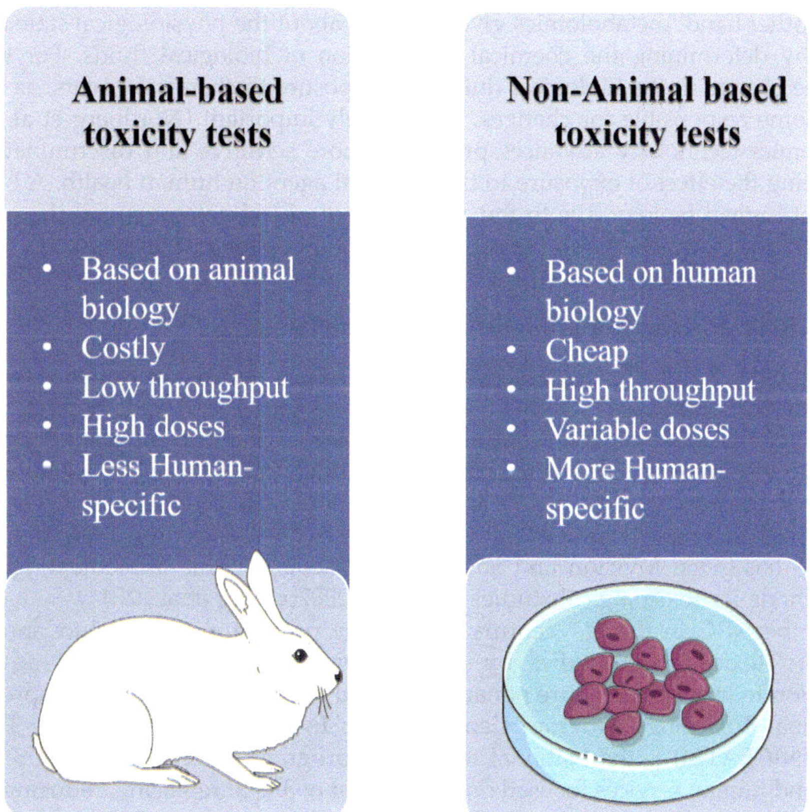

FIGURE 26.1 Comparison between animal-based and non-animal-based toxicity testing.

in molecular biology help not only in understanding the cellular network and pathways of toxicity but also assist in developing a model for testing directly related to human biology.

In starting of the 21st century, the publication of the human genome draft sequence made gene expression profiling possible (Consortium, 2001). Toxicogenomics is the subbranch of genomics that amalgamate toxicology with information-dense genomic technology to understand the response of the genome to hazardous chemical exposure (Duffus et al., 2007). Transcriptomics, proteomics, and metabolomics are the three major branches under the umbrella of omics technologies used by toxicogenomics. Transcriptomics deals with the expression of messenger ribonucleic acid (mRNA) levels in a cell population using various high throughput technologies and deoxyribonucleic acid (DNA) microarray. In contrast, gene expression profiling deals with mRNA expression, which is connecting step between genes and proteins, and it is used to understand whether genes are active or silent (Council, 2007a). Additionally, in omics study, proteomics is the next step after transcriptomics, which deals with the expression of proteins encoded by ribonucleic acid (RNA). Proteomics is more complicated than genomics because a particular genome is approximately constant, but proteins produced in the cell may vary from time to time. Therefore, proteomes can also act as a toxicity signature owing to the expression of distinct proteins on toxicants exposure (Council, 2007a; Merrick and Bruno, 2004).

On the other hand, metabolomics gives the idea about the physiological state of the organ or tissue by determining the chemical composition of biological fluids. For toxicological studies, the change in the biological fluid after exposure to chemical agents, as well as part of the genome responsible for changes, is extremely important (Nordberg et al., 2004). In a nutshell, omics technology advances provide a more sensitive and discriminating method for predicting the effect of exposure to the chemical agent on human health. A better understanding of human biology due to the advancement of technology paved the way for high throughput, cheap, quicker, and human-specific methods for toxicity studies.

26.3.2 Vision for the nonanimal-based toxicity testing

To overcome the challenges associated with toxicity testing of animal models and to develop low-cost, quick, highly robust, and human biology-based toxicity tests, various government agencies and scientific communities reviewed the current testing strategies and developed a vision for nonanimal-based toxicity testing. In 2007, the United States (US) Environmental Protection Agency (EPA), in collaboration with US National Research Council (NRC), published a report entitled "Toxicity Testing in the 21st Century: A Vision and a Strategy." NRC has given a vision and strategy to toxicologists for implementing nonanimal-based methods for toxicological studies (Council, 2007b; Berg et al., 2011).

As per the NRC in the 21st century, this is the peak time to introduce innovative approaches in toxicological studies by implementing recent technological advancements. NRC's vision to implement future nonanimal-based toxicity testing has widespread support. The National Toxicology Program Center for the Evaluation of Alternative Toxicological Methods (NICEATM) is the National toxicology program office under the US department of health and human services focused on the concept of 3Rs of replacing, reducing, or refining animal use in toxicological studies (NIEHS, 2021).

Many elements of the US NRC vision were also familiar with European initiatives aimed at the development of nonanimal-based methods. The European Union (EU) introduced registration, evaluation, authorization, and restriction of chemical (REACH) substances programs for the chemical industry. As per the REACH, the program industry must prefer animal testing as the last option for toxicity testing. REACH emphasizes doing relevant in vitro testing, and if animal testing is done, then it must be designed in such a way that it fills the existing knowledge gap (Lilienblum et al., 2008; Locke et al., 2017).

26.3.3 Pitfalls associated with nonanimal-based toxicity testing

In vitro toxicity testing and various computational models emerged as high throughput, cheap, quicker, and human-specific methods for toxicity studies; however, they are associated with some challenges, which need to be addressed for the implementation of nonanimal-based toxicity testing vision (Fig. 26.2).

26.3.3.1 Lack of cell lines with physiological relevance

To understand the molecular basis of toxicity, the cell line must mimic the condition required to initiate the toxicity pathway (in vivo). The development of an in vitro model, which entirely mimics in vivo conditions, is quite unrealistic and challenging. Providing a microenvironment mimicking cell-compound interactions and cell-cell interaction is complicated (Krewski et al., 2020).

26.3.3.2 Intra- and interlaboratory variability

Intra- and interlaboratory variability leads to poor reliability of cell-based toxicity testing. Different standard operating procedures and differences in qualitative observation may be

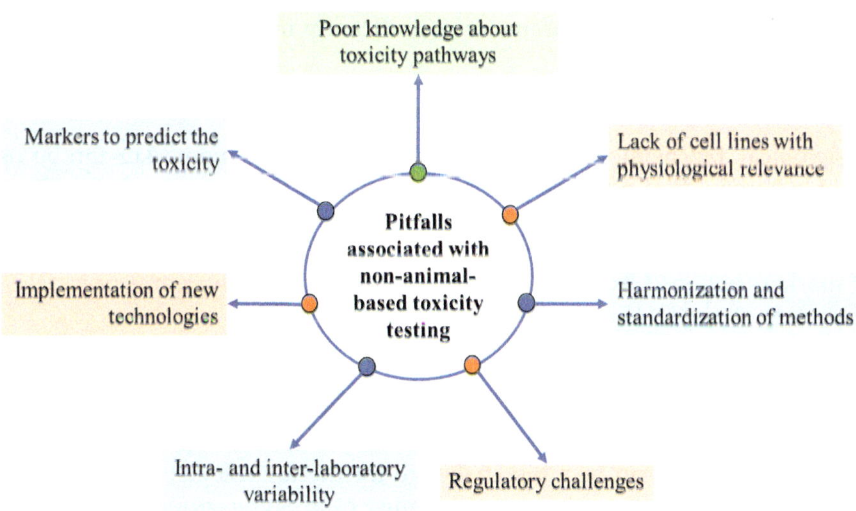

FIGURE 26.2 Pitfalls associated with nonanimal-based toxicity testing.

responsible for laboratory variability, which results in the deviation of final results (Berg et al., 2011).

26.3.3.3 Poor knowledge about toxicity pathways

The pathway between molecular initiating event to perturbation of cellular response also results in an adverse effect and is termed a toxicity pathway. Initiating events is the starting point of the interaction of the chemical agent with a biological system of the organism (Council, 2007b). To understand the toxicity pathway and determine the endpoints of the toxicological studies, the available in vivo data still provide inadequate information about the correlation between diseased (e.g., diabetics, cancer, etc.) and healthy states (Desai et al., 2021). Apart from the pharmaceuticals, in vivo data for comparison is rare for other chemical agents (Berg et al., 2011; Rajpoot et al., 2020c; Kumawat et al., 2020).

26.3.3.4 Implementation of new technologies

Expeditious implementation of new emerging technology is necessary to convert the vision of nonanimal-based toxicity testing into reality, but applying these new technologies also faces several hurdles. For instance, to understand the mode of toxicology by gene expression profiling, there must be a link between the mode of toxicity and gene regulation events. As a massive amount of data is generated by gene expression profiling, its extracting desired information from the sheer weight of the data, which is also a challenge for the toxicologist (Orphanides, 2003; Smith, 2001; Bassett et al., 1999; Sauer et al., 2017). This advancement in computational toxicity (CompTox) by US EPA evaluates more than thousands of chemical agents in a concise period and produces a large amount of data. However, integrating this massive data from CompTox is also challenging for the toxicologist (Thomas et al., 2019).

26.3.3.5 Harmonization and standardization of methods

Identifying critical factors for the reliability of an assay is a big challenge in front of a toxicologist. For in vitro toxicological studies, both culture media and biological reagents must be selected carefully because these parameters significantly impact the in vitro toxicity testing results (Locke et al., 2017).

26.3.3.6 Markers to predict the toxicity

A physiological, biochemical, or histological change in the biomarker can be used as an indicator of a pathological response or pharmacological process to a chemical agent (Jain, 2010). Therefore, before conducting any toxicological studies, the relevance of markers must be established. For the prediction of endpoints in clinical toxicological studies, optimization of markers obtained from a human-specific in vitro test system is necessary (Krewski et al., 2020; Berg et al., 2011).

26.3.3.7 Regulatory challenges

The nature of data obtained from nonanimal-based toxicity testing is highly different from the current data evaluated by the regulatory system. Hence, the regulatory acceptance of this nonanimal-based toxicity can be a big challenge for the toxicologist. As per the Toxic Substances Control Act (TSCA) guidelines, data must clear some ground rules for regulatory acceptance testing. From the business point of view, the development of new nonanimal-based toxicological studies will be hindered if the data generated by these methods will not be accepted. Hence, toxicological studies reliant on cell-based data demand a scientific discussion between toxicologists and regulatory bodies to bridge the gap between new cellular-based data and current data (Locke et al., 2017; Prior et al., 2019).

26.4 Nanoscience brings a new challenge for the toxicologist

In the 21st century, nanotechnology is one of the most emerging and promising fields of science (Gadekar et al., 2021; Ditani et al., 2021; Ganguly et al., 2018; Bahadar et al., 2016). Nanotechnology is defined as the design, production, and characterization of materials with unique properties by controlling the size in the nanoscale range (Tekade et al., 2017; Bayda et al., 2020). The unique property offered by nanomaterials due to their small size has been exploited in various areas like engineering, medicine, computer science, and material science (Bayda et al., 2020; Pandey et al., 2020; Patel et al., 2020; Rajani et al., 2020). In addition, nanotechnology has also shown its presence in regenerating human tissues/organs and three-dimensional printing products/devices for replacing different defective body parts (Rajpoot et al. 2020a, 2020d, 2020e). These transplanted devices can also have the possibility of producing toxicity owing to their rejection by the body. Hence, this rapid progression of nanotechnology is accompanied by new challenges for the toxicologist, especially in medicine (Achanta et al., 2021; Anup et al. 2021a, 2021c; Polaka et al., 2021; Bahadar et al., 2016; Ganguly et al., 2018).

Environmental toxicity studies for occupational health workers at the workplace is a challenging task for the toxicologist (Sahu and Hayes, 2017). During the energetic process, the nanoparticles (NPs) aerosolization is attained, which could be due to the low density and small size of the NPs. Therefore, risk assessment of the airborne nanomaterial waste generated during manufacturing at the workplace is necessary for the safety of workers (Geraci and Castranova, 2010; Maynard and Kuempel, 2005). Developing exposure limits and conducting the risk assessment of the NPs for the workers at a place where NPs are produced or handled is also a considerable challenge for the toxicologist. Reflection of particle size and exposure level at the workplace in the bioassay system to carry out toxicological studies is a complex task for the toxicologist (Geraci and Castranova, 2010; Kuempel et al., 2012).

Toxicological studies of nanomaterials used in the treatment of various diseases are crucial for the toxicologist due to the unique properties of the nanoformulations (Sreeharsha et al., 2020; Rajpoot et al. 2020d, 2020e, 2021c; Rajpoot and Tekade, 2019). Physiochemical properties of the NPs strongly differ from the bulk material through which the NPs is composed because the property of nanomaterials is highly dependent upon the size, shape, and coating of the nanomaterials (Guisbiers et al., 2012; Haase et al., 2012; Rajpoot et al. 2020b, 2020f; Padiyar et al., 2020). Nanotoxicology is a complex domain to work. Unlike conventional toxicology, the biological effect of NPs made from one particular composition can't be generalized because the toxicity of nanomaterial depends not only on the composition but also on shape, size, and nanomaterial surface. Hence, if there is any change in NPs' shape, size, and surface characteristics, then all toxicity tests must be carried out for those NPs. Therefore, in the case of nanomaterial toxicity, characterization of the nanomaterial is critical, as depicted in Fig. 26.3 (Sharifi et al., 2012).

NPs size, shape, surface area, polydispersity, and structural properties play an essential role in nanotoxicology. Sometimes, bulk material from which NPs is formed cannot enter the cell. Still, at the same time, NPs of that material can enter the cells via ion channels due to their small size and may be responsible for inducing toxicity. The polydispersity of the particle is critical to understand whether toxicity is due to the large or small particles (Dhawan and Sharma, 2010; Dhawan et al., 2009). Many studies demonstrated that the shape of the NPs also alters the toxicity activity. Hamilton and the group reported that titanium dioxide nanospheres were less bioactive in both cellular and animal models compared to nanowires of the same composition and diameter (Porter et al., 2008; Hamilton et al., 2009).

The large surface area of the NPs is responsible for the high reactivity of the NPs. Further, the structure, as well as physicochemical properties of NPs, can have a significant influence on the different pharmacokinetic parameters like absorption, distribution, metabolism, and

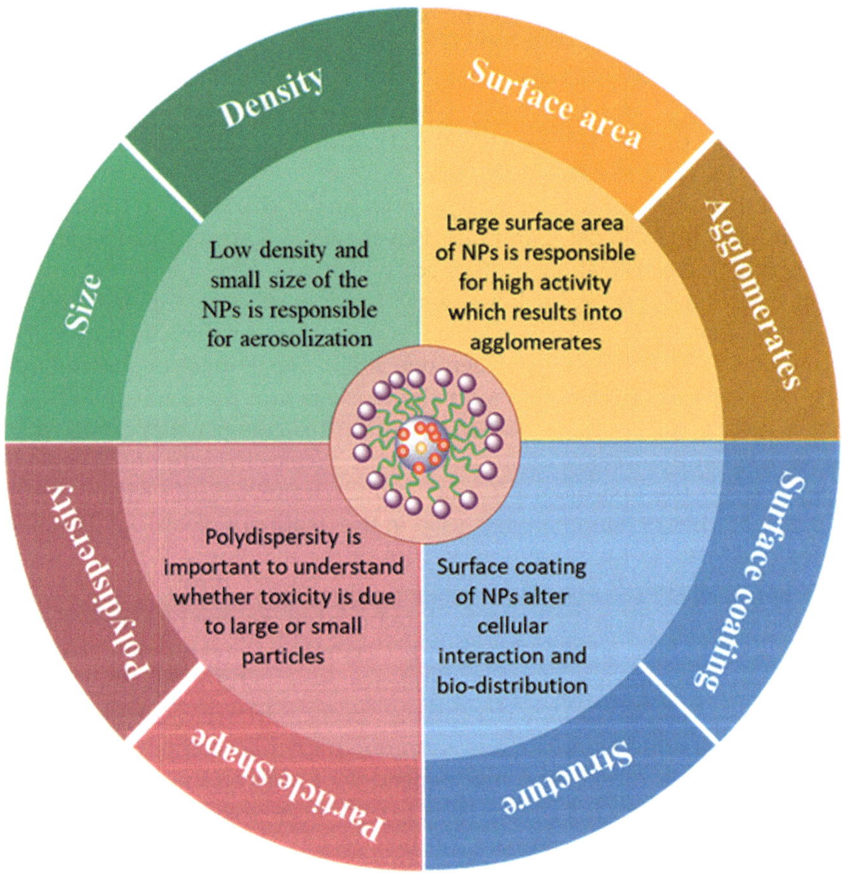

FIGURE 26.3 Nanomaterial characteristics play a critical role in interpreting toxicological studies.

excretion of these toxic agents through the body (Tambe et al. 2021b, 2021e; Rajpoot et al. 2021a, 2021b). In in vitro, toxicological studies found that NPs bind to the proteins already present in suspension media due to their high surface activity and interfere with the evaluation of the cytotoxicity of NPs (Lynch and Dawson, 2020). The degree of NPs dispersion is critical for the biological activity of the NPs. In this regard, Wang and the group demonstrated that poorly dispersed single-walled carbon nanotubes (SWCNTs) showed no effect on the lung fibroblasts in culture.

In contrast, well-dispersed SWCNT showed proliferation of the fibroblasts (Wang et al., 2010). During in vivo studies, when NPs are suspended in biological media like phosphate-buffered saline (PBS), NPs tend to agglomerate into larger particles, which alters the bioactivity of NPs (Geraci and Castranova, 2010). Challenges associated with in vitro and in vivo toxicological studies of nanomaterials are described in Fig. 26.4 (Dhawan and Sharma, 2010).

26.5 Challenges associated with risk communications

Risk communication is an interactive process in which information and point of views on probabilities and the extent of risk is exchanged among toxicologists, risk assessors, and various interested parties (Organization, 2018). The vital role of the toxicologist is to assess the risks rationally for the benefit of human health and provide information related to this risk to the general public. The major challenge in front of the toxicologist is to explain scientific risk issues and their legal context to the public in laymen's language (Wallace, 2011). In the internet era, the overflooded and distorted information raises contradictory concerns among the public, and it's a challenge for the toxicologist to banish the myths about the subject and to achieve the trust of the public. For risk communication, product information on the label also plays an important role. The challenge for toxicologists and risk experts is to provide written information in a short but comprehensive manner with all official requirements specified by laws and regulations (Lilienblum and Lilienblum, 2020).

26.6 Challenges posed by rare and newly emerging diseases

As per the US, a rare disease affects less than two lakh individuals (USFDA, 2021). As a small human population is affected by a rare disease, therefore, a small sample size can be collected, which is a major issue to treat the rare disease. A small sample population in rare diseases leads to poor quality statistics data, which provide incomplete information about the toxicity caused by a chemical agent and is a big issue for the toxicologist (Mitani and Haneuse, 2020). Apart from the rare disease, the dynamics and landscape of new and emerging diseases like COVID-19 is a major challenge for the toxicologist (Esser et al., 2020).

26.7 Challenges posed by limited access to information

Pharmaceuticals and agrochemicals come under highly regulated markets because these industries are directly related to the health of the human population, due to which product

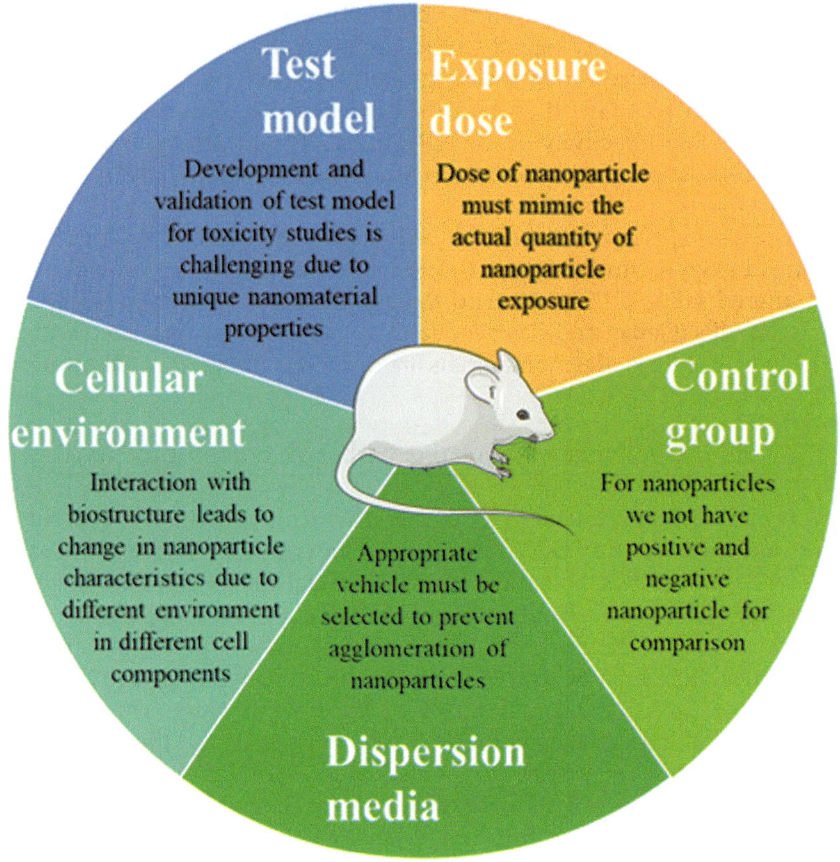

FIGURE 26.4 Challenges associated with in vitro and in vivo toxicological studies of nanomaterials.

efficacy and safety are of supreme importance. To secure regulatory approval, extensive data is generated to prove the safety and efficacy of the product. A lot of time and money is typically invested to generate this data. To motivate research and pay off the investment, regulatory authorities and Trade-Related Aspects of Intellectual Property Rights (TRIPS) recognized the need for data protection. Therefore, regulatory data protection becomes crucial in a highly regulated market dealing with product safety and efficacy (Cook, 2007; Armouti and Nsour, 2016).

This protection of safety data by regulatory data protection, patenting acts, and copyright leads to limited access to information for the toxicologist to evaluate the toxicity potential of chemical agents. Advancement in emerging technologies leads to the collecting of large amounts of in vitro toxicology data. For the initial evaluation, this data must be compared with already available animal and human toxicology data to reach some conclusion but limited access to this data is a major hurdle for the toxicologist to establish a relationship between in vitro and in vivo toxicology data available for animal and human (Locke et al., 2017). To overcome this challenge, there is a need for "open data," which is freely available for the evaluation of the toxicity potential of the compound. There is a good initiative by the US EPA to provide EPA computational toxicology data without any copyright restriction for the evaluation of the toxicity potential of the chemical agent (EPA, 2021).

26.8 Approaches to overcome these challenges

Toxicologists can overcome some of the above-discussed challenges by applying different tactics (Fig. 26.5). For instance, in the case of nonanimal-based toxicity studies, cell lines with high relevancy to in vivo conditions can be developed by sufficiently understanding molecular aspects of in vivo process. Understanding the in vivo condition helps to develop a proper microenvironment for the in vitro model. Strict compliance with the standard operating procedure is a must to overcome variability in cytotoxicity studies. For the harmonization and standardization of toxicity testing methods, parameters necessary for the reproducibility and reliability of toxicity assay should be addressed systematically (Berg et al., 2011).

The major challenge in front of toxicologists for nanotoxicology is the availability of a vast number of NPs to be tested to check their toxicity potential. Therefore, to overcome this challenge, interdisciplinary collaboration is required to develop a matrix relationship between NPs' physiochemical properties and toxicological response. This matrix relationship can be developed by establishing a collaboration between formulation scientists and toxicologists. In this regard, the formulation scientists would formulate groups of NPs with desired physicochemical properties, and toxicologists check the biological activity of all sets to develop a relationship matrix from which toxicity of a similar set of NPs can be predicated without carrying out complete toxicity studies (Geraci and Castranova, 2010). Additionally, some novel

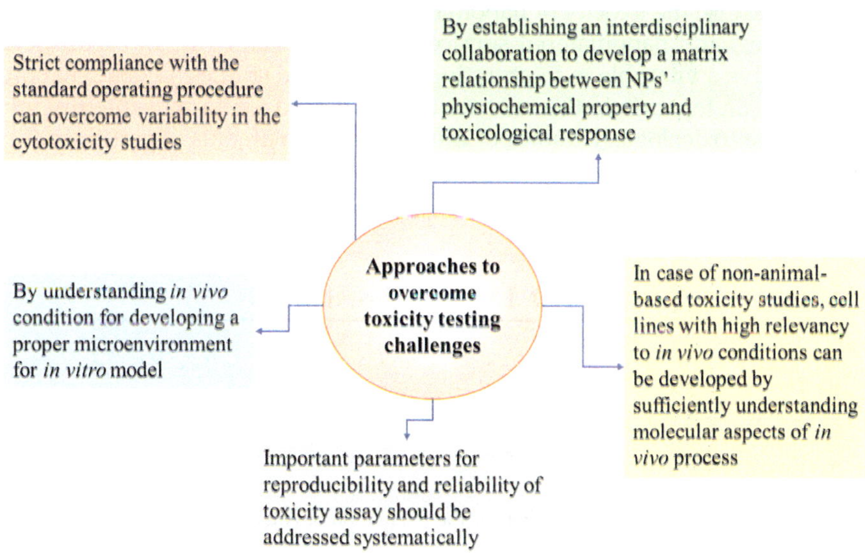

FIGURE 26.5 Various approaches to overcome toxicity testing challenges.

computational approaches and models are also used for predicting the toxicity of a chemical agent (Tambe et al. 2021a, 2021c, 2021d). In this regard, several software are employed for pharmacokinetic and toxicokinetic analysis of chemical agents (Anup et al., 2021b).

26.9 Conclusion

Toxicologist deals with testing drugs, pesticides, and many other chemical products to check their potential to cause harmful and adverse effects on health. Thus, toxicologist plays an essential role in ensuring the safety of the human population. Traditionally, animal-based toxicological studies are conducted to check toxicity potential, but some challenges are also associated with animal-based toxicity testing. Extrapolation of animal toxicity data to humans, low human specificity, restricted use of animals, and growing ethical concerns are some of the challenges associated with animal-based toxicity studies.

In the 21st century, technological advances like omics, biotechnology, computational biology, and molecular biology paved the pathway for high throughput, less costly, rapid, and human-specific nonanimal-based toxicological studies. Implementing these new emerging technologies for nonanimal-based toxicological studies is challenging. Various government agencies and scientific communities developed a vision and road map for the implementation of nonanimal-based toxicological studies in reality. Still, the implementation of this vision into reality is quite challenging. The development of in vitro model, which entirely mimics in vivo conditions, is the critical challenge associated with nonanimal-based toxicological studies.

Nanotechnology has emerged as one of the most promising fields of science in the 21st century. Nanomaterial toxicity testing is challenging due to its unique characteristics. Unlike conventional toxicology, the biological effect of NPs made from one particular composition can't be generalized because the toxicity of nanomaterial depends not only on the composition but also on shape, size, and nanomaterial surface properties. Therefore, the characterization of nanomaterials plays a vital role in interpreting toxicological studies. Overall, nanotoxicology is a complex domain to work. In this context, there is a need for various interdisciplinary collaborations for the toxicological studies of these complex materials. Apart from this, limited access to information due to regulatory data protection, patenting acts, and copyright restriction is a crucial challenge for the toxicologist.

26.10 List of abbreviations

3RS replacing, reducing, or refining
DNA deoxyribonucleic acid
EPA Environmental Protection Agency
EU European Union
mRNA messenger RNA
MTD maximum tolerated dose
NICEATM National Toxicology Program Center for the Evaluation of Alternative Toxicological Methods
NPs nanoparticles
NRC National Research Council

PBS phosphate-buffered saline
REACH registration, evaluation, authorization, and restriction of chemical
RNA ribonucleic acid
SWCNT single-walled carbon nanotubes
TRIPS Trade-Related Aspects of Intellectual Property Rights
TSCA Toxic Substances Control Act
US United States

References

Achanta, N.S.K., Rajpoot, K., Tekade, R.K., 2021. Drug metabolic kinetics. In: Tekade, R.K. (Ed.), Biopharmaceutics and Pharmacokinetics Considerations. Elsevier, Academic Press, pp. 1–19.

Andersen, M.E., Krewski, D., 2009. Toxicity testing in the 21st century: bringing the vision to life. Toxicol. Sci. 107 (2), 324–330.

Anup, N., Desai, N., Rajpoot, K., Tekade, R.K., 2021a. Kinetics of maternal-fetal drug transfer. In: Tekade, R.K. (Ed.), Biopharmaceutics and Pharmacokinetics Considerations, pp. 1–18.

Anup, N., Gadeval, A., Rajpoot, K., Tekade, R.K., 2021b. Software used in ADME computation. In: Tekade, R.K. (Ed.), Biopharmaceutics and Pharmacokinetics Elsevier. Academic Press, pp. 1–10.

Anup, N., Rajpoot, K., Tekade, R.K., 2021c. Overview of biopharmaceutics and pharmacokinetics. In: Tekade, R.K. (Ed.), Biopharmaceutics and Pharmacokinetics Considerations. Elsevier, Academic Press, pp. 1–23.

Armouti, W., Nsour, M.F., 2016. Test data protection: different approaches and implementation in pharmaceuticals. Marquette Intellect. Prop. Law Rev. 20, 267.

Bahadar, H., Maqbool, F., Niaz, K., Abdollahi, M., 2016. Toxicity of nanoparticles and an overview of current experimental models. Iran. Biomed. J. 20 (1), 1–11.

Bassett, D.E., Eisen, M.B., Boguski, M.S., 1999. Gene expression informatics—it's all in your mine. Nat. Genet. 21 (1), 51–55.

Bayda, S., Adeel, M., Tuccinardi, T., Cordani, M., Rizzolio, F., 2020. The history of nanoscience and nanotechnology: from chemical–physical applications to nanomedicine. Molecules 25 (1), 112.

Berg, N., De Wever, B., Fuchs, H.W., Gaca, M., Krul, C., Roggen, E.L., 2011. Toxicology in the 21st century–working our way towards a visionary reality. Toxicol. Vitro 25 (4), 874–881.

Borzelleca, J.F., 2000. Paracelsus: herald of modern toxicology. Toxicol. Sci. 53 (1), 2–4.

Chevret, S., 2014. Maximum Tolerable Dose (MTD). Wiley StatsRef: Statistics Reference Online.

Chung, H., Choe, S., 2019. Challenges in forensic toxicology. Aust. J. Forensic Sci. 51 (6), 665–673.

Consortium, I.H.G.S., 2001. Initial sequencing and analysis of the human genome. Nature 409 (6822), 860–921.

Cook, T., 2007. Regulatory data protection in pharmaceuticals and other sectors. Intellectual Property Management in Health and Agricultural Innovation: A Handbook of Best Practices, Volumes 1 and 2, pp. 437–455.

Council, N.R., 2006. Toxicity Testing for Assessment of Environmental Agents: Interim Report.

Council, N.R., 2007a. Applications of Toxicogenomic Technologies to Predictive Toxicology and Risk Assessment.

Council, N.R., 2007b. Toxicity Testing in the 21st Century: A Vision and a Strategy. National Academies Press.

Desai, N., Koppisetti, H., Rajpoot, K., Tekade, M., Sharma, M.C., Tekade, R.K., 2021. Influence of fever on pharmacokinetics of drugs. In: Tekade, R.K. (Ed.), Biopharmaceutics and Pharmacokinetics Considerations, first ed. Elsevier, pp. 1–13.

Dhawan, A., Sharma, V., 2010. Toxicity assessment of nanomaterials: methods and challenges. Anal. Bioanal. Chem. 398 (2), 589–605.

Dhawan, A., Sharma, V., Parmar, D., 2009. Nanomaterials: a challenge for toxicologists. Nanotoxicology 3 (1), 1–9.

Ditani, A.S., Mallick, P.P., Anup, N., Tambe, V., Polaka, S., Sengupta, P., Rajpoot, K., Tekade, R.K., 2021. Biosimilars accessible in the market for the treatment of cancer. J. Contr. Release 336, 112–129.

Duffus, J.H., Nordberg, M., Templeton, D.M., 2007. Glossary of terms used in toxicology, (IUPAC Recommendations 2007). Pure Appl. Chem. 79 (7), 1153–1344.

EPA, 2021. https://www.epa.gov/chemical-research/downloadable-computational-toxicology-data.

Esser, C., Hochrath, K., Schikowski, T., Haarmann-Stemmann, T., 2020. COVID-19 research: toxicological input urgently needed. Arch. Toxicol. 94 (7), 2547–2548.

Gadekar, V., Borade, Y., Kannaujia, S., Rajpoot, K., Anup, N., Tambe, V., Kalia, K., Tekade, R.K., 2021. Nanomedicines accessible in the market for clinical interventions. J. Contr. Release 330, 372–397.

Ganguly, P., Breen, A., Pillai, S.C., 2018. Toxicity of nanomaterials: exposure, pathways, assessment, and recent advances. ACS Biomater. Sci. Eng. 4 (7), 2237–2275.

Geraci, C.L., Castranova, V., 2010. Challenges in assessing nanomaterial toxicology: a personal perspective. Wiley Interdiscipl. Rev. Nanomed. Nanobiotechnol. 2 (6), 569–577.

Guisbiers, G., Mejía-Rosales, S., Leonard Deepak, F., 2012. Nanomaterial Properties: Size and Shape Dependencies. Hindawi.

Haase, A., Tentschert, J., Luch, A., 2012. Nanomaterials: a challenge for toxicological risk assessment?. In: Molecular, Clinical and Environmental Toxicology. Springer, pp. 219–250.

Hamilton, R.F., Wu, N., Porter, D., Buford, M., Wolfarth, M., Holian, A., 2009. Particle length-dependent titanium dioxide nanomaterials toxicity and bioactivity. Part. Fibre Toxicol. 6 (1), 35.

Jain, K.K., 2010. The Handbook of Biomarkers, first ed. Humana Press, Springer, Totowa, New Jersey, United States.

Krewski, D., Andersen, M.E., Tyshenko, M.G., Krishnan, K., Hartung, T., Boekelheide, K., Wambaugh, J.F., Jones, D., Whelan, M., Thomas, R., Yauk, C., Barton-Maclaren, T., Cote, I., 2020. Toxicity testing in the 21st century: progress in the past decade and future perspectives. Arch. Toxicol. 94 (1), 1–58.

Kuempel, E.D., Geraci, C.L., Schulte, P.A., 2012. Risk assessment and risk management of nanomaterials in the workplace: translating research to practice. Ann. Occup. Hyg. 56 (5), 491–505.

Kumawat, A., Raval, N., Reddy, G., Rajpoot, K., Tekade, R.K., 2020. Gene delivery to tackle diabetic nephropathy. In: Tekade, R.K. (Ed.), The Future of Pharmaceutical Product Development and Research. Academic Press, pp. 515–537.

Lilienblum, W., Dekant, W., Foth, H., Gebel, T., Hengstler, J.G., Kahl, R., Kramer, P.J., Schweinfurth, H., Wollin, K.M., 2008. Alternative methods to safety studies in experimental animals: role in the risk assessment of chemicals under the new European Chemicals Legislation (REACH). Arch. Toxicol. 82 (4), 211–236.

Lilienblum, W., Lilienblum, M., 2020. Risk communication: challenges for toxicologists and other risk experts. Regulat. Toxicol. 1–13.

Locke, P.A., Westphal, M., Tischler, J., Hessler, K., Frasch, P., Myers, B., Krewski, D., 2017. Implementing toxicity testing in the 21st century: challenges and opportunities. Int. J. Risk Assess. Manag. 20 (1–3), 198–225.

Lynch, I., Dawson, K.A., 2020. Protein–nanoparticle interactions. Nano-Enabled Med. Appl. 231–250.

Maynard, A.D., Kuempel, E.D., 2005. Airborne nanostructured particles and occupational health. J. Nanoparticle Res. 7 (6), 587–614.

Merrick, B.A., Bruno, M.E., 2004. Genomic and proteomic profiling for biomarkers and signature profiles of toxicity. Curr. Opin. Mol. Therapeut. 6 (6), 600–607.

Mitani, A.A., Haneuse, S., 2020. Small data challenges of studying rare diseases. JAMA Netw. Open 3 (3), e201965.

NIEHS, 2021. https://www.niehs.nih.gov/health/topics/science/sya-iccvam/index.cfm.

Nordberg, M., Duffus, J., Templeton, D.M., 2004. Glossary of terms used in toxicokinetics (IUPAC Recommendations 2003). Pure Appl. Chem. 76 (5), 1033–1082.

Organization, W.H., 2018. Risk Communication Applied to Food Safety: Handbook. Food & Agriculture Org.

Orphanides, G., 2003. Toxicogenomics: challenges and opportunities. Toxicol. Lett. 140–141, 145–148.

Padiyar, A., Agrawal, O.P., Rajpoot, K., Tekade, R.K., 2020. Hydrotropy, mixed hydrotropy, and mixed solvency as trending concept for solubilization of lipophilic drugs. In: Tekade, R.K. (Ed.), The Future of Pharmaceutical Product Development and Research. Academic Press, pp. 145–178.

Pamies, D., Hartung, T., 2017. 21st century cell culture for 21st century toxicology. Chem. Res. Toxicol. 30 (1), 43–52.

Pandey, V., Ganeshpurkar, A., Thakur, A., Sharma, M., Rajpoot, K., Tekade, M., Sreeharsha, N., Tekade, R.K., 2020. Gold nanoparticles: an advanced drug delivery and diagnostic tool. In: Tekade, R.K. (Ed.), The Future of Pharmaceutical Product Development and Research. Academic Press, pp. 609–669.

Patel, V., Rajani, C., Paul, D., Borisa, P., Rajpoot, K., Youngren-Ortiz, S.R., Tekade, R.K., 2020. Dendrimers as novel drug-delivery system and its applications. In: Tekade, R.K. (Ed.), Drug Delivery Systems. Academic Press, pp. 333–392.

Polaka, S., Swetha, K.L., Dittakavi, S., Rajpoot, K., Tekade, R.K., 2021. Bioanalytical method development and validation for establishing bioavailability and bioequivalence. In: Tekade, R.K. (Ed.), Biopharmaceutics and Pharmacokinetics Considerations. Elsevier, pp. 1–30.

Porter, D., Holian, A., Sriram, K., Wu, N., Wolfarth, M., Hamilton, R., Buford, M., 2008. Engineered titanium dioxide nanowire toxicity in vitro and in vivo. Toxicologist 102, A1492.

Prior, H., Casey, W., Kimber, I., Whelan, M., Sewell, F., 2019. Reflections on the progress towards non-animal methods for acute toxicity testing of chemicals. Regul. Toxicol. Pharmacol. 102, 30–33.

Rajani, C., Borisa, P., Karanwad, T., Borade, Y., Patel, V., Rajpoot, K., Tekade, R.K., 2020. Cancer-targeted chemotherapy: emerging role of the folate anchored dendrimer as drug delivery nanocarrier. In: Chauhan, A., Kulhari, H. (Eds.), Pharmaceutical Applications of Dendrimers. Elsevier, pp. 151–198.

Rajpoot, K., Safavi, M., Sreeharsha, N., Tekade, R.K., 2020a. Recent advances in regenerative medicine. In: Tekade, R.K. (Ed.), The Future of Pharmaceutical Product Development and Research. Academic Press, pp. 367–412.

Rajpoot, K., Tekade, M., Pandey, V., Nagaraja, S., Youngren-Ortiz, S.R., Tekade, R.K., 2020b. Self-microemulsifying drug-delivery system: ongoing challenges and future ahead. In: Tekade, R.K. (Ed.), Drug Delivery Systems. Academic Press, pp. 393–454.

Rajpoot, K., Tekade, M., Sharma, M.C., Molugulu, N., Tekade, R.K., 2020c. New advances in insulin products. In: Tekade, R.K. (Ed.), The Future of Pharmaceutical Product Development and Research. Academic Press, pp. 483–514.

Rajpoot, K., Tekade, M., Sharma, M.C., Sreeharsha, N., Arafat, B., Tekade, R.K., 2020d. 3D printing as an emerging tool in pharmaceutical product development. In: Tekade, R.K. (Ed.), The Future of Pharmaceutical Product Development and Research. Academic Press, pp. 27–71.

Rajpoot, K., Tekade, M., Sharma, M.C., Sreeharsha, N., Sharma, A., Tekade, R.K., 2020e. Recombinant blood products and therapeutic enzymes: an update. In: Tekade, R.K. (Ed.), The Future of Pharmaceutical Product Development and Research. Academic Press, pp. 447–482.

Rajpoot, K., Tekade, M., Sreeharsha, N., Sharma, M.C., Tekade, R.K., 2020f. Recent advancements in solubilization of hydrophobic drugs. In: Tekade, R.K. (Ed.), The Future of Pharmaceutical Product Development and Research. Academic Press, pp. 109–144.

Rajpoot, K., Tekade, R.K., 2019. Microemulsion as drug and gene delivery vehicle: an inside story. In: Tekade, R.K. (Ed.), Drug Delivery Systems. Academic Press, pp. 455–520.

Rajpoot, K., Tekade, R.K., Chatterjee, B., Sharma, M.C., Tekade, M., 2021a. Biopharmaceutical considerations in the pediatric and geriatric formulation development. In: Tekade, R.K. (Ed.), Biopharmaceutics and Pharmacokinetics Considerations. Elsevier, Academic Press, pp. 1–36.

Rajpoot, K., Tekade, R.K., Sharma, M.C., Safavi, M., Tekade, M., 2021b. Pharmacokinetics modeling in drug delivery. In: Tekade, R.K. (Ed.), Biopharmaceutics and Pharmacokinetics Considerations. Elsevier, Academic Press, pp. 1–56.

Rajpoot, K., Tekade, R.K., Sharma, M.C., Tekade, M., 2021c. Pharmacokinetics and biopharmaceutics: "a leader or attendant". In: Tekade, R.K. (Ed.), Biopharmaceutics and Pharmacokinetics Considerations. Elsevier, Academic Press, pp. 1–11.

Sahu, S.C., Hayes, A.W., 2017. Toxicity of nanomaterials found in human environment: a literature review. Toxicol. Res. Appl. 1, 2397847317726352.

Sauer, U.G., Deferme, L., Gribaldo, L., Hackermüller, J., Tralau, T., van Ravenzwaay, B., Yauk, C., Poole, A., Tong, W., Gant, T.W., 2017. The challenge of the application of'omics technologies in chemicals risk assessment: background and outlook. Regul. Toxicol. Pharmacol. 91, S14–S26.

Sharifi, S., Behzadi, S., Laurent, S., Forrest, M.L., Stroeve, P., Mahmoudi, M., 2012. Toxicity of nanomaterials. Chem. Soc. Rev. 41 (6), 2323–2343.

Smith, L.L., 2001. Key challenges for toxicologists in the 21st century. Trends Pharmacol. Sci. 22 (6), 281–285.

Smith, L.L., 2006. Future challenges for toxicologists. Toxicol. Lett. 164, S38–S39.

Sreeharsha, N., Rajpoot, K., Tekade, M., Kalyane, D., Nair, A.B., Venugopala, K.N., Tekade, R.K., 2020. Development of metronidazole loaded chitosan nanoparticles using QbD approach-a novel and potential antibacterial formulation. Pharmaceutics 12 (10).

Sun, H., Xia, M., Austin, C.P., Huang, R., 2012. Paradigm shift in toxicity testing and modeling. AAPS J. 14 (3), 473–480.

Tambe, V., Desai, N., Rajpoot, K., Tekade, R.K., 2021a. "Organ-on-a-chip"-based physiologically relevant pharmacokinetic models. In: Tekade, R.K. (Ed.), Biopharmaceutics and Pharmacokinetics Considerations, first ed. Elsevier, pp. 1–31.

Tambe, V., Ditani, A., Rajpoot, K., Tekade, R.K., 2021b. Pharmacokinetics aspects of structural modifications in drug design and therapy. In: Tekade, R.K. (Ed.), Biopharmaceutics and Pharmacokinetics Considerations. Elsevier, Academic Press, pp. 1–27.

Tambe, V., Kathkar, U., Raval, N., Rajpoot, K., Shilpi, S., Khatri, K., Tekade, R.K., 2021c. Positron emission tomography as a noninvasive tool in pharmacokinetics studies. In: Tekade, R.K. (Ed.), Biopharmaceutics and Pharmacokinetics Considerations. Elsevier, Academic Press, pp. 1–25.

Tambe, V., Pande, S., Gadeval, A., Rajpoot, K., Raval, N., Tekade, R.K., 2021d. Microdialysis: an emerging technique for pharmacokinetic-pharmacodynamic profiling. In: Tekade, R.K. (Ed.), Biopharmaceutics and Pharmacokinetics Considerations, first ed. Elsevier, pp. 1–16.

Tambe, V., Shukla, H., Rajpoot, K., Pandey, M.M., Tekade, R.K., 2021e. Pharmacokinetics aspects of biotechnological products. In: Tekade, R.K. (Ed.), Biopharmaceutics and Pharmacokinetics Considerations. Elsevier, Academic Press, pp. 1–27.

Tambe, V., Sirsat, B., Rajpoot, K., Gadeval, A., Tekade, R.K., 2021f. Pharmacogenomics and drug metabolism. In: Tekade, R.K. (Ed.), Biopharmaceutics and Pharmacokinetics Considerations. Elsevier, Academic Press, pp. 1–31.

Tekade, R.K., Maheshwari, R., Soni, N., Tekade, M., Chougule, M.B., 2017. Nanotechnology for the development of nanomedicine. In: Nanotechnology-based Approaches for Targeting and Delivery of Drugs and Genes. Elsevier, pp. 3–61.

Thomas, R.S., Bahadori, T., Buckley, T.J., Cowden, J., Deisenroth, C., Dionisio, K.L., Frithsen, J.B., Grulke, C.M., Gwinn, M.R., Harrill, J.A., 2019. The next generation blueprint of computational toxicology at the US Environmental Protection Agency. Toxicol. Sci. 169 (2), 317–332.

USFDA, 2021. US Food and Drug Administration. Developing Products for Rare Diseases and Conditions. https://www.fda.gov/industry/developing-products-rare-diseases-conditions. (Accessed 22 May 2021).

Wallace, H.M., 2011. Risk perception in toxicology—part II: toxicology must Be the solution not the problem. Toxicol. Sci. 121 (1), 7–10.

Wang, L., Mercer, R.R., Rojanasakul, Y., Qiu, A., Lu, Y., Scabilloni, J.F., Wu, N., Castranova, V., 2010. Direct fibrogenic effects of dispersed single-walled carbon nanotubes on human lung fibroblasts. J. Toxicol. Environ. Health 73 (5), 410–422.

Wexler, P., Anderson, B.D., Gad, S.C., Hakkinen, P.B., Kamrin, M., De Peyster, A., Locey, B., Pope, C., Mehendale, H.M., Shugart, L.R., 2005. Encyclopedia of Toxicology, vol. 1. Academic Press.

Worth, A.P., 2019. Types of toxicity and applications of toxicity testing. In: The History of Alternative Test Methods in Toxicology. Elsevier, pp. 7–10.

Index

'*Note:* Page numbers followed by "f" indicate figures and "t" indicate tables.'

E

N

O

9780443158407